Neoplastic Diseases of the Blood

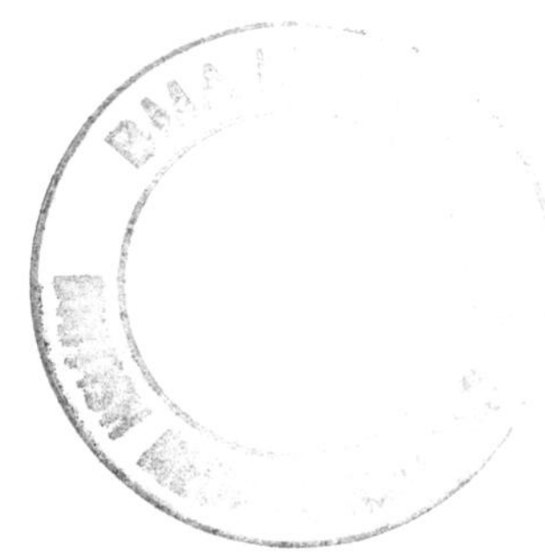

Peter H. Wiernik • Janice P. Dutcher
Morie A. Gertz
Editors

Neoplastic Diseases of the Blood

Sixth Edition

Volume 1

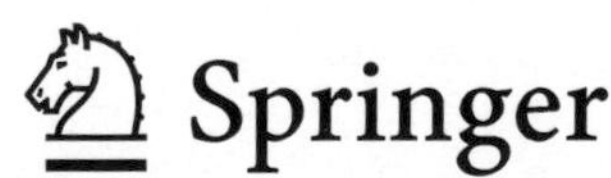

Editors
Peter H. Wiernik
Cancer Research Foundation
Chappaqua, NY
USA

Janice P. Dutcher
Cancer Research Foundation
Chappaqua, NY
USA

Morie A. Gertz
Department of Hematology
Mayo Clinic Department of Hematology
Rochester, MN
USA

ISBN 978-3-319-64262-8 ISBN 978-3-319-64263-5 (eBook)
DOI 10.1007/978-3-319-64263-5

Library of Congress Control Number: 2017962622

Printed on acid-free paper

This Springer imprint is published by Springer Nature
The registered company is Springer International Publishing AG
The registered company address is: Gewerbestrasse 11, 6330 Cham, Switzerland

The editors of the sixth edition of this book dedicate it to our families; to our mentors; to the hundreds of fellows we have trained over the years, many of whom have gone on to lead major cancer research and treatment programs on several continents; and to the thousands of patients we have had the privilege to care for and learn from over the decades. We also honor the continuing influence on this edition by former editors of previous editions, Drs. George P. Canellos, John M, Goldman, Robert A, Kyle and Charles A. Schiffer.

Preface

The sixth edition of *Neoplastic Diseases of the Blood* is long overdue despite the fact that the fifth edition was published only five years ago, due to the fact that major progress in our understanding of the nature of hematologic malignancies and their treatment has occurred in the interim. This edition is current and up to date, drawing heavily on recent references, and is designed to be a readable, encyclopedic resource for established hematologists and oncologists as well as for trainees in our disciplines.

The chapter structure of the book follows essentially that of the fifth edition, with the addition of some new chapters in the myeloma section. This edition is also divided into five sections like previous editions, each developed and managed by an editor: Chronic Leukemias and Related Disorders (Peter H. Wiernik), Acute Leukemias (Peter H. Wiernik), Myeloma and Related Disorders (Morrie Gertz), Lymphomas (Peter H. Wiernik), and Supportive Care (Janice P. Dutcher). Over 100 authors, many new to this edition, have contributed their expertise to this work.

Our sincere hope is that patients with hematologic malignancies will directly benefit from our work. This hope drove us to take on and complete this huge task that is the creation of this book.

We thank the publisher, Springer Medicine, for invaluable assistance during all phases of the development of the book. Special thanks to Maureen Alexander, Developmental Editor at Springer, for her highly professional continual interactions with the editors and all authors that was instrumental in bringing this project to a close in a timely manner, and to Andy Kwan, Editor, Clinical Medicine for Springer, for overseeing the project from beginning to end.

Chappaqua, NY, USA	Peter H. Wiernik
Chappaqua, NY, USA	Janice P. Dutcher
Rochester, MN, USA	Morie A. Gertz

The Editors

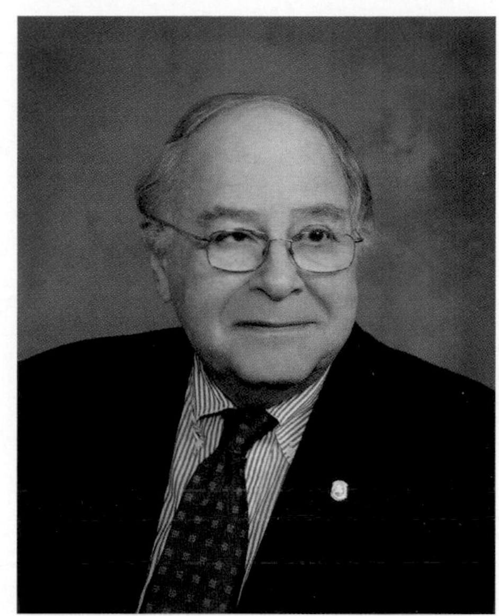

Peter H. Wiernik, M.D.

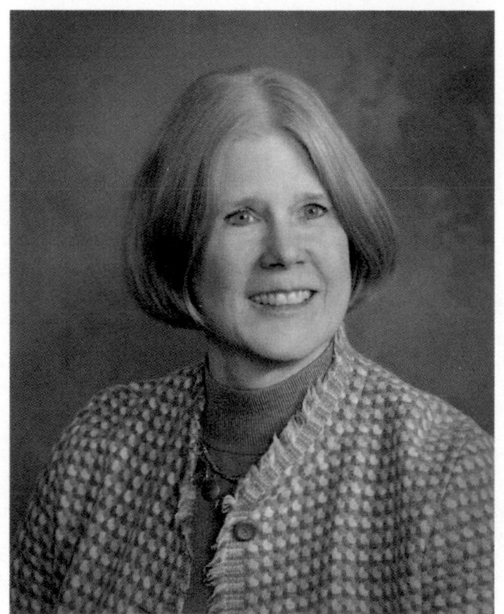

Janice P. Dutcher, M.D.

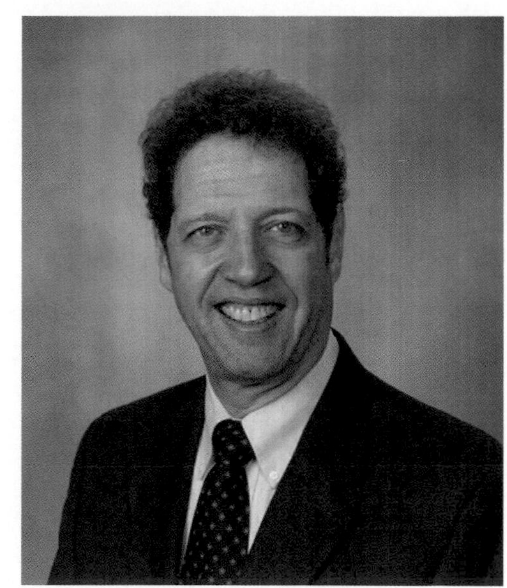

Morie A. Gertz, M.D.

Contents

Contributors

Syed A. Abutalib, M.D. Hematology and Hematopoietic Cell Transplant and Cell Therapy Programs, Cancer Treatment Centers of America, Midwestern Regional Medical Center, Zion, IL, USA

Sarah Alexander, M.D. Division of Pediatric Hematology/Oncology, Hospital for Sick Children, University of Toronto, Toronto, ON, Canada

Sonia Ali, M.D. Division of Hematology/Oncology, Scripps Clinic, La Jolla, CA, USA

Elias J. Anaissie Medical Director, CTI Clinical Trial and Consulting Services, Covington, KY, USA

Mir Basharath Alikhan, M.D. Department of Pathology, University of Chicago, Chicago, IL, USA

Claudio Anasetti, M.D. Department of Blood and Marrow Transplantation, Moffitt Cancer Center, Tampa, FL, USA

James O. Armitage, M.D. Division of Oncology/Hematology, Department of Internal Medicine, University of Nebraska Medical Center, Omaha, NE, USA

Belinda R. Avalos, M.D. Department of Hematologic Oncology and Blood Disorders, Levine Cancer Institute—Carolinas Healthcare System, Charlotte, NC, USA

Hervé Avet-Loiseau, M.D., Ph.D. Laboratoire UGM, IUC-Oncopole, Toulouse, France

Barbara J. Bain, M.B.B.S., F.R.A.C.P., F.R.C.Path Department of Haematology, St. Mary's Hospital, Imperial College London, London, UK

John M. Bennett, M.D. Pathology and Laboratory Medicine, Emeritus, Department of Pathology, University of Rochester Medical Center, Rochester, NY, USA

Joan Bladé, M.D., Ph.D. Amyloidosis and Myeloma Unit, Department of Hematology, Clinic Barcelona, Barcelona, Spain

Esteban Braggio, Ph.D. Department of Hematology/Oncology, Mayo Clinic, Scottsdale, AZ, USA

Francis K. Buadi, M.B., Ch.B. Division of Hematology, Mayo Clinic, Rochester, MN, USA

Lynda J. Campbell, M.B.B.S., F.R.C.P.A., F.H.G.S.A. Victorian Cancer Cytogenetics Service, St. Vincent's Hospital Melbourne, Fitzroy, VIC, Australia

Department of Medicine (St. Vincent's Hospital Melbourne), University of Melbourne, Fitzroy, VIC, Australia

George P. Canellos, M.D., D.Sc., F.R.C.P. Harvard Medical School, Dana Farber Cancer Institute, Boston, MA, USA

Alfonso Quintás Cardama, M.D. Department of Leukemia, MD Anderson Cancer Center, Houston, TX, USA

Daniel Catovsky, M.D., D.Sc., F.R.C.Path, F.R.C.P, F.Med.Sci Division of Molecular Pathology, The Institute of Cancer Research, Surrey, London, UK

James R. Cerhan, M.D., Ph.D. Department of Health Sciences Research, Mayo Clinic, Rochester, MN, USA

Rajshekhar Chakraborty, M.D. Department of Hematology/Oncology, Cleveland Clinic Foundation, Cleveland, OH, USA

Edward A. Copelan, M.D., F.A.C.P. Department of Hematologic Oncology and Blood Disorders, Levine Cancer Institute—Carolinas Healthcare System, Charlotte, NC, USA

Jill Corre, Pharm.D., Ph.D. Hematological Laboratory, UGM, University Hospital, IUC, Toulouse, France

Jorge Cortes, M.D. Department of Leukemia, MD Anderson Cancer Center, Houston, TX, USA

David G. Crockett, M.D. Division of Oncology/Hematology, Department of Internal Medicine, University of Nebraska Medical Center, Omaha, NE, USA

Jennifer Crombie, M.D. Department of Medical Oncology, Dana Farber Cancer Center, Boston, MA, USA

Judith Cukor, Ph.D. Department of Psychiatry, Weill Cornell Medicine, Psychiatry Collaborative Care Center, New York, NY, USA

Matthew S. Davids, M.D., M.M.Sc. Harvard Medical School, Dana Farber Cancer Institute, Boston, MA, USA

H. Joachim Deeg, M.D. Clinical Research Division, Fred Hutchinson Cancer Research Center and the University of Washington, Seattle, WA, USA

Barbara A. Degar, M.D. Dana-Farber/Boston Children's Cancer and Blood Disorders Clinic, Boston, MA, USA

Thomas G. DeLoughery, M.D., M.A.C.P., F.A.W.M. Division of Hematology/Oncology, Oregon Health Sciences University, Portland, OR, USA

Medicine, Pathology, and Pediatrics, Department of Hematology MC L586, Oregon Health Sciences University, Portland, OR, USA

Meletios Dimopoulos, M.D. Department of Experimental Therapeutics, University of Athens, Athens, Greece

Angela Dispenzieri, M.D. Division of Hematology and Internal Medicine, Mayo Clinic, Rochester, MN, USA

Mayo Medical School, Rochester, MN, USA

Simit Mahesh Doshi, M.D., M.P.H. Department of Nephrology, IUH University Hospital, Indianapolis, IN, USA

Janice P. Dutcher, M.D. Cancer Research Foundation of New York, Chappaqua, NY, USA

Omotayo Fasan, M.D., M.R.C.P. Department of Hematologic Oncology and Blood Disorders, Levine Cancer Institute—Carolinas Healthcare System, Charlotte, NC, USA

Maria Pia Franco, M.D. Department of Medicine, Division of Infectious Disease and International Medicine, Program in Adult Transplant Infectious Disease, University of Minnesota, Minneapolis, MN, USA

Medicine/Infectious Disease, Mayo Memorial Building, Minneapolis, MN, USA

Emil J Freireich, M.D. Department of Leukemia, University of Texas MD Anderson Cancer Center, Houston, TX, USA

Robert E. Gallagher, M.D. Albert Einstein Cancer Center, New York, NY, USA

Morie A. Gertz, M.D. Department of Medicine, Mayo Clinic, Rochester, MN, USA

Sergio Giralt, M.D. Chief, Adult Bone Marrow Transplant Service, Memorial Sloan Kettering Cancer Center, New York, NY, USA

Eli Glatstein, M.D. Department of Radiation Oncology, University of Pennsylvania, Philadelphia, PA, USA

Nicola Gökbuget, M.D. Department of Medicine II, Goethe University Hospital, Frankfurt, Germany

Jamie S. Green, M.D. Department of Medicine, Division of Infectious Disease and International Medicine, Program in Adult Transplant Infectious Disease, University of Minnesota, Minneapolis, MN, USA

Medicine/Infectious Disease, Mayo Memorial Building, Minneapolis, MN, USA

Seymour Grufferman, M.D., M.P.H., S.M., Dr. P.H Consultant in Epidemiology, Sante Fe, NM, USA

John A. Hansen, M.D. Fred Hutchinson Cancer Research Center, Seattle, WA, USA

Division of Clinical Research, Department of Medicine, University of Washington, Seattle, WA, USA

Joerg Hasford, M.D. Department for Medical Informatics, Biometry, and Epidemiology, Ludwig-Maximilians-Universitaet, Munich, Germany

Nyla A. Heerema, Ph.D., F.A.C.M.G. Department of Pathology, The Ohio State Wexner Medical Center, Columbus, OH, USA

Shelly Heimfeld, Ph.D. Clinical Research Division, Fred Hutchinson Cancer Research Center and the University of Washington, Seattle, WA, USA

John W. Hiemenz, M.D. Division of Hematology/Oncology, University of Florida Health, Gainesville, FL, USA

Dieter Hoelzer, M.D., Ph.D. Department of Medicine II, Goethe University Hospital, Frankfurt, Germany

Richard S. Houlston, M.D., Ph.D., D.Sc., F.R.S., F.Med.Sci. Division of Genetics and Epidemiology, The Institute of Cancer Research, Surrey, UK

Division of Molecular Pathology, The Institute of Cancer Research, Sutton, Surrey, UK

Jack W. Hsu, M.D. Division of Hematology/Oncology, University of Florida College of Medicine, Gainesville, FL, USA

Malin Hultcrantz, M.D., Ph.D. Myeloma Service, Department of Medicine, Memorial Sloan Kettering Cancer Center, New York, NY, USA

Ryan W. Jacobs, M.D. Department of Hematologic Oncology and Blood Disorders, Levine Cancer Institute—Carolinas Healthcare System, Charlotte, NC, USA

Deepa Jeyakumar, M.D. Division of Hematology/Oncology, Department of Medicine, UC Irvine Medical Center/Chao Family Comprehensive Cancer Center, Orange, CA, USA

Nisha S. Joseph, M.D. Department of Hematology and Medical Oncology, Winship Cancer Institute, Emory University, School of Medicine, Atlanta, GA, USA

Hagop Kantarjian, M.D. Department of Leukemia, MD Anderson Cancer Center, Houston, TX, USA

Rebecca Kehm, M.P.H. Division of Epidemiology and Clinical Research, Department of Pediatrics, University of Minnesota Medical School, Minneapolis, MN, USA

Mena Kinal, M.Sc. Segal Cancer Centre and Lady Davis Institute, Jewish General Hospital, Department of Oncology, McGill University, Montréal, QC, Canada

Karen E. King, M.D. Department of Pathology, Johns Hopkins University School of Medicine, Baltimore, MD, USA

H. Phillip Koeffler, M.D. Department of Medicine/Hematology-Oncology, UCLA/Cedars-Sinai Medical Center, Los Angeles, CA, USA

Marina Konopleva, M.D., Ph.D. Department of Leukemia, MD Anderson Cancer Center, Houston, TX, USA

Robert A. Kyle, M.D. Laboratory of Medicine and Pathology, Department of Hematology, Mayo Clinic, Rochester, MN, USA

Heather Landau, M.D. Weill Cornell Medical College, New York, NY, USA

Department of Medicine, Adult BMT Service, Memorial Sloan Kettering Cancer Center, New York, NY, USA

Ola Landgren, M.D., Ph.D. Myeloma Service, Department of Medicine, Memorial Sloan Kettering Cancer Center, New York, NY, USA

Alessandra Larocca, M.D. Department of Hematology, Azienda Ospedaliero-Universitaria Città della Salute e della Scienza di Torino, University of Torino, Torino, Italy

Hillard M. Lazarus, M.D., F.A.C.P. Department of Medicine, Case Western Reserve University School of Medicine, Cleveland, OH, USA

Helen Leather, B. Pharm. Division of Hematology/Oncology, Department of Medicine, University of Florida, Gainesville, FL, USA

Tomer Levin T. Levin, M.B.B.S. Department of Psychiatry, Weill Cornell Medicine, Psychiatry Collaborative Care Center, New York, NY, USA

Marshall A. Lichtman, M.D. James P. Wilmot Cancer Institute, University of Rochester Medical Center, Rochester, NY, USA

Dan L. Longo, M.D. Harvard Medical School, Brigham and Women's Hospital, Boston, MA, USA

Sagar Lonial, M.D. Department of Hematology and Medical Oncology, Winship Cancer Institute, Emory University School of Medicine, Atlanta, GA, USA

Brenton G. Mar, M.D., Ph.D. Dana Farber/Boston Children's Cancer and Blood Disorders Center, Boston, MA, USA

Erin L. Marcotte, M.P.H., Ph.D. Division of Epidemiology and Clinical Research, Department of Pediatrics, University of Minnesota Medical School, Minneapolis, MN, USA

Paul J. Martin, M.D. Department of Medicine, University of Washington, Seattle, WA, USA

Fred Hutchinson Cancer Research Center, Seattle, WA, USA

María-Victoria Mateos, M.D., Ph.D. Department of Hematology, Complejo Asistencial Universitario de Salamanca/Instituto Biosanitario de Salamanca (CAUSA/IBSAL), Salamanca, Spain

L. Jeffrey Medeiros, M.D. Department of Hematopathology, University of Texas MD Anderson Cancer Center, Houston, TX, USA

Giampaolo Merlini, M.D. Department of Medicine, Center for Research and Treatment of Systematic Amyloidoses, University of Pavia, University Hospital Policlinico San Matteo, Pavia, Italy

Filippo Milano, M.D., Ph.D. Clinical Research Division, Fred Hutchinson Cancer Research Center, and the University of Washington, Seattle, WA, USA

Kenneth Miller, M.D. Department of Hematology/Oncology, Tufts Medical Center, Boston, MA, USA

Wilson H. Miller Jr. M.D., Ph.D. Segal Cancer Centre and Lady Davis Institute, Jewish General Hospital, Department of Oncology, McGill University, Montréal, QC, Canada

Paul M. Ness, M.D. Department of Pathology, Johns Hopkins University School of Medicine, Baltimore, MD, USA

Jessica N. Nichol, Ph.D. Segal Cancer Centre and Lady Davis Institute, Jewish General Hospital, Department of Oncology, McGill University, Montréal, QC, Canada

Tom Tomer Noff, M.D. Department of Neurology, University of Indiana School of Medicine, Indianapolis, IN, USA

Anne J. Novak, Ph.D. Department of Internal Medicine, Mayo Clinic, Rochester, MN, USA

Marcio Nucci, M.D. Department of Internal Medicine—Hematology, University Hospital, Federal University of Rio de Janeiro, Rio de Janeiro, Brazil

Susan O'Brien, M.D. Department of Medicine, Sue and Ralph Stern Center for Cancer, Chao Family Comprehensive Cancer Center, UC Irvine Health, Orange, CA, USA

David G. Oscier, M.A., M.B., F.R.C.P., F.R.C.Path., Faculty of Medicine, Cancer Genomics, Academic Unit of Cancer Sciences, Southampton General Hospital, University of Southampton, Southampton, UK

Department of Hematology, Royal Bournemouth Hospital, Bournemouth, UK

Howard Ozer, M.D., Ph.D. Department of Hematology/Oncology, UI Cancer Center, University of Illinois at Chicago,, Chicago, IL, USA

Elisabeth Paietta, Ph.D. Department of Oncology, Albert Einstein College of Medicine, Montefiore Medical Center, Bronx, NY, USA

Antonio Palumbo, M.D. Department of Hematology, Azienda Ospedaliero-Universitaria Città della Salute e della Scienza di Torino, Torino, Italy

Melinda Pauly, M.D. Division of Hematology/Oncology, Department of Pediatrics, Emory University, Aflac Cancer and Blood Disorder's Center, Atlanta, GA, USA

Effie W. Petersdorf, M.D. Division of Medical Oncology, Division of Clinical Research, Department of Clinical Research, Fred Hutchinson Cancer Research Center, Seattle, WA, USA

Department of Medicine, University of Washington, Seattle, WA, USA

Monika Pilichowska, M.D., Ph.D. Department of Pathology, Tufts Medical Center, Boston, MA, USA

John P. Plastaras, M.D. Division of Epidemiology and Clinical Research, Department of Radiation Oncology, University of Pennsylvania, Philadelphia, PA, USA

Jenny N. Poynter, Ph.D. Division of Epidemiology and Clinical Research, Department of Pediatrics, University of Minnesota Medical School, Minneapolis, MN, USA

Susana Catalina Raimondi, Ph.D., F.A.C.M.G. Department of Pathology, St Jude Children Research Hospital, Memphis, TN, USA

Sébastien Robiou-Du-Pont, Ph.D. UGM—CRCT Team 13, Toulouse University Hospital—IUCT, Toulouse, France

Maren Rohrbacher, M.D. Pharmacovigilance, Mannheim, Germany

G. David Roodman, M.D., Ph.D. Department of Hematology and Oncology, Indiana University School of Medicine, Indianapolis, IN, USA

Laura Rosiñol, M.D., Ph.D. Department of Hematology, Hospital Clinic, Barcelona, Spain

Jesús F. San-Miguel, M.D., Ph.D. Clínica Universidad de Navarra, Navarra, Spain

Alan Saven, M.D. Division of Hematology/Oncology, Scripps Clinic, La Jolla, CA, USA

Robyn Scherber, M.D., M.P.H. Division of Hematology/Oncology, Oregon Health Sciences University, Portland, OR, USA

Charles A. Schiffer, M.D. Department of Oncology, Karmanos Cancer Institute, Wayne State University School of Medicine, Detroit, MI, USA

Christopher Sequeira, M.D. Division of Hematology/Oncology, UI Cancer Center, University of Illinois at Chicago, Chicago, IL, USA

Joseph J. Shatzel, M.D. Division of Hematology/Oncology, Oregon Health Sciences University, Portland, OR, USA

Taimur Sher, M.D. Department of Hematology, Mayo Clinic, Jacksonville, FL, USA

Lewis B. Silverman, M.D. Division of Pediatric Hematology-Oncology, Department of Pediatric Oncology, Dana-Farber Cancer Institute, Boston Children's Hospital, Boston, MA, USA

Susan L. Slager, Ph.D. Department of Health Sciences Research, Mayo Clinic, Rochester, MN, USA

Logan G. Spector, Ph.D. Division of Epidemiology and Clinical Research, Department of Pediatrics, University of Minnesota Medical School, Minneapolis, MN, USA

Helen E. Speedy, Ph.D. Division of Genetics and Epidemiology, The Institute of Cancer Research, Surrey, London, UK

David P. Steensma, M.D. Department of Medical Oncology, Dana-Farber Cancer Institute, Boston, MA, USA

Jonathan C. Strefford, B.Sc., P.C.C.C., Ph.D. Faculty of Medicine, Cancer Genomics, Academic Unit of Cancer Sciences, Southampton General Hospital, University of Southampton, Southampton, UK

Hyung Chan Suh, M.D., Ph.D. Division of Hematology Oncology, David Geffen School of Medicine at UCLA, Los Angeles, CA, USA

Martin S. Tallman, M.D. Memorial Sloan Kettering Cancer Center, Weill Cornell Medical College, New York, NY, USA

Steven P. Treon, M.D., Ph.D. Department of Medicine, Harvard Medical School, Dana Farber Cancer Institute, Boston, MA, USA

Tony H. Truong, M.D., M.P.H. Division of Pediatric Oncology, Blood and Marrow Transplant, Alberta Children's Hospital, University of Calgary, Calgary, AB, Canada

N. Nukhet Tuzuner, M.D. Department of Pathology, Cerrahpasa Medical Faculty, Istanbul, Turkey

Girish Venkataraman, M.B.B.S., M.D. Department of Pathology, Section of Hematopathology, University of Chicago, Chicago, IL, USA

Julie M. Vose, M.D., M.B.A. Division of Oncology/Hematology, Department of Internal Medicine, University of Nebraska Medical Center, Omaha, NE, USA

Renata Walewska, M.B.Ch.B., F.R.C.Path., Ph.D. Department of Haematology, Royal Bournemouth Hospital, Bournemouth, UK

Meaghan Wall, M.B.B.S., Ph.D., F.R.A.C.P., F.R.C.P.A. Victorian Cancer Cytogenetics Service, St. Vincent's Hospital Melbourne, Fitzroy, VIC, Australia

Department of Medicine (St. Vincent's Hospital Melbourne), University of Melbourne, Fitzroy, VIC, Australia

Sheila Weitzman, M.B.B.Ch., F.R.C.P.(C) Division of Pediatric Hematology/Oncology, Hospital for Sick Children, University of Toronto, Toronto, ON, Canada

Peter H. Wiernik, M.D., D.hc., F.A.S.C.O. Cancer Research Foundation, Chappaqua, NY, USA

John R. Wingard, M.D. Division of Hematology/Oncology, University of Florida College of Medicine, Gainesville, FL, USA

Mariko Yabe, M.D., Ph.D. Department of Hematopathology, University of Texas MD Anderson Cancer Center, Houston, TX, USA

Jo-Anne H. Young, M.D. Department of Medicine, Division of Infectious Disease and International Medicine, Program in Adult Transplant Infectious Disease, University of Minnesota, Minneapolis, MN, USA

Medicine/Infectious Disease, Mayo Memorial Building, Minneapolis, MN, USA

Part I

Chronic Leukemias and Related Disorders

A History of the Chronic Leukemias

1

George P. Canellos and Matthew S. Davids

Introduction

Leukemias, both chronic and acute, were not described separately. Historically, the state of excessive quantities of blood cells and secondary organ involvement is attributed to Velpeau in 1827 [1]; although initial observations suggested that the excess of corpuscles in the blood was related to suppuration, it appeared that those cases were more likely to be what is now known as chronic leukemia because of the duration of disease and systemic enlargement noted [2]. Virchow in 1845 introduced the term of white blood of "leukaemie." He accumulated nine cases and doubted that infection was an explanation for the process [3]. The first reported case in America was in 1852. Virchow also differentiated the leukemias according to "splenic" or "lymphatic" leukemia [4]. By 1870, Neumann proposed that splenic leukemias were derived from cells originating in the bone marrow [5]. Further separation of acute versus chronic leukemias was made by Ebstein (1889) introducing the term "acute leukemia," a disease with a very short survival [6]. It remained for Ehrlich to begin staining cells to separate granulocytes from lymphoid cells. This provided a test to classify leukemia even further than prior unstained descriptions [7]. The primitive cells, known as blasts, were further clarified by Naegeli in 1900 separating to some extent myeloblastic from lymphoblasts [8]. However, Turk in 1903 assembled all the "lymphoid" diseases under one classification known as lymphomatoses [9]. However, the true neoplastic nature of these disorders was confirmed when they could be induced in experimental animals by toxic chemical injection.

G.P. Canellos, M.D., D.Sc., (Hon.) F.R.C.P. (✉)
M.S. Davids, M.D., M.M.Sc.
Division of Medical Oncology, Department of Medicine, Dana-Farber Cancer Institute, Harvard Medical School, 450 Brookline Ave, Boston, MA 02215, USA
e-mail: George_canellos@dfci.harvard.edu

Chronic Myeloid Leukemia

Chronic myeloid leukemia remained as defined by early investigations until 1960 when Nowell and Hungerford using the new technology of cytogenetics described a marker chromosome with deletion of genetic material known as the Philadelphia chromosome. This provided a test which defined CML as a clonal disorder [10]. This was further supported by studying patients who were heterozygous for isochromosomes of glucose-6-phosphate dehydrogenase which further defined the clonal origins of a number of other disorders [11]. In the 1970s, a greater understanding of the Philadelphia chromosome evolved. It was demonstrated by DeKlein that the human analog of the murine v-abl oncogene was translocated from its normal location on chromosome 9 to chromosome 22 and soon after that the reciprocal translocation of genetic material from chromosome 22 to chromosome 9 was described, resulting in a fusion gene BCR-ABL on chromosome 22 [12]. Two molecular rearrangements on BCR-ABL are possible but both result in a hybrid messenger RNA and thus a protein kinase [13, p. 210]. Modern molecular technology now allows for reassessment of minute quantities of the gene and facilitates the assessment of new therapeutics in assessing remission of the disease. A number of other features of CML have been attributed to the gene including proliferation, less apoptosis, and diminished cellular adhesion. The early therapeutic history of CML probably began with the use of arsenic trioxide (1% solution known as Fowler's solution). It was used on occasion in the nineteenth century with some transient benefit until the discovery of X-rays which were used to radiate the enlarged spleens. This resulted in significant improvements in signs and symptoms as well as blood counts [14]. The modern chemotherapy era for CML began with the demonstrations of the cytotoxic effects of nitrogen mustard [15]. An oral derivative of alkylating agent research was busulfan, which was introduced in 1953 and was, for a considerable period, the standard oral therapy of CML [16]. Other agents, such as chlorambucil and thiopurines as well as colchicine

P.H. Wiernik et al. (eds.), *Neoplastic Diseases of the Blood*, DOI 10.1007/978-3-319-64263-5_1

derivatives, were used. Because of the unpredictable and sometimes extensive bone marrow suppression with busulfan, another antimetabolite, hydroxyurea, was introduced and shown to be active [17]. The blastic phase of CML was quite refractory to effective treatment regimens used for acute myeloid leukemia and almost never resulted in a remission. Transient, but complete, remissions were however achieved when the blastic phase assumed lymphoid characteristics [18]. Vincristine and prednisone could produce remissions lasting months. The lymphoid nature of the blastic cells was confirmed by immunologic and cytologic tests [19]. Treatment also included interferon for a period before the introduction of the specific tyrosine kinase inhibitors directed at the BCR-ABL protein tyrosine kinase [20]. There was an initial success in producing hematologic as well as molecular remissions, and resurrecting the suppressed normal hemopoietic elements resulting in prolonged remissions [21]. The initial agent was imatinib but new mutations resulted in disease relapse and other more potent ABL inhibitors such as nilotinib, dasatinib, and ponatinib were introduced [22, 23]. The actions of these agents have dramatically altered the natural history and resulted in prolongation of survival obviating the need for allogeneic transplantation which was also a component of the treatment plan for some prior to the introduction of the tyrosine kinase inhibitors. Allotransplantation in its time was potentially curative, providing that there was a compatible donor, tolerance to graft-versus-host disease, and a survival from septicemia. Nonetheless, this could be curative and basically a manifestation of effective immunotherapy by allogeneic T cells against leukemic stem cells. Few patients are now candidates for this treatment as the new kinase inhibitors have had an overwhelming effect on the natural history of CML. It remains an effective therapy for those intolerant to all tyrosine kinase inhibitors (TKI) or with mutations conferring resistance to effect TKI therapy [24]. Allogeneic transplants were successful in the past when performed in the chronic phase with 12-year survival of 60–70%. The introduction of tyrosine kinase inhibitors, such as imatinib, has resulted in 8-year survivals of over 90% when used in the chronic phase. However, although uncommon, point mutations can occur and confer resistance to at least generations of inhibitors. The gatekeeper mutation, T3151, is the offender, but even for this mutation a recent TKI, ponatinib, has been introduced.

Chronic Lymphocytic Leukemia

The early histories of treating CML and CLL have much in common due to the limited availability of treatment options and the inability to distinguish the diseases with any degree of accuracy. In the 1940s and 1950s, Osgood [25–27] tested the hypothesis that whole-body external irradiation or administration of radioactive phosphorus could be titrated to control the leukocyte count at a level below 30×10^9/L. He claimed that this strategy was effective in patients with slowly progressing disease and that it could increase the chance of survival to 20 years. However, his results were not confirmed in later randomized trials comparing irradiation with chlorambucil and other alkylating agents [28, 29].

Progress in the clinical management of patients with CML has relied on improved understanding of the different types of disease and on improved prognosis. In the past, diseases diagnosed as CLL would have included a mixture of T- and B-cell leukemias, hairy cell leukemia, and a variety of other conditions associated with lymphocytosis. In contrast, the cells can now be identified accurately by cellular morphology, immunophenotype, cytogenetics, and other features [30] so that subtypes of disease can be grouped together and informative clinical trials can be designed.

It has been recognized for many years that cases of CLL have variable clinical courses [31]. The wide range of survival times for patient with CLL, from a few years to more than a decade, made treatment decisions difficult, particularly because some patients remained well even if they were not treated. This led to the development of staging systems, based on prognostic indicators and other criteria, to facilitate the choice of therapy for individual patients. The long list of prognostic indicators in CLL now includes age, sex, lymphocyte doubling time, cell morphology, and cytogenetic abnormalities [30]. In particular, patients with del(17p), del(11q), or complex cytogenetics have a poorer overall survival, whereas those with del(13q), trisomy 12, or normal cytogenetics have a better prognosis [32]. Patients whose CLL cells are positive for ZAP-70 tend to have a shorter time to treatment [33]. Testing for the mutational status of the immunoglobulin heavy-chain variable region (*IGHV*) also has significant prognostic impact, as patients with <2% similarity to germline DNA ("mutated") have a more indolent course and longer survival compared to those with >2% ("unmutated") [34, 35]. Recently, the presence of somatic mutations such as *TP53, NOTCH1, SF3B1*, and others has allowed further subgrouping of CLL [36, 37].

With regard to CLL therapy, most patients can be observed for a prolonged period of time after diagnosis without the need for treatment. This has been studied in several randomized clinical trials of early intervention with chemotherapy versus delaying therapy until patients meet treatment indications [38]. These indications as per the 2008 IW-CLL criteria include progressive cytopenias due to bone marrow infiltration by CLL, progressive organ-threatening, bulky lymphadenopathy, or progressive constitutional symptoms in the setting of progressive disease [39]. In the absence of these signs or symptoms, an overall survival advantage to early intervention with chemotherapy has never been demonstrated.

Once patients do meet treatment indications, numerous therapeutic options are available. Long-term low-dose treatment with the oral alkylating agent chlorambucil was a mainstay of CLL therapy for decades. For patients with more indolent forms of CLL, this approach regulated the size of the malignant B-cell clone without inducing major cytopenias or other toxicities [40]. The purine analog fludarabine was subsequently found to induce a higher rate of complete remission and a longer progression-free survival than chlorambucil, but as monotherapy it did not confer an overall survival advantage in a randomized trial [41]. Fludarabine plus the intravenous alkylating agent cyclophosphamide (FC) became a new standard of care when it was shown to induce deeper and more durable remissions than fludarabine alone [42]. In the 2000s, rituximab was added to FC to make the FCR regimen, which was pioneered by Keating and colleagues at MD Anderson Cancer Center [43, 44]. The promising results of their initial studies were subsequently confirmed by the German CLL Study Group in their CLL8 trial, which showed an overall survival advantage to FCR over FC as initial therapy for younger, fit patients with CLL [45]. This trial is notable for being the first randomized trial to demonstrate an overall survival benefit in CLL. More recently, a regimen comprised of the alkylating agent bendamustine with rituximab (BR) has become popular for frontline CLL therapy due to its high level of efficacy and generally favorable tolerability [46]. CLL10 is a large, randomized phase III trial that randomized previously untreated patients to FCR vs. BR [47]. The results demonstrated that FCR induced a higher rate of complete remission, more minimal residual disease (MRD) negativity, and a longer PFS than BR. However, an overall survival benefit has not yet emerged, and BR also provided excellent efficacy and tolerability. In particular, older, frailer patients had less severe cytopenias and infectious complications with BR compared to FCR, and therefore BR can be considered a standard regimen in this population. In patients under 65, FCR provided deeper and more durable remissions with relatively comparable toxicity, making it still the standard of care for this group. Recently published data by both the MD Anderson and German CLL groups on the long-term results of FCR treatment suggest that a substantial number of patients with mutated IGHV CLL will be cured by initial therapy with FCR [48, 49].

Patients who become refractory to chemoimmunotherapy and those with high-risk disease markers such as del(17p) or unmutated *IGHV* typically have less durable responses to chemoimmunotherapy. Several approaches have been used to manage these high-risk patients. The monoclonal antibody alemtuzumab (Campath I-H, anti-CD52) was shown to have a high rate of response in patients with del(17p) CLL and was found to be particularly useful in patients with the bulk of disease in the blood and bone marrow and minimal lymphadenopathy [50]. High-dose methylprednisolone was shown to induce a high rate of remission in high-risk patients and was most useful in those with bulky lymphadenopathy [51, 52]. The UK group attempted to combine these two approaches in their CLL206 trial, which gave concurrent alemtuzumab and methylprednisolone to TP53-deleted CLL [53]. Although their response rates, PFS, and OS were substantial for this population, the toxicity of this highly immunosuppressive approach was also apparent, with grade 3–4 infections occurring in half of the patients.

Given the significant unmet medical need for patients with high-risk CLL, particularly those who became refractory to chemoimmunotherapy, there was an urgent need for the development of novel agents to treat this disease. Years of laboratory research had revealed that two of the "Achilles heels" of CLL pathophysiology were the B-cell receptor (BCR) pathway and the intrinsic mitochondrial pathway of apoptosis, with its key anti-apoptotic protein B-cell leukemia/lymphoma-2 (BCL-2). The first effort to target the BCR pathway in CLL examined the Syk inhibitor fostamatinib. CLL patients treated with fostamatinib had significant shrinkage of lymphadenopathy while at the same time showing a rising lymphocyte count, which was initially concerning for disease progression [54]. Fostamatinib also had several off-target effects which led to significant toxicities and the development of this drug in CLL did not move forward. Shortly after this, two drugs entered into clinical trials which would forever change the history of CLL treatment, ibrutinib, the oral inhibitor of Bruton's Tyrosine Kinase (BTK) [55], and idelalisib [56], an oral inhibitor of the delta-isoform of phosphoinositide-3-kinase (PI3K), which is selectively expressed in lymphocytes. In early-phase clinical trials, both of these drugs demonstrated an initial lymphocytosis and as with fostamatinib, at the same time nodal disease and cytopenias were improving. This phenomenon was later named "lymphocyte redistribution," as it was recognized that through disruption of integrin signaling in the stromal microenvironment, CLL cells were being released from the lymph nodes and marrow and into the blood of patients and then subsequently undergoing apoptosis. The recognition that this epiphenomenon was not disease progression but quite the opposite—a sign of disease response—led to a consensus statement that lymphocyte redistribution should not constitute progression and a new category of response known as partial response with lymphocytosis (PR-L) or nodal response should be used to classify these patients [57].

Both ibrutinib and idelalisib were found to be highly active in early-phase trials, and remarkably patients had equivalent response rates irrespective of traditional high-risk markers such as del(17p) or unmutated IGHV [58, 59]. In phase III randomized trials, ibrutinib was found to have an overall survival benefit compared to the anti-CD20 antibody ofatumumab, leading to its FDA approval in relapsed/refractory

CLL [60]. Idelalisib plus rituximab was found to have an OS benefit compared to rituximab alone, leading to its approval in relapsed/refractory CLL [61]. Ibrutinib went on to receive frontline approval for CLL based on an overall survival benefit demonstrated in a phase III study comparing it to chlorambucil for initial therapy in older, frail patients [62]. Idelalisib was also being studied in several frontline trials in CLL and other indications, but due to an increased risk of mortality due to infectious complications as well as significant autoimmune toxicities, its development for frontline CLL therapy came to a halt in 2016 [63].

The other key pathway for CLL cell survival is the intrinsic mitochondrial pathway of apoptosis. CLL is well known to express high levels of the anti-apoptotic protein BCL-2, on which the malignant cells depend for their survival. An early attempt to target this pathway was the oral BCL-2/BCL-XL/BCL-w inhibitor navitoclax [64]. Although substantial efficacy was seen with navitoclax in CLL, there was also significant thrombocytopenia observed, which was thought to be on target toxicity due to inhibition of BCL-XL, which is important for platelet survival [65, 66]. A second-generation BCL-2 inhibitor was developed known as venetoclax, which is highly selective for BCL-2 with minimal activity against BCL-XL [67]. In the phase I first in human study, venetoclax was found to be so active against CLL cells that there were several cases of tumor lysis syndrome including one mortality due to this [68]. After lowering the initial starting dose and doing a gradual intrapatient dose ramp-up, the rates of tumor lysis syndrome dropped substantially and there were no further clinical sequelae. As with the BCR inhibitors, venetoclax induced a high rate of response even in patients refractory to fludarabine or harboring ominous prognostic markers such as del(17p). Unlike the BCR inhibitors, the responses induced by venetoclax included a significant number of patients achieving complete response with some patients achieving minimal residual disease negativity. A subsequent pivotal phase II study of venetoclax in patients with del(17p) confirmed these initial results [69] and led to FDA approval of venetoclax for relapsed/refractory CLL with del(17p) in 2016.

Although an exciting development, the novel therapies recently developed for CLL are unlikely to be curative on their own and therefore must be continued for ongoing therapy. Current clinical trials are looking at combination strategies to facilitate time-limited therapy, in some cases with curative intent. These promising trials involve novel agents plus chemotherapy, novel agents plus a monoclonal antibody, and novel agent-only combination approaches, all of which appear to be promising.

To date, the only consistently curative strategy for CLL has been allogeneic bone marrow transplantation. Many CLL patients are older and frail with significant comorbidities and do not tolerate myeloablative conditioning regimens well. Non-myeloablative conditioning regimens (also known as reduced-intensity conditioning) for transplantation have substantial efficacy with less toxicity, and appear to be equally effective for patients with high-risk disease [70]. Rates of success for allotransplant appear to be highest in patients who are maximally cytoreduced prior to transplant. Overall there is about a 40% rate of long-term progression-free survival in CLL patients treated with reduced-intensity allogeneic transplantation, although rates of graft vs. host disease and treatment-related mortality remain substantial. To build on this immunologic approach to treating CLL with less toxicity than allotransplant, several groups have recently presented data on a novel approach known as chimeric antigen receptor (CAR) T cell therapy. This approach utilizes autologous T cells from the patient and ex vivo introduces a CD19 antigen receptor. The T cells are then reinfused back into the patient where they can proceed to eradicate residual CLL. Several dramatic responses have been observed in refractory CLL patients treated with CAR-T cells, and some of these responses have had substantial longevity [71]. Toxicities include a cytokine release syndrome and neurotoxicity. Ongoing studies of this promising new approach in CLL will help define the optimal use of this technology in CLL.

Although there have been many exciting developments in CLL research over the last several years, there are several areas of unmet medical needs. These include patients with high-risk disease such as del(17p) or complex cytogenetics, whose responses to novel agents are less durable, patients who develop Richter's syndrome for which therapy remains inadequate, and patients who desire time-limited therapy with curative potential. Many clinical trials have launched recently to answer these questions, and these promising new approaches suggest that the future outcomes for patients with CLL will only continue to improve in time.

References

1. Velpeau A. Sur la resorption du puseat sur l'alteration du sang dans les maladies clinique de persection nenemant. Premier observation. Rev Med. 1827;2:216.
2. Bennett JH. Case of hypertrophy of the spleen and liver in which death took place from suppuration of the blood. Edinb Med Surg J. 1845;64:413.
3. Virchow R. Weisses Blut und Milztumoren Med Z. 1846;15:157.
4. Virchow R. Zur pathologischen Physiologie des Bluts: Die Bedeutung der milz- und Lymph-Drusen-Krankheiten fur die Blutmischung (Leukaemia). Virchows Arch. 1853;5:43.
5. Neumann E. Ein Fall von Leukamie mit Erkrankung des Knochenmarkes. Arch Heilk. 1870;11:1.
6. Ebstein W. Ueber die acute Leukamie und Pseudoleukamie. Duet Arch Klin Med. 1889;44:343.
7. Ehrlich P. Parbenanalytische Untersuchungen zur Histologie und Klinik des Blutes. Berlin: Hirschwald; 1891.
8. Naegeli O. Uber rothes Knochenmark und Myeloblasten. Deut Med Wochenschr. 1900;18:287.
9. Turk W. Ein System der Lymphomatosen. Wien Klin Wochenschr. 1903;16:1073.

10. Nowell PC, Hungerford DA. A minute chromosome in human granulocytic leukemia. Science. 1960;132:1497.
11. Fialkow PJ, Martin PJ, Najfeld V, Penfold GK, Jacobson RJ, Hansen JA. Evidence for a multistep pathogenesis of chronic myelogenous leukemia. Blood. 1981;58:159.
12. De Klein A, Van Kessel A, Grosveld G, Bartram CR, Hagemeijer A, Bootsma D, Spurr NK, Heisterkamp N, Groffen J, Stephenson JR. A cellular oncogene is translocated to the Philadelphia chromosome in chronic myelocytic leukaemia. Nature. 1982;300:765.
13. Ben-Neriah Y, Daley GQ, Mes-Masson A-M, Witte ON, Baltimore D. The chronic myelogenous leukemia specific p210 protein is the product of the bcr/abl hybrid gene. Science. 1986;223:212.
14. Lissauer H. Zwei Falle von Leukaemie. Berl Klin Wochenschr. 1865;2:403.
15. Goodman LS, Wintrobe MM, Dameshek W, Goodman MJ, Gilman A, McLennan MT. Nitrogen mustard therapy. JAMA. 1946;132:126.
16. Haddow A, Timmis GM. Myleran in chronic myeloid leukaemia: chemical composition and biological function. Lancet. 1953;i:207.
17. Schwartz JH, Canellos GP. Hydroxyurea in the management of the hematologic complications of chronic granulocytic leukemia. Blood. 1975;46:11.
18. Canellos GP, DeVita VT, Whang-Peng J, Carbone PP. Hematologic and cytogenetic remission of blastic transformation in chronic granulocytic leukemia. Blood. 1971;38:671.
19. McCaffrey R, Smolen R, Baltimore D. Terminal deoxynucleotidyl transferase in a case of childhood acute lymphoblastic leukemia. PNAS. 19731;70:521.
20. Talpaz M, McCredie KB, Malvigit GM, Gutterman JU. Leukocyte interferon-induced myeloid cytoreduction in chronic myelogenous leukaemia. Br Med J. 1983;1:201.
21. Druker B, Talpaz M, Resta DJ, et al. Efficacy and safety of a specific inhibitor of the BCR-ABL tyrosine kinase in chronic myeloid leukemia. N Engl J Med. 2001;344:1031.
22. Saglio G, Kim D-W, Issaragrisil S, et al. Nilotinib versus imatinib for newly diagnosed chronic myeloid leukemia. N Engl J Med. 2010;362:2251.
23. Cortes JE, Kantarjian H, Shah NP, et al. Ponatinib in refractory Philadelphia chromosome-positive leukemias. N Engl J Med. 2012;367:2075.
24. Ralich J. Stem cell transplant for chronic myeloid leukemia in the imatinib era. Semin Hematol. 2010;47:354.
25. Osgood EE. Titrated, regularly spaced radioactive phosphorus or spray roentgen therapy of leukemias. AMA Arch Intern Med. 1951;87(3):329–48.
26. Osgood EE, Koler RD. The results of the 15-year program of treatment of chronic leukemias with titrated regularly spaced total-body irradiation with phosphorus 32 or X-ray. In: Proceedings of the sixth international society of hematology (Boston 1956); 1958. p. 44.
27. Osgood EE. Treatment of chronic leukemias. J Nucl Med. 1964;5:139–53.
28. Huguley CM Jr. Long-term study of chronic lymphocytic leukemia: interim report after 45 months. Cancer Cheother Rep. 1962;16:241.
29. Rubin P, Bennett JM, Begg C, Bozdech MJ, Silber R. The comparison of total body irradiation vs chlorambucil and prednisone for remission induction of active chronic lymphocytic leukemia: an ECOG study. Part I: Total body irradiation-response and toxicity. Int J Radiat Oncol Biol Phys. 1981;7(12):1623–32.
30. Zweibel JA, Cheson BD. Chronic lymphocytic leukemia: staging and prognostic factors. Semin Oncol. 1998;25:42.
31. Dameshek W. Chronic lymphocytic leukemia—an accumulative disease of immunolgically incompetent lymphocytes. Blood. 1967;29(Suppl 4):566–84.
32. Dohner H, Stilgenbauer S, Benner A, et al. Genomic aberrations and survival in chronic lymphocytic leukemia. N Engl J Med. 2000;343(26):1910–6.
33. Wiestner A, Rosenwald A, Barry TS, et al. ZAP-70 expression identifies a chronic lymphocytic leukemia subtype with unmutated immunoglobulin genes, inferior clinical outcome, and distinct gene expression profile. Blood. 2003;101(12):4944–51.
34. Hamblin TJ, Davis Z, Gardiner A, Oscier DG, Stevenson FK. Unmutated Ig V(H) genes are associated with a more aggressive form of chronic lymphocytic leukemia. Blood. 1999;94(6):1848–54.
35. Damle RN, Wasil T, Fais F, et al. Ig V gene mutation status and CD38 expression as novel prognostic indicators in chronic lymphocytic leukemia. Blood. 1999;94(6):1840–7.
36. Puente XS, Pinyol M, Quesada V, et al. Whole-genome sequencing identifies recurrent mutations in chronic lymphocytic leukaemia. Nature. 2011;475(7354):101–5.
37. Wang L, Lawrence MS, Wan Y, et al. SF3B1 and other novel cancer genes in chronic lymphocytic leukemia. N Engl J Med. 2011;365(26):2497–506.
38. CLL Trialists' Collaborative Group. Chemotherapeutic options in chronic lymphocytic leukemia: a meta-analysis of the randomized trials. J Natl Cancer Inst. 1999;91(10):861–8.
39. Hallek M, Cheson BD, Catovsky D, et al. Guidelines for the diagnosis and treatment of chronic lymphocytic leukemia: a report from the International Workshop on Chronic Lymphocytic Leukemia updating the National Cancer Institute-Working Group 1996 guidelines. Blood. 2008;111(12):5446–56.
40. Sawitsky A, Rai KR, Glidewell O, Silver RT. Comparison of daily versus intermittent chlorambucil and prednisone therapy in the treatment of patients with chronic lymphocytic leukemia. Blood. 1977;50(6):1049–59.
41. Rai KR, Peterson BL, Appelbaum FR, et al. Fludarabine compared with chlorambucil as primary therapy for chronic lymphocytic leukemia. N Engl J Med. 2000;343(24):1750–7.
42. Eichhorst BF, Busch R, Hopfinger G, et al. Fludarabine plus cyclophosphamide versus fludarabine alone in first-line therapy of younger patients with chronic lymphocytic leukemia. Blood. 2006;107(3):885–91.
43. Wierda W, O'Brien S, Wen S, et al. Chemoimmunotherapy with fludarabine, cyclophosphamide, and rituximab for relapsed and refractory chronic lymphocytic leukemia. J Clin Oncol. 2005;23(18):4070–8.
44. Keating MJ, O'Brien S, Albitar M, et al. Early results of a chemoimmunotherapy regimen of fludarabine, cyclophosphamide, and rituximab as initial therapy for chronic lymphocytic leukemia. J Clin Oncol. 2005;23(18):4079–88.
45. Hallek M, Fischer K, Fingerle-Rowson G, et al. Addition of rituximab to fludarabine and cyclophosphamide in patients with chronic lymphocytic leukaemia: a randomised, open-label, phase 3 trial. Lancet. 2010;376(9747):1164–74.
46. Fischer K, Cramer P, Busch R, et al. Bendamustine in combination with rituximab for previously untreated patients with chronic lymphocytic leukemia: a multicenter phase II trial of the German Chronic Lymphocytic Leukemia Study Group. J Clin Oncol. 2012;30(26):3209–16.
47. Eichhorst B, Robak T, Montserrat E, et al. Appendix 6: Chronic lymphocytic leukaemia: eUpdate published online September 2016 (http://www.esmo.org/Guidelines/Haematological-Malignancies). Ann Oncol. 2016;27(Suppl 5):v143–4.
48. Thompson PA, Wierda WG. Eliminating minimal residual disease as a therapeutic end point: working toward cure for patients with CLL. Blood. 2016;127(3):279–86.
49. Fischer K, Bahlo J, Fink AM, et al. Long-term remissions after FCR chemoimmunotherapy in previously untreated patients with CLL: updated results of the CLL8 trial. Blood. 2016;127(2):208–15.
50. Stilgenbauer S, Zenz T, Winkler D, et al. Subcutaneous alemtuzumab in fludarabine-refractory chronic lymphocytic leukemia: clinical results and prognostic marker analyses from the CLL2H study of the German Chronic Lymphocytic Leukemia Study Group. J Clin Oncol. 2009;27(24):3994–4001.

51. Castro JE, James DF, Sandoval-Sus JD, et al. Rituximab in combination with high-dose methylprednisolone for the treatment of chronic lymphocytic leukemia. Leukemia. 2009;23(10):1779–89.
52. Castro JE, Sandoval-Sus JD, Bole J, Rassenti L, Kipps TJ. Rituximab in combination with high-dose methylprednisolone for the treatment of fludarabine refractory high-risk chronic lymphocytic leukemia. Leukemia. 2008;22(11):2048–53.
53. Pettitt AR, Jackson R, Carruthers S, et al. Alemtuzumab in combination with methylprednisolone is a highly effective induction regimen for patients with chronic lymphocytic leukemia and deletion of TP53: final results of the national cancer research institute CLL206 trial. J Clin Oncol. 2012;30(14):1647–55.
54. Friedberg JW, Sharman J, Sweetenham J, et al. Inhibition of Syk with fostamatinib disodium has significant clinical activity in non-Hodgkin lymphoma and chronic lymphocytic leukemia. Blood. 2010;115(13):2578–85.
55. Honigberg LA, Smith AM, Sirisawad M, et al. The Bruton tyrosine kinase inhibitor PCI-32765 blocks B-cell activation and is efficacious in models of autoimmune disease and B-cell malignancy. Proc Natl Acad Sci U S A. 2010;107(29):13075–80.
56. Herman SE, Gordon AL, Wagner AJ, et al. Phosphatidylinositol 3-kinase-delta inhibitor CAL-101 shows promising preclinical activity in chronic lymphocytic leukemia by antagonizing intrinsic and extrinsic cellular survival signals. Blood. 2010;116(12):2078–88.
57. Cheson BD, Byrd JC, Rai KR, et al. Novel targeted agents and the need to refine clinical end points in chronic lymphocytic leukemia. J Clin Oncol. 2012;30(23):2820–2.
58. Brown JR, Byrd JC, Coutre SE, et al. Idelalisib, an inhibitor of phosphatidylinositol 3-kinase p110delta, for relapsed/refractory chronic lymphocytic leukemia. Blood. 2014;123(22):3390–7.
59. Byrd JC, O'Brien S, James DF. Ibrutinib in relapsed chronic lymphocytic leukemia. N Engl J Med. 2013;369(13):1278–9.
60. Byrd JC, Brown JR, O'Brien S, et al. Ibrutinib versus ofatumumab in previously treated chronic lymphoid leukemia. N Engl J Med. 2014;371(3):213–23.
61. Furman RR, Cheng S, Lu P, et al. Ibrutinib resistance in chronic lymphocytic leukemia. N Engl J Med. 2014;370(24):2352–4.
62. Burger JA, Tedeschi A, Barr PM, et al. Ibrutinib as initial therapy for patients with chronic lymphocytic leukemia. N Engl J Med. 2015;373(25):2425–37.
63. Lampson BL, Kasar SN, Matos TR, et al. Idelalisib given front-line for treatment of chronic lymphocytic leukemia causes frequent immune-mediated hepatotoxicity. Blood. 2016;128(2):195–203.
64. Tse C, Shoemaker AR, Adickes J, et al. ABT-263: a potent and orally bioavailable Bcl-2 family inhibitor. Cancer Res. 2008;68(9):3421–8.
65. Wilson WH, O'Connor OA, Czuczman MS, et al. Navitoclax, a targeted high-affinity inhibitor of BCL-2, in lymphoid malignancies: a phase 1 dose-escalation study of safety, pharmacokinetics, pharmacodynamics, and antitumour activity. Lancet Oncol. 2010;11(12):1149–59.
66. Vogler M, Hamali HA, Sun XM, et al. BCL2/BCL-X(L) inhibition induces apoptosis, disrupts cellular calcium homeostasis, and prevents platelet activation. Blood. 2011;117(26):7145–54.
67. Souers AJ, Leverson JD, Boghaert ER, et al. ABT-199, a potent and selective BCL-2 inhibitor, achieves antitumor activity while sparing platelets. Nat Med. 2013;19(2):202–8.
68. Roberts AW, Davids MS, Seymour JF. New agents to treat chronic lymphocytic leukemia. N Engl J Med. 2016;374(22):2186–7.
69. Stilgenbauer S, Eichhorst B, Schetelig J, et al. Venetoclax in relapsed or refractory chronic lymphocytic leukaemia with 17p deletion: a multicentre, open-label, phase 2 study. Lancet Oncol. 2016;17(6):768–78.
70. Dreger P, Dohner H, Ritgen M, et al. Allogeneic stem cell transplantation provides durable disease control in poor-risk chronic lymphocytic leukemia: long-term clinical and MRD results of the German CLL Study Group CLL3X trial. Blood. 2010;116(14):2438–47.
71. Porter DL, Levine BL, Kalos M, Bagg A, June CH. Chimeric antigen receptor-modified T cells in chronic lymphoid leukemia. N Engl J Med. 2011;365(8):725–33.

Epidemiology and Etiology of Chronic Myeloid Leukemia

2

Maren Rohrbacher and Joerg Hasford

Introduction

Epidemiology can be defined as the study of the frequency, distribution, and causes of diseases in populations, mainly with observational designs. In recent years the traditional spectrum of epidemiology was extended to a variety of so-called hyphenated epidemiological subdisciplines like genetic, environmental, pharmaco, and healthcare epidemiology. Epidemiology has become an important multidisciplinary science and is essential for the identification of risk factors, assessment of the burden of disease, development of preventive actions, and promotion of public health. Chronic myeloid disease has been identified as a disease entity for the first time in 1845 independently by Virchow and Bennett [1, 2]. In 1973, Rowley published that the so-called Philadelphia (Ph) chromosome, which is pathognomonic for Ph-positive (Ph+) chronic myeloid leukemia (CML), is the result of a translocation between the chromosomes 9 and 22 [3]. From a commonly fatal disease CML has become, with the introduction of tyrosine kinase inhibitors (TKIs) since 2001, for most patients a kind of chronic disease. More recent studies report that the life expectancy of patients with CML approximates the one of the normal population [4, 5].

As CML is a very rare disease and the diagnosis requires elaborate diagnostic tools like cytogentic tests, FISH, or PCR techniques, it remained outside of the focus of most cancer registries and epidemiologists. Thus, reliable epidemiological information on Ph/BCR-ABL-positive CML is still limited, but much better compared to the situation 15 years ago. The aim of this chapter is to review the current knowledge regarding etiology, incidence, prevalence and survival rates, secondary malignancies, health care, and issues of the daily CML practice.

M. Rohrbacher, M.D.
Pharmacovigilance, Mannheim 68161, Germany
e-mail: m.rohrbacher@web.de

J. Hasford, M.D. (✉)
Department for Medical Informatics, Biometry, and Epidemiology, Ludwig-Maximilians-Universitaet, Marchioninistrasse 15, Munich 81377, Germany
e-mail: has@ibe.med.uni-muenchen.de

Etiology

CML is caused by a chromosome abnormality, the BCR-ABL fusion oncogene [Philadelphia chromosome (Ph)] [6, 7]. This oncogene is imperative for a Ph/BCR-ABL-positive CML. Specific genetic or environmental factors can result in the fusion of breakpoints of chromosome 9 in the ABL gene with certain breakpoints on chromosome 22 in the BCR gene [7].

No evidence for genetic predisposition in individual persons has been provided, and case reports of familial CML are rare [7–12]. Lifestyle factors such as smoking and a high body mass index have been identified as possible risk factors for CML [13–16].

An association between chemical exposure to benzene, organic solvents, alkylating agents, topoisomerase II inhibitors or other chemotherapeutic agents, and de novo CML has been shown repeatedly, but the evidence was not entirely consistent [7, 17–21]. An increased CML incidence has been seen among workers exposed to benzene or benzene-containing solvents [17, 20]. Benzene itself is not considered genotoxic, but its major hepatic metabolites, phenol, hydroxyquinone, and 1,2,4-benzenetriol and their metabolic products (e.g., 1,4-benzoquinone and semiquinone) are suspected to induce DNA damages in bone marrow cells as well as alkylating agents and topoisomerase inhibitors [22–25]. The benzene metabolite, trans-muconaldehyde, although genotoxic, seemed to get inactivated in the liver by glutathione. Thus, the active form could not reach sufficient levels in the marrow to harm hematopoietic cell chromosomes [7]. In cell line cultures, benzene-related metabolites, alkylating agents, or topoisomerase II inhibitors caused abnormalities of chromosomes 5 (monosomy or del(5q31)), 7 (monosomy), and 8 (trisomy), often causally associated with secondary acute

P.H. Wiernik et al. (eds.), *Neoplastic Diseases of the Blood*, DOI 10.1007/978-3-319-64263-5_2

myelogenous leukemia after cytotoxic therapy [7, 17, 22–24, 26–28]. Neither relevant breaks in chromosomes 9 or 22 nor the formation of the BCR-ABL fusion gene were observed in in vitro tests [7, 22, 24, 27–29]. Studies of late effects of chemotherapy for a variety of malignancies did not show an increased risk for secondary CML [7].

In comparison to chemical exposures, leukemogenic effects of acute, high-dose ionizing radiation exposure have been identified by the Atomic Bomb Casualty Commission in Japan after World War II in extensive epidemiological studies [20, 30–32]. The latest published data indicated that 20% of all leukemias were classified as CML based on an analysis between 1950 and end of 2001 [33, 34].

Also the incidence of CML among the Chernobyl cleanup workers increased in the last 20 years after the Chernobyl Nuclear Power Plant accident [35]. In the United States, CML represents about 17% of the potentially radiation-induced new cases of leukemia per year [7]. Biological plausibility further strengthened the compelling epidemiological evidence for radiation-induced CML by hematopoietic cell line cultures: The BCR-ABL oncogene could result from high-dose X-ray or gamma irradiation and the subsequent transcription of BCR-ABL message in such cells [36, 37]. High-dose radiation exposure can directly generate leukemia-specific fusion genes [37].

Incidence

Knowledge on clinical and molecular features of Ph/BCR-ABL-positive CML is extensive, but the epidemiology has still not been studied in detail [34, 38]. Sources of these data are mortality statistics [39], cancer population-based registries such as the Swedish Cancer Registry [40, 41], the Saarland Registry [42, 43] in Germany, the database of the Surveillance, Epidemiology and End Results (SEERs) Program of the United States National Cancer Institute [44, 45], or surveys such as the European Treatment and Outcome Study CML-Registry (EUTOS) [46].

Worldwide CML incidence rates vary from 0.6 to 2.8 cases per 100,000 inhabitants with an obvious increase in age [38, 40–52] (Table 2.1). CML occurs with greater frequency in men than in women as shown in male-to-female ratios ranging between 1.2 and 1.8 [34, 38, 40–47, 49, 53, 54].

The most recently published results from the EUTOS population-based CML-registry which collected incidence data from 20 European countries reported a raw incidence of 0.39/100,000/year in people 20–29 years old, and of 1.52 in those >70 years old, showing a maximum of 1.39 in Italy and a minimum of 0.69 in Poland [46]. Here, the median age at the time of diagnosis was about 56 (range 50–64) years. With a male-to-female ratio of 1.16 men were more often affected. Interestingly, a majority (53.5%) of the patients presented no palpable spleen at diagnosis, and 88.2% were classified as EUTOS score low-risk patients [46]. Some geographic and/or ethnic variations and different diagnostic accurateness might contribute to the variability of the reported incidences.

Table 2.1 Crude and standardized CML incidences of population-based registries and surveys

	Time of observation	Number of patients	Incidence crude	Incidence (WSP)[a]
SEER [44, 45]	1998–2000	–	–	1.8[b]
	2003–2007	4653	–	1.7[b]
	2008–2012	5955	–	1.8[b]
EUTOS registry[c] [46]	2008–2012	2904	1.0	0.9
France [51]	1985–2006	906	–	0.8
France [52]	1998–2009	781	–	0.8
Swedish Cancer Registry [40, 41]	1998–2000	260	1.0	0.7
	2001–2008	704	1.0	0.7
	2009–2014	633	1.1	0.7
Scotland Leukemia Registry[c] [48]	1999–2000	64	0.6	–
Thames Registry [47]	1999–2000	180	–	0.8
Leukemia Research Fund [49]	1984–1993	1115	–	0.6
Cancer Registry of Saarland [42, 43]	1998–2000	65	2.0	1.0
	2001–2007	142	1.9	0.9
	2008–2012	140	2.8	1.2
Southwest Germany[c] [54]	1998–2000	172	0.6	–
Southeast Germany [50]	2004	201	1.9	1.3

Modified with permission from Rohrbacher and Hasford [38]
[a]World Standard Population
[b]United States Standard Population
[c]CML cases with known Ph/BCR-ABL-positive status

A crude incidence of Ph/BCR-ABL-positive CML of 0.6 per 100,000 is available from the Scotland Leukaemia Registry [48] and from a survey in the Southwest of Germany [54] (Table 2.1). Both studies covered a population size of about 9 million inhabitants. In the German study the incidence of all reported 218 CML cases including negative and unknown Ph/BCR-ABL status was 0.8, and of CML and CMML (0.2) combined 1.0 [54]. As the Ph/BCR-ABL status was only available for 87.2% of the German CML patients and not for any of the 61 patients with a diagnosis of CMML, incidence estimates provided there probably represent the lower margin of the true CML incidence. The variations of incidences seen might indicate geographic and/or ethnic variability beyond technical artifacts [34, 38, 55]. Some registries try to increase data comparability by standardization according to the age structure of the world standard population (WSP). WSP weighs age-specific incidences in populations with higher proportions of younger people than in the European standard population [56].

All publications considered in Table 2.1 are from northern Europe [40–43, 46–49, 54] or the United States [44, 45]. There seems to be variability of incidences of geographic areas even in the same country as exemplified by the Swedish National Cancer Registry [49] and the Goteborg Central Disease Registry [57] which reported incidences for polycythemia vera and primary myelofibrosis differing by a factor of up to more than two [38]. This is of interest, as differences in the CML risk group composition between southern (Italy) and northern European countries (Poland, the United Kingdom, Austria, Germany) were reported [46, 58, 59]. However, the recently observed data of the EUTOS registry could not identify a particular regional clustering of high and low incidences among Europe [46].

Between 1993 and 2004 the second Edition of the International Classification of Diseases for Oncology (ICD-O) (WHO Geneva 1990) for coding CML cases was commonly used, which did not differentiate true CML, Ph- and BCR-ABL-negative CML, chronic myelomonocytic leukemia (CMML), or subacute myeloid leukemia [38]. Since 2005, the discriminate coding of the molecular BCR-ABL-negative and -positive status has been possible on the basis of the new third Edition of ICD-O (WHO Geneva 2000) [38]. Basic data, stratified for BCR-ABL status, have not been shown in the latest cancer reports (Table 2.1). Consequently, the published incidences for CML may be higher than the true ones as BCR-ABL-negative cases are included. Up to 5% of patients with chronic myelogenous leukemia do not have the Ph-translocation t(9;22)(q34;q11) or a BCR-ABL molecular rearrangement [60].

Prevalence and Survival Rates

Prevalence of chronic, life-threatening, and costly disease has a major impact on the healthcare systems [61–63]. By the targeted treatment with TKIs a long-term survival is observed [62, 63]. An 8-year overall survival (OS) of 89% was recently published which approximates a normal life expectation [64]. Thus, this improved life expectation under the treatment of TKIs directly increases prevalence rates.

CML prevalence data itself remain scarce as population-based registries mostly provide "CML" data in a general category of "Leukemia" [41, 43, 45]. Nevertheless, some estimations are available from France, Sweden, the United States, and Germany: Within a French survey 906 newly diagnosed CML cases were identified in a population of about four million inhabitants for the period of 1985 to 2006 [51]. The calculated prevalence rate had increased from 5.8/100,000 during 1998 to 6.8 (2002) to 7.3 (2003) and to 10.4 in 2007. In another French survey based on 781 CML patients from population-based registries, the following data were presented [52]: The 5-year relative survival (RS) rates among patients with (Ph+) CML were 44% when diagnosed in 1980–1986, 64% in 1987–1999, and 89% in 2000–2009. The 8-year RS rate of patients with Ph+ CML diagnosed was 83% in 2000–2009.

For the Swedish population, prevalence data from 1985 to 2012 showed an increase from 3.9 to 11.9 per 100,000 inhabitants, and as an assumption 22.0 per 100,000 inhabitants by 2060 [5, 62]. The 5-year OS increased from 0.18 to 0.82, and the 5-year RS between 2006 and 2012 was close to a normal 40-year-old, but lower for 80-year-old CML patients (0.95 and 0.63).

For the US population the following data were available [63, 65, 66]: Estimated prevalence was about 70,000 CML patients in 2010, 112,000 in 2020, 144,000 in 2030, 167,000 in 2040, and 181,000 in 2050 against the backdrop of an annual incidence of 4800 CML patients [63]. A mortality ratio of CML patients (in their first 10 years since the diagnosis of CML) vs. the general population with the same age distribution was calculated to be 1.53 [63]. Using the SEERs database, the 5-year OS was improved for all patients between 2000 and 2005 [65]. Compared with patients who were diagnosed in 2000, the 5-year survival improved among patients aged 15–44 years (hazard ratio (HR) for mortality 0.43), aged 45–64 years (HR 0.716), and aged 65–74 years (HR 0.692), and patients aged 75–84 years had an increased 5-year OS rate from 19% in 2000 to 36% in 2005 (HR 0.568). These data were retrieved from 5138 patients [65]. SEERs data were also used to compare ethnic survival rates among Caucasian, African-Americans, and other races and within each race to see survival differences from the pre-imatinib (1973–2000) to post-imatinib eras (2002–2008) [66]. Here, the RS was significantly improved in the imatinib era, but these improvements were modest in the population-based data compared to those reported from clinical trials [66]. Interestingly, young (<50-year-old) female African-American CML patients have a lower RS in the imatinib era compared to young female Caucasian CML patients.

Considering the situation in Germany, the authors based their study on population-based data of about 10.5 million people in the statutory health insurance system in Bavaria for the years 2008–2013 [67]. Survival rates were adapted from the literature. The mean estimated age-standardized (Old European Standard Population) incidence rates per 100,000 inhabitants were 1.300 and 1.768 for women and men. Based on the population data, a total number of about 9000 CML patients was estimated in Germany for 2012, and it was expected that the number of CML patients would increase further until at least 2040 to 2050 with a maximum of more than 20,000 CML patients as the most probable scenario [67].

As a consequence of this considerable increase of the CML prevalence, the burden for the healthcare systems will rise with respect to costs and clinical services used.

Secondary Malignancy

The observed rise of the prevalence rates, associated with a long-term survival for the patients with TKI treatment, is still under investigation especially focusing on the risk of secondary malignancies [68, 69]. So far, a significant higher occurrence of secondary solid tumors such as gastrointestinal, nose, and throat cancer was observed in the imatinib era than in the pre-imatinib era [69].

Population-based data from 868 CML patients diagnosed between 2002 and 2011 in the Swedish Cancer registry and from 5511 CML patients in the SEERs database indicate that CML patients treated in the TKI era had an increased risk of developing a second (non-hematological) malignancy compared to the general population [68, 69]. In detail, the risk of second malignancies was higher in the CML cohort ($N = 868$) compared to the general population, with a standardized incidence ratio (SIR) of 1.52 (95% CI 1.13–1.99). Here, the SIR before and after the second year following diagnosis of CML was 1.58 and 1.47 [68]. Among the 8511 adult CML patients, 446 patients developed 473 secondary malignancies. The SIR for secondary malignancies in CML patients was significantly higher with the observed/expected ratio 1.27 ($P < 0.05$) and absolute excess risk of 32.09 per 10,000 person years compared to the general population [69]. The rate of secondary malignancies of all sites in the post-imatinib era was significantly higher compared to the pre-imatinib era with the observed/expected ratio of 1.48 versus 1.06 ($P = 0.03$) [69]. The authors assumed that the estimated elevated risk is more likely linked to the underlying CML disease than to the TKI therapy [68].

The occurrence of these secondary cancer entities in TKI-treated CML patients in comparison to the general population is the focus of ongoing research.

Health Care and Daily Practice

Patient's survival depends on the available national healthcare system [70–77]. There, aspects of medicines' costs play an important role in treatment decisions, and may also be the reason behind different treatment recommendations in different countries [77]. The growing life expectancy is in addition an influencing factor for the daily clinical practice. Especially, an age disparity for elderly patients in the administration of TKI therapy has been observed as an issue.

For the approved TKIs such as imatinib, dasatinib, and nilotinib, there are high healthcare costs noticed [76, 77]. In the United States the price for imatinib has been increased threefold from initially $30,000 per year in 2001 to $92,000 per year in 2012 [76, 77]. At the same time in 2012, three new drugs were approved by the US Food and Drug Administration (FDA) with pricing levels at $28,000 (omacetaxine), $118,000 (bosutinib), and $138,000 (ponatinib) per year.

The reason for the high TKI therapy prices can be the expensive developmental costs for new targeted, effective, safe, and tolerable medicines, but the negative clinical aspects of the pricing have also to be discussed. A forum of CML experts emphasized that this economic model of high therapy costs can cause a comprised access of needy patients to the targeted drugs with the clinical consequence of a less effective therapy and a poorer survival outcome [77]. Additionally, this pricing model can potentially harm the sustainability of healthcare systems [77].

Examples of the pharmacoeconomic/epidemiologic associations between national healthcare systems, patient's individual access to targeted CML treatment, and patients' survival rates are shortly described in the following: US patients have to pay an average of 20% of the drug prices out of their own pocket (about $20,000–$30,000 per year) which may induce a personal bankruptcy depending on the private household budget. These circumstances can be reasons for poor compliance, drug discontinuation, and worse outcome: It was observed that 10% of the US patients failed to take prescribed drugs mostly due to costs. By evaluating the survival rates in the United States, the estimated 5-year survival rate is currently still 60% although there was an improvement since the imatinib release in 2001 [77]. This suggests a lower TKI treatment penetration rates in the United States compared to higher TKI treatment penetration and compliance rates in Europe, e.g., in Sweden with an estimated 10-year survival rates of 80% where patients have an access to lifesaving CML drugs via the national healthcare policy [77].

Consequently, there are further discussions needed whether lowering the TKI prices would improve treatment penetration rates, increase compliance, and expand CML patient population living longer and continuing on TKI therapy. This concept would paradoxically increase revenues to pharmaceutical companies from sales of TKIs [77].

Focusing on the clinical practice, CML experts from, e.g., the European LeukemiaNet (ELN) (http://www.leukemia-net.org) have developed recommendations for the medical management of patients of all ages with CML including the definition of CML phases, the appropriate use of TKIs, the evaluation of cytogenetic and molecular responses, and optimized treatment strategies [78–82]. The patient's age at the time of diagnosis and the individual concomitant comorbidities are factors influencing treatment decisions. It was observed that especially elderly patients received either a reduced dose of imatinib in case of concomitant comorbidities or another therapy but not the targeted TKI treatment with the benefit of a better survival [80–84]. This was confirmed by the validated EUTOS score demonstrating that under TKI treatment increasing age did not play a significant negative role for the probability to achieve a complete cytogenetic remission and a long progression-free survival [85, 86].

However, based on published data, there seems to be an age disparity in imatinib-containing treatments being probably associated with a worse survival for especially elderly CML patients: The use of imatinib was inversely associated with patient's age: 90, 75, and 46% for patients aged 20–59, 60–79, and ≥80 in a study based on SEERs and population-based data with 423 CML patients diagnosed in 2003 [84]. Elderly patients who received imatinib survived significantly longer than those who did not. After adjusting for the patient's age, the imatinib use did not vary significantly by race/ethnicity, socioeconomic status, urban/rural residence, presence of comorbid conditions, or insurance status [84].

Further examples for age disparity in CML treatment: In Lithuania, survival data and the TKI treatment penetrance from 601 CML patients were analyzed [87]. The patients' data were retrieved from the national haematological disease-monitoring system being diagnosed between 2000 and 2013 [87]. The reported median age at diagnosis was 62 years. A 5-year RS rate increased from 0.33 (95% CI, 0.27–0.40, in 2000–2004) to 0.55 (95% CI, 0.47–0.63, in 2005–2009), but the 5-year RS survival rates for patients aged 65–74 years and ≥75 years were only 0.33 (95% CI, 0.24–0.42) and 0.18 (95% CI 0.07–0.23). The TKI penetrance rate for the patients grew from 1.5% (in 2000–2004) to 30.6% (in 2005–2009) and 69.1% (in 2010–2013); however, the TKI penetrance rate was lower in the older age groups (60% for the 65–74, and 19% for the ≥75 years patient group, in 2010–2013). Hence, the RS for elderly patients remained poorer as this patient population rarely received TKIs for their CML treatment [87].

In Sweden, the cancer registry provided data from 779 CML patients for an observed period between 2002 and 2010 [5]. The population's median age here was 60 years. Regarding the TKI penetration rate, nearly 50% of the patients received a TKI, a proportion that increased to 94% for younger (<70 years) and 79% for older (>80 years) patients during 2007–2009. The estimated 5-year RS was close to 1.0 for patients younger than 60 years, 0.9 for those aged 60–80 years, and only 0.6 for elderly patients (>80 years) [5]. Despite respective treatment recommendations, the majority of elderly CML patients received non-imatinib-containing regimens as first-line treatment during 2002–2004. From 2006 a change in imatinib therapy for elderly patients was observed, but nevertheless, this population was less likely to be treated with TKIs than younger patients.

Besides the described TKI treatment age disparity in daily practice, it is known that elderly patients are underrepresented in most investigational clinical trials. This was shown in a comparison between multicenter trials and population-based registries during the last decades [38]: The median age in multicenter trials [58, 88–109] (Table 2.2b) is 49 years, even in trials without age limitation as an inclusion criterion [89, 95, 104]. In contrast, the median age is up to 67 years in population-based registries [44–46, 110–112] (Table 2.2a), concluding that data of clinical trials underestimate the true age of the CML population. Within a German survey it was determinated that the chance for a CML patient <65 years to be enrolled in a clinical study was 3.8 times higher than for a CML patient ≥65 years [54].

Table 2.2 Age at diagnosis of CML patients in population-based registries and clinical trials

	Number of cases	Age (years), mean ± SD/ median (range)
(A) Registries [Ref. No.], data period		
EUTOS registry, 2002–2006 [46]	2904	56 (18–99) tbc
Czech Republic/Slovakia CAMELIA registry, 2000–2008 [110]	661	51 (15–83)
Thames Cancer Registry, UK, 1999–2000 [47]	180	65 (20–98)
Austrian CML registry, <2000 to 2009 [111]	179	53 (17–88)
SEER Cancer Statistics Review, 2003–2007 for whites [44]	4653	Median age 67 (n.a.)[a]
SEER Cancer Statistics Review, 2008–2012 for whites [44]	5955	Median age 66 (n.a.)
SEER Cancer Statistics Review, 1973–1998 for all races [112]	8229	Median age 64 (n.a.)
SEER Cancer Statistics Review, 2008–2012 for all races [45]	7441	Median age 64 (n.a.)
(B) Clinical Trials [Ref. No.]		
The Italian Cooperative Study Group on Chronic Myeloid Leukemia, N Engl J Med 1994 [90]	322	48 ± 14
Hehlmann et al., Blood 1994 [83]	513	48 (17–85)
Allan et al., Lancet 1995 [59]	587	47 (15–84)
Guilhot et al., N Engl J Med 1997 [108]	754	50 (7–70)
Hasford et al., JNCI 1998 [109]	1303	49 (10–85)
The Benelux CML Study Group, Blood 1998 [91]	195	56 (20–83)
Bonifazi et al., Blood 2001 [106]	317	49 (9–73)
Baccarani et al., Blood 2002 [105]	538	45 ± 13
Hehlmann et al., Leukemia 2003 [88]	534	48 (10–83)
Kluin-Nelemans et al., Blood 2004 [92][b]	407	60 (20–81)

(continued)

Table 2.2 (continued)

	Number of cases	Age (years), mean ± SD/ median (range)
Druker et al., N Engl J Med 2006 [107]	1106	50 (18–70)
Kantarjian et al., Blood 2006 [93]	929	48/43 (15–84)
Hehlmann et al., Blood 2007 [89]	621	49 (11–90)
Jabbour et al., Blood 2009 [94]	169	50 (17–94)
Saussele et al., Blood 2010 [95][c]	84	37 (16–62)
Palandri et al., Haematologica 2010 [96]	495	49 (18–80)
Efficace et al., Blood 2011 [97]	448	57 (19–87)
Hanfstein et al., Leukemia 2012 [98][c]	1223	52 (16–85)
Marin et al., J Clin Oncol 2012 [99]	282	46 (13–86)
Cortes et al., J Clin Oncol 2012 [100]	502	48 (18-91)
Jabbour et al., Leukemia 2013 [101]	315	58 (21–85)
Castagnetti et al., Annals of oncology 2015 [102]	2784	50 (18–87)
Saussele et al., Blood 2015 [103][c]	1519	63 (16–88)

Modified with permission from Rohrbacher and Hasford [38]

[a]n.a. = range not available

[b]This study comprises mostly elderly patients since younger patients were recruited for transplantation studies

[c]The referenced publications [95, 98, 103] retrieved their data from the CML IV Study

Another practical aspect in daily CML management is the association between the frequency of molecular monitoring and the risk of progression and progression-free survival (PFS). This was evaluated in a US study with 402 CML patients being on first-line imatinib therapy [113]. There, it has been shown that patients who had on average three to four qPCR tests per year had a lower risk of progression and longer PFS compared to patients who had no qPCR monitoring. These results were also observed in in those patients being monitored with one to two qPCR tests per year compared to those without any molecular monitoring [113]. Thus, patients can benefit from regularly scheduled qPCR testings which is in accordance to current CML recommendations.

Furthermore, it seems that patients treated in teaching hospitals achieve better outcomes: Based on 1491 patients of the German CML Study IV, the authors compared the outcomes of patients from teaching hospitals with those from municipal hospitals and office-based physicians [114]. Adjusting for age, EUTOS score, Karnofsky performance status, year of diagnosis, and experience with CML, a significant survival advantage for teaching hospital patients (HR 0.63–0.61) was found. In particular, when treated in teaching hospitals, patients with blast crisis showed a superior outcome (2-year survival rate: 47.7% vs. 22.3% vs. 25.0%) [114].

Some of the current issues in CML health care and daily clinical practices have been highlighted. More efforts are necessary that all CML patients get access to the targeted TKI treatment and benefit from the reported better survival associated with regular molecular monitoring. Especially, for the population of elderly patients the age disparity in TKI-containing treatment and the exclusion in investigational trials should be reduced by continuous education and implementation of the proposed recommendations.

Summary

Epidemiological information on Ph/BCR-ABL-positive CML is still limited. Available CML incidence rates vary from 0.6 to 2.8 cases per 100,000 inhabitants with an obvious increase in age. Some geographic and/or ethnic variations might contribute to this variability, but there are also differences in diagnostic accurateness. The observed prevalence rates increase with the widespread use of TKIs improving patients' survival and quality of life. Consequencently, an estimated 8-year OS of 89% has recently been determinated indicating an almost normal life expectation for the CML patients.

This outstanding therapeutic achievement asks for further research on the occurrence of secondary malignancies, other therapy-related risks, the treatment of elderly patients, the economic impact on healthcare systems by the expensive long-term treatment, and the chances to stop treatment with TKIs in patients with complete remission without risking relapse of CML.

References

1. Virchow R. Weisses Blut. Frorieps Notizen. 1845;36:151–6.
2. Bennett JH. Case of hypertrophy of the spleen and liver, in which death took place from suppuration of the blood. Edinburgh Med Surg J. 1845;64:413–23.
3. Rowley JD. A new consistent chromosomal abnormality in chronic myelogenous leukaemia identified by quinacrine fluorescence and Giemsa staining. Nature. 1973;243:290–3.
4. Gambacorti-Passerini C, Antolini L, Mahon FX, et al. Multicenter independent assessment of outcomes in chronic myeloid leukemia patients treated with imatinib. J Natl Cancer Inst. 2011;103:553–61.
5. Hoglund M, Sandin F, Hellstrom K, et al. Tyrosine kinase inhibitor usage, treatment outcome, and prognostic scores in CML: report from the population-based Swedish CML registry. Blood. 2013;122(7):1284–92.
6. Apperley JF. Chronic myeloid leukaemia. Lancet. 2015;385:1447–59.
7. Lichtman MA. Is there an entity of chemically induced BCR-ABL-positive chronic myelogenous leukemia? Oncologist. 2008;13(6):645–54.

8. Segel GB, Lichtman MA. Familial (inherited) leukemia, lymphoma, and myeloma: an overview. Blood Cells Mol Dis. 2004;32:246–61.
9. Hemminki K, Jiang Y. Familial myeloid leukemias from the Swedish Family-Cancer Database. Leuk Res. 2002;26:611–3.
10. Wiernik P. Familial leukemias. Curr Treat Options Oncol. 2015;16:2–11.
11. Björkholm M, Kristinsson SY, Landgren O, et al. No familial aggregation in chronic myeloid leukemia. Blood. 2013;122:460–1.
12. Lillicrap DA, Sterndale H. Familial chronic myeloid leukaemia. Lancet. 1984;2(8404):699.
13. Kasim K, Levallois P, Abdous B, et al. Lifestyle factors and the risk of adult leukemia in Canada. Cancer Causes Control. 2005;16(5):489–500.
14. Strom SS, Yamamura Y, Kantarjian HM, et al. Obesity, weight gain, and risk of chronic myeloid leukemia. Cancer Epidemiol Biomarkers Prev. 2009;18(5):1501–6.
15. Kabat GC, Wu JW, Moore S, et al. Cancer Epidemiol Biomarkers Prev. 2013;22(5):848–54.
16. Musselman J, Blair C, Cerhan JR, et al. Risk of adult acute and chronic myeloid leukemia with cigarette smoking and cessation. Cancer Epidemiol. 2013;37(4):1–15.
17. Mehlman MA. Dangerous and cancer-causing properties of products and chemicals in the oil refining and petrochemical industries. Part XXX: causal relationship between chronic myelogenous leukemia and benzene-containing solvents. Ann N Y Acad Sci. 2006;1076:110–9.
18. Lamm SH, Engel A, Joshi KP, Byrd DM 3rd, Chen R. Chronic myelogenous leukemia and benzene exposure: a systematic review and meta-analysis of the case-control literature. Chem Biol Interact. 2009;182(2-3):93–7.
19. Björk J, Albin M, Welinder H, et al. Are occupational, hobby, or lifestyle exposures associated with Philadelphia chromosome positive chronic myeloid leukaemia? Occup Environ Med. 2001;58(11):722–7.
20. Brandt L. Environmental factors and leukaemia. Med Oncol Tumor Pharmacother. 1985;2(1):7–10.
21. Schnatter AR, Rosamilia K, et al. Review of the literature on benzene exposure and leukemia subtypes. Chem Biol Interact. 2005;153–154:9–21.
22. Smith MT. The mechanism of benzene-induced leukemia: a hypothesis and speculations on the cause of leukemia. Environ Health Perspect. 2007;104(Suppl 6):1219–25.
23. Whysner J, Reddy MV, Ross PM, et al. Genotoxicity of benzene and its metabolites. Mutat Res. 2004;566:99–130.
24. Escobar PA, Smith MT, Vasishta A, et al. Leukaemia-specific chromosome damage detected by comet with fluorescence in situ hybridization (comet-FISH). Mutagenesis. 2007;22:321–7.
25. Lindsey RH Jr, Bender RP, Osheroff N. Effects of benzene metabolites on DNA cleavage mediated by human topoisomerase II alpha: 1,4-hydroquinone is a topoisomerase II poison. Chem Res Toxicol. 2005;18:761–70.
26. Zhang L, Yang W, Hubbard AE, et al. Nonrandom aneuploidy of chromosomes 1, 5, 6, 7, 8, 9, 11, 12, and 21 induced by the benzene metabolites hydroquinone and benzenetriol. Environ Mol Mutagen. 2005;45:388–96.
27. Mamuris Z, Prieur M, Dutrillaux B, et al. The chemotherapeutic drug melphalan induces breakage of chromosomes regions rearranged in secondary leukemia. Cancer Genet Cytogenet. 1989;37:65–77.
28. Beranek DT. Distribution of methyl and ethyl adducts following alkylation with monofunctional alkylating agents. Mutat Res. 1990;231:11–30.
29. Albertini R, Vacek P, Walker VE, et al. 1,3-Butadiene, CML and the t(9:22) translocation: a reality check. Chem Biol Interact. 2015;241:32–9.
30. Preston DL, Kusumi S, Tomonaga M, et al. Cancer incidence in atomic bomb survivors. Part III. Leukemia, lymphoma and multiple myeloma, 1950–1987. Radiat Res. 1994;137(Suppl 2):S68–97.
31. Finch SC. Radiation-induced leukemia: lessons from history. Best Pract Res Clin Haematol. 2007;20:109–18.
32. Ichimaru M, Tomonaga M, Amenomori T, et al. Atomic bomb and leukemia. J Radiat Res (Tokyo). 1991;32(Suppl 2):14–9.
33. Hsu WL, Preston DL, Soda M, et al. The incidence of leukemia, lymphoma and multiple myeloma among atomic bomb survivors: 1950–2001. Radiat Res. 2013 Mar;179(3):361–82.
34. Hoglund M, Sandin F, Simonsson B. Epidemiology of chronic myeloid leukaemia: an update. Ann Hematol. 2015;94(Suppl 2):S241–7.
35. Gluzman D, Imamura N, Sklyarenko L, et al. Patterns of hematological malignancies in Chernobyl clean-up workers (1996–2005). Exp Oncol. 2006;28(1):60–3.
36. Ito T, Seyama T, Mizuno T, et al. Induction of BCR-ABL fusion genes by in vitro X-irradiation. Jpn J Cancer Res. 1993;84:105–9.
37. Deininger MW, Bose S, Gora-Tybor J, et al. Selective induction of leukemia-associated fusion genes by high-dose ionizing radiation. Cancer Res. 1998;58:421–5.
38. Rohrbacher M, Hasford J. Epidemiology of chronic myeloid leukaemia (CML). Best Pract Res Clin Haematol. 2009;22(3):295–302.
39. Parkin DM. The evolution of the population-based cancer registry. Nat Rev Cancer. 2006;6:603–12.
40. Swedish Cancer Registry, 1998–2008, Annual report publications of the Centre of Epidemiology at the National Board of Health and Welfare. http://www.socialstyrelsen.se/Statistik/statistik_amne/Cancer. Accessed May 2010.
41. Swedish Cancer Registry, 2009–2014, Annual report publications of the Centre of Epidemiology at the National Board of Health and Welfare. http://www.socialstyrelsen.se/statistics/statisticaldatabase/cancer. Accessed March 2016.
42. Krebsregister Saarland, 1998–2007, Germany. http://www.krebsregister.saarland.de. Accessed May 2010.
43. Krebsregister Saarland, 2008–2012, Germany. http://www.krebsregister.saarland.de/datenbank/datenbank.html. Accessed March 2016.
44. Altekruse SF, Kosary CL, Krapcho M, et al. SEER cancer statistics review, 1975–2007. Bethesda: National Cancer Institute. http://seer.cancer.gov/csr/1975_2007/. Accessed May 2010.
45. Howlader N, Noone AM, Krapcho M, et al. Cancer statistics review, 1975–2012, Bethesda: National Cancer Institute http://seer.cancer.gov/csr/2009_2012/. Accessed April 2016.
46. Hoffmann VS, Baccarani M, Hasford J, et al. The EUTOS population-based registry: incidence and clinical characteristics of 2904 CML patients in 20 European Countries. Leukemia. 2015;29(6):1336–43.
47. Phekoo KJ, Richards MA, Moller H, Schey SA. The incidence and outcome of myeloid malignancies in 2,112 adult patients in south East-England. Haematologica. 2006;91:1400–4.
48. Harrison SJ, Johnson PRE, Holyoake TL. The Scotland Leukaemia Registry audit of incidence, diagnosis and clinical management of new patients with chronic myeloid leukaemia in 1999 and 2000. Scott Med J. 2004;49:87–90.
49. McNally RJ, Rowland D, Roman E, Cartwright RA. Age and sex distributions of hematological malignancies in the U.K. Hematol Oncol. 1997;15:173–89.
50. Hasford J, Tauscher M, Hochhaus A. Incidence, comorbidity and treatment survey of chronic myeloid leukemia in Germany. Blood (ASH Annual Meeting Abstracts). 2007;110:Abstract 2964
51. Corm S, Micol J, Leroyer A, et al. Kinetic of chronic myeloid leukaemia (CML) prevalence in Northern France since the introduction of imatinib. J Clin Oncol. 2008;26(Suppl.):Abstract 7088
52. Penot A, Preux PM, Le Guyader S, et al. Incidence of chronic myeloid leukemia and patient survival: results of five French

population-based cancer registries 1980–2009. Leuk Lymphoma. 2015;56(6):1771–7.

53. Lee J, Birnstein E, Masiello D, Yang D, et al. Gender and ethnic differences in chronic myelogenous leukemia prognosis and treatment response: a single-institution retrospective study. J Hematol Oncol. 2009;2:30.
54. Rohrbacher M, Berger U, Hochhaus A, et al. Clinical trials underestimate age of chronic myeloid leukemia (CML) patients. incidence and median age of Ph/BCR-ABL positive CML and other chronic myeloproliferative disorders in a representative area in Germany. Leukemia. 2008;23:602–4.
55. Mendizabal A, Younes N, Levine PH. Geographic and income variations in age at diagnosis and incidence of chronic myeloid leukemia. Int J Hematol. 2016;103(1):70–8.
56. Ahmad O, Boschi-Pinto C, Lopez A, et al. Age standardization of rates: a new WHO standard. GPE Discussion paper Series: No. 31. http://www.who.int/infobase/help. Accessed May 2010.
57. Ridell B, Carneskog J, Wedel H, et al. Incidence of chronic myeloproliferative disorders in the city of Göteborg, Sweden 1983–1992. Eur J Haematol. 2000;65:267–71.
58. Hasford J, Baccarani M, Hehlmann R, et al. Interferon-a and hydroxyurea in early chronic myeloid leukemia: a comparative analysis of the Italian and German chronic myeloid leukemia trials with interferon-a. Blood. 1996;88:5384–91.
59. Allan NC, Richards SM, Shepherd PC. UK Medical Research Council randomised, multicentre trial of interferon-alpha n1 for chronic myeloid leukaemia: improved survival irrespective of cytogenetic response. The UK medical research council's working parties for therapeutic trials in adult leukaemia. Lancet. 1995;345:1392–7.
60. Onida F, Ball G, Kantarjian HM, et al. Characteristics and outcome of patients with Philadelphia chromosome negative, bcr/abl negative chronic myelogenous leukemia. Cancer. 2002;95(8):1673–84.
61. Micheli A, Mugno E, Krogh V, et al. Cancer prevalence in European registry areas. Ann Oncol. 2002;13:840–65.
62. Gunnarsson N, Sjalander A, Sandin F, et al. Population-based assessment of chronic myeloid leukemia in Sweden: striking increase in survival and prevalence. Eur J Haematol. 2016;97(4):387–92.
63. Huang X, Cortes J, Kantarjian H. Estimations of the increasing prevalence and plateau prevalence of chronic myeloid leukemia in the era of tyrosine kinase inhibitor therapy. Cancer. 2012;118(12):3123–7.
64. Pfirrmann M, Hoffmann VS, Hasford J, et al. Prognosis of long-term survival considering disease-specific death in patients with chronic myeloid leukemia. Leukemia. 2016;30(1):48–56.
65. Brunner AM, Campigotto F, Sadrzadeh H, et al. Trends in all-cause mortality among patients with chronic myeloid leukemia: a Surveillance, Epidemiology, and End Results database analysis. Cancer. 2013;119(14):2620–9.
66. Mandal R, Bolt DM, Shah B. Disparities in chronic myeloid leukemia survival by age, gender, and ethnicity in pre- and post-imatinib eras in the US. Acta Oncol. 2013;52(4):837–41.
67. Lauseker M, Gerlach R, Tauscher M, Hasford J. Improved survival boosts the prevalence of chronic myeloid leukemia: predictions from a population-based study. J Cancer Res Clin Oncol. 2016;142(7):1441–7.
68. Gunnarsson N, Wallvik J, Sjalander A, et al. Second malignancies following treatment of chronic myeloid leukaemia in the tyrosine kinase inhibitor era. Br J Haematol. 2015;169(5):683–8.
69. Shah BK, Ghimire KB. Second primary malignancies in chronic myeloid leukemia. Indian J Hematol Blood Transfus. 2014;30(4):236–40.
70. Tardieu S, Brun-Strang C, Berthaud P, et al. Management of chronic myeloid leukemia in France: a multicentered cross-sectional study on 538 patients. Pharmacoepidemiol Drug Saf. 2005;14:545–53.
71. Verdecchia A, Baili P, Quaglia A, et al. Patient survival for all cancers combined as indicator of cancer control in Europe. Eur J Public Health. 2008;18:527–32.
72. Menzin J, Lang K, Earle CC, et al. Treatment patterns, outcomes and costs among elderly patients with chronic myeloid leukaemia: a population-based analysis. Drugs Aging. 2004;21(11):737–46.
73. Darkow T, Henk HJ, Thomas SK, et al. Treatment interruptions and non-adherence with imatinib and associated healthcare costs: a retrospective analysis among managed care patients with chronic myelogenous leukaemia. Pharmacoeconomics. 2007;25(6):481–96.
74. Dalziel K, Round A, Stein K, et al. Effectiveness and cost-effectiveness of imatinib for first-line treatment of chronic myeloid leukaemia in chronic phase: a systematic review and economic analysis. Health Technol Assess. 2004;8(28):iii. 1–120
75. Micheli A, Capocaccia R, Martinez C, et al. Cancer control in Europe: a proposed set of European cancer health indicators. Eur J Public Health. 2003;13:116–8.
76. Conti RM, Padula WV, Larson RA. Changing the cost of care for chronic myeloid leukemia: the availability of generic imatinib in the USA and the EU. Ann Hematol. 2015;94(Suppl 2):S249–57.
77. Experts in Chronic Myeloid Leukemia. The price of drugs for chronic myeloid leukemia (CML) is a reflection of the unsustainable prices of cancer drugs: from the perspective of a large group of CML experts. Blood. 2013;121(22):4439–42.
78. Baccarani M, Saglio G, Goldman J, et al. Evolving concepts in the management of chronic myeloid leukemia. Recommendations from an expert panel on behalf of the European LeukemiaNet. Blood. 2006;108:1809–20.
79. Baccarani M, Cortes J, Pane F, et al. Chronic myeloid leukemia: an update of concepts and management recommendations of European LeukemiaNet. J Clin Oncol. 2009;27(35):6041–51.
80. Breccia M, Luigiana L, Latagliata R, et al. Age influences initial dose and compliance to imatinib in chronic myeloid leukemia elderly patients but concomitant comorbidities appear to influence overall and event-free survival. Leuk Res. 2014;38(10):1173–6.
81. Gugliotta G, Castagnetti F, Apolinari M, et al. First-line treatment of newly diagnosed elderly patients with chronic myeloid leukemia: current and emerging strategies. Drugs. 2014;74(6):627–43.
82. Seiter K. Considerations in the management of elderly patients with chronic myeloid leukemia. Clin Lymphoma Myeloma Leuk. 2012;12(1):12–9.
83. Russo D, Malagola M, Skert C, et al. Treatment of chronic myeloid leukemia elderly patients in the tyrosine kinase inhibitor era. Curr Cancer Drug Targets. 2013;13(7):755–67.
84. Wiggins C, Harlan L, Nelson H, et al. Age disparity in the dissemination of imatinib for treating chronic myeloid leukemia. Am J Med. 2010;123(8):764.e1–9.
85. Hasford J, Baccarani M, Hoffmann V, et al. Predicting complete cytogenetic response and subsequent progression-free survival in 2060 patients with CML on imatinib treatment: the EUTOS score. Blood. 2011;118:686–92.
86. Hoffmann VS, Baccarani M, Lindoerfer D, et al. The EUTOS prognostic score: review and validation in 1288 patients with CML treated frontline with imatinib. Leukemia. 2013;27:2016–22.
87. Beinortas T, Tavorienė I, Tadas Žvirblis T, et al. Chronic myeloid leukemia incidence, survival and accessibility of tyrosine kinase inhibitors: a report from population-based Lithuanian haematological disease registry 2000–2013. BMC Cancer. 2016;16:198.
88. Hehlmann R, Berger U, Pfirrmann M, et al. Randomized comparison of interferon a and hydroxyurea with hydroxyurea monotherapy in chronic myeloid leukemia (CML-Study II): prolongation of survival by the combination of interferon a and hydroxyurea. Leukemia. 2003;17:1529–37.
89. Hehlmann R, Berger U, Pfirrmann M, et al. Drug treatment is superior to allografting as first line therapy in chronic myeloid leukemia. Blood. 2007;109:4686–92.

90. The Italian Cooperative Study Group on Chronic Myeloid Leukemia. Interferon alfa-2a as compared with conventional chemotherapy for the treatment of chronic myeloid leukemia. N Engl J Med. 1994;330:820–5.
91. The Benelux CML Study Group. Randomized study on hydroxyurea alone versus hydroxyurea combined with low-dose interferon-a2b for chronic myeloid leukemia. Blood. 1998;91:2713–21.
92. Kluin-Nelemans HC, Buck G, Le Cessie S, et al. Randomized comparison of low-dose versus high-dose interferon-alfa in chronic myeloid leukemia: prospective collaboration of 3 joint trials by the MRC and HOVON groups. Blood. 2004;103:4408–15.
93. Kantarjian HM, Talpaz M, O'Brien S, et al. Survival benefit with imatinib mesylate versus interferon alpha-based regimens in newly diagnosed chronic phase chronic myelogenous leukemia. Blood. 2006;108:1835–40.
94. Jabbour E, Daniel Jones D, Kantarjian HM, et al. Long-term outcome of patients with chronic myeloid leukemia treated with second-generation tyrosine kinase inhibitors after imatinib failure is predicted by the in vitro sensitivity of BCR-ABL kinase domain mutations. Blood. 2009;114:2037–43.
95. Saussele S, Lauseker M, Gratwohl A, et al. Allogeneic hematopoietic stem cell transplantation (allo SCT) for chronic myeloid leukemia in the imatinib era: evaluation of its impact within a subgroup of the randomized German CML Study IV. Blood. 2010;115(10):1880–5.
96. Palandri F, Castagnetti F, Iacobucci I, et al. The response to imatinib and interferon-{alpha} is more rapid than the response to imatinib alone: a retrospective analysis of 495 Philadelphia-positive chronic myeloid leukemia patients in early chronic phase. Haematologica. 2010;95(8):1415–9.
97. Efficace F, Baccarani M, Breccia M. Health-related quality of life in chronic myeloid leukemia patients receiving long-term therapy with imatinib compared with the general population. Blood. 2011;118:4554–60.
98. Hanfstein B, Müller MC, Hehlmann R, the SAKK, the German CML Study Group, et al. Early molecular and cytogenetic response is predictive for long-term progression-free and overall survival in chronic myeloid leukemia (CML). Leukemia. 2012;26:2096–102.
99. Marin D, Ibrahim AR, Lucas C, et al. Assessment of BCR-ABL1 transcript levels at 3 months is the only requirement for predicting outcome for patients with chronic myeloid leukemia treated with tyrosine kinase inhibitors. J Clin Oncol. 2012;30:232–8.
100. Cortes JE, Kim DW, Kantarjian HM, et al. Bosutinib versus imatinib in newly diagnosed chronic-phase chronic myeloid leukemia: results from the BELA trial. J Clin Oncol. 2012;30:3486–92.
101. Jabbour E, le Coutre PD, Cortes J, et al. Prediction of outcomes in patients with Ph+ chronic myeloid leukemia in chronic phase treated with nilotinib after imatinib resistance/intolerance. Leukemia. 2013;27:907–13.
102. Castagnetti F, Gugliotta G, de Vivo A. Differences among young adults, adults and elderly chronic myeloid leukemia patients. Ann Oncol. 2015;26:185–92.
103. Saussele S, Krauss MP, Hehlmann R, et al. Impact of comorbidities on overall survival in patients with chronic myeloid leukemia: results of the randomized CML study IV. Blood. 2015;126(1):42–9.
104. Hehlmann R, Heimpel H, Hasford J, et al. Randomized comparison of interferon-alpha with busulfan and hydroxyurea in chronic myelogenous leukemia. Blood. 1994;84:4064–77.
105. Baccarani M, Rosti G, De Vivo A, et al. A randomized study of interferon-alpha versus interferon-alpha and low-dose arabinosyl cytosine in chronic myeloid leukemia. Blood. 2002;99:1527–35.
106. Bonifazi F, De Vivo A, Rosti G, et al. Chronic myeloid leukemia and interferon-alpha: a study of complete cytogenetic responders. Blood. 2001;98:3074–81.
107. Druker BJ, Guilhot F, O'Brien SG, et al. Five-year follow-up of patients receiving imatinib for chronic myeloid leukemia. N Engl J Med. 2006;355:2408–17.
108. Guilhot F, Chastang C, Michallet M, et al. Interferon alpha2b (IFN) combined with cytarabine versus interferon alone in chronic myelogenous leukemia. N Engl J Med. 1997;337:223–9.
109. Hasford J, Pfirrmann M, Hehlmann R, et al. A new prognostic score for the survival of patients with chronic myeloid leukemia treated with interferon alfa. J Natl Cancer Inst. 1998;90:850–8.
110. Faber E, Koza V, Jarosova M, et al. Treatment of consecutive patients with chronic myeloid leukaemia in the cooperating centres from the Czech Republic and the whole of Slovakia after 2000—a report from the population-based CAMELIA Registry. Eur J Haematol. 2011;87(2):157–68.
111. Schmidt S, Wolf D, Gastl G, et al. Wien Klin Wochenschr. 2010;122(19–20):558–66.
112. Xie Y, Davies SM, Xiang Y, Robison LL, Ross JA. Trends in leukemia incidence and survival in the United States (1973–1998). Cancer. 2003;97:2229–35.
113. Goldberg SL, Chen L, Guerin A, et al. Association between molecular monitoring and long-term outcomes in chronic myelogenous leukemia patients treated with first line imatinib. Curr Med Res Opin. 2013;29:1075–82.
114. Lauseker M, Hasford J, Pfirrmann M, Hehlmann R, German CML Study Group, et al. The impact of health care settings on survival time of patients with chronic myeloid leukemia. Blood. 2014;123:2494–6.

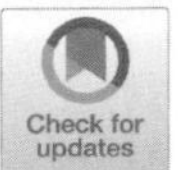

Pathology of the Chronic Myeloid Leukemias

3

Barbara J. Bain

Introduction

The chronic myeloid leukemias are a group of hematological neoplasms resulting from mutation in either a pluripotent (lymphoid-myeloid) stem cell or in a multipotent myeloid progenitor or stem cell. The former group of leukemias are actually, or potentially, of mixed phenotype while the latter have a purely myeloid phenotype.

Diagnosis of these conditions is based on clinical and hematological features with genetic analysis being crucial for the recognition of some categories. Genetic analysis has been incorporated, as far as current knowledge permits, into the classification of the chronic myeloid leukemias, in the 2016 update of the 2008 World Health Organization (WHO) *Classification of Tumours of Haematopoietic and Lymphoid Tissues* [1]. Depending on their typical hematological features and any relevant genetic abnormality, they are assigned to the categories: (a) myeloproliferative neoplasm; (b) myelodysplastic/myeloproliferative neoplasm; and (c) myeloid or lymphoid neoplasm with rearrangement of *PDGFRA*, *PDGFRB*, or *FGFR1*or with *PCM1-JAK2*.

In making a morphological diagnosis, the peripheral blood features are often of critical importance. The bone marrow aspirate and trephine biopsy sections give useful supplementary information. Flow cytometric immunophenotyping is only of diagnostic importance when there is presentation with acute-phase disease or when acute transformation subsequently occurs. Immunohistochemistry on trephine biopsy sections can be useful, particularly in the recognition of dysplastic megakaryocytes and for confirmation of the presence of dysplastic mast cells. Cytochemistry is now of little importance in diagnosis; the neutrophil alkaline phosphatase score is redundant when genetic analysis is available and immunophenotyping is superior to cytochemistry for the recognition of the lineage involved in acute transformation.

Chronic Myelogenous Leukemia

Chronic myelogenous leukemia (CML) results from a mutation in a pluripotent hematopoietic stem cell that leads to formation of a *BCR-ABL1* fusion gene [2]. The associated acquired cytogenetic abnormality is usually t(9;22)(q34.1;q11.2), but there are other mechanisms, including variant and complex translocations (see Chap. 6). The derivative chromosome 22 is known as the Philadelphia (Ph) chromosome. Alternative designations of this condition are chronic granulocytic leukemia and chronic myeloid leukemia, but it should be noted that the latter term, although very widely used and now favored by the WHO, is open to misinterpretation since it is also used as a generic term for all the chronic myeloid leukemias.

This disease occurs at all ages, but incidence increases steadily with age and is somewhat higher in men than in women. Common clinical features are weight loss, low-grade fever, sweating, splenomegaly, and, when disease is advanced, hepatomegaly [3]. Lymphadenopathy is only a feature when acute transformation occurs. Patients with a very high white cell count can have features of leukostasis, such as blurred vision and priapism. Many patients are now diagnosed as a result of an incidental blood count when they are asymptomatic.

The natural history of CML is that the chronic phase of the disease is followed by acute transformation (myeloid, lymphoid, or mixed), which may be preceded by an accelerated phase. The abrupt onset of acute transformation without a preceding accelerated phase is more common in lymphoid transformation.

Peripheral Blood Count and Cytology

The peripheral blood count in *chronic-phase CML* typically shows leukocytosis and anemia. Usually there is also

B.J. Bain, M.B.B.S., F.R.A.C.P., F.R.C.Path
Department of Hematology, St. Mary's Hospital Campus of Imperial College Faculty of Medicine, St Mary's Hospital, Praed Street, London W2 1NY, UK
e-mail: b.bain@ic.ac.uk

P.H. Wiernik et al. (eds.), *Neoplastic Diseases of the Blood*, DOI 10.1007/978-3-319-64263-5_3

thrombocytosis although the platelet count can be normal or reduced. Some patients have thrombocytosis without leukocytosis. Such *BCR-ABL1*-positive cases should be recognized as a variant of CML [2]. The blood film characteristically shows a particular increase in myelocytes and neutrophils (Fig. 3.1). Basophils are almost invariably increased and eosinophils usually so [4]. Eosinophil and basophil myelocytes may also be present. The absolute monocyte count is increased but not in proportion to the increase in granulocytes. The number of blast cells and promyelocytes is proportionate to the number of myelocytes. Cells of the granulocyte lineages do not show dysplastic features. Platelets show anisocytosis with some giant forms. There may be occasional circulating megakaryocyte nuclei with scanty cytoplasm ("bare" megakaryocyte nuclei). Red cells may show nonspecific abnormalities, such as anisocytosis and mild poikilocytosis. There may be circulating nucleated red blood cells. Neutrophil alkaline phosphatase is reduced in the great majority of patients, but this test is redundant when cytogenetic and molecular analyses are available.

Peripheral blood features of the *accelerated phase* of CML may include leukocytosis or thrombocytosis that is refractory to treatment; an increasing basophil count; a disproportionate increase in blast cells; the appearance of dysplastic features such as hypolobulated neutrophils and circulating micromegakaryocytes; thrombocytopenia; and increasing anemia. A disproportionate increase in eosinophils can occur but is much less common than marked basophilia. Poikilocytosis may become more marked and there may be teardrop poikilocytes.

In *blast transformation* there is usually an increase in blast cells in the peripheral blood (Fig. 3.2). Usually these are myeloblasts, megakaryoblasts, or lymphoblasts. When transformation is megakaryoblastic, there may also be circulating micromegakaryocytes. Less common forms of transformation (determined by the underlying further mutations that have occurred) include mixed phenotype, monoblastic, eosinophilic, erythroblastic, and hypergranular promyelocytic.

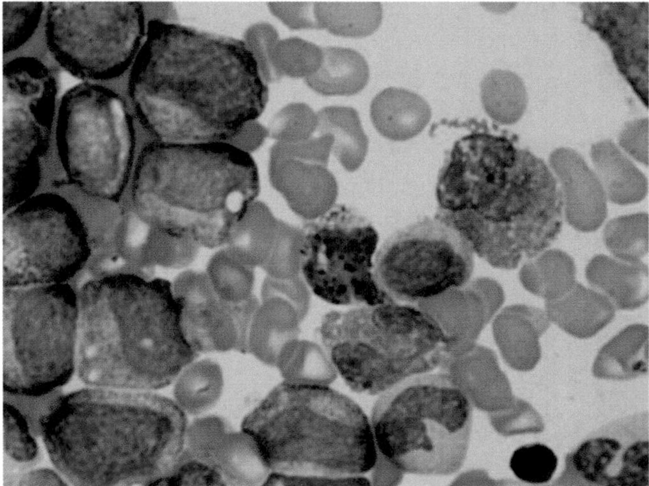

Fig. 3.1 Peripheral blood (PB) film from a patient with chronic myelogenous leukemia with an unusually high white cell count showing an increase of neutrophils, eosinophils, basophils, and granulocyte precursors. May-Grünwald-Giemsa stain (MGG), high power

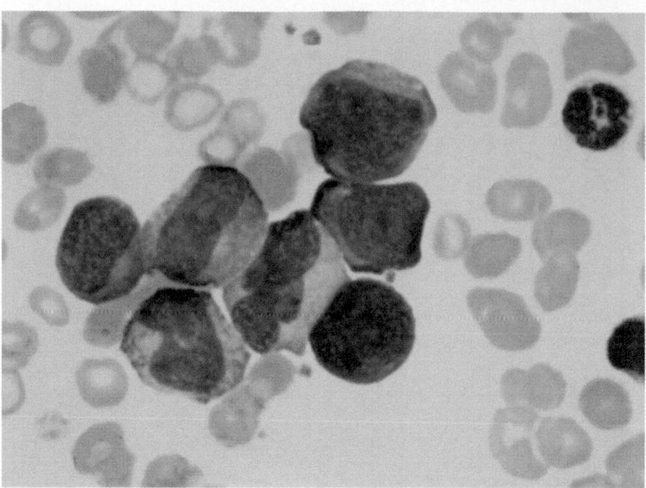

Fig. 3.2 PB film from a patient with transformation of chronic myelogenous leukemia showing three blast cells, granulocyte precursors, and several dysplastic cells of neutrophil lineage. MGG, high power

Bone Marrow Cytology

The bone marrow aspirate in *chronic-phase CML* shows marked hypercellularity due to an increase in granulocytes and their precursors (Fig. 3.3). The myeloid:erythroid ratio is almost always greater than 10:1 and often of the order of 25:1. Megakaryocytes are usually increased with a tendency to be smaller than normal with reduced nuclear lobulation, reflecting a decrease in ploidy. However, micromegakaryocytes, such as those seen in the myelodysplastic syndromes, are not a feature of chronic-phase disease. Sometimes there is an increase in storage cells—pseudo-Gaucher cells and sea blue histiocytes.

In the *accelerated phase*, the aspirate may show increased blast cells, increased basophils, and dysplastic features in the cells of any lineage.

In *blast transformation*, the bone marrow shows increased blast cells, except in the minority of cases in which transformation is first detected at an extramedullary site. Myeloblasts are often agranular and Auer rods are usually absent. In the case of myeloid or mixed lineage transformation, there are usually dysplastic features, particularly in the megakaryocyte lineage (Fig. 3.4).

Flow Cytometric Immunophenotyping

Immunophenotyping is not diagnostically useful in chronic-phase disease.

Genetics

Cytogenetic and genetic features are discussed in Chap. 6.

Histology

In *chronic-phase CML*, trephine biopsy sections show an increase in cells of all granulocyte lineages but, apart from the loss of fat cells, with retention of normal bone marrow architecture (Fig. 3.5) [5–7]. There is an expansion of the band of myeloblasts and promyelocytes that is usually detected against the bony spicule and around arterioles. Eosinophils are readily detected, but basophils are not specifically identifiable on hematoxylin and eosin (H&E) stains as granules are dissolved during processing. Megakaryocytes are increased in number with a reduction in average size and nuclear lobulation. They are normally located and do not form large clusters. Erythropoiesis is decreased. Mast cells and plasma cells are often increased. Increased storage cells may be apparent (Fig. 3.6). Bone marrow vascularity is increased (neoangiogenesis). Reticulin is usually normal or only mildly increased.

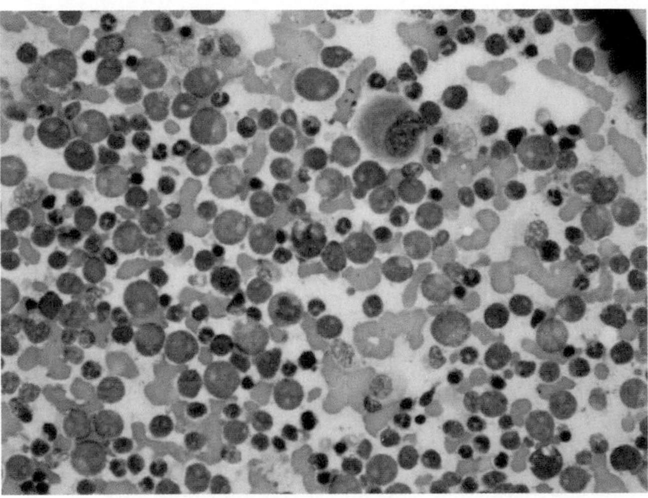

Fig. 3.3 Bone marrow film from a patient with chronic myelogenous leukemia showing increased granulopoiesis and a hypolobated megakaryocyte. MGG, low power

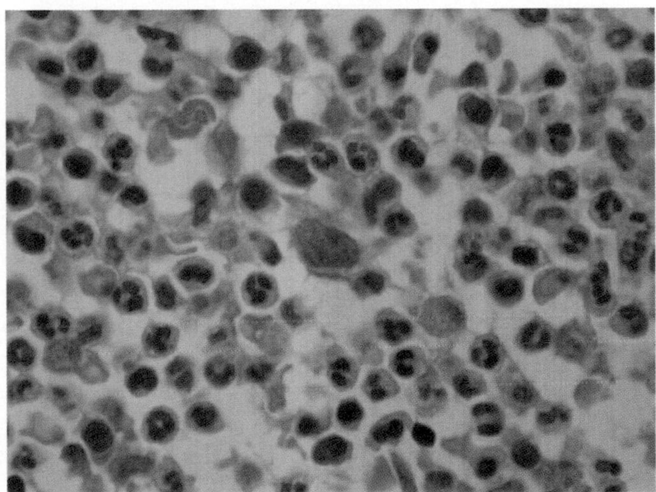

Fig. 3.5 Bone marrow trephine biopsy section from a patient with chronic myelogenous leukemia showing increased granulopoiesis and a relatively small, hypolobated megakaryocyte. Hematoxylin and eosin stain (H&E), low power

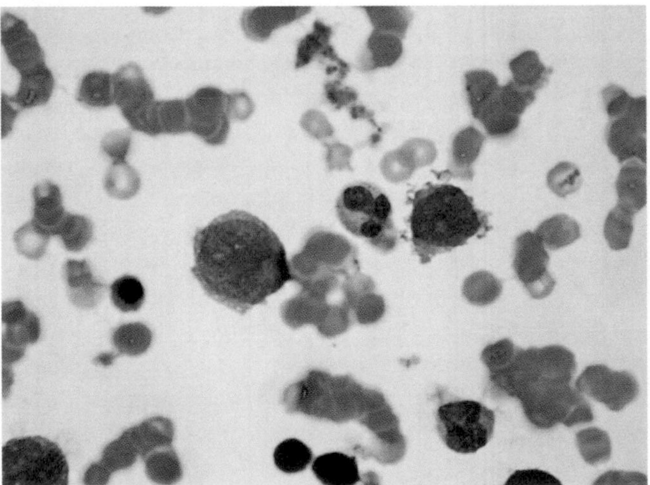

Fig. 3.4 Bone marrow film from a patient with megakaryoblastic transformation showing a neutrophil flanked by a blast cell (*left*) and a micromegakaryocyte (*right*). MGG, high power

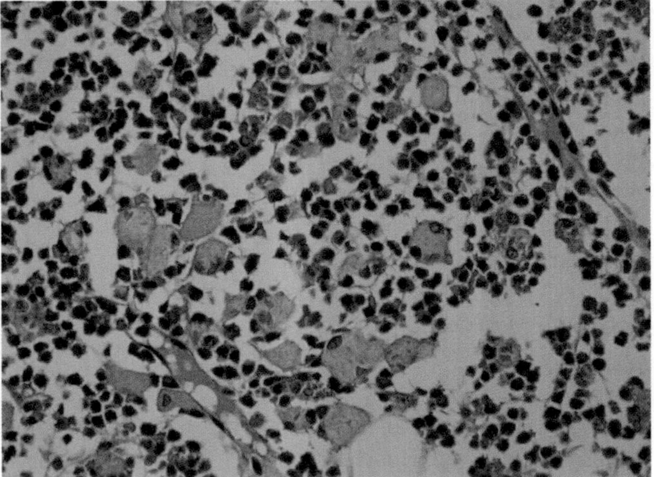

Fig. 3.6 Bone marrow trephine biopsy section from a patient with chronic-phase myelogenous leukemia showing numerous pseudo-Gaucher cells. H&E, low power

In *accelerated phase*, the changes that would be expected from the bone marrow aspirate are present. In addition, the bone marrow architecture may be abnormal, e.g., with megakaryocytes located adjacent to bony spicules or forming large clusters. Intravascular hemopoiesis and bone marrow necrosis can occur. Reticulin may be increased. Sometimes the increase in reticulin is marked and there is also collagen fibrosis and osteosclerosis (Fig. 3.7).

Immunohistochemistry with CD42b or CD61 monoclonal antibodies can be used to identify dysplastic megakaryocytes. CD34 antibodies can identify blast cells and endothelial cells of new vessels.

In *blast transformation*, there is an increase in the blast cells of one or more lineages. In myeloid transformation, there can also be a marked increase of dysplastic megakaryocytes, often in large clusters or sheets. The pattern of blast infiltration may initially be random focal, but subsequently blast cells obliterate maturing hematopoietic cells. Reticulin and collagen fibrosis are common, particularly when there is an increase in megakaryoblasts and dysplastic megakaryocytes.

Immunohistochemistry can be used to identify myeloblastic crisis (CD68, lysozyme), megakaryoblastic crisis (CD42b, CD61), erythroblastic crisis (antiglycophorin—CD235a or CD236R), and B-lymphoblastic crisis (CD79a is more generally positive than CD20). CD34 immunohistochemistry can help in the quantification of blast cells.

In extramedullary transformation, there is initially infiltration of another tissue or organ, e.g., a lymph node, with subsequent spread to the marrow. In extramedullary transformation, immunohistochemistry is useful for confirmation of the diagnosis.

Atypical (Ph-Negative) Chronic Myeloid Leukemia

Atypical chronic myeloid leukemia (aCML) is an uncommon, Ph-negative, *BCR-ABL1*-negative chronic myeloid leukemia, which is categorized in the WHO classification as an MDS/MPN [8–10]. Clinical features are similar to those of CML, but the prognosis is worse. Death may result from bone marrow failure or evolution to acute myeloid leukemia (AML). Atypical CML is mainly a disease of adults, particularly elderly adults with a similar incidence in men and women.

Peripheral Blood Count and Cytology

The peripheral blood shows leukocytosis and anemia (Fig. 3.8). The WHO classification has a white cell count (WBC) of at least 13×10^9/L as a diagnostic criterion. There may be anisocytosis, poikilocytosis, macrocytosis, or dimorphism. The platelet count is often reduced but may be normal or increased. In comparison with CML, anemia tends to be more severe and thrombocytopenia more common. There is an increase in neutrophils and their precursors. Eosinophils and basophils are often increased but less consistently than in CML. Basophils are usually less than 2% of leucocytes. However, some patients have prominent eosinophilia. The monocyte count is relatively higher than in CML; it may be more than 1×10^9/L, but monocytes are less than 10% of leucocytes. Granulocyte precursors are also present. In comparison with chronic myelomonocytic leukemia, promyelocytes, myelocytes, and metamyelocytes are at least 10% of leukocytes and

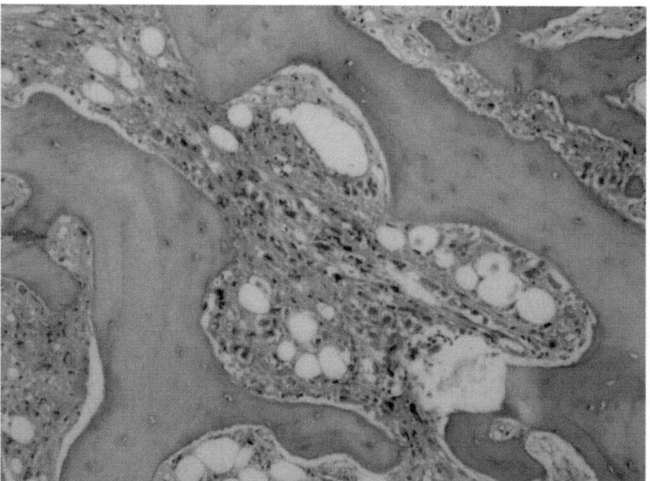

Fig. 3.7 Bone marrow trephine biopsy section from a patient with accelerated phase of chronic myelogenous leukemia showing myelofibrosis and osteosclerosis. There are numerous dysplastic megakaryocytes embedded in the loose fibrous tissue. H&E, low power

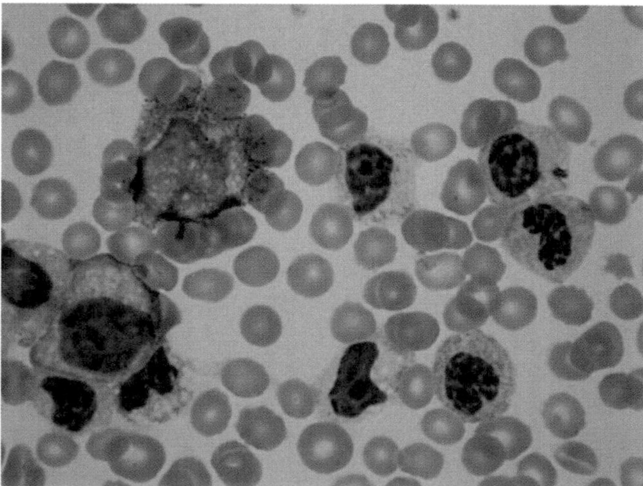

Fig. 3.8 PB film from a patient with atypical chronic myeloid leukemia showing neutrophil precursors and dysplastic neutrophils (hypolobated, nuclear clumping, and hypogranularity). MGG, high power

sometimes 15% or higher. These may include blast cells but, by definition, blast cells (plus promonocytes) are less than 20% in the blood (and the bone marrow). Dysplastic features are present in neutrophils; hypolobation, abnormal nuclear shapes, increased chromatin clumping, and reduced granularity may be seen. Monocytes may also be dysplastic, showing hyperlobation or hypolobation, increased cytoplasmic basophilia, and increased granularity. The neutrophil alkaline phosphatase score is variable and is not diagnostically useful.

Bone Marrow Cytology

The bone marrow aspirate shows increased cellularity with an increase mainly in neutrophils and their precursors. Monocytes and their precursors may be increased and a nonspecific esterase stain can help in their detection. Megakaryocytes may be present in normal numbers or may be decreased or increased. There is dysplasia, which is often of trilineage. Dysgranulopoiesis is usual, but there may also be ring sideroblasts and other features of dyserythropoiesis, hypolobated megakaryocytes, and micromegakaryocytes.

Flow Cytometric Immunophenotyping

Immunophenotyping is not known to be diagnostically useful.

Genetics

Karyotypic abnormalities are common and can include trisomy 8, 20q−, and i(17q) and abnormalities of chromosomes 12, 13, 14, 17, and 19. *SETBP1*, *ETNK1*, *NRAS*, *KRAS*, *CBL*, and *TET2* may be mutated. *CSF3R* mutation has been reported but its presence favors a diagnosis of chronic neutrophilic leukemia. Patients with *BCR-ABL1*, rearrangement of *PDGFRA*, *PDGFRB*, or *FGFR1*, or *PCM1-JAK2* are specifically excluded from this diagnostic category.

Histology

Cellularity is increased as a result of an increase in neutrophils and precursors and a variable increase in monocyte precursors. There is dysplasia and the architecture is disorganized. Reticulin may be increased and collagen fibrosis and osteosclerosis occasionally occur. Immunohistochemistry is useful to highlight dysplastic megakaryocytes (CD42b and CD61) and increased monocytes (CD14 and CD68R).

Chronic Myelomonocytic Leukemia

This is Ph-negative chronic myeloid leukemia that is categorized in the WHO classification as an MDS/MPN [11, 12]. The most prominent clinical features are anemia and splenomegaly, but skin and lymph node infiltration and pleural, peritoneal, and pericardial effusions can also be seen. It is mainly a disease of the middle aged and elderly and shows a male predominance. Transformation to AML occurs in up to a quarter of the patients.

Peripheral Blood Count and Cytology

The peripheral blood shows a normocytic or macrocytic anemia. Red cells are sometimes dimorphic. Leukocytosis is usual but not invariable. There is monocytosis with, by definition, a monocyte count of more than 1×10^9/L (Fig. 3.9). Neutrophils may be increased, normal, or decreased. Neutrophil precursors may be present but, in contrast to aCML, they are less than 10% of the cells and usually less than 5%. There may be small numbers of blast cells and promonocytes; by definition, they total less than 20% of leukocytes, but they are usually much less. The number of blast cells (plus promonocytes) in the blood is of prognostic significance and the presence of 5% or more leads to a classification as CMML-2. A minority of patients have prominent eosinophilia. The platelet count is often reduced but can be normal or high.

Dysplastic features may be present, but are usually less prominent than in aCML. Monocytes may be immature (cytoplasmic basophilia, reduced chromatin condensation, or reduced nuclear lobulation).

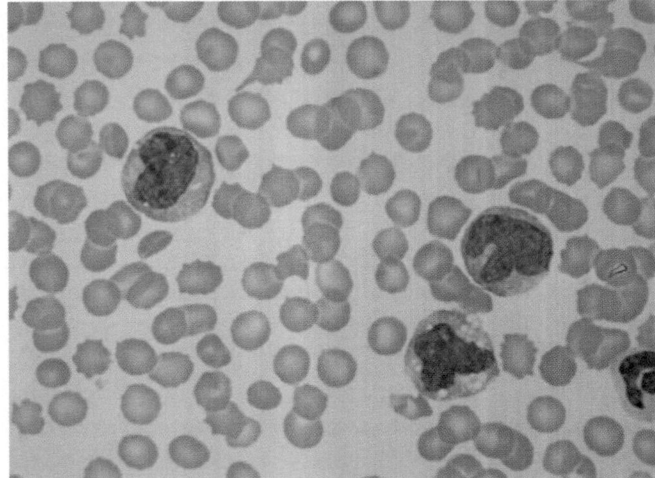

Fig. 3.9 PB film from a patient with chronic myelomonocytic leukemia showing thrombocytopenia and three immature, abnormal monocytes. MGG, high power

Bone Marrow Cytology

The bone marrow shows increased cellularity due to an increase of neutrophils and monocytes and their precursors but a nonspecific esterase stain may be necessary to demonstrate the increase in cells of monocyte lineage. Blasts plus promonocytes are less than 20%. The number of blast cells (plus promonocytes) in the marrow is of prognostic significance and the presence of 10% or more leads to the classification as CMML-2. Auer rods are rarely present but, when present, also lead to classification as CMML-2; a myeloperoxidase or Sudan black B stain is useful for their detection. Some patients have an increase of eosinophils and precursors. There is variable dysplasia, which may include ring sideroblasts.

Flow Cytometric Immunophenotyping

Immunophenotyping may show monocytes to be phenotypically abnormal with reduced, increased, or aberrant expression of various antigens. An abnormal phenotype may be the result of immaturity of monocytes (e.g., reduced CD14 expression) or of aberrant antigen expression (e.g., expression of CD2).

Genetics

Karyotypic abnormalities are detected in a quarter to a half of patients. They include trisomy 8, monosomy 7 and 7q−, and rearrangements with a 12p breakpoint. Common molecular changes include mutations of *RAS* group genes, *RUNX1*, *TET2*, *SRSF2*, *ASXL1*, *SETBP1*, and *CBL*. By definition, *BCR-ABL1*, rearrangement of *PDGFRA, PDGFRB* and *FGFR1*, and *PCM1-JAK2* are absent.

Histology

Trephine biopsy sections show the changes that would be expected from the aspirate. Hypercellularity is usual and results from an increase in the cells of both neutrophil and monocyte lineages. Immunohistochemistry (CD14, CD68R, or CD163) may be necessary to demonstrate the increase in the cells of monocyte lineage. Erythropoiesis may be quantitatively normal or increased. There may be nodules of plasmacytoid dendritic cells, confirmed by immunohistochemistry for CD4, CD14, CD68R, and CD123 [13, 14]. Reticulin deposition is often increased.

Chronic Eosinophilic Leukemia

Chronic eosinophilic leukemias, in the WHO classification, are categorized either as chronic eosinophilic leukemia (CEL), not otherwise specified [15], or as chronic myeloid or lymphoid neoplasm associated with rearrangement of *PDGFRA*, *PDGFRB*, or *FGFR1*, or with *PCM1-JAK2* [16–18]. Diagnosis and categorization require both cytogenetic and molecular analyses, the latter to detect the most frequent rearrangement of *PDGFRA*, a *FIP1L1-PDGFRA* fusion gene resulting from a cryptic deletion at 4q12. Diagnosis of CEL requires an eosinophil count of at least 1.5×10^9/L and some evidence that the process is leukemic in nature, such as a clonal cytogenetic or molecular abnormality or an increase in blast cells.

Leukemias with rearrangement of *PDGFRA* can present as CEL, AML with eosinophilia, or T-lineage acute lymphoblastic leukemia (ALL) with eosinophilia [17, 19]. Leukemias with rearrangement of *PDGFRB* can present as CEL or as either CMML or aCML with eosinophilia. Leukemias with rearrangement of *FGFR1* can present as CEL, AML with eosinophilia, or acute lymphoblastic leukemia/lymphoma (ALL) with eosinophilia; ALL is most often of T lineage but can be of B lineage [17]. Leukemias with *PCM1-JAK2* can be CEL or aCML but some patients have had the features of primary myelofibrosis [18]. In all these disorders, patients who present with chronic phase disease can subsequently suffer acute transformation.

Clinical presentation can be with features suggestive of leukemia (such as anemia, splenomegaly, and sometimes lymphadenopathy) or features reflecting tissue damage by eosinophils (such as cardiac, respiratory, and neurological symptoms). CEL associated with *FIP1L1-PDGFRA* shows a remarkable male predominance. Cases with *PCM1-JAK2* also show a marked male predominance [18]. CEL associated with *PDGFRB* or *FGFR1* rearrangement is also more common in males. CEL associated with rearrangement of *PDGFRA* or *PDGFRB* is sensitive to imatinib and making these specific diagnoses is therefore important. Cases with *PCM1-JAK2* show some responsiveness to ruxolitinib.

Elevation of serum vitamin B_{12} and serum tryptase is usual in patients with CEL associated with *FIP1L1-PDGFRA*.

Peripheral Blood Count and Cytology

The peripheral blood shows an increase in eosinophils, which may be cytologically fairly normal or may show reduced or increased nuclear lobulation, loss of granules, darkly staining (purple) granules, or cytoplasmic vacuolation (Fig. 3.10). There may be eosinophil precursors and blast cells. By definition, blast cells are less than 20%. Some patients also have an increase in neutrophils or monocytes, anemia, or thrombocytopenia.

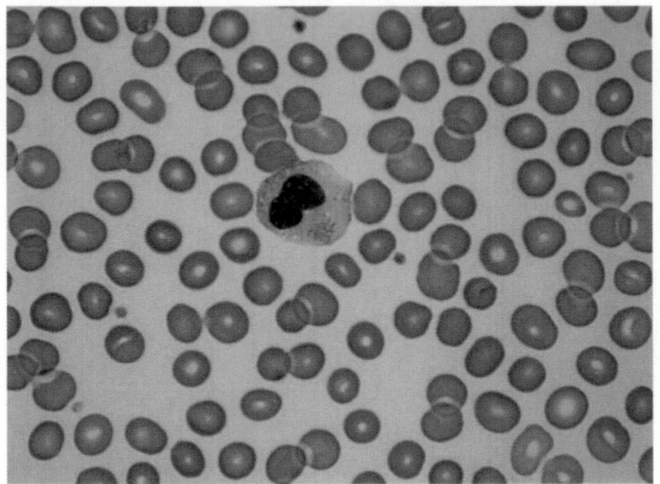

Fig. 3.10 PB film from a patient with chronic eosinophilic leukemia associated with *FIP1L1-PDGFRA* fusion showing an eosinophil with a poorly lobulated nucleus, a few vacuoles, and only a small cluster of granules. MGG, high power

Bone Marrow Cytology

The bone marrow shows an increase in eosinophils and their precursors plus a variable increase in precursors of monocytes and neutrophils. Blast cells may be increased but are less than 20%.

Flow Cytometric Immunophenotyping

Immunophenotyping is occasionally needed to show the lineage of blast cells and thus distinguish CEL and related conditions from ALL with reactive eosinophilia. It must be noted that in the case of CEL associated with rearrangement of *PDGFRA* or *FGFR1*, there may be either presentation as ALL or a lymphoblastic transformation; usually but not invariably the lymphoid component is of T lineage.

Genetics

Karyotypic analysis may show t(5;12)(q31~q33;p12) or another translocation with a 5q31-32 breakpoint involving *PDGFRB*. Rarely there is a translocation with a 4q12 breakpoint involving *PDGFRA*, but usually rearrangement of this gene is cryptic, resulting from an interstitial deletion. *FGFR1* rearrangement most often results from t(8;13)(p11;q12), leading to a *ZMYM2-FGFR1* fusion gene. *PCM1-JAK2* fusion results from the t(8;9)(p22;p24.1) translocation. Other nonspecific chromosomal abnormalities may be found including trisomy 8, 20q–, monosomy 7, and i(17q). The demonstration of t(8;21)(q22;q22.1), inv(16)(p13.1q22), or t(16;16)(p13.1;q22) excludes a diagnosis of CEL and leads to a diagnosis of AML regardless of the blast percentage.

The most important molecular abnormality that must be sought in suspected CEL is the *FIP1L1-PDGFRA* fusion gene, which can be demonstrated either by fluorescence in situ hybridization (FISH) analysis or by PCR (nested PCR often being needed) [16]. Occasionally patients with *FIP1L1-PDGFRA*-associated CEL develop a further mutation in the fusion gene, sometimes associated with imatinib resistance or transformation to AML [19].

Histology

Trephine biopsy sections show the expected increase in eosinophils and precursors and a variable increase in the cells of neutrophil or monocyte lineages. Charcot–Leyden crystals are also sometimes seen [20]. Cases associated with rearrangement of *PDGFRA* or *PDGFRB* may show an increase of mast cells, which are sometimes spindle shaped and clustered. Their presence can be highlighted by immunohistochemistry for mast cell tryptase. The mast cells may show aberrant expression of CD25 and sometimes of CD2, whereas the neoplastic cells of systemic mastocytosis usually show aberrant expression of both CD2 and CD25.

Chronic Neutrophilic Leukemia

Chronic neutrophilic leukemia is a rare myeloproliferative neoplasm that occurs mainly in adults [21]. It is characterized by increased neutrophil production, splenomegaly, and sometimes hepatomegaly. Transformation to AML can occur and at this stage the neutrophil count may fall [22]. Older adults are mainly affected with no gender difference.

Peripheral Blood Count and Cytology

There is leukocytosis and neutrophilia (Fig. 3.11). The WHO classification requires a white cell count of at least 25×10^9/L for this diagnosis. Neutrophils may be heavily granulated and Döhle bodies are sometimes present, but there are no dysplastic features and there are only small numbers of neutrophil precursors [23]. With disease progression there may be anemia and thrombocytopenia.

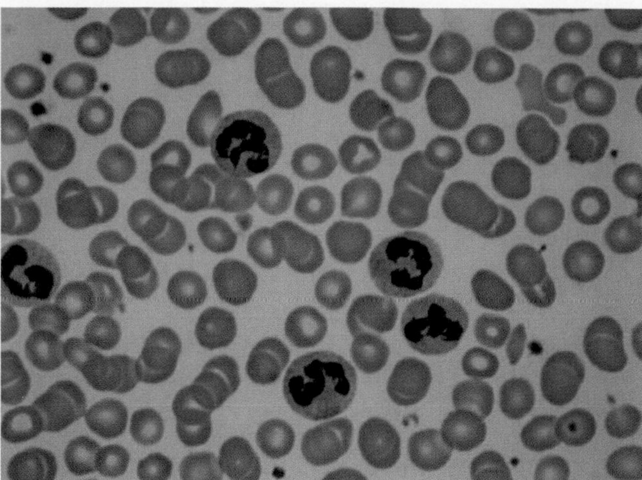

Fig. 3.11 PB film from a patient with chronic neutrophilic leukemia showing cytologically normal neutrophils. MGG, high power

Bone Marrow Cytology

The bone marrow aspirate shows an increase of neutrophils and their precursors without dysplastic features or any increase in the blast cells. The bone marrow must be carefully examined to exclude a plasma cell neoplasm since reactive neutrophilia due to multiple myeloma or monoclonal gammopathy of undetermined significance is an important differential diagnosis [23].

Flow Cytometric Immunophenotyping

Immunophenotyping has no role in diagnosis.

Genetics

Cytogenetic analysis is usually normal. A minority of patients have karyotypic abnormalities typical of myeloid neoplasms such as trisomy 8, trisomy 9, trisomy 21, 11q–, 12p–, or 20q–. Nullisomy 17, a complex karyotype and several nonrecurrent translocations have also been reported. Sometimes an initially normal karyotype becomes abnormal, with acute transformation [22]. There is a strong association with an activating mutation in the proximal membrane domain of *CSF3R* [24]. There is also often an associated mutation of *SETBP1* or *ASXL1*. Occasional patients have a *JAK2* V617F mutation, which may be homozygous [23]. By definition, there is no *BCR-ABL1* fusion gene.

Histology

Trephine biopsy sections show increased granulopoiesis.

Juvenile Myelomonocytic Leukemia

This is a rare myelodysplastic/myeloproliferative neoplasm of children [25–29]. Peak incidence is under the age of 3 years and the condition is twice as common in boys. Predisposing conditions include neurofibromatosis type 1 (*NF1* mutated), Noonan syndrome (*PTPN11* mutated), and *CBL*-mutation associated syndrome. Clinical features can include fever, cough, splenomegaly, hepatomegaly, often lymphadenopathy, skin lesions (an eczematous or maculopapular rash or xanthomas), and a bleeding tendency. Respiratory tract infections are common. In patients with underlying neurofibromatosis there may be café-au-lait spots whereas patients with Noonan syndrome have facial dysmorphism and congenital cardiac anomalies. A hallmark of the disease is increased sensitivity in vitro to granulocyte-macrophage colony-stimulating factor as a result of increased signaling through the RAS-MAPK pathway. The rate of disease progression is quite variable, but prognosis is generally poor unless hematopoietic stem cell transplantation is carried out. Transformation to AML occurs in about 15% of the patients [28]. Occasional patients have had transformation to B-cell precursor ALL and the same acquired genetic lesion has sometimes been found in T-lymphoid and myeloid cells, suggesting that the leukemic clone may be derived from a pluripotent lymphoid-myeloid stem cell [28].

Peripheral Blood Count and Cytology

The peripheral blood shows leukocytosis, monocytosis, and neutrophilia with a lesser increase in granulocyte precursors (Fig. 3.12). Eosinophilia and basophilia are less common than neutrophilia. WHO criteria include a monocyte count of at least 1×10^9/L. There is a variable degree of dysplasia. Blast cells (plus promonocytes) are usually

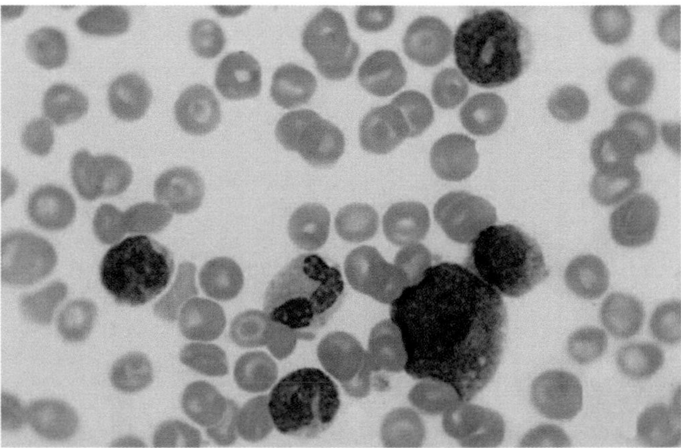

Fig. 3.12 PB film from a patient with juvenile myelomonocytic leukemia showing a neutrophil, a promyelocyte, and dysplastic cells, mainly of monocyte lineage. MGG, high power

low and, by definition, never more than 20% in the blood or bone marrow. Anemia and thrombocytopenia are usual. There may be circulating nucleated red blood cells or neutrophil precursors and some patients have macrocytosis. There is often increased rouleaux formation.

Blood tests show other abnormalities. Polyclonal hypergammaglobulinemia is common and the erythrocyte sedimentation rate is increased. There may be autoantibodies including anti-erythrocyte antibodies. The hemoglobin F percentage is usually increased in comparison with age-matched healthy children and there may be other features suggesting reversion to fetal-type erythropoiesis, such as increased expression of the i antigen and decreased expression of the I antigen, carbonic anhydrase, and hemoglobin A_2.

Bone Marrow Cytology

The bone marrow is hypercellular as a result of increased granulopoiesis. Blast cells (plus promonocytes) are less than 20%. Megakaryocytes are often reduced.

Flow Cytometric Immunophenotyping

Immunophenotyping is not diagnostically useful.

Genetics

There is no specific chromosomal abnormality and cytogenetic analysis is often normal. Some patients have monosomy 7, trisomy 8, or a complex karyotypic abnormality. Chromosomal analysis may be initially normal but become abnormal during the course of the illness. Genetic analysis shows four nonoverlapping groups of patients with loss-of-function mutation in *NF1* (inherited or acquired) or mutation in *PTPN11* (inherited or acquired) [30], *CBL* [31], or a *RAS* group gene (*NRAS* or *KRAS*) [32]; a mutation in one of these genes is found in 85% of cases. In children with neurofibromatosis there may be homozygosity for the mutant gene as a result of acquired uniparental disomy or there may be somatic mutation in the initially normal allele [33, 34]. Similarly, patients with an inherited *CBL* mutation usually show loss of heterozygosity.

Histology

The bone marrow is hypercellular as a result of increased granulopoiesis and a variable increase in monocytopoiesis and erythropoiesis. Reticulin may be increased.

Conclusions

The chronic myeloid leukemias are a heterogeneous group of hematopoietic neoplasms, some with mainly proliferative features and others with myelodysplastic/myeloproliferative characteristics. Origin may be in a pluripotent lymphoid-myeloid stem cell or in a committed myeloid cell. Since leukemias with a *BCR-ABL1* fusion gene or rearrangement of *PDGFRA* or *PDGFRB* are sensitive to tyrosine kinase inhibitors, precise diagnosis is of considerable importance.

References

1. Swerdlow SH, Campo E, Harris NL, Jaffe ES, Pileri SA, Stein H, Thiele J, editors. World Health Organization Classification of tumours of haematopoietic and lymphoid tissue. Revised 4th ed. Lyon: IARC Press; 2017.
2. Vardiman J, Melo J, Baccarani M, Radich J, Thiele J. Chronic myeloid leukaemia, *BCR-ABL1*-positive. In: Swerdlow SH, Campo E, Harris NL, Jaffe ES, Pileri SA, Stein H, Thiele J, editors. World Health Organization Classification of tumours of haematopoietic and lymphoid tissue. Revised 4th ed. Lyon: IARC Press; 2017.
3. Savage DG, Szydlo RM, Goldman JM. Clinical features at diagnosis in 430 patients with chronic myeloid leukaemia seen at a referral centre over a 16-year period. Br J Haematol. 1997;96:111–6.
4. Spiers AS, Bain BJ, Turner JE. The peripheral blood in chronic granulocytic leukaemia. Study of 50 untreated Philadelphia-positive cases. Scand J Haematol. 1977;18:25–38.
5. Schmid C, Frisch B, Beham A, Jäger K, Kettner G. Comparison of bone marrow histology in early chronic granulocytic leukemia and in leukemoid reaction. Eur J Haematol. 1990;44:154–8.
6. Thiele J, Kvasnicka HM, Schmitt-Graeff A, Zirbes TK, Birnbaum F, Kressmann C, et al. Bone marrow features and clinical findings in chronic myeloid leukemia—a comparative, multicenter, immunohistochemical and morphometric study of 614 patients. Leuk Lymphoma. 2000;36:295–308.
7. Bain BJ, Clark D, Wilkins BS. Bone marrow pathology. 4th ed. Oxford: Wiley-Blackwell; 2010. p. 243–7.
8. Kantarjian HM, Keating MJ, Walters RS, McCredie KB, Smith TL, Talpaz M, et al. Clinical and prognostic features of Philadelphia chromosome-negative chronic myelogenous leukemia. Cancer. 1986;58:2023–30.
9. Martiat P, Michaux JL, Rodhain J. Philadelphia-negative (Ph-) chronic myeloid leukemia (CML): comparison with Ph+ CML and chronic myelomonocytic leukemia. The Groupe Francais de Cytogenetique Hematologique. Blood. 1991;78:205–11.
10. Orazi A, Bennett JM, Bain BJ, Brunning RD, Thiele J. Atypical chronic myeloid leukaemia, *BCR-ABL1*-negative. In: Swerdlow SH, Campo E, Harris NL, Jaffe ES, Pileri SA, Stein H, Thiele J, editors. World Health Organization classification of tumours of haematopoietic and lymphoid tissue. Revised 4th ed. Lyon: IARC Press; 2017.
11. Bennett JM, Catovsky D, Daniel MT, Flandrin G, Galton DA, Gralnick HR, et al. Proposals for the classification of the myelodysplastic syndromes. Br J Haematol. 1982;51:189–99.
12. Orazi A, Bennett J, Germing U, Brunning RD, Bain BJ, Cazzola M, Foucar K, Thiele J. Chronic myelomonocytic leukaemia. In: Swerdlow SH, Campo E, Harris NL, Jaffe ES, Pileri SA, Stein H, Thiele J, editors. World Health Organization Classification of tumours of haematopoietic and lymphoid tissue. Revised 4th ed. Lyon: IARC Press; 2017.
13. Chen Y-C, Chou J-M, Letendre L, Li CY. Clinical importance of bone marrow monocytic nodules in patients with myelodysplasia: retrospective analysis of 21 cases. Am J Hematol. 2005;79:329–31.

14. Orazi A, Chiu R, O'Malley DP, Czader M, Allen SL, An C, et al. Chronic myelomonocytic leukemia: the role of bone marrow biopsy immunohistology. Mod Pathol. 2006;19:1536–45.
15. Bain BJ, Horny H-P, Hasserjian RP, Orazi O. Chronic eosinophilic leukaemia, NOS. In: Swerdlow SH, Campo E, Harris NL, Jaffe ES, Pileri SA, Stein H, Thiele J, editors. World Health Organization Classification of tumours of haematopoietic and lymphoid tissue. Revised 4th ed. Lyon: IARC Press; 2017.
16. Cools J, DeAngelo DJ, Gotlib J, Stover EH, Legare RD, Cortes J, et al. A tyrosine kinase created by fusion of the *PDGFRA* and *FIP1L1* genes is a therapeutic target of imatinib in idiopathic hypereosinophilic syndrome. N Engl J Med. 2003;348:1201–14.
17. Bain BJ, Horny H-P, Arber DA, Tefferi A, Hasserjian RP. Myeloid/lymphoid neoplasms with eosinophilia and rearrangements of *PDGFRA*, *PDGFRB* or *FGFR1* or with *PCM1-JAK2*. In: Swerdlow SH, Campo E, Harris NL, Jaffe ES, Pileri SA, Stein H, Thiele J, editors. World Health Organization Classification of tumours of haematopoietic and lymphoid tissue. Revised 4th ed. Lyon: IARC Press; 2017.
18. Bain BJ, Ahmed S. Should myeloid and lymphoid neoplasms with *PCM1-JAK2* and other rearrangements of *JAK2* be recognised as specific entities? Br J Haematol. 2014;166:809–17.
19. Sorour Y, Dalley CD, Snowden JA, Cross NC, Reilly JT. Acute myeloid leukaemia with associated eosinophilia: justification for *FIP1L1-PDGFRA* screening in cases lacking the *CBFB-MYH11* fusion gene. Br J Haematol. 2009;146:225–7.
20. Lyall H, O'Connor S, Clark D. Charcot–Leyden crystals in the trephine biopsy of a patient with *FIP1L1-PDGFRA*—positive myeloproliferative disorder. Br J Haematol. 2007;138:405.
21. Bain BJ, Brunning RD, Orazi O, Thiele J. Chronic neutrophilic leukaemia. In: Swerdlow SH, Campo E, Harris NL, Jaffe ES, Pileri SA, Stein H, Thiele J, editors. World Health Organization Classification of tumours of haematopoietic and lymphoid tissue. Revised 4th ed. Lyon: IARC Press; 2017.
22. Amato D, Memon S, Wang C. Myeloblastic transformation of chronic neutrophilic leukaemia. Br J Haematol. 2008;142:148.
23. Bain BJ, Ahmad S. Chronic neutrophilic leukaemia and plasma cell-related neutrophilic leukaemoid reactions. Br J Haematol. 2015;171:400–10.
24. Maxon JE, Gotlib J, Pollyea DA, Fleischman AG, Agarwal A, Eide CA, et al. Oncogenic CSF3R mutations in chronic neutrophilic leukemia anf atypical CML. N Engl J Med. 2013;368:1781–90.
25. Neimeyer CM, Aricó M, Basso G, members of the European Working Group on Myelodysplastic Syndromes in Childhood (EWOG-MDS), et al. Chronic myelomonocytic leukemia in childhood: a retrospective analysis of 110 cases. Blood. 1997;89:3534–43.
26. Aricò M, Biondi A, Pui C-H. Juvenile myelomonocytic leukemia. Blood. 1997;90:479–88.
27. Niemeyer CM, Kratz CP. Paediatric myelodysplastic syndromes and juvenile myelomonocytic leukaemia: molecular classification and treatment options. Br J Haematol. 2008;140:610–24.
28. Koike K, Matsuda K. Recent advances in pathogenesis and management of juvenile myelomonocytic leukaemia. Br J Haematol. 2008;141:567–75.
29. Baumann I, Bennett JM, Niemeyer CM, Thiele J. Juvenile myelomonocytic leukaemia. In: Swerdlow SH, Campo E, Harris NL, Jaffe ES, Pileri SA, Stein H, Thiele J, editors. World Health Organization Classification of tumours of haematopoietic and lymphoid tissue. Revised 4th ed. Lyon: IARC Press; 2017.
30. Kratz CP, Niemeyer CM, Castleberry RP, Cetin M, Bergsträsser E, Emanuel PD, et al. The mutational spectrum of PTPN11 in juvenile myelomonocytic leukemia and Noonan syndrome/myeloproliferative disease. Blood. 2005;106:2183–5.
31. Loh ML, Sakai DS, Flotho C, Kang M, Fliegaf M, Archambeault S, et al. Mutations in *CBL* occur frequently in juvenile myelomonocytic leukemia. Blood. 2009;114:1859–63.
32. Lauchle JO, Braun BS, Loh ML, Shannon K. Inherited predispositions and hyperactive Ras in myeloid leukemogenesis. Pediatr Blood Cancer. 2006;46:579–85.
33. Shannon KM, O'Connell P, Martin GA, Paderanga D, Olson K, Dinndorf P, et al. Loss of the normal *NF1* allele from the bone marrow of children with type 1 neurofibromatosis and malignant myeloid disorders. N Engl J Med. 1994;330:597–601.
34. Flotho C, Steinemann D, Mullighan CG, et al. Genome-wide single nucleotide polymorphism analysis in juvenile myelomonocytic leukemia identifies uniparental disomy surrounding the NF1 locus in cases associated with neurofibromatosis but not in cases with mutant RAS or PTPN11. Oncogene. 2007;26:5816–21.

4 Molecular Biology and Cytogenetics of Chronic Myeloid Leukemia

Marina Konopleva, Alfonso Quintás Cardama, Hagop Kantarjian, and Jorge Cortes

Introduction

Chronic myeloid leukemia (CML) is a clonal myeloproliferative neoplasia characterized by the t(9;22)(q34;q11) balanced reciprocal translocation that causes the fusion of a portion of chromosome 9 to chromosome 22 (der22), thereby replacing a fragment of chromosome 22 which fuses to chromosome 9 (der9). The resultant minute chromosome der22, designated as the Philadelphia chromosome (Ph), is the hallmark of CML [1]. The molecular event resulting from this translocation is the hybrid *BCR-ABL1* oncogene, which encodes the constitutively active BCR-ABL1 protein kinase [1]. The BCR-ABL1 oncoprotein can transform cells through phosphorylation of tyrosine residues on a variety of intermediary proteins that transmit signals from the cytoplasm to the nucleus. The ultimate proof that BCR-ABL1 kinase expression can induce CML was provided by experiments in which murine bone marrow was transfected with a retrovirus encoding *BCR-ABL1* and transplanted into irradiated syngeneic recipients. Transplanted recipients developed several hematologic malignancies, most frequently a myeloproliferative syndrome that resembles very closely chronic-phase CML [2]. The demonstration that BCR-ABL1 kinase activity played a critical role in cellular transformation provided the rationale for developing molecules aimed at targeting such activity. Kinase-based assays demonstrated that imatinib, the first tyrosine kinase inhibitor (TKI) developed for the treatment of CML, potently inhibited ABL1 kinase [3, 4]. This inhibitory activity translated into impressive clinical activity [5]. The remarkable clinical success of imatinib propelled the rational design and development of other TKIs (e.g., nilotinib, dasatinib, bosutinib, ponatinib) aided by structural biology and high-throughput medicinal chemistry methods. Despite these agents' clinical activity, many patients with CML receiving TKI therapy frequently manifest measurable amounts of residual disease, and in some the TKI therapy eventually fails. Among patients with accelerated-phase (AP) or blastic phase (BP) CML, responses are less frequent and often short-lived [6]. These shortcomings of TKI therapy have resulted in research efforts aimed at understanding the behavior of CML stem cells, the molecular basis of transformation to AP and BP, and the mechanisms of resistance to TKIs.

The *BCR-ABL1* Oncogene

The breakpoints within *ABL1* map either upstream of exon Ib, downstream of exon Ia, or, more frequently, between exons Ib and Ia [7]. In most patients with CML and in one-third of adults with Ph-positive B-cell acute lymphoblastic leukemia (Ph + B-ALL), the breakpoints within *BCR* map to a 5.8-kb area spanning exons e12–e16 (formerly b1–b5), referred to as the *major breakpoint cluster region* (M-*bcr*). Alternative splicing produces fusion transcripts with either e13a2 or e14a2 junctions that give rise to a 210 kDa protein ($p210^{BCR\text{-}ABL1}$) [8]. In two-thirds of adults with Ph + B-ALL and in occasional cases of CML, the *BCR* breakpoint localizes to a 54.4-kb area between exons e2′ and e2 (*minor breakpoint cluster region* or m-*bcr*), which produces an e1a2 transcript that translates into $p190^{BCR\text{-}ABL1}$ and is associated with a more aggressive CML course. A third breakpoint cluster region (μ-*bcr*) gives rise to a 230 kDa fusion protein ($p230^{BCR\text{-}ABL1}$) that is associated with a very indolent course of CML [9].

Several experimental models, such as *BCR-ABL1*-expressing CD34+ cells in culture [10, 11] or retrovirally transduced *BCR-ABL1*-positive mouse cells [2, 12], have helped establish a direct causality between BCR-ABL1 and CML. A lysine-to-arginine substitution at residue 1176 (K1176R) in the ATP-binding pocket of ABL1 inactivates

M. Konopleva, M.D., Ph.D. (✉) • A.Q. Cardama, M.D.
H. Kantarjian, M.D. • J. Cortes, M.D.
Department of Leukemia, MD Anderson Cancer Center, 1515 Holcombe Blvd, Faculty Center Tower, Unit 428, Houston, TX 77030, USA
e-mail: mkonople@mdanderson.org; alfonso.quintas@novartis.com; hkantarj@mdanderson.org; jcortes@mdanderson.org

P.H. Wiernik et al. (eds.), *Neoplastic Diseases of the Blood*, DOI 10.1007/978-3-319-64263-5_4

the kinase activity of BCR-ABL1 and prevents the development of leukemia in mice, even when *BCR-ABL1*^{K1176R} is expressed in hematopoietic stem cells (HSCs) [13]. Further proof of the central role of *BCR-ABL1* as the pathogenetic driver in CML was provided by developing transgenic mice in which the tetracycline-responsive element (tet-O) inducibly drives *BCR-ABL1* expression specifically in HSCs. SCL-tTA/BCR-ABL-tetO mice, resulting from crossing *BCR-ABL1* tet-O mice with mice expressing the tetracycline transactivator (tTA) under the control of the murine stem cell leukemia (SCL) gene 3′ enhancer, developed a myeloproliferative disease that recapitulated multiple features of human CML upon tetracycline withdrawal [14]. The clinical success of imatinib, a small molecule that inhibits the kinase activity of BCR-ABL1, has further confirmed the oncogenic role of this protein kinase.

Autoregulation of the *BCR-ABL1* Protein Kinase

BCR-ABL1 kinase is a multidomain protein (Fig. 4.1). The N-terminus of BCR-ABL1 includes the "Cap" region, present in two different isoforms, 1a and 1b, as a consequence of alternative splicing of the first exon. The ABL1b isoform contains a C_{14} myristoyl moiety covalently linked to the N-terminus and is expressed at higher levels than type 1a, which is not myristoylated. ABL1 also contains highly conserved Src-homology-2 (SH2) and SH3 domains and a tyrosine kinase domain [15]. The SH2 domain interacts with and phosphorylates signaling proteins, including p62dok, c-Cbl, Rin-1, Tub, and mDab1. Mutations within the SH2 domain have been found to delay the onset of, but fail to prevent, BCR-ABL1-induced myeloproliferation [16]. The last ABL1 exon region contains several distinct domains, including four proline-rich SH3 motifs (which act as docking sites for SH3 domains of adaptor proteins such as Crk, GRB2 [growth-factor-receptor-bound 2], and Nck) [17, 18], a DNA-binding domain, an actin-binding domain, three nuclear localization signals, and one nuclear export signal, which determines the subcellular localization of ABL1 (Fig. 4.1). BCR also exhibits a complex spatial modularity that includes a coiled-coil oligomerization domain, a serine/threonine kinase domain, a Dbl/CDC24 guanine–nucleotide exchange factor homology domain, a pleckstrin homology domain, a calcium-dependent lipid-binding site, and a RAC guanosine triphosphatase-activating protein domain. Tyr177 at BCR serves as docking site for GRB2, GRB10, 14-3-3, and ABL1 proteins through its SH2 domain [19]. The myristoyl modification at the end of the N-terminal segment of ABL1b engages the C-terminal lobe of the ABL1 catalytic domain and facilitates the docking of the SH2 and SH3 domains onto the kinase domain [20, 21]. The absence of the myristoyl group results in constitutive tyrosine kinase activity [15]. In the inactive conformation of the kinase domain, the rotation of the helix αC displaces critical catalytic residues out of the active site, thus hampering ATP access to the active site [15]. The X-ray crystal structure of the oligomerization domain of BCR-ABL1 (residues 1–72 or BCR_{1-72}) showed that two monomers associate in an antiparallel

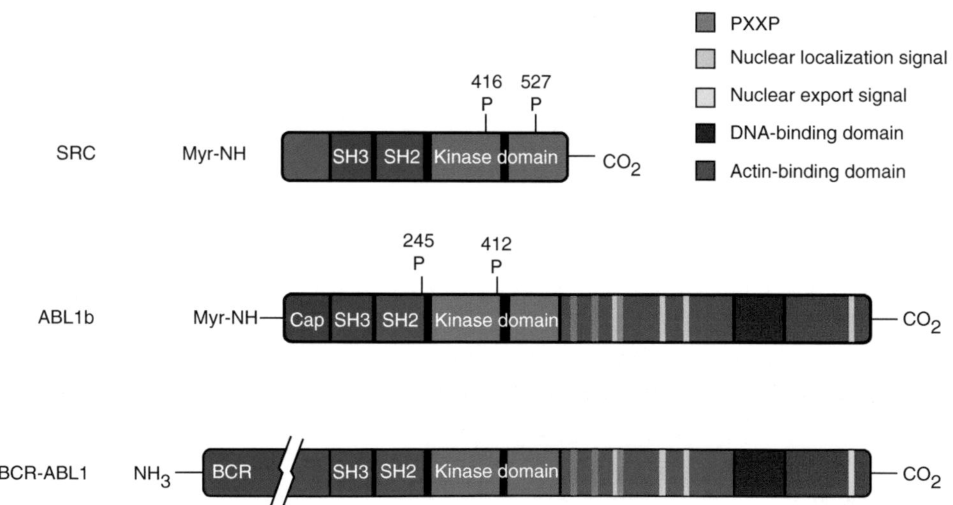

Fig. 4.1 Modular structure of the BCR-ABL1 protein. The modular structure of BCR-ABL1 is lined up against those of SRC and ABL1b kinases, which share a common central core that includes a tyrosine kinase domain, a SRC-homology-2 (SH2) domain, and an SH3 domain. The NH2 terminus in ABL1 and BCR-ABL1 kinases is the "Cap" region. Alternative splicing of the first ABL1 exon yields two ABL1 isoforms (a and b). ABL1b contains a myristate site (Myr-NH) at the extreme end of the amino-terminal segment, which binds to the kinase domain and keeps the SH2–SH3 autoinhibitory structure in place (i.e., in the "off state")

dimer, which in turn stacks to form a tetramer [22]. Mutations at the coiled-coil domain impairing BCR-ABL1 oligomerization drastically compromise the kinase activity and the leukemogenic potential of BCR-ABL1 [23].

Signaling Pathways Stemming from BCR-ABL1 Kinase

BCR-ABL1 activates numerous downstream signaling pathways (Fig. 4.2). Such activation stems from a multiprotein complex formed by BCR-ABL1 kinase and an array of substrates and adaptor proteins, which include GRB2, CrkL, c-CBL, and p62(DOK). Signaling emanating from this complex leads to cellular transformation. The phosphorylation of the tyrosine residue 177 (Tyr177) of BCR is essential for BCR-ABL1-mediated leukemogenesis [24]. A tyrosine-to-phenylalanine substitution at this residue (Tyr177Phe) impairs GRB2 binding and markedly diminishes BCR-ABL1-induced RAS activation [25], which impedes the transformation of primary bone marrow cultured in the presence of ABL1 kinase activity [25]. Transfection of a mutant *BCR-ABL1* isoform carrying the Tyr177Phe mutation prevents the induction of a myeloproliferative disorder in a murine stem cell transplantation model of CML [25]. Tyr177 functions as a high-affinity docking site for the SH2 domain of GRB2, which in turn recruits SOS (a guanine–nucleotide exchanger of *RAS*), resulting in activation of RAS [19] and the scaffold adapter GRB2-associated binding protein 2 (GAB2) [19]. The importance of GAB2 is illustrated by the fact that BCR-ABL1 fails to transform primary myeloid cells from *GAB2*$^{-/-}$ mice [26]. The GRB2/GAB2 complex activates phosphatidylinositol 3-kinase (PI3K)/AKT [27] and ERK in primary CML cells. Interestingly, MEK-ERK activation is cytokine dependent in chronic phase (CP) but becomes constitutively activated in CML BP and is readily detectable in CD34+ progenitors [28]. Mutation of BCR-ABL1 protein at any of three of the direct binding sites for GRB2, namely CBL, p62(DOK), and CRKL, resulted in defective transformation of primary hematopoietic cells in a mouse model of CML because of decreased activation of the MAP kinase and PI3K pathways but not of the transcription factor signal transducer and activation of transcription 5 (STAT5) [29]. Overall, these data indicate that disruption of the interaction between BCR-ABL1 and BCR-ABL1 substrates may result in abrogation of leukemogenesis.

Other important proteins phosphorylated by BCR-ABL1 kinase are the SRC family kinases (SFKs) HCK, LYN, and FGR. LYN kinase is activated indirectly upon activation of JAK2 kinase by BCR-ABL1. Inhibition of JAK2 reduces the level of the SET protein and increases serine/threonine phosphatase 2A (PP2A) and tyrosine phosphatase 1 (SHP1) activities, which decrease the levels of activated LYN [30]. In turn, phosphorylated HCK recruits STAT5 [19, 31], which upregulates cyclin D1. This in turn induces cell cycle progression from G_1 to S

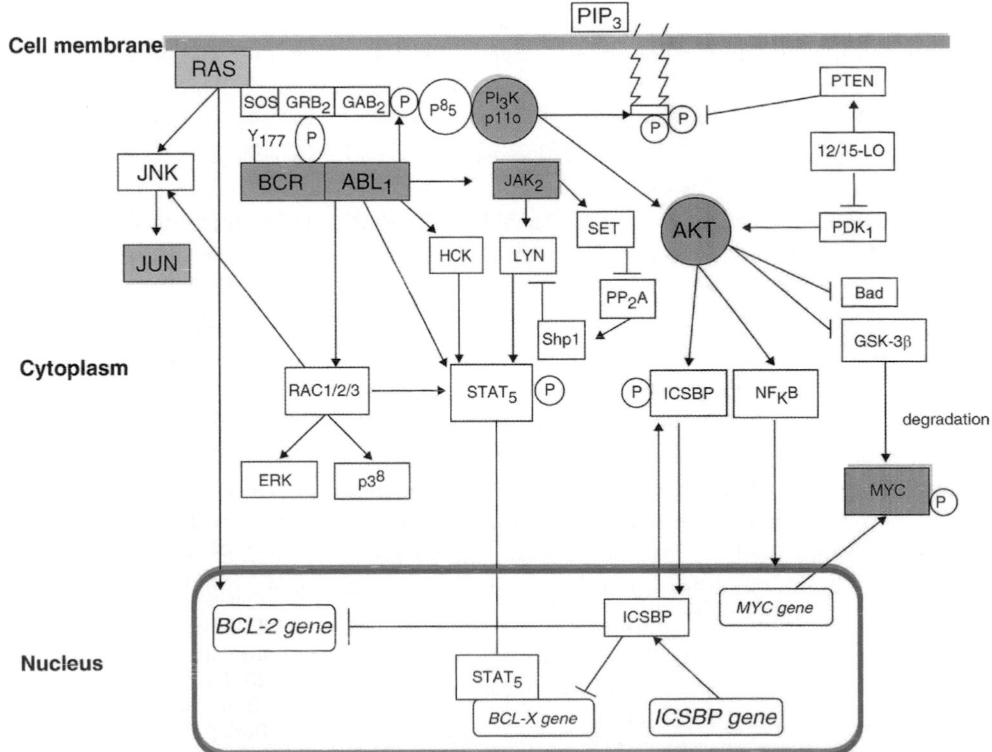

Fig. 4.2 Signaling pathways stemming from BCR-ABL1 kinase. BCR-ABL1 kinase phosphorylates a series of intracellular substrates, thus activating several signaling pathways that promote cell proliferation and inhibition of apoptosis

phase [32]. However, whether Src kinases are indispensable for BCR-ABL1-mediated leukemogenesis remains controversial, since *BCR-ABL1* can cause a CML-like picture in bone marrow of mice lacking *Lyn, Hck, and Fgr* [33]. In turn, the generation of acute lymphoid disease is mitigated in the same model [33], and knocking down LYN by siRNA impairs survival of CML lymphoid blasts [34], indicating that the requirement of SFKs is greater in CML lymphoid transformation than in CP.

STAT5 is constitutively activated in CML. STAT5 downregulation mediated by siRNA in primary CML samples markedly impairs Ph + myeloid colony formation. Fetal liver hematopoietic progenitors from *STAT5a*$^{-/-}$:: *STAT5b*$^{-/-}$ mice retrovirally transduced with BCR-ABL1 failed to induce leukemia in recipient mice [35]. Conditional deletion of STAT5 in purified stem cells from p210$^{BCR/ABL}$ mice failed to initiate CML in mice [36]. Furthermore, the anti-apoptotic protein BCL-X, which is repressed by the transcription factor interferon consensus sequence-binding protein (ICSBP) [37], is transcriptionally activated by STAT5 [38].

Although the individual contribution of some BCR-ABL1 downstream pathways may appear negligible when evaluated individually, a cooperative interplay may be necessary for the full realization of the leukemogenic potential of BCR-ABL1. For instance, when *BCR-ABL1*-positive K562 cells were induced to express dominant negative forms of RAS, PI3K, or STAT5, marked apoptosis was observed in cells expressing two of the three dominant negative mutants in any combination [39].

RAC guanosine triphosphatases (GTPases) are activated in primary CML cells [40]. In a murine model of p210$^{BCR\text{-}ABL1}$-induced myeloproliferative disease, targeting of *RAC1* and *RAC2* genes, which encode the GTPases RAC1 and RAC2, markedly delayed myeloproliferation and abrogated the phosphorylation of the BCR-ABL1 downstream signaling molecules CrKL, JNK, ERK, and p38 [40]. This suggests that BCR-ABL1 signaling is highly dependent on RAC GTPases. This contention is supported by experiments using NSC23766, a specific RAC1/RAC2 inhibitor [41].

JUNB is a transcription factor that belongs to the activator protein 1 family. It functions as a tumor suppressor in myeloid cells [42]. JUNB exerts its tumor-suppressor activity by abrogating cell proliferation and survival through inhibition of the RAS downstream target JUN. Transgenic mice lacking the *JUNB* gene in the myeloid lineage (*JunB*$^{-/-}$Ubi-*JunB* mice) develop myeloproliferation that closely resembles CML; a fraction of these animals progress to BP [43, 44]. Granulocyte-macrophage colony-stimulating factor (GM-CSF)-mediated proliferation and survival of *JUNB*-deficient granulocyte/macrophage progenitors (GMPs) are associated with changes in anti-apoptotic proteins such as Bcl2 and Bclx and in cell cycle regulators p16ink4a and *c-Jun* [43].

Mice lacking the enzyme 12/15-lipoxygenase (12/15-LO) develop a myeloproliferative disorder with 100% penetrance that progresses to transplantable leukemia independent from ABL1 dysregulation [45]. Cells isolated from chronic-stage 12/15-LO-deficient mice (*Alox15*) exhibit increased PI3K/AKT activation as well as ICSBP, which results in decreased direct DNA binding, limiting the ability of ICSBP to repress BCL-2 gene transcription and promoting leukemic cell survival (Fig. 4.2) [45]. ICSBP is a negative regulator of granulocyte differentiation. *ICSBP*$^{-/-}$ and *ICSBP*$^{+/-}$ mice exhibit deregulated hematopoiesis manifested as a CML-like myeloproliferative disorder [46]. Forced expression of ICSBP inhibited *BCR-ABL1*-induced CML-like disease in vivo [47]. All the effects observed in *Alox15* mice were reversed upon treatment with a PI3K inhibitor. This suggests that 12/15-LO is an important suppressor of myeloproliferation [45]. Additionally, the arachidonate 5-lipoxygenase (5-LO) gene (Alox5) was identified as a critical regulator for CML LSC. BCR-ABL failed to transform bone marrow from Alox5-deficient mice, and both genetic or pharmacologic inhibition of Alox5 impaired the function of leukemic stem cells (LSCs) [48].

Progression to Advanced-Phase CML

The understanding of the mechanisms associated with the progression from CP to AP and BP has been dramatically hampered by the lack of animal models that faithfully recapitulate the process of CML transformation in vivo, which is almost invariably preceded by a protracted "chronic" myeloproliferative phase. However, several factors have been identified in samples from patients with AP CML as central to the process of transformation (Fig. 4.3). Genome-wide analysis of gene expression profiles may aid in characterizing gene candidates responsible for disease progression. Unfortunately, most studies have failed to provide clear-cut answers, likely because of differences in types of samples, array platforms, and/or statistical methodologies employed [49–54]. DNA microarray analysis comparing the gene expression in 91 cases of CML in all phases found striking similarities between gene expression in AP and BP. This suggests that CML might conform to a biphasic rather than a classic triphasic model of progression [54]. Genes potentially involved in AP/BP compared to CP included cytokines (IL3RA, SOCS2), alternative RAS pathways (Rras2), DNA-damage response genes, and genes involved in HSC self-renewal and interaction with the bone marrow stroma, such as those that encode effectors in the Wnt pathway (e.g., β-catenin) [54]. A genome-wide screening using single-nucleotide polymorphism (SNP) arrays identified only 0.47 copy number alterations per CML CP case (range 0–8), suggesting that *BCR-ABL1* is sufficient to induce CML. In contrast, a mean

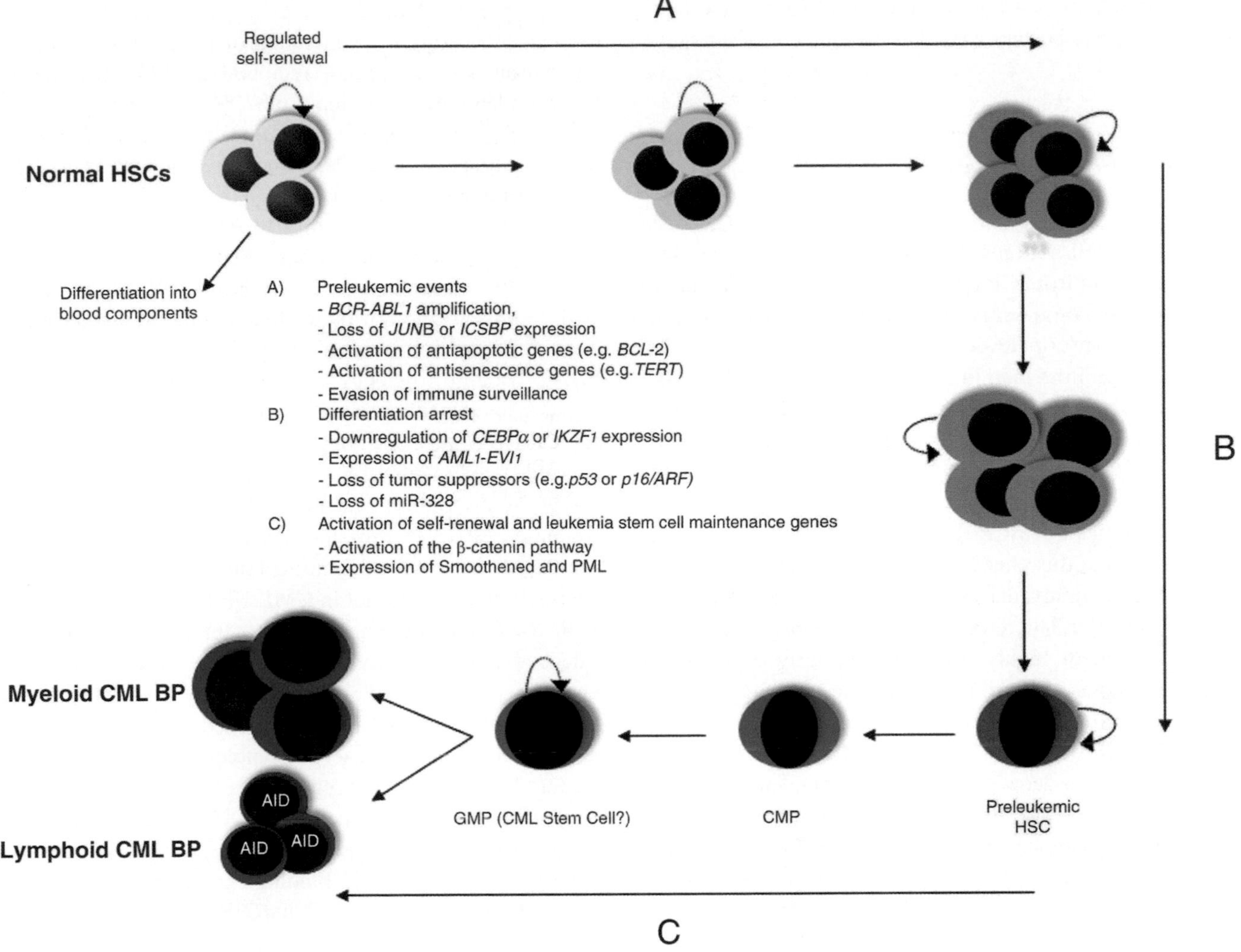

Fig. 4.3 Progression to blastic phase. In CML, hematopoietic stem cells (HSCs) accumulate genetic abnormalities that result in enhanced proliferation, survival advantage, cytokine independence, immune evasion, decreased apoptosis, and differentiation arrest. Granulocyte–monocyte progenitors (GMP) carrying such abnormalities are endowed with self-renewal potential, feed the leukemic pool during disease progression, and facilitate the emergence of clonal leukemic stem cells (LSCs) that drive the transition to blast-phase (BP) CML. Expression of activation-induced deaminase (AID) drives CML progression toward the lymphoid lineage

of 7.8 copy number alterations were detected per CML BP case (range 0–28), indicating that progression requires the acquisition of additional genomic alterations [55].

Blastic Phase Arises from Primitive CML Progenitors

In CML, CD34^{+}CD38^{-}Lin^{-} LSCs express high *BCR-ABL1* transcript levels [56]. LSCs acquire additional genetic and/or epigenetic abnormalities during the transition from CP to BP that confer resistance to apoptosis, extended replicative life span, and consequently a survival advantage [57, 58]. Mice genetically null for the *JUNB* [43] or *ICSBP* alleles develop a CML-like myeloproliferative disorder that, in the case of *JUNB*, arises from the HSC compartment and in some cases progresses to BP. JunB inactivation increases the proliferation of long-term repopulating HSCs in vivo without impairing their self-renewal potential [59]. Whether *BCR-ABL1* directly abrogates or cooperates with JunB expression to promote myeloproliferation during CML progression warrants further investigation, as does the determination of the cell of origin from which the BP clone arises. While transforming clones appear to arise from the HSC compartment in *JUNB*$^{-/-}$ mice, some reports suggest that the acquisition of self-renewal properties by a subset of committed progenitors may result in a CML-like phenotype that includes progression to BP in a mouse model in which the hMRP8p210$^{BCR\text{-}ABL1}$ transgene is expressed specifically by GMPs and their myelomonocytic progeny but not by HSCs [60]. These data suggest that BP may result from the progressive acquisition of genetic alterations within progenitors downstream of the

HSC that acquire self-renewal properties [60]. Importantly, GMPs have also been proposed as candidate LSCs in human CML BP [56].

CML BP Cells Overexpress BCR-ABL1

The continuous and unrestrained activity of BCR-ABL1 kinase is central not only for CML maintenance but also in the progression from CP to BP. *BCR-ABL1* mRNA and protein levels are consistently higher in BP than in CP [61, 62]. *BCR-ABL1* transcript levels may be 200-fold greater in CML CD34+ progenitors than in more differentiated *BCR-ABL1*-positive cells [63]. *BCR-ABL1* has been shown to promote clonogenicity [63, 64], growth factor independence [63], protection against apoptosis [64], cell motility [63], and disease latency in a dose-dependent manner [63]. The reason for the increment of *BCR-ABL1* transcript levels is not well understood, but this phenomenon is likely a consequence of the proliferative advantage resulting from high BCR-ABL1 kinase activity and therefore from selective pressure favoring the expansion of highly proliferative/poorly differentiated leukemic clones. Experimental evidence has demonstrated that levels of *BCR-ABL1* mRNA in the CD34+ GMPs were higher in CML BP than in CML CP [56]. *BCR-ABL1*-positive GMPs have been demonstrated to be expanded in CML BP [56]. Alternatively, it has been proposed that the BCR-ABL1 oncoprotein promotes the expression of *BCR-ABL1* transcripts and/or that *BCR-ABL1* transcript degradation may be selectively downregulated in CD34+ CML progenitors [65]. *BCR-ABL1*-independent mechanisms may also play an important role in CML progression. For instance, overexpression and/or activation of the SFKs HCK, LYN, and FYN has been linked to CML progression and imatinib resistance [66–69]. *BCR-ABL1* retrovirally transduced into bone marrow cells derived from *LYN*$^{-/-}$*HCK*$^{-/-}$*FGR*$^{-/-}$ mice efficiently induced CML but not B-ALL in recipient mice, which suggests that SFKs may play an important role in the pathogenesis of Ph + B-ALL and lymphoid CML BP [33, 70]. BCR-ABL1-independent activation of LYN was noted in patients with imatinib-resistant CML expressing unmutated *BCR-ABL1* [71]. Anti-SFK therapy may therefore be beneficial in advanced-phase CML [70].

Arrest of Differentiation

Progressive corruption of the differentiation program characterizes CML progression. BCR-ABL1 modulates the activity of transcription factors that regulate the expression of several differentiation-related genes (Fig. 4.3) [72, 73]. The *IKZF1* gene, which encodes the transcription factor Ikaros, is essential for lymphoid lineage specification. Ikaros isoforms lacking the DNA-binding domain act in a dominant negative fashion, preventing the generation of the earliest lymphoid progenitors and of mature lymphocytes [74]. SNP array analysis identified the presence of *IKZF1* deletions (typically monoallelic deletions of exons 3–6) in more than 80% of patients with Ph + ALL. Deletions were not present in CML CP cases but were found in 66–75% of CML CP cases transformed to lymphoid (but never to myeloid) CML BP [55, 75]. Downregulation of Ikaros expression causes partial block of B-cell maturation at the pro-B-cell stage in mice [76], and inactivation of Ikaros function blocks the development of B-lymphoid progenitors at the pre-B-cell stage [77]. *IKZF1* haploinsufficiency or the expression of dominant negative Ikaros isoforms may contribute to the pathogenesis of *BCR-ABL1*-positive lymphoid malignancies by inducing arrested B-cell maturation.

The transcription factor CCAAT/enhancer binding protein-α (CEBPα), a master regulator of myeloid differentiation [78], is expressed in normal bone marrow cells and in CML CP samples but not in CML BP [79]. Transplantation of *BCR-ABL1*-expressing CEBPα$^{-/-}$ fetal liver cells fails to induce myeloproliferative disease in mice. Rather, it induces an immature, lethal transplantable erythroleukemia. Transplantation of CEBPα-transduced cells consistently yielded a disease that closely resembles CML CP [80], suggesting that CEBPα downregulation abrogates cell commitment toward a myeloid cell fate. Differentiation arrest in myeloid CML BP is driven by BCR-ABL1/MAPK-induced activity of the poly(rC)-binding protein heterogeneous nuclear ribonucleoprotein E2 (hnRNP E2), which regulates the translation of specific mRNAs [79]. Expression of hnRNP E2 is low or undetectable in CML CP but is high in CML BP CD34+ bone marrow progenitors. Upon interaction with the 5′-untranslated region of *CEBPA* mRNA causes suppression of CEBPα [79]. MicroRNAs (miRNAs), small noncoding RNAs that have been shown to be important regulators of oncogene and tumor-suppressor gene expression in human cancer, can also inhibit the activity of RNA-binding proteins [81]. Indeed, miR-328 binds hnRNP E2, likely through its C-rich clusters in a seed sequence-independent manner, and as a consequence prevents the binding of hnRNP E2 to *CEBPA* mRNA, thus rescuing *CEBPA* mRNA translation and myeloid maturation. Not surprisingly, miR-328 expression is lost in CML BP in a BCR-ABL1 dose- and kinase-dependent manner through the MAPK-hnRNP E2 pathway. Restoration of miR-328 rescued differentiation and impaired the survival of *BCR-ABL1*-positive blast cells, partly by targeting the survival factor PIM [81].

Hybrid dominant negative transcription factors arising from chromosomal translocations such as *NUP98-HOXA9* [82] or *AML1-EVI1* [83] have been implicated in the pathogenesis of CML BP. NUP98-HOXA9 alters the balance between symmetric and asymmetric renewal division, favoring the former and causing preferential growth of immature precursors, while *AML1-EVI1* has been shown to cause differentiation blockade, in both cases facilitating the transition to CML BP [84]. NUP98-HOXA9 induces expression of the RNA-binding protein Musashi2 (Msi2), which in turn represses differentiation factor Numb, known to be expressed at low levels in CML BP [85]. Msi2, normally highly expressed in HSCs and overexpressed in advanced CML, is associated with poor survival. In a mouse model, it cooperates with BCR-ABL1 to induce an aggressive leukemia [86].

Genomic Instability and DNA Repair

BCR-ABL1 expression has been associated with increased production of endogenous reactive oxygen species (ROS) that result in chronic oxidative DNA damage, double-strand breaks (DSBs) in S and G_2/M cell cycle phases, and mutagenesis [87]. DNA damage surveillance is faulty in CML owing to inhibited ataxia telangiectasia and RAD3-related (ATR) nuclear protein kinase signaling, which attenuates the activation of checkpoint kinase 1 (CHK1) and abrogates the intra-S-phase cell cycle checkpoint [88]. Nonhomologous end-joining and homologous recombination as well as nucleotide excision repair exhibit unfaithful repair of DSBs induced by ROS [87] and γ-irradiation [89] as a consequence of BCR-ABL1 kinase activity [87]. As a result, G/C-to A/T-transitions and G/C-to-T/A transversions in the coding regions of multiple genes (including the kinase domain of *BCR-ABL1*) have been demonstrated in CML cells but not in *BCR-ABL1*-negative cells [87, 90]. It has been shown that lymphoid (but not myeloid) CML BP cells express the B-cell-specific mutator enzyme activation-induced deaminase (AID), which contributes to genetic instability by hypermutation of tumor suppressor and DNA repair genes and to induction of mutations in the kinase domain of *BCR-ABL1* [91]. These results indicate that ROS generated by BCR-ABL1, in addition to aberrant regulation of DNA repair, contribute to a mutator phenotype in CML cells and lead to genomic instability that results in cytogenetic aberrations, point mutations, and consequently TKI resistance [90, 92]. Indeed, *BCR-ABL* has been shown to disrupt proteins involved in DNA DSB repair [93–95] and to cause cell cycle arrest in G_2/M in cells treated with DNA-damaging agents [96].

Chromosomal Abnormalities in CML

Approximately 80% of patients with CML develop additional nonrandom cytogenetic aberrations in Ph + cells, an occurrence known as "clonal evolution," which is a reflection of the genetic instability that characterizes the transition to advanced-phase CML [97]. In some reports, clonal evolution has been reported in advanced-phase CML at higher frequencies than *BCR-ABL1* mutations [98]. The most frequent cytogenetic abnormalities associated with clonal evolution are trisomy 8 (34%), isochromosome 17 (20%), and duplicate Ph chromosome (38%) [90, 99], which have been linked to c-*Myc* overexpression, loss of 17p (which results in *p53* loss), and *BCR-ABL1* overexpression, respectively [61, 100, 101]. Other cytogenetic abnormalities, such as trisomy 21, trisomy 17, and deletion 7, have been identified in less than 10% of cases of clonal evolution [102]. Also, 10–15% of patients with CML present with deletions within the derivative chromosome 9, which may lead to more rapid progression to BP [103]. In patients with 3q26.2 rearrangements (approximately 5%), the disease fails to respond to TKI treatment, exhibits a high rate of transformation to BP, and has a poor outcome [104, 105]. 3q26.2 gene rearrangements cause overexpression of a proto-oncogene, transcription factor EVI1 [106, 107]. Co-occurrence of RAS/receptor tyrosine kinase mutations contributes to leukemic transformation in myeloid malignancies [108]. Clonal evolution may therefore reflect a state of genetic instability that is frequently associated with advanced phases of CML and appears to play a pivotal role in CML progression. In the era of TKI therapy, single chromosomal change that includes trisomy 8, -Y, and an extra copy of Ph confers overall good response to therapy and favorable prognosis, while i(17)(q10), -7/7q (-7/del7q), and 3q26.2 rearrangements or concurrent emergence of more than two additional chromosomal abnormalities is associated with poor survival [109]. Cytogenetic abnormalities have also been detected in Ph-negative metaphases of 2–17% of patients with CML and have been occasionally linked with development of myelodysplasia or acute myeloid leukemia (AML) [110]. The SNP array findings that patients with CP CML harbored a mean 0.47 copy number alterations while those with BP CML harbored a mean 7.8 copy number alterations [55] further support the idea that multiple genomic aberrations accumulate during progression to BP CML.

Inactivation of Tumor-Suppressor Genes

The most frequently mutated tumor suppressor in human cancer is *p53*. In CML, *p53* can be found mutated during progression to BP in 25–30% of patients with myeloid CML BP. In addition to *p53*, exon 2 of the *INK4A/ARF* locus is deleted in 50% of cases of lymphoid CML BP [111], leading to loss of *p16* and *p14/ARF* expression, which regulates the G_1/S checkpoint by inhibiting the G_1-phase cyclin D-Cdk4/Cdk6 and by downregulating p53, respectively [100]. Deletion of the *P19ARF* gene in mice alters the nature of leukemia-initiating cells, rendering common lymphoid progenitors and precursor B-lymphocytes susceptible to transformation by BCR-ABL [112]. Because ARF enhances p53 levels by interfering with the activity of MDM2, the principal negative regulator of p53, homozygous deletion at the *p16/ARF* locus represents a functional equivalent of *p53* mutation in myeloid CML BP. Clones of CML cells carrying such deletions are likely to be selected during CML progression [100]. Retroviral transduction of *BCR-ABL1* into *ARF*-null murine bone marrow cells rapidly generates polyclonal expansion of self-renewing pre-B cells [113]. Given the impact of p53 in disease progression, it is intuitive to think that alterations in the p53 pathway may also play a role in response to TKI therapy. Imatinib therapy causes p53 activation that is a direct consequence of BCR-ABL1 kinase inhibition [114]. By contrast, p53 inactivation has been shown to impair imatinib activity in vivo, suggesting that a mutated p53 pathway may contribute to imatinib resistance in advanced-phase CML [114].

The *RUNX* family of transcription factors has also been implicated in imatinib response in CML [115]. In mice transplanted with bone marrow cells retrovirally infected with *BCR-ABL1* and subsequently treated with imatinib to select for leukemic cells in which the proviral integration had affected genes modulating imatinib response, clonal outgrowth of cells carrying similar integration sites has been shown. Proviral integration near the *RUNX3* promoter induced expression of RUNX3, and *BCR-ABL1*-positive cell lines with stable or inducible expression of RUNX1 or RUNX3 were protected from apoptosis induced by imatinib treatment [115]. Imatinib therapy was also selected for *RUNX1*-expressing cells in vivo after infection of primary bone marrow cells with both *BCR-ABL1* and *RUNX1* [115], suggesting that *RUNX1* contributes to disease persistence.

Several miRNAs have been shown to act as tumor suppressors in CML and therefore they are subjected to a strong selection pressure. miRNA 203, which maps to 14q42, is frequently lost in lymphoid CML BP. Both *ABL1* and *BCR-ABL1* genes contain miR-203 target sequences. It has been shown that miR-203 is silenced through genetic (loss of one allele) and epigenetic (promoter CpG hypermethylation in the remaining allele) mechanisms, which suggests the existence of enormous selective pressure in CML cells to silence miR-203 in order to gain a proliferative advantage [116]. These data suggest that loss of miR-203 may play a critical role in CML progression. Decreased expression of other miRNAs such as miR-10a [117] and the miR-17-92 cluster [118] has also been associated with a gain in proliferative potential and possible transformation to CML BP. The RNA-binding protein Lin28 is highly expressed in CML BP, causing repression of miRNA let-7 and activation of let-7 targets, including signaling pathways important for CML proliferation [119].

PP2A functions as a tumor suppressor by antagonizing BCR-ABL1 [120]. BCR-ABL1 kinase inhibits PP2A by upregulating SET, a phosphoprotein that inhibits PP2A [120]. In turn, PP2A activates SHP1, which abrogates BCR-ABL1 phosphorylation and targets it for proteasomal degradation [120]. Both SET inhibition and PP2A activation represent potential therapeutic strategies. The PP2A activator fingolimod (FTY720) [121] induces apoptosis and impairs the clonogenic potential of the TKI-resistant 32D-p210(T315I)$^{BCR\text{-}ABL1}$ cell line and of primary bone marrow cells from patients with BP CML or Ph + B-ALL [122]. Fingolimod induced molecular remissions in severe combined immunodeficiency (SCID) mice transplanted with myeloid or lymphoid progenitors transformed with p210$^{BCR\text{-}ABL1}$ or p190$^{BCR\text{-}ABL1}$, respectively [122].

In summary, multiple lines of evidence suggest that the increased survival, proliferation, and differentiation arrest of CML BP cells relies upon the intimate cooperation of BCR-ABL1 with an array of genes deregulated during disease progression. A better understanding of these abnormalities and the generation of more faithful CML animal models will likely facilitate the development of more effective therapies for CML BP.

CML Stem Cells

The existence of LSCs was first demonstrated in AML, when upon transplantation into nonobese diabetic (NOD)–SCID mice, only the CD34 + CD38− population was capable of propagating AML in a new host [123]. These cells encompass <1% of the total number of AML cells. LSCs were then demonstrated in CML [124] and shown to contain two distinct populations of cells: a very small set consisting of highly quiescent diploid cells in the G_0 phase, and a larger one consisting of cells in $G_1/S/G_2/M$ [125]. While solid experimental data support the existence of a subset of leukemic cells capable of giving rise to new leukemic cells, thus promoting the proliferation of the malignant clone, the precise origin of such cells remains unclear. Ph + stem cells isolated from patients with CML treated with imatinib are able to repopulate immunocompromised mice, suggesting that TKIs are unable to eliminate quiescent CML stem cells [126]. Yet, approximately 40% of CML patients in the "Stop Imatinib Trial" (STIM) who achieved a complete molecular response were able to discontinue imatinib and maintain molecular remission [127], indicating either that CML stem cells are eliminated over time by the TKI or that minimal residual disease is eliminated through immune surveillance.

Quiescence and Persistence

One of the main features that sets *BCR-ABL1*-expressing LSCs apart from more committed leukemic progenitors is that LSCs are innately resistant to chemotherapeutic agents, radiation [128], and BCR-ABL1 TKIs [129–131]. Mathematical models have shown that, when exposed to imatinib or other TKIs, CML cells decline in number in a biphasic pattern. During the initial stages of treatment, TKIs induce brisk and acute clearance of *BCR-ABL1* transcripts, likely a reflection of the elimination of the most differentiated CML cells. This is followed by a second slope of slower decline of *BCR-ABL1* transcripts, reflecting the targeting of more primitive CML progenitors, including CML LSCs, typically resulting in persistent residual disease [132, 133]. The factors underlying resistance of *BCR-ABL1*-positive LSCs to TKI therapy are not yet clearly defined. Factors invoked to explain this phenomenon include the following: (a) enhanced expression by CML stem cells of interleukin-3 (IL-3) and granulocyte colony-stimulating factor, which correlate with the primitive status of LSCs; (b) downregulation of the influx transporter human organic cation transporter-1 (hOCT1) and upregulation of the adenosine triphosphate-binding cassette transporter ABCB1 (MDR-1) and ABCG2, responsible for the influx and efflux of imatinib, respectively [65]; (c) increased expression of *BCR-ABL1* mRNA, protein, and kinase activity, which suggests that TKI-induced killing of CML LSCs requires doses much higher than those required to eliminate more mature *BCR-ABL1*-positive progenitors [134–136]; and (d) increased instability of the *BCR-ABL1* oncogene, which has been linked to increased levels of ROS and oxidative DNA damage, resulting in a higher rate of BCR-ABL1 kinase domain mutations in *BCR-ABL1*-positive LSCs even before exposure to therapy [137, 138]. There is therefore ample evidence that CML stem cells are resistant to the pro-apoptotic effects of TKIs, which may set the stage for CML relapse. However, other possibilities must be taken into account. For instance, in addition to imatinib, CML stem cells have proven highly resistant to the potent TKIs nilotinib and dasatinib [134–136]. In these cells, MAPK, PI3K, and STAT5 remain active despite BCR-ABL1 kinase inhibition [136]. Although CML LSCs express BCR-ABL [139], blockade of BCR-ABL activity by TKIs fails to eradicate CML stem cells [140, 141]. These observations suggest the interesting possibility that primitive quiescent CML stem cells may not depend on BCR-ABL1 kinase activation for survival. This would explain the TKIs' lack of activity against CML stem cells. An even more intriguing possibility is that TKI-induced BCR-ABL1 inhibition in CML stem cells might reverse the LSC phenotype to a "normal HSC" phenotype, thus calling into question the clinical importance of eradicating this subset of cells.

A potential way to eradicate LSCs is to stimulate their entry into the cell cycle [142, 143]. Interferon alpha (IFNα) has been shown to have this effect in quiescent CML stem cells. Upon binding to its receptor, IFNα induces STAT1 and STAT2 phosphorylation, which activates HSCs through the phosphorylation of AKT1 [142] and other factors involved in proliferation and by forming a complex with interferon regulator factor 9 (IRF9), which binds to the interferon-stimulated responsive element (ISRE) in genes whose transcription is regulated by IFNα. The negative regulator IRF2 competes with IRF9 for binding to ISRE, and its inactivation causes constitutive IFNα activity that causes HSCs to exit G_0 and enter an active cell cycle [142] that results in the depletion of the dormant HSC pool [144]. Therefore, while chronic activation of the IFNα pathway causes HSC depletion and compromises HSC function, acute INFα administration causes proliferation of dormant HSCs [142].

Stem Cell Maintenance Pathways

Several signaling pathways involved in embryonic development processes (tissue patterning, cell proliferation, differentiation) have been implicated in stem cell maintenance. These pathways have been shown to be involved in the pathogenesis of human cancer as they confer growth and/or survival advantage. The β-catenin pathway is key for HSC self-renewal in mice. Upon translocation to the nucleus, β-catenin interacts with its transcriptional coactivator lymphoid enhancer factor/T-cell factor (LEF/TCF) to modulate the transcription of genes such as *MYC* and *cyclin D1*. The transition from CP to BP in humans is characterized by a six- to tenfold expansion of GMPs rather than expansion of the HSC pool. Transfection of axin, a specific inhibitor of the β-catenin pathway, abrogates leukemic GMP replating and results in similar levels of β-catenin and LEF/TCF in HSCs in both normal controls and patients with CP or BP CML. Increased levels of β-catenin, LEF/TCF, and *BCR-ABL1* transcripts can be detected in GMPs isolated from patients in BP CML. The latter are endowed with increased self-renewal capabilities and stemness in vitro (as assessed by serial replating assays), compared with normal GMPs [56]. These data indicate the coexistence of two distinct self-renewing cell populations: one mainly consisting of GMPs that express high *BCR-ABL1* transcripts and enhanced nuclear β-catenin, which would be responsible for the transition to BP CML, and a second one involving *BCR-ABL1*-positive HSCs with a quiescent cell cycle, which would be responsible for the expansion and maintenance of the disease in CP. In this context, the role of the *BCR-ABL1* oncogene is not entirely clear, as this oncogene, unlike other leukemogenic fusion oncogenes such as *MLL-ENL* or *MOZ-TIF2*, can transform HSCs but is not sufficient to transform committed myeloid progenitors lacking inherent self-renewal capacity [145]. Additional pathways must therefore be implicated in LSC maintenance in CML.

The hedgehog (Hh) pathway is important during embryonic and postnatal development and in cancer [146]. Mutations in genes encoding proteins involved in the Hh pathway, such as *patched-1* (*PTCH1*) and *smoothened* (*SMO*), have been reported in several malignancies

[146–148]. Hh has been shown to play a role in primitive and adult hematopoiesis and is activated in LSCs [149–151]. Smo is a transmembrane receptor negatively regulated by the Hh receptor patched, which, in turn, is alleviated upon binding of the Hh proteins Shh, Ihh, or Dhh to patched [152]. In a murine model of CML, *BCR-ABL1*-expressing cells exhibited Smo upregulation, which was partially decreased upon treatment with imatinib or nilotinib [150]. Smo loss impairs HSC renewal, attenuates *BCR-ABL1*-induced CML, and depletes CML stem cells, likely through activation of Numb [152]. When *Smo*$^{-/-}$ cells transduced with *BCR-ABL1* were transplanted into irradiated mice, the number of LSCs was significantly lower than in control mice. Constitutively active Smo stimulates the propagation of CML stem cells and causes disease progression, supporting the important role of the Hh pathway in CML stem cells [152]. Pharmacological inhibition of Hh signaling with cyclopamine, which stabilizes Smo in its inactive form, abrogated the propagation of *BCR-ABL1*-positive cells and prolonged survival in a CML mouse model. These results, as well as recent data demonstrating the acquisition of *SMO* mutations that impair the binding of the Smo protein to Smo small-molecule inhibitors [153], highlight the importance of the Hh pathway in the pathogenesis of human cancer, and support the use of drugs that inhibit Hh signaling to eradicate LSCs in CML.

Blast cells obtained from patients with CML CP express high levels of the promyelocytic leukemia (PML) tumor-suppressor protein, which cannot be detected in more committed progenitors [154]. Genetic deletion of PML in mice or PML downregulation by arsenic trioxide resulted in increased cell cycling and ultimately exhaustion of HSCs that impaired hematopoietic reconstitution in recipient mice. CML leukemia-initiating cells (LICs) were generated by transduction of *p210*$^{BCR\text{-}ABL1}$ into *Pml*$^{-/-}$ HSCs. PML is therefore required for LIC mitotic quiescence and maintenance and this is accomplished through mTOR repression. Activation of mTOR with arsenic trioxide hampers HSC and LIC maintenance. Therefore, Hh inhibitors, mTOR activators, and IFNα are potential therapeutic strategies to eradicate LSCs in CML as they compromise LSC propagation, maintenance, and function. However, these may not be the only alternatives to effectively targeting LSCs, as other pathways appear to play a critical role in LSC homeostasis in CML. It has been shown that BCR-ABL1 kinase activates Akt signaling, which abrogates the forkhead O transcription factors (FOXO), resulting in proliferation and inhibition of apoptosis of CML cells [155]. By using a syngeneic transplantation system of immature bone marrow cells retrovirally transduced with *BCR-ABL1*, LICs have been found to be characterized by nuclear localization of FoxO3a and low Akt phosphorylation, both phenomena critically modulated by transforming growth factor-beta (TGF-β). In serial transplantation experiments utilizing LICs derived from *Foxo3a*$^{+/+}$ and *Foxo3a*$^{-/-}$ mice, genetic deficiency of Foxo3a remarkably limited the ability of LICs to induce a leukemic phenotype. In keeping with these results, TGF-β inhibitor therapy impaired the colony-forming ability of human CD34^{+}CD38^{-}Lin^{-} CML cells in vitro [155], which suggests that the TGF-β–FOXO pathway has an essential role in the maintenance of CML LICs. Similarly, *ALOX5*, the arachidonate 5-lipoxygenase (5-LO) gene, has been identified as a critical regulator of LSCs in CML [156]. Alox5 deficiency renders BCR-ABL1 unable to induce CML in mice by impairing differentiation, cell division, and survival of LSCs but not normal HSCs. BCR-ABL suppresses Blk (encoding B-lymphoid kinase), which functions as a tumor suppressor in CML stem cells through an upstream regulator, Pax5, and a downstream effector, p27 [157].

Regulation of quiescence in LSC and insensitivity to TKIs is modulated by a pathway of peroxisome proliferator-activated receptor gamma (PPARγ) and its downstream targets STAT5 and HIF2α/CITED2, known to facilitate LSC dormancy [158]. In turn, activation of PPARγ by this antidiabetic glitazone drugs decreased STAT5 expression and reduced the LSC pool, causing stem cells to exit quiescence and eliminating disease when combined with TKIs. Additional pathways and transcriptional regulators implicated in CML stem cell maintenance include BCL-6 [159], MPL/JAK [160, 161], SIRT1 [162], Notch [163], Bmi1 [164], IL2/CD25 signaling [165], and autophagy [166]. Interactions between LSCs and bone marrow microenvironment may also influence the success of CML therapy [167, 168], and approaches targeting LSC-niche interactions have been shown to be effective in preclinical model systems [169, 170]. Additionally, the hypoxic nature of the marrow niche has been proposed to offer LSC maintenance and protection from TKIs [171].

BCR-ABL1 Kinase Domain Mutations and TKI Resistance

CML may fail to respond or may lose its response to TKI therapy through a series of BCR-ABL1-dependent or -independent mechanisms of resistance including TKI compliance and bioavailability, pharmacodynamics, genetic changes, *BCR-ABL1* kinase domain mutations, or BCR-ABL1 overexpression. The most frequent and clinically relevant mechanism of resistance to TKI therapy is the acquisition of mutations within the kinase domain of *BCR-ABL1* (Fig. 4.4). Mutations have been reported at frequencies ranging from 40 to 90% among patients with imatinib-resistant CML [172–177]. Kinases are plastic multimodular structures that oscillate between an active and an inactive conformation. Different TKIs bind different conformations of the BCR-ABL1 kinase. For instance, imatinib and

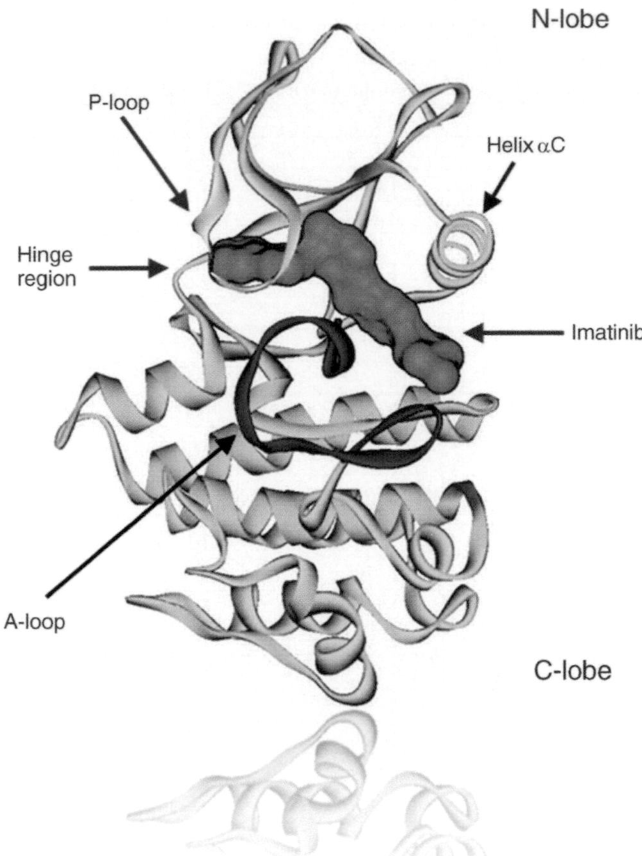

Fig. 4.4 3D structure of the ABL1 kinase domain in complex with imatinib. The ATP-binding site in the ABL1 kinase domain is located between the activation loop (A-loop) and the phosphate-binding loop (P-loop). The A-loop controls the ABL1 catalytic activity by switching between the active and the inactive conformations of the kinase. Imatinib inserts its pyridinyl group underneath the helix αC in the NH2-terminal lobe of ABL1 kinase, displacing ATP and freezing the kinase in its inactive conformation. Mutations mapping at the P-loop, the A-loop, and imatinib contact sites are the most common causes of acquired resistance to imatinib therapy

nilotinib bind the inactive conformation of ABL1 kinase, in which the highly conserved Asp-Phe-Gly (DFG) residues are swung out of the catalytic cleft ("DFG-out") [178, 179]. Imatinib extends deeply into the catalytic domain, and its pyridinyl group locates underneath the αC helix in the NH_2-terminal lobe of ABL1 kinase [178]. On the other hand, X-ray crystallography [180] and NMR spectroscopy [181] have shown that dasatinib binds the active ("DFG-in") conformation of ABL1.

Over 100 different point mutations encoding single-amino acid substitutions within the kinase domain of *BCR-ABL1* have been detected in patients with imatinib-resistant CML [20, 177, 178, 182, 183], and others have been generated in vitro by random mutagenesis of *BCR-ABL1* [182, 184]. Imatinib-resistant mutations tend to cluster at specific regions within ABL1 kinase. One such region, the P-loop region (residues 248–255) of the kinase domain, serves as a docking site for phosphate moieties of ATP [185–187]. While some studies linked P-loop mutations to a poorer clinical outcome [188, 189], others have not confirmed this observation [190]. In fact, not all P-loop mutations have the same transformation potency or sensitivity to different TKIs. Second-generation TKIs such as dasatinib, bosutinib, and, to a lesser extent, nilotinib are active against some P-loop mutations (Table 4.1). Other areas within ABL1 kinase frequently affected by mutations include the activation (A) loop (residues 381–402), whose mutations prevent the kinase from adopting the inactive conformation to which imatinib binds, and the catalytic (C) domain (residues 350–363). Particularly worrisome are those mutations that affect ATP-contact sites within the ATP-binding region (e.g., T315I, F317L, V299L). Selected ATP-binding loop mutations such as Y253F increase intrinsic BCR-ABL kinase activity [191, 192]. The gatekeeper residue Thr315 sits at the periphery of the nucleotide-binding site of ABL1 and forms an H-bond with imatinib and dasatinib [183]. Mutation of Thr315 to isoleucine (T315I) disrupts this H-bond interaction, which, in addition to the steric hindrance imposed by the isoleucine side chain and the stabilization of the kinase in the active conformation, impairs imatinib binding, causes complete insensitivity to this compound as well as to second-generation TKIs, and promotes malignant transformation [6, 174, 179, 193–197]. T315I mutation has been reported in approximately 15% of patients after failure of imatinib therapy [198]. For patients with a gatekeeper T315 mutation, the only TKI approved for clinical use is ponatinib [199]. Ponatinib is a type II inhibitor that avoids T315 by inclusion of a rigid triple-carbon bond. Ponatinib at higher concentrations is capable of inhibiting other BCR-ABL mutations (such as E225V), and these levels are clinically achievable, accounting for higher response rates to ponatinib in CML patients with multiple mutations [200]. The F317L and V299L mutations almost invariably arise during dasatinib therapy but retain sensitivity against nilotinib [201]. Mutations occurring at a subset of residues (Q253, Y253, E255, T315, E459, and F486) are more frequently detected in patients with advanced-phase CML [202].

Despite the wide variety of *BCR-ABL1* point mutations, most mutants are rare, with mutations involving residues Gly250, Tyr253, Glu255, Thr315, Met351, and Phe359 accounting for 60–70% of all mutations [203]. The presence of T315-inclusive compound mutations, i.e., two or more mutations within the same BCR-ABL molecule, confers resistance to all currently available TKIs [204] and has been found in patients in whom ponatinib failed [200, 205]. This is not the case for non-T315I compound mutations, which are variably sensitive to several TKIs. Over 60 different BCR-ABL1 compound mutations have been reported in association with sequential TKI use and resistance [206–208]. Clones with the E225K/T315 compound mutation

Table 4.1 Sensitivity of BCR-ABL1 kinase domain mutations to imatinib and the second-generation tyrosine kinase inhibitors nilotinib, dasatinib, and ponatinib

	BCR-ABL$_1$ isoform	Imatinib (nM)	Nilotinib (nM)	Dasatinib (nM)	Ponatinib (nM) [199]
	Native	260	13	0.8	0.5
P-loop	$M_{244}V$	2000	38	1.3	2.2
	$G_{250}E$	1350	48	1.8	4.1
	$Q_{252}H$	1325	70	3.4	2.2
	$Y_{253}H$	>6400	450	1.3	6.2
	$Y_{253}F$	3475	125	1.4	2.8
	$E_{255}K$	5200	200	5.6	14
	$E_{255}V$	>6400	430	11	36
	$V_{299}L$	540	NA	18	NT
ATP-binding site	$F_{311}L$	480	23	1.3	NT
	$T_{315}I$	>6400	>2000	>200	11
	$T_{315}A$	971	61	125	1.6
	$F_{317}L$	1050	50	7.4	1.1
	$F_{317}V$	350	NA	53	10
Catalytic domain	$M_{351}T$	880	15	1.1	1.5
	$E_{355}G$	2300	NA	1.8	NT
	$F_{359}V$	1825	175	2.2	10
	$V_{379}I$	1630	51	0.8	NT
A-loop	$L_{387}M$	1000	49	2	NT
	$H_{396}R$	1750	41	1.3	NT
	$H_{396}P$	850	41	0.6	1.1

NA not applicable, *NT* not tested

were shown in vitro to produce paracrine factor IL-3, which promotes survival of bystander non-mutated cells through the MEK/ERK and JAK2/STAT5 pathways [209]. Novel allosteric BCR-ABL inhibitors binding in non-ATP pocket sites have entered clinical trials and have been shown in preclinical studies to restore the sensitivity to conventional TKIs of the T315I mutant [210]. Whether such inhibitors can block compound mutations remains to be determined.

It is worth emphasizing that different mutations are endowed with different transforming capabilities that are not tightly related to their kinase activity. In pre-B-cell transformation assays, T315I (which has weaker kinase activity than p210$^{BCR\text{-}ABL1}$) and E255K consistently showed a 10–20% increase in oncogenic potency relative to that of p210$^{BCR\text{-}ABL1}$; whereas the P-loop mutants Y253F and E255V had potencies similar to those of p210$^{BCR\text{-}ABL1}$ and Y253H, T315A, F317L, and M351T were markedly weaker [192]. Relative to unmutated *BCR-ABL1*, Y253F and E255K mutants have higher transformation potency, whereas M351T and H396P mutants are less potent. The kinase activity of E255K, H396P, and T315I did not correlate with transforming potency. Analysis of the phosphotyrosine proteome by mass spectroscopy confirmed the presence of different phosphorylation signatures among the different mutants, confirming that different mutations determine substrate specificity leading to activation of different downstream pathways [191]. Importantly, some patients with CML tend to accumulate more than one BCR-ABL1 mutation, frequently within the same *BCR-ABL1* allele, when they experience sequential TKI therapy failure, and this accumulation of mutations was associated with greater oncogenic potency than each individual mutation [206].

BCR-ABL1 kinase-independent mechanisms of resistance are thought to involve activation of alternative signaling pathways and might involve multiple mechanisms. For example, activation of pSTAT3, STAT5, MAPK, JAK2, LYN, SYK, PI3K, and XPO1/CRM1 has been implicated in kinase-independent resistance to TKIs [68, 211–219]. Other mechanisms of resistance include impaired inhibitor influx or increased drug efflux, such as cation transporter OCT1 for imatinib resistance [220, 221] and MDR1 for nilotinib resistance [222].

Concluding Remarks

The central role of *BCR-ABL1* as the causative agent in the pathogenesis of CML is firmly established. Cells expressing *BCR-ABL1* acquire growth factor independence and exhibit deregulated cell proliferation and increased resistance to apoptosis. These capabilities are acquired and sustained by a complex network of signals that emanate from the constitutive kinase activity of BCR-ABL1. Such signals result initially in unbridled myeloproliferation of mature myeloid elements; over time CML cells exhibit a marked loss of differentiation and growth arrest at the very early steps of myeloid maturation, which, in the absence of appropriate therapy, results in the transformation to BP. The initial steps of the pathogenesis of CML are directly choreographed by BCR-ABL1. Its activity during transformation, while necessary, is no longer sufficient. The mechanisms that govern the transformation process are not well understood, but research advances in this area have unveiled the previously unknown involvement of a series of transcription factors, miRNAs, and tumor suppressors in this process. Accordingly, blocking the constitutive activation of BCR-ABL1 kinase with TKIs such as imatinib results in high rates of response and a dramatic prolongation of survival among patients with CML CP. However, this strategy is not durably effective in patients with CML BP. It is therefore important to continue unraveling the intimate molecular mechanisms of transformation to better devise therapeutic strategies for patients with advanced-phase CML. In addition, while current TKI therapy for CML CP is highly effective, it does not fully eradicate the leukemic clones in most patients. The persistence of circulating and bone marrow-based CML cells is likely a consequence of the lack of sensitivity of primitive progenitors and CML stem cells to TKIs. A better understanding of the mechanisms that regulate CML stem cell homeostasis would facilitate the development of molecularly curative strategies for patients with CML.

References

1. Quintas-Cardama A, Cortes J. Molecular biology of bcr-abl1-positive chronic myeloid leukemia. Blood. 2009;113(8):1619–30.
2. Daley GQ, Van Etten RA, Baltimore D. Induction of chronic myelogenous leukemia in mice by the P210bcr/abl gene of the Philadelphia chromosome. Science. 1990;247(4944):824–30.
3. Buchdunger E, Zimmermann J, Mett H, Meyer T, Muller M, Druker BJ, et al. Inhibition of the Abl protein-tyrosine kinase in vitro and in vivo by a 2-phenylaminopyrimidine derivative. Cancer Res. 1996;56(1):100–4.
4. Druker BJ, Tamura S, Buchdunger E, Ohno S, Segal GM, Fanning S, et al. Effects of a selective inhibitor of the Abl tyrosine kinase on the growth of Bcr-Abl positive cells. Nat Med. 1996;2(5):561–6.
5. O'Brien SG, Guilhot F, Larson RA, Gathmann I, Baccarani M, Cervantes F, et al. Imatinib compared with interferon and low-dose cytarabine for newly diagnosed chronic-phase chronic myeloid leukemia. N Engl J Med. 2003;348(11):994–1004.
6. Druker BJ, Sawyers CL, Kantarjian H, Resta DJ, Reese SF, Ford JM, et al. Activity of a specific inhibitor of the BCR-ABL tyrosine kinase in the blast crisis of chronic myeloid leukemia and acute lymphoblastic leukemia with the Philadelphia chromosome. N Engl J Med. 2001;344(14):1038–42.
7. Melo JV. The diversity of BCR-ABL fusion proteins and their relationship to leukemia phenotype. Blood. 1996;88(7):2375–84.
8. Faderl S, Talpaz M, Estrov Z, O'Brien S, Kurzrock R, Kantarjian HM. The biology of chronic myeloid leukemia. N Engl J Med. 1999;341(3):164–72.
9. Pane F, Frigeri F, Sindona M, Luciano L, Ferrara F, Cimino R, et al. Neutrophilic-chronic myeloid leukemia: a distinct disease with a specific molecular marker (BCR/ABL with C3/A2 junction). Blood. 1996;88(7):2410–4.
10. Ramaraj P, Singh H, Niu N, Chu S, Holtz M, Yee JK, et al. Effect of mutational inactivation of tyrosine kinase activity on BCR/ABL-induced abnormalities in cell growth and adhesion in human hematopoietic progenitors. Cancer Res. 2004;64(15):5322–31.
11. Zhao RC, Jiang Y, Verfaillie CM. A model of human p210(bcr/ABL)-mediated chronic myelogenous leukemia by transduction of primary normal human CD34(+) cells with a BCR/ABL-containing retroviral vector. Blood. 2001;97(8):2406–12.
12. Heisterkamp N, Jenster G, ten Hoeve J, Zovich D, Pattengale PK, Groffen J. Acute leukaemia in bcr/abl transgenic mice. Nature. 1990;344(6263):251–3.
13. Zhang X, Ren R. Bcr-Abl efficiently induces a myeloproliferative disease and production of excess interleukin-3 and granulocyte-macrophage colony-stimulating factor in mice: a novel model for chronic myelogenous leukemia. Blood. 1998;92(10):3829–40.
14. Koschmieder S, Gottgens B, Zhang P, Iwasaki-Arai J, Akashi K, Kutok JL, et al. Inducible chronic phase of myeloid leukemia with expansion of hematopoietic stem cells in a transgenic model of BCR-ABL leukemogenesis. Blood. 2005;105(1):324–34.
15. Hantschel O, Superti-Furga G. Regulation of the c-Abl and Bcr-Abl tyrosine kinases. Nat Rev Mol Cell Biol. 2004;5(1):33–44.
16. Zhang X, Wong R, Hao SX, Pear WS, Ren R. The SH2 domain of bcr-Abl is not required to induce a murine myeloproliferative disease; however, SH2 signaling influences disease latency and phenotype. Blood. 2001;97(1):277–87.
17. Feller SM, Knudsen B, Hanafusa H. c-Abl kinase regulates the protein binding activity of c-Crk. EMBO J. 1994;13(10):2341–51.
18. Smith JM, Katz S, Mayer BJ. Activation of the Abl tyrosine kinase in vivo by Src homology 3 domains from the Src homology 2/Src homology 3 adaptor Nck. J Biol Chem. 1999;274(39):27956–62.
19. Ren R. Mechanisms of BCR-ABL in the pathogenesis of chronic myelogenous leukaemia. Nat Rev Cancer. 2005;5(3):172–83.
20. Hantschel O, Nagar B, Guettler S, Kretzschmar J, Dorey K, Kuriyan J, et al. A myristoyl/phosphotyrosine switch regulates c-Abl. Cell. 2003;112(6):845–57.
21. Nagar B, Hantschel O, Young MA, Scheffzek K, Veach D, Bornmann W, et al. Structural basis for the autoinhibition of c-Abl tyrosine kinase. Cell. 2003;112(6):859–71.
22. Zhao X, Ghaffari S, Lodish H, Malashkevich VN, Kim PS. Structure of the Bcr-Abl oncoprotein oligomerization domain. Nat Struct Biol. 2002;9(2):117–20.
23. Smith KM, Yacobi R, Van Etten RA. Autoinhibition of Bcr-Abl through its SH3 domain. Mol Cell. 2003;12(1):27–37.
24. Zhang X, Subrahmanyam R, Wong R, Gross AW, Ren R. The NH(2)-terminal coiled-coil domain and tyrosine 177 play important roles in induction of a myeloproliferative disease in mice by Bcr-Abl. Mol Cell Biol. 2001;21(3):840–53.
25. Pendergast AM, Quilliam LA, Cripe LD, Bassing CH, Dai Z, Li N, et al. BCR-ABL-induced oncogenesis is mediated by direct interaction with the SH2 domain of the GRB-2 adaptor protein. Cell. 1993;75(1):175–85.
26. Sattler M, Mohi MG, Pride YB, Quinnan LR, Malouf NA, Podar K, et al. Critical role for Gab2 in transformation by BCR/ABL. Cancer Cell. 2002;1(5):479–92.
27. Skorski T, Kanakaraj P, Nieborowska-Skorska M, Ratajczak MZ, Wen SC, Zon G, et al. Phosphatidylinositol-3 kinase activity is regulated by BCR/ABL and is required for the growth of Philadelphia chromosome-positive cells. Blood. 1995;86(2):726–36.
28. Notari M, Neviani P, Santhanam R, Blaser BW, Chang JS, Galietta A, et al. A MAPK/HNRPK pathway controls BCR/ABL oncogenic potential by regulating MYC mRNA translation. Blood. 2006;107(6):2507–16.

29. Johnson KJ, Griswold IJ, O'Hare T, Corbin AS, Loriaux M, Deininger MW, et al. A BCR-ABL mutant lacking direct binding sites for the GRB2, CBL and CRKL adapter proteins fails to induce leukemia in mice. PLoS One. 2009;4(10):e7439.
30. Samanta AK, Chakraborty SN, Wang Y, Kantarjian H, Sun X, Hood J, et al. Jak2 inhibition deactivates Lyn kinase through the SET-PP2A-SHP1 pathway, causing apoptosis in drug-resistant cells from chronic myelogenous leukemia patients. Oncogene. 2009;28(14):1669–81.
31. Ilaria RL Jr, Van Etten RA. P210 and P190(BCR/ABL) induce the tyrosine phosphorylation and DNA binding activity of multiple specific STAT family members. J Biol Chem. 1996;271(49):31704 10.
32. Nosaka T, Kawashima T, Misawa K, Ikuta K, Mui AL, Kitamura T. STAT5 as a molecular regulator of proliferation, differentiation and apoptosis in hematopoietic cells. EMBO J. 1999;18(17):4754–65.
33. Hu Y, Liu Y, Pelletier S, Buchdunger E, Warmuth M, Fabbro D, et al. Requirement of Src kinases Lyn, Hck and Fgr for BCR-ABL1-induced B-lymphoblastic leukemia but not chronic myeloid leukemia. Nat Genet. 2004;36(5):453–61.
34. Ptasznik A, Nakata Y, Kalota A, Emerson SG, Gewirtz AM. Short interfering RNA (siRNA) targeting the Lyn kinase induces apoptosis in primary, and drug-resistant, BCR-ABL1(+) leukemia cells. Nat Med. 2004;10(11):1187–9.
35. Hoelbl A, Schuster C, Kovacic B, Zhu B, Wickre M, Hoelzl MA, et al. Stat5 is indispensable for the maintenance of bcr/abl-positive leukaemia. EMBO Mol Med. 2010;2(3):98–110.
36. Kovacic B, Hoelbl A, Litos G, Alacakaptan M, Schuster C, Fischhuber KM, et al. Diverging fates of cells of origin in acute and chronic leukaemia. EMBO Mol Med. 2012;4(4):283–97.
37. Gabriele L, Phung J, Fukumoto J, Segal D, Wang IM, Giannakakou P, et al. Regulation of apoptosis in myeloid cells by interferon consensus sequence-binding protein. J Exp Med. 1999;190(3):411–21.
38. Gesbert F, Griffin JD. Bcr/Abl activates transcription of the Bcl-X gene through STAT5. Blood. 2000;96(6):2269–76.
39. Sonoyama J, Matsumura I, Ezoe S, Satoh Y, Zhang X, Kataoka Y, et al. Functional cooperation among Ras, STAT5, and phosphatidylinositol 3-kinase is required for full oncogenic activities of BCR/ABL in K562 cells. J Biol Chem. 2002;277(10):8076–82.
40. Thomas EK, Cancelas JA, Chae HD, Cox AD, Keller PJ, Perrotti D, et al. Rac guanosine triphosphatases represent integrating molecular therapeutic targets for BCR-ABL-induced myeloproliferative disease. Cancer Cell. 2007;12(5):467–78.
41. Cancelas JA, Lee AW, Prabhakar R, Stringer KF, Zheng Y, Williams DA. Rac GTPases differentially integrate signals regulating hematopoietic stem cell localization. Nat Med. 2005;11(8):886–91.
42. Angel P, Karin M. The role of Jun, Fos and the AP-1 complex in cell-proliferation and transformation. Biochim Biophys Acta. 1991;1072(2–3):129–57.
43. Passegue E, Wagner EF, Weissman IL. JunB deficiency leads to a myeloproliferative disorder arising from hematopoietic stem cells. Cell. 2004;119(3):431–43.
44. Passegue E, Jochum W, Schorpp-Kistner M, Mohle-Steinlein U, Wagner EF. Chronic myeloid leukemia with increased granulocyte progenitors in mice lacking junB expression in the myeloid lineage. Cell. 2001;104(1):21–32.
45. Middleton MK, Zukas AM, Rubinstein T, Jacob M, Zhu P, Zhao L, et al. Identification of 12/15-lipoxygenase as a suppressor of myeloproliferative disease. J Exp Med. 2006;203(11):2529–40.
46. Holtschke T, Lohler J, Kanno Y, Fehr T, Giese N, Rosenbauer F, et al. Immunodeficiency and chronic myelogenous leukemia-like syndrome in mice with a targeted mutation of the ICSBP gene. Cell. 1996;87(2):307–17.
47. Hao SX, Ren R. Expression of interferon consensus sequence binding protein (ICSBP) is downregulated in Bcr-Abl-induced murine chronic myelogenous leukemia-like disease, and forced coexpression of ICSBP inhibits Bcr-Abl-induced myeloproliferative disorder. Mol Cell Biol. 2000;20(4):1149–61.
48. Chen Y, Hu Y, Zhang H, Peng C, Li S. Loss of the Alox5 gene impairs leukemia stem cells and prevents chronic myeloid leukemia. Nat Genet. 2009;41(7):783–92.
49. Zheng C, Li L, Haak M, Brors B, Frank O, Giehl M, et al. Gene expression profiling of CD34+ cells identifies a molecular signature of chronic myeloid leukemia blast crisis. Leukemia. 2006;20(6):1028–34.
50. Nowicki MO, Pawlowski P, Fischer T, Hess G, Pawlowski T, Skorski T. Chronic myelogenous leukemia molecular signature. Oncogene. 2003;22(25):3952–63.
51. Kaneta Y, Kagami Y, Tsunoda T, Ohno R, Nakamura Y, Katagiri T. Genome-wide analysis of gene-expression profiles in chronic myeloid leukemia cells using a cDNA microarray. Int J Oncol. 2003;23(3):681–91.
52. Kronenwett R, Butterweck U, Steidl U, Kliszewski S, Neumann F, Bork S, et al. Distinct molecular phenotype of malignant CD34(+) hematopoietic stem and progenitor cells in chronic myelogenous leukemia. Oncogene. 2005;24(34):5313–24.
53. Yong AS, Szydlo RM, Goldman JM, Apperley JF, Melo JV. Molecular profiling of CD34+ cells identifies low expression of CD7, along with high expression of proteinase 3 or elastase, as predictors of longer survival in patients with CML. Blood. 2006;107(1):205–12.
54. Radich JP, Dai H, Mao M, Oehler V, Schelter J, Druker B, et al. Gene expression changes associated with progression and response in chronic myeloid leukemia. Proc Natl Acad Sci U S A. 2006;103(8):2794–9.
55. Mullighan CG, Miller CB, Radtke I, Phillips LA, Dalton J, Ma J, et al. BCR-ABL1 lymphoblastic leukaemia is characterized by the deletion of Ikaros. Nature. 2008;453(7191):110–4.
56. Jamieson CH, Ailles LE, Dylla SJ, Muijtjens M, Jones C, Zehnder JL, et al. Granulocyte-macrophage progenitors as candidate leukemic stem cells in blast-crisis CML. N Engl J Med. 2004;351(7):657–67.
57. Jamieson CH, Weissman IL, Passegue E. Chronic versus acute myelogenous leukemia: a question of self-renewal. Cancer Cell. 2004;6(6):531–3.
58. Weissman I. Stem cell research: paths to cancer therapies and regenerative medicine. JAMA. 2005;294(11):1359–66.
59. Santaguida M, Schepers K, King B, Sabnis AJ, Forsberg EC, Attema JL, et al. JunB protects against myeloid malignancies by limiting hematopoietic stem cell proliferation and differentiation without affecting self-renewal. Cancer Cell. 2009;15(4):341–52.
60. Jaiswal S, Traver D, Miyamoto T, Akashi K, Lagasse E, Weissman IL. Expression of BCR/ABL and BCL-2 in myeloid progenitors leads to myeloid leukemias. Proc Natl Acad Sci U S A. 2003;100(17):10002–7.
61. Gaiger A, Henn T, Horth E, Geissler K, Mitterbauer G, Maier-Dobersberger T, et al. Increase of bcr-abl chimeric mRNA expression in tumor cells of patients with chronic myeloid leukemia precedes disease progression. Blood. 1995;86(6):2371–8.
62. Guo JQ, Wang JY, Arlinghaus RB. Detection of BCR-ABL proteins in blood cells of benign phase chronic myelogenous leukemia patients. Cancer Res. 1991;51(11):3048–51.
63. Barnes DJ, Schultheis B, Adedeji S, Melo JV. Dose-dependent effects of Bcr-Abl in cell line models of different stages of chronic myeloid leukemia. Oncogene. 2005;24(42):6432–40.
64. Cambier N, Chopra R, Strasser A, Metcalf D, Elefanty AG. BCR-ABL activates pathways mediating cytokine independence and protection against apoptosis in murine hematopoietic cells in a dose-dependent manner. Oncogene. 1998;16(3):335–48.
65. Jiang X, Zhao Y, Smith C, Gasparetto M, Turhan A, Eaves A, et al. Chronic myeloid leukemia stem cells possess multiple unique

features of resistance to BCR-ABL targeted therapies. Leukemia. 2007;21(5):926–35.
66. Ban K, Gao Y, Amin HM, Howard A, Miller C, Lin Q, et al. BCR-ABL1 mediates up-regulation of Fyn in chronic myelogenous leukemia. Blood. 2008;111(5):2904–8.
67. Dai Y, Rahmani M, Corey SJ, Dent P, Grant S. A Bcr/Abl-independent, Lyn-dependent form of imatinib mesylate (STI-571) resistance is associated with altered expression of Bcl-2. J Biol Chem. 2004;279(33):34227–39.
68. Donato NJ, Wu JY, Stapley J, Gallick G, Lin H, Arlinghaus R, et al. BCR-ABL independence and LYN kinase overexpression in chronic myelogenous leukemia cells selected for resistance to STI571. Blood. 2003;101(2):690–8.
69. Donato NJ, Wu JY, Stapley J, Lin H, Arlinghaus R, Aggarwal BB, et al. Imatinib mesylate resistance through BCR-ABL independence in chronic myelogenous leukemia. Cancer Res. 2004;64(2):672–7.
70. Hu Y, Swerdlow S, Duffy TM, Weinmann R, Lee FY, Li S. Targeting multiple kinase pathways in leukemic progenitors and stem cells is essential for improved treatment of Ph+ leukemia in mice. Proc Natl Acad Sci U S A. 2006;103(45):16870–5.
71. Wu J, Meng F, Kong LY, Peng Z, Ying Y, Bornmann WG, et al. Association between imatinib-resistant BCR-ABL mutation-negative leukemia and persistent activation of LYN kinase. J Natl Cancer Inst. 2008;100(13):926–39.
72. Carlesso N, Frank DA, Griffin JD. Tyrosyl phosphorylation and DNA binding activity of signal transducers and activators of transcription (STAT) proteins in hematopoietic cell lines transformed by Bcr/Abl. J Exp Med. 1996;183(3):811–20.
73. Perrotti D, Bonatti S, Trotta R, Martinez R, Skorski T, Salomoni P, et al. TLS/FUS, a pro-oncogene involved in multiple chromosomal translocations, is a novel regulator of BCR/ABL-mediated leukemogenesis. EMBO J. 1998;17(15):4442–55.
74. Winandy S, Wu P, Georgopoulos K. A dominant mutation in the Ikaros gene leads to rapid development of leukemia and lymphoma. Cell. 1995;83(2):289–99.
75. Iacobucci I, Storlazzi CT, Cilloni D, Lonetti A, Ottaviani E, Soverini S, et al. Identification and molecular characterization of recurrent genomic deletions on 7p12 in the IKZF1 gene in a large cohort of BCR-ABL1-positive acute lymphoblastic leukemia patients: on behalf of Gruppo Italiano Malattie Ematologiche dell'Adulto Acute Leukemia Working Party (GIMEMA AL WP). Blood. 2009;114(10):2159–67.
76. Kirstetter P, Thomas M, Dierich A, Kastner P, Chan S. Ikaros is critical for B cell differentiation and function. Eur J Immunol. 2002;32(3):720–30.
77. Joshi I, Yoshida T, Jena N, Qi X, Zhang J, Van Etten RA, et al. Loss of Ikaros DNA-binding function confers integrin-dependent survival on pre-B cells and progression to acute lymphoblastic leukemia. Nat Immunol. 2014;15(3):294–304.
78. Tenen DG. Disruption of differentiation in human cancer: AML shows the way. Nat Rev Cancer. 2003;3(2):89–101.
79. Perrotti D, Cesi V, Trotta R, Guerzoni C, Santilli G, Campbell K, et al. BCR-ABL suppresses C/EBPalpha expression through inhibitory action of hnRNP E2. Nat Genet. 2002;30(1):48–58.
80. Wagner K, Zhang P, Rosenbauer F, Drescher B, Kobayashi S, Radomska HS, et al. Absence of the transcription factor CCAAT enhancer binding protein alpha results in loss of myeloid identity in bcr/abl-induced malignancy. Proc Natl Acad Sci U S A. 2006;103(16):6338–43.
81. Eiring AM, Harb JG, Neviani P, Garton C, Oaks JJ, Spizzo R, et al. miR-328 functions as an RNA decoy to modulate hnRNP E2 regulation of mRNA translation in leukemic blasts. Cell. 2010;140(5):652–65.
82. Dash AB, Williams IR, Kutok JL, Tomasson MH, Anastasiadou E, Lindahl K, et al. A murine model of CML blast crisis induced by cooperation between BCR/ABL and NUP98/HOXA9. Proc Natl Acad Sci U S A. 2002;99(11):7622–7.
83. Nucifora G, Birn DJ, Espinosa R 3rd, Erickson P, LeBeau MM, Roulston D, et al. Involvement of the AML1 gene in the t(3;21) in therapy-related leukemia and in chronic myeloid leukemia in blast crisis. Blood. 1993;81(10):2728–34.
84. Wu M, Kwon HY, Rattis F, Blum J, Zhao C, Ashkenazi R, et al. Imaging hematopoietic precursor division in real time. Cell Stem Cell. 2007;1(5):541–54.
85. Ito T, Kwon HY, Zimdahl B, Congdon KL, Blum J, Lento WE, et al. Regulation of myeloid leukaemia by the cell-fate determinant Musashi. Nature. 2010;466(7307):765–8.
86. Kharas MG, Lengner CJ, Al-Shahrour F, Bullinger L, Ball B, Zaidi S, et al. Musashi-2 regulates normal hematopoiesis and promotes aggressive myeloid leukemia. Nat Med. 2010;16(8):903–8.
87. Nowicki MO, Falinski R, Koptyra M, Slupianek A, Stoklosa T, Gloc E, et al. BCR/ABL oncogenic kinase promotes unfaithful repair of the reactive oxygen species-dependent DNA double-strand breaks. Blood. 2004;104(12):3746–53.
88. Melo JV, Barnes DJ. Chronic myeloid leukaemia as a model of disease evolution in human cancer. Nat Rev Cancer. 2007;7(6):441–53.
89. Slupianek A, Nowicki MO, Koptyra M, Skorski T. BCR/ABL modifies the kinetics and fidelity of DNA double-strand breaks repair in hematopoietic cells. DNA Repair. 2006;5(2):243–50.
90. Koptyra M, Falinski R, Nowicki MO, Stoklosa T, Majsterek I, Nieborowska-Skorska M, et al. BCR/ABL kinase induces self-mutagenesis via reactive oxygen species to encode imatinib resistance. Blood. 2006;108(1):319–27.
91. Klemm L, Duy C, Iacobucci I, Kuchen S, von Levetzow G, Feldhahn N, et al. The B cell mutator AID promotes B lymphoid blast crisis and drug resistance in chronic myeloid leukemia. Cancer Cell. 2009;16(3):232–45.
92. Canitrot Y, Lautier D, Laurent G, Frechet M, Ahmed A, Turhan AG, et al. Mutator phenotype of BCR--ABL transfected Ba/F3 cell lines and its association with enhanced expression of DNA polymerase beta. Oncogene. 1999;18(17):2676–80.
93. Deutsch E, Dugray A, AbdulKarim B, Marangoni E, Maggiorella L, Vaganay S, et al. BCR-ABL down-regulates the DNA repair protein DNA-PKcs. Blood. 2001;97(7):2084–90.
94. Slupianek A, Poplawski T, Jozwiakowski SK, Cramer K, Pytel D, Stoczynska E, et al. BCR/ABL stimulates WRN to promote survival and genomic instability. Cancer Res. 2011;71(3):842–51.
95. Slupianek A, Dasgupta Y, Ren SY, Gurdek E, Donlin M, Nieborowska-Skorska M, et al. Targeting RAD51 phosphotyrosine-315 to prevent unfaithful recombination repair in BCR-ABL1 leukemia. Blood. 2011;118(4):1062–8.
96. Slupianek A, Hoser G, Majsterek I, Bronisz A, Malecki M, Blasiak J, et al. Fusion tyrosine kinases induce drug resistance by stimulation of homology-dependent recombination repair, prolongation of G(2)/M phase, and protection from apoptosis. Mol Cell Biol. 2002;22(12):4189–201.
97. Cortes J, O'Dwyer ME. Clonal evolution in chronic myelogenous leukemia. Hematol Oncol Clin North Am. 2004;18(3):671–84, x.
98. Lahaye T, Riehm B, Berger U, Paschka P, Muller MC, Kreil S, et al. Response and resistance in 300 patients with BCR-ABL-positive leukemias treated with imatinib in a single center: a 4.5-year follow-up. Cancer. 2005;103(8):1659–69.
99. Johansson B, Fioretos T, Mitelman F. Cytogenetic and molecular genetic evolution of chronic myeloid leukemia. Acta Haematol. 2002;107(2):76–94.
100. Calabretta B, Perrotti D. The biology of CML blast crisis. Blood. 2004;103(11):4010–22.
101. Jennings BA, Mills KI. c-myc locus amplification and the acquisition of trisomy 8 in the evolution of chronic myeloid leukaemia. Leuk Res. 1998;22(10):899–903.

102. Quintas-Cardama A, Cortes JE. Chronic myeloid leukemia: diagnosis and treatment. Mayo Clin Proc. 2006;81(7):973–88.
103. Huntly BJ, Bench A, Green AR. Double jeopardy from a single translocation: deletions of the derivative chromosome 9 in chronic myeloid leukemia. Blood. 2003;102(4):1160–8.
104. Wang W, Cortes JE, Lin P, Beaty MW, Ai D, Amin HM, et al. Clinical and prognostic significance of 3q26.2 and other chromosome 3 abnormalities in CML in the era of tyrosine kinase inhibitors. Blood. 2015;126(14):1699–706.
105. Theil KS, Cotta CV. The prognostic significance of an inv(3)(q21q26.2) in addition to a t(9;22)(q34;q11.2) in patients treated with tyrosine kinase inhibitors. Cancer Genet. 2014;207(5):171–6.
106. Yamazaki H, Suzuki M, Otsuki A, Shimizu R, Bresnick EH, Engel JD, et al. A remote GATA2 hematopoietic enhancer drives leukemogenesis in inv(3)(q21;q26) by activating EVI1 expression. Cancer Cell. 2014;25(4):415–27.
107. Groschel S, Sanders MA, Hoogenboezem R, de Wit E, Bouwman BA, Erpelinck C, et al. A single oncogenic enhancer rearrangement causes concomitant EVI1 and GATA2 deregulation in leukemia. Cell. 2014;157(2):369–81.
108. Groschel S, Sanders MA, Hoogenboezem R, Zeilemaker A, Havermans M, Erpelinck C, et al. Mutational spectrum of myeloid malignancies with inv(3)/t(3;3) reveals a predominant involvement of RAS/RTK signaling pathways. Blood. 2015;125(1):133–9.
109. Wang W, Cortes JE, Tang G, Khoury JD, Wang S, Bueso-Ramos CE, et al. Risk stratification of chromosomal abnormalities in chronic myelogenous leukemia in the era of tyrosine kinase inhibitor therapy. Blood. 2016;127(22):2742–50.
110. Kovitz C, Kantarjian H, Garcia-Manero G, Abruzzo LV, Cortes J. Myelodysplastic syndromes and acute leukemia developing after imatinib mesylate therapy for chronic myeloid leukemia. Blood. 2006;108(8):2811–3.
111. Sill H, Goldman JM, Cross NC. Homozygous deletions of the p16 tumor-suppressor gene are associated with lymphoid transformation of chronic myeloid leukemia. Blood. 1995;85(8):2013–6.
112. Wang PY, Young F, Chen CY, Stevens BM, Neering SJ, Rossi RM, et al. The biologic properties of leukemias arising from BCR/ABL-mediated transformation vary as a function of developmental origin and activity of the p19ARF gene. Blood. 2008;112(10):4184–92.
113. Williams RT, den Besten W, Sherr CJ. Cytokine-dependent imatinib resistance in mouse BCR-ABL+, Arf-null lymphoblastic leukemia. Genes Dev. 2007;21(18):2283–7.
114. Wendel HG, de Stanchina E, Cepero E, Ray S, Emig M, Fridman JS, et al. Loss of p53 impedes the antileukemic response to BCR-ABL inhibition. Proc Natl Acad Sci U S A. 2006;103(19):7444–9.
115. Miething C, Grundler R, Mugler C, Brero S, Hoepfl J, Geigl J, et al. Retroviral insertional mutagenesis identifies RUNX genes involved in chronic myeloid leukemia disease persistence under imatinib treatment. Proc Natl Acad Sci U S A. 2007;104(11):4594–9.
116. Bueno MJ, Perez de Castro I, Gomez de Cedron M, Santos J, Calin GA, Cigudosa JC, et al. Genetic and epigenetic silencing of microRNA-203 enhances ABL1 and BCR-ABL1 oncogene expression. Cancer Cell. 2008;13(6):496–506.
117. Agirre X, Jimenez-Velasco A, San Jose-Eneriz E, Garate L, Bandres E, Cordeu L, et al. Down-regulation of hsa-miR-10a in chronic myeloid leukemia CD34+ cells increases USF2-mediated cell growth. Mol Cancer Res. 2008;6(12):1830–40.
118. Venturini L, Battmer K, Castoldi M, Schultheis B, Hochhaus A, Muckenthaler MU, et al. Expression of the miR-17-92 polycistron in chronic myeloid leukemia (CML) CD34+ cells. Blood. 2007;109(10):4399–405.
119. Viswanathan SR, Powers JT, Einhorn W, Hoshida Y, Ng TL, Toffanin S, et al. Lin28 promotes transformation and is associated with advanced human malignancies. Nat Genet. 2009;41(7):843–8.
120. Neviani P, Santhanam R, Trotta R, Notari M, Blaser BW, Liu S, et al. The tumor suppressor PP2A is functionally inactivated in blast crisis CML through the inhibitory activity of the BCR/ABL-regulated SET protein. Cancer Cell. 2005;8(5):355–68.
121. Kappos L, Antel J, Comi G, Montalban X, O'Connor P, Polman CH, et al. Oral fingolimod (FTY720) for relapsing multiple sclerosis. N Engl J Med. 2006;355(11):1124–40.
122. Neviani P, Santhanam R, Oaks JJ, Eiring AM, Notari M, Blaser BW, et al. FTY720, a new alternative for treating blast crisis chronic myelogenous leukemia and Philadelphia chromosome-positive acute lymphocytic leukemia. J Clin Invest. 2007;117(9):2408–21.
123. Bonnet D, Dick JE. Human acute myeloid leukemia is organized as a hierarchy that originates from a primitive hematopoietic cell. Nat Med. 1997;3(7):730–7.
124. Sirard C, Lapidot T, Vormoor J, Cashman JD, Doedens M, Murdoch B, et al. Normal and leukemic SCID-repopulating cells (SRC) coexist in the bone marrow and peripheral blood from CML patients in chronic phase, whereas leukemic SRC are detected in blast crisis. Blood. 1996;87(4):1539–48.
125. Holyoake T, Jiang X, Eaves C, Eaves A. Isolation of a highly quiescent subpopulation of primitive leukemic cells in chronic myeloid leukemia. Blood. 1999;94(6):2056–64.
126. Chu S, McDonald T, Lin A, Chakraborty S, Huang Q, Snyder DS, et al. Persistence of leukemia stem cells in chronic myelogenous leukemia patients in prolonged remission with imatinib treatment. Blood. 2011;118(20):5565–72.
127. Mahon FX, Rea D, Guilhot J, Guilhot F, Huguet F, Nicolini F, et al. Discontinuation of imatinib in patients with chronic myeloid leukaemia who have maintained complete molecular remission for at least 2 years: the prospective, multicentre Stop Imatinib (STIM) trial. Lancet Oncol. 2010;11(11):1029–35.
128. Neering SJ, Bushnell T, Sozer S, Ashton J, Rossi RM, Wang PY, et al. Leukemia stem cells in a genetically defined murine model of blast-crisis CML. Blood. 2007;110(7):2578–85.
129. Graham SM, Jorgensen HG, Allan E, Pearson C, Alcorn MJ, Richmond L, et al. Primitive, quiescent, Philadelphia-positive stem cells from patients with chronic myeloid leukemia are insensitive to STI571 in vitro. Blood. 2002;99(1):319–25.
130. Holtz MS, Forman SJ, Bhatia R. Nonproliferating CML CD34+ progenitors are resistant to apoptosis induced by a wide range of proapoptotic stimuli. Leukemia. 2005;19(6):1034–41.
131. Holtz MS, Slovak ML, Zhang F, Sawyers CL, Forman SJ, Bhatia R. Imatinib mesylate (STI571) inhibits growth of primitive malignant progenitors in chronic myelogenous leukemia through reversal of abnormally increased proliferation. Blood. 2002;99(10):3792–800.
132. Michor F, Hughes TP, Iwasa Y, Branford S, Shah NP, Sawyers CL, et al. Dynamics of chronic myeloid leukaemia. Nature. 2005;435(7046):1267–70.
133. Roeder I, Horn M, Glauche I, Hochhaus A, Mueller MC, Loeffler M. Dynamic modeling of imatinib-treated chronic myeloid leukemia: functional insights and clinical implications. Nat Med. 2006;12(10):1181–4.
134. Copland M, Hamilton A, Elrick LJ, Baird JW, Allan EK, Jordanides N, et al. Dasatinib (BMS-354825) targets an earlier progenitor population than imatinib in primary CML but does not eliminate the quiescent fraction. Blood. 2006;107(11):4532–9.
135. Jorgensen HG, Allan EK, Jordanides NE, Mountford JC, Holyoake TL. Nilotinib exerts equipotent antiproliferative effects to imatinib and does not induce apoptosis in CD34+ CML cells. Blood. 2007;109(9):4016–9.
136. Konig H, Holtz M, Modi H, Manley P, Holyoake TL, Forman SJ, et al. Enhanced BCR-ABL kinase inhibition does not result in increased inhibition of downstream signaling pathways or increased growth suppression in CML progenitors. Leukemia. 2008;22(4):748–55.

137. Barnes DJ, Palaiologou D, Panousopoulou E, Schultheis B, Yong AS, Wong A, et al. Bcr-Abl expression levels determine the rate of development of resistance to imatinib mesylate in chronic myeloid leukemia. Cancer Res. 2005;65(19):8912–9.
138. Jiang X, Saw KM, Eaves A, Eaves C. Instability of BCR-ABL gene in primary and cultured chronic myeloid leukemia stem cells. J Natl Cancer Inst. 2007;99(9):680–93.
139. Kumari A, Brendel C, Hochhaus A, Neubauer A, Burchert A. Low BCR-ABL expression levels in hematopoietic precursor cells enable persistence of chronic myeloid leukemia under imatinib. Blood. 2012;119(2):530–9.
140. Corbin AS, Agarwal A, Loriaux M, Cortes J, Deininger MW, Druker BJ. Human chronic myeloid leukemia stem cells are insensitive to imatinib despite inhibition of BCR-ABL activity. J Clin Invest. 2011;121(1):396–409.
141. Hamilton A, Helgason GV, Schemionek M, Zhang B, Myssina S, Allan EK, et al. Chronic myeloid leukemia stem cells are not dependent on Bcr-Abl kinase activity for their survival. Blood. 2012;119(6):1501–10.
142. Essers MA, Offner S, Blanco-Bose WE, Waibler Z, Kalinke U, Duchosal MA, et al. IFNalpha activates dormant haematopoietic stem cells in vivo. Nature. 2009;458(7240):904–8.
143. Passegue E, Ernst P. IFN-alpha wakes up sleeping hematopoietic stem cells. Nat Med. 2009;15(6):612–3.
144. Passegue E, Rafii S, Herlyn M. Cancer stem cells are everywhere. Nat Med. 2009;15(1):23.
145. Huntly BJ, Shigematsu H, Deguchi K, Lee BH, Mizuno S, Duclos N, et al. MOZ-TIF2, but not BCR-ABL, confers properties of leukemic stem cells to committed murine hematopoietic progenitors. Cancer Cell. 2004;6(6):587–96.
146. Evangelista M, Tian H, de Sauvage FJ. The hedgehog signaling pathway in cancer. Clin Cancer Res. 2006;12(20 Pt 1):5924–8.
147. Fogarty MP, Kessler JD, Wechsler-Reya RJ. Morphing into cancer: the role of developmental signaling pathways in brain tumor formation. J Neurobiol. 2005;64(4):458–75.
148. Gorlin RJ. Nevoid basal cell carcinoma syndrome. Dermatol Clin. 1995;13(1):113–25.
149. Byrd N, Becker S, Maye P, Narasimhaiah R, St-Jacques B, Zhang X, et al. Hedgehog is required for murine yolk sac angiogenesis. Development. 2002;129(2):361–72.
150. Dierks C, Beigi R, Guo GR, Zirlik K, Stegert MR, Manley P, et al. Expansion of Bcr-Abl-positive leukemic stem cells is dependent on Hedgehog pathway activation. Cancer Cell. 2008;14(3):238–49.
151. Trowbridge JJ, Scott MP, Bhatia M. Hedgehog modulates cell cycle regulators in stem cells to control hematopoietic regeneration. Proc Natl Acad Sci U S A. 2006;103(38):14134–9.
152. Zhao C, Chen A, Jamieson CH, Fereshteh M, Abrahamsson A, Blum J, et al. Hedgehog signalling is essential for maintenance of cancer stem cells in myeloid leukaemia. Nature. 2009;458(7239):776–9.
153. Yauch RL, Dijkgraaf GJ, Alicke B, Januario T, Ahn CP, Holcomb T, et al. Smoothened mutation confers resistance to a Hedgehog pathway inhibitor in medulloblastoma. Science. 2009;326(5952):572–4.
154. Ito K, Bernardi R, Morotti A, Matsuoka S, Saglio G, Ikeda Y, et al. PML targeting eradicates quiescent leukaemia-initiating cells. Nature. 2008;453(7198):1072–8.
155. Naka K, Hoshii T, Muraguchi T, Tadokoro Y, Ooshio T, Kondo Y, et al. TGF-beta-FOXO signalling maintains leukaemia-initiating cells in chronic myeloid leukaemia. Nature. 2010;463(7281):676–80.
156. Chen Y, Peng C, Abraham SA, Shan Y, Guo Z, Desouza N, et al. Arachidonate 15-lipoxygenase is required for chronic myeloid leukemia stem cell survival. J Clin Invest. 2014;124(9):3847–62.
157. Zhang H, Peng C, Hu Y, Li H, Sheng Z, Chen Y, et al. The Blk pathway functions as a tumor suppressor in chronic myeloid leukemia stem cells. Nat Genet. 2012;44(8):861–71.
158. Prost S, Relouzat F, Spentchian M, Ouzegdouh Y, Saliba J, Massonnet G, et al. Erosion of the chronic myeloid leukaemia stem cell pool by PPARgamma agonists. Nature. 2015;525(7569):380–3.
159. Hurtz C, Hatzi K, Cerchietti L, Braig M, Park E, Kim YM, et al. BCL6-mediated repression of p53 is critical for leukemia stem cell survival in chronic myeloid leukemia. J Exp Med. 2011;208(11):2163–74.
160. Gallipoli P, Cook A, Rhodes S, Hopcroft L, Wheadon H, Whetton AD, et al. JAK2/STAT5 inhibition by nilotinib with ruxolitinib contributes to the elimination of CML CD34+ cells in vitro and in vivo. Blood. 2014;124(9):1492–501.
161. Zhang B, Li L, Ho Y, Li M, Marcucci G, Tong W, et al. Heterogeneity of leukemia-initiating capacity of chronic myelogenous leukemia stem cells. J Clin Invest. 2016;126(3):975–91.
162. Li L, Wang L, Li L, Wang Z, Ho Y, McDonald T, et al. Activation of p53 by SIRT1 inhibition enhances elimination of CML leukemia stem cells in combination with imatinib. Cancer Cell. 2012;21(2):266–81.
163. Aljedai A, Buckle AM, Hiwarkar P, Syed F. Potential role of Notch signalling in CD34+ chronic myeloid leukaemia cells: cross-talk between Notch and BCR-ABL. PLoS One. 2015;10(4):e0123016.
164. Rizo A, Horton SJ, Olthof S, Dontje B, Ausema A, van Os R, et al. BMI1 collaborates with BCR-ABL in leukemic transformation of human CD34+ cells. Blood. 2010;116(22):4621–30.
165. Kobayashi CI, Takubo K, Kobayashi H, Nakamura-Ishizu A, Honda H, Kataoka K, et al. The IL-2/CD25 axis maintains distinct subsets of chronic myeloid leukemia-initiating cells. Blood. 2014;123(16):2540–9.
166. Bellodi C, Lidonnici MR, Hamilton A, Helgason GV, Soliera AR, Ronchetti M, et al. Targeting autophagy potentiates tyrosine kinase inhibitor-induced cell death in Philadelphia chromosome-positive cells, including primary CML stem cells. J Clin Invest. 2009;119(5):1109–23.
167. MacLean AL, Filippi S, Stumpf MP. The ecology in the hematopoietic stem cell niche determines the clinical outcome in chronic myeloid leukemia. Proc Natl Acad Sci U S A. 2014;111(10):3883–8.
168. Zhang B, Li M, McDonald T, Holyoake TL, Moon RT, Campana D, et al. Microenvironmental protection of CML stem and progenitor cells from tyrosine kinase inhibitors through N-cadherin and Wnt-beta-catenin signaling. Blood. 2013;121(10):1824–38.
169. Krause DS, Lazarides K, Lewis JB, von Andrian UH, Van Etten RA. Selectins and their ligands are required for homing and engraftment of BCR-ABL1+ leukemic stem cells in the bone marrow niche. Blood. 2014;123(9):1361–71.
170. Zhang J, Ren X, Shi W, Wang S, Chen H, Zhang B, et al. Small molecule Me6TREN mobilizes hematopoietic stem/progenitor cells by activating MMP-9 expression and disrupting SDF-1/CXCR4 axis. Blood. 2014;123(3):428–41.
171. Ng KP, Manjeri A, Lee KL, Huang W, Tan SY, Chuah CT, et al. Physiologic hypoxia promotes maintenance of CML stem cells despite effective BCR-ABL1 inhibition. Blood. 2014;123(21):3316–26.
172. Corbin AS, La Rosee P, Stoffregen EP, Druker BJ, Deininger MW. Several Bcr-Abl kinase domain mutants associated with imatinib mesylate resistance remain sensitive to imatinib. Blood. 2003;101(11):4611–4.
173. Gambacorti-Passerini CB, Gunby RH, Piazza R, Galietta A, Rostagno R, Scapozza L. Molecular mechanisms of resistance to imatinib in Philadelphia-chromosome-positive leukaemias. Lancet Oncol. 2003;4(2):75–85.
174. Gorre ME, Mohammed M, Ellwood K, Hsu N, Paquette R, Rao PN, et al. Clinical resistance to STI-571 cancer therapy caused by BCR-ABL gene mutation or amplification. Science. 2001;293(5531):876–80.

175. Hochhaus A, La Rosee P. Imatinib therapy in chronic myelogenous leukemia: strategies to avoid and overcome resistance. Leukemia. 2004;18(8):1321–31.
176. Lowenberg B. Minimal residual disease in chronic myeloid leukemia. N Engl J Med. 2003;349(15):1399–401.
177. Shah NP, Nicoll JM, Nagar B, Gorre ME, Paquette RL, Kuriyan J, et al. Multiple BCR-ABL kinase domain mutations confer polyclonal resistance to the tyrosine kinase inhibitor imatinib (STI571) in chronic phase and blast crisis chronic myeloid leukemia. Cancer Cell. 2002;2(2):117–25.
178. Schindler T, Bornmann W, Pellicena P, Miller WT, Clarkson B, Kuriyan J. Structural mechanism for STI 571 inhibition of abelson tyrosine kinase. Science. 2000;289(5486):1938–42.
179. Weisberg E, Manley PW, Breitenstein W, Bruggen J, Cowan-Jacob SW, Ray A, et al. Characterization of AMN107, a selective inhibitor of native and mutant Bcr-Abl. Cancer Cell. 2005;7(2):129–41.
180. Tokarski JS, Newitt JA, Chang CY, Cheng JD, Wittekind M, Kiefer SE, et al. The structure of Dasatinib (BMS-354825) bound to activated ABL kinase domain elucidates its inhibitory activity against imatinib-resistant ABL mutants. Cancer Res. 2006;66(11):5790–7.
181. Vajpai N, Strauss A, Fendrich G, Cowan-Jacob SW, Manley PW, Grzesiek S, et al. Solution conformations and dynamics of ABL kinase-inhibitor complexes determined by NMR substantiate the different binding modes of imatinib/nilotinib and dasatinib. J Biol Chem. 2008;283(26):18292–302.
182. Azam M, Latek RR, Daley GQ. Mechanisms of autoinhibition and STI-571/imatinib resistance revealed by mutagenesis of BCR-ABL. Cell. 2003;112(6):831–43.
183. Nagar B, Bornmann WG, Pellicena P, Schindler T, Veach DR, Miller WT, et al. Crystal structures of the kinase domain of c-Abl in complex with the small molecule inhibitors PD173955 and imatinib (STI-571). Cancer Res. 2002;62(15):4236–43.
184. Hochhaus A, Kreil S, Corbin AS, La Rosee P, Muller MC, Lahaye T, et al. Molecular and chromosomal mechanisms of resistance to imatinib (STI571) therapy. Leukemia. 2002;16(11):2190–6.
185. Carter TA, Wodicka LM, Shah NP, Velasco AM, Fabian MA, Treiber DK, et al. Inhibition of drug-resistant mutants of ABL, KIT, and EGF receptor kinases. Proc Natl Acad Sci U S A. 2005;102(31):11011–6.
186. Deininger M, Buchdunger E, Druker BJ. The development of imatinib as a therapeutic agent for chronic myeloid leukemia. Blood. 2005;105(7):2640–53.
187. O'Hare T, Walters DK, Stoffregen EP, Jia T, Manley PW, Mestan J, et al. In vitro activity of Bcr-Abl inhibitors AMN107 and BMS-354825 against clinically relevant imatinib-resistant Abl kinase domain mutants. Cancer Res. 2005;65(11):4500–5.
188. Branford S, Rudzki Z, Walsh S, Parkinson I, Grigg A, Szer J, et al. Detection of BCR-ABL mutations in patients with CML treated with imatinib is virtually always accompanied by clinical resistance, and mutations in the ATP phosphate-binding loop (P-loop) are associated with a poor prognosis. Blood. 2003;102(1):276–83.
189. Soverini S, Martinelli G, Rosti G, Bassi S, Amabile M, Poerio A, et al. ABL mutations in late chronic phase chronic myeloid leukemia patients with up-front cytogenetic resistance to imatinib are associated with a greater likelihood of progression to blast crisis and shorter survival: a study by the GIMEMA Working Party on Chronic Myeloid Leukemia. J Clin Oncol. 2005;23(18):4100–9.
190. Jabbour E, Kantarjian H, Jones D, Talpaz M, Bekele N, O'Brien S, et al. Frequency and clinical significance of BCR-ABL mutations in patients with chronic myeloid leukemia treated with imatinib mesylate. Leukemia. 2006;20(10):1767–73.
191. Griswold IJ, MacPartlin M, Bumm T, Goss VL, O'Hare T, Lee KA, et al. Kinase domain mutants of Bcr-Abl exhibit altered transformation potency, kinase activity, and substrate utilization, irrespective of sensitivity to imatinib. Mol Cell Biol. 2006;26(16):6082–93.
192. Skaggs BJ, Gorre ME, Ryvkin A, Burgess MR, Xie Y, Han Y, et al. Phosphorylation of the ATP-binding loop directs oncogenicity of drug-resistant BCR-ABL mutants. Proc Natl Acad Sci U S A. 2006;103(51):19466–71.
193. Azam M, Seeliger MA, Gray NS, Kuriyan J, Daley GQ. Activation of tyrosine kinases by mutation of the gatekeeper threonine. Nat Struct Mol Biol. 2008;15(10):1109–18.
194. Kantarjian H, Giles F, Wunderle L, Bhalla K, O'Brien S, Wassmann B, et al. Nilotinib in imatinib-resistant CML and Philadelphia chromosome-positive ALL. N Engl J Med. 2006;354(24):2542–51.
195. Lombardo LJ, Lee FY, Chen P, Norris D, Barrish JC, Behnia K, et al. Discovery of N-(2-chloro-6-methyl- phenyl)-2-(6-(4-(2-hydroxyethyl)- piperazin-1-yl)-2-methylpyrimidin-4- ylamino) thiazole-5-carboxamide (BMS-354825), a dual Src/Abl kinase inhibitor with potent antitumor activity in preclinical assays. J Med Chem. 2004;47(27):6658–61.
196. Shah NP, Tran C, Lee FY, Chen P, Norris D, Sawyers CL. Overriding imatinib resistance with a novel ABL kinase inhibitor. Science. 2004;305(5682):399–401.
197. Talpaz M, Shah NP, Kantarjian H, Donato N, Nicoll J, Paquette R, et al. Dasatinib in imatinib-resistant Philadelphia chromosome-positive leukemias. N Engl J Med. 2006;354(24):2531–41.
198. Cortes J, Jabbour E, Kantarjian H, Yin CC, Shan J, O'Brien S, et al. Dynamics of BCR-ABL kinase domain mutations in chronic myeloid leukemia after sequential treatment with multiple tyrosine kinase inhibitors. Blood. 2007;110(12):4005–11.
199. O'Hare T, Shakespeare WC, Zhu X, Eide CA, Rivera VM, Wang F, et al. AP24534, a pan-BCR-ABL inhibitor for chronic myeloid leukemia, potently inhibits the T315I mutant and overcomes mutation-based resistance. Cancer Cell. 2009;16(5):401–12.
200. Cortes JE, Kim DW, Pinilla-Ibarz J, le Coutre P, Paquette R, Chuah C, et al. A phase 2 trial of ponatinib in Philadelphia chromosome-positive leukemias. N Engl J Med. 2013;369(19):1783–96.
201. Soverini S, Martinelli G, Colarossi S, Gnani A, Castagnetti F, Rosti G, et al. Presence or the emergence of a F317L BCR-ABL mutation may be associated with resistance to dasatinib in Philadelphia chromosome-positive leukemia. J Clin Oncol. 2006;24(33):e51–2.
202. Apperley JF. Part I: mechanisms of resistance to imatinib in chronic myeloid leukaemia. Lancet Oncol. 2007;8(11):1018–29.
203. Weisberg E, Manley PW, Cowan-Jacob SW, Hochhaus A, Griffin JD. Second generation inhibitors of BCR-ABL for the treatment of imatinib-resistant chronic myeloid leukaemia. Nat Rev Cancer. 2007;7(5):345–56.
204. Gibbons DL, Pricl S, Posocco P, Laurini E, Fermeglia M, Sun H, et al. Molecular dynamics reveal BCR-ABL1 polymutants as a unique mechanism of resistance to PAN-BCR-ABL1 kinase inhibitor therapy. Proc Natl Acad Sci U S A. 2014;111(9):3550–5.
205. Zabriskie MS, Eide CA, Tantravahi SK, Vellore NA, Estrada J, Nicolini FE, et al. BCR-ABL1 compound mutations combining key kinase domain positions confer clinical resistance to ponatinib in Ph chromosome-positive leukemia. Cancer Cell. 2014;26(3):428–42.
206. Shah NP, Skaggs BJ, Branford S, Hughes TP, Nicoll JM, Paquette RL, et al. Sequential ABL kinase inhibitor therapy selects for compound drug-resistant BCR-ABL mutations with altered oncogenic potency. J Clin Invest. 2007;117(9):2562–9.
207. Khorashad JS, Kelley TW, Szankasi P, Mason CC, Soverini S, Adrian LT, et al. BCR-ABL1 compound mutations in tyrosine kinase inhibitor-resistant CML: frequency and clonal relationships. Blood. 2013;121(3):489–98.
208. Soverini S, De Benedittis C, Machova Polakova K, Brouckova A, Horner D, Iacono M, et al. Unraveling the complexity of tyrosine kinase inhibitor-resistant populations by ultra-deep sequencing of the BCR-ABL kinase domain. Blood. 2013;122(9):1634–48.

209. Liu J, Joha S, Idziorek T, Corm S, Hetuin D, Philippe N, et al. BCR-ABL mutants spread resistance to non-mutated cells through a paracrine mechanism. Leukemia. 2008;22(4):791–9.
210. Zhang J, Adrian FJ, Jahnke W, Cowan-Jacob SW, Li AG, Iacob RE, et al. Targeting Bcr-Abl by combining allosteric with ATP-binding-site inhibitors. Nature. 2010;463(7280):501–6.
211. Eiring AM, Page BD, Kraft IL, Mason CC, Vellore NA, Resetca D, et al. Combined STAT3 and BCR-ABL1 inhibition induces synthetic lethality in therapy-resistant chronic myeloid leukemia. Leukemia. 2015;29(3):586–97.
212. Warsch W, Kollmann K, Eckelhart E, Fajmann S, Cerny-Reiterer S, Holbl A, et al. High STAT5 levels mediate imatinib resistance and indicate disease progression in chronic myeloid leukemia. Blood. 2011;117(12):3409–20.
213. Aceves-Luquero CI, Agarwal A, Callejas-Valera JL, Arias-Gonzalez L, Esparis-Ogando A, del Peso OL, et al. ERK2, but not ERK1, mediates acquired and "de novo" resistance to imatinib mesylate: implication for CML therapy. PLoS One. 2009;4(7):e6124.
214. Burchert A, Wang Y, Cai D, von Bubnoff N, Paschka P, Muller-Brusselbach S, et al. Compensatory PI3-kinase/Akt/mTor activation regulates imatinib resistance development. Leukemia. 2005;19(10):1774–82.
215. Gioia R, Leroy C, Drullion C, Lagarde V, Etienne G, Dulucq S, et al. Quantitative phosphoproteomics revealed interplay between Syk and Lyn in the resistance to nilotinib in chronic myeloid leukemia cells. Blood. 2011;118(8):2211–21.
216. Khorashad JS, Eiring AM, Mason CC, Gantz KC, Bowler AD, Redwine HM, et al. shRNA library screening identifies nucleocytoplasmic transport as a mediator of BCR-ABL1 kinase-independent resistance. Blood. 2015;125(11):1772–81.
217. Walker CJ, Oaks JJ, Santhanam R, Neviani P, Harb JG, Ferenchak G, et al. Preclinical and clinical efficacy of XPO1/CRM1 inhibition by the karyopherin inhibitor KPT-330 in Ph+ leukemias. Blood. 2013;122(17):3034–44.
218. Ma L, Shan Y, Bai R, Xue L, Eide CA, Ou J, et al. A therapeutically targetable mechanism of BCR-ABL-independent imatinib resistance in chronic myeloid leukemia. Sci Transl Med. 2014;6(252):252ra121.
219. Wang Y, Cai D, Brendel C, Barett C, Erben P, Manley PW, et al. Adaptive secretion of granulocyte-macrophage colony-stimulating factor (GM-CSF) mediates imatinib and nilotinib resistance in BCR/ABL+ progenitors via JAK-2/STAT-5 pathway activation. Blood. 2007;109(5):2147–55.
220. White DL, Saunders VA, Dang P, Engler J, Zannettino AC, Cambareri AC, et al. OCT-1-mediated influx is a key determinant of the intracellular uptake of imatinib but not nilotinib (AMN107): reduced OCT-1 activity is the cause of low in vitro sensitivity to imatinib. Blood. 2006;108(2):697–704.
221. White DL, Dang P, Engler J, Frede A, Zrim S, Osborn M, et al. Functional activity of the OCT-1 protein is predictive of long-term outcome in patients with chronic-phase chronic myeloid leukemia treated with imatinib. J Clin Oncol. 2010;28(16):2761–7.
222. Agrawal M, Hanfstein B, Erben P, Wolf D, Ernst T, Fabarius A, et al. MDR1 expression predicts outcome of Ph+ chronic phase CML patients on second-line nilotinib therapy after imatinib failure. Leukemia. 2014;28(7):1478–85.

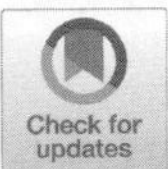

5 Diagnosis and Treatment of Chronic Myeloid Leukemia

Charles A. Schiffer

Introduction

The original recognition of leukemia in the nineteenth century and the story of our progressive understanding of the biology and the development of treatment of chronic myeloid leukemia (CML) have been well reviewed in recent years [1–3]. Today, the diagnosis of CML usually presents few problems. In contrast, planning a therapeutic strategy for a patient who presents in chronic phase and monitoring a patient who starts treatment with a tyrosine kinase inhibitor (TKI) present a number of challenges. The same is true for a patient in chronic phase whose disease proves resistant to initial treatment with a TKI. Even more difficult may be the issue of how best to treat a patient presenting in or progressing to an advanced phase of CML. In this chapter, we review some of the essentials of diagnosis of CML with the main focus on the results of available treatment options and guidance on therapeutic strategy.

Diagnosis

Definition, Diagnostic Criteria, and Differential Diagnosis

CML is a clonal myeloproliferative expansion of transformed primitive hematopoietic progenitor cells involving myeloid, monocytic, erythroid, megakaryocytic, B-lymphoid, and occasionally T-lymphoid lineages [4]. Since 1960 when Nowell and Hungerford [5] described the specific karyotypic abnormality, a G group chromosomal abnormality that came to be known as the Philadelphia (Ph[1] or Ph) chromosome, there has been rapid progress in our understanding of the pathogenesis of the leukemia, providing us with the means to easily diagnose and monitor the disease. Subsequent studies further characterized the Ph to be the result of a balanced translocation between chromosomes 9 and 22 (t(9;22)(q34;q11)) [6]. A series of subsequent studies demonstrated that this resulted in a fusion gene involving the *BCR* (breakpoint cluster region) gene from chromosome 22 and the Abelson cellular oncogene, *ABL* from chromosome 9, which produces a chimeric protein which is responsible for the constitutive proliferation of myeloid cells [9]. Mice transfected with the *BCR-ABL1* fusion gene develop a myeloproliferative disorder resembling human CML or other Ph1 acute leukemias [1, 7–9].

The detection of the BCR-ABL1 fusion gene is the pathognomonic feature of almost all cases of CML. A few conditions demonstrate overlapping clinical features, the most common being a "leukemoid reaction" which occurs usually in response to severe infection. In contrast, however, the presence of splenomegaly and a low leukocyte alkaline phosphatase score (a test which is no longer performed routinely) suggest a diagnosis of CML. The presence of the characteristic Ph chromosome will allow the distinction of CML from disorders such as primary proliferative polycythemia, idiopathic myelofibrosis, and primary thrombocythemia, which can occasionally have a somewhat overlapping clinical presentation. The identification of *BCR-ABL1* in a peripheral blood sample by reverse transcriptase-polymerase chain reaction (RT-PCR) techniques or by fluorescence in situ hybridization (FISH) will give the definitive answer, though approximately 5% of patients with a blood picture resembling CML are negative for the Ph chromosome by cytogenetics [10, 11].

Among such Ph-negative patients, there is a preponderance of males and older patients, with lower leukocyte counts and thrombocytopenia being more typical of this subgroup. Of those patients who lack a Ph chromosome, about half are also *BCR-ABL1* negative; they are sometimes designated as "atypical CML" and their prognosis is poorer than that of patients with *BCR-ABL1*-positive leukemia

C.A. Schiffer, M.D.
Department of Oncology, Karmanos Cancer Institute, Wayne State University School of Medicine, 4100 John R., HWCR 4th Floor, Detroit, MI 48201, USA
e-mail: schiffer@karmanos.org

P.H. Wiernik et al. (eds.), *Neoplastic Diseases of the Blood*, DOI 10.1007/978-3-319-64263-5_5

[10]. The other half have cryptic *BCR-ABL1* fusion gene on a normal-appearing chromosome 22 and such patients are usually designated Ph-negative, *BCR-ABL1*-positive CML. Their clinical features and response to treatment with TKIs differ little, if at all, from those of patients with a Ph chromosome. Specific mention should also be made of those patients who appear to have primary thrombocythemia but with a Ph chromosome and a *BCR-ABL1* gene. Such patients should be considered to have CML and should be managed as if they had classic CML. It is therefore recommended that all patients with apparent primary thrombocytosis should be tested for the Ph translocation and/or *BCR-ABL1* by RT-PCR.

Evaluation of a Suspected Case of CML

The specifics of the investigation of a newly presenting patient with CML are detailed in Table 5.1. In the presenting history, it is helpful to ask about certain features, such as the presence of night sweats or bone pain, as they may indicate transforming disease. Symptoms suggestive of hyperviscosity such as headaches, confusion, and visual disturbances are important to identify, but occur infrequently even in patients with very elevated WBC. It may be helpful to determine exposure to potential mutagens, especially high levels of ionizing irradiation, although it is very unusual for CML to develop as a "secondary" leukemia. There was a transient increase in the incidence of CML in Japanese survivors in the first decade after the atomic bomb exposure [12–14], but it is not clear that irradiation in the doses used for therapy of other cancers results in CML. Examination should particularly focus on retinal examination and lymph node areas, and include documenting the size of the spleen and liver. It is important to reassure the patient and family that the disease is not inherited, and to establish whether the patient has any siblings and hence potential for allografting.

Table 5.1 Investigations to be performed in suspected cases of CML

• CBC with differential and review of blood film
• Biochemistry screen including uric acid
• Bone marrow aspirate and trephine biopsy for:
Morphology (assess cellularity and degree of fibrosis on biopsy) • Cytogenetics (fluorescent in situ hybridization [FISH] if metaphase cultures fail) • Sample for immunophenotyping (process only if blast crisis is evident morphologically; not necessary if typical chronic phase) • Samples stored for research purposes if appropriate locally or for mailing to research group • RT-PCR if not available from peripheral blood (needed to define breakpoint for future monitoring)
Consider CMV serology and HLA type patient and siblings if allograft is being considered

A complete blood count and film review are critical in establishing the prognostic score (discussed later), and the number of blasts, basophils, and eosinophils should be calculated for this purpose. Immunophenotyping is only relevant to classify blast crisis. The trephine biopsy should be assessed for cellularity and the degree of fibrosis. Complete karyotypic analysis is necessary to assess for the presence of additional cytogenetic abnormalities in the Ph clone since FISH and RT-PCR will not detect abnormalities on chromosomes other than 9 and 22. It should be noted that all of these studies, save the assessment of marrow fibrosis, can be done on peripheral blood, since, because of the presence of circulating immature elements, chromosome analysis can generally be done successfully. Hence, some clinicians forego bone marrow evaluation in patients with typical, early-stage disease.

Clinical Presentation and Phases of Disease

Savage et al. [15] described a series of 430 consecutive cases presenting to one center for consideration of allogeneic transplant and these data are the first description of the presenting features of such a large group of CML patients in the modern era (Table 5.2). Approximately 20% of the patients were diagnosed when a blood sample was taken for other reasons. It is likely a higher fraction of people in developed countries are currently diagnosed "incidentally" given the increased use of "routine" screening blood tests. Some cases were diagnosed during pregnancy, while donating blood, or undergoing routine surgery.

Of those presenting with symptoms, the 10 most commonly recorded are shown in Table 5.2. In retrospect, patients may describe fatigue, weakness, or a sense of fullness in the left upper quadrant with early satiety after meals. Other symptoms including visual disturbance, weakness, arthralgia, cough, malaise, dizziness, nausea/vomiting, ankle edema, priapism, and mental changes occurred in less than 5% of the cases. Thrombocytosis with a count above 1×10^{12}/L was found in 25% of cases, although there did not appear to be any correlation between abnormal bleeding and the level of thrombocytosis. Splenomegaly and purpura were the most common physical signs at presentation, at 75% and 16%, respectively.

Ninety-three percent of the patients presented in chronic phase, i.e., with fewer than 5% blasts in the bone marrow. It is sometimes difficult, particularly if the marrow or blood smear staining is not done well, to confuse younger myeloid elements with true blasts, and it is not unusual to have the appearance of a somewhat higher percentage of blasts at presentation, although it eventually becomes clear that the

Table 5.2 Clinical presentation of 430 patients referred to the Hammersmith Hospital for consideration of transplantation from 1981 [15]

• 80% of the patients were symptomatic at the time of presentation, although most symptoms were mild to moderate in severity	
• 20% of the patients had the diagnosis of CML made incidentally on routine CBC	
• 93% of the patients presented with chronic-phase disease	
• Thrombosis and leukostasis were rare even with very high platelet/white blood cell counts	
Median CBC values (range):	
WBC	174 (5.0–850.0) × 10^9/L
Hemoglobin	10.3 (4.9–16.6) g/dL
Platelets	430 (17–3182) × 10^9/L
• 19% of the patients presented with a WBC >350 × 10^9/L	
• 25% of the patients presented with platelets >1 × 10^{12}/L	
Most common symptoms at presentation	
Fatigue and lethargy	33%
Weight loss	20%
Abdominal mass or fullness	15%
Bone pain	7%
Headache	6%
Bleeding	21%
Splenic discomfort	19%
Sweats	15%
Infection	6%
Dyspnea	~5%
Most common findings on physical examination	
Spleen palpable	75%
1–10 cm	37%
>10 cm	39%
Purpura	16%
Palpable liver	2%

The median age of 34 years was somewhat younger than CML in general because these were patients referred for transplantation

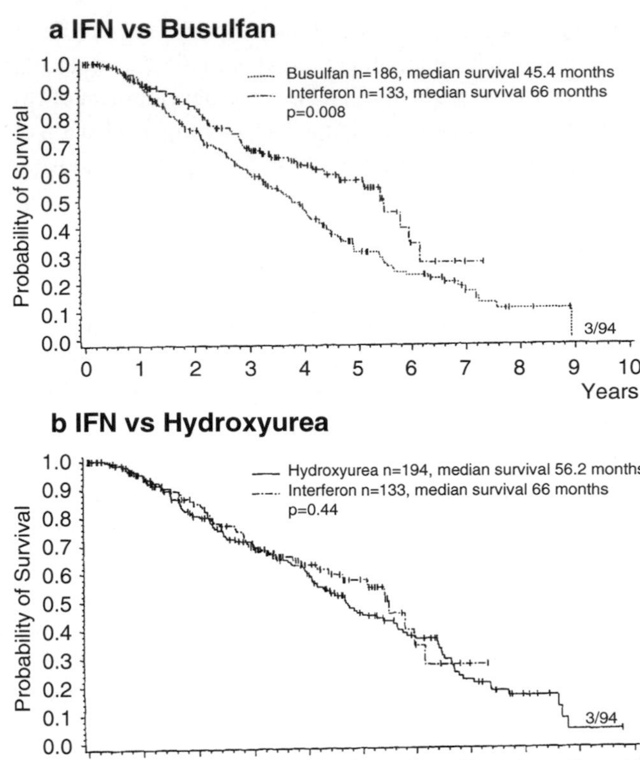

Fig. 5.1 These survival curves demonstrate the inexorable rate of death due to blastic transformation in patients not undergoing allogeneic transplantation in the pre-TKI era. Reprinted with permission [43]

patient was truly in chronic phase after observing the response to treatment.

Before the introduction of tyrosine kinase inhibitors (TKI), the duration of chronic phase was usually between 3 and 8 years (median 4–5 years in most series), although exceptions occurred, with some patients evolving rapidly to blast crisis, whereas others did not progress for 15 or more years (Fig. 5.1). In the past, the disease inevitably progressed from this "benign" chronic stage to the accelerated phase and ultimately to a fatal blast crisis. The situation is now very different. Patients who respond to treatment with a TKI and achieve a complete cytogenetic response (CCyR) may maintain this response for many years and possibly indefinitely, provided that they continue to take a TKI on a regular basis. Thus, the progression from chronic phase to advanced phase that seemed in the past to be inevitable now appears to be preventable.

Table 5.3 Criteria used in defining phases of disease in CML

WHO criteria for accelerated phase 2016 [17]
• >10–19% blasts in blood or marrow
Persistent or increasing WBC (>10 × 10^9/L), unresponsive to therapy
• >20% basophils in blood
• Thrombocytopenia (<100 × 10^9/L) unrelated to therapy
• Persistent thrombocytosis (>1000 × 10^9/L) unresponsive to therapy

Accelerated Phase

The definition of *accelerated phase* is vague, and different criteria have been used in the past by different groups [16]. A recent definition proposed by the World Health Organization [17] is summarized in Table 5.3, with anemia, increasing basophils or eosinophils, thrombocytopenia (or occasionally thrombocytosis), or increasing proportion of blasts being the most common findings. Clinical features suggesting "acceleration" supplement these laboratory findings and commonly include fever, night sweats, weight loss, bone pain, increasing splenomegaly despite therapy, and development of extramedullary disease (chloromas).

Failure to achieve a hematologic response to initial therapy with a TKI, hematological, cytogenetic, or molecular resistance to two sequential TKIs, or the development of two mutations in BCR-ABL1 during TKI therapy, is also a worrisome feature, in the absence of the findings listed above.

Blast Phase

The definition of *blastic transformation* (also referred to as blast phase or blast crisis) is based on the presence of more than 20% blasts in the peripheral blood or bone marrow, or the demonstration of extramedullary infiltration by blast cells. In two-thirds of the cases, the blasts are myeloid with one-third of B-lymphoid lineage. The blasts are often undifferentiated morphologically and immunophenotyping is therefore recommended in all cases. Transformation to lymphoid blast crisis can occur suddenly, sometimes even early in the course of chronic phase, and carries a marginally better prognosis than myeloid transformation. Both are usually fatal despite intensive treatment and have a median survival from diagnosis of blast crisis of only 3–6 months, unless remission can be achieved and followed by allogeneic transplantation.

It can be difficult to distinguish patients presenting initially with Ph-positive acute myeloid leukemia (AML) or acute lymphoblastic leukemia (ALL) from those with blast crisis of CML. For patients with Ph + ALL, the presence of significant splenomegaly is more in keeping with preexisting, undiagnosed CML, whereas the presence of $p190^{BCR\text{-}ABL1}$ suggests de novo ALL while $p210^{BCR\text{-}ABL1}$ might suggest preexisting CML. It is possible, in both children and adults with CML, to develop blast transformation with mixed lineages, i.e., both lymphoid and myeloid surface markers detectable on the same cells [18] or distinct subpopulations of blasts with either lymphoid or myeloid characteristics [19]. T-lymphoid blast transformation is rare, but there are several cases showing both the *BCR-ABL1* fusion gene and T-cell receptor (TCR) gene rearrangements [20].

Cytogenetic and molecular changes are well recognized in 50–80% of the patients during transformation to accelerated or blast phase. So-called minor cytogenetic changes include monosomies of chromosomes 7 and 17, loss of the Y chromosome, and trisomies of chromosomes 17 and 21 [21]. Major cytogenetic changes, which suggest a more aggressive clinical course, include a double-Ph chromosome, trisomy 8, isochromosome i(17q), trisomy 19, and translocations of chromosome 3 with chromosome 21, t(3;21)(q26;q22) [22–24]. Alterations of the p53 gene on the long arm of chromosome 17 by deletion, rearrangement, or mutation, occurring predominantly with myeloid blast crisis, have been identified in up to 30% of CML patients entering the blast phase [25, 26]. Even before clinical manifestations, it is sometimes possible to detect these cytogenetic changes in the bone marrow, extramedullary masses, or splenectomy specimens [27].

Clinical signs of blastic transformation may be due to the rapid increase in blasts in the peripheral blood. The most significant areas compromised are the cerebral and respiratory circulations, resulting in multifocal bleeding, dyspnea, and hypoxemia [28]. Tumors due to the deposition of blast cells, known as chloromas or granulocytic sarcomas, may be visible before the detection of blasts in the peripheral blood. It is important to distinguish such tumors from undifferentiated carcinomas and diffuse large-cell non-Hodgkin's lymphoma, which may require immunohistochemical staining. Commonly, the tumors are detected in lymph nodes, cutaneous tissue, or as lucent bone deposits on X-ray. Meningeal deposition may result in cord compression or a variety of neurologic symptoms [29].

Prognostic Scores

Prognostic models aim to categorize patients into different risk groups at diagnosis. These scores all require examination of the first blood film made on the newly diagnosed patient, and the subsequent loss of this blood film is the most common reason for an incomplete score. Prognostic scores have traditionally been utilized in the context of analyzing large clinical trials and thus they should be applied to the individual patient with some caution. Small variations in the parameters described can make a significant difference to the final score; accurate determination of these blood values is therefore crucial. Older scores were proposed by Tura et al. [30], and subsequently in 1982 by Cervantes and Rozman [31]. More contemporary systems are described in Table 5.4. It should be noted that the outcomes for the Sokal and Hasford scores evaluated patients in the pre-TKI era whereas the EUTOS score included 2060 patients treated with imatinib between 2002 and 2006.

Gratwohl et al. [35] devised a simple scoring system based on five main factors following analysis of 3142 patients who had undergone allogeneic stem cell transplantation for CML between 1989 and 1997. The combined score for these factors (donor/recipient histocompatibility, stage of disease, patient and donor age and sex, and time from diagnosis) in an individual patient predicted the probability of survival after allografting and was helpful in the counseling of patients. Although many of these factors are probably still relevant, it is difficult to use this formula with precision now, given the major improvements in transplant methodology which have decreased transplant-related mortality, as well as possible improved outlook in patients treated predominantly with TKIs.

Table 5.4 Prognostic scores commonly used in CML

Sokal score (1984) [32]
• Criteria required at presentation (prior to treatment): 1. Age 2. Spleen size (cm below costal margin measured clinically with a tape) 3. Platelet count prior to any treatment 4. Blast percentage in peripheral blood (preferably 500 cells counted, but at least 200)
• Formula: Exp[0.0116(age—43.4) + 0.0345(spleen—7.51) + 0.188 (platelets/700) 2—0.563) + 0.0887 (% blasts—2.1)] Good prognosis <0.8 Moderate prognosis 0.8–1.2 Poor prognosis >1.2
Hasford (Euro) score (1998) [33]
• Data analyzed on 1573 patients
• Criteria required at presentation (prior to treatment): Same as Sokal score with the addition of: – Eosinophil percentage in peripheral blood (same no. of cells counted) – Basophil percentage in peripheral blood (same no. of cells counted)
• Formula: (0.6666 × age [0 when <50 years; otherwise 1]) +0.0420 × spleen size [cm from costal margin] +1.0956 × platelet count [0 when platelets <1500; otherwise 1] +0.0584 × blasts [%] +0.0413 × eosinophils [%] +0.2039 × basophils [0 when basophils <3%; otherwise 1] multiplied by 1000 Low risk ≤780—median survival 100 months Intermediate risk >780 < 1480—median survival 69 months High risk >1480—median survival 45 months
EUTOS score [34]
• Formula: (7 × basophil [%]) + (4 × spleen [cm]) Low risk <87 (79% of patients) High risk ≥87 (21% Of patients)

An online calculator for the most commonly used scores is available at http://bloodref.com/myeloid/cml/sokal-hasford

Treatment

The introduction of the tyrosine kinase inhibitors in 1998 fundamentally changed the treatment of CML. Until that time it has been widely accepted that an allogeneic stem cell transplant, if the patient had a suitable donor and if the procedure was successful, could cure CML, whereas other therapies were essentially palliative and would modestly prolong life, if at all. Early studies with imatinib mesylate, the original TKI, showed that it could reduce Ph-negative hematopoiesis in patients shown previously to be resistant to interferon-alpha [36], and subsequent studies demonstrated that it had the capacity to induce durable CCyR in 60% or more of the patients presenting in chronic phase. It is now widely accepted that CML presenting in chronic phase should be treated initially with a TKI. The choice of which TKI to use is still a matter of discussion, as described below. Treatment decisions for patients presenting in advanced phases of CML are more difficult.

Immediate Management of Newly Diagnosed Patients

The immediate management of a newly presenting patient with possible CML involves the initial history taking and investigations described in the previous sections. The next step is to control any immediate life-threatening complications such as leukostasis, hemorrhage, or infection, before appropriate antileukemic chemotherapy. Tumor lysis syndrome is relatively rare in patients in chronic phase, but nonetheless, it is prudent to commence allopurinol 300 mg daily and encourage plentiful oral fluid intake. Once the leukocyte count has been reduced below 30×10^9/L, allopurinol should no longer be required unless the patient has a history of gout or continues to be hyperuricemic. On some occasions it may be necessary to reduce the leukocyte load more urgently, especially if there is evidence of leukostasis causing the clinical manifestations previously described. This may be achieved by the temporary use of large doses of hydroxyurea, on the order of 3–6 g daily, and/or by leukapheresis. Leukapheresis may also be considered as a useful temporizing treatment during pregnancy [37, 38].

Prior to the initiation of antileukemic therapy, it is important to discuss and document the implications for future fertility with the patient and possibly his or her partner. It is possible to arrange cryopreservation of spermatocytes and sometimes oocytes, and this is preferably done in liaison with a center specializing in fertility medicine. Although unusual, if blood products are required, CMV-negative products should be administered until the CMV status is available.

Historically, before the development of TKIs, patients were treated with either hydroxyurea or busulfan, both for initial cytoreductions and for long-term control. Although generally well tolerated, therapy was palliative, and neither drug was able to reduce or eliminate the Ph clone and neither changed the inexorable evolution to blast crisis (Fig. 5.1). Hence, all suitable patients were considered for allogeneic transplantation. Trials with interferon-alpha, alone or in combination, were initiated in the early 1980s. The results with these older therapy will be reviewed briefly before detailed discussion of treatment with TKIs, initially studied in the late 1990s and widely available a few years later.

Hydroxyurea (Hydroxycarbamide)/Busulfan (Myleran)

Hydroxyurea, in doses of 2–3 g/day, may be given for a few days or weeks if a TKI is not immediately available [39, 40]. The dose is decreased as the WBC declines. Since its introduction in 1972 and until 2000, hydroxyurea was the "workhorse" therapy for CML. It is highly effective in controlling the hematological abnormalities of this disorder but does not produce any useful cytogenetic responses, even at high dose [40]. It has the advantage of relatively few side effects but has to be given continuously. Busulfan was also used by many clinicians and had the potential advantage that it could be given intermittently. A randomized comparison suggested an advantage for hydroxyurea [41].

Interferon-Alpha

Since the first reports of its activity in CML in 1983 [42], interferon-alpha has been widely investigated both as a single agent and in combination [43] (Fig. 5.1). There are no convincing data that there were significant differences between Roferon (Roche) and Intron A (Schering Plough). Both products are available in a pen device similar to those used for delivering insulin and a pegylated version which can be given weekly is now available. The precise mechanism of action is unclear although many possible mechanisms have been proposed [44, 45].

A meta-analysis by the CML Trialists' Collaborative Group of seven randomized trials [46, 47] demonstrated a statistically significant survival advantage of IFN (57% at 5 years) over either hydroxyurea or busulfan (42% at 5 years). The initial adverse effects of IFN administered daily include fevers, chills, malaise, arthralgia, and myalgia, sometimes summarized as "flu-like," whereas chronic toxicities include autoimmune-type phenomena, hypothyroidism, Raynaud's phenomenon, connective tissue disorder, and neuropsychiatric disorders. Patients commonly feel very tired and depressed. Elevations of liver enzymes and triglycerides are common.

Interferon in combination with cytarabine has been evaluated in a number of studies. Guilhot et al. reported data from a multicenter randomized trial comparing IFN+ low-dose cytarabine with IFN alone [48]. They reported a significant increase in the rate of major cytogenetic response (41% vs. 24%) and improved survival (85.7% vs. 79.1% at 3 years) in chronic-phase CML patients treated with the combination. The rate of CCyR was low. The main problem was discontinuation of the combined therapy due to side effects. Other investigators have also demonstrated the efficacy of this regimen [49], but other studies have failed to confirm a survival advantage. Interestingly, although most cytogenetic responses were partial, a small fraction of interferon-treated patients achieved persistent complete cytogenetic responses. This combination served as the control arm in the IRIS study which evaluated the benefit of imatinib as initial treatment in chronic phase [50].

Imatinib Mesylate for CML in Chronic Phase

The tyrosine kinase activity of the *BCR-ABL1* oncogene is required for malignant transformation of hematopoietic cells in CML [9, 51, 52]. Imatinib mesylate is a 2′-phenylaminopyrimidine compound designed to inhibit the binding of phosphate donor ATP to the kinase domain (SH1) of the protein. This activity prevents the downstream phosphorylation of the signal transduction proteins involved in leukemogenesis [51, 53–56]. Imatinib inhibits *BCR-ABL1*, *TEL-ABL*, and *ABL* kinase activity and inhibits growth and viability of cells transformed by any of these *ABL* oncogenes. In addition, it was found to inhibit other tyrosine kinases encoded by *PDGF-R* and *c-KIT* as well as cells expressing the p210 BCR-ABL1 protein tyrosine kinase found in Ph + ALL.

Imatinib was developed by Lydon and Druker [57] in collaboration with Ciba-Geigy (now Novartis) in the early 1990s. The compound entered clinical trials in June 1998 and by the end of 1999 it had become clear that imatinib was active in controlling the hematological and clinical features of CML, with high bioavailability as an oral compound. A phase I study demonstrated that at a dosage level of over 300 mg/day by mouth, the drug was able to restore the leukocyte count to normal in patients with IFN-resistant CML in chronic phase with a few patients achieving Ph negativity [36]. The drug was also active in controlling the blast cell count in patients in myeloid blast and lymphoid transformation, but the majority relapsed within 6 months [58].

A series of large phase II studies in interferon-refractory or -intolerant chronic-phase patients confirmed the remarkable efficacy of 400 mg imatinib daily, with high rates of durable CCyR with excellent overall tolerance, resulting in regulatory approval in this patient population [59], as well as in patients with more advanced disease [60–62]. Subsequently, a phase III prospective randomized trial (the so-called IRIS study) was conducted in 1106 previously untreated patients, comparing interferon and cytarabine as per the previous French regimen [48], with imatinib at a dose of 400 mg daily [50]. Fourteen and one-half percent of the patients receiving interferon and low-dose cytarabine achieved a CCyR as opposed to 76% of the patients in the imatinib arm. These differences were highly significant and in terms of side effect profile, tolerability, and quality-of-life measures and rate of major molecular response (MMR) [63], there again were major and significant differences in favor of imatinib [63]. Other trials [64–67], as well as longer term follow-up of the IRIS patients [68, 69], confirmed the durability of these benefits with an estimated event-free survival at 6 years of 83%, and freedom from progression to accelerated or blast phase of 93% on the IRIS trial (Fig. 5.2). Furthermore, responding patients whose disease had not progressed in their first 3 years were extremely unlikely to relapse at a later time and also unlikely to suffer from late-onset side effects. These results were the first to validate the achievement of CCyR as a surrogate for significant and durable long-term benefit of TKI treatment in newly diagnosed patients. Historical comparisons showed a survival advantage from imatinib treatment compared to interferon-based therapies [70, 71].

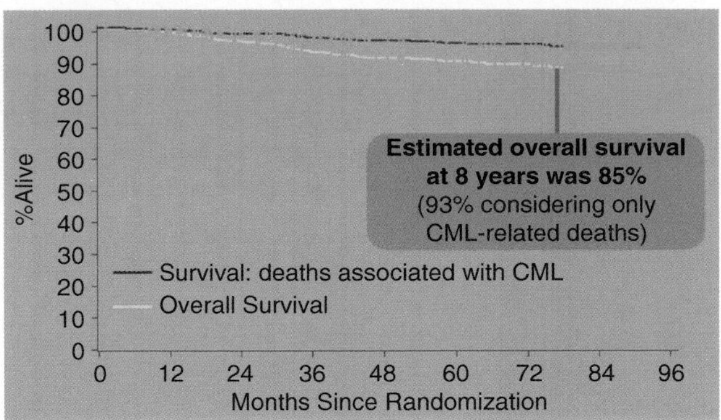

Fig. 5.2 Survival of imatinib-treated patients on the IRIS trial (reprinted with permission from O'Brien SG, Guilhot F, Goldman JM, Hochhaus A, Hughes TP, Radich JP et al. International Randomized Study of Interferon versus STI571 (IRIS) 7-year follow-up: sustained survival, low rate of transformation and increased rate of major molecular response (MMR) in patients (pts) with newly diagnosed chronic myeloid leukemia in chronic phase (CML-CP) treated with imatinib (IM). Blood 2008; 112: 76 (Abstract #186))

Imatinib Dose

Investigators at the MD Anderson Cancer Center in Houston reasoned that clinical results might be improved by starting treatment with a higher dose of imatinib and therefore designed a study in which newly diagnosed patients started treatment with imatinib at 800 mg daily [72]. Many patients are unable to tolerate this higher dosage, but comparison with the results of the standard 400 mg daily showed that CCyRs and major molecular responses (MMR), defined as a 3-log reduction in *BCR-ABL1* transcripts on the International Scale (IS—see below), were achieved more rapidly with the higher dose of imatinib. This experience led other investigators to design studies to compare prospectively 400 mg daily with 600 or 800 mg daily [64, 66, 73, 74]. The large German CML IV trial extended these observations showing that a higher fraction of patients treated with the higher dose achieved a 4.5-log reduction with the higher dose [66]. It does, however, appear that whereas response to the higher dose is clearly more rapid, the longer term results show less convincing superiority for the higher dose and no survival benefit has been demonstrated, likely in part because of the effect of potent second-generation TKIs given after initial imatinib treatment. Thus, at this time, there seems no good reason to alter the "standard" 400 mg initial dosage for adults. Parenthetically, pediatricians have opted to adapt imatinib dosage based on the child's body weight or body surface area [75].

Side Effects of Imatinib

Though patients taking imatinib are spared the more unpleasant side effects associated with conventional cytotoxic drugs, imatinib can still cause a variety of unwanted adverse reactions and some are severe enough to necessitate reducing dosage or discontinuing the drug [76–78]. Among the most prominent non-hematologic side effects are nausea, fluid retention, weight gain, diarrhea, bone pains, rashes, and disturbances of liver function. Most of these symptoms occur early in the treatment course, are of low grade, and can resolve over time. Imatinib can also cause significant cytopenias which almost always improves; occasional patients with anemia may benefit from administration of erythropoietin. An international consortium evaluated more than 800 patients in CyCR for greater than 2 years and then followed for a median of ~6 years. Fatigue and muscle cramps were the most prominent longer term side effects. The findings were very reassuring in that there was no increase in the occurrence of cardiovascular events, organ dysfunction, or other cancers. The overall survival of these patients was identical to that of age-matched normal controls [79]. Another long-term evaluation showed that other medical comorbidities did not influence response or CML-related survival [80]. In children, prolonged use of imatinib may cause skeletal growth velocity and comprehensive long-term follow-up studies are desirable, given the likelihood that most patients will be receiving imatinib indefinitely [81].

Monitoring Responses to Treatment with TKIs

The first evidence of response is reduction of the elevated leukocyte count and resolution of splenomegaly, followed by normalization of a more sensitive measure of residual leukemia, namely the number of Ph-positive metaphases in the bone marrow. The most sensitive test for low levels of leukemia is to measure *BCR-ABL1* transcript numbers in the blood or marrow using a real-time quantitative reverse transcriptase-PCR (RT-PCR or RQ-PCR) [82–84]. Analysis of blood gives results equivalent to those derived from bone marrow, but the specimen needs to be processed within 48 h of collection. Fluorescence in situ hybridization (FISH) used to identify a *BCR-ABL1* fusion gene in interphase cells is more sensitive than metaphase cytogenetics but less sensitive than RT-PCR. Peripheral blood FISH, which correlates very well with marrow cytogenetics, may be used if RQ-PCR for *BCR-ABL1* is not available [85]. In the past, the standard approach was to monitor marrow metaphase cytogenetics until a patient achieves CCyR and then to monitor RQ-PCR for *BCR-ABL1* transcripts at regular intervals to quantify the depth of reduction and to recognize incipient relapse. In patients with a clear-cut marked reduction in RT-PCR levels to a level consistent with at least a CCyR, some clinicians no longer do bone marrows for cytogenetic analysis.

Although RQ-PCR to quantify *BCR-ABL1* transcript numbers is now widely available, it must be remembered that the technique is demanding and can give both false-positive results (if for example the specimen is accidentally contaminated with material from another patient) and false-negative results (if for example the patient's specimen is degraded during collection and processing). The measurement of a control gene, usually *ABL1*, can assess whether the sample is adequate for analysis and results are expressed as the ratio of BCR-ABL1 to levels of the control gene. Initially, the methods by which results are expressed in different laboratories were not standardized, although most laboratories now express results as a log reduction using the International Scale (IS) which uses a correction factor applied to the "raw" results which are unique to individual laboratories and kits, and which provides standardization and comparability of results among different testing laboratories [86–88].

The IS arbitrarily assigns a baseline value of 100% to each patient [86]. A two-log reduction on the IS (i.e., a value of 1%) roughly corresponds to a CCyR while a greater-than-three-log reduction is termed a "major molecular response" (MMR). Both CCyR and MMR have been used as endpoints in clinical trials (see below). Current PCR technologies permit detection of a single CML cell among ~10^5 normal cells with corresponding IS values of 4.5- to 5-log reductions. In contrast, cytogenetics can detect ~1 Ph + cell among 20 normals and FISH ~1/200 normal cells. If transcripts are not detectable, the term "complete molecular response (CMR)" is sometimes used although this result is still consistent with the survival in a patient's body of perhaps 1×10^7 leukemia cells [88, 89], some of which may be resistant to all currently available TKIs. At very low levels of residual leukemia, the use of a DNA-based PCR technique may be more sensitive than one based on cDNA [89]. Lastly, although highly quantitative, there can be variation in QT-PCR values in duplicate specimen analyzed in the same laboratory, and hence, it is recommended that values be repeated before making decisions about changing therapy.

Resistance to Imatinib

A small proportion of patients who start imatinib in chronic phase, but a larger proportion of those who start the drug in advanced phases, do not respond well initially and require treatment with alternative agents. This is defined as primary resistance. Other patients can respond initially, achieving either a hematological response or a cytogenetic response followed by loss of response. This is defined as secondary resistance. The overall incidence of resistance is obviously time dependent but is of the order of 20–30% in patients who start treatment in chronic phase. The risk of developing secondary resistance appears to diminish with time and patients who have been in CCyR for more than 2 years, and who continue to take imatinib, seem to have an exceedingly low risk of relapse. Treatment failure occurs more commonly in patients with more "advanced" chronic phase as assessed by clinical measures such as the Sokal score, an observation consistent with the lower response rates in patients in accelerated phase. Patients with higher scores who do respond well, however, have long-term outcomes similar to other responding patients.

Resistance can also be classified according to whether it is associated with continuing inhibition of kinase activity of the *BCR-ABL1* oncoprotein or reversal of this inhibition. The mechanisms associated with this reversal of inhibition are not well defined, but some patients have cytogenetic evidence of clonal evolution and occasional examples of amplification of the *BCR-ABL1* gene in patients resistant to imatinib have been identified. The best characterized molecular event in patients with imatinib resistance is the acquisition of point mutations in the kinase domain of the *BCR-ABL1* gene, most commonly evaluated by Sanger sequencing, such that a mutant oncoprotein is produced. The prototype is the T315I mutation whereby a threonine at position 315 in the *BCR-ABL1* protein is replaced by an isoleucine which impedes binding of imatinib in the ATP-binding pocket of the enzyme [90–93]. Other mutations in residues that make contact with imatinib in the P-loop of the enzyme can also be associated with clinical resistance. More than 50 different mutations have been identified in patients who have lost their response to imatinib and other TKIs [94], although such mutations are found in at most 50% of such patients, indicating that other as-yet unidentified molecular events are the direct cause of resistance. Testing for mutations in *BCR-ABL1* should be done whenever a change in therapy is contemplated because of resistance to treatment, since occasionally the mutational profile would suggest using a particular TKI [95, 96]. Mutations are more common in advanced stages of CML and multiple mutations, consistent with progressive genetic instability, can sometimes be identified at the time of progression. In contrast, *BCR-ABL1* mutations are rarely found at diagnosis in chronic phase and mutational testing is not advised at this stage.

Another possible mechanism of resistance is related to increased expression of the P-glycoprotein (Pgp) efflux pump affecting the transmembrane transport of imatinib [97, 98]. Conversely, imatinib is transported into cells by the human OCT1 transporter and low levels of OCT1 have also been linked with poor clinical response to imatinib [99]. In practice, acquired resistance is likely to be multifactorial and mechanisms may differ in different patients. One study identified a gene signature suggestive of disease progression which could be found in patients in clinical chronic phase prior to their disease progression although this approach is currently not in use clinically [100].

In vitro measurement of the concentration of imatinib that will inhibit proliferation by 50% (IC50) of an individual patient's cells has been studied in an attempt to predict the desirable in vivo imatinib concentration [101]. Two studies suggested that low plasma "trough" levels of imatinib, as defined as the lowest level before the next scheduled dose of imatinib, can correlate with a lower probability of achieving a CCyR [102, 103]. Such low trough levels might be an indication for increasing the prescribed dose of imatinib. There was considerable overlap between the levels in good and less robust responders, and neither approach can be recommended for use in individual patients.

Perhaps most importantly, it must be appreciated that a major cause of an inadequate response or loss of initial response to imatinib may be the simple fact that some patients may not take the prescribed dose on a regular basis, for which there may be a variety of reasons, including forgetfulness, desire to lessen side effects, or desire to save money in countries where the patient has to pay for the drug themselves [104, 105]. Moreover, casual questioning of the patient about his or her adherence to the prescribed dosage may not always yield reliable answers. It is imperative to carefully question patients about compliance before switching treatment or increasing dosage.

Evaluation of Response to Imatinib: European LeukemiaNet Recommendations

In order to optimize the treatment benefit from imatinib, molecular and/or cytogenetic responses should be monitored serially so that changes in therapy can be recommended as needed. The European LeukemiaNet has presented the consensus recommendations of a panel of experts who agreed on a series of criteria for CP patients who started imatinib at 400 mg daily to define treatment "failure," "optimal response," and an intermediate "warning" group who require closer monitoring [106]. The most recent iteration of these recommendations, published in 2013 [107], is summarized in Table 5.5 with an updated version currently being assembled. It must be emphasized that fluctuations in values are common over time and that there is also considerable inherent variability in the tests themselves. Thus, values near these somewhat arbitrary "cutoffs" should be repeated before changes in therapy are considered. These guidelines may also be used to evaluate the effectiveness of treatment with other TKIs, used either as initial or salvage therapy. Similar guidelines have been offered by the National Comprehensive Cancer Network in the USA (http://www.nccn.org). In earlier years, the treatment change usually involved an increase in imatinib dosage to 600 or 800 mg/day; more recently, switches to newer, more potent TKIs are usually recommended. This approach is supported by a randomized phase II trial which demonstrated superior outcomes with the use of dasatinib in this setting when compared with increased doses of imatinib [108].

Perhaps the most debated aspect of the ELN recommendation concerns the "warning" should patients not achieve BCR-ABL1 ≤ 10% at 3 or 6 months. Numerous studies have shown that a > 1-log reduction (i.e., <10%) is associated with an excellent long-term outcome with few long-term treatment failures, assuming continued compliance with the medication [66, 69, 109–113]. The results are poorer in patients who remain >10% at 3 months, although still >80% of these patients are long-term survivors with continued therapy with either imatinib or other TKIs [66]. Although the temptation is to switch therapy rapidly in patients with slower responses, the only trial which evaluated this approach systematically failed to demonstrate benefit from earlier switching from imatinib to nilotinib [114]. In addition, the 10% number is not an absolute dichotomous decision point in that values of 11% and 9%, for example, are within the range of tests of the same sample done in duplicate. Similarly, the implications of 11% vs. 50% (both >10% on the IS) are certainly different. Thus, tests should be repeated and a pattern or trend established, before therapy is switched to another TKI, particularly at the 3- and 6-month time points.

Some recent studies have suggested that the rate at which the transcripts decrease in the first few months after

Table 5.5 Criteria for definition of response based on European LeukemiaNet recommendations [107]

	Failure	Warning	Optimal response
3 months	Non-CHR and/or Ph+ >95%	BCR-ABL1 > 10% and/or Ph + 36–95%	BCR-ABL1 ≤ 10% and/or Ph + ≤35%
6 months	BCR-ABL1 > 10% and/or Ph+ >35%	BCR-ABL1 1–10% and/or Ph + 1–35%	BCR-ABL1 < 1% and/or Ph + 0
12 Months	BCR-ABL1 > 1% and/or Ph+ >0	BCR-ABL1 > 0.1–1%	BCR-ABL1 ≤ 0.1%
18 months	Less than CCyR		MMR (3-log reduction in transcripts)
Any time	Loss of CHR	CCA/Ph– (–7, or 7q–)	BCR-ABL1 ≤ 0.1%
	Loss of CCyR		
	Kinase domain mutation insensitive to Imatinib		
	Confirmed loss of MMR		
	Clonal evolution		

CHR complete hematological response, *CyR* cytogenetic response, *CCyR* complete cytogenetic response, *MMR* major molecular response

TKI therapy is begun, sometimes termed the "velocity of elimination," might be a more sensitive means of distinguishing between good and poor responders. This approach requires better standardization of the transcript levels at the time of diagnosis and is not broadly applicable at this time [111, 115].

Managing the Patient in Whom Imatinib Has Not Been Sufficiently Effective

Changes in therapy after treatment with imatinib can be prompted by the development of intolerable side effects, failure to obtain adequate reduction in BCR-ABL1 transcripts as defined above, or less commonly obvious disease progression. It is critical to assess patient compliance with the imatinib before attributing treatment failure to drug resistance [104]. If a switch in therapy is contemplated, assessment of BCR-ABL1 mutations should be done because occasionally the type of mutation will suggest the use of a specific TKI with better activity against that particular conformational change in the BCR-ABL1 [116–118]. Most often however, either no mutation is detected or the sensitivities to other TKIs are predicted to be similar, and the choice of second TKI is predicated on issues such as convenience of therapy and side effect spectrum.

So-called second-generation TKIs were synthesized and entered the clinic remarkably rapidly after the discovery of imatinib. All of these agents are orally bioavailable, were initially evaluated and approved by regulatory agencies for use in patients with treatment failure or intolerance to imatinib, and were subsequently tested in comparative trials with imatinib as initial therapy. All are administered orally. These agents have never been directly compared with each other in randomized trials, but the overall response rates of dasatinib, bosutinib, and nilotinib are similar in imatinib-relapsed/refractory/intolerant patients. CCyR rates of ~40–50% which, if achieved, are generally sustained for many years, can be anticipated, with the highest response rates, as might be expected, in patients switched for intolerance [119–125]. Response rates are lower with "third-line" TKI treatment although sustained responses can also be achieved with a switch to an alternative TKI. Ponatinib is the most potent of these drugs when used in the more advanced setting but has a very high rate of cardiovascular side effects as described below [126, 127]. Because of the lower response rates with second-line treatment, many clinicians evaluate for possible allogeneic transplant, reserving transplant for patients poorly responsive to the subsequent treatment.

The side effect profile varies considerably among the different TKIs, presumably because all inhibit multiple tyrosine kinase pathways in addition to BCR-ABL1 signaling. All can be associated with usually transient rash, diarrhea, fatigue, headache, elevations of liver transaminases, and pancreatic enzymes, with occasional overt pancreatitis, but each also can produce side effects relatively unique to that agent.

Dasatinib

Dasatinib (Sprycel) is an inhibitor with activity against a range of tyrosine kinases including SRC and SRC family kinases. In vitro studies showed that it was 325 times as potent as imatinib against BCR-ABL1 [128]. It is effective in producing major cytogenetic responses in ~40% of the patients still in chronic phase who develop resistance to imatinib [108, 129]. A randomized study evaluating different doses and schedules of dasatinib identified 100 mg/day as the preferred starting dose, although many patients wind up taking lower doses long term with continued effectiveness [122]. These responses can be sustained, and with follow-up of 7 years, the PFS and OS were ~42% and 65%, respectively, using the 100 mg dose [130].

Dasatinib causes more profound cytopenias than does imatinib, and can be associated with QTc prolongation, and pleural effusions can develop in more than 20% of patients [108, 130]. Effusions are more common in patients with more advanced CML and those with prior cardiac disease. Most are asymptomatic and can resolve spontaneously or with dose reduction, but some require thoracentesis and occasionally a switch to another TKI. Effusions are usually detected within the first few months of dasatinib treatment but can occur after many months or years of treatment and patients should be advised to contact their CML care giver should symptoms of shortness of breath or chest discomfort develop. Pericardial effusions have also been noted and a small number of patients have been described with pulmonary hypertension, clinically indistinguishable from "primary" pulmonary hypertension. These can resolve with dasatinib discontinuation but fatalities have been reported [131, 132]. The mechanism(s) responsible for these fluid retention and vascular changes are not known. Lastly, ~30% of CML patients develop a proliferation of T/NK cells within the first few months of treatment which in some patients can persist for years [133–136]. There is a suggestion that the rates of CyCR and PFS may be higher in such patients, suggesting an immunomodulatory effect [137], but these findings need further confirmation.

Nilotinib

Nilotinib (Tasigna) is a chemically modified form of imatinib with greater potency and selectivity for *BCR-ABL1* than imatinib [138]. A large phase 2 study in 321 patients resistant to or intolerant of imatinib demonstrated a 45% CyCR rate with PFS of 57% and OS of 78% after 4 years of follow-up using a dose of 400 mg twice daily [139, 140]. Nilotinib should be taken on an empty stomach, at least 2 h apart from meals. More recent trials have suggested that the recommended dose should be 300 mg twice daily [141].

Although nilotinib is well tolerated overall, patients have to be monitored carefully during the first 1–2 months for hepatic transaminase elevations and for clinical or subclinical pancreatitis manifested by elevations of lipase and amylase. These abnormalities are usually transient and subclinical, and most patients can be restarted on nilotinib after the values normalize. There is a "black box" warning on the nilotinib label because of a few cases of sudden death occurring early in the nilotinib trials. Fortunately, this was a very rare event in the thousands of patients treated subsequently, although monitoring of the QTc interval is recommended after nilotinib is started. Lastly, the more recent randomized ENESTnd trial in newly diagnosed patients with CML trials demonstrated a somewhat alarming incidence of >15% of cardiovascular events including myocardial and cerebrovascular ischemia and infarction as well as peripheral arterial occlusive disease [141, 142]. The incidence of these problems in imatinib-treated patients was ~1%. This experience confirmed earlier case reports describing peripheral arterial occlusive disease in nilotinib recipients [143]. The mechanism is not known although nilotinib can precipitate or exacerbate diabetes. These issues need to be considered in individual patients when deciding among different TKIs and patients receiving nilotinib should have other vascular risk factors such as hypertension, hypercholesteremia, smoking cessation, and diabetes monitored and treated as needed. Many clinicians also prescribe prophylaxis with aspirin, although there are no prospective data supporting this approach [144].

Bosutinib

Bosutinib (SKI-606, Bosulif), a 7-alkoxy-3-quinolinecarbonitrile, functions as a dual inhibitor of SRC and ABL kinases, and preclinical studies demonstrated a high antiproliferative activity in human and murine CML cell lines [145, 146]. Bosutinib was recently approved in the USA for the treatment of imatinib-resistant/intolerant patients as well as some patients refractory to either nilotinib or dasatinib, based on a phase 2 trial using a dose of 500 mg/day, which demonstrated a major cytogenetic response rate of 40% and OS of 78% with approximately 4 years of follow-up [119, 123, 124, 147]. Newer studies with bosutinib utilize a dose of 400 mg/day. Diarrhea and transaminase elevations occurring during the first few months of treatment are the most common toxicities, sometimes requiring dose reductions and/or temporary cessation of therapy [148].

Ponatinib

Ponatinib is a potent *BCR-ABL1* developed as a scaffold (unlike the other TKIs) designed to make a hydrogen bond with the T315 mutant oncoprotein [91, 127, 149, 150]. Ponatinib adapts to such steric hindrance by virtue of a long and flexible ethynyl tricarbon linker. X-ray crystallographic analysis of the ponatinib-murine T315I ABL complex revealed that the compound binds to the complex in the inactive conformation, similar to imatinib, and interacts via hydrogen bonds at five distinct amino acid residues. In vitro studies demonstrated potent activity against cell lines resistant to other TKIs and large phase 2 studies were conducted in patients resistant to therapy with nilotinib or dasatinib. The phase 2 PACE trial reported major cytogenetic responses in 51% of the 203 patients with chronic-phase CML resistant or intolerant to dasatinib or nilotinib and in 70% of the 64 patients in chronic phase with T315I mutations. Approximately 90% of responses were sustained at 1 year and the drug was effective across a broad range of *BCR-ABL1* mutations [126].

Ponatinib was approved for use in this patient population as well as for patients in more advanced-stage CML. Short-term toxicities included skin rash, hypertension, and occasional pancreatitis. However, longer term follow-up demonstrated a disturbing incidence of predominantly arterial cardiovascular events including strokes, myocardial infarction, peripheral arterial occlusive disease, and heart failure [144]. At least 27% of study participants experienced such side effects and although cardiovascular events were more common in older patients with predisposing risk factors, some younger patients without apparent vascular issues were also affected [151]. The original studies used a dose of 45 mg/day and more recent studies are in progress evaluating lower doses and/or rapid reduction of dose as soon as responses are detected. The mechanism of the vascular toxicity is not known [144]. The drug was initially withdrawn from the market but is now available for use in highly selected patients and in particular those with the T315I mutation for which there is no other effective therapy [152, 153]. If patients are responding, the lowest effective dose should be used and the author follows some patients in sustained molecular response using 15 mg/day.

Omacetaxine (Homoharringtonine)

Omacetaxine mepesuccinate (Homoharringtonine HHT) is a novel plant cephalotaxine alkaloid originally derived from the *Cephalotaxus fortunei* tree [154–156]. Omacetaxine is approved in the USA for the treatment of chronic-phase CMl resistant to two TKIs, including patients with the T315I mutation. The recommended dose and schedule are 1.25 mg/m^2

subcutaneous injection twice daily for 14 days of a 28-day cycle for the induction phase and 1.25 mg/m^2 subcutaneous injection twice daily for 7 days of a 28-day cycle for maintenance. Rates of complete hematologic, major cytogenetic, and complete cytogenetic response were 77%, 23%, and 16%, respectively [109, 157]. The main side effects include significant cytopenias, infection, diarrheas, fatigue, and fever. Median PFS was ~7 months. Omacetaxine is sometimes used as a bridge to transplantation in patients in more advanced stages, although hydrea and myleran are also used for disease control and palliation in this situation.

Initial Therapy of Chronic Phase with Newer TKIs

Shortly after approval of the second-generation TKIs for imatinib refractory patients, randomized trials were initiated using these drugs as initial treatment in chronic phase. In the Dasision study, previously untreated patients were randomized to receive either 100 mg daily of dasatinib or imatinib, 400 mg daily [110, 158]. In the ENESTnd study, two different doses of nilotinib, 300 mg twice daily and 400 mg twice daily, were compared with imatinib 400 mg daily [141, 142, 159]. The primary endpoints were CCyR and MMR after 12 months of treatment. In both studies, cytogenetic and molecular responses were achieved more rapidly than with imatinib and in both studies the early rate of progression from CP to advanced phase was higher in the imatinib arm than in any of the three test arms. Based on these results, both dasatinib and nilotinib were approved by regulatory agencies as initial treatment in chronic phase.

A trial of similar design (BELA) evaluating bosutinib was also completed, and although overall results were actually very similar to the other trials, bosutinib has not yet been approved as initial therapy [160, 161]. A repeat trial using a dose of 400 mg of bosutinib was recently completed and demonstrated higher rates of CyCR in the bosutinib treated patients.

Lastly, a trial comparing ponatinib and imatinib was stopped before completion when the cardiovascular side effects of ponatinib became apparent [162]. Even in this trial, with only short follow-up, 6% of ponatinib-treated patients experienced severe cardiovascular events (Table 5.6).

These studies have appropriately influenced discussions of the preferable first-line treatment of chronic phase. Cross-study comparisons cannot be done because of some differences in statistical methods, definitions of endpoints, duration of follow-up, and most importantly variability in the details of follow-up and types of treatment after patients went "off study" or switched from their original randomized treatment. All of these trials were sponsored by pharmaceutical companies. A study comparing imatinib and dasatinib done in the USA, and coordinated by the Southwest Oncology Group, was similar in design to Dasision and reported very similar results [113].

The overall results of these studies are very similar and a number of general statements can be made:

- OS was very high with no differences according to initial treatment, although most studies reported slightly higher rates of "CML-related" deaths in the imatinib-treated patients.
- With longer follow-up, 40–50% of patients were no longer receiving their initial treatment. Switches were made because of side effects and occasionally for disease progression (somewhat more commonly in the imatinib groups) and presumably most of these patients received alternative TKIs. Details of secondary treatment are generally not available, but it is important to emphasize that one must consider the totality of initial and subsequent therapy in evaluating overall results. Given the excellent OS and low rates of progression, it is clear that subsequent treatment has a critical role in achieving these outcomes.
- Transformation to AP/BP occurred more frequently with imatinib treatment. Almost all these events occurred within the first 1–2 years and were quite uncommon with longer follow-up, although the overall rate of transformation was low with all treatments. Information about whether transformations developed primarily in patients with "advanced" chronic phase with high-risk features is not available. This is important because many experi-

Table 5.6 Summary of long-term results

	Dasision (*n* = 519) (Minimum of 5 years of follow-up)		ENESTnd (*n* = 846) (Minimum of 5 years of follow-up)			BELA (*n* = 502) (Minimum of 2 years of follow-up)	
	IMAT	DAS	IMAT	NIL 300	NIL400	IMAT	BOS
CyCR (%)	80%	85% @ 18 months	77%	87% @ 24 months		79%	80% @ 24 months
MMR (%)	64%	76	60%	77	77	49%	59% @ 24 months
AP/BC (%)	7.3	4.6	4.8	1.3	0.7	5.5	1.6
PFS (%)	85	86	91	95.8	92.2	88	92
OS (%)	90	91	91.7	93.7	96.2	95	97
Receiving initial therapy (%)	63	61	50%	60	62	71	63

enced clinicians now utilize second-generation TKIs in preference to imatinib in such patients, based on the results of the randomized trials.
- All studies showed that results were inferior in patients with transcripts >10% at 3 months, independent of treatment arm, although a higher fraction of patients achieved this "milestone" with the second-generation TKIs. There is no information about subsequent approaches to treatment in such patients and the problems of relying on a single IS value to change treatment have been described above.
- The "depth" of molecular response continued to improve over time and all studies noted lower rates of "deep" reductions >4 and 4.5 logs in imatinib-treated patients. There is speculation that this may permit more patients treated with second-generation TKIs to successfully discontinue treatment but there are as yet no data addressing this issue. It should also be noted that all the response rates reported in the table utilized the cumulative incidence statistic and information as to whether these deep responses persisted on repeated testing is not available.

The decision about which TKI is preferable as initial therapy must also consider the unique toxicity profiles of the drugs. Some notable issues include the following:

- There was an appreciable incidence of **cardiovascular events** of approximately 15–20% in nilotinib-treated patients which continues to increase over time, compared to 3–4% in imatinib-treated patients. Rates in the Dasision trial were ~5% vs. 2% in dasatinib- and imatinib-treated patients, respectively. Glucose intolerance and hypercholesteremia were also more common with nilotinib compared to imatinib. Recommendations about concurrent treatment of cardiovascular risk factors and patient selection for treatment with nilotinib have recently been published [163–165], but it is not known if these approaches will be effective in reducing the incidence of cardiovascular side effects.
- **Pleural effusions** developed in ~28% of dasatinib-treated patients compared to 0.1% in the imatinib group. Most such patients could continue dasatinib with temporary discontinuations and dose adjustments. **Pulmonary hypertension** with clinical manifestations was detected in 5% of dasatinib-treated patients.
- Eleven **infectious deaths** were reported in the dasatinib group in the Dasision trial, compared to one in the imatinib group. There is no apparent explanation for this discrepancy.

The debate about the best initial treatment continues [166]. It is apparent from these studies that the second-generation TKIs are more potent than imatinib in that the rate of initial response is faster, and the depth of response may be greater with a likely lower (albeit still very low) rate of initial disease progression, but with equivalent overall survival. Longer term toxicity data with bosutinib are lacking, but it is clear that both nilotinib and dasatinib have important issues unique to each agent, whereas the long-term follow-up data with imatinib are very reassuring [79, 80, 106]. Certainly, preexisting medical problems in individual patients have to be an important consideration. In any event, it is likely that with the increasing availability of generic imatinib, insurers and other payors will be directing, if not mandating, initial treatment with imatinib. Fortunately, the results of these randomized trials provide reassurance that this is a most reasonable approach for the overwhelming majority of newly diagnosed patients. In addition, a large trial of ~1500 patients conducted by the German CML group which evaluated different approaches using imatinib confirmed these excellent long-term outcomes [66].

Stopping Imatinib in Responding Patients: The Concept of "Treatment-Free Remission"

A small number of patients treated with interferon-alpha in the 1990s achieved durable CCyR which has continued for many years after the interferon was stopped [47]. In 2007, Rousselot and colleagues reported details of 12 CML patients in France who received imatinib as primary treatment or after prior treatment with interferon and achieved CMR [167]. These patients had stopped their imatinib for different reasons after 2 or more years in CMR; six had relapsed at the molecular level and six were still in CMR at the time of the report. These observations were extended in the STIM ("Stop Imatinib") study of 100 patients who had undetectable transcripts over a number of years using highly sensitive PCR assays. Approximately 50% of patients had a molecular relapse, almost all within 6 months of treatment cessation [168]. All relapsing patients promptly responded to reintroduction of imatinib which was restarted when MMR was lost (>0.1 on the IS) [169, 170]. Remarkably, only rare recurrences were detected in the remainder of the patients, with the latest update at a median follow-up of 4 years. The relapse rate was lower in patients who were PCR undetectable for >8 years. Other studies have shown similar results [171]. Importantly, discontinuation should only be considered in patients with consistently very low to undetectable transcript levels for at least a few years and many trials, some of which use different durations and depth of "negativity" prior to cessation, are in progress. All trials mandate careful molecular monitoring for the first 12 months with continued intermittent long-term monitoring thereafter, because it is not known if very late relapses will occur. It has been postulated that the long remissions may be due to immunologic control of any residual CML stem cells, but the precise mechanisms are unknown.

Whether such patients can really be regarded as "cured" is debatable but undoubtedly one major target today should be to find strategies that will enable us to increase the proportion of patients who may safely stop treatment [172, 173].

An interesting "withdrawal syndrome" characterized by musculoskeletal and articular discomfort and pain has been described in an appreciable fraction of patients who discontinued TKIs. The symptoms are usually mild and transient and easily managed with nonsteroidal anti-inflammatory agents, although persistence of clinically significant achiness can occur in a few patients, which may or may not improve with restarting TKIs [174, 175].

Imatinib and Other TKIs During Pregnancy

Preclinical studies based on animal data suggested that imatinib and other TKIs could be teratogenic in certain circumstances and women taking imatinib have been routinely advised to take steps to avoid conception. Nonetheless, some women have conceived while taking imatinib and in most cases where the pregnancy went to term the baby appeared to have been normal. However, certain specific developmental abnormalities including hypospadias, exomphalos, and defective skeletal formation have been seen more often than would have been expected in women not taking imatinib [176, 177] and the advice to avoid pregnancy while being treated with the drug must be upheld.

Therefore, counseling a woman already on imatinib who wants to start or to enlarge her family is difficult, and generally clinicians continue to advise against pregnancy. If the patient has achieved a deep response, stopping imatinib to allow the patient to conceive and carry the child without exposure to imatinib is a consideration, but this approach almost certainly puts the patient at increased risk of relapse and possibly disease progression. Interferon-alpha is not known to be teratogenic and has been considered to be an alternative, particularly for women who become pregnant while receiving a TKI. There are few published data evaluating this approach, however. Women who become pregnant while receiving imatinib should contact their physicians immediately. Available evidence suggests that patients who stop imatinib and then relapse respond as well to reintroduction of imatinib as they did originally [170]. Less is known about the possible harmful effect of imatinib on male spermatogenesis and small case series have shown a very low rate of fetal abnormalities in children whose fathers were taking imatinib [178].

Advanced-Phase Disease

In the past, patients who presented in accelerated and blastic phases were treated with a higher starting dose of imatinib of 600 mg daily [61], although the use of dasatinib or nilotinib is now preferred in such patients. In general, advanced-phase patients respond much less well to imatinib than those who start treatment in chronic phase with low rates of CyCR and high rates of relapse should response be achieved. However, patients who satisfy the criteria for "acceleration" are in fact heterogeneous: at one end of the spectrum the term covers patients whose leukemia is only slightly more advanced than late chronic phase while in others the leukemia may be verging on blastic phase. Patients with "early" accelerated phase may obtain long-term responses to imatinib as a single agent, while others usually have much shorter responses [61]. Patients presenting in blastic transformation need a much more aggressive initial strategy. All patients in AP/BP should be evaluated for allogeneic stem cell transplantation while they are receiving their initial TKI treatment.

It can sometimes be difficult to distinguish between patients in lymphoid blast phase at the time of diagnosis, from de novo Ph + acute lymphoblastic leukemia (ALL). Combining a TKI with standard anti-ALL treatment is the best initial approach [179]. Once remission is achieved, maintenance treatment with cytotoxic drugs together with a TKI can then be continued. Neuroprophylaxis is also advisable. For patients presenting in myeloid blast phase, the combined use of a TKI with therapy appropriate to AML may be the best approach. AML-like chemotherapy alone produces few complete remissions [180]. In both circumstances, allogeneic stem cell transplantation should be done in all suitable patients, preferably while the patient is in complete remission. Most centers continue the use of a TKI after engraftment, but no comprehensive studies about the duration of such maintenance TKI are available.

Allogeneic Stem Cell Transplantation

Until the advent of TKIs, allogeneic stem cell transplantation was the recommended initial approach for patients who were relatively young and had suitable donors, with rates of disease-free survival approximating 70%, with very few late relapses [181]. Currently, allogeneic SCT is reserved for those with advanced-stage disease or those in whom treatment with second-generation TKIs was not successful. More details about conditioning regimens and donor selection are presented in other chapters. *BCR-ABL1* transcripts should be monitored serially for the first few years after transplant. It is important to recognize that there can be transient *BCR-ABL1* positivity in the first year posttransplant in patients who are ultimately destined *not* to proceed to overt relapse [181]. Two or more consecutive samples with increasing numbers of *BCR-ABL1* transcripts are required at a minimum to establish a relapse. For patients with confirmed relapse after allogeneic SCT, options for treatment include the withdrawal of immunosuppression, use of a TKI to which the patient has not previously been exposed, and/or donor lymphocyte infusions.

Summary

The therapy of CML has been revolutionized over the last 15 years with the advent of TKI therapy, such that the survival of chronic-phase patients responding to TKI treatment approximates that of age-matched controls. There is now the prospect that some patients might be able to stop TKI therapy and remain in remission and possibly even be cured in the longer term. Over the next decade, research will focus on evaluating how to use the various TKIs in the most cost-effective way to further improve the long-term outcome and quality of life of patients with CML. Stem cell transplantation has a minor, but still important, role in the small number of patients for whom TKIs are not effective or tolerated.

Acknowledgments This section is an extensive update of the chapter from the earlier edition authored by Drs. Stephen O'Brien and John Goldman and is dedicated to the memory of John Goldman who was a pioneer and leader in our understanding of the biology and therapy of CML and a valued friend and colleague.

References

1. Goldman JM. Chronic myeloid leukemia: a historical perspective. Semin Hematol. 2010;47(4):302–11.
2. Cortes J, Kantarjian H. How I treat newly diagnosed chronic phase CML. Blood. 2012;120(7):1390–7.
3. Hehlmann R. How I treat CML blast crisis. Blood. 2012;120(4):737–47.
4. Fialkow PJ, Jacobson RJ, Papayannopoulou T. Chronic myelocytic leukemia: clonal origin in a stem cell common to the granulocyte, erythrocyte, platelet and monocyte/macrophage. Am J Med. 1977;63(1):125–30.
5. Nowell PC, Hungerford DA. Chromosome studies on normal and leukemic human leukocytes. J Natl Cancer Inst. 1960;25:85–109.
6. Rowley JD. Letter: a new consistent chromosomal abnormality in chronic myelogenous leukaemia identified by quinacrine fluorescence and Giemsa staining. Nature. 1973;243(5405):290–3.
7. Daley GQ, Van Etten RA, Baltimore D. Induction of chronic myelogenous leukemia in mice by the P210bcr/abl gene of the Philadelphia chromosome. Science. 1990;247(4944):824–30.
8. Daley GQ, Van Etten RA, Baltimore D. Blast crisis in a murine model of chronic myelogenous leukemia. Proc Natl Acad Sci U S A. 1991;88(24):11335–8.
9. Lugo TG, Pendergast AM, Muller AJ, Witte ON. Tyrosine kinase activity and transformation potency of bcr-abl oncogene products. Science. 1990;247(4946):1079–82.
10. Kurzrock R, Bueso-Ramos CE, Kantarjian H, Freireich E, Tucker SL, Siciliano M, et al. BCR rearrangement-negative chronic myelogenous leukemia revisited. J Clin Oncol. 2001;19(11):2915–26.
11. Ezdinli EZ, Sokal JE, Crosswhite L, Sandberg AA. Philadelphia-chromosome-positive and -negative chronic myelocytic leukemia. Ann Intern Med. 1970;72(2):175–82.
12. Bizzozero OJ Jr, Johnson KG, Ciocco A. Radiation-related leukemia in Hiroshima and Nagasaki, 1946-1964. I. Distribution, incidence and appearance time. N Engl J Med. 1966;274(20):1095–101.
13. Ichimaru M, Ishimaru T, Belsky JL. Incidence of leukemia in atomic bomb survivors belonging to a fixed cohort in Hiroshima and Nagasaki, 1950--71. Radiation dose, years after exposure, age at exposure, and type of leukemia. J Radiat Res. 1978;19(3):262–82.
14. Wald N. Leukemia in Hiroshima City atomic bomb survivors. Science. 1958;127(3300):699–700.
15. Savage DG, Szydlo RM, Goldman JM. Clinical features at diagnosis in 430 patients with chronic myeloid leukaemia seen at a referral centre over a 16-year period. Br J Haematol. 1997;96(1):111–6.
16. Kantarjian HM, Dixon D, Keating MJ, Talpaz M, Walters RS, McCredie KB, et al. Characteristics of accelerated disease in chronic myelogenous leukemia. Cancer. 1988;61(7):1441–6.
17. Arber DA, Orazi A, Hasserjian R, Thiele J, Borowitz MJ, Le Beau MM, et al. The 2016 revision to the World Health Organization classification of myeloid neoplasms and acute leukemia. Blood. 2016;127(20):2391–405.
18. Shumak KH, Baker MA, Taub RN, Coleman MS. Myeloblastic and lymphoblastic markers in acute undifferentiated leukemia and chronic myelogenous leukemia in blast crisis. Cancer Res. 1980;40(11):4048–52.
19. Forman EN, Padre-Mendoza T, Smith PS, Barker BE, Farnes P. Ph1-positive childhood leukemias: spectrum of lymphoid-myeloid expressions. Blood. 1977;49(4):549–58.
20. Chan LC, Furley AJ, Ford AM, Yardumian DA, Greaves MF. Clonal rearrangement and expression of the T cell receptor beta gene and involvement of the breakpoint cluster region in blast crisis of CGL. Blood. 1986;67(2):533–6.
21. Speed DE, Lawler SD. Chronic granulocytic Leukaemia. The chromosomes and the disease. Lancet. 1964;1(7330):403–8.
22. Kantarjian HM, Keating MJ, Talpaz M, Walters RS, Smith TL, Cork A, et al. Chronic myelogenous leukemia in blast crisis. Analysis of 242 patients. Am J Med. 1987;83(3):445–54.
23. Mitelman F. The cytogenetic scenario of chronic myeloid leukemia. Leuk Lymphoma. 1993;11(Suppl 1):11–5.
24. Fabarius A, Kalmanti L, Dietz CT, Lauseker M, Rinaldetti S, Haferlach C, et al. Impact of unbalanced minor route versus major route karyotypes at diagnosis on prognosis of CML. Ann Hematol. 2015;94(12):2015–24.
25. Stuppia L, Calabrese G, Peila R, Guanciali-Franchi P, Morizio E, Spadano A, et al. p53 loss and point mutations are associated with suppression of apoptosis and progression of CML into myeloid blastic crisis. Cancer Genet Cytogenet. 1997;98(1):28–35.
26. Ahuja H, Bar-Eli M, Advani SH, Benchimol S, Cline MJ. Alterations in the p53 gene and the clonal evolution of the blast crisis of chronic myelocytic leukemia. Proc Natl Acad Sci U S A. 1989;86(17):6783–7.
27. Stoll C, Oberling F, Flori E. Chromosome analysis of spleen and/or lymph nodes of patients with chronic myeloid leukemia (CML). Blood. 1978;52(4):828–38.
28. Vernant JP, Brun B, Mannoni P, Dreyfus B. Respiratory distress of hyperleukocytic granulocytic leukemias. Cancer. 1979;44(1):264–8.
29. Schwartz JH, Canellos GP, Young RC, DeVita VT Jr. Meningeal leukemia in the blastic phase of chronic granulocytic leukemia. Am J Med. 1975;59(6):819–28.
30. Tura S, Baccarani M, Corbelli G. Staging of chronic myeloid leukaemia. Br J Haematol. 1981;47(1):105–19.
31. Cervantes F, Rozman C. A multivariate analysis of prognostic factors in chronic myeloid leukemia. Blood. 1982;60(6):1298–304.
32. Sokal JE, Baccarani M, Russo D, Tura S. Staging and prognosis in chronic myelogenous leukemia. Semin Hematol. 1988;25(1):49–61.
33. Hasford J, Pfirrmann M, Hehlmann R, Allan NC, Baccarani M, Kluin-Nelemans JC, et al. A new prognostic score for survival of patients with chronic myeloid leukemia treated with interferon alfa. Writing Committee for the Collaborative CML Prognostic Factors Project Group. J Natl Cancer Inst. 1998;90(11):850–8.

34. Hasford J, Baccarani M, Hoffmann V, Guilhot J, Saussele S, Rosti G, et al. Predicting complete cytogenetic response and subsequent progression-free survival in 2060 patients with CML on imatinib treatment: the EUTOS score. Blood. 2011;118(3):686–92.
35. Gratwohl A, Hermans J, Goldman JM, Arcese W, Carreras E, Devergie A, et al. Risk assessment for patients with chronic myeloid leukaemia before allogeneic blood or marrow transplantation. Chronic Leukemia Working Party of the European Group for Blood and Marrow Transplantation. Lancet. 1998;352(9134):1087–92.
36. Druker BJ, Talpaz M, Resta DJ, Peng B, Buchdunger E, Ford JM, et al. Efficacy and safety of a specific inhibitor of the BCR-ABL tyrosine kinase in chronic myeloid leukemia. N Engl J Med. 2001;344(14):1031–7.
37. Caplan SN, Coco FV, Berkman EM. Management of chronic myelocytic leukemia in pregnancy by cell pheresis. Transfusion. 1978;18(1):120–4.
38. Fitzgerald D, Rowe JM, Heal J. Leukapheresis for control of chronic myelogenous leukemia during pregnancy. Am J Hematol. 1986;22(2):213–8.
39. Kennedy BJ. Hydroxyurea therapy in chronic myelogenous leukemia. Cancer. 1972;29(4):1052–6.
40. Kolitz JE, Kempin SJ, Schluger A, Wong GY, Berman E, Jhanwar S, et al. A phase II pilot trial of high-dose hydroxyurea in chronic myelogenous leukemia. Semin Oncol. 1992;19(3 Suppl 9):27–33.
41. Hehlmann R, Heimpel H, Hasford J, Kolb HJ, Pralle H, Hossfeld DK, et al. Randomized comparison of busulfan and hydroxyurea in chronic myelogenous leukemia: prolongation of survival by hydroxyurea. The German CML Study Group. Blood. 1993;82(2):398–407.
42. Talpaz M, McCredie K, Kantarjian H, Trujillo J, Keating M, Gutterman J. Chronic myelogenous leukaemia: haematological remissions with alpha interferon. Br J Haematol. 1986;64(1):87–95.
43. Hehlmann R, Heimpel H, Hasford J, Kolb HJ, Pralle H, Hossfeld DK, et al. Randomized comparison of interferon-alpha with busulfan and hydroxyurea in chronic myelogenous leukemia. The German CML Study Group. Blood. 1994;84(12):4064–77.
44. Talpaz M. Interferon-alfa-based treatment of chronic myeloid leukemia and implications of signal transduction inhibition. Semin Hematol. 2001;38(3 Suppl 8):22–7.
45. Guilhot F, Lacotte-Thierry L. Interferon-alpha: mechanisms of action in chronic myelogenous leukemia in chronic phase. Hematol Cell Ther. 1998;40(5):237–9.
46. Interferon alfa versus chemotherapy for chronic myeloid leukemia: a meta-analysis of seven randomized trials: chronic Myeloid Leukemia Trialists' Collaborative Group. J Natl Cancer Inst. 1997;89(21):1616–20.
47. Bonifazi F, de Vivo A, Rosti G, Guilhot F, Guilhot J, Trabacchi E, et al. Chronic myeloid leukemia and interferon-alpha: a study of complete cytogenetic responders. Blood. 2001;98(10):3074–81.
48. Guilhot F, Chastang C, Michallet M, Guerci A, Harousseau JL, Maloisel F, et al. Interferon alfa-2b combined with cytarabine versus interferon alone in chronic myelogenous leukemia. French Chronic Myeloid Leukemia Study Group. N Engl J Med. 1997;337(4):223–9.
49. Kantarjian HM, O'Brien S, Smith TL, Rios MB, Cortes J, Beran M, et al. Treatment of Philadelphia chromosome-positive early chronic phase chronic myelogenous leukemia with daily doses of interferon alpha and low-dose cytarabine. J Clin Oncol. 1999;17(1):284–92.
50. O'Brien SG, Guilhot F, Larson RA, Gathmann I, Baccarani M, Cervantes F, et al. Imatinib compared with interferon and low-dose cytarabine for newly diagnosed chronic-phase chronic myeloid leukemia. N Engl J Med. 2003;348(11):994–1004.
51. Druker BJ, Tamura S, Buchdunger E, Ohno S, Segal GM, Fanning S, et al. Effects of a selective inhibitor of the Abl tyrosine kinase on the growth of Bcr-Abl positive cells. Nat Med. 1996;2(5):561–6.
52. Oda T, Tamura S, Matsuguchi T, Griffin JD, Druker BJ. The SH2 domain of ABL is not required for factor-independent growth induced by BCR-ABL in a murine myeloid cell line. Leukemia. 1995;9(2):295–301.
53. Beran M, Cao X, Estrov Z, Jeha S, Jin G, O'Brien S, et al. Selective inhibition of cell proliferation and BCR-ABL phosphorylation in acute lymphoblastic leukemia cells expressing Mr 190,000 BCR-ABL protein by a tyrosine kinase inhibitor (CGP-57148). Clin Cancer Res. 1998;4(7):1661–72.
54. Carroll M, Ohno-Jones S, Tamura S, Buchdunger E, Zimmermann J, Lydon NB, et al. CGP 57148, a tyrosine kinase inhibitor, inhibits the growth of cells expressing BCR-ABL, TEL-ABL, and TEL-PDGFR fusion proteins. Blood. 1997;90(12):4947–52.
55. Deininger MW, Goldman JM, Lydon N, Melo JV. The tyrosine kinase inhibitor CGP57148B selectively inhibits the growth of BCR-ABL-positive cells. Blood. 1997;90(9):3691–8.
56. Gambacorti-Passerini C, le Coutre P, Mologni L, Fanelli M, Bertazzoli C, Marchesi E, et al. Inhibition of the ABL kinase activity blocks the proliferation of BCR/ABL+ leukemic cells and induces apoptosis. Blood Cells Mol Dis. 1997;23(3):380–94.
57. Druker BJ, Lydon NB. Lessons learned from the development of an abl tyrosine kinase inhibitor for chronic myelogenous leukemia. J Clin Invest. 2000;105(1):3–7.
58. Druker BJ, Sawyers CL, Kantarjian H, Resta DJ, Reese SF, Ford JM, et al. Activity of a specific inhibitor of the BCR-ABL tyrosine kinase in the blast crisis of chronic myeloid leukemia and acute lymphoblastic leukemia with the Philadelphia chromosome. N Engl J Med. 2001;344(14):1038–42.
59. Kantarjian H, Sawyers C, Hochhaus A, Guilhot F, Schiffer C, Gambacorti-Passerini C, et al. Hematologic and cytogenetic responses to imatinib mesylate in chronic myelogenous leukemia. N Engl J Med. 2002;346(9):645–52.
60. Ottmann OG, Druker BJ, Sawyers CL, Goldman JM, Reiffers J, Silver RT, et al. A phase 2 study of imatinib in patients with relapsed or refractory Philadelphia chromosome-positive acute lymphoid leukemias. Blood. 2002;100(6):1965–71.
61. Talpaz M, Silver RT, Druker BJ, Goldman JM, Gambacorti-Passerini C, Guilhot F, et al. Imatinib induces durable hematologic and cytogenetic responses in patients with accelerated phase chronic myeloid leukemia: results of a phase 2 study. Blood. 2002;99(6):1928–37.
62. Sawyers CL, Hochhaus A, Feldman E, Goldman JM, Miller CB, Ottmann OG, et al. Imatinib induces hematologic and cytogenetic responses in patients with chronic myelogenous leukemia in myeloid blast crisis: results of a phase II study. Blood. 2002;99(10):3530–9.
63. Hughes TP, Kaeda J, Branford S, Rudzki Z, Hochhaus A, Hensley ML, et al. Frequency of major molecular responses to imatinib or interferon alfa plus cytarabine in newly diagnosed chronic myeloid leukemia. N Engl J Med. 2003;349(15):1423–32.
64. Baccarani M, Rosti G, Castagnetti F, Haznedaroglu I, Porkka K, Abruzzese E, et al. Comparison of imatinib 400 mg and 800 mg daily in the front-line treatment of high-risk, Philadelphia-positive chronic myeloid leukemia: a European LeukemiaNet Study. Blood. 2009;113(19):4497–504.
65. Gugliotta G, Castagnetti F, Palandri F, Breccia M, Intermesoli T, Capucci A, et al. Frontline imatinib treatment of chronic myeloid leukemia: no impact of age on outcome, a survey by the GIMEMA CML Working Party. Blood. 2011;117(21):5591–9.
66. Hehlmann R, Muller MC, Lauseker M, Hanfstein B, Fabarius A, Schreiber A, et al. Deep molecular response is reached by the majority of patients treated with imatinib, predicts survival, and is achieved more quickly by optimized high-dose imatinib: results from the randomized CML-study IV. J Clin Oncol. 2014;32(5):415–23.
67. Jain P, Kantarjian H, Alattar ML, Jabbour E, Sasaki K, Nogueras Gonzalez G, et al. Long-term molecular and cytogenetic response

and survival outcomes with imatinib 400 mg, imatinib 800 mg, dasatinib, and nilotinib in patients with chronic-phase chronic myeloid leukaemia: retrospective analysis of patient data from five clinical trials. Lancet Haematol. 2015;2(3):e118–28.
68. Druker BJ, Guilhot F, O'Brien SG, Gathmann I, Kantarjian H, Gattermann N, et al. Five-year follow-up of patients receiving imatinib for chronic myeloid leukemia. N Engl J Med. 2006;355(23):2408–17.
69. Hochhaus A, Larson RA, Guilhot F, Radich JP, Branford S, et al. Long-Term Outcomes of Imatinib Treatment for Chronic Myeloid Leukemia. N Engl J Med. 2017; 376(10):917–27.
70. Kantarjian HM, Talpaz M, O'Brien S, Jones D, Giles F, Garcia-Manero G, et al. Survival benefit with imatinib mesylate versus interferon-alpha-based regimens in newly diagnosed chronic-phase chronic myelogenous leukemia. Blood. 2006;108(6):1835–40.
71. Roy L, Guilhot J, Krahnke T, Guerci-Bresler A, Druker BJ, Larson RA, et al. Survival advantage from imatinib compared with the combination interferon-alpha plus cytarabine in chronic-phase chronic myelogenous leukemia: historical comparison between two phase 3 trials. Blood. 2006;108(5):1478–84.
72. Kantarjian H, Talpaz M, O'Brien S, Garcia-Manero G, Verstovsek S, Giles F, et al. High-dose imatinib mesylate therapy in newly diagnosed Philadelphia chromosome-positive chronic phase chronic myeloid leukemia. Blood. 2004;103(8):2873–8.
73. Hughes TP, Branford S, White DL, Reynolds J, Koelmeyer R, Seymour JF, et al. Impact of early dose intensity on cytogenetic and molecular responses in chronic- phase CML patients receiving 600 mg/day of imatinib as initial therapy. Blood. 2008;112(10):3965–73.
74. Baccarani M, Druker BJ, Branford S, Kim DW, Pane F, Mongay L, et al. Long-term response to imatinib is not affected by the initial dose in patients with Philadelphia chromosome-positive chronic myeloid leukemia in chronic phase: final update from the Tyrosine Kinase Inhibitor Optimization and Selectivity (TOPS) study. Int J Hematol. 2014;99(5):616–24.
75. Millot F, Guilhot J, Nelken B, Leblanc T, De Bont ES, Bekassy AN, et al. Imatinib mesylate is effective in children with chronic myelogenous leukemia in late chronic and advanced phase and in relapse after stem cell transplantation. Leukemia. 2006;20(2):187–92.
76. Deininger MW, O'Brien SG, Ford JM, Druker BJ. Practical management of patients with chronic myeloid leukemia receiving imatinib. J Clin Oncol. 2003;21(8):1637–47.
77. Marin D, Marktel S, Bua M, Armstrong L, Goldman JM, Apperley JF, et al. The use of imatinib (STI571) in chronic myelod leukemia: some practical considerations. Haematologica. 2002;87(9):979–88.
78. Steegmann JL, Baccarani M, Breccia M, Casado LF, Garcia-Gutierrez V, Hochhaus A, et al. European LeukemiaNet recommendations for the management and avoidance of adverse events of treatment in chronic myeloid leukaemia. Leukemia. 2016;30(8):1648–71.
79. Gambacorti-Passerini C, Antolini L, Mahon FX, Guilhot F, Deininger M, Fava C, et al. Multicenter independent assessment of outcomes in chronic myeloid leukemia patients treated with imatinib. J Natl Cancer Inst. 2011;103(7):553–61.
80. Saussele S, Krauss MP, Hehlmann R, Lauseker M, Proetel U, Kalmanti L, et al. Impact of comorbidities on overall survival in patients with chronic myeloid leukemia: results of the randomized CML study IV. Blood. 2015;126(1):42–9.
81. Millot F, Claviez A, Leverger G, Corbaciglu S, Groll AH, Suttorp M. Imatinib cessation in children and adolescents with chronic myeloid leukemia in chronic phase. Pediatr Blood Cancer. 2014;61(2):355–7.
82. Hughes T, Branford S. Molecular monitoring of BCR-ABL as a guide to clinical management in chronic myeloid leukaemia. Blood Rev. 2006;20(1):29–41.
83. Kaeda J, Chase A, Goldman JM. Cytogenetic and molecular monitoring of residual disease in chronic myeloid leukaemia. Acta Haematol. 2002;107(2):64–75.
84. Hughes T, Deininger M, Hochhaus A, Branford S, Radich J, Kaeda J, et al. Monitoring CML patients responding to treatment with tyrosine kinase inhibitors: review and recommendations for harmonizing current methodology for detecting BCR-ABL transcripts and kinase domain mutations and for expressing results. Blood. 2006;108(1):28–37.
85. Reinhold U, Hennig E, Leiblein S, Niederwieser D, Deininger MW. FISH for BCR-ABL on interphases of peripheral blood neutrophils but not of unselected white cells correlates with bone marrow cytogenetics in CML patients treated with imatinib. Leukemia. 2003;17(10):1925–9.
86. Branford S, Fletcher L, Cross NC, Muller MC, Hochhaus A, Kim DW, et al. Desirable performance characteristics for BCR-ABL measurement on an international reporting scale to allow consistent interpretation of individual patient response and comparison of response rates between clinical trials. Blood. 2008;112(8):3330–8.
87. Cross NC, White HE, Ernst T, Welden L, Dietz C, Saglio G, et al. Development and evaluation of a secondary reference panel for BCR-ABL1 quantification on the International Scale. Leukemia. 2016;30(9):1844–52.
88. White HE, Matejtschuk P, Rigsby P, Gabert J, Lin F, Lynn Wang Y, et al. Establishment of the first World Health Organization International Genetic Reference Panel for quantitation of BCR-ABL mRNA. Blood. 2010;116(22):e111–7.
89. Bartley PA, Ross DM, Latham S, Martin-Harris MH, Budgen B, Wilczek V, et al. Sensitive detection and quantification of minimal residual disease in chronic myeloid leukaemia using nested quantitative PCR for BCR-ABL DNA. Int J Lab Hematol. 2010;32(6 Pt 1):e222–8.
90. Modugno M, Casale E, Soncini C, Rosettani P, Colombo R, Lupi R, et al. Crystal structure of the T315I Abl mutant in complex with the aurora kinases inhibitor PHA-739358. Cancer Res. 2007;67(17):7987–90.
91. Shah NP. Ponatinib: targeting the T315I mutation in chronic myelogenous leukemia. Clin Adv Hematol Oncol. 2011;9(12):925–6.
92. Soverini S, Iacobucci I, Baccarani M, Martinelli G. Targeted therapy and the T315I mutation in Philadelphia-positive leukemias. Haematologica. 2007;92(4):437–9.
93. Gorre ME, Mohammed M, Ellwood K, Hsu N, Paquette R, Rao PN, et al. Clinical resistance to STI-571 cancer therapy caused by BCR-ABL gene mutation or amplification. Science. 2001;293(5531):876–80.
94. Corbin AS, La Rosee P, Stoffregen EP, Druker BJ, Deininger MW. Several Bcr-Abl kinase domain mutants associated with imatinib mesylate resistance remain sensitive to imatinib. Blood. 2003;101(11):4611–4.
95. O'Hare T, Deininger MW, Eide CA, Clackson T, Druker BJ. Targeting the BCR-ABL signaling pathway in therapy-resistant Philadelphia chromosome-positive leukemia. Clin Cancer Res. 2011;17(2):212–21.
96. O'Hare T, Walters DK, Stoffregen EP, Jia T, Manley PW, Mestan J, et al. In vitro activity of Bcr-Abl inhibitors AMN107 and BMS-354825 against clinically relevant imatinib-resistant Abl kinase domain mutants. Cancer Res. 2005;65(11):4500–5.
97. Mahon FX, Belloc F, Lagarde V, Chollet C, Moreau-Gaudry F, Reiffers J, et al. MDR1 gene overexpression confers resistance to imatinib mesylate in leukemia cell line models. Blood. 2003;101(6):2368–73.
98. Thomas J, Wang L, Clark RE, Pirmohamed M. Active transport of imatinib into and out of cells: implications for drug resistance. Blood. 2004;104(12):3739–45.

99. Watkins DB, Hughes TP, White DL. OCT1 and imatinib transport in CML: is it clinically relevant? Leukemia. 2015;29(10):1960–9.
100. Radich JP, Dai H, Mao M, Oehler V, Schelter J, Druker B, et al. Gene expression changes associated with progression and response in chronic myeloid leukemia. Proc Natl Acad Sci U S A. 2006;103(8):2794–9.
101. White D, Saunders V, Lyons AB, Branford S, Grigg A, To LB, et al. In vitro sensitivity to imatinib-induced inhibition of ABL kinase activity is predictive of molecular response in patients with de novo CML. Blood. 2005;106(7):2520–6.
102. Larson RA, Druker BJ, Guilhot F, O'Brien SG, Riviere GJ, Krahnke T, et al. Imatinib pharmacokinetics and its correlation with response and safety in chronic-phase chronic myeloid leukemia: a subanalysis of the IRIS study. Blood. 2008;111(8):4022–8.
103. Picard S, Titier K, Etienne G, Teilhet E, Ducint D, Bernard MA, et al. Trough imatinib plasma levels are associated with both cytogenetic and molecular responses to standard-dose imatinib in chronic myeloid leukemia. Blood. 2007;109(8):3496–9.
104. Marin D, Bazeos A, Mahon FX, Eliasson L, Milojkovic D, Bua M, et al. Adherence is the critical factor for achieving molecular responses in patients with chronic myeloid leukemia who achieve complete cytogenetic responses on imatinib. J Clin Oncol. 2010;28(14):2381–8.
105. Tefferi A, Kantarjian H, Rajkumar SV, Baker LH, Abkowitz JL, Adamson JW, et al. In support of a patient-driven initiative and petition to lower the high price of cancer drugs. Mayo Clin Proc. 2015;90(8):996–1000.
106. Baccarani M, Cortes J, Pane F, Niederwieser D, Saglio G, Apperley J, et al. Chronic myeloid leukemia: an update of concepts and management recommendations of European LeukemiaNet. J Clin Oncol. 2009;27(35):6041–51.
107. Baccarani M, Deininger MW, Rosti G, Hochhaus A, Soverini S, Apperley JF, et al. European LeukemiaNet recommendations for the management of chronic myeloid leukemia: 2013. Blood. 2013;122(6):872–84.
108. Kantarjian H, Pasquini R, Hamerschlak N, Rousselot P, Holowiecki J, Jootar S, et al. Dasatinib or high-dose imatinib for chronic-phase chronic myeloid leukemia after failure of first-line imatinib: a randomized phase 2 trial. Blood. 2007;109(12):5143–50.
109. Cortes JE, Kantarjian HM, Rea D, Wetzler M, Lipton JH, Akard L, et al. Final analysis of the efficacy and safety of omacetaxine mepesuccinate in patients with chronic- or accelerated-phase chronic myeloid leukemia: results with 24 months of follow-up. Cancer. 2015;121(10):1637–44.
110. Cortes JE, Saglio G, Kantarjian HM, Baccarani M, Mayer J, Boque C, et al. Final 5-year study results of DASISION: the dasatinib versus imatinib study in treatment-naive chronic myeloid leukemia patients trial. J Clin Oncol. 2016;34(20):2333–40.
111. Hanfstein B, Shlyakhto V, Lauseker M, Hehlmann R, Saussele S, Dietz C, et al. Velocity of early BCR-ABL transcript elimination as an optimized predictor of outcome in chronic myeloid leukemia (CML) patients in chronic phase on treatment with imatinib. Leukemia. 2014;28(10):1988–92.
112. Milojkovic D, Nicholson E, Apperley JF, Holyoake TL, Shepherd P, Drummond MW, et al. Early prediction of success or failure of treatment with second-generation tyrosine kinase inhibitors in patients with chronic myeloid leukemia. Haematologica. 2010;95(2):224–31.
113. Radich JP, Kopecky KJ, Appelbaum FR, Kamel-Reid S, Stock W, Malnassy G, et al. A randomized trial of dasatinib 100 mg versus imatinib 400 mg in newly diagnosed chronic-phase chronic myeloid leukemia. Blood. 2012;120(19):3898–905.
114. Yeung DT, Osborn MP, White DL, Branford S, Braley J, Herschtal A, et al. TIDEL-II: first-line use of imatinib in CML with early switch to nilotinib for failure to achieve time-dependent molecular targets. Blood. 2015;125(6):915–23.
115. Branford S, Yeung DT, Parker WT, Roberts ND, Purins L, Braley JA, et al. Prognosis for patients with CML and >10% BCR-ABL1 after 3 months of imatinib depends on the rate of BCR-ABL1 decline. Blood. 2014;124(4):511–8.
116. Branford S, Rudzki Z, Walsh S, Parkinson I, Grigg A, Szer J, et al. Detection of BCR-ABL mutations in patients with CML treated with imatinib is virtually always accompanied by clinical resistance, and mutations in the ATP phosphate-binding loop (P-loop) are associated with a poor prognosis. Blood. 2003;102(1):276–83.
117. Shah NP, Nicoll JM, Nagar B, Gorre ME, Paquette RL, Kuriyan J, et al. Multiple BCR-ABL kinase domain mutations confer polyclonal resistance to the tyrosine kinase inhibitor imatinib (STI571) in chronic phase and blast crisis chronic myeloid leukemia. Cancer Cell. 2002;2(2):117–25.
118. Soverini S, Gnani A, Colarossi S, Castagnetti F, Abruzzese E, Paolini S, et al. Philadelphia-positive patients who already harbor imatinib-resistant Bcr-Abl kinase domain mutations have a higher likelihood of developing additional mutations associated with resistance to second- or third-line tyrosine kinase inhibitors. Blood. 2009;114(10):2168–71.
119. Cortes JE, Khoury HJ, Kantarjian HM, Lipton JH, Kim DW, Schafhausen P, et al. Long-term bosutinib for chronic phase chronic myeloid leukemia after failure of imatinib plus dasatinib and/or nilotinib. Am J Hematol. 2016;91(12):1206–14.
120. Kantarjian H, Giles F, Wunderle L, Bhalla K, O'Brien S, Wassmann B, et al. Nilotinib in imatinib-resistant CML and Philadelphia chromosome-positive ALL. N Engl J Med. 2006;354(24):2542–51.
121. Kantarjian HM, Giles FJ, Bhalla KN, Pinilla-Ibarz J, Larson RA, Gattermann N, et al. Nilotinib is effective in patients with chronic myeloid leukemia in chronic phase after imatinib resistance or intolerance: 24-month follow-up results. Blood. 2011;117(4):1141–5.
122. Kantarjian H, Cortes J, Kim DW, Dorlhiac-Llacer P, Pasquini R, DiPersio J, et al. Phase 3 study of dasatinib 140 mg once daily versus 70 mg twice daily in patients with chronic myeloid leukemia in accelerated phase resistant or intolerant to imatinib: 15-month median follow-up. Blood. 2009;113(25):6322–9.
123. Khoury HJ, Cortes JE, Kantarjian HM, Gambacorti-Passerini C, Baccarani M, Kim DW, et al. Bosutinib is active in chronic phase chronic myeloid leukemia after imatinib and dasatinib and/or nilotinib therapy failure. Blood. 2012;119(15):3403–12.
124. Redaelli S, Piazza R, Rostagno R, Magistroni V, Perini P, Marega M, et al. Activity of bosutinib, dasatinib, and nilotinib against 18 imatinib-resistant BCR/ABL mutants. J Clin Oncol. 2009;27(3):469–71.
125. Shah NP, Guilhot F, Cortes JE, Schiffer CA, le Coutre P, Brummendorf TH, et al. Long-term outcome with dasatinib after imatinib failure in chronic-phase chronic myeloid leukemia: follow-up of a phase 3 study. Blood. 2014;123(15):2317–24.
126. Cortes JE, Kantarjian H, Shah NP, Bixby D, Mauro MJ, Flinn I, et al. Ponatinib in refractory Philadelphia chromosome-positive leukemias. N Engl J Med. 2012;367(22):2075–88.
127. Tanneeru K, Guruprasad L. Ponatinib is a pan-BCR-ABL kinase inhibitor: MD simulations and SIE study. PLoS One. 2013;8(11):e78556.
128. Lombardo LJ, Lee FY, Chen P, Norris D, Barrish JC, Behnia K, et al. Discovery of N-(2-chloro-6-methyl- phenyl)-2-(6-(4-(2-hydroxyethyl)- piperazin-1-yl)-2-methylpyrimidin-4- ylamino) thiazole-5-carboxamide (BMS-354825), a dual Src/Abl kinase inhibitor with potent antitumor activity in preclinical assays. J Med Chem. 2004;47(27):6658–61.
129. Talpaz M, Shah NP, Kantarjian H, Donato N, Nicoll J, Paquette R, et al. Dasatinib in imatinib-resistant Philadelphia chromosome-positive leukemias. N Engl J Med. 2006;354(24):2531–41.
130. Shah NP, Rousselot P, Schiffer C, Rea D, Cortes JE, Milone J, et al. Dasatinib in imatinib-resistant or -intolerant chronic-phase,

chronic myeloid leukemia patients: 7-year follow-up of study CA180-034. Am J Hematol. 2016;91(9):869–74.

131. Rasheed W, Flaim B, Seymour JF. Reversible severe pulmonary hypertension secondary to dasatinib in a patient with chronic myeloid leukemia. Leuk Res. 2009;33(6):861–4.
132. Shah NP, Wallis N, Farber HW, Mauro MJ, Wolf RA, Mattei D, et al. Clinical features of pulmonary arterial hypertension in patients receiving dasatinib. Am J Hematol. 2015;90(11):1060–4.
133. Kreutzman A, Juvonen V, Kairisto V, Ekblom M, Stenke L, Seggewiss R, et al. Mono/oligoclonal T and NK cells are common in chronic myeloid leukemia patients at diagnosis and expand during dasatinib therapy. Blood. 2010;116(5):772–82.
134. Kreutzman A, Ladell K, Koechel C, Gostick E, Ekblom M, Stenke L, et al. Expansion of highly differentiated CD8+ T-cells or NK-cells in patients treated with dasatinib is associated with cytomegalovirus reactivation. Leukemia. 2011;25(10):1587–97.
135. Mustjoki S, Ekblom M, Arstila TP, Dybedal I, Epling-Burnette PK, Guilhot F, et al. Clonal expansion of T/NK-cells during tyrosine kinase inhibitor dasatinib therapy. Leukemia. 2009;23(8):1398–405.
136. Valent JN, Schiffer CA. Prevalence of large granular lymphocytosis in patients with chronic myelogenous leukemia (CML) treated with dasatinib. Leuk Res. 2011;35(1):e1–3.
137. Schiffer CA, Cortes JE, Hochhaus A, Saglio G, le Coutre P, Porkka K, et al. Lymphocytosis after treatment with dasatinib in chronic myeloid leukemia: effects on response and toxicity. Cancer. 2016;122(9):1398–407.
138. Weisberg E, Manley PW, Breitenstein W, Bruggen J, Cowan-Jacob SW, Ray A, et al. Characterization of AMN107, a selective inhibitor of native and mutant Bcr-Abl. Cancer Cell. 2005;7(2):129–41.
139. Kantarjian HM, Giles F, Gattermann N, Bhalla K, Alimena G, Palandri F, et al. Nilotinib (formerly AMN107), a highly selective BCR-ABL tyrosine kinase inhibitor, is effective in patients with Philadelphia chromosome-positive chronic myelogenous leukemia in chronic phase following imatinib resistance and intolerance. Blood. 2007;110(10):3540–6.
140. Giles FJ, le Coutre PD, Pinilla-Ibarz J, Larson RA, Gattermann N, Ottmann OG, et al. Nilotinib in imatinib-resistant or imatinib-intolerant patients with chronic myeloid leukemia in chronic phase: 48-month follow-up results of a phase II study. Leukemia. 2013;27(1):107–12.
141. Kantarjian HM, Hochhaus A, Saglio G, De Souza C, Flinn IW, Stenke L, et al. Nilotinib versus imatinib for the treatment of patients with newly diagnosed chronic phase, Philadelphia chromosome-positive, chronic myeloid leukaemia: 24-month minimum follow-up of the phase 3 randomised ENESTnd trial. Lancet Oncol. 2011;12(9):841–51.
142. Hochhaus A, Saglio G, Hughes TP, Larson RA, Kim DW, Issaragrisil S, et al. Long-term benefits and risks of frontline nilotinib vs imatinib for chronic myeloid leukemia in chronic phase: 5-year update of the randomized ENESTnd trial. Leukemia. 2016;30(5):1044–54.
143. Le Coutre P, Rea D, Abruzzese E, Dombret H, Trawinska MM, Herndlhofer S, et al. Severe peripheral arterial disease during nilotinib therapy. J Natl Cancer Inst. 2011;103(17):1347–8.
144. Valent P, Hadzijusufovic E, Schernthaner GH, Wolf D, Rea D, le Coutre P. Vascular safety issues in CML patients treated with BCR/ABL1 kinase inhibitors. Blood. 2015;125(6):901–6.
145. Golas JM, Arndt K, Etienne C, Lucas J, Nardin D, Gibbons J, et al. SKI-606, a 4-anilino-3-quinolinecarbonitrile dual inhibitor of Src and Abl kinases, is a potent antiproliferative agent against chronic myelogenous leukemia cells in culture and causes regression of K562 xenografts in nude mice. Cancer Res. 2003;63(2):375–81.
146. Puttini M, Coluccia AM, Boschelli F, Cleris L, Marchesi E, Donella-Deana A, et al. In vitro and in vivo activity of SKI-606, a novel Src-Abl inhibitor, against imatinib-resistant Bcr-Abl+ neoplastic cells. Cancer Res. 2006;66(23):11314–22.
147. Cortes JE, Kantarjian HM, Brummendorf TH, Kim DW, Turkina AG, Shen ZX, et al. Safety and efficacy of bosutinib (SKI-606) in chronic phase Philadelphia chromosome-positive chronic myeloid leukemia patients with resistance or intolerance to imatinib. Blood. 2011;118(17):4567–76.
148. Gambacorti-Passerini C, Cortes JE, Lipton JH, Dmoszynska A, Wong RS, Rossiev V, et al. Safety of bosutinib versus imatinib in the phase 3 BELA trial in newly diagnosed chronic phase chronic myeloid leukemia. Am J Hematol. 2014;89(10):947–53.
149. Buffa P, Romano C, Pandini A, Massimino M, Tirro E, Di Raimondo F, et al. BCR-ABL residues interacting with ponatinib are critical to preserve the tumorigenic potential of the oncoprotein. FASEB J. 2014;28(3):1221–36.
150. O'Hare T, Shakespeare WC, Zhu X, Eide CA, Rivera VM, Wang F, et al. AP24534, a pan-BCR-ABL inhibitor for chronic myeloid leukemia, potently inhibits the T315I mutant and overcomes mutation-based resistance. Cancer Cell. 2009;16(5):401–12.
151. Cortes JE, Talpaz M, Kantarjian H. Ponatinib in Philadelphia chromosome-positive leukemias. N Engl J Med. 2014;370(6):577.
152. Dalzell MD. Ponatinib pulled off market over safety issues. Manag Care. 2013;22(12):42–3.
153. Breccia M, Pregno P, Spallarossa P, Arboscello E, Ciceri F, Giorgi M, et al. Identification, prevention and management of cardiovascular risk in chronic myeloid leukaemia patients candidate to ponatinib: an expert opinion. Ann Hematol. 2016;96(4):549–58.
154. Gandhi V, Plunkett W, Cortes JE. Omacetaxine: a protein translation inhibitor for treatment of chronic myelogenous leukemia. Clin Cancer Res. 2014;20(7):1735–40.
155. O'Brien S, Kantarjian H, Keating M, Beran M, Koller C, Robertson LE, et al. Homoharringtonine therapy induces responses in patients with chronic myelogenous leukemia in late chronic phase. Blood. 1995;86(9):3322–6.
156. O'Brien S, Kantarjian H, Koller C, Feldman E, Beran M, Andreeff M, et al. Sequential homoharringtonine and interferon-alpha in the treatment of early chronic phase chronic myelogenous leukemia. Blood. 1999;93(12):4149–53.
157. Cortes J, Lipton JH, Rea D, Digumarti R, Chuah C, Nanda N, et al. Phase 2 study of subcutaneous omacetaxine mepesuccinate after TKI failure in patients with chronic-phase CML with T315I mutation. Blood. 2012;120(13):2573–80.
158. Kantarjian HM, Shah NP, Cortes JE, Baccarani M, Agarwal MB, Undurraga MS, et al. Dasatinib or imatinib in newly diagnosed chronic-phase chronic myeloid leukemia: 2-year follow-up from a randomized phase 3 trial (DASISION). Blood. 2012;119(5):1123–9.
159. Saglio G, Kim DW, Issaragrisil S, le Coutre P, Etienne G, Lobo C, et al. Nilotinib versus imatinib for newly diagnosed chronic myeloid leukemia. N Engl J Med. 2010;362(24):2251–9.
160. Brummendorf TH, Cortes JE, de Souza CA, Guilhot F, Duvillie L, Pavlov D, et al. Bosutinib versus imatinib in newly diagnosed chronic-phase chronic myeloid leukaemia: results from the 24-month follow-up of the BELA trial. Br J Haematol. 2015;168(1):69–81.
161. Cortes JE, Kim DW, Kantarjian HM, Brummendorf TH, Dyagil I, Griskevicius L, et al. Bosutinib versus imatinib in newly diagnosed chronic-phase chronic myeloid leukemia: results from the BELA trial. J Clin Oncol. 2012;30(28):3486–92.
162. Lipton JH, Chuah C, Guerci-Bresler A, Rosti G, Simpson D, Assouline S, et al. Ponatinib versus imatinib for newly diagnosed chronic myeloid leukaemia: an international, randomised, open-label, phase 3 trial. Lancet Oncol. 2016;17(5):612–21.
163. Breccia M, Arboscello E, Bellodi A, Colafigli G, Molica M, Bergamaschi M, et al. Proposal for a tailored stratification at baseline and monitoring of cardiovascular effects during follow-up

in chronic phase chronic myeloid leukemia patients treated with nilotinib frontline. Crit Rev Oncol Hematol. 2016;107:190–8.
164. Breccia M, Colafigli G, Molica M, Alimena G. Cardiovascular risk assessments in chronic myeloid leukemia allow identification of patients at high risk of cardiovascular events during treatment with nilotinib. Am J Hematol. 2015;90(5):E100–1.
165. Rea D, Mirault T, Raffoux E, Boissel N, Andreoli AL, Rousselot P, et al. Usefulness of the 2012 European CVD risk assessment model to identify patients at high risk of cardiovascular events during nilotinib therapy in chronic myeloid leukemia. Leukemia. 2015;29(5):1206–9.
166. Schiffer CA. First-line treatment for patients with CML in chronic phase: why imatinib is an appropriate choice. Oncology (Williston Park). 2013;27(8):780, 825.
167. Rousselot P, Huguet F, Rea D, Legros L, Cayuela JM, Maarek O, et al. Imatinib mesylate discontinuation in patients with chronic myelogenous leukemia in complete molecular remission for more than 2 years. Blood. 2007;109(1):58–60.
168. Mahon FX, Rea D, Guilhot J, Guilhot F, Huguet F, Nicolini F, et al. Discontinuation of imatinib in patients with chronic myeloid leukaemia who have maintained complete molecular remission for at least 2 years: the prospective, multicentre Stop Imatinib (STIM) trial. Lancet Oncol. 2010;11(11):1029–35.
169. Rousselot P, Charbonnier A, Cony-Makhoul P, Agape P, Nicolini FE, Varet B, et al. Loss of major molecular response as a trigger for restarting tyrosine kinase inhibitor therapy in patients with chronic-phase chronic myelogenous leukemia who have stopped imatinib after durable undetectable disease. J Clin Oncol. 2014;32(5):424–30.
170. Goh HG, Kim YJ, Kim DW, Kim HJ, Kim SH, Jang SE, et al. Previous best responses can be re-achieved by resumption after imatinib discontinuation in patients with chronic myeloid leukemia: implication for intermittent imatinib therapy. Leuk Lymphoma. 2009;50(6):944–51.
171. Ross DM, Branford S, Seymour JF, Schwarer AP, Arthur C, Yeung DT, et al. Safety and efficacy of imatinib cessation for CML patients with stable undetectable minimal residual disease: results from the TWISTER study. Blood. 2013;122(4):515–22.
172. Hughes TP, Ross DM. Moving treatment-free remission into mainstream clinical practice in CML. Blood. 2016;128(1):17–23.
173. Ross DM, Hughes TP. How I determine if and when to recommend stopping tyrosine kinase inhibitor treatment for chronic myeloid leukaemia. Br J Haematol. 2014;166(1):3–11.
174. Lee SE, Choi SY, Song HY, Kim SH, Choi MY, Park JS, et al. Imatinib withdrawal syndrome and longer duration of imatinib have a close association with a lower molecular relapse after treatment discontinuation: the KID study. Haematologica. 2016;101(6):717–23.
175. Richter J, Soderlund S, Lubking A, Dreimane A, Lotfi K, Markevarn B, et al. Musculoskeletal pain in patients with chronic myeloid leukemia after discontinuation of imatinib: a tyrosine kinase inhibitor withdrawal syndrome? J Clin Oncol. 2014;32(25):2821–3.
176. Milojkovic D, Apperley JF. How I treat leukemia during pregnancy. Blood. 2014;123(7):974–84.
177. Pye SM, Cortes J, Ault P, Hatfield A, Kantarjian H, Pilot R, et al. The effects of imatinib on pregnancy outcome. Blood. 2008;111(12):5505–8.
178. Ault P, Kantarjian H, O'Brien S, Faderl S, Beran M, Rios MB, et al. Pregnancy among patients with chronic myeloid leukemia treated with imatinib. J Clin Oncol. 2006;24(7):1204–8.
179. Ravandi F, O'Brien SM, Cortes JE, Thomas DM, Garris R, Faderl S, et al. Long-term follow-up of a phase 2 study of chemotherapy plus dasatinib for the initial treatment of patients with Philadelphia chromosome-positive acute lymphoblastic leukemia. Cancer. 2015;121(23):4158–64.
180. Sacchi S, Kantarjian HM, O'Brien S, Cortes J, Rios MB, Giles FJ, et al. Chronic myelogenous leukemia in nonlymphoid blastic phase: analysis of the results of first salvage therapy with three different treatment approaches for 162 patients. Cancer. 1999;86(12):2632–41.
181. Goldman JM, Majhail NS, Klein JP, Wang Z, Sobocinski KA, Arora M, et al. Relapse and late mortality in 5-year survivors of myeloablative allogeneic hematopoietic cell transplantation for chronic myeloid leukemia in first chronic phase. J Clin Oncol. 2010;28(11):1888–95.

Etiology and Epidemiology of Chronic Lymphocytic Leukemia

6

Helen E. Speedy, Daniel Catovsky, and Richard S. Houlston

Introduction

Chronic lymphocytic leukemia (CLL) is an indolent malignancy resulting from an accumulation of CD5-positive neoplastic B-cells, characterized by a low rate of proliferation. CLL accounts for approximately 30% of all newly diagnosed leukemia cases each year and is the most common form of adult leukemia in Western countries [1]. Although still an incurable malignancy, recent studies have identified over 30 common genetic variants that are associated with the risk of developing CLL. Deciphering the mechanisms by which these variants influence disease risk represents the next challenge in studies of CLL susceptibility and will be key in advancing our understanding of its biological basis.

Descriptive Epidemiology

CLL is primarily a disease of later life with a median age of diagnosis in European populations of around 70 [1]. Two key features of the disease have hampered the acquisition of descriptive data on CLL. Firstly, CLL is often encountered as a chance (and often late) diagnosis and this in turn can be merely a consequence of healthcare provision rather than any true difference in disease incidence between countries. Secondly, many epidemiological studies have failed to distinguish B-cell disease including prolymphocytic leukemia and possibly lymphocytic lymphomas as part of CLL. Even accepting these caveats it is apparent that the CLL incidence rates are nearly twice as high in men as in women and that rates vary considerably throughout the world.

CLL occurrence is highest in Europe and European populations elsewhere in the world, with low rates in South and East Asia and sub-Saharan Africa (Table 6.1). The lowest recorded rates of CLL come from Japan. The observed

H.E. Speedy, Ph.D.
Division of Genetics and Epidemiology, The Institute of Cancer Research, Sutton, Surrey, London SM2 5NG, UK
e-mail: helen.speedy@icr.ac.uk

D. Catovsky, M.D., D.Sc., F.R.C.Path, F.R.C.P, F.Med.Sci
Division of Molecular Pathology, The Institute of Cancer Research, Sutton, Surrey, London SM2 5NG, UK
e-mail: daniel.catovsky@icr.ac.uk

R.S. Houlston, M.D., Ph.D., D.Sc., F.R.S., F.Med.Sci (✉)
Division of Genetics and Epidemiology, The Institute of Cancer Research, Sutton, Surrey, London SM2 5NG, UK

Division of Molecular Pathology, The Institute of Cancer Research, Sutton, Surrey, London SM2 5NG, UK
e-mail: richard.Houlston@icr.ac.uk

Table 6.1 World incidence rates of chronic lymphocytic leukemia

Race/ethnicity	Male	Female
All races	6.3	3.3
White	6.7	3.5
Black	4.9	2.4
Hispanic	2.7	1.6
Asian/Pacific Islander	1.7	0.7
American-Indian/Alaska Native	1.7	1.3
Country	**Male**	**Female**
Canada	3.7	1.8
Denmark	3.4	1.5
New Zealand	3.0	1.5
New South Wales, Australia	2.8	1.4
Tarragona, Spain	2.4	0.9
England and Wales, UK	2.3	1.1
The Netherlands	2.2	1.0
Turin, Italy	2.2	0.9
Israel Jews	2.1	1.1
Harare, Zimbabwe, Africa	1.7	1.3
Mumbai, India	0.6	0.3
Cali, Colombia	0.5	0.2
Shanghai, China	0.2	0.1
Osaka, Japan	0.1	0.0

The incidence rates are age adjusted and show cases per 100,000 per year. Race/ethnicity rates are based on Surveillance Epidemiology and End Results data on cases diagnosed in 2009–2013. Data for the incidence rates by country used with permission from Parkin DM, Whelan SL, Ferlay J, Ragmand L, Young J (eds): Cancer Incidence in Five Continents, Volume VII. IARC Sci. Publ., 1997

P.H. Wiernik et al. (eds.), *Neoplastic Diseases of the Blood*, DOI 10.1007/978-3-319-64263-5_6

30-fold variation in national rates has led many researchers to investigate a genetic basis for CLL risk. This notion is reinforced by the observation that the incidence of CLL remains low in Asians, even in those born in the United States, suggesting that genetic susceptibility rather than environmental or lifestyle factors are the greater determinant of risk [2, 3].

Environmental-Lifestyle Risk Factors

Although several environmental risk factors for acute myeloid leukemia are well recognized, such as exposure to benzene [4], smoking [5], and ionizing radiation [6], information regarding the role of chemical exposures in the development of CLL is very limited and no robust associations have so far been documented. In fact, there does not seem to be a clear association between CLL risk and any of the exposures that commonly cause other types of cancer.

Links with agricultural occupations or agricultural chemicals probably provide the strongest leads to date for environmental risk factors [7, 8]. These associations have been observed in several studies of different designs and in different geographical locations, but very few have evaluated specific agricultural agents. Excesses of CLL noted in studies of the rubber [9] and petroleum [10, 11] industries have raised the possibility of links with benzene and other solvents, but such associations remain essentially unvalidated. Other occupations that have been considered as potential risk sources for CLL include mining [12], or those with exposure to asbestos [13] and certain chemicals [14], but again no conclusive etiologic links exist.

Ionizing radiation has been implicated as a cause of most forms of leukemia for several decades, but a number of studies of highly exposed populations have not indicated an association with CLL. The justification for concluding that the risk of CLL is increased by exposure to ionizing radiation has been challenged owing to considerations such as the low background incidence rate of CLL in some studies on which the presumption is based, and the anticipated long latency between initiation and death from CLL [15]. However, a follow-up study specifically taking into account these and other confounding factors did not find a consistent association between radiation and CLL [16].

Immune Dysfunction as a Risk Factor

Intuitively, links between genetics and immune dysfunction as a possible basis for CLL are highly attractive. One study reported that infection is a constant risk in CLL that is associated with shortened survival [17]. It seems apparent that CLL tumor cells utilize immunosuppressive mechanisms to evade immune recognition. Although CLL cells express tumor antigens that can be presented by major histocompatibility complex class I and class II molecules, an effective immune response is not elicited against the tumor cells [18, 19]. However, there is no compelling evidence linking infection by human T-cell lymphotropic virus, human immunodeficiency virus, or immunosuppression following organ transplantation with CLL [20].

A variety of prior medical conditions have been reported to confer an increased risk of CLL including scarlet fever, bronchitis, and rheumatoid arthritis [21]. However, no consistent association has yet emerged and these assertions must be considered as unreliable.

Familial Clustering of CLL

Over the last seven decades more than 100 families have been reported in the literature in which clustering of CLL has been documented. While not exclusively a consequence of genetic predisposition, familial aggregation provides strong evidence for inherited genetic factors playing a role in disease development. In a number of the families reported, CLL co-segregates with other B-cell lymphoproliferative disorders (LPD), such as Hodgkin's lymphoma (HL), suggesting that part of the familial predisposition could be mediated through pleiotropic mechanisms [22–24].

Eight epidemiological case-control and cohort studies have systematically enumerated the risk of relatives of CLL patients developing CLL or other LPDs [21, 22, 25–29]. The largest and most comprehensive of these was based on an analysis of 9717 CLL cases and 38,159 controls ascertained through the Swedish Cancer Registry [27]. This study firmly underscored the notion that CLL is characterized by a high familial relative risk (RR); the RR of CLL in first-degree relatives of cases was increased 8.5-fold. Furthermore, the risk of other non-Hodgkin lymphoma (NHL) in these relatives was increased 1.9-fold. Evaluating NHL subtypes revealed a striking excess of indolent B-cell NHL, specifically lymphoplasmacytic lymphoma/Waldenström macroglobulinemia and hairy cell leukemia [27]. These findings substantiate a relationship between the risk of CLL and other LPDs which has anecdotally previously been noted in case reports of single families and that may reflect the pleiotropic effects of an inherited predisposition.

In familial CLL, the proportion of affected females is higher when compared to sporadic CLL. Females might therefore have more predisposition genes or their genes might be more penetrant than those of males. The relatives of affected females probably share the same predisposition genes, which increase their genetic liability, accounting for the higher proportion of familial cases among females compared to males.

The phenotype of earlier age of onset and increased risk of second tumors is a classical feature of many familial cancers. An early survey of 28 CLL families suggested that familial cases present around 10 years earlier than sporadic cases, implying a more aggressive clonal expansion [30]; however, more recent studies provide little support for such an assertion [31]. Anticipation, the phenomenon of intensified clinical severity and earlier age of onset with each successive generation, has been reported for CLL, with mean declines between parents and offspring being as many as 22 years [32–34]. However, findings were based on data from families ascertained for genetic studies, which are enriched for younger cases, thereby introducing bias through censoring or cohort effects. In a study using Swedish registry data where corrections were made for possible sources of bias there was little evidence to support anticipation in CLL [35].

Models of Inherited Genetic Susceptibility

The observation of large families segregating CLL in an apparent Mendelian fashion provided a strong rationale for searching for moderate–high-risk gene mutations. To date, five linkage scans of CLL families have been performed [36–40]; however none has provided robust evidence for the existence of a single major locus conferring susceptibility to the disease. The premise of these studies is that in a proportion of families with CLL, chromosomal regions that harbor mutations conferring a substantive disease risk will segregate with the affected family members.

The failure of linkage analysis to identify a high-impact CLL risk locus led to a reappraisal of the inheritance pattern in CLL and an increased interest in a polygenic model of disease susceptibility (Fig. 6.1).

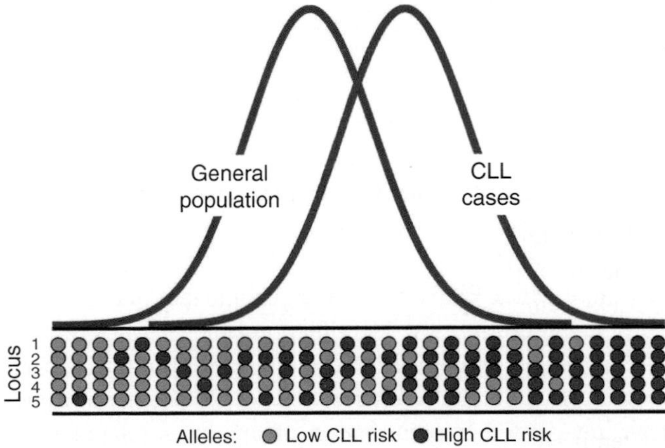

Fig. 6.1 The polygenic model of disease susceptibility. The distribution of alleles at CLL risk loci in both cases and controls follows a normal distribution. However in cases there is a shift toward an increased number of high-risk alleles. For clarity, only five risk loci are illustrated

This model, which is based on disease risk being a function of the inheritance of multiple low-risk variants, is amenable to interrogation by a genome-wide association study (GWAS) design. This approach has proved particularly successful in determining genetic risk factors for CLL and is discussed in detail below.

Common Genetic Susceptibility to CLL

The search for low-risk alleles for CLL has centered on association studies, where the frequencies of common variants (usually single-nucleotide polymorphisms, SNPs) are compared between cases and controls. Initial efforts were small-scale studies that employed a candidate gene-based approach. No susceptibility alleles have been unequivocally identified by this method which is hampered by the inherent statistical uncertainty that results from studying just a few hundred cases and controls and has only limited power to reliably identify genetic determinants conferring modest but potentially important risks [41]. Furthermore, without a clear understanding of the biology of predisposition the definition of suitable genes for the disease is inherently problematic making an unbiased approach to loci selection highly desirable.

The publication of International HapMap Consortium catalog of common human genetic variation [42] and the subsequent widespread manufacture of high-density SNP genotyping arrays revolutionized the case-control association study design. The GWAS approach assesses disease association in an unbiased manner, by comparing the frequencies of thousands of SNPs, surveyed across the genome, in a large number of cases and controls. In the past 8 years, GWAS have identified 35 independent variants at 31 genetic loci that are significantly associated with CLL risk (Table 6.2, [43–51]).

The effect size of the individual variants identified by GWAS is modest, with relative risks in the order of 1.16–1.87 per allele (Table 6.2). However, it is worth noting that the common occurrence of the risk alleles (>5% frequency) means that their cumulative burden in the population and contribution to disease incidence is high. Moreover, the burden increases with increasing numbers of variant alleles and for the 2% of the population who carry 13 or more risk alleles; the risk of CLL is increased approximately eightfold. Grouping cases and controls according to the number of risk alleles carried illustrates that the effect of these loci fits the polygenic model of inheritance (Fig. 6.1), with the number of risk alleles following a normal distribution in both cases and controls, but with a shift toward a higher number of risk alleles in cases [45].

Latest estimates suggest that common variation can explain up to 57% of the familial risk of CLL. To date, the

Table 6.2 SNPs associated with CLL risk in published genome-wide association studies

Locus	Published SNP	Nearest gene(s)	Study	SNP type	Reported OR[a]
2p22.2	rs3770745	*QPCT*	[44]	Intronic	1.24
2q13	rs13401811	*ACOXL, BCL2L11*	[44]	Intronic (*ACOXL*)	1.41
	rs17483466	*ACOXL, BCL2L11*	[47]	Intronic (*ACOXL*)	1.39
	rs9308731	*ACOXL, BCL2L11*	[43]	Intronic (*BCL2L11*)	1.19
2q33.1	rs3769825	*CASP8*	[44]	Intronic	1.19
2q37.1	rs13397985	*SP140*	[47]	Intronic	1.41
2q37.3	rs757978	*FARP2*	[45]	Missense	1.39
3p24.1	rs9880772	*EOMES*	[43]	Intergenic	1.19
3q26.2	rs10936599	*MYNN*	[51]	Synonymous	1.26
3q28	rs9815073	*LPP*	[43]	Intronic	1.18
4q25	rs898518	*LEF1*	[44]	Intronic	1.20
4q26	rs6858698	*CAMK2D*	[51]	Intergenic	1.31
5p15.33	rs10069690	*TERT*	[51]	Intronic	1.20
6p25.3	rs872071	*IRF4*	[47]	3′-UTR	1.54
6p25.2	rs73718779	*SERPINB6*	[43]	Intronic	1.26
6p21.32	rs674313	*HLA-DRB1*	[49]	Intergenic	1.87
6p21.31	rs210142	*BAK1*	[50]	Intronic	1.37
6q25.2	rs2236256	*IPCEF1, OPRM1*	[51]	3′-UTR	1.23
7q31.33	rs17246404	*POT1*	[51]	3′-UTR	1.22
8q22.3	rs2511714	*ODF1*	[51]	Intergenic	1.16
8q24.21	rs2456449	*CASC19*	[45]	Intergenic	1.26
9p21.3	rs1679013	*CDKN2B-AS1*	[44]	Intergenic	1.19
10q23.31	rs4406737	*ACTA2, FAS*	[44]	Intronic	1.27
11p15.5	rs7944004	*C11orf21*	[44]	Intergenic	1.20
11q24.1	rs735665	*GRAMD1B*	[47]	Intergenic	1.45
12q24.13	rs10735079	*OAS3, OAS1*	[48]	Intronic	1.18
15q15.1	rs8024033	*BMF*	[44]	Intergenic	1.22
15q21.3	rs7169431	*RFX7*	[45]	Intergenic	1.36
15q23	rs7176508	*PCAT29*	[47]	Intergenic	1.37
16q24.1	rs391525	*IRF8*	[49]	Intronic	1.82
	rs305061	*IRF8*	[45]	Intergenic	1.22
18q21.32	rs4368253	*PMAIP1*	[44]	Intergenic	1.19
18q21.33	rs4987855	*BCL2*	[44]	3′-UTR	1.47
	rs4987852	*BCL2*	[44]	3′-UTR	1.41
19q13.3	rs11083846	*PRKD2*	[47]	Intronic	1.35

OR odds ratio
[a]OR given is as reported in referenced study

variants identified by GWAS account for approximately 16.5% of the familial risk [43]. Therefore it seems likely that new larger studies or meta-analysis of existing datasets will provide the power to identify further common genetic variants that contribute to CLL risk. Furthermore, it is possible that some of the "missing heritability" may be explained by low-frequency variants (<1%) of intermediate effect size. The advent of next-generation sequencing, which allows high-throughput examination of whole-exome and whole-genome DNA sequences, should extend our capabilities to examine the impact of these germline variants on CLL risk.

Using Genetic Associations to Understand CLL Biology

With more than 30 regions of the genome that play a role in CLL susceptibility now identified, a somewhat clearer picture of the key biological processes involved in CLL development is beginning to emerge. Network-based approaches have revealed that perturbation of apoptosis-related pathways is an important factor in CLL with SNPs close to *BCL2L11*, *BMF*, *BCL2*, *PMAIP1*, and *BAK1* (part of the intrinsic BCL2-regulated apoptosis pathway) as well as *FAS* and *CASP8* (part of the extrinsic death receptor-led pathway) being robustly associated with CLL risk (Fig. 6.2). It is noteworthy that BH3 mimetics such as Venetoclax [52] inhibit the pro-survival BCL2 proteins, facilitating apoptosis of CLL cells, thus illustrating how GWAS discoveries could prove useful in identifying future CLL treatment targets.

GWAS findings also implicate dysfunctional lymphocyte proliferation and immune response in CLL susceptibility. *IRF4* is a strong candidate for involvement in CLL risk a priori, being a key regulator of lymphocyte development and proliferation. Moreover, *IRF4* expression is involved in the development of CLL [53] and multiple myeloma [54]. Through interaction with transcription factors including PU.1, IRF4 controls the termination of pre-B-cell receptor signaling and promotes the differentiation of pro-B-cells to small B-cells. Furthermore, via BLIMP1 and BCL6, IRF4 controls the transition of memory B-cells, thought to be a precursor cell type for CLL, to plasma cells [55–57]. A model of disease etiology based on the causal variant impairing transition of memory B-cells through reduced IRF4 expression is supported by the association of the risk allele with lower *IRF4* mRNA levels in Epstein–Barr virus (EBV)-transformed lymphocytes [47].

Variation in *IRF8* also represents a strong candidate for the association with CLL risk through its regulation of the α (alpha)- and β (beta)-interferon response. Moreover, *IRF8* is involved in B-cell lineage specification, with IRF8 deficiency skewing development of progenitor cells toward myeloid lineages at the expense of B-cells [58]. Additionally, IRF8 is implicated in immunoglobulin rearrangement and the selection of high-affinity B-cell receptor clones in the germinal center [59, 60]. It has also been shown to negatively regulate the differentiation of plasmablasts, antagonizing the actions of IRF4 [59, 61], and is a mediator of the extrinsic apoptosis pathway [62, 63].

SP140 is the lymphoid-restricted homolog of *SP100* expressed in all mature B-cells and plasma cell lines, as well as some T-cells [64, 65]. SP100 is a major mediator of EBV-encoded nuclear antigen leader protein co-activation, which is important for establishment of latent viral infections and B-cell immortalization [66]. *SP140* expression has also been

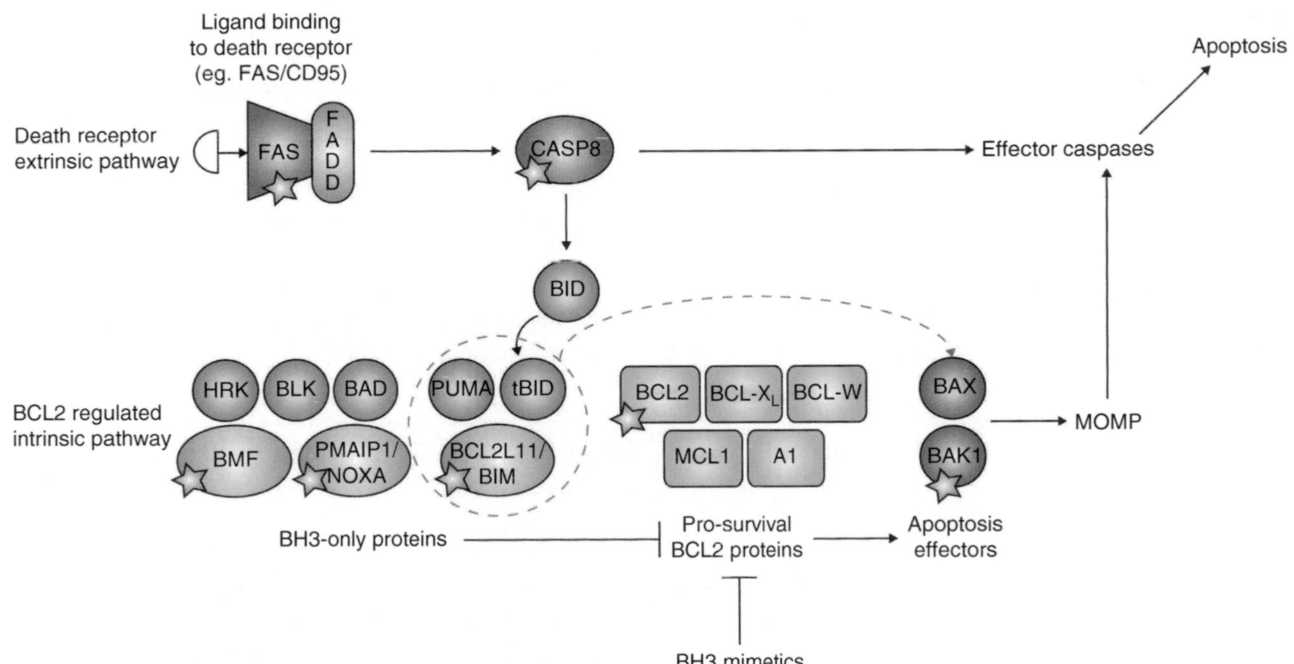

Fig. 6.2 Variation in components of the intrinsic and extrinsic apoptosis pathways is implicated in CLL predisposition. Apoptosis in humans can occur via the intrinsic or extrinsic pathway. In the intrinsic pathway, apoptotic stimuli activate the pro-apoptotic BH3-only proteins which can sequester the pro-survival B-cell CLL/lymphoma 2 (BCL2) family members, thus enabling activation of pro-apoptotic effectors BCL2-associated X protein (BAX) and BCL2-antagonist/killer 1 (BAK1). Some BH3-only proteins (surrounded by dotted line) may also directly activate BAX and BAK1, while therapeutic BH3 mimetics function by inhibiting BCL2 proteins. The pro-apoptosis effectors facilitate mitochondrial outer membrane permeabilization (MOMP), which leads to a cascade of effector caspases that culminates in cell death. The extrinsic apoptosis pathway is activated by binding of a death receptor ligand to its receptor. One such receptor is FAS (also known as CD95). Ligand-receptor engagement leads to CASP8 (caspase 8) activation via the FAS-associated death domain (FADD). Active CASP8 links to the intrinsic pathway by converting the BH3-only protein, BH3 interacting domain death agonist (BID) to truncated BID (tBID), and also feeds into the effector caspases which catalyze cellular destruction. GWAS have identified SNPs near to *BMF*, *PMAIP1*, *BCL2L11*, *BCL2*, *BAK1*, *FAS*, and *CASP8* that are associated with CLL risk, demonstrating that dysfunctional apoptosis is likely to play an important role in disease susceptibility

implicated in host response to immunodeficiency virus type 1 [67]. Another CLL susceptibility locus resides close to *OAS3* and *OAS1*. The *OAS* genes encode enzymes that produce 2′–5′-linked oligoadenylates, which in turn activate the RNaseL system to limit viral replication following infection [68]. It is therefore possible that CLL risk is increased by alterations in the immune response to viral challenge.

LEF1, encoding lymphocyte enhancer factor-1, is a member of the LEF-1/TCF family of transcription factors which acts via the Wnt signaling pathway. LEF1 is vital for the proliferation and survival of B-cells and T-cells and overexpressed in CLL compared to normal mature B-cell subsets [69, 70]. *EOMES* (eomesodermin) plays a role in CD8+ T-cell differentiation [71] and the relative levels of CD8+ T-cells expressing high levels of *EOMES* are critical in maintaining the antiviral T-cell response to chronic infection [72]. SNPs at the *EOMES* locus have also been associated with Hodgkin's lymphoma [73], as well as two autoimmune disorders: multiple sclerosis [74] and rheumatoid arthritis [75].

Mechanisms of Effect of CLL Risk Variants

Although the proximity of CLL risk variants to biologically plausible genes implicates these genes in the etiology of CLL, it remains to be elucidated exactly how the change of a single-nucleotide of DNA sequence can modulate an individual's susceptibility to CLL. Only one of the published SNPs is a missense variant. SNP rs757978 results in the substitution of threonine for isoleucine at amino acid 260 in *FARP2* (FERM, RhoGEF, and Pleckstrin Domain Protein 2) and is predicted to be deleterious by the SIFT algorithm [76].

The majority of published CLL GWAS SNPs reside within noncoding regions of the genome and it is likely that they exert their effects on CLL risk through *cis*-regulation of nearby genes. Indeed, correlations between SNP genotype and mRNA levels have been shown for a number of the risk SNPs including rs872071 and *IRF4*; rs13397985 and *SP140*; rs210134 and *BAK1;* rs10936599 and *TERC*; as well as rs10735079 and *OAS1/2/3* [77–79].

The mechanisms by which these SNPs modulate gene expression might involve mediation of chromatin accessibility, differential transcription factor binding, and/or formation of looping chromatin interactions. Such effects have recently been described for SNPs associated with type 2 diabetes [80], prostate cancer [81], and neuroblastoma [82] although perhaps the archetypal model for a noncoding variant mediating a long-range regulatory effect is demonstrated by previous work on the 8q24.21 interval in colorectal cancer. In this instance the associated SNP, rs6983267, resides 335 kb upstream of *MYC*; however the risk locus is characterized by enhancer-related histone modifications and can form chromatin loop to the *MYC* promoter and the risk variant is shown to increase binding of the transcription factor TCF4 [83–85]. Given that 8q24.21 also harbors a risk variant for CLL, which resides some 565 kb upstream of *MYC* [45], it is appealing to predict a similar mode of action. This is especially relevant because MYC and IRF4 form an auto-regulatory loop during B-cell activation [54].

Monoclonal B-cell Lymphocytosis as a Precursor Condition

The recognition that common variants influence the risk of CLL raises the possibility that, while clinically diagnosed CLL may be uncommon in the population, susceptibility may be far more common. Intriguingly this assertion is supported by the observation that CLL-phenotype B-cells (CD5+, CD23+, CD20low, sIgMlow) of monoclonal B-cell lymphocytosis (MBL) are detectable in ~3% of adults in the general population [86] and that they are essentially indistinguishable from CLL B-cells in terms of chromosomal abnormalities and *IGHV* mutation status.

The recent report that MBL develops into CLL at a rate of 1.1% per year provides direct evidence that MBL is a precursor lesion for CLL [87]. These data coupled with the observation that approximately 10% of relatives of familial CLL patients have MBL support the assertion that MBL is a surrogate marker for genetic predisposition. In an evaluation of 10 CLL risk variants in 419 MBL cases and 1753 controls, six of the risk SNPs were also significantly associated with MBL, thus providing further evidence for MBL being a precursor condition to CLL [88].

Links Between Germline Variants and the Tumor

A small number of GWAS SNPs have been associated with clinical features of CLL. For example, the *IRF8* variant rs305061 was associated with IGHV mutational status, with the risk allele correlating with poor prognosis unmutated CLL [45]. In a separate study of 840 CLL cases, carriers of the risk allele of the *IRF4* 3′UTR variant rs872071 had a significantly shorter treatment-free survival time than non-carriers [89].

Recent next-generation sequencing efforts of tumor DNA from CLL patients [90–92] have identified recurrent somatic mutations in two genes (*POT1* and *IRF4)* which also harbor common germline predisposition variants. As studies of the tumor DNA are extended, it will be of interest to note whether further overlap with germline risk factors is identified or to determine whether germline factors might predispose to particular somatic changes.

Conclusions and Reflections

Our knowledge of the role of germline genetic factors in CLL predisposition is rapidly progressing. It is now well established that the disease is characterized by having amongst the highest familial risks of any malignancy. Moreover, the observation that MBL represents a progenitor lesion offers considerable opportunities for understanding the key events in the development of CLL.

Using the GWAS approach, over 30 susceptibility loci for CLL have been identified. Further investigation of these regions to identify the causal genetic variants is likely to yield mechanistic insights into the biological basis of CLL. Building on our current understanding that impaired apoptotic processes and a dysfunctional immune response are important in disease predisposition could also help identify potential therapeutic targets.

Despite the success of GWAS, a substantial proportion of the familial risk of CLL remains unexplained. In part this may be accounted for by the presence of low-frequency variants of moderate effect size, too rare to be captured by GWAS but with lower effect sizes than would be expected in Mendelian disease. To this end, utilization of whole-exome and whole-genome sequencing strategies could help to identify additional genes involved in CLL predisposition and further advance our knowledge of this complex disease.

References

1. SEER Stat Fact Sheets. Chronic Lymphocytic Leukemia (CLL) http://seer.cancer.gov/statfacts/html/clyl.html 1975–2013 [cited 2016].
2. Gale RP, Cozen W, Goodman MT, Wang FF, Bernstein L. Decreased chronic lymphocytic leukemia incidence in Asians in Los Angeles County. Leuk Res. 2000;24(8):665–9.
3. Haenszel W, Kurihara M. Studies of Japanese migrants. I. Mortality from cancer and other diseases among Japanese in the United States. J Natl Cancer Inst. 1968;40(1):43–68.
4. Vigliani EC. Leukemia associated with benzene exposure. Ann N Y Acad Sci. 1976;271:143–51.
5. Brown LM, Gibson R, Blair A, Burmeister LF, Schuman LM, Cantor KP, et al. Smoking and risk of leukemia. Am J Epidemiol. 1992;135(7):763–8.
6. Preston DL, Kusumi S, Tomonaga M, Izumi S, Ron E, Kuramoto A, et al. Cancer incidence in atomic bomb survivors. Part III. Leukemia, lymphoma and multiple myeloma, 1950-1987. Radiat Res. 1994;137(2 Suppl):S68–97.
7. Amadori D, Nanni O, Falcini F, Saragoni A, Tison V, Callea A, et al. Chronic lymphocytic leukaemias and non-Hodgkin's lymphomas by histological type in farming-animal breeding workers: a population case-control study based on job titles. Occup Environ Med. 1995;52(6):374–9.
8. Blair A, White DW. Leukemia cell types and agricultural practices in Nebraska. Arch Environ Health. 1985;40(4):211–4.
9. Delzell E, Sathiakumar N, Graff J, Macaluso M, Maldonado G, Matthews R, et al. An updated study of mortality among North American synthetic rubber industry workers. Res Rep Health Eff Inst. 2006;132:1–63. discussion 5-74
10. Huebner WW, Chen VW, Friedlander BR, Wu XC, Jorgensen G, Bhojani FA, et al. Incidence of lymphohaematopoietic malignancies in a petrochemical industry cohort: 1983–94 follow up. Occup Environ Med. 2000;57(9):605–14.
11. Raabe GK, Wong O. Leukemia mortality by cell type in petroleum workers with potential exposure to benzene. Environ Health Perspect. 1996;104(Suppl 6):1381–92.
12. Gilman PA, Ames RG, McCawley MA. Leukemia risk among U.S. white male coal miners. A case-control study. J Occup Med. 1985;27(9):669–71.
13. Schwartz DA, Vaughan TL, Heyer NJ, Koepsell TD, Lyon JL, Swanson GM, et al. B cell neoplasms and occupational asbestos exposure. Am J Ind Med. 1988;14(6):661–71.
14. Blair A, Purdue MP, Weisenburger DD, Baris D. Chemical exposures and risk of chronic lymphocytic leukaemia. Br J Haematol. 2007;139(5):753–61.
15. Richardson DB, Wing S, Schroeder J, Schmitz-Feuerhake I, Hoffmann W. Ionizing radiation and chronic lymphocytic leukemia. Environ Health Perspect. 2005;113(1):1–5.
16. Schubauer-Berigan MK, Daniels RD, Fleming DA, Markey AM, Couch JR, Ahrenholz SH, et al. Chronic lymphocytic leukaemia and radiation: findings among workers at five US nuclear facilities and a review of the recent literature. Br J Haematol. 2007;139(5):799–808.
17. Molica S. Infections in chronic lymphocytic leukemia: risk factors, and impact on survival, and treatment. Leuk Lymphoma. 1994;13(3–4):203–14.
18. Krackhardt AM, Harig S, Witzens M, Broderick R, Barrett P, Gribben JG. T-cell responses against chronic lymphocytic leukemia cells: implications for immunotherapy. Blood. 2002;100(1):167–73.
19. Krackhardt AM, Witzens M, Harig S, Hodi FS, Zauls AJ, Chessia M, et al. Identification of tumor-associated antigens in chronic lymphocytic leukemia by SEREX. Blood. 2002;100(6):2123–31.
20. Analo HI, Akanmu AS, Akinsete I, Njoku OS, Okany CC. Seroprevalence study of HTLV-1 and HIV infection in blood donors and patients with lymphoid malignancies in Lagos, Nigeria. Cent Afr J Med. 1998;44(5):130–4.
21. Cartwright RA, Bernard SM, Bird CC, Darwin CM, O'Brien C, Richards ID, et al. Chronic lymphocytic leukaemia: case control epidemiological study in Yorkshire. Br J Cancer. 1987;56(1):79–82.
22. Goldin LR, Pfeiffer RM, Li X, Hemminki K. Familial risk of lymphoproliferative tumors in families of patients with chronic lymphocytic leukemia: results from the Swedish Family-Cancer Database. Blood. 2004;104(6):1850–4.
23. Jonsson V, Houlston RS, Catovsky D, Yuille MR, Hilden J, Olsen JH, et al. CLL family 'Pedigree 14' revisited: 1947–2004. Leukemia. 2005;19(6):1025–8.
24. Linet MS, Van Natta ML, Brookmeyer R, Khoury MJ, McCaffrey LD, Humphrey RL, et al. Familial cancer history and chronic lymphocytic leukemia. A case-control study. Am J Epidemiol. 1989;130(4):655–64.
25. Giles GG, Lickiss JN, Baikie MJ, Lowenthal RM, Panton J. Myeloproliferative and lymphoproliferative disorders in Tasmania, 1972–80: occupational and familial aspects. J Natl Cancer Inst. 1984;72(6):1233–40.
26. Goldgar DE, Easton DF, Cannon-Albright LA, Skolnick MH. Systematic population-based assessment of cancer risk in first-degree relatives of cancer probands. J Natl Cancer Inst. 1994;86(21):1600–8.
27. Goldin LR, Bjorkholm M, Kristinsson SY, Turesson I, Landgren O. Elevated risk of chronic lymphocytic leukemia and other indolent non-Hodgkin's lymphomas among relatives of patients with chronic lymphocytic leukemia. Haematologica. 2009;94(5):647–53.
28. Gunz FW, Gunz JP, Veale AM, Chapman CJ, Houston IB. Familial leukaemia: a study of 909 families. Scand J Haematol. 1975;15(2):117–31.

29. Pottern LM, Linet M, Blair A, Dick F, Burmeister LF, Gibson R, et al. Familial cancers associated with subtypes of leukemia and non-Hodgkin's lymphoma. Leuk Res. 1991;15(5):305–14.
30. Ishibe N, Sgambati MT, Fontaine L, Goldin LR, Jain N, Weissman N, et al. Clinical characteristics of familial B-CLL in the National Cancer Institute Familial Registry. Leuk Lymphoma. 2001;42(1–2):99–108.
31. Crowther-Swanepoel D, Wild R, Sellick G, Dyer MJ, Mauro FR, Cuthbert RJ, et al. Insight into the pathogenesis of chronic lymphocytic leukemia (CLL) through analysis of IgVH gene usage and mutation status in familial CLL. Blood. 2008;111(12):5691–3.
32. Horwitz M, Goode EL, Jarvik GP. Anticipation in familial leukemia. Am J Hum Genet. 1996;59(5):990–8.
33. Wiernik PH, Ashwin M, Hu XP, Paietta E, Brown K. Anticipation in familial chronic lymphocytic leukaemia. Br J Haematol. 2001;113(2):407–14.
34. Yuille MR, Houlston RS, Catovsky D. Anticipation in familial chronic lymphocytic leukaemia. Leukemia. 1998;12(11):1696–8.
35. Daugherty SE, Pfeiffer RM, Mellemkjaer L, Hemminki K, Goldin LR. No evidence for anticipation in lymphoproliferative tumors in population-based samples. Cancer Epidemiol Biomark Prev. 2005;14(5):1245–50.
36. Fuller SJ, Papaemmanuil E, McKinnon L, Webb E, Sellick GS, Dao-Ung LP, et al. Analysis of a large multi-generational family provides insight into the genetics of chronic lymphocytic leukemia. Br J Haematol. 2008;142(2):238–45.
37. Goldin LR, Ishibe N, Sgambati M, Marti GE, Fontaine L, Lee MP, et al. A genome scan of 18 families with chronic lymphocytic leukaemia. Br J Haematol. 2003;121(6):866–73.
38. Raval A, Tanner SM, Byrd JC, Angerman EB, Perko JD, Chen SS, et al. Downregulation of death-associated protein kinase 1 (DAPK1) in chronic lymphocytic leukemia. Cell. 2007;129(5):879–90.
39. Sellick GS, Goldin LR, Wild RW, Slager SL, Ressenti L, Strom SS, et al. A high-density SNP genome-wide linkage search of 206 families identifies susceptibility loci for chronic lymphocytic leukemia. Blood. 2007;110(9):3326–33.
40. Sellick GS, Webb EL, Allinson R, Matutes E, Dyer MJ, Jonsson V, et al. A high-density SNP genomewide linkage scan for chronic lymphocytic leukemia-susceptibility loci. Am J Hum Genet. 2005;77(3):420–9.
41. Sava GP, Speedy HE, Houlston RS. Candidate gene association studies and risk of chronic lymphocytic leukemia: a systematic review and meta-analysis. Leuk Lymphoma. 2014;55(1):160–7.
42. The International HapMap Consortium. A haplotype map of the human genome. Nature. 2005;437(7063):1299–320.
43. Berndt SI, Camp NJ, Skibola CF, Vijai J, Wang Z, Gu J, et al. Meta-analysis of genome-wide association studies discovers multiple loci for chronic lymphocytic leukemia. Nat Commun. 2016;7:10933.
44. Berndt SI, Skibola CF, Joseph V, Camp NJ, Nieters A, Wang Z, et al. Genome-wide association study identifies multiple risk loci for chronic lymphocytic leukemia. Nat Genet. 2013;45(8):868–76.
45. Crowther-Swanepoel D, Broderick P, Di Bernardo MC, Dobbins SE, Torres M, Mansouri M, et al. Common variants at 2q37.3, 8q24.21, 15q21.3 and 16q24.1 influence chronic lymphocytic leukemia risk. Nat Genet. 2010;42(2):132–6.
46. Crowther-Swanepoel D, Di Bernardo MC, Jamroziak K, Karabon L, Frydecka I, Deaglio S, et al. Common genetic variation at 15q25.2 impacts on chronic lymphocytic leukaemia risk. Br J Haematol. 2011;154(2):229–33.
47. Di Bernardo MC, Crowther-Swanepoel D, Broderick P, Webb E, Sellick G, Wild R, et al. A genome-wide association study identifies six susceptibility loci for chronic lymphocytic leukemia. Nat Genet. 2008;40(10):1204–10.
48. Sava GP, Speedy HE, Di Bernardo MC, Dyer MJ, Holroyd A, Sunter NJ, et al. Common variation at 12q24.13 (OAS3) influences chronic lymphocytic leukemia risk. Leukemia. 2015;29(3):748–51.
49. Slager SL, Rabe KG, Achenbach SJ, Vachon CM, Goldin LR, Strom SS, et al. Genome-wide association study identifies a novel susceptibility locus at 6p21.3 among familial CLL. Blood. 2011;117(6):1911–6.
50. Slager SL, Skibola CF, Di Bernardo MC, Conde L, Broderick P, McDonnell SK, et al. Common variation at 6p21.31 (BAK1) influences the risk of chronic lymphocytic leukemia. Blood. 2012;120(4):843–6.
51. Speedy HE, Di Bernardo MC, Sava GP, Dyer MJ, Holroyd A, Wang Y, et al. A genome-wide association study identifies multiple susceptibility loci for chronic lymphocytic leukemia. Nat Genet. 2014;46(1):56–60.
52. Souers AJ, Leverson JD, Boghaert ER, Ackler SL, Catron ND, Chen J, et al. ABT-199, a potent and selective BCL-2 inhibitor, achieves antitumor activity while sparing platelets. Nat Med. 2013;19(2):202–8.
53. Shukla V, Ma S, Hardy RR, Joshi SS, Lu R. A role for IRF4 in the development of CLL. Blood. 2013;122(16):2848–55.
54. Shaffer AL, Emre NC, Lamy L, Ngo VN, Wright G, Xiao W, et al. IRF4 addiction in multiple myeloma. Nature. 2008;454(7201):226–31.
55. Busslinger M. Transcriptional control of early B cell development. Annu Rev Immunol. 2004;22:55–79.
56. Klein U, Casola S, Cattoretti G, Shen Q, Lia M, Mo T, et al. Transcription factor IRF4 controls plasma cell differentiation and class-switch recombination. Nat Immunol. 2006;7(7):773–82.
57. Shapiro-Shelef M, Calame K. Regulation of plasma-cell development. Nat Rev Immunol. 2005;5(3):230–42.
58. Wang H, Lee CH, Qi C, Tailor P, Feng J, Abbasi S, et al. IRF8 regulates B-cell lineage specification, commitment, and differentiation. Blood. 2008;112(10):4028–38.
59. Xu H, Chaudhri VK, Wu Z, Biliouris K, Dienger-Stambaugh K, Rochman Y, et al. Regulation of bifurcating B cell trajectories by mutual antagonism between transcription factors IRF4 and IRF8. Nat Immunol. 2015;16(12):1274–81.
60. Lee CH, Melchers M, Wang H, Torrey TA, Slota R, Qi CF, et al. Regulation of the germinal center gene program by interferon (IFN) regulatory factor 8/IFN consensus sequence-binding protein. J Exp Med. 2006;203(1):63–72.
61. Carotta S, Willis SN, Hasbold J, Inouye M, Pang SH, Emslie D, et al. The transcription factors IRF8 and PU.1 negatively regulate plasma cell differentiation. J Exp Med. 2014;211(11):2169–81.
62. Burchert A, Cai D, Hofbauer LC, Samuelsson MK, Slater EP, Duyster J, et al. Interferon consensus sequence binding protein (ICSBP; IRF-8) antagonizes BCR/ABL and down-regulates bcl-2. Blood. 2004;103(9):3480–9.
63. Yang D, Thangaraju M, Browning DD, Dong Z, Korchin B, Lev DC, et al. IFN regulatory factor 8 mediates apoptosis in nonhemopoietic tumor cells via regulation of Fas expression. J Immunol. 2007;179(7):4775–82.
64. Bloch DB, de la Monte SM, Guigaouri P, Filippov A, Bloch KD. Identification and characterization of a leukocyte-specific component of the nuclear body. J Biol Chem. 1996;271(46):29198–204.
65. Dent AL, Yewdell J, Puvion-Dutilleul F, Koken MH, de The H, Staudt LM. LYSP100-associated nuclear domains (LANDs): description of a new class of subnuclear structures and their relationship to PML nuclear bodies. Blood. 1996;88(4):1423–6.
66. Ling PD, Peng RS, Nakajima A, Yu JH, Tan J, Moses SM, et al. Mediation of Epstein-Barr virus EBNA-LP transcriptional coactivation by Sp100. EMBO J. 2005;24(20):3565–75.
67. Madani N, Millette R, Platt EJ, Marin M, Kozak SL, Bloch DB, et al. Implication of the lymphocyte-specific nuclear body protein Sp140 in an innate response to human immunodeficiency virus type 1. J Virol. 2002;76(21):11133–8.
68. Sadler AJ, Williams BR. Interferon-inducible antiviral effectors. Nat Rev Immunol. 2008;8(7):559–68.

69. Reya T, O'Riordan M, Okamura R, Devaney E, Willert K, Nusse R, et al. Wnt signaling regulates B lymphocyte proliferation through a LEF-1 dependent mechanism. Immunity. 2000;13(1):15–24.
70. Tandon B, Peterson L, Gao J, Nelson B, Ma S, Rosen S, et al. Nuclear overexpression of lymphoid-enhancer-binding factor 1 identifies chronic lymphocytic leukemia/small lymphocytic lymphoma in small B-cell lymphomas. Mod Pathol. 2011;24(11):1433–43.
71. Pearce EL, Mullen AC, Martins GA, Krawczyk CM, Hutchins AS, Zediak VP, et al. Control of effector CD8+ T cell function by the transcription factor Eomesodermin. Science. 2003;302(5647):1041–3.
72. Buggert M, Tauriainen J, Yamamoto T, Frederiksen J, Ivarsson MA, Michaelsson J, et al. T-bet and Eomes are differentially linked to the exhausted phenotype of CD8+ T cells in HIV infection. PLoS Pathog. 2014;10(7):e1004251.
73. Frampton M, da Silva Filho MI, Broderick P, Thomsen H, Forsti A, Vijayakrishnan J, et al. Variation at 3p24.1 and 6q23.3 influences the risk of Hodgkin's lymphoma. Nat Commun. 2013;4:2549.
74. Patsopoulos NA, Bayer Pharma MS Genetics Working Group, Steering Committees of Studies Evaluating IFNβ-1b and a CCR1-Antagonist, ANZgene Consortium, GeneMsa, et al. Genome-wide meta-analysis identifies novel multiple sclerosis susceptibility loci. Ann Neurol. 2011;70(6):897–912.
75. Okada Y, Wu D, Trynka G, Raj T, Terao C, Ikari K, et al. Genetics of rheumatoid arthritis contributes to biology and drug discovery. Nature. 2014;506(7488):376–81.
76. Ng PC, Henikoff S. SIFT: Predicting amino acid changes that affect protein function. Nucleic Acids Res. 2003;31(13):3812–4.
77. Grundberg E, Small KS, Hedman AK, Nica AC, Buil A, Keildson S, et al. Mapping cis- and trans-regulatory effects across multiple tissues in twins. Nat Genet. 2012;44(10):1084–9.
78. Nica AC, Parts L, Glass D, Nisbet J, Barrett A, Sekowska M, et al. The architecture of gene regulatory variation across multiple human tissues: the MuTHER study. PLoS Genet. 2011;7(2):e1002003.
79. Westra HJ, Peters MJ, Esko T, Yaghootkar H, Schurmann C, Kettunen J, et al. Systematic identification of trans eQTLs as putative drivers of known disease associations. Nat Genet. 2013;45(10):1238–43.
80. Gaulton KJ, Ferreira T, Lee Y, Raimondo A, Magi R, Reschen ME, et al. Genetic fine mapping and genomic annotation defines causal mechanisms at type 2 diabetes susceptibility loci. Nat Genet. 2015;47(12):1415–25.
81. Whitington T, Gao P, Song W, Ross-Adams H, Lamb AD, Yang Y, et al. Gene regulatory mechanisms underpinning prostate cancer susceptibility. Nat Genet. 2016;48(4):387–97.
82. Oldridge DA, Wood AC, Weichert-Leahey N, Crimmins I, Sussman R, Winter C, et al. Genetic predisposition to neuroblastoma mediated by a LMO1 super-enhancer polymorphism. Nature. 2015;528(7582):418–21.
83. Pomerantz MM, Ahmadiyeh N, Jia L, Herman P, Verzi MP, Doddapaneni H, et al. The 8q24 cancer risk variant rs6983267 shows long-range interaction with MYC in colorectal cancer. Nat Genet. 2009;41(8):882–4.
84. Tuupanen S, Turunen M, Lehtonen R, Hallikas O, Vanharanta S, Kivioja T, et al. The common colorectal cancer predisposition SNP rs6983267 at chromosome 8q24 confers potential to enhanced Wnt signaling. Nat Genet. 2009;41(8):885–90.
85. Wright JB, Brown SJ, Cole MD. Upregulation of c-MYC in cis through a large chromatin loop linked to a cancer risk-associated single-nucleotide polymorphism in colorectal cancer cells. Mol Cell Biol. 2010;30(6):1411–20.
86. Rawstron AC, Green MJ, Kuzmicki A, Kennedy B, Fenton JA, Evans PA, et al. Monoclonal B lymphocytes with the characteristics of "indolent" chronic lymphocytic leukemia are present in 3.5% of adults with normal blood counts. Blood. 2002;100(2):635–9.
87. Rawstron AC, Bennett FL, O'Connor SJ, Kwok M, Fenton JA, Plummer M, et al. Monoclonal B-cell lymphocytosis and chronic lymphocytic leukemia. N Engl J Med. 2008;359(6):575–83.
88. Crowther-Swanepoel D, Corre T, Lloyd A, Gaidano G, Olver B, Bennett FL, et al. Inherited genetic susceptibility to monoclonal B-cell lymphocytosis. Blood. 2010;116(26):5957–60.
89. Allan JM, Sunter NJ, Bailey JR, Pettitt AR, Harris RJ, Pepper C, et al. Variant IRF4/MUM1 associates with CD38 status and treatment-free survival in chronic lymphocytic leukaemia. Leukemia. 2010;24(4):877–81.
90. Landau DA, Tausch E, Taylor-Weiner AN, Stewart C, Reiter JG, Bahlo J, et al. Mutations driving CLL and their evolution in progression and relapse. Nature. 2015;526(7574):525–30.
91. Puente XS, Bea S, Valdes-Mas R, Villamor N, Gutierrez-Abril J, Martin-Subero JI, et al. Non-coding recurrent mutations in chronic lymphocytic leukaemia. Nature. 2015;526(7574):519–24.
92. Ramsay AJ, Quesada V, Foronda M, Conde L, Martinez-Trillos A, Villamor N, et al. POT1 mutations cause telomere dysfunction in chronic lymphocytic leukemia. Nat Genet. 2013;45(5):526–30.

Morphology and Immunophenotype of Chronic Lymphocytic Leukemia

7

Mir Basharath Alikhan and Girish Venkataraman

Introduction

Chronic lymphocytic leukemia (CLL) is a low-grade, mature B-cell lymphoproliferative disorder (LPD) characterized by proliferation of small lymphocytes in the bone marrow and peripheral blood, often with extramedullary involvement in lymphoid tissues, such as lymph nodes and spleen [1]. The most common mature B-cell lymphoma, particularly in Western countries, CLL was first clinically described in 1845 and morphologically characterized by Minot and Isaacs in 1924 [2, 3]. Since these initial descriptions, the diagnosis of CLL is now often made by a combination of characteristic morphologic and immunophenotypic features. While the diagnosis of CLL is often straightforward based on these criteria, distinction from other mature B-cell lymphomas or reactive conditions may sometimes be challenging. Monoclonal B cell lymphocytosis is a related entity now thought to represent the precursor to overt CLL, and consists of "low-count" and "high-count" variants; the two have significant clinical and prognostic differences [4]. Recent advances in the molecular genetics of CLL necessitate further ancillary studies to ensure timely and adequate treatment, including targeted therapies, for patients requiring intervention. Although CLL is best characterized as an indolent neoplasm, progression to an aggressive lymphoma, most often either large-cell transformation or less commonly Hodgkin lymphoma transformation, occurs in 1–12% of patients [5–7]. Determination of *IGHV* mutation status, detection of certain chromosome aberrations, and positivity for immunohistochemical markers (such as CD38 and ZAP-70) can help to prognosticate patients and guide therapy.

M.B. Alikhan, M.D.
Department of Pathology, University of Chicago, 5841 S. Maryland Ave, Chicago, IL 60637, USA

G. Venkataraman, M.B.B.S., M.D. (✉)
Department of Pathology, Section of Hematopathology, University of Chicago, 5841 S Maryland Ave. TW055B, MC0008, Chicago, IL 60637, USA
e-mail: girish.venkataraman@uchospitals.edu

Definitions

CLL is a neoplasm of mature B-cells that primarily affects the bone marrow and peripheral blood, and often shows involvement of extramedullary tissues such as lymph node and spleen. According to the World Health Organization (WHO) classification criteria based on the 2008 International Workshop on Chronic Lymphocytic leukemia (IWCLL), the diagnosis of CLL can only be made in the presence of an absolute B-cell monocytosis of ≥5000 B-lymphocytes/μL in the peripheral blood for at least 3 months [1, 8]. Although most cases of CLL show a characteristic immunophenotype (B-cells with CD5 and CD23 co-expression), these features are not always present and thus not strictly required for the diagnosis [9].

The term "small lymphocytic lymphoma (SLL)" is given to neoplasms which lack a significant leukemic component and show a predominant extramedullary disease distribution, often in lymph nodes and spleen. Patients present with lymphadenopathy in the absence of any cytopenias or significant lymphocytosis. In these cases, the degree of lymphocytosis does not meet the criteria of CLL (e.g., absolute B-lymphocytosis is <5000 B-cells/μL).

On the other hand, patients with a smaller population of circulating monoclonal B-cells that do not meet the criteria for CLL and are asymptomatic (i.e., without lymphadenopathy, cytopenias, or autoimmune disease) are classified as having monoclonal B-cell lymphocytosis (MBL) [4, 10] (see Table 7.1 for timeline of important studies in MBL). This is a heterogeneous entity wherein otherwise healthy patients are found to have small populations of clonal B-cells in the peripheral blood. The term "lymphocytosis" does not refer to overall absolute lymphocytosis, but only to the monoclonal B-cells. Indeed, patients with MBL may have normal white cell peripheral blood counts. These populations of clonal B-cells are essentially absent in healthy individuals.

MBL is subclassified into three immunophenotypic categories and two clinical subtypes. With regard to the immunophenotypic subtypes of MBL, the vast majority have a typical

P.H. Wiernik et al. (eds.), *Neoplastic Diseases of the Blood*, DOI 10.1007/978-3-319-64263-5_7

Table 7.1 Timeline summary of major MBL-related studies leading up to the WHO 2016 revision

Author (year)	Comment
Marti G (2005) [10]	Publication of consensus guidelines of MBL: definition of absolute B-cell count (ABCC) <5000/μL in the absence of signs and symptoms of lymphoproliferative disorder or autoimmune disease
Swerdlow (2008) [11]; Hallek M (2008) [8]	Adoption of 2005 consensus guidelines by WHO and International Workshop on CLL
Rawstron AC (2008) [12]	Identification that cases with ABCC <1900/μL had a very low rate of progression to CLL
Rawstron AC (2010) [13]	Meta-analysis noting bimodal distribution of clonal B-cells within MBL with one peak between 0.1 and 10 B-cells/μL and another at >500/μL
Gibson (2011) [14] & Ghia (2011) [15]	Recognition of "nodal counterpart" of MBL
Vardia A (2013) [16]	Closer immunogenetic relationship of HC-MBL to Rai stage 0 CLL based on similar somatic hypermutation and BCR stereotypy
Swerdlow (2016) [17]	WHO 2016 revision emphasizing the need for closer follow-up of HC-MBL cases; disallows ability to diagnose CLL with ABCC <5000/μL with cytopenias in the absence of clinical signs or symptoms

CLL-type immunoprofile, with expression of B-cell marker CD19, co-expression of CD5 and CD23, and dim expression of CD20 and surface light and heavy chain [18]. Other, less common subtypes include the non-CLL phenotype, without expression of CD5, and atypical CLL phenotype, with co-expression of CD5 but with strong expression of CD20 and/or negative or low expression of CD23. Mantle cell lymphoma (MCL) should be excluded in those with atypical CLL phenotype while those with the non-CLL profile may be related to marginal zone or lymphoplasmacytic lymphomas [19].

More clinically important is the distinction between high-count MBL (HC-MBL) and low-count MBL (LC-MBL), based on the concentration of circulating clonal B-cells. The cutoff most widely applied to distinguish the two subtypes is 500 clonal B-cells/μL. LC-MBL is generally detected in asymptomatic patients without lymphocytosis, often as an incidental finding or in the setting of population-based studies, using high-sensitivity flow cytometry techniques. Employing eight-color flow cytometry analysis in population studies showed that CLL-like clonal B-cells are present in up to 12% of the general population, more often in the elderly [20]. In contrast, patients with HC-MBL present with lymphocytosis and are recognized in a clinical setting.

The biologic relationship between HC-MBL and CLL is significant, as 1–4% of patients with HC-MBL per year go on to develop overt CLL, highlighting the importance of lifelong follow-up of lymphocytosis [12, 21] as well as the notion that HC-MBL is an obligate precursor of CLL. LC-MBL, conversely, does not require follow-up as the risk of progression is quite low and is not considered a pre-leukemic condition [16].

Another line of evidence that supports the relationship between HC-MBL and CLL is the analysis of immunoglobulin gene repertoires. LC-MBL often shows rearrangement of the *IGHV4-59/61* gene which is rarely observed in CLL. In contrast, HC-MBL shows a repertoire more similar to CLL, such as expression of *IGHV3-23* and *IGHV4-34* [16]. Additionally, mutational analysis using massive parallel deep sequencing found similar acquired genetic mutations between HC-MBL and CLL (such as *NOTCH* and *Wnt*) [22] and was unable to distinguish between HC-MBL and Rai stage 0 CLL. Factors related to progression from HC-MBL to CLL remain largely elusive, with some suggesting that noncoding mRNAs, particularly microRNAs such as miR-155, have a role to play [23].

Finally, it is important to note that although most MBL are CLL-like with regard to immunophenotype, non-CLL forms exist. In these cases, the diagnostic considerations include mantle cell lymphoma (in CD5+, CD23− cases; atypical CLL-like) or marginal zone lymphoma (in CD5− cases; non-CLL) [24]. Appropriate ancillary studies should be carried out to exclude these entities.

Epidemiology and Clinical Aspects

CLL is the most common adult mature B-cell leukemia in the Western world, where it accounts for 30% of all leukemias in this population. The incidence increases in the elderly and the median age at diagnosis is about 70 years [25]. Similarly, the incidence of MBL also increases with advanced age, paralleling CLL. Familial cases of CLL have also been described [26]. It is estimated that in 2016, the about 19,000 new cases of CLL will be diagnosed in the United States and about 5000 patients will die of the disease [25]. SLL accounts for about 7% of all non-Hodgkin lymphomas and also tends to occur in elderly males.

Due to more accurate and sensitive diagnostic techniques, the vast majority of CLL patients (up to 70%) are asymptomatic at presentation [27, 28], and the disease is often detected as an incidental finding on routine complete blood counts, which, in most cases, will show preserved hematopoietic cell lineages. Symptomatic patients may show cytopenias, which is most often due to infiltration of the bone marrow by leukemic cells. Autoimmune cytopenias are fairly frequently described in CLL and may affect all three cell lines. Anemia may also be attributed to immune-mediated destruction of red blood cells or red cell precursors (pure red cell aplasia). Although multiple mechanisms are postulated, one line of evidence suggests that CLL B-cells may act as antigen-processing cells which take up red cell antigens, and induce a secondary T-cell activation which in turn leads to activation of normal B-cells resulting in red cell antibody production and consequent destruction of red cells [29]. Hypogammaglobulinemia may also be present at the time of diagnosis in up to half of cases.

Extramedullary disease in CLL/SLL comes to clinical attention most often as lymphadenopathy and, less commonly, splenomegaly. Not uncommonly, it is diagnosed on lymphadenectomy specimens excised for other tumors, such as carcinomas [30]. Lymphocytic infiltrates can be found in a variety of other anatomic sites, such as gastrointestinal tract, kidney, liver [31], and skin. However, with the exception of possibly the latter two sites, these often do not manifest clinically and are detected as part of routine workup. Cutaneous involvement by CLL can present at localized disease or generalized erythematous papules, plaques, nodules, or tumors [32]. Rare sites of involvement include Waldeyer's ring, thyroid, lung, gallbladder, prostate, central nervous system, leptomeninges, serosal surfaces, and other sites [33–38].

Cell of Origin and Pathogenesis

The understanding of CLL leukemogenesis has undergone considerable modifications in the past few years. Most now agree that CLL derives from an antigen-experienced B-cell that can be of two general subtypes: either with somatic mutations in the variable genes of the immunoglobulin heavy-chain gene (*IGHV*), termed "mutated CLL" which are derived from CD5+/CD27+ post-germinal center B-cells, or with germline configuration (or low-level somatic hypermutation) of the gene, referred to as unmutated CLL which in turn are derived from CD5+/CD27− mature B-cells.

At a molecular level, unmutated CLL is defined as having at least 98% sequence homology to the germline [39]. Mutated CLL characterizes the majority of cases. In both subtypes, initial inducing mutations in the B-cell provide a growth advantage [40]. Unmutated CLL cells express surface immunoglobulin receptors with relatively more intact/functional BCR signaling pathway that can be activated by multiple antigens such as auto-antigens and carbohydrate components of microbes. Repetitive stimulation of the induced B-cells by these antigens results in clonal proliferation and leukemia. In contrast, CLL cells with mutated *IGHV* genes do not have the polyreactivity seen in unmutated CLL cells, and their ability to proliferate is relatively diminished compared to the latter. In some cases, anergy develops due to excessive B-cell receptor stimulation, leading to compromise of antigen binding and subsequent apoptosis.

However, changes in the B-cell receptor signaling pathway promote expansion of the leukemic clone and development of CLL. In particular, CLL cells overexpress Toll-like receptor 9 (TLR9), an innate immune receptor that responds to bacterial unmethylated cytosine guanine dinucleotide (CpG) oligodeoxynucleotides (ODNs) [41]. When stimulated, TLR9, through coregulation with MYD88, induces the NF-κB pathway, resulting in apoptosis. Some have suggested that this pathway may be exploited through TLR9 stimulators, such as CpG ODNs [42]. Zeta-associated protein 70 (ZAP70, see below) is often seen in unmutated CLL. In such cases, activation of TLR9 leads to ZAP70-dependent activation of spleen tyrosine kinase (Syk). This results in the degradation of proapoptotic protein Bim, leading to survival of the CLL clone. Additionally, activation of Syk leads to downstream production of autoreactive IgM, which binds the B-cell receptor complex and, in an autocrine manner, causes a continual positive feedback loop [43]. This model may explain why unmutated status of CLL has a poor prognosis compared to the mutated type, as the former is subject to constant antigenic stimulation and production of leukemic subclones [44] as well as increased tumor cell survival. Interestingly, up to 30% of unmutated CLL show similar B-cell receptors, suggesting that a unique set of antigens is responsible for clonal expansion. One may speculate that stimulation at the pre-CLL stage by antigens such as an environmental agent, i.e., a virus or commensal bacteria, or specific autoantigen is responsible for leukemic proliferation [45–47].

Additional lines of evidence that supports the derivation of CLL cells from activated B-cells as opposed to naïve B-cells as was previously thought include similar gene expression profiling data to memory B-cells, presence of mRNA for various cytokines, and expression of memory cell markers such as CD27, regardless of mutational status [48, 49]. The activated B-cell may arise from the marginal zone of follicles or from germinal centers. Those arising from germinal centers require T-cell activation and mutation of *IGHV* genes. In contrast, CLL cells from the marginal zones may or may not require T-cell activation, and only a subset show mutation of *IGHV* genes.

Although the putative normal counterpart of the CLL cell is thought to be an antigen-experienced memory B-cell as outlined above, some studies have shown that the earliest genetic changes leading to CLL can be found in hematopoietic stem cell (HSC). In particular, HSCs from patient will CLL were successfully engrafted into immunodeficient mice and resulted in clonal B-cell lymphoproliferations [50]. The data suggest that these HSCs are primed towards the B-cell lineage and subsequent clonal proliferation.

Morphology of CLL/SLL

Peripheral Blood

Involvement of peripheral blood is required in the diagnosis of CLL and is often the initial mode of diagnosis. As mentioned above, there is absolute lymphocytosis with monoclonal B-cells exceeding a concentration of 5000/μL. The overall white cell count may be normal or elevated. Patients may be anemic, which is most often attributed to leukemic infiltration of the bone marrow, although autoimmune erythrocyte destruction is also common at the time of diagnosis.

The circulating leukemic cells of CLL are often monotonous, small- to medium-sized lymphocytes with fairly round and even nuclear membranes, scant agranular, basophilic cytoplasm, inconspicuous nucleoli, and exaggerated clumping of nuclear chromatin. This latter feature is often characterized as a "cracked mud," "chocolate chip cookie," or "soccer ball" appearance of the nuclei on well-stained smears (Fig. 7.1). The cytoplasm may contain vacuoles or crystals and can occasionally be more abundant. Cytoplasmic inclusions containing immunoglobulin have also been described [51]. Smudge cells (Fig. 7.1) are often observed due to the tendency of leukemic cells to be easily disrupted during smear preparation. This is an important clue to the diagnosis of CLL as this feature is lacking or rare in most other B-cell leukemias when analyzing well-prepared smears. The addition of albumin to the peripheral blood can prevent the disruption of leukemic cells and the presence of smudge cells on the smear [52].

Cells with more abundant cytoplasm and a prominent single nucleolus are termed *prolymphocytes* and often constitute less than 10% of the total leukemic cells (Fig. 7.1). If they predominate, the diagnosis of B-cell prolymphocytic leukemia (B-PLL) should be considered, which is defined as a mature B-cell leukemia with greater than 55% prolymphocytes. A patient diagnosed with typical CLL who is found to have rising numbers of prolymphocytes on follow-up smears may represent transformation to a higher grade leukemia. Other patients may present with large numbers of prolym-

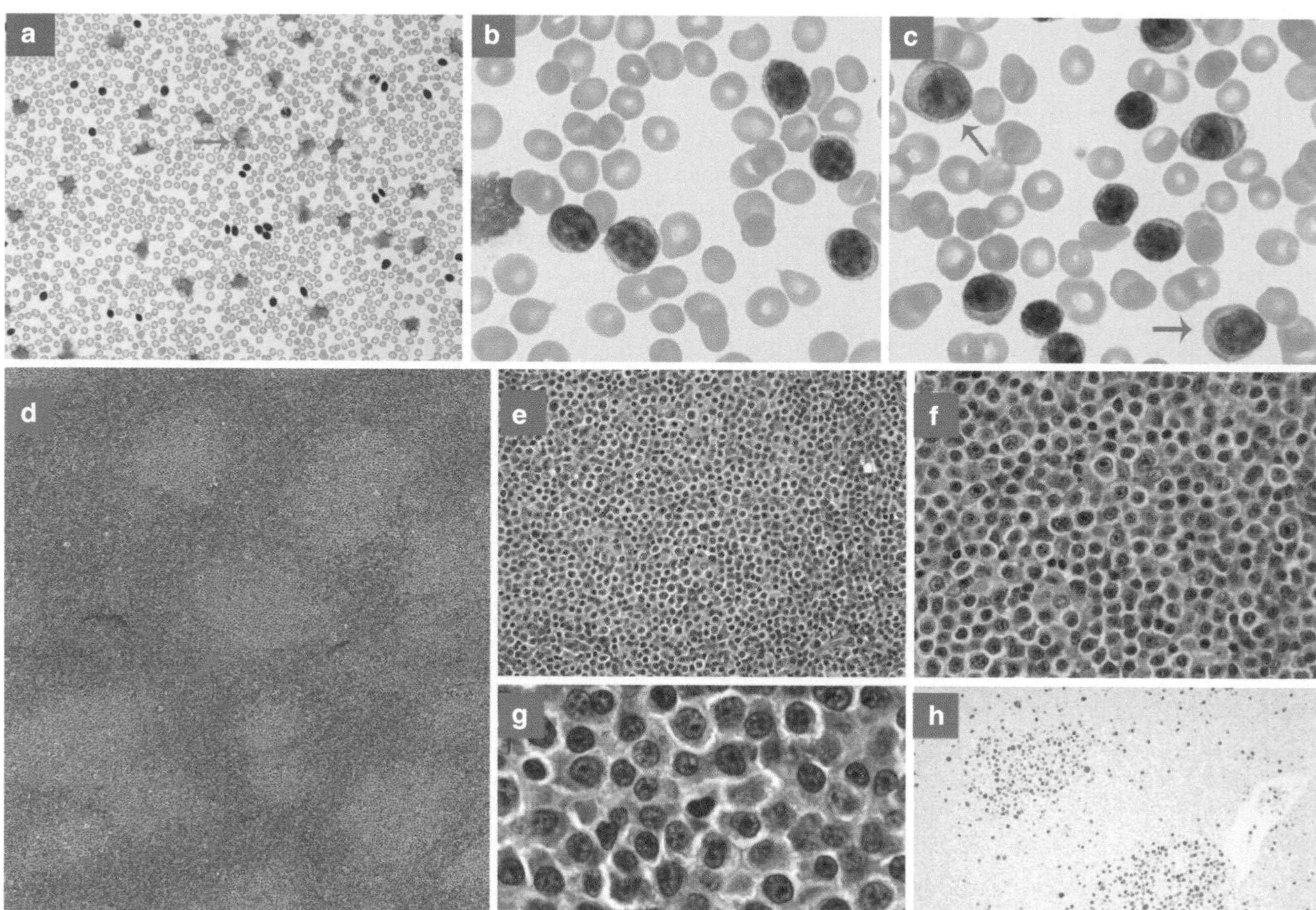

Fig. 7.1 CLL morphology in peripheral blood and lymph nodes: (**a**) Peripheral blood with absolute lymphocytosis and numerous smudge cells (*arrow*) which are sheared CLL cells with fragile cytoplasmic membranes. This smudging can be prevented by incubating the cells with bovine albumin before preparing the smear. (**b**) High power of CLL cells in peripheral blood demonstrated small CLL cells with typical "cracked-mud" chromatin and inconspicuous nucleoli. (**c**) CLL with trisomy 12 demonstrating increased number of larger cells with prominent nucleoli consistent with prolymphocytes. (**d**) Low-power histology of CLL with diffuse sheets of small lymphoid cells and associated nodular clusters of pale areas called "growth centers/proliferation centers." CLL is probably unique in being the only lymphoma exhibiting such proliferation. (**e, f**) High-power views of a growth center with scattered prolymphocytes and paraimmunoblasts that are larger cells with prominent nucleoli (H&E stain). (**g**) High-power view of CLL cells in lymph node demonstrating clumped nuclear chromatin and inconspicuous nucleoli. (**h**) Growth centers with proliferating cells (Ki-67 immunostain)

phocytes in the blood that remain stable throughout the disease course. A recent study found that increased circulating prolymphocytes at presentation with distinct immunohistochemical and genetic variation from classic CLL was an independent adverse prognostic factor with frequent progressive disease to Richter transformation and shorter overall survival [53].

Slight differences in the classic morphology may be observed. The nuclear contours can sometimes be irregular and mildly indented and/or the lymphoid cells are larger. In cases of typical CLL, these account for less than 2% of the leukemic cells. When they are more abundant, the diagnosis of *atypical* CLL should be considered (see below). In such cases, cytogenetic analysis should be performed as specific findings have been linked with atypical morphology, particularly trisomy 12, which can present with slightly higher numbers of prolymphocytes or CLL cells with atypical morphology (Fig. 7.1) [39, 54–56].

Plasmacytoid differentiation can also be observed in atypical CLL and has morphologic overlap with lymphoplasmacytic lymphoma. Patients may present with an IgM paraprotein, but levels often do not exceed 3 g/dL. The morphologic features often lead to diagnostic difficulty, but the presence of prolymphocytes/paraimmunoblasts, proliferation centers, and typical CLL/SLL immunophenotype aids in the diagnosis of CLL/SLL over lymphoplasmacytic lymphoma in such cases [57]. Some have suggested a possible association with del(7)(q32) [58].

Uncommonly, Reed-Sternberg-like cells can be observed in otherwise typical cases of CLL/SLL, characterized by the presence of rare or occasionally large, pleomorphic cells. Only if a distinct region of the biopsy has typical Hodgkin inflammatory background can the diagnosis of transformation to Hodgkin lymphoma be rendered [59]; sparse presence of R-S-like cells in otherwise extensive small lymphocytic proliferation is not diagnostic of transformation. Epstein-Barr virus is often detected in these cases.

A recent study suggests that increased circulating monocyte-derived cells promote CLL survival through cell-cell interactions and secreted factors and thus worse patient outcomes. Indeed, increased monocytes were found to be an adverse prognostic factor leading to decreased time to first therapy and overall survival [60].

In all cases of atypical CLL, cytogenetic analysis should be performed, as studies have consistently shown adverse prognosis, more severe cytopenias, worse lymphocytosis at presentation, and more rapid disease progression [61]. Such cases can also show immunohistochemical differences from classic CLL and the results can overlap with other B-cell lymphoproliferative disorders such as mantle cell lymphoma, lymphoplasmacytic lymphoma, and marginal zone lymphoma [62].

Bone Marrow

Although the bone marrow is invariably involved in virtually all cases of CLL, bone marrow biopsy examination is not required to render the diagnosis. However, the biopsy may be helpful in assessing the degree of involvement and aid in correlation with peripheral blood cell counts in cases presenting with cytopenias. Leukemic cells in the marrow aspirate are morphologically similar to those in the peripheral blood (Fig. 7.2) and often comprise greater than 30% of all nucleated cells. However, the percentage of CLL cells may differ, due to the multifocal nature of the disease in the marrow. In view of this, examination of an adequate bone marrow trephine biopsy (greater than 10 mm in length, but preferably up to 20 mm, taken from the posterior iliac crest) provides more useful information with regard to the extent of involvement [63]. Additionally, the histologic pattern of involvement can aid in the diagnosis of CLL and help exclude other lymphomas in the differential.

Various patterns of CLL infiltration may be observed, and multiple patterns can be observed within the same bone marrow biopsy. The most common architectural pattern seen is multifocal, interstitial nodular involvement (Fig. 7.2). Importantly, the nodules are non-paratrabecular, in contrast to bone marrow infiltrates of follicular lymphoma, which characteristically show paratrabecular localization. On low-power examination of the biopsy, the nodular interstitial infiltrates are readily identifiable due to their darker appearance compared to the surrounding hematopoietic marrow. On higher magnification, the cells are small with round nuclei, inconspicuous nucleoli, and a clumped chromatin pattern. The edges of the nodules may show diffusion of the leukemic cells into the marrow interstitium. Proliferation centers that harbor prolymphocytoid cells are common in lymph nodes involved by CLL/SLL, but not usually observed in the marrow. The presence of germinal centers (interfollicular pattern) is quite rare; their presence should prompt exclusion of other lymphomas [64].

Other common patterns include a more diffuse interstitial infiltrate wherein the leukemic cells are in close association with and interspersed between the normal hematopoietic marrow elements with effacement of the overall marrow architecture. These areas are more difficult to identify on low-power examination than the nodular infiltrates. However, they often impart a slightly darker appearance than the surrounding normal marrow elements. Less commonly, solid growth of leukemic cells replacing the marrow elements can be seen. In such cases, peripheral cytopenias are expected, which can predict a more aggressive disease and worse overall outcome. Some studies have demonstrated that a solid growth pattern is linked with expression of the 70-kDa zeta-associated protein (ZAP-70) and unmutated status of *IGHV*, which is thought to confer a worse prognosis [65, 66].

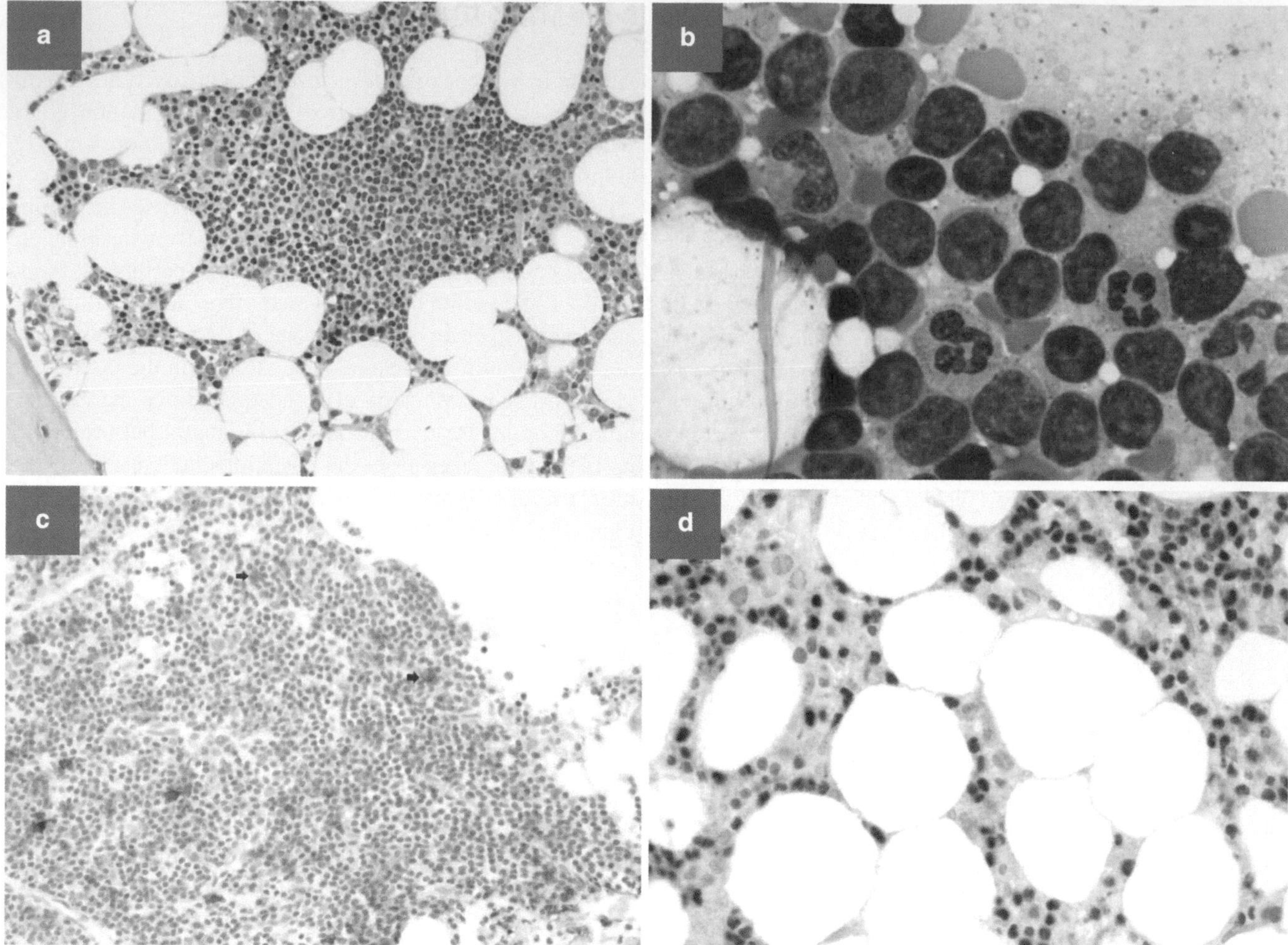

Fig. 7.2 Bone marrow in CLL: (**a**) Nodular infiltrate of small lymphoid cells of CLL involving the interstitial areas of the marrow. (**b**) High-power view of CLL cells in the marrow aspirate. (**c**) CD20 immunostain in a CLL with very dim expression in a subset of the B-cells (*arrow*). CD20 may also be downregulated after rituximab-containing regimens such as fludarabine, cyclophosphamide, and rituximab (FCR). In such cases, Pax5 may be more helpful. (**d**) Pax5 immunostain highlights prominent interstitial infiltrate of CLL cells

Marrow involvement can be detected in most MBL cases and with three different patterns described (focal interstial, nodular and diffuse interstitial) in one study examining 26 MBL cases (CLL-like, atypical CLL-like, and non-MBL types). In this study focal interstitial pattern was the most common pattern observed in most CLL-like and atypical CLL-like MBL. Uncommonly, the bone marrow may be the first detected site of involvement by transformed CLL, showing enlarged, atypical lymphoid cells that differ from the usual small cells of classic CLL [67].

Marrow biopsy is often performed to assess the underlying cause of cytopenias which may be secondary to diffuse involvement of the marrow by leukemic cells or autoimmune destruction of one or more cell lineages. The presence of erythroid hyperplasia in an anemic patient may suggest peripheral red cell destruction due to autoimmune disease, which is not an uncommon presentation in CLL patients [68]. Anemia without a marrow response can indicate the rare instance of pure red cell aplasia [69]. In turn, red cell aplasia can result as a result of direct immune destruction by activated B-cells or evolve as a result of secondary T-large granular lymphocyte expansion in the context of CLL.

Another advantage of assessing the bone marrow biopsy is the ability to perform immunohistochemical stains, particularly when fresh cells are not available for flow cytometric analysis. The immunophenotype by immunohistochemistry would be similar to results of flow cytometry (see below). However, some important caveats when assessing immunohistochemistry results include careful evaluation of CD20 staining. As in flow cytometry, CD20 expression can be dimmer than the surrounding normal B-cells (Fig. 7.2). In patients that have undergone anti-CD20 immunotherapy, CD20 expression can be lost and hence may not be reliable in picking up the CLL population. In these cases, staining with PAX5 (Fig. 7.2) can be helpful to determine B-cell lineage.

Lymph Node

The predominant pattern of lymph node involvement by CLL/SLL is diffuse effacement of the nodal architecture. The lymph node follicles and sinuses are often obliterated, and the neoplastic cells can extend into the surrounding adipose tissue. The predominant neoplastic cell is small to medium sized with clumped chromatin, inconspicuous nucleoli, and scant cytoplasm (Fig. 7.1), imparting a dark appearance to most of the affected lymph node. The nucleus is most often round, but can have some irregularity or cleaving which may cause diagnostic confusion with follicular lymphoma or mantle cell lymphoma.

Characteristically, proliferation centers (so-called pseudofollicles) are present throughout the node as part of the diffuse architectural effacement and are characterized by paler staining areas compared to the darker zones of the remainder of the neoplasm (Fig. 7.1). The lighter staining is due to involvement of the proliferation centers by larger lymphoid cells: prolymphocytes and paraimmunoblasts (see below and Fig. 7.1). Prolymphocytes in the lymph node are medium-sized cells with more abundant cytoplasm and a more prominent nucleolus compared to the predominant CLL cells. Paraimmunoblasts are larger, with a wider rim of cytoplasm, dispersed chromatin, and a distinct central eosinophilic nucleolus.

The more abundant cytoplasm of these cells causes separation between the tumor nuclei and imparts the lighter appearance. The contrast can be better appreciated at low-power light microscopy if the light is dimmed. Proliferation centers can also be assessed using a marker of DNA synthesis, such as Ki-67, which would be high in the proliferation centers and virtually negative in the remainder of the lymphoma (Fig. 7.1). If such areas dominate the lymph node histology, concern for high-grade transformation to a large-cell lymphoma should be considered.

Proliferation centers can mimic germinal centers of a normal follicle. However, the absence of a distinct mantle zone and apoptotic debris can be histologic clues of a proliferation center rather than a germinal center. Additionally, immunohistochemical study would show that the cells of proliferation centers are CD10−, Bcl6−, and Bcl2+, in contrast to normal germinal centers [70]. Rarely proliferation centers may also express cyclin D1 but there is no underlying *IgH/CCND1* translocation in these cases [71].

Variant patterns of lymph node involvement are less common and include an interfollicular architecture where the neoplastic cells surround remnant reactive lymph node follicles [72]. A perifollicular pattern is also described. These may lead to diagnostic confusion with follicular lymphoma, marginal zone lymphoma, or mantle cell lymphoma. Helpful features in the diagnosis of CLL/SLL include presence of proliferation centers, absence of cyclin D1 immunostaining, and characteristic immunoprofile (see below). As mentioned above, Reed-Sternberg-like cells can be observed in cases of CLL/SLL. If rare or occasional, they are not considered to represent transformation to Hodgkin lymphoma (HL). However, if more abundant and present with the typical milieu seen in HL, the concern for transformation is much higher.

Spleen

Splenic involvement by CLL is almost always present as part of the generalized disease. However, the degree of involvement is variable. Spleens are almost always enlarged, sometimes to massive weights, but the capsule is usually not compromised [73]. On gross examination, there is a miliary pattern of involvement, with 0.2–1.5 cm micronodules present throughout the cut surface. Histologically, the white pulp is replaced and expanded by proliferation of the small leukemic cells of CLL, similar to the predominant cells seen in the lymph nodes. In contrast to the lymph node morphology, proliferation centers with prolymphocytes and paraimmunoblasts are not usually observed. The tumor often infiltrates into the red pulp cords and sinuses and will extend along the periarteriolar lymphoid sheaths and splenic trabeculae [74, 75].

Other Organs

Although the liver is commonly involved in CLL, clinically apparent hepatic dysfunction is not common [76]. The leukemic cells often infiltrate the portal tracts and less commonly the sinuses can also be involved. The neoplasm can be mistaken for inflammatory infiltrates of hepatitis, for example. However, the monotonous nature of the lymphoid cells and characteristic immunophenotype can help to distinguish the two entities.

Cutaneous involvement can present in a variety for different clinical forms, including plaques, nodules, or tumors. Histologically, the dermis shows leukemic infiltrates that tend to be localized around vascular and adnexal structures [32].

The gastrointestinal tract, central nervous system, and other organs can also be involved, albeit rarely, and are often seen only on autopsy specimens as "case reports" in the literature [77–79].

Immunophenotype of CLL

Immunophenotyping of CLL is one of the most essential aspects of diagnosis and prognosis of the disease, allowing for differentiation between reactive conditions and other lymphoproliferative disorders as well as assessment of adverse prognostic markers. The most useful, rapid, and efficient method of immunophenotyping is multicolor flow cytometry, which allows for multiparameter testing with multiple antibodies, and facilitates determination of the strength of antigen expression. Most tissues can be submitted for flow cytometry, the easiest being peripheral blood, but also bone marrow aspirates and freshly procured solid tissues such as lymph nodes, following disaggregation. Immunophenotyping on solid, fixed tissues with immunohistochemistry can also be useful in cases when fresh tissue or peripheral blood is not available for analysis.

In the typical form of CLL, neoplastic cells show moderate expression of CD19 and the nuclear B-cell transcription factor PAX5, supporting a B-lymphocytes lineage [80]. Other B-cell antigens are characteristically downregulated (Fig. 7.3) and show weak/dim expression, such as CD20, CD79a/b, and surface immunoglobulin (Fig. 7.3), which is usually IgD with or without IgM. Expression of other immunoglobulin heavy chains (IgG or IgA) is uncommon. This low expression of CD20 and Ig is quite unique to CLL and is an important differentiating clue between this and other B-cell lymphoproliferative disorders [8, 28]. Mechanistically, the low sIg levels in CLL are thought to result from altered glycosylation and folding of the CD79a and μ chains although the BCR signaling remains intact [81].

Another important marker is the co-expression of CD5, a T-cell antigen (Fig. 7.3). Compared to the background T-cells, CD5 expression is slightly weaker. CD5+ B cells can be found normally in the mantle zones of secondary follicles. Additionally, regenerating naïve B-cell can also express CD5 [82]. The co-expression of CD5 can also be observed in mantle cell lymphoma. However, MCL does not show the weak expression of most B-cell markers as does CLL, and often does not express CD23. Immunohistochemistry for cyclin D1 is present in most cases of MCL, in contrast to typical cases of CLL.

CD23 is a low-affinity receptor for IgE and an adhesion molecule that is expressed by naïve B-cells. It is normally

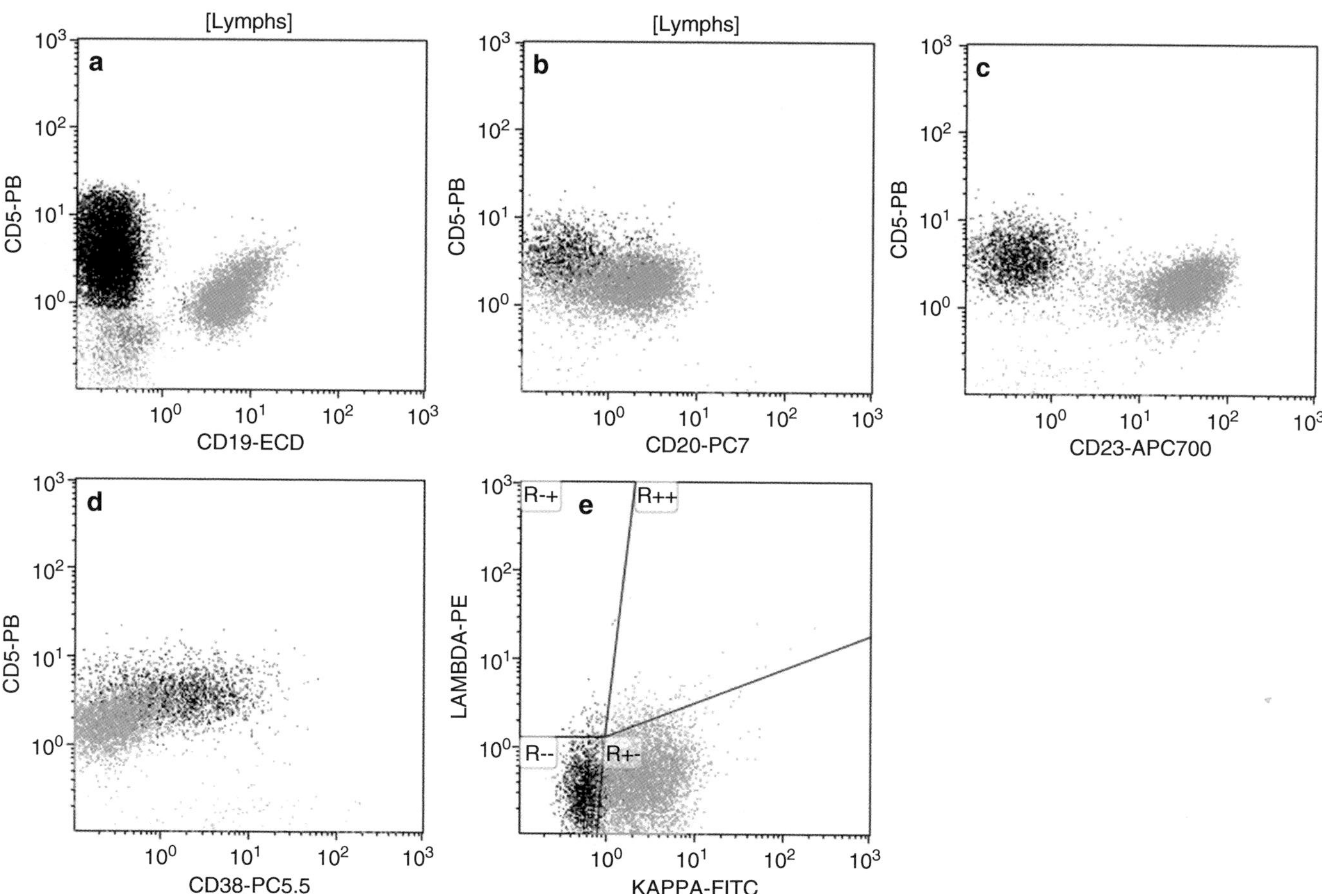

Fig. 7.3 Flow cytometry of CLL: (**a**) The CLL cells are marked *green* and express CD19 (**b**) The CD5 + CLL cells express dim-negative CD20 with slightly dimmer CD5 compared to the T-cells (*violet*). (**c**) There is co-expression of CD23, but the CLL cells are negative for CD38 (**d**) and express dim surface-restricted kappa immunoglobulin light chain (expression level is barely more than the background light chain-negative T-cells) (**e**)

lost after the germinal center reaction in the process of memory B-cell formation. Some have suggested that CD23 correlates with proliferative activity in CLL [83]. Most cases of CLL show expression of CD23 (Fig. 7.3), in contrast to other B-cell neoplasms, such as mantle cell lymphoma. FMC7, an epitope on the CD20 molecule that is expressed by most MCL, is often negative in CLL, although up to 15% of cases can be positive for this marker [84, 85], especially in cases with bright CD20 and Ig positivity.

Bcl-2 is overexpressed in CLL and is related to resistance of apoptosis in the tumor cells, conferring a survival advantage [86]. The mechanism of overexpression in follicular lymphoma is related to the recurrent translocation t(14;18). This is not the case with CLL; rather, hypomethylation of DNA is felt to be the mechanism driving Bcl-2 overexpression [87]. With the advent of selective inhibitors of Bcl-2, the overexpression of the molecule on CLL cells is now more clinically relevant [88, 89].

CD11c, a marker often seen in hairy cell leukemia and B-cell prolymphocytic leukemia, can be observed in CLL. However, the intensity of positivity in cases of CLL, when evaluated by flow cytometry, is usually less than what is observed in hairy cell leukemia (dim negative in most cases), providing a clue to differentiate the two neoplasms using this marker [90].

Among CLL prognostic markers, CD38 and ZAP-70 are the most studied and prognostically important. CD38 is a membrane protein that functions as an adenosine diphosphate ribosyl cyclase. Downstream, this enzymatically controls intracellular calcium levels and is a marker for cell activation [91]. Analysis by flow cytometry would yield three patterns of CD38 positivity: uniformly negative (Fig. 7.3), uniformly positive, and a bimodal pattern with only a subset of the CLL population showing expression [92]. The latter two patterns are associated with unmutated *IGHV* in most cases, which is implicated in poor prognosis. Although a cutoff of 20% positive cells in the tumor has been proposed by some authors, the presence of smaller CD38+ subpopulations (e.g., <10%) may be significant to predict unmutated *IGHV* status. A subset of cases, up to 30% in some studies, shows discordant results with *IGHV* mutation status. In this regard, CD38 positivity is thought to be an independent prognostic factor in CLL [93, 94].

ZAP-70 is not normally expressed in B-cells, but is a tyrosine kinase involved in T-cell receptor signal transduction [95]. The expression of ZAP-70 facilitates the recruitment of Syk to the BCR complex resulting in additional increased BCR signaling. Compared to CD38 expression, ZAP-70 shows more concordance with unmutated *IGHV* status, with up to 97% of ZAP-70-positive cases showing unmutated *IGHV* [95, 96]. Protein expression can be tested by either flow cytometry or immunohistochemistry. In flow cytometry analysis, ZAP-70 in CLL is considered positive when over 20% of tumor cells show expression [97]. In conjunction with CD38 and mutational analysis, three prognostic subgroups can be determined: those with concordant results (ZAP-70+, CD38+, unmutated *IGHV*) have the worst prognosis, while patients without ZAP-70 or CD38 expression and mutated *IGHV* have better prognosis. Those with discordant results have a prognosis intermediate between the two [98, 99]. It is now known that CD38, CD44, CD49d, and matrix metalloproteinase-9 (MMP-9) expressed on ZAP-70+ CLL cells form a macromolecular complex which promotes cross talk between BCR signaling and CD44 further affecting CLL cell migration and homing [100].

A small subset of CLL cases can exhibit variant immunophenotypes and are sometimes termed "atypical" CLL. Some cases can show bright CD20 or sIg expression, and have been correlated with the presence of trisomy 12 [101, 102]. As mentioned above, about 15% of cases can be positive for FMC7. Lack of CD5 co-expression has also been reported, and thought to confer a worse prognosis than CD5+ cases [103].

On the other hand, the classic immunophenotype of CLL can be seen in other lymphomas, including MCL and MZL [104, 105]. Thus, the typical findings on flow cytometry and/or immunohistochemistry are not entirely sensitive nor specific. Indeed CD5 positivity has been described in all other non-CLL small B-cell lymphomas [106]. This highlights the importance of morphologic correlation when evaluating all cases of B-cell lymphoproliferations.

Some of the more recent immunohistochemical markers of CLL include CD200 and lymphoid enhancer binding factor 1 (LEF1). CD200 is a glycoprotein belonging to the immunoglobulin superfamily. It is expressed in most cases of CLL in contrast to MCL, giving it diagnostic utility in cases where the immunophenotyping results may be overlapping between the two entities [107]. Some have suggested a prognostic utility as well, with cases showing strong expression of CD200 having a better overall survival and longer time to treatment [108]. LEF1, on the other hand, is a transcription factor related to the Wnt pathway that helps to regulate genes associated with cell death and survival [109]. LEF1 expression was also found in CD19+/CD5+ B-cells in patients with monoclonal B-cell lymphocytosis, suggesting that this pathway may play an early role in the leukemogenesis of CLL. Most cases of CLL show expression of LEF1 in contrast to MCL [110, 111]. Recent studies also show that strong expression of LEF1 is an adverse prognostic factor [112].

In addition to these diagnostic and prognostic markers, CD2 and CD13 have both been aberrantly described to be expressed in cases of familial CLL [113]. Given the immune derangements consequent to CLL, expansions of certain unusual T-cell populations have been noted in CLL including CD4 + CD8+ populations in line with evidence indicating expansions of these population in elderly patients and CLL-like MBL [114, 115].

Transformation in CLL

The development of an aggressive lymphoma either synchronously or subsequent to a diagnosis of chronic lymphocytic leukemia (CLL) is called "Richter transformation" (RT) and is the accepted definition in the 2008 (and 2016 revision) WHO classification of hematopoietic tumors [11, 17, 116]. Two distinct pathologic variants are described, namely diffuse large B-cell lymphoma (DLBCL) variant (90% of all RT) and the less common Hodgkin lymphoma (HL) variant (10% of all RT) [117]. The former occurs ~2 years after a CLL diagnosis (including in treated and untreated patients) while the latter occurs at a median of 6 years subsequent to a diagnosis of CLL mostly in treated patients [118, 119].

Diffuse Large B-Cell Lymphoma-Richter Transformation (DLBCL-RT)

General Considerations

CLL patients with significant lymphadenopathy, certain genetic polymorphism, and somatic *NOTCH1* carry an increased risk of transformation [7, 120–123]. While the diagnosis of DLBCL-RT is fairly straightforward in most instances, there are three situations in which a diagnosis of DLBCL-RT should not be rendered: (1) Cases of CLL with numerous expansive and at times confluent growth centers: While such "accelerated" cases exhibit more aggressive clinical course with a median overall survival intermediate between typical CLL and DLBCL-RT, the current upcoming revisions note that these cases should not be termed as DLBCL-RT [124]. (2) The occurrence of EBV+ aggressive lymphomas after T-cell-depleting therapies for CLL including alemtuzumab, and as such these malignancies are considered to be secondary to iatrogenic immunosuppression and do not warrant a diagnosis of DLBCL-RT [125]. However, clonally identical B-cells have been reported to be detected in the both the CLL component prior to therapy and the post-alemtuzumab B-cell lymphoproliferation [126]. (3) Lastly, identification of small CD5+ B-cell clones in staging marrows of patients with extramedullary DLBCL without prior/concurrent history of CLL is likely unrelated biologically to the DLBCL and such cases are best considered as de novo DLBCLs.

Histopathology

DLBCL-RT occurs typically as a nodal disease but may also involve extranodal tissues including peripheral blood and bone marrow (Fig. 7.4). Involved lymph nodes show partial or total effacement of the nodal architecture by a DLBCL component with variable amounts of associated CLL component, which is spatially separate or intimately admixed with the DLBCL component. Cytologically, the DLBCL exhibits immunoblastic cytomorphology (with prominent eosinophilic nucleoli and moderate amount of cytoplasm, Fig. 7.4) but cases with centroblastic morphology and in rare instances plasmablastic/plasmacytic morphology has also been described [127–129]. A small proportion of cases may be positive for EBV with coexistent herpes simplex infection, which may be apparent as areas of extensive necrosis with typical Cowdry Type A inclusions. Prior fludarabine exposure increases the risk of HSV infection. Immunophenotypically, the DLBCL-RT exhibits non-GCB phenotype (CD10-, BC6-, MUM1/IRF4+) phenotype in 62–100% of cases based on the Hans classifier with variable expression of CD5 (32–77%) and CD23 (14–80%) [7, 130] (Fig. 7.4). Expression of Mum-1/IRF4 is in keeping with the phenotype of activated B-cell (ABC)/IRF-4- DLBCLs which have worse outcome compared to cases of de novo DLBCLs (Fig. 7.4). Specifically among DLBCL-RTs, there is overrepresentation of non-germinal center B-cell phenotype compared to de novo DLBCLs where the frequency is much lower [131–133].

Given the prognostic relevance of ZAP-70 and p53 in CLL, there has been interest in relevance of these two proteins in the DLBCL-RT. One recent study including 34 DLBCL-RTs noted that ZAP-70 expression by immunohistochemistry in DLBCL-RT (Fig. 7.4) was less frequent (13% of all DLBCLs tested) compared to the CLL component (66%) [130]. However, ZAP-70 status did not have any prognostic value. However, a significant proportion of DLBCL-RT in this study expressed p53 [130]. This observation is in congruence with reported genomic studies corroborating overrepresentation of *TP53* mutations in CLL and their corresponding DLBCL-RT tissues compared to CLLs that have not transformed to DLBCL with reported *TP53* disruption and *CDKN2A* as a main mechanism of transformation in CLL [134]. This study further identified a second major subgroup characterized by the presence of trisomy 12 comprising a third of the cases in the series indicating the existence of distinct pathways of transformation to DLBCL in CLL.

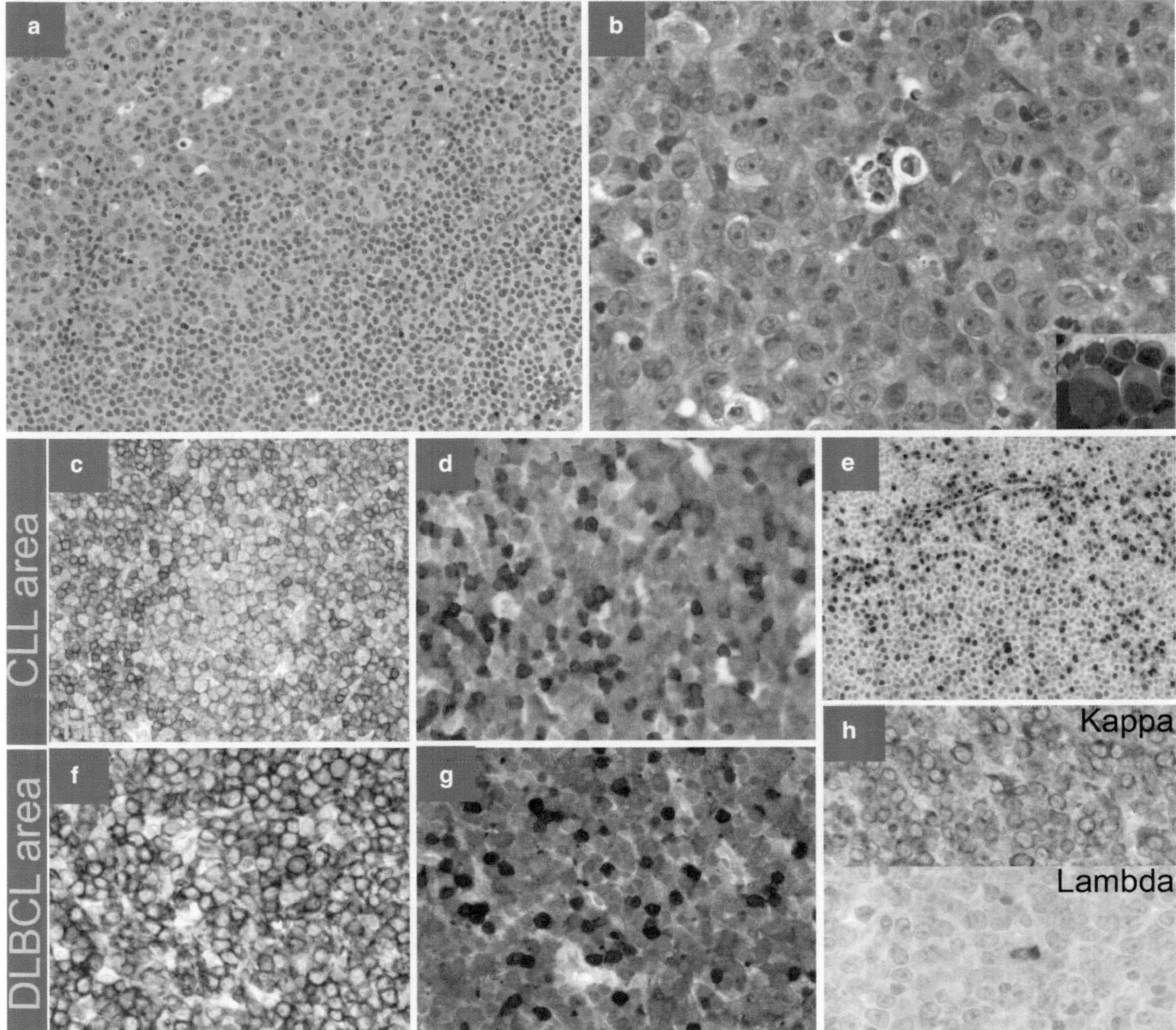

Fig. 7.4 Diffuse large B-cell lymphoma-Richter transformation (**a**). Bone marrow with spatially distinct large cell (*top left*) and CLL component (*bottom right*). (**b**) Large cell area at high power with prominent immunoblastic cytomorphology (inset shows large cells on marrow aspirate smears). (**c**, **f**) demonstrate CD5 immunostain in the CLL (proliferation centers) and DLBCL areas. Both components in this case are CD5 positive and ZAP-70 positive (**d**, **g**) In both stains, background T-cells express bright CD5 and ZAP-70. (**e**) Mum-1/IRF4+ staining within growth centers (*lower half of figure*) with an associated plasmacytic component at the periphery (*upper half of figure*). (**h**) The large-cell component shows restricted kappa light chain by immunohistochemistry (*top panel*)

Clonality Studies and Differential Diagnostic Considerations

Despite the frequently differing immunophenotype of DLBCL-RT in comparison with the prior CLL, clonality studies of IG genes and *IGHV* segment usage indicate that both components are frequently clonally related in up to 80% of cases [123, 130]. Also, with respect to *IGHV* status and cell of origin status, de novo DLBCLs differ from DLBCL-RT in frequently carrying mutated *IGHV* genes as opposed to DLBCL-RT which harbor unmutated *IGHV* genes. Another important differential in this setting is de novo CD5+ DLBCL since CD5 expression is otherwise unusual for de novo DLBCLs. However, CD5+ DLBCLs, despite being clinically/immunophenotypically similar (advanced age and stage at presentation, non-GC phenotype) to DLBCL-RT, in contrast carry mutated *IGHV* (up to 80% of cases) and are frequently CD23 negative as opposed to CD5+ transformation of B-CLL which is unmutated in most instances [135–137].

Clonally unrelated DLBCL-RT were noted to harbor less frequent *TP53* mutations, less frequent B-cell receptor stereotypy, and longer outcome compared to clonally related cases, nearly 47% of which harbored *TP53* aberrations [123]. This study noted MYC aberrations in up to 26% of DLBCL-RT cases. It is unclear as yet if MYC IHC positivity/aberrations in DLBCL-RT are independently prognostic or are only reflective of an aggressive *TP53* mutation-driven biology. There is some evidence that it is implicated in transformation [123, 138, 139]. One recent study noted that *MYC* aberrations are frequently acquired during the course of the disease and when present as part of a complex karyotype were associated with the development of RT and adverse outcome in contrast to cases harboring *MYC* aberrations as a part of a non-complex karyotype which responded well to standard risk-adapted therapy [140].

Classical Hodgkin Lymphoma-Richter Transformation (CHL-RT)

This variant of CLL transformation is 10–20 times less common than DLBCL-RT and occurs in less than 1% of CLL patients [118, 141–143]. In one of the first studies from Mayo Clinic looking at the incidence of CHL-RT in CLL patients within a prospective and a nested cohort (including only the subset with newly diagnosed CLL within the study period 1995–2011), the 10-year risk of CHL was 0.5% [118]. Compared to de novo CHL patients, CHL-RT patients in this study exhibited shorter overall survival and frequently presented at higher IPS stage and furthermore patients receiving any CLL therapy prior to the CHL transformation did worse compared to those who did not. Although 67% of cases in this series developed EBV+ CHL-RT, it was not possible to draw conclusions on outcome stratified by EBV status due to confounding prior nucleoside analog therapy in most patients within the EBV+ subset.

Two different histologic patterns of CHL have been described in the context of CHL-RT [59, 144, 145]. "Type I" pattern referred to the occurrence of isolated Hodgkin/Reed-Sternberg (HRS) cells scattered in a background of CLL lacking the typical polymorphous cellular milieu of CHL (viz. fibrosis, eosinophils, and neutrophils). "Type II" denoted cases with HRS cells scattered within typical CHL microenvironmental milieu (Fig. 7.5). These lesions may demonstrate synchronous composite histology with CLL and

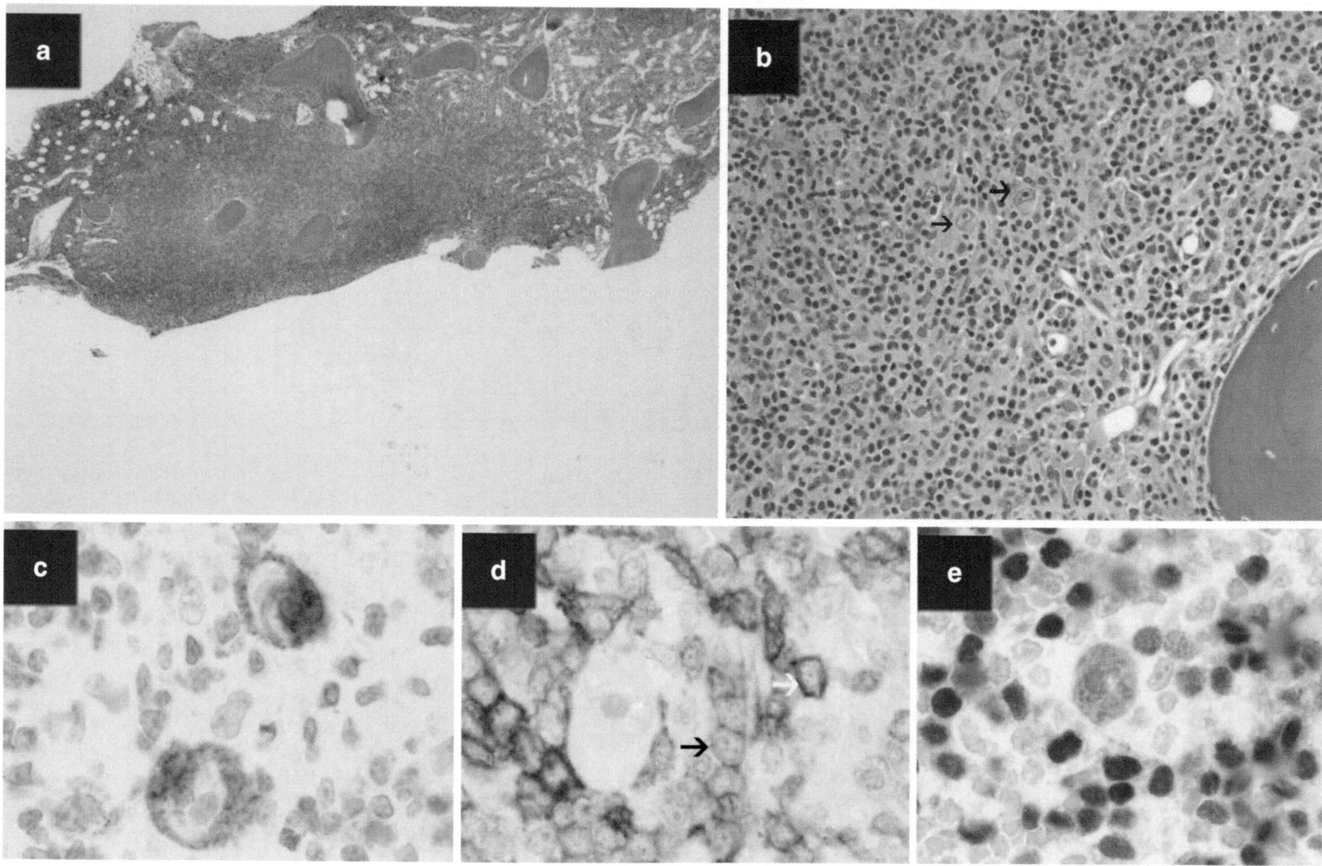

Fig. 7.5 Hodgkin lymphoma-Richter transformation in a CLL patient with two prior treatments including fludarabine, cyclophosphamide, and ofatumumab as well as acalabrutinib (irreversible Btk inhibitor) with progressive lymphadenopathy in whom bone marrow biopsy was performed for cytopenias. (**a**) Low-power view of marrow core biopsy showing nodular interstitial lymphohistiocytic aggregates which at high power (**b**) shows scattered HRS cells (*arrows*) amidst a polymorphous cellular milieu comprising lymphocytes, histiocytes, and few eosinophils. (**c**) The HRS cells express CD30 and are rimmed by CD5+ T-cells. (**d**) The CD5 immunostain shows T-cells with bright CD5 (*white arrow*) and CD5-dim lymphoid cells corresponding to CLL cells (*black arrow*) better highlighted on Pax5 immunostain (**e**)

Hodgkin components (either in the same node or different sites) or as metachronous development of CHL subsequent to CLL diagnosis. Progression from type I to type II histology may occur in some instances.

Immunophenotypically, the HRS cells exhibit a similar phenotype as seen in de novo classical Hodgkin lymphoma (CD30+, CD15+/variable, CD45-, weak Pax-5) (Fig. 7.5) with variable downregulation of other B-cell markers (CD20, CD79a, Oct-2, Bob.1) [117]. Most cases are usually positive for EBV (71%) in the HRS cells by in situ hybridization or EBV-LMP1 immunohistochemistry [141, 146]. While earlier biologic studies informed us regarding the occurrence of some clonally related and other clonally unrelated cases with inverse association of EBV and clonal relatedness, these were mostly single reports and small case series where results were not generalizable [59, 144, 145, 147]. In one of the largest series of such cases published recently including 26 type I Hodgkin-like lesions, the authors examined the EBV status, clonal relatedness (of both CLL and CHL components), and ZAP-70 status [146]. In this study, the authors noted that the CHL component was clonally related in about 40% of cases and interestingly all CLL negative for ZAP-70 were clonally related to the paired CHL component. This is in contrast to DLBCL-RT wherein all or most cases of DLBCL-RT are clonally related to the CLL component regardless of *IGHV* status. Only age > 70 years was predictive of adverse outcome in this study. While it was controversial from earlier studies whether type I lesions should be considered transformation, the study by Chen noted that cases with type I histology had an overall survival similar to cases with type II histology.

Minimal Residual Disease Testing in CLL by Flow Cytometry

With the progress made with combinations of chemotherapy and immunotherapy in CLL, there is growing recognition of association of MRD-negative status and other outcome measures. Several studies have demonstrated the utility of MRD-based flow cytometric testing in a variety of clinical settings including first-line, salvage/high-risk, and post-allogeneic transplant settings and it is thought that it may perhaps be useful even as a clinical trial endpoint with novel immunotherapy agents [148].

While earlier studies examined MRD status using two-, three-, or four-color tubes including CD19, CD5, and Kappa/lambda [149–152], the first major approach to standardized combinations was proposed by the European Research initiative in CLL (ERIC) which examined 728 paired blood and marrow samples and demonstrated that there was a high concordance between blood and marrow although marrow FC was required for definitive assessment of MRD-negative status 3 months after alemtuzumab therapy. There was concordance of the FC-based MRD status and real-time quantitative allele-specific oligonucleotide (RQ-ASO) immunoglobulin heavy-chain gene (IgH) polymerase chain reaction (PCR) [153]. This study identified specific useful four-color FC combinations including CD19/CD5 with CD20/CD38, CD81/CD22, and CD79b/CD43 as the most useful combination for detecting MRD at the 0.01% level. These observations were then extended in a follow-up study demonstrating equivalence of a harmonized six-color panel with the previously proposed four-color panel in detecting residual CLL at the 0.01% level utilizing the same marker combinations including CD20, CD22, CD38, CD43, CD79b, and CD81 [154]. This latter study utilized a threshold of at least 50 events to define a CLL population with the need for CD3 for determining the limit of detection. Very recently, a combination of markers proposed by ERIC were tested in an eight-color panel with the ability to detect MRD at 0.007% level [155].

Differential Diagnosis

In the assessment of a patient with B-cell lymphocytosis, the differential diagnosis can be broad and range from benign, reactive conditions to a number of B-cell lymphomas. An important and useful first step in differentiating between these conditions is a systematic assessment of lymphocyte morphology. Generally, uniformly small-to-medium cells in the peripheral blood is suggestive of CLL, while variability in cell size and shape is more indicative of a reactive condition or another lymphoma. Clinical history is also important, as lymphocytosis in a young patient is more likely to represent an infectious process, such as a viral illness, rather than lymphoma. Polyclonal B-cell lymphocytosis, a rare condition more common in young female smokers and associated with HLA DR7 [156], may also enter the differential. It is characterized by a persistent B-cell lymphocytosis of mostly small, round lymphocytes with only mild morphologic variability, closely resembling CLL. Often, flow cytometry and/or clonality studies may be necessary to exclude lymphoma.

Distinction between CLL and other mature B-cell neoplasms can be more difficult especially when the morphology of CLL is atypical. In the early 1990s, a flow cytometric scoring system was proposed by Matutes and coworkers which examined the expression levels of CD5, CD22, CD23, FMC7, and surface immunoglobulin. CLL with a typical expression pattern (CD5+, CD23+, FMC7-, dim sIg, and dim CD22) were assigned a score of 5 [157]. However, in these cases, particular attention to morphologic features, along with correlation with immunophenotype, can aid in arriving at the correct diagnosis.

Mantle cell lymphoma, particularly the small-cell variant, is possibly the most important differential diagnosis, due to some similar morphologic and immunophenotypic features with CLL, despite its significantly poorer prognosis. Leukemic presentation can occur in MCL [158] and the cells can resemble CLL, namely medium-sized cells with scant cytoplasm. However, the nuclei in MCL are often cleaved and the chromatin usually is more dispersed. In tissue sections, proliferation centers that are characteristic of CLL are notably absent in MCL. Additionally, prolymphocytes are not found in cases of MCL. Although both lymphomas share expression of CD5, in contrast with CLL, MCL shows strong expression of CD20 and CD79b. A key differentiating factor is the expression of cyclin D1 in MCL, which is correlated with the presence of t(11;14)(q13;q32). In cases where cyclin D1 is absent, SOX11 is present in most cases [159]. Absence of SOX11 was found to confer better survival and a more indolent form of MCL [160].

Uncommonly, CLL can exhibit plasmacytoid features, morphologically resembling lymphoplasmacytic lymphoma (LPL). The latter contains a mixture of plasma cells, plasmacytoid cells, and small lymphocytes. The peripheral blood may also exhibit red cell agglutination, indicative of the presence of antibodies on the red cell surface (Fig. 7.6). The bone marrow may show diffuse infiltration (Fig. 7.6). Mast cells are typically increased in LPL. Proliferation centers are absent and CD5 is generally not expressed although CD10 can rarely be expressed in LPL. Expression of CD20, surface immunoglobulin, and CD79a is usually higher than in CLL. Testing for serum IgM paraprotein and presence of concurrent *MYD88* L265P mutation (which is now known to be present in almost all LPL) allows confirmation of LPL [161].

CLL with increased prolymphocytes or in prolymphocytic transformation can resemble B-cell prolymphocytic lymphoma (B-PLL). However, as defined by the WHO, the diagnosis of B-PLL requires that the neoplastic cells comprise 55% or more of the peripheral white blood cells (Fig. 7.6). Although lymph node involvement is uncommon in B-PLL, if present, proliferation centers are not observed. CD20 expression in B-PLL is typically bright, in contrast to most cases of CLL.

The distinction between follicular lymphoma and CLL is often straightforward. Although at times the pseudofollicles of CLL can resemble the true neoplastic follicles of follicular lymphoma and the neoplastic cells can appear slightly cleaved, attention to all architectural and morphologic features, along with immunophenotypic profiles, would aid in the diagnosis. When evaluating bone marrow samples, follicular lymphoma typically occupies the paratrabecular spaces, rather than interstitial or diffuse involvement that is characteristic of CLL.

Splenic marginal zone lymphoma presents with peripheral blood and spleen involvement without significant lymphadenopathy. The neoplastic cells characteristically have polar villi (Fig. 7.6) with a chromatin pattern quite similar to CLL cells. The bone marrow shows intra-sinusoidal infiltrates (Fig. 7.6), which are very unusual in CLL. Immunophenotypically, there is strong expression of FMC7 and B-cell markers, in contrast to CLL cells. CD5 can be expressed in some cases of splenic marginal zone lymphomas, and some suggest that cases with this immunophenotype present with higher levels of lymphocytosis. However, there was no difference in overall outcome in CD5+ lymphomas as compared to CD5-negative cases [162].

Differentiation of hairy cell leukemia (HCL) from CLL is usually not very challenging. HCL often presents in the peripheral blood, spleen, and bone marrow, without significant peripheral lymph node involvement. The classic cytomorphology of HCL cells is medium-sized lymphoid cells with circumferential hairlike cytoplasmic projections (Fig. 7.6). The nuclear membrane is often oval or indented and the chromatin is slightly more dispersed than the clumpy chromatin pattern seen in CLL cells. Examination of the bone marrow often shows diffuse involvement and a "fried-egg" appearance of the neoplastic cells (Fig. 7.6). Immunophenotypically, HCL cells have strong expression of sIg and B-cell antigens, such as CD20. More specific hairy cell markers such as CD103, CD25, and CD123 are often present. Immunohistochemical stains for annexin A1, tartrate-resistant acid phosphatase (TRAP) (Fig. 7.6), and DBA.44 on tissue sections can also be helpful. CD5 is often negative.

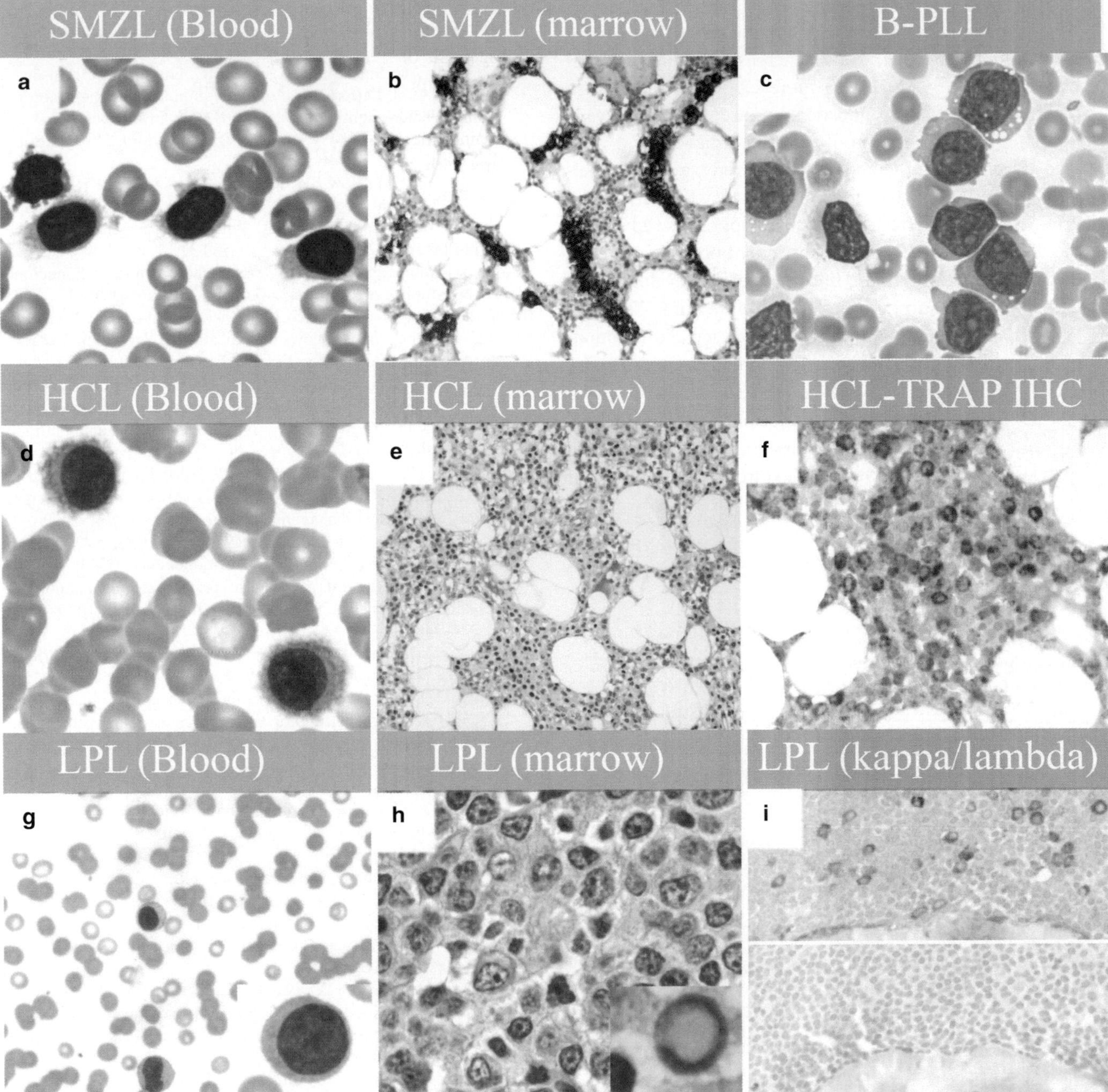

Fig. 7.6 Differential diagnostic considerations. (**a**) Splenic marginal zone lymphoma (SMZL) involving peripheral blood with polar villous projections (**b**) SMZL in marrow characteristically shows intrasinusoidal infiltration pattern of lymphoma cells more frequently which is a useful diagnostic feature (CD20 immunoperoxidase stain). There is often heterogeneity of cell size in such cases but typical clumped nuclear chromatin and smudge cells as seen in CLL are not present. (**c**) B-Prolymphocytic leukemia (B-PLL) containing uniform population of large cells with distinct nucleoli and moderate amount of cytoplasm. With growing understanding, very few of such cases represent CLL in prolymphocytic transformation. (**d**) Hairy cell leukemia (HCL) involving peripheral blood with typical hairy cytomorphology. (**e**) HCL involving bone marrow core biopsy with typical fried-egg appearance (**f**) Tartrate-resistant acid phosphatase (TRAP) immunohistochemistry strongly positive in HCL. (**g**) Lymphoplasmacytic lymphoma involving peripheral blood with marked red cell agglutination (*inset:* typical cell with morphology intermediate between lymphocytes and plasma cells). (**h**) Core biopsy of LPL showing extensive infiltration by LPL cells (*inset:* Dutcher body, defined as intranuclear inclusions of cytoplasmic immunoglobulin) (**i**) Kappa light-chain restriction with LPL cells demonstrated via IHC on core biopsy. Although the morphologic distinction is easy in most instances, HCL, SMZL, and B-PLL may variably express CD5 and CD23 in a significant proportion of cases and may pose diagnostic confusion from a flow cytometric perspective

Conclusion

As our understanding of the pathogenesis of CLL grows, "bench-side" discoveries are increasingly finding their way to the "bedside," with more examples of targeted therapy and precise prognostication discovered each year. The molecular genetic profile of each tumor can aid clinicians in providing the appropriate therapy, a delicate balance between effective medicine against the tumor and minimizing any toxic side effects. Despite these advances, the diagnosis of CLL is still dependent on analysis using the classic, ageless light microscope and evaluation of characteristic morphologic and architectural features. With the additional help of flow cytometry and immunohistochemistry, CLL can be differentiated from its mimics and a precise diagnosis can be rendered by the pathologist. Only after this point do molecular tests have meaning and a context can be drawn that links the basic science discoveries in CLL to the practical treatment and care of the patients we serve.

References

1. Muller-Hermelink H, Montserrat E, Catovsky D. Chronic lymphocytic leukaemia/small lymphocytic lymphoma. WHO classification of tumours of haematopoietic and lymphoid tissues. 4th ed. Lyon, France: International Agency for Research on Cancer Press; 2008. p. 180–2.
2. Minot B, Issacs R. Lymphatic leukemia: age, incidence, duration and benefit derived from irradiation. Boston Med Surg J. 1924;1:1–9.
3. Rai KR. Progress in chronic lymphocytic leukaemia: a historical perspective. Baillieres Clin Haematol. 1993;6:757–65.
4. Scarfò L, Ghia P. What does it mean I have a monoclonal B-cell lymphocytosis? Recent insights and new challenges. Semin Oncol. 2016;43:201–8.
5. Omoti CE, Omoti AE. Richter syndrome: a review of clinical, ocular, neurological and other manifestations. Br J Haematol. 2008;142:709–16.
6. Rossi D, Cerri M, Capello D, Deambrogi C, Rossi FM, Zucchetto A, et al. Biological and clinical risk factors of chronic lymphocytic leukaemia transformation to Richter syndrome. Br J Haematol. 2008;142:202–15.
7. Rossi D, Gaidano G. Richter syndrome: pathogenesis and management. Semin Oncol. 2016;43:311–9.
8. Hallek M, Cheson BD, Catovsky D, Caligaris-Cappio F, Dighiero G, Döhner H, et al. Guidelines for the diagnosis and treatment of chronic lymphocytic leukemia: a report from the International Workshop on Chronic Lymphocytic Leukemia updating the National Cancer Institute-Working Group 1996 guidelines. Blood. 2008;111:5446–56.
9. Romano C, Sellitto A, Chiurazzi F, Simeone L, De Fanis U, Raia M, et al. Clinical and phenotypic features of CD5-negative B cell chronic lymphoproliferative disease resembling chronic lymphocytic leukemia. Int J Hematol. 2015;101:67–74.
10. Marti GE, Rawstron AC, Ghia P, Hillmen P, Houlston RS, Kay N, et al. Diagnostic criteria for monoclonal B-cell lymphocytosis. Br J Haematol. 2005;130:325–32.
11. Swerdlow SH, Campo E, Harris NL, Jaffe ES, Pileri S, Stein H, et al. WHO classification of tumours of haematopoietic and lymphoid tissues. 4th ed. Lyon, France: International Agency for Research on Cancer; 2008.
12. Rawstron AC, Bennett FL, O'Connor SJM, Kwok M, Fenton JAL, Plummer M, et al. Monoclonal B-cell lymphocytosis and chronic lymphocytic leukemia. N Engl J Med. 2008;359:575–83.
13. Rawstron AC, Shanafelt T, Lanasa MC, Landgren O, Hanson C, Orfao A, et al. Different biology and clinical outcome according to the absolute numbers of clonal B-cells in monoclonal B-cell lymphocytosis (MBL). Cytometry B Clin Cytom. 2010;78(Suppl 1):S19–23.
14. Gibson SE, Swerdlow SH, Ferry JA, Surti U, Dal Cin P, Harris NL, et al. Reassessment of small lymphocytic lymphoma in the era of monoclonal B-cell lymphocytosis. Haematologica. 2011;96:1144–52.
15. Ghia P. Another piece of the puzzle: is there a "nodal" monoclonal B-cell lymphocytosis? Haematologica. 2011;96:1089–91.
16. Vardi A, Dagklis A, Scarfò L, Jelinek D, Newton D, Bennett F, et al. Immunogenetics shows that not all MBL are equal: the larger the clone, the more similar to CLL. Blood. 2013;121:4521–8.
17. Swerdlow SH, Campo E, Pileri SA, Harris NL, Stein H, Siebert R, et al. The 2016 revision of the World Health Organization (WHO) classification of lymphoid neoplasms. Blood. 2016;127(20):2375–90.
18. Shanafelt TD, Ghia P, Lanasa MC, Landgren O, Rawstron AC. Monoclonal B-cell lymphocytosis (MBL): biology, natural history and clinical management. Leukemia. 2010;24:512–20.
19. Nieto WG, Teodosio C, López A, Rodríguez-Caballero A, Romero A, Bárcena P, et al. Non-CLL-like monoclonal B-cell lymphocytosis in the general population: prevalence and phenotypic/genetic characteristics. Cytometry B Clin Cytom. 2010;78(Suppl 1):S24–34.
20. Nieto WG, Almeida J, Romero A, Teodosio C, López A, Henriques AF, et al. Increased frequency (12%) of circulating chronic lymphocytic leukemia-like B-cell clones in healthy subjects using a highly sensitive multicolor flow cytometry approach. Blood. 2009;114:33–7.
21. Shanafelt TD, Kay NE, Rabe KG, Call TG, Zent CS, Maddocks K, et al. Brief report: natural history of individuals with clinically recognized monoclonal B-cell lymphocytosis compared with patients with Rai 0 chronic lymphocytic leukemia. J Clin Oncol. 2009;27:3959–63.
22. Morabito F, Mosca L, Cutrona G, Agnelli L, Tuana G, Ferracin M, et al. Clinical monoclonal B lymphocytosis versus Rai 0 chronic lymphocytic leukemia: a comparison of cellular, cytogenetic, molecular, and clinical features. Clin Cancer Res. 2013;19:5890–900.
23. Ferrajoli A, Shanafelt TD, Ivan C, Shimizu M, Rabe KG, Nouraee N, et al. Prognostic value of miR-155 in individuals with monoclonal B-cell lymphocytosis and patients with B chronic lymphocytic leukemia. Blood. 2013;122:1891–9.
24. Xochelli A, Kalpadakis C, Gardiner A, Baliakas P, Vassilakopoulos TP, Mould S, et al. Clonal B-cell lymphocytosis exhibiting immunophenotypic features consistent with a marginal-zone origin: is this a distinct entity? Blood. 2014;123:1199–206.
25. National Cancer Institute. SEER stat fact sheets: Chronic Lymphocytic Leukemia (CLL). https://seer.cancer.gov/statfacts/html/clyl.html.
26. Ng D, Toure O, Wei M-H, Arthur DC, Abbasi F, Fontaine L, et al. Identification of a novel chromosome region, 13q21.33-q22.2, for susceptibility genes in familial chronic lymphocytic leukemia. Blood. 2007;109:916–25.
27. Rozman C, Montserrat E. Chronic lymphocytic leukemia. N Engl J Med. 1995;333:1052–7.
28. Montserrat E, Moreno C. Chronic lymphocytic leukaemia: a short overview. Ann Oncol. 2008;19(Suppl 7):vii320–5.
29. Hodgson K, Ferrer G, Montserrat E, Moreno C. Chronic lymphocytic leukemia and autoimmunity: a systematic review. Haematologica. 2011;96:752–61.

30. Weir EG, Epstein JI. Incidental small lymphocytic lymphoma/chronic lymphocytic leukemia in pelvic lymph nodes excised at radical prostatectomy. Arch Pathol Lab Med. 2003;127:567–72.
31. Baumhoer D, Tzankov A, Dirnhofer S, Tornillo L, Terracciano LM. Patterns of liver infiltration in lymphoproliferative disease. Histopathology. 2008;53:81–90.
32. Cerroni L, Zenahlik P, Höfler G, Kaddu S, Smolle J, Kerl H. Specific cutaneous infiltrates of B-cell chronic lymphocytic leukemia: a clinicopathologic and prognostic study of 42 patients. Am J Surg Pathol. 1996;20:1000–10.
33. Graff-Baker A, Sosa JA, Roman SA. Primary thyroid lymphoma: a review of recent developments in diagnosis and histology-driven treatment. Curr Opin Oncol. 2010;22:17–22.
34. Vega F, Padula A, Valbuena JR, Stancu M, Jones D, Medeiros LJ. Lymphomas involving the pleura: a clinicopathologic study of 34 cases diagnosed by pleural biopsy. Arch Pathol Lab Med. 2006;130:1497–502.
35. Benekli M, Büyükaşik Y, Haznedaroğlu IC, Savaş MC, Ozcebe OI. Chronic lymphocytic leukemia presenting as acute urinary retention due to leukemic infiltration of the prostate. Ann Hematol. 1996;73:143–4.
36. Trisolini R, Lazzari Agli L, Poletti V. Bronchiolocentric pulmonary involvement due to chronic lymphocytic leukemia. Haematologica. 2000;85:1097.
37. Garofalo M, Murali R, Halperin I, Magardician K, Moussouris HF, Masdeu JC. Chronic lymphocytic leukemia with hypothalamic invasion. Cancer. 1989;64:1714–6.
38. Morrison C, Shah S, Flinn IW. Leptomeningeal involvement in chronic lymphocytic leukemia. Cancer Pract. 1998;6:223–8.
39. Hamblin TJ, Davis Z, Gardiner A, Oscier DG, Stevenson FK. Unmutated Ig V(H) genes are associated with a more aggressive form of chronic lymphocytic leukemia. Blood. 1999;94:1848–54.
40. Chiorazzi N, Rai KR, Ferrarini M. Chronic lymphocytic leukemia. N Engl J Med. 2005;352:804–15.
41. Liang X, Moseman EA, Farrar MA, Bachanova V, Weisdorf DJ, Blazar BR, et al. Toll-like receptor 9 signaling by CpG-B oligodeoxynucleotides induces an apoptotic pathway in human chronic lymphocytic leukemia B cells. Blood. 2010;115:5041–52.
42. Grandjenette C, Kennel A, Faure GC, Béné MC, Feugier P. Expression of functional toll-like receptors by B-chronic lymphocytic leukemia cells. Haematologica. 2007;92:1279–81.
43. Wagner M, Oelsner M, Moore A, Götte F, Kuhn P-H, Haferlach T, et al. Integration of innate into adaptive immune responses in ZAP-70-positive chronic lymphocytic leukemia. Blood. 2016;127:436–48.
44. Colombo M, Cutrona G, Reverberi D, Fabris S, Neri A, Fabbi M, et al. Intraclonal cell expansion and selection driven by B cell receptor in chronic lymphocytic leukemia. Mol Med. 2011;17:834–9.
45. Ghiotto F, Fais F, Valetto A, Albesiano E, Hashimoto S, Dono M, et al. Remarkably similar antigen receptors among a subset of patients with chronic lymphocytic leukemia. J Clin Invest. 2004;113:1008–16.
46. Messmer BT, Albesiano E, Efremov DG, Ghiotto F, Allen SL, Kolitz J, et al. Multiple distinct sets of stereotyped antigen receptors indicate a role for antigen in promoting chronic lymphocytic leukemia. J Exp Med. 2004;200:519–25.
47. Schwartz RS, Stollar BD. Heavy-chain directed B-cell maturation: continuous clonal selection beginning at the pre-B cell stage. Immunol Today. 1994;15:27–32.
48. Klein U, Tu Y, Stolovitzky GA, Mattioli M, Cattoretti G, Husson H, et al. Gene expression profiling of B cell chronic lymphocytic leukemia reveals a homogeneous phenotype related to memory B cells. J Exp Med. 2001;194:1625–38.
49. Rosenwald A, Alizadeh AA, Widhopf G, Simon R, Davis RE, Yu X, et al. Relation of gene expression phenotype to immunoglobulin mutation genotype in B cell chronic lymphocytic leukemia. J Exp Med. 2001;194:1639–47.
50. Kikushige Y, Ishikawa F, Miyamoto T, Shima T, Urata S, Yoshimoto G, et al. Self-renewing hematopoietic stem cell is the primary target in pathogenesis of human chronic lymphocytic leukemia. Cancer Cell. 2011;20:246–59.
51. den Ottolander GJ, Brederoo P, Schuurman RK, Teeuwsen VJ, Schuit HR, van der Meulen J, et al. Intracellular immunoglobulin G "pseudocrystals" in a patient with chronic B-cell leukemia. Cancer. 1986;58:43–51.
52. Lunning MA, Zenger VE, Dreyfuss R, Stetler-Stevenson M, Rick ME, White TA, et al. Albumin enhanced morphometric image analysis in CLL. Cytometry B Clin Cytom. 2004;57:7–14.
53. Oscier D, Else M, Matutes E, Morilla R, Strefford JC, Catovsky D. The morphology of CLL revisited: the clinical significance of prolymphocytes and correlations with prognostic/molecular markers in the LRF CLL4 trial. Br J Haematol. 2016;174(5):767–75.
54. Matutes E, Oscier D, Garcia-Marco J, Ellis J, Copplestone A, Gillingham R, et al. Trisomy 12 defines a group of CLL with atypical morphology: correlation between cytogenetic, clinical and laboratory features in 544 patients. Br J Haematol. 1996;92:382–8.
55. Cordone I, Matutes E, Catovsky D. Monoclonal antibody Ki-67 identifies B and T cells in cycle in chronic lymphocytic leukemia: correlation with disease activity. Leukemia. 1992;6:902–6.
56. Criel A, Wlodarska I, Meeus P, Stul M, Louwagie A, Van Hoof A, et al. Trisomy 12 is uncommon in typical chronic lymphocytic leukaemias. Br J Haematol. 1994;87:523–8.
57. Lin P, Hao S, Handy BC, Bueso-Ramos CE, Medeiros LJ. Lymphoid neoplasms associated with IgM paraprotein: a study of 382 patients. Am J Clin Pathol. 2005;123:200–5.
58. Offit K, Louie DC, Parsa NZ, Noy A, Chaganti RS. Del (7)(q32) is associated with a subset of small lymphocytic lymphoma with plasmacytoid features. Blood. 1995;86:2365–70.
59. Ohno T, Smir BN, Weisenburger DD, Gascoyne RD, Hinrichs SD, Chan WC. Origin of the Hodgkin/Reed-Sternberg cells in chronic lymphocytic leukemia with "Hodgkin's transformation.". Blood. 1998;91:1757–61.
60. Friedman DR, Sibley AB, Owzar K, Chaffee KG, Slager S, Kay NE, et al. Relationship of blood monocytes with chronic lymphocytic leukemia aggressiveness and outcomes: a multi-institutional study. Am J Hematol. 2016;91:687–91.
61. Oscier DG, Matutes E, Copplestone A, Pickering RM, Chapman R, Gillingham R, et al. Atypical lymphocyte morphology: an adverse prognostic factor for disease progression in stage A CLL independent of trisomy 12. Br J Haematol. 1997;98:934–9.
62. Frater JL, McCarron KF, Hammel JP, Shapiro JL, Miller ML, Tubbs RR, et al. Typical and atypical chronic lymphocytic leukemia differ clinically and immunophenotypically. Am J Clin Pathol. 2001;116:655–64.
63. Montserrat E, Villamor N, Reverter JC, Brugués RM, Tàssies D, Bosch F, et al. Bone marrow assessment in B-cell chronic lymphocytic leukaemia: aspirate or biopsy? A comparative study in 258 patients. Br J Haematol. 1996;93:111–6.
64. Kim YS, Ford RJ, Faber JA, Bell RH, Elenitoba-Johnson KS, Medeiros LJ. B-cell chronic lymphocytic leukemia/small lymphocytic lymphoma involving bone marrow with an interfollicular pattern. Am J Clin Pathol. 2000;114:41–6.
65. Schade U, Bock O, Vornhusen S, Jäger A, Büsche G, Lehmann U, et al. Bone marrow infiltration pattern in B-cell chronic lymphocytic leukemia is related to immunoglobulin heavy-chain variable region mutation status and expression of 70-kd zeta-associated protein (ZAP-70). Hum Pathol. 2006;37:1153–61.

66. Zanotti R, Ambrosetti A, Lestani M, Ghia P, Pattaro C, Remo A, et al. ZAP-70 expression, as detected by immunohistochemistry on bone marrow biopsies from early-phase CLL patients, is a strong adverse prognostic factor. Leukemia. 2007;21:102–9.
67. Randen U, Tierens AM, Tjønnfjord GE, Delabie J. Bone marrow histology in monoclonal B-cell lymphocytosis shows various B-cell infiltration patterns. Am J Clin Pathol. 2013;139:390–5.
68. Kipps TJ, Carson DA. Autoantibodies in chronic lymphocytic leukemia and related systemic autoimmune diseases. Blood. 1993;81:2475–87.
69. Yoo D, Pierce LE, Lessin LS. Acquired pure red cell aplasia associated with chronic lymphocytic leukemia. Cancer. 1983;51:844–50.
70. Schmid C, Isaacson PG. Proliferation centres in B-cell malignant lymphoma, lymphocytic (B-CLL): an immunophenotypic study. Histopathology. 1994;24:445–51.
71. Gradowski JF, Sargent RL, Craig FE, Cieply K, Fuhrer K, Sherer C, et al. Chronic lymphocytic leukemia/small lymphocytic lymphoma with cyclin D1 positive proliferation centers do not have CCND1 translocations or gains and lack SOX11 expression. Am J Clin Pathol. 2012;138:132–9.
72. Gupta D, Lim MS, Medeiros LJ, Elenitoba-Johnson KS. Small lymphocytic lymphoma with perifollicular, marginal zone, or interfollicular distribution. Mod Pathol. 2000;13:1161–6.
73. Narang S, Wolf BC, Neiman RS. Malignant lymphoma presenting with prominent splenomegaly. A clinicopathologic study with special reference to intermediate cell lymphoma. Cancer. 1985;55:1948–57.
74. Edelman M, Evans L, Zee S, Gnass R, Ratech H. Splenic microanatomical localization of small lymphocytic lymphoma/chronic lymphocytic leukemia using a novel combined silver nitrate and immunoperoxidase technique. Am J Surg Pathol. 1997;21:445–52.
75. Arber DA, Rappaport H, Weiss LM. Non-Hodgkin's lymphoproliferative disorders involving the spleen. Mod Pathol. 1997;10:18–32.
76. Schwartz JB, Shamsuddin AM. The effects of leukemic infiltrates in various organs in chronic lymphocytic leukemia. Hum Pathol. 1981;12:432–40.
77. Garicochea B, Cliquet MG, Melo N, del Giglio A, Dorlhiac-Llacer PE, Chamone DA. Leptomeningeal involvement in chronic lymphocytic leukemia identified by polymerase chain reaction in stored slides: a case report. Mod Pathol. 1997;10:500–3.
78. Kuse R, Lueb H. Gastrointestinal involvement in patients with chronic lymphocytic leukemia. Leukemia. 1997;11(Suppl 2):S50–1.
79. Elliott MA, Letendre L, Li CY, Hoyer JD, Hammack JE. Chronic lymphocytic leukaemia with symptomatic diffuse central nervous system infiltration responding to therapy with systemic fludarabine. Br J Haematol. 1999;104:689–94.
80. Mhawech-Fauceglia P, Saxena R, Zhang S, Terracciano L, Sauter G, Chadhuri A, et al. Pax-5 immunoexpression in various types of benign and malignant tumours: a high-throughput tissue microarray analysis. J Clin Pathol. 2007;60:709–14.
81. Vuillier F, Dumas G, Magnac C, Prevost M-C, Lalanne AI, Oppezzo P, et al. Lower levels of surface B-cell-receptor expression in chronic lymphocytic leukemia are associated with glycosylation and folding defects of the mu and CD79a chains. Blood. 2005;105:2933–40.
82. Bomberger C, Singh-Jairam M, Rodey G, Guerriero A, Yeager AM, Fleming WH, et al. Lymphoid reconstitution after autologous PBSC transplantation with FACS-sorted CD34+ hematopoietic progenitors. Blood. 1998;91:2588–600.
83. Bennett F, Rawstron A, Plummer M, de Tute R, Moreton P, Jack A, et al. B-cell chronic lymphocytic leukaemia cells show specific changes in membrane protein expression during different stages of cell cycle. Br J Haematol. 2007;139:600–4.
84. Asplund SL, McKenna RW, Doolittle JE, Kroft SH. CD5-positive B-cell neoplasms of indeterminate immunophenotype: a clinicopathologic analysis of 26 cases. Appl Immunohistochem Mol Morphol. 2005;13:311–7.
85. Craig FE, Foon KA. Flow cytometric immunophenotyping for hematologic neoplasms. Blood. 2008;111:3941–67.
86. Papageorgiou SG, Kontos CK, Pappa V, Thomadaki H, Kontsioti F, Dervenoulas J, et al. The novel member of the BCL2 gene family, BCL2L12, is substantially elevated in chronic lymphocytic leukemia patients, supporting its value as a significant biomarker. Oncologist. 2011;16:1280–91.
87. Hanada M, Delia D, Aiello A, Stadtmauer E, Reed JC. bcl-2 gene hypomethylation and high-level expression in B-cell chronic lymphocytic leukemia. Blood. 1993;82:1820–8.
88. Anderson MA, Deng J, Seymour JF, Tam C, Kim SY, Fein J, et al. The BCL2 selective inhibitor venetoclax induces rapid onset apoptosis of CLL cells in patients via a TP53 independent mechanism. Blood. 2016;127(25):3215–24.
89. Roberts AW, Davids MS, Pagel JM, Kahl BS, Puvvada SD, Gerecitano JF, et al. Targeting BCL2 with venetoclax in relapsed chronic lymphocytic leukemia. N Engl J Med. 2016;374:311–22.
90. Marotta G, Raspadori D, Sestigiani C, Scalia G, Bigazzi C, Lauria F. Expression of the CD11c antigen in B-cell chronic lymphoproliferative disorders. Leuk Lymphoma. 2000;37:145–9.
91. Malavasi F, Deaglio S, Funaro A, Ferrero E, Horenstein AL, Ortolan E, et al. Evolution and function of the ADP ribosyl cyclase/CD38 gene family in physiology and pathology. Physiol Rev. 2008;88:841–86.
92. Ghia P, Guida G, Stella S, Gottardi D, Geuna M, Strola G, et al. The pattern of CD38 expression defines a distinct subset of chronic lymphocytic leukemia (CLL) patients at risk of disease progression. Blood. 2003;101:1262–9.
93. Jelinek DF, Tschumper RC, Geyer SM, Bone ND, Dewald GW, Hanson CA, et al. Analysis of clonal B-cell CD38 and immunoglobulin variable region sequence status in relation to clinical outcome for B-chronic lymphocytic leukaemia. Br J Haematol. 2001;115:854–61.
94. Hamblin TJ, Orchard JA, Ibbotson RE, Davis Z, Thomas PW, Stevenson FK, et al. CD38 expression and immunoglobulin variable region mutations are independent prognostic variables in chronic lymphocytic leukemia, but CD38 expression may vary during the course of the disease. Blood. 2002;99:1023–9.
95. Crespo M, Bosch F, Villamor N, Bellosillo B, Colomer D, Rozman M, et al. ZAP-70 expression as a surrogate for immunoglobulin-variable-region mutations in chronic lymphocytic leukemia. N Engl J Med. 2003;348:1764–75.
96. Orchard JA, Ibbotson RE, Davis Z, Wiestner A, Rosenwald A, Thomas PW, et al. ZAP-70 expression and prognosis in chronic lymphocytic leukaemia. Lancet. 2004;363:105–11.
97. Wilhelm C, Neubauer A, Brendel C. Discordant results of flow cytometric ZAP-70 expression status in B-CLL samples if different gating strategies are applied. Cytometry B Clin Cytom. 2006;70:242–50.
98. Schroers R, Griesinger F, Trümper L, Haase D, Kulle B, Klein-Hitpass L, et al. Combined analysis of ZAP-70 and CD38 expression as a predictor of disease progression in B-cell chronic lymphocytic leukemia. Leukemia. 2005;19:750–8.
99. D'Arena G, Tarnani M, Rumi C, Vaisitti T, Aydin S, De Filippi R, et al. Prognostic significance of combined analysis of ZAP-70 and CD38 in chronic lymphocytic leukemia. Am J Hematol. 2007;82:787–91.
100. Buggins AGS, Levi A, Gohil S, Fishlock K, Patten PEM, Calle Y, et al. Evidence for a macromolecular complex in poor prognosis CLL that contains CD38, CD49d, CD44 and MMP-9. Br J Haematol. 2011;154:216–22.

101. Ho AK, Hill S, Preobrazhensky SN, Miller ME, Chen Z, Bahler DW. Small B-cell neoplasms with typical mantle cell lymphoma immunophenotypes often include chronic lymphocytic leukemias. Am J Clin Pathol. 2009;131:27–32.
102. Tam CS, Otero-Palacios J, Abruzzo LV, Jorgensen JL, Ferrajoli A, Wierda WG, et al. Chronic lymphocytic leukaemia CD20 expression is dependent on the genetic subtype: a study of quantitative flow cytometry and fluorescent in-situ hybridization in 510 patients. Br J Haematol. 2008;141:36–40.
103. Huang JC, Finn WG, Goolsby CL, Variakojis D, Peterson LC. CD5- small B-cell leukemias are rarely classifiable as chronic lymphocytic leukemia. Am J Clin Pathol. 1999;111:123–30.
104. Schlette E, Fu K, Medeiros LJ. CD23 expression in mantle cell lymphoma: clinicopathologic features of 18 cases. Am J Clin Pathol. 2003;120:760–6.
105. Matutes E, Polliack A. Morphological and immunophenotypic features of chronic lymphocytic leukemia. Rev Clin Exp Hematol. 2000;4:22–47.
106. Dronca RS, Jevremovic D, Hanson CA, Rabe KG, Shanafelt TD, Morice WG, et al. CD5-positive chronic B-cell lymphoproliferative disorders: diagnosis and prognosis of a heterogeneous disease entity. Cytometry B Clin Cytom. 2010;78(Suppl 1):S35–41.
107. Palumbo GA, Parrinello N, Fargione G, Cardillo K, Chiarenza A, Berretta S, et al. CD200 expression may help in differential diagnosis between mantle cell lymphoma and B-cell chronic lymphocytic leukemia. Leuk Res. 2009;33:1212–6.
108. Miao Y, Fan L, Wu Y-J, Xia Y, Qiao C, Wang Y, et al. Low expression of CD200 predicts shorter time-to-treatment in chronic lymphocytic leukemia. Oncotarget. 2016;7:13551–62.
109. Gutierrez A, Tschumper RC, Wu X, Shanafelt TD, Eckel-Passow J, Huddleston PM, et al. LEF-1 is a prosurvival factor in chronic lymphocytic leukemia and is expressed in the preleukemic state of monoclonal B-cell lymphocytosis. Blood. 2010;116:2975–83.
110. Amador-Ortiz C, Goolsby CL, Peterson LC, Wolniak KL, McLaughlin JL, Gao J, et al. Flow cytometric analysis of lymphoid enhancer-binding factor 1 in diagnosis of chronic lymphocytic leukemia/small lymphocytic lymphoma. Am J Clin Pathol. 2015;143:214–22.
111. Menter T, Dirnhofer S, Tzankov A. LEF1: a highly specific marker for the diagnosis of chronic lymphocytic B cell leukaemia/small lymphocytic B cell lymphoma. J Clin Pathol. 2015;68:473–8.
112. Wu W, Zhu H, Fu Y, Shen W, Miao K, Hong M, et al. High LEF1 expression predicts adverse prognosis in chronic lymphocytic leukemia and may be targeted by ethacrynic acid. Oncotarget. 2016;7(16):21631–43.
113. Ahmad E, Steinberg SM, Goldin L, Hess CJ, Caporaso N, Kreitman RJ, et al. Immunophenotypic features distinguishing familial chronic lymphocytic leukemia from sporadic chronic lymphocytic leukemia. Cytometry B Clin Cytom. 2008;74:221–6.
114. Ghia P, Prato G, Stella S, Scielzo C, Geuna M, Caligaris-Cappio F. Age-dependent accumulation of monoclonal CD4+CD8+ double positive T lymphocytes in the peripheral blood of the elderly. Br J Haematol. 2007;139:780–90.
115. Fazi C, Scarfò L, Pecciarini L, Cottini F, Dagklis A, Janus A, et al. General population low-count CLL-like MBL persists over time without clinical progression, although carrying the same cytogenetic abnormalities of CLL. Blood. 2011;118:6618–25.
116. Lortholary P, Ripault M, Boiron M. Richter's syndrome. Nouv Rev Fr Hematol. 1964;4:456–7.
117. Brecher M, Banks PM. Hodgkin's disease variant of Richter's syndrome. Report of eight cases. Am J Clin Pathol. 1990;93:333–9.
118. Parikh SA, Habermann TM, Chaffee KG, Call TG, Ding W, Leis JF, et al. Hodgkin transformation of chronic lymphocytic leukemia: incidence, outcomes, and comparison to de novo Hodgkin lymphoma. Am J Hematol. 2015;90:334–8.
119. Parikh SA, Rabe KG, Call TG, Zent CS, Habermann TM, Ding W, et al. Diffuse large B-cell lymphoma (Richter syndrome) in patients with chronic lymphocytic leukaemia (CLL): a cohort study of newly diagnosed patients. Br J Haematol. 2013;162:774–82.
120. Fabbri G, Rasi S, Rossi D, Trifonov V, Khiabanian H, Ma J, et al. Analysis of the chronic lymphocytic leukemia coding genome: role of NOTCH1 mutational activation. J Exp Med. 2011;208:1389–401.
121. Aydin S, Rossi D, Bergui L, D'Arena G, Ferrero E, Bonello L, et al. CD38 gene polymorphism and chronic lymphocytic leukemia: a role in transformation to Richter syndrome? Blood. 2008;111:5646–53.
122. Rossi D, Spina V, Cerri M, Rasi S, Deambrogi C, De Paoli L, et al. Stereotyped B-cell receptor is an independent risk factor of chronic lymphocytic leukemia transformation to Richter syndrome. Clin Cancer Res. 2009;15:4415–22.
123. Rossi D, Spina V, Deambrogi C, Rasi S, Laurenti L, Stamatopoulos K, et al. The genetics of Richter syndrome reveals disease heterogeneity and predicts survival after transformation. Blood. 2011;117:3391–401.
124. Giné E, Martinez A, Villamor N, López-Guillermo A, Camos M, Martinez D, et al. Expanded and highly active proliferation centers identify a histological subtype of chronic lymphocytic leukemia ("accelerated" chronic lymphocytic leukemia) with aggressive clinical behavior. Haematologica. 2010;95:1526–33.
125. Lepretre S, Aurran T, Mahé B, Cazin B, Tournilhac O, Maisonneuve H, et al. Excess mortality after treatment with fludarabine and cyclophosphamide in combination with alemtuzumab in previously untreated patients with chronic lymphocytic leukemia in a randomized phase 3 trial. Blood. 2012;119:5104–10.
126. Janssens A, Berth M, De Paepe P, Verhasselt B, Van Roy N, Noens L, et al. EBV negative Richter's syndrome from a coexistent clone after salvage treatment with alemtuzumab in a CLL patient. Am J Hematol. 2006;81:706–12.
127. Martinez D, Valera A, Perez NS, Sua Villegas LF, Gonzalez-Farre B, Sole C, et al. Plasmablastic transformation of low-grade B-cell lymphomas: report on 6 cases. Am J Surg Pathol. 2013;37:272–81.
128. Robak T, Urbańska-Ryś H, Strzelecka B, Krykowski E, Bartkowiak J, Błoński JZ, et al. Plasmablastic lymphoma in a patient with chronic lymphocytic leukemia heavily pretreated with cladribine (2-CdA): an unusual variant of Richter's syndrome. Eur J Haematol. 2001;67:322–7.
129. Hsi ED, Lorsbach RB, Fend F, Dogan A. Plasmablastic lymphoma and related disorders. Am J Clin Pathol. 2011;136:183–94.
130. Mao Z, Quintanilla-Martinez L, Raffeld M, Richter M, Krugmann J, Burek C, et al. IgVH mutational status and clonality analysis of Richter's transformation: diffuse large B-cell lymphoma and Hodgkin lymphoma in association with B-cell chronic lymphocytic leukemia (B-CLL) represent 2 different pathways of disease evolution. Am J Surg Pathol. 2007;31:1605–14.
131. Hans CP, Weisenburger DD, Greiner TC, Gascoyne RD, Delabie J, Ott G, et al. Confirmation of the molecular classification of diffuse large B-cell lymphoma by immunohistochemistry using a tissue microarray. Blood. 2004;103:275–82.
132. Rosenwald A, Wright G, Chan WC, Connors JM, Campo E, Fisher RI, et al. The use of molecular profiling to predict survival after chemotherapy for diffuse large-B-cell lymphoma. N Engl J Med. 2002;346:1937–47.
133. Berglund M, Thunberg U, Amini R-M, Book M, Roos G, Erlanson M, et al. Evaluation of immunophenotype in diffuse large B-cell lymphoma and its impact on prognosis. Mod Pathol. 2005;18:1113–20.
134. Chigrinova E, Rinaldi A, Kwee I, Rossi D, Rancoita PMV, Strefford JC, et al. Two main genetic pathways lead to the transformation of chronic lymphocytic leukemia to Richter syndrome. Blood. 2013;122:2673–82.

135. Yamaguchi M, Seto M, Okamoto M, Ichinohasama R, Nakamura N, Yoshino T, et al. De novo CD5+ diffuse large B-cell lymphoma: a clinicopathologic study of 109 patients. Blood. 2002;99:815–21.
136. Nakamura N, Nakamura S, Yamaguchi M, Ichinohasama R, Yoshino T, Kuze T, et al. CD5+ diffuse large B-cell lymphoma consists of germline cases and hypermutated cases in the immunoglobulin heavy chain gene variable region. Int J Hematol. 2005;81:58–61.
137. Taniguchi M, Oka K, Hiasa A, Yamaguchi M, Ohno T, Kita K, et al. De novo CD5+ diffuse large B-cell lymphomas express VH genes with somatic mutation. Blood. 1998;91:1145–51.
138. Landau DA, Tausch E, Taylor-Weiner AN, Stewart C, Reiter JG, Bahlo J, et al. Mutations driving CLL and their evolution in progression and relapse. Nature. 2015;526:525–30.
139. Put N, Van Roosbroeck K, Konings P, Meeus P, Brusselmans C, Rack K, et al. Chronic lymphocytic leukemia and prolymphocytic leukemia with MYC translocations: a subgroup with an aggressive disease course. Ann Hematol. 2012;91:863–73.
140. Li Y, Hu S, Wang SA, Li S, Huh YO, Tang Z, et al. The clinical significance of 8q24/MYC rearrangement in chronic lymphocytic leukemia. Mod Pathol. 2016;29:444–51.
141. Tsimberidou A-M, O'Brien S, Kantarjian HM, Koller C, Hagemeister FB, Fayad L, et al. Hodgkin transformation of chronic lymphocytic leukemia: the M. D. Anderson Cancer Center experience. Cancer. 2006;107:1294–302.
142. Bockorny B, Codreanu I, Dasanu CA. Hodgkin lymphoma as Richter transformation in chronic lymphocytic leukaemia: a retrospective analysis of world literature. Br J Haematol. 2012;156:50–66.
143. Jamroziak K, Tadmor T, Robak T, Polliack A. Richter syndrome in chronic lymphocytic leukemia: updates on biology, clinical features and therapy. Leuk Lymphoma. 2015;56:1949–58.
144. Pescarmona E, Pignoloni P, Mauro FR, Cerretti R, Anselmo AP, Mandelli F, et al. Hodgkin/Reed-Sternberg cells and Hodgkin's disease in patients with B-cell chronic lymphocytic leukaemia: an immunohistological, molecular and clinical study of four cases suggesting a heterogeneous pathogenetic background. Virchows Arch. 2000;437:129–32.
145. de Leval L, Vivario M, De Prijck B, Zhou Y, Boniver J, Harris NL, et al. Distinct clonal origin in two cases of Hodgkin's lymphoma variant of Richter's syndrome associated with EBV infection. Am J Surg Pathol. 2004;28:679–86.
146. Xiao W, Chen WW, Sorbara L, Davies-Hill T, Pittaluga S, Raffeld M, et al. Hodgkin lymphoma variant of Richter transformation: morphology, EBV status, clonality and survival analysis-with comparison to Hodgkin-like Lesion. Hum Pathol. 2016;55:108–16.
147. Tzankov A, Fong D. Hodgkin's disease variant of Richter's syndrome clonally related to chronic lymphocytic leukemia arises in ZAP-70 negative mutated CLL. Med Hypotheses. 2006;66:577–9.
148. Thompson PA, Wierda WG. Eliminating minimal residual disease as a therapeutic end point: working toward cure for patients with CLL. Blood. 2016;127:279–86.
149. Vuillier F, Claisse JF, Vandenvelde C, Travade P, Magnac C, Chevret S, et al. Evaluation of residual disease in B-cell chronic lymphocytic leukemia patients in clinical and bone-marrow remission using CD5-CD19 markers and PCR study of gene rearrangements. Leuk Lymphoma. 1992;7:195–204.
150. Maloum K, Sutton L, Baudet S, Laurent C, Bonnemye P, Magnac C, et al. Novel flow-cytometric analysis based on BCD5+ subpopulations for the evaluation of minimal residual disease in chronic lymphocytic leukaemia. Br J Haematol. 2002;119:970–5.
151. Gupta R, Jain P, Deo SVS, Sharma A. Flow cytometric analysis of CD5+ B cells: a frame of reference for minimal residual disease analysis in chronic lymphocytic leukemia. Am J Clin Pathol. 2004;121:368–72.
152. Hillmen P. MRD in CLL. Clin Adv Hematol Oncol. 2006;4:6–7; discussion 10; suppl 12.
153. Rawstron AC, Villamor N, Ritgen M, Böttcher S, Ghia P, Zehnder JL, et al. International standardized approach for flow cytometric residual disease monitoring in chronic lymphocytic leukaemia. Leukemia. 2007;21:956–64.
154. Rawstron AC, Böttcher S, Letestu R, Villamor N, Fazi C, Kartsios H, et al. Improving efficiency and sensitivity: European Research Initiative in CLL (ERIC) update on the international harmonised approach for flow cytometric residual disease monitoring in CLL. Leukemia. 2013;27:142–9.
155. Dowling AK, Liptrot SD, O'Brien D, Vandenberghe E. Optimization and validation of an 8-color single-tube assay for the sensitive detection of minimal residual disease in B-cell chronic lymphocytic leukemia detected via flow cytometry. Lab Med. 2016;47:103–11.
156. Delage R, Jacques L, Massinga-Loembe M, Poulin J, Bilodeau D, Mignault C, et al. Persistent polyclonal B-cell lymphocytosis: further evidence for a genetic disorder associated with B-cell abnormalities. Br J Haematol. 2001;114:666–70.
157. Matutes E, Owusu-Ankomah K, Morilla R, Garcia Marco J, Houlihan A, Que TH, et al. The immunological profile of B-cell disorders and proposal of a scoring system for the diagnosis of CLL. Leukemia. 1994;8:1640–5.
158. Ferrer A, Salaverria I, Bosch F, Villamor N, Rozman M, Beà S, et al. Leukemic involvement is a common feature in mantle cell lymphoma. Cancer. 2007;109:2473–80.
159. Salaverria I, Royo C, Carvajal-Cuenca A, Clot G, Navarro A, Valera A, et al. CCND2 rearrangements are the most frequent genetic events in cyclin D1(-) mantle cell lymphoma. Blood. 2013;121:1394–402.
160. Fernàndez V, Salamero O, Espinet B, Solé F, Royo C, Navarro A, et al. Genomic and gene expression profiling defines indolent forms of mantle cell lymphoma. Cancer Res. 2010;70:1408–18.
161. Treon SP, Xu L, Yang G, Zhou Y, Liu X, Cao Y, et al. MYD88 L265P somatic mutation in Waldenström's macroglobulinemia. N Engl J Med. 2012;367:826–33.
162. Baseggio L, Traverse-Glehen A, Petinataud F, Callet-Bauchu E, Berger F, French M, et al. CD5 expression identifies a subset of splenic marginal zone lymphomas with higher lymphocytosis: a clinico-pathological, cytogenetic and molecular study of 24 cases. Haematologica. 2010;95:604–12.

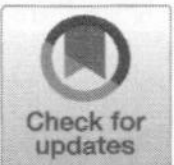

8 The Genomic and Epigenomic Landscape of Chronic Lymphocytic Leukemia

Jonathan C. Strefford, Renata Walewska, and David G. Oscier

Introduction

Since the previous edition of this book, our understanding of the cytogenetics and genomics of chronic lymphocytic leukemia has taken a quantum leap forward, principally the result of seminal technological advances (Fig. 8.1). In the 1970s, the development of polyclonal B-cell mitogens culminated with the discovery of the first cytogenetic abnormality in CLL, trisomy 12, in 1980, shortly followed by the interstitial deletion of 13q14 [1, 2]. With the advent of more effective mitogens, most recently CpG oligonucleotides combined with interleukin 2 [3, 4], the majority of cases of CLL yield metaphase preparation and clonal abnormalities are identifiable in approximately 80% [5]. In contrast to many other mature B-cell tumors, recurrent reciprocal translocations are uncommon in CLL, whereas copy number changes, particularly deletion events such as those affecting 11q, 13q, and 17p, and trisomy of chromosome 12 occur frequently.

In the 1980s, fluorescent *in situ* hybridization (FISH) approaches overcame the need for dividing cells, thereby permitting the analysis of interphase nuclei. The seminal study by Döhner and colleagues established the relative prognostic significance of a panel of recurrent copy number changes, based on the presence of 17p, 11q, and 13q deletions, and trisomy 12, with 13q deletions (as a sole abnormality) and 17p deletion being the markers of best and worst prognosis, respectively [6]. Similar data can now be obtained using either multiplex ligation-dependent probe amplification (MLPA) or quantitative PCR [7–10], although these approaches are rarely used in the clinical setting.

The development of comparative genomic hybridization (CGH) initially with a chromosome template [11], but later with an array-based template [12], allowed the entire genome to be screened for copy number alterations (CNAs) in a single experiment. Currently, copy number changes and loss of heterozygosity (LOH) events can be detected using arrays with more than two million unique genomic features, enabling the identification of genomic alterations of 10–100Kb in size. These studies have identified novel recurrent regions of copy number changes and permitted the gene content of more established lesions to be accurately delineated.

While early molecular studies, employing traditional approaches, identified important mutated cancer genes in CLL, such as *TP53* and *ATM* genes occurring in approximately 80% of patients with *TP53* loss and 40% of patients with *ATM* loss, respectively [13, 14], it was the development of high-throughput massively parallel sequencing that permitted the analysis of the entire CLL genome [15]. Whole-genome (WGS) and -exome (WES) sequencing of more than 1000 CLL patients has led to the discovery of novel mutated cancer genes, positioned within key biological pathways, and has allowed the aforementioned "Döhner" prognostic model to be nuanced with both gene mutation and immunogenetic data [16]. Furthermore, these experiments can be performed with much greater resolution, allowing clinically relevant low-level subclonal mutations to be identified and providing insights into the nature and extent of intraclonal heterogeneity [17, 18]. Indeed, single cells can be isolated using modern flow cytometry or microfluidic approaches and analyzed using next-generation sequencing (NGS) techniques, providing even greater resolution of the clonal architecture of human neoplasms. Methodological advances are also contributing to a greater understanding of the methylome

J.C. Strefford, B.Sc., P.C.C.C., Ph.D. (✉)
Faculty of Medicine, Cancer Genomics, Academic Unit of Cancer Sciences, Southampton General Hospital, University of Southampton, Tremona Road, Southampton SO16 6YD, UK
e-mail: jcs@soton.ac.uk

R. Walewska, M.B.Ch.B., F.R.C.Path., Ph.D.
Department of Haematology, Royal Bournemouth Hospital, Castle Lane East, Bournemouth BH7 7DW, UK

D.G. Oscier, M.A., M.B., F.R.C.P., F.R.C.Path.
Faculty of Medicine, Cancer Genomics, Academic Unit of Cancer Sciences, Southampton General Hospital, University of Southampton, Tremona Road, Southampton SO16 6YD, UK

Department of Haematology, Royal Bournemouth Hospital, Castle Lane East, Bournemouth BH7 7DW, UK

P.H. Wiernik et al. (eds.), *Neoplastic Diseases of the Blood*, DOI 10.1007/978-3-319-64263-5_8

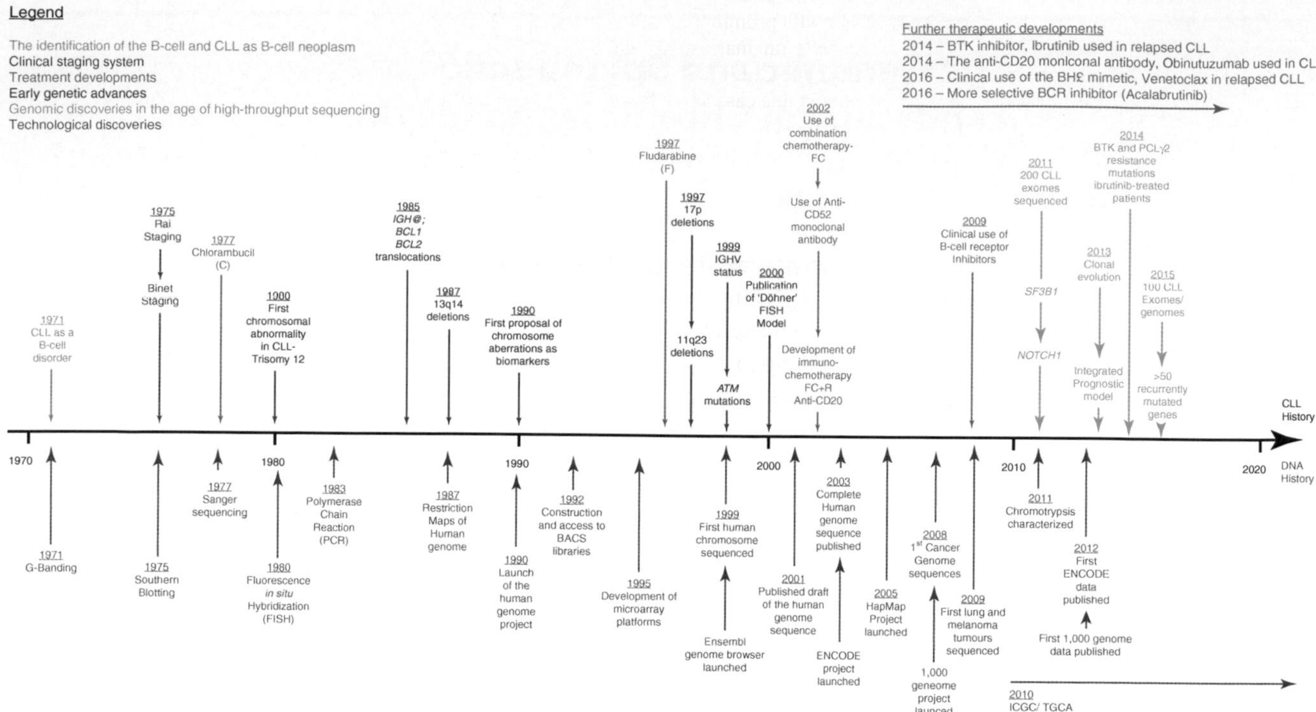

Fig. 8.1 Historical overview of the developments in the field of genomics, and the advancing understanding of the molecular pathogenesis and treatment of CLL

and chromatin landscape in CLL and their relationship to the putative cells of origin of *IGHV*-mutated and unmutated CLL [19–22]. While a complete annotation of the CLL genome and epigenome is in sight, ongoing analysis of the CLL proteome, transcriptome including microRNA expression, and functional consequences of specific genomic and epigenetic abnormalities are beginning to unravel the drivers for clonal selection while also providing prognostic data and identifying therapeutic targets.

In the remainder of this chapter we provide an overview of the genomic landscape, and discuss the commonest genomic abnormalities found in both CLL (Tables 8.1 and 8.2) and Richter's transformation, epigenetic abnormalities, genetic predisposition to CLL, and finally the clinical importance of genomic abnormalities in the management of patients with CLL.

Table 8.1 Recurrent copy number changes in CLL

Gene name	Prevalence (%)	Principal candidate genes	Other candidate genes	References
del(13q)	60–80	*miR-15a/16-1*, *DLEU2*	*RB1*, *DLEU7*	[2, 23, 24]
del(11q)	10–20	*ATM*	*BIRC3*, *MRE11*, *H2AFX*	[25]
del(17p)	5–50	*TP53*	–	[6]
Trisomy 12	10–15	Unknown	–	[26]
del(6q)	5	Unknown	–	[27]
dup(2p)	5–28	*REL*, *BCL11A*, *XPO1*	*MYCN*	[28, 29]
dup(8q)	5	*CMYC*	–	[30]
del(15q)	4	*MGA*	–	[30, 31]
del(3p)	3	*SETD2*	–	[32]

Chromosomal Abnormalities

Deletion of Chromosomal Band, 13q14

Deletion of 13q14.3 is the commonest cytogenetic abnormality in CLL, seen in 50–60% of patients (Table 8.1). Recent WGS data demonstrates the result of interstitial deletions in approximately 60% of patients and translocations involving numerous, sometimes recurring, partner chromosomes (e.g., chromosomes 1, 2, and 14) in the remainder [48]. Approximately 10% of 13q deletions are the result of a complex chain of genomic lesions targeting several chromosomes, characteristic of chromoplexy [49]. 13q14 deletions may be heterozygous (in 70% of cases) or homozygous, where the latter can be the result of copy number-neutral LOH in rare cases [23].

The size of the 13q14 deletion is highly heterogenous in both size and gene content, but a minimally deleted region which includes exons from *DLEU2*, a long noncoding RNA, *DLEU1*, and miRNA 15a/16-1 cluster has been reported [50]. The importance of these genes is demonstrated most strikingly by a transgenic mouse model, in which either the minimally deleted region encompassing both *DLEU2* and miR 15a/16-1 or miR 15a/16-1 alone was deleted [51]. In both models a clonal B-cell population proliferated in approximately 30% of mice. In the majority of cases the histology and immunophenotype of these B-cell expansions resembled human CD5-positive monoclonal B-cell lymphocytosis (MBL), CLL, or small lymphocytic lymphoma (SLL). A minority of mice developed clonal CD5-negative lymphomas. Bi-allelic deletions and deletions of both *DLEU2* and miR 15a/16-1 were associated with more aggressive disease [51]. In this model, the miRNA cluster regulates the expression of a series of cell cycle genes including *CCND1, CCND2, CCNE1, CDK4*, and *CDK6* which, in turn, regulate transition from G0 to G1 to S phase [51].

Table 8.2 Recurrent mutation genes in CLL, whose importance is evidenced by validation across independent cohorts with associated biological or clinical correlations

Gene name	Gene nomenclature	Approximate frequency (%)	References
Tumor protein p53	*TP53*	5–27	[13]
Ataxia telangiectasia mutated	*ATM*	9–14	[14]
Notch 1	*NOTCH1*	3–24	[33–35]
Splicing factor 3b, subunit 1, 155 kDa	*SF3B1*	5–17	[34, 36]
Nuclear factor of kappa light polypeptide gene enhancer in B-cell inhibitor, epsilon	*NFKBIE*	10	[37]
Paired box 5	*PAX5*	9	[38]-
Ribosomal protein S15	*RPS15*	5–20	[17, 39]
Early growth response 2	*EGR2*	1–8	[18, 37]
Baculoviral IAP repeat containing 3	*BIRC3*	1.5–6	[40]
Chromodomain helicase DNA-binding protein 2	*CHD2*	5	[34]
Mediator complex subunit 12	*MED12*	2–5	[18, 41]
Protection of telomeres 1	*POT1*	5	[34]
Myeloid differentiation primary response gene 88	*MYD88*	3–5	[34, 42]
SET domain containing 2	*SETD2*	4	[32, 38]
F-box and WD repeat domain containing 7, E3 ubiquitin protein ligase	*FBXW7*	4	[36]
SAM domain and HD domain 1	*SAMHD1*	3	[18, 43]
Sucrase-isomaltase (alpha-glucosidase)	*SI*	3	[44]
Exportin 1	*XPO1*	2.5	[42]
V-raf murine sarcoma viral oncogene homolog B1	*BRAF*	2–4	[17, 45]
V-Ki-ras2 Kirsten rat sarcoma viral oncogene homolog	*KRAS*	2	[18, 46]
Interferon regulatory factor 4	*IRF4*	1.5	[17, 38, 47]

Several other studies have shown a correlation between downregulation of miR 15a/16b and upregulation of BCL2 expression [52, 53]. The consequences of loss of DLEU2 and other genes outside the minimally deleted region which nevertheless are deleted in most cases with 13q14 loss are areas of intensive research, where it is clear that 13q deletion size has significant biological and clinical consequences [23, 54, 55].

Genomic Lesions Targeting 11q23

Structural abnormalities of the long arm of chromosome 11 are frequent in CLL, occurring in approximately 20% of patients (Table 8.1). The incidence is higher in advanced- than in early-stage disease and patients frequently have widespread bulky lymphadenopathy. Cytogenetic studies show that most cases with an 11q abnormality have a deletion involving 11q23. Deletions vary in size usually occurring within the 11q21–q25 region. Balanced translocations in this region are rare [54].

The great majority of 11q deletions in CLL result in loss of the ataxia telangiectasia-mutated (*ATM*) gene and approximately 40% of patients with *ATM* loss carry a mutation of the remaining allele (Table 8.2) [55, 56]. Approximately 12% of patients have an *ATM* mutation without an accompanying 11q deletion [57]. In patients with bi-allelic *ATM* abnormalities, the mutation may either precede or follow the deletion of the other allele [40]

As only 40% of 11q deleted cases carry an inactivating mutation of *ATM*, and in vitro studies of the function of the double-stranded DNA repair pathway appear to be preserved in patients with an 11q deletion without an *ATM* mutation, it has been postulated that other genes on 11q may impact disease pathogenesis [40]. The postulated role of other genes on 11q has not been supported by the analysis of genes within the well-defined MDR on 11q, where studies have shown reduced expression of these genes, but have not identified deleterious mutations [57]. However, genomic profiling approaches have shown that 11q deletions are heterogeneous in both size and location, and it has been proposed that other genes involved in DNA damage response, such as Mre11 and *H2AFX*, deleted in 50% and 18% of cases with an 11q deletion, respectively, might also contribute to leukemogenesis [58].

Another gene on 11q of potential importance is *BIRC3*, a negative regulator of NF-κB signaling. *BIRC3* deletions occur in approx. 80% of cases with 11q loss, where they are always concomitant with *ATM* deletion [56, 57]. Mutation occurs in approx. 2% of cases, where they associate with constitutive noncanonical NF-κB activation in fludarabine-refractory CLL patients with these mutations [40]. However, *ATM* and *BIRC3* lesions often coexist in the same patient, and it is an *ATM* mutation that is most associated with poor outcome in del(11q) CLL [57]. 11q deletions can also include the microRNA (miR) cluster that included miR-34b and miR-34c. These miRs interact with p53, with reduced expression and hypermethylation of miR-34b/c locus occurring preferentially in non-11q deleted cases [58].

Deletion and Mutations of the Tumor-Suppressor Gene, *TP53*

Structural abnormalities of chromosome 17p, including deletions, translocations (usually unbalanced), and isochromosome 17q, are detectable cytogenetically in less than 5% of patients with early-stage CLL rising to over 30% in patients with advanced chemo-refractory disease (Table 8.1). In routine practice it is usual to screen for 17p loss using a FISH probe encompassing the *TP53* gene. Factors that can influence interphase FISH results such as the choice of probe, number of cells counted, scoring of all lymphocytes or just clonal B cells, and choice of cutoff are of particular importance for TP53 screening in view of the clinical significance of *TP53* loss. 80–90% of cases with *TP53* loss have a mutation of the remaining allele (Table 8.2). 3–5% of patients acquire a *TP53* mutation without loss of the other allele [59–62]. Bi-allelic *TP53* mutation also occurs in rare cases, due to either a second unique mutation or the presence of 17p copy number-neutral loss of heterozygosity [59].

Using traditional molecular screening approaches, *TP53* mutations can be identified in approximately 9% of untreated CLL cases, with loss of the second allele seen in the majority of mutated cases (Table 8.2). Differences in the incidence of *TP53* loss and/or mutation among series reflect differences in patient populations and methods for screening for *TP53* mutations. The majority of *TP53* mutations are missense and located within the DNA-binding domain of p53 encoded by exons 5–8. Approximately 20% of mutations occur within 6 "hot spots." The *TP53* mutation profile is similar in both previously untreated and treated patients suggesting that chemotherapy selects preexisting small p53 mutated clones [59]. The presence of a *TP53* mutation, thought to be an event preceding clonal evolution [60], is a strong independent marker of adverse survival and a powerful predictor of poor response to chemo-immunotherapy, and therefore has direct implications on treatment decisions [61]. Low-level subclonal mutations, beyond the resolution of Sanger sequencing (down to 0.3% of the cancer cells), reside in approximately 9% of untreated CLL, mutations that expand to become more clonal in sequential samples from patients that ultimately relapse [61, 62]. Patients with these subclonal *TP53* mutations show the same clinical phenotype and poor survival [61] as patients with clonal mutations and carry a higher risk of mutation selection by therapy. Identifying *TP53* defects early in their evolution may enable improved clinical management of high-risk CLL. It is important to mention a rare subset of early-stage CLL patients with mutated *IGHV* genes and *TP53* abnormalities do exhibit a more stable disease course [63].

Functional studies in which double-stranded DNA breaks are induced in leukemic cells in vitro and the expression of p53 and its downstream targets such as p21 and miR34a are measured are also able to detect TP53 abnormalities in CLL [63]. More recent studies suggest that primary abnormalities of p21 and miR34a expression in patients with no detectable TP53 abnormality may also cause p53 dysfunction and can be associated with poor clinical outcome [30, 32]. *TP53* abnormalities are frequently associated with complex genomic abnormalities and a poor outcome as discussed below.

Trisomy 12

Trisomy 12 is the most frequent numerical chromosome abnormality in CLL occurring in approximately 10% of patients (Table 8.1). It is usually the primary cytogenetic abnormality detectable at diagnosis; acquisition of trisomy 12 during the course of disease is extremely rare. There is a strong but as-yet unexplained association between trisomy 12 and both atypical lymphocyte morphology and an atypical immunophenotype [64]. The role of trisomy 12 in the pathogenesis of CLL remains unclear. Structural abnormalities of chromosome 12 may result in a partial trisomy 12 with duplication of the region between q13 and q22. This region includes the MDM2 gene which is overexpressed in patients with trisomy 12 [65]. Trisomy 12 may occur as the sole cytogenetic abnormality in CLL but is frequently accompanied by additional trisomies, particularly of chromosomes 19 and 18 [66], deletion of 13q14, or immunoglobulin gene translocations, as discussed below.

Other Copy Number Aberrations

In addition to chromosomal rearrangements, a number of rare, but recurrent, copy number changes are present in the genome of CLL patients (Table 8.1). Interstitial deletions of 14q are rare and deletion break points are clustered and may juxtapose the immunoglobulin enhancer to an as-yet unidentified gene. Deletions of 6q can be detected in approximately

5% of patients with CLL, but multiple minimally deleted regions have been identified or candidate gene has been proposed. The clinical significance of 6q loss is uncertain but has been associated with atypical lymphocyte morphology-extensive lymphadenopathy but not chemoresistance. Overrepresentation of chromosome 2p has been consistently reported as a genomic abnormality in CLL in studies using CGH and SNP arrays. Overall occurrence has been reported in 5% of early-stage CLL patients, rising to 28% in stage B and C disease. Conventional cytogenetics shows a variety of mechanisms resulting in duplication. However, 2p duplication rarely occurs in isolation and is often associated with adverse genetic abnormalities: del(11q) and del(17p) and unmutated *IGHV* genes. The duplicated region most commonly reported includes the oncogenes *REL* and *MYCN*. Expression of NMYC has been shown to be elevated in the presence of a 2p24 duplication suggesting that this gene may be of significance in disease progression. Other regions targeted by recurrent copy number changes at a low incidence include duplications of 8q24, and deletions of 15q15.1 (4% of cases) and 3p21 (3% of cases), with *c-MYC*, *MGA*, and *SETD2* as candidate genes, respectively [30, 32].

Structural Chromosomal Rearrangements

Translocations involving the immunoglobulin gene loci are rare in CLL (<5%) and result in juxtaposition of a number of recurring partner genes to the transcriptional control of the immunoglobulin locus. The most common partner genes are *BCL2* (18q22) and *BCL3* (19q13) and more rarely *BCL11A* (2p15), *CCND3* (6p21), *CMYC* (8q24), and *CCND1* (11q13). The t(14;19)(q32;q13) is usually associated with trisomy 12 and most patients have atypical lymphocyte morphology, an atypical immunophenotype, and unmutated IGHV genes. The clinical course is usually progressive and the response to standard chemotherapy is poor. The t(11;14) translocation has been described as a rare secondary aberration in patients relapsing after therapy [64]. The clinical importance of the t(14;18) is uncertain, and it occurs as a primary or secondary event, commonly concomitant trisomy 12. The t(2;14)(p16;q32) is extremely rare and is associated with atypical morphology, immunophenotype, and bulky disease [67]. Translocations involving *CMYC* and a variety of partners including the immunoglobulin gene loci are associated with increased prolymphocytes, complex cytogenetic abnormalities, and a poor prognosis.

Patterns and Mechanisms of Genomic Complexity

Growing evidence suggests that the presence of genomic complexity [5, 65], defined by the presence of increased numbers of chromosomal lesions, can predict short overall survival [5, 65], independent of the presence of 17p deletions [66]. Indeed, interest has recently refocused on the presence of karyotypic complexity, defined by chromosomal banding analysis, as it represents a powerful independent predictor of poor response to the kinase inhibitor, ibrutinib [68].

As genomic complexity is often observed in patients with *ATM* and *TP53* gene lesion [69], it may be that these defects allow telomeres to shorten below the length at which apoptosis or senescence is normally triggered, thus leading to further telomere attrition and accumulation of short telomeres [70, 71], enabling uncapped telomeres to fuse, resulting in genomic instability. While DNA damage can be accumulated over time, high levels of DNA damage can also be acquired rapidly. One example is chromothripsis, a catastrophic process involving genome shattering that occurs during a single mitotic cycle resulting in a pattern of oscillating DNA copy number changes along a single chromosome, or a few chromosomes [67]. The frequency of chromothripsis is approximately 3–5% of human cancers, was first identified in a CLL patient [30, 67], and is the result of a partitioned chromosome(s) in a micronucleus that becomes damaged and is reintegrated into the daughter nuclei [72, 73]. Chromothripsis occurs preferentially in patients with unmutated *IGHV* genes and high-risk genomic aberrations [30], such as mutations in *TP53*, suggesting that a defective DNA damage response is critical to the process of chromothripsis, or the tolerance of the genomic damage [74]. While patients with chromothripsis exhibit both inferior OS and PFS, it is unclear if this is independent of the aforementioned poor-risk genomic lesions [30]. The acquisition of multiple single-nucleotide variants can also occur in a single mitotic explosion, termed kataegis [75], and has also been observed in the genome of CLL patients. This process drives cytosine-specific mutagenesis, often in regions flanking sites of genomic rearrangement, and can result in up to several thousand base-pair substitutions occurring rapidly [76].

In CLL, the biological and clinical importance of telomere structure has been well studied. Telomeres cap the ends of chromosomes, playing a crucial role in the maintenance of genomic integrity. Telomere length is a critical determining factor of telomere function, with critically eroded telomeres being subjected to aberrant DNA repair leading to telomere fusion and genomic instability. The presence of shortened telomere length (TL) is associated with poor clinical survival when assessed by a variety of techniques, as with terminal restriction fragment analysis, FISH-based approaches, and quantitative PCR, with a strong association between short TL and unmutated *IGHV* status [77–81]. The application of STELA (single telomere length analysis) to detect very short telomeres showed that shortening TL in CLL patients can result in loss of their end capping function and make them subject to telomere fusion [82]. Clinically, the acute telomere attrition can precede disease progression, providing further evidence that TL in asymptomatic disease may have powerful predictive value [83].

The Mutational Landscape of CLL

NGS technology has permitted the interrogation of the entire cancer genome for sequence changes at base-pair resolution. WGS and WES data has been collected on more than a thousand CLL patients [17, 18, 33, 34, 36, 38, 42, 84, 85]. However, papers from Landau et al. [17] and Puente et al. [38] published in 2015 provide the most comprehensive and current depiction of the mutational landscape of CLL. Based on the six possible base substitutions and information on the bases immediately 3′ and 5′ to the mutated base, 30 distinct mutational signatures have been identified across all cancer types [76]. Five different signatures have been recognized in CLL. Two (signatures 1 and 5) show a correlation between the number of mutations and increasing age, while two (signatures 2 and 13) have been attributed to activation of AID/POBEC cytidine deaminases. Signature 9 is confined to B-cell tumors that have undergone somatic hypermutation of variable region immunoglobulin genes and is attributed to DNA polymerase η-mediated repair of AID-induced lesions [76, 86]. Understanding underlying mutational mechanisms has clear clinical utility. Modifying the age-related mutational signatures may delay cancer initiation. Furthermore, the recognition of key signatures in asymptomatic patients may facilitate early diagnosis or quantify genotoxic exposure levels.

CLL cases have a median of 0.6–0.87 mutations per megabase (Mb) of genomic DNA which is low compared to solid tumors. Landau et al. and Puente et al. identified an average of 15.3 and 26.9 somatic mutations per patient, respectively [18, 38]. There is a level of discordance between the recurrently mutated genes identified by these two studies. These discrepancies probably reflect the relatively small cohort size and therefore consequent statistical power to identify rare mutated cancer genes, but may also be attributable to the different cohort composition, sequencing platforms, and bioinformatics pipelines used. For example, 22 recurrently mutated genes were implicated in both studies (including *BIRC3*, *CHD2*, *XPO1*, and *EGR2*), while genes only identified by a single study include *SETD2*, *ARID1A*, *NFKBIE* [38], *KRAS*, and *SAMHD1* [17]. While these two studies and indeed a plethora of others have failed to identify a unifying mutation in all patients, and it is unlikely that such a mutation exists at the genomic level, four genes are recurrently mutated at relatively high frequencies across multiple studies. In addition to the aforementioned genes, *TP53* and *ATM*, the other prevalent mutated genes are *NOTCH1* and *SF3B1* (Fig. 8.2). In addition, a glut of additional mutated genes occur at a frequency of approx. 5%, and lead to the dysfunction of eight key cellular processes: (1) cell cycle regulation, (2) DNA damage response, (3) apoptosis, (4) NOTCH1 signaling, (5) RNA metabolism, (6) NF-kB signaling, (7) chromatin remodeling, and (8) BCR signaling (54)

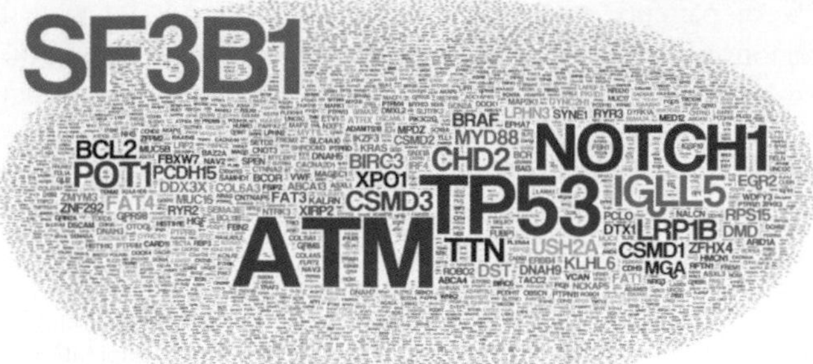

Fig. 8.2 Recurrently mutated cancer genes identified in CLL. This word cloud represents the presence and prevalence of gene mutations in CLL, where the font size represents the mutational frequency of a given gene. The mutation data was obtained from the Sanger Institute Catalogue of Somatic Mutations in Cancer web site, http://cancer.sanger.ac.uk/cosmic [87], with permission

(Tables 8.2 and 8.3, Fig. 8.3). These mutations can be present in the entire cancer cell population (clonal) or found in only a small "subclonal" population of cells. Deep sequencing approaches can detect low-level subclonal mutations present in as little as 0.3% of cancer cells [61] beyond the resolution of standard Sanger sequencing [89].

Mutations of *NOTCH1* and Associated Proteins

In CLL, the importance of Notch signaling is well established where activation confers apoptosis resistance and cell survival in CLL cells [90] and Notch1-signaling inhibitors, such as γ-secretase inhibitors, accelerate B-CLL cell apoptosis by proteasome inhibition and endoplasmic reticulum stress enhancement [91]. The role that gene mutations play in activating Notch signaling and mutations was first described in a small cohort of 43 patients, where 2 patients (4.6%) harbored a heterozygous 2 bp frame-shift deletion (ΔCT7544–7545, P2515Rfs*4) within the PEST domain of *NOTCH1* [35]. The Spanish CLL Genome Consortium confirmed these early observations and demonstrated that this variant creates a premature stop codon, the removal of the PEST sequence from C-terminal protein domain that ultimately results in the accumulation of an active Notch1 isoform in tumor cells [42]. Subsequent studies show that mutations across exon 34 of *NOTCH1* [33, 34, 36, 42], and even within the 3′ UTR of the gene, where noncoding mutations create aberrant splicing events, result in the loss of the *NOTCH1* PEST domain, and consequent constitutive Notch1 activation [38]. *NOTCH1* mutations associate with unmutated *IGHV* CLL, expression of CD38 and ZAP-70, the presence of trisomy 12, short telomeres, and increased prevalence of prolymphocytes [81, 92, 93]. Mutation frequency varies enormously based on the stage of the disease analyzed, ranging from 3% in MBL and 6–10% at CLL diagnosis to >20%

Table 8.3 Recurrently mutated genes in CLL, without biological or clinical evidence

Gene name	Gene nomenclature	Approximate frequency (%)	References
FAT atypical cadherin 1	*FAT1*	10	[88]
Low-density lipoprotein receptor-related protein 1B	*LRP1B*	5	[34]
MGA, MAX dimerization protein	*MGA*	5	[17]
Zinc finger protein 292	*ZNF292*	5	[38]
Zinc finger, MYM-type 3	*ZMYM3*	4	[36]
DEAD (Asp-Glu-Ala-Asp) box polypeptide 3, X-linked	*DDX3X*	3	[18, 36]
Mitogen-activated protein kinase 1	*MAPK1*	3	[36]
IKAROS family zinc finger 3	*IKZF3*	3	[17]
Bromodomain adjacent to zinc finger domain 2A	*BAZ2A*	3	[17]
Histone cluster 1, H1e	*HIST1H1E*	3	[18]
BCL6 corepressor	*BCOR*	3	[18, 38]
Receptor (TNFRSF)-interacting serine-threonine kinase 1	*RIPK1*	3	[18]
Caspase recruitment domain family member 11	*CARD11*	3	[17]
Kelch-like family member 6	*KLHL6*	2	[42]
Nuclear RNA export factor 1	*NXF1*	2	[17, 38]
Nuclear factor kappa B subunit 2	*NFKB2*	2	[38]
Cyclin D2	*CCND2*	2	[38]
Spectrin repeat containing nuclear envelope protein 1	*SYNE1*	2	[38]
AT-rich interaction domain 1A	*ARID1A*	2	[38]
CCR4-NOT transcription complex subunit 3	*CNOT3*	2	[38]
Dual-specificity tyrosine phosphorylation-regulated kinase 1A	*DYRK1A*	2	[17]
Mitogen-activated protein kinase kinase 1	*MAP2K1*	2	[17]
Inositol-trisphosphate 3-kinase B	*ITPKB*	2	[18]
TNF receptor-associated factor 2	*TRAF2*	2	[17]
Far upstream element-binding protein 1	*FUBP1*	1.9	[17]
Exportin 4	*XPO4*	1.8	[17]
Neuroblastoma RAS viral (v-ras) oncogene homolog	*NRAS*	1–3	[18, 45]
Protein tyrosine phosphatase, non-receptor type 11	*PTPN11*	1	[17, 38]
SET domain containing 1A	*SETD1A*	1	[38]
E74 like ETS transcription factor 4	*ELF4*	1	[17]
BRCA1/BRCA2-containing complex subunit 3	*BRCC3*	1	[17]
EWS RNA-binding protein 1	*EWSR1*	1	[17]
ATRX, chromatin remodeler	*ATRX*	1	[38]
Family with sequence similarity 50 member A	*FAM50A*	1	[17]
TNF receptor-associated factor 3	*TRAF3*	1	[17, 38]
Additional sex combs like 1, transcriptional regulator	*ASXL1*	1	[17, 38]
Checkpoint kinase 2	*CHEK2*	1	[17]
G protein subunit beta 1	*GNB1*	1	[17]
Histone cluster 1 H1 family member b	*HIST1H1B*	1	[17]
Pim-1 proto-oncogene, serine/threonine kinase	*PIM1*	1	[17]
Retinoblastoma 1	*RB1*	2[a]	[24]

[a]Frequency in those patients with large 13q deletions which include the *RB1* locus. Defined as "type II" deletions [55]

of patients with alkylating agent or purine analogue-refractory disease [33, 94]. An additional 3% of CLL patients harbor the noncoding 3′UTR mutation [38, 62, 95]. Patients with a mutant *NOTCH1* have inferior survival compared to wild-type patients, compared to 11q deleted patients [16, 92]. The mutational frequency of *NOTCH1* is higher in CLL lymph nodes than in matched peripheral CLL B-cells (24%) and the Notch pathway is frequently activated in lymph node cases independently of *NOTCH1* mutational status, suggesting the existence of other initiating mechanisms, such as ligand activation [96]. Functionally, microenvironmental interactions appear to be required for Notch activation in mutated cases, where these interactions foster conditions that may favor drug resistance [97], but may be overcome with the use of γ-secretase inhibitors, particularly in combination with fludarabine [98]. Mutations in other Notch signaling

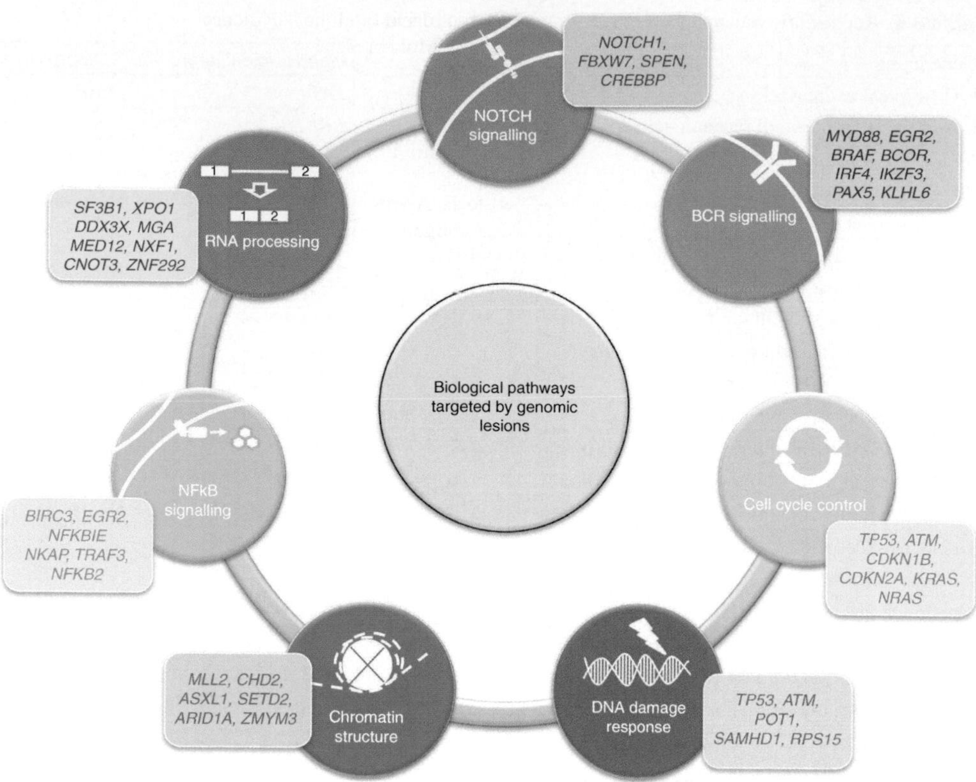

Fig. 8.3 The biological pathways deregulated in CLL by somatic gene mutations. The key biologically relevant genes recurrently mutated in CLL, and the pathways and processes to which they contribute. Genes with functional diversity are represented in the pathway to which they most significantly contribute

proteins have been identified in CLL. For example, *FBXW7*, which targets activated *NOTCH1* for degradation, is mutated in ~2.5% of patients and may provide another mechanism for activated Notch signaling [99].

SF3B1 Mutations and RNA Processing

SF3B1, an important component of the RNA splicing machinery that achieves successful transcription and guarantees the functional diversity of protein species using alternative splicing, is recurrently mutated in CLL but not in other chronic B-cell lymphoproliferative neoplasms [34, 36, 85]. 5–17% of CLL patients harbor *SF3B1* mutations where they are associated with advanced clinical stage, 11q23 deletions, presence of stereotyped IGHV usage (subset #2), and fludarabine-refractory disease in cases with no *TP53* abnormality. Furthermore, they predict reduced TFTT and OS independent of other prognostic variables [34, 36, 85, 99–101].

Using targeted and global experimental approaches, early studies showed that *SF3B1* mutations result in aberrant splicing [34, 36] that is driven by the use of a different branch point sequence in mutant *SF3B1* patients [102]. Initial studies identified a highly expressed truncated *FOXP1* transcript, *FOXP1w* in *SF3B1*-mutated CLL, that lacks two putative PEST domain sequences involved in protein degradation [34]. A subsequent RNA-Seq study implicated an aberrant spliced *ATM* transcript [103] and it is now evident that *SF3B1* mutations may impact DNA damage response [104]. Aberrant splicing of genes involved in B-cell differentiation, Hippo signaling, and NF-κB activation has also been implicated in *SF3B1*-mutated CLL [103]. The identification of mutations within the spliceosome complexes raises the possibility that CLL tumor cells may be sensitive to spliceosome inhibitors. Indeed, *SF3B1* mutations confer sensitivity to the splicing modulator sudemycin, promoting an anti-tumor effect with the BTK inhibitor, ibrutinib [105], and the SF3B1 inhibitor spliceostatin A induces cell death in CLL cells through Mcl-1 downregulation, most markedly in combination with Bcl-2/Bcl-XL antagonists [106].

Another gene involved in RNA processing has also been implicated in CLL pathogenesis, *XPO1*, which encodes the nuclear exporter, Exportin-1, responsible for controlling the directional movement of 100 s proteins and RNA species from the nucleus to the cytoplasm. 4.6% of *IGHV*-unmutated CLL cases harbor somatic mutations in *XPO1* [42], and cause increased Exportin-1 levels in tumor cells, and consequent externalization of key TSP, compromising a cell's ability to respond to DNA damage [107]. Inhibitors of XPO1 may restore apoptotic pathways and chemosensitivity in CLL cells by facilitating nuclear export of key proteins [107, 108].

Other Mutations

Other recurrently mutated genes have emerged, and are continuing to emerge, from high-throughput sequencing projects, albeit at low frequencies (Tables 8.2 and 8.3) [18, 36, 42].

As previously noted, these genes often act within key biological pathways (Fig. 8.3) [18, 34, 36]. Some of the most established are outlined below:

1. **NFKB Signaling**. Recurrently mutated genes have been identified in both the canonical and noncanonical NFκB signaling pathways, where they can result in activation signaling [37, 56, 109, 110]. In addition to aforementioned involvement of the *BIRC3* gene, up to 10% of CLL cases have mutations targeting *NFKBIE*, which encodes NFκB inhibitor epsilon (IKBE). Cellular studies show reduced IKBE expression in mutant cases, decreased IKBE-p65 interactions and increased nuclear p65 levels, and constitutive NFκB activity [110].
2. **B-cell Receptor Signaling.** *MYD88*, a crucial adaptor of the Toll-like receptor (TLR) complex, is mutated in approx. 5% of CLL cases, occurring exclusively in patients with mutated *IGHV* genes. Upon TLR ligand binding, a homodimer of MYD88 is recruited to the receptor, forms a complex with IRAK4, activates IRAK1 and 2, and ultimately leads to TRAF6 activation, phosphorylation of IκBα, and activation of NF-κB [111]. In CLL, the L265P mutation provides constitutive activation of NF-κB activity, by imposing MYD88-IRAK signaling even when ligand receptor binding is absent [42]. However, the clinical impact of MYD88 mutations remains controversial, as conclusive evidence demonstrating independent prognostic significance is lacking [112, 113]. The transcription factor, *EGR2*, is activated by B-cell stimulation and also mutated in 8% of advanced-stage CLL. *BRAF* mutations have a postulated role in fludarabine sensitivity and are associated with reduced time to first treatment [37, 38, 114].
3. **Cell cycle, Apoptosis, DNA Damage.** In addition to the well-studied involvement of the *TP53* and *ATM* loci, other genes with a role in these processes have been recently implicated. *RPS15,* which encodes a component of the 40S ribosomal subunit, is mutated in 20% of CLL patients relapsing post-chemo-immunotherapy [39]. *RPS15* mutations are early clonal events, associated with reduced survival, the functional consequences of which are defective p53 stability and increased degradation [39]. Mutations in the nuclease *SAMHD1* are reported in 3% of patients at diagnosis and are enriched in therapy-refractory patients [43]. Preliminary data suggests that mutations may promote tumorigenesis by deregulation of DNA repair [43]. *POT1*, a component of the shelterin complex, plays a critical role in the protection of telomeres. At diagnosis, mutations occur in approx. 3% of patients [84, 115] rising to 8.1% in patients receiving chlorambucil-based therapy, where they are associated with a shorter survival [46]. In *POT1*-mutated cell lines, chromosomes become fragile, with numerous telomeric and structural aberrations implicating these mutations in promoting genomic instability [84]; this association is not supported by the study of primary CLL tumors [115].
4. **Chromatin Modifiers.** *CHD2*, a chromatin modifier, is mutated in 5.3% of patients, principally in *IGHV*-mutated tumors. Mutations are principally truncating or target functional domains and functional experiments demonstrate alteration of the nuclear distribution of *CHD2* and protein association with actively transcribed genes in mutated patients [116]. Histone methyltransferases (HMTs) are essential epigenetic regulators of chromatin modification and recurrent mutations targeting such genes have only recently been documented in CLL [38]. *SETD2*, the histone methyltransferase non-redundantly responsible for the trimethylation of lysine 36 on histone 3 (H3K36me3), is mutated in up to 4% of patients, and likely to be an early loss-of-function event associated with aggressive disease [32].
5. **Noncoding mutations.** In addition to the aforementioned *NOTCH1* 3′UTR mutations, a second recurrent noncoding mutation has been reported, resulting in deregulation of *PAX5*. In CLL, mutations located within a telomeric enhancer element, 330Kb from the *PAX5* locus, result in reduced *PAX5* expression, and were the only recurrent mutation in a subset of IGHV-unmutated CLL patients, suggesting that these mutations may contribute to disease pathophysiology [38].

Clonal Evolution

Historically, we often consider genomic heterogeneity to exist between patients (inter-tumor), in part explaining the biological and clinical variability that exists between individuals with the same disease. However, it is evident that considerable "intra-tumoral" heterogeneity also exists, such that a tumor can contain many genetically and biologically unique subclonal populations of cancer cells. This cellular plasticity is a prerequisite for Darwinian selection that ultimately selects cellular populations with favorable biological traits, driven by the pressure of therapy and even the tumor microenvironment. In CLL, researchers working with FISH and SNP arrays have long observed the acquisition of genomic aberrations during disease course, with the suggestion that the diagnostic and relapse disease can be genetically distinct [117–120]. However, it has been the application of NGS to temporally and even anatomically discrete cancer specimens from the same CLL patient that has conclusively revealed the composition of clonal expansion [121]. Clonal evolution can occur quickly, or over a more protracted period of time, and follows two simple evolutionary models [122]. Firstly, tumor evolution can develop in a linear fashion, with the maintenance of a founder clone with successive acquisition of new mutations. Secondly, competition between different cancer subclones can persist, resulting in a more complex branching anatomy. In the context of a branching evolution, convergence can occur, where independent mutations in the same genes can be acquired in different subclones [123].

Landau and coauthors [18] showed that passenger events accumulate before the acquisition of recurrent driver mutations (e.g., del(13q), tri12, and *MYD88* mutations) with subsequent malignant initiation. During CLL progression, later subclonal driver mutations target cancer genes like *ATM*, *TP53*, and *RAS* and undergo clonal expansion. The authors also showed an elevated prevalence of clonal evolution in treated patients, and linked the presence of subclones to adverse survival [18]. Subsequent studies demonstrated genomic heterogeneity between different anatomical compartments with mutations expanding in the lymph node and repopulating the peripheral blood compartment at relapse following positive selection by therapy [122, 124, 125]. Rose-Zerilli et al. reported a CLL patient whom at diagnosis presented with mutated immunoglobulin genes, but who developed a fatal *IGHV*-unmutated CLL clone years later, not evident at diagnosis with traditional molecular approaches, but detectable with modern NGS approaches. These observations have important clinical implications and support a model in which low-level subclonal mutations present in early-stage disease can anticipate the evolutionary course of the disease [17].

Epigenetic Abnormalities

There is increasing evidence that epigenetic abnormalities are both frequent and important in the initiation and progression of human malignancies, including CLL. Epigenetic mechanisms that are deregulated in cancer include changes to higher order chromatin structure, such as histone modifications, and DNA methylation, both of which are crucial layers of epigenetic programming that regulates gene transcription and genome stability, and contribute to normal B-cell development. DNA methylation, which occurs predominantly at the cytosine residue of CpG dinucleotides, is the most well-studied epigenetic mechanism in CLL [19, 20, 126, 127]. Candidate gene approaches identified differential methylation at promoters and CpG islands of genes including *DAPK1*, TCL1, *ZAP70*, *HoxA4*, *TWIST2*, as well as CLL-associated microRNAs and long intervening noncoding RNAs [128, 129]. Although DNA methylation and gene expression are frequently poorly correlated, a strong association was noted between the methylation status of *ZAP70*. The methylation status of a single ZAP70 CpG site was subsequently shown to have prognostic significance [130, 131].

New insights have emerged from global methylation profiling of normal B-cell subsets and large CLL cohorts, using both methylation arrays and whole-genome bisulfite sequencing [19, 20, 126, 132]. Normal B-cell maturation from naive to memory B-cells is accompanied by prominent hypomethylation, especially of enhancer and promoter regions and gene bodies together with hypermethylation in regions of transcriptional elongation [20, 132]. The methylation profile of CLL closely recapitulates that seen in normal B cells, such that IGHV-mutated and unmutated CLL maintain the epigenetic signature of memory B-cells (MBC) and naive B-cells (NBC), respectively. Interestingly, both studies identified a third epigenetic CLL subgroup with an intermediate methylation signature enriched for M-CLL with fewer somatic IGHV mutations [126]. These three CLL epitypes exhibit different clinico-biological features, with the MBC-like CLL cases exhibiting a more indolent clinical course. As a result of these studies, an assay has been developed to assess the methylation status of 5 CpG dinucleotides that can identify these three prognostically relevant groups in a simple manner [127].

Despite the similarity of CLL methylation signatures to their likely cells of origin, aberrant methylation is also observed, for example in the binding sites for key transcription factor families [20]. The mechanisms underlying aberrant methylation and its importance in the pathogenesis of CLL are under investigation. Although initial observations showed that global DNA methylation tends to remain temporally stable in sequential tumor samples [133], more recent studies have identified intra-tumor epigenetic heterogeneity. This is associated with subclonal genomic heterogeneity and an adverse outcome [19, 126].

Genetic Predisposition to CLL

Epidemiological surveys have shown that CLL has one of the highest familial risks of any cancer, with an 8.5-fold increased risk among first-degree relatives for developing CLL and a 1.9-fold risk for other B-cell chronic lymphoproliferative disorders, especially lymphoplasmacytic lymphoma and hairy cell leukemia [134, 135]. Genome-wide association studies undertaken in over 5000 patients with CLL and 12,000 controls have identified over 30 loci associated with increased susceptibility to CLL [136–140]. The susceptibility to CLL associated with each variant single-nucleotide polymorphism (SNP) is low, but increases if multiple risk variants are co-inherited. Most SNPs map to noncoding regions of the genome, frequently close to or within genes involved in apoptosis, B-cell differentiation, or telomere function suggesting that they may act by influencing the expression of these genes. This mechanism was recently confirmed at the susceptibility locus located at 15q15.1. A SNP (rs539846) within this locus maps to a super-enhancer in intron 3 of the B-cell lymphoma 2 modifying factor gene (*BMF*), a pro-apoptotic BH3 protein which binds to, and neutralizes, the anti-apoptotic protein BCL2. The rs539846 risk allele modifies a transcription binding site for the transcription factor RELA, reducing BMF expression and potentially attenuating the apoptotic response [141].

Although the somatically acquired genomic mutations associated with sporadic CLL have rarely been implicated in genetic susceptibility to CLL, inactivating germline mutations in shelterin genes, especially POT1, critical for telomere function, have recently been discovered in CLL patients with strong family histories of CLL, consistent with the GWAS data. The authors estimated that 11% of familial CLL may be ascribed to mutations in this class of genes [142].

The Molecular Pathogenesis of Richter's Syndrome

Richter's syndrome (RS) denotes the histological diagnosis of either diffuse large B-cell lymphoma (DLBCL) or more rarely Hodgkin's lymphoma in a patient known to have CLL. In most cases the lymphoma is clonally related to the CLL but clonally unrelated lymphomas are also well documented. Preliminary investigations into the molecular mechanism of transformation to clonally related DLBCL have been performed [143, 144], but considerably less is currently known about the transformation process of other clonally related lymphoma subtypes or in patients who transform to clonally unrelated DLBCL.

In clonally related transformed DLBCL, the BCR is likely to play an important role in the transformation process, as clonally related DLBCL cases show remarkable bias in BCR usage, with enrichment of stereotyped "subset 8" cases (Fig. 8.4). This suggests that a restricted panel of antigenic epitopes are important in the transformation process. Deletions and/or mutations of the TP53 genes are the most prevalent genetic lesions found in clonally related DLBCL, identified in approx. 60% of cases [143]. The chemo-refractory phenotype that predominates in this disease is likely to be determined by loss of *TP53* function, and the resultant loss of cell cycle control that mediates resistance to chemotherapeutic agents. Approximately 40% of cases with clonally related DLBCL transformation show evidence of *MYC* aberrations, often acquired at transformation [143, 144]. In 30% of cases, *MYC* is targeted by structural rearrangements, including juxtaposition of *MYC* to the *IGHV* locus, genomic gain of 8q24, or activating point mutations [143]. Mutually exclusive to *MYC* abnormalities are activating mutations within the PEST domain of *NOTCH1* occurring in approximately 30% of cases, resulting in constitutively activated Notch signaling. While rare in diagnostic CLL cohorts, *CDKN2A* deletions can be identified in 30% of DLBCL transformed patients, and are likely to emerge in the tumor clone at transformation [143, 144].

Risk factors for the acquisition of a clonally related DLCBL principally focus on CLL cases with "subset 8" IGHV usage [145], who have a very high risk of transformation, approximately 80% at 10 years, and those that harbor a *NOTCH1* mutation; *NOTCH1*-mutated CLL cases have a cumulative probability of Richter transformation of 45% (compared to 4% for wild-type *NOTCH1* cases) [146]. Post-transformation, patients lacking TP53 lesions display more

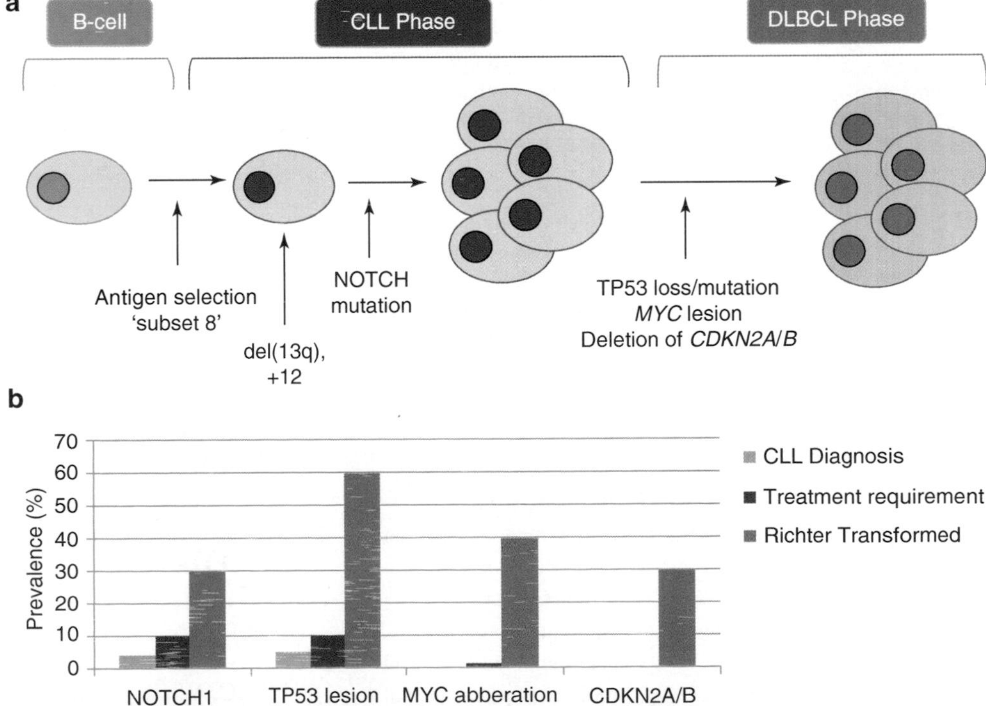

Fig. 8.4 The molecular pathogenesis of Richter's syndrome. (**a**) shows the accumulation of genomic lesions through the process of CLL development, progression, and transformation. (**b**) shows the prevalence of key genomic aberrations through the process of CLL development, progression, and transformation that are causally implicated in Richter transformation

favorable outcome than TP53-deleted or -mutated cases [147]. The changing therapeutic landscape for CLL will likely mold the epidemiology of transformation, as the non-genotoxic nature of modern treatment modalities will exert a different selective pressure on the tumor clone. Given the high prevalence of *TP53* lesions in transformed DLBCL, the prediction is that fewer *TP53*-driven transformation events will occur. However, it will be important to study transformation mechanisms in the context of new therapies, as clonal selection will sculpture the molecular mechanisms of transformation. Using targeted therapeutics against the molecular pathways that are disrupted in transformed CLL may show promise in the management of these tumors, such as the BCR, gamma secretase, bromodomain and cyclin-dependent kinase inhibitors, and novel compounds gaining traction for the management of aggressive lymphoma, such as immune checkpoint and XPO1 inhibitors.

Genomic Abnormalities in Clinical Practice

Genomic abnormalities are one of an increasing number of biomarkers that have clinical relevance in the management of patients with CLL. Although the diagnosis of CLL is based on immunophenotypic and morphological criteria, genomic abnormalities have both prognostic value in calculating the natural history of CLL patients and predictive value in determining the response to therapy. Furthermore, genomic screening can identify mechanisms of drug resistance and finally genomic abnormalities may act as therapeutic targets. Table 8.4 lists examples of the genomic abnormalities reported to have adverse prognostic significance in CLL in either large patient cohorts or clinical trials.

Predicting Natural History

Over 80% of CLL patients are asymptomatic at diagnosis and have a low tumor burden. Precisely identifying those likely to progress has the potential to inform patients and their families, and influence the need for and timing of follow-up and the timing and selection of optimal treatment. Following the recognition that individual copy number abnormalities, genomic mutations, and genomic complexity could influence both time to first treatment (TTFT) and overall survival when measured at or close to diagnosis, a variety of models have been developed which encompass the most frequent genomic abnormalities alone or in combination with other biomarkers.

A large study by Davide Rossi and colleagues has proposed a prognostic algorithm for overall survival through the integration of gene mutations and chromosomal abnormalities [16]. The authors analyzed CLL patients for FISH abnormalities and sequence mutations and offered four

Table 8.4 Genome lesions of clinical importance

Genomic abnormality	Clinical context	TTFT	PFS	OS	References
Genomic complexity (GC)	At diagnosis	X			[148, 149]
	Chemo-immunotherapy trial			X	[46]
	Ibrutinib for R/R disease			X	[68]
Chromothripsis	Chemo-immunotherapy trial		X	X	[30]
del(11q)	At diagnosis				[25]
	CT trial		X	X	[150]
TP53 abnormalities	At diagnosis	X		X	[6, 13]
	CT, Chemo-immunotherapy trials		X	X	[150–152]
	Chemo-immunotherapy for relapse/ refractory disease			X	[153, 154]
	Ibrutinib trial for previously untreated or relapsed disease		X		[155]
Subclonal drivers	Pre-chemo-immunotherapy (all drivers)	X	X		[17, 18]
	TP53 pretreatment	X		X	[61, 62]
Multiple drivers	Pretreatment	X			[38]
SF3B1	At diagnosis	X			[156]
	Chemotherapy trial			X	[92]
	Chemo-immunotherapy trial		X	X	[153]
NOTCH1	At diagnosis	X			[156]
	Chemotherapy trial			X	[92]
	Chemo-immunotherapy		X	X	[153]
RPS15	Chemo-immunotherapy trial		X		[17]

Time to first treatment (TTFT), progression-free (PFS) and overall survival risk classifications: (1) high-risk patients with either *TP53* defects and/or *BIRC3* disruption; (2) intermediate-risk, harboring *NOTCH1* and/or *SF3B1* mutations and/or del(11q); (3) low-risk, harboring trisomy 12 or a normal profile; and perhaps most importantly (4) a very-low-risk group with del(13q) only, whose survival did not differ from that of a matched general population. This model added significantly to the "Döhner" model [157], due to the coexistence of poor-risk gene mutations in low-risk groups defined purely based on FISH and retained prognostic significance over time regardless of clonal evolution. However subsequent similar large studies which also used TTFT as an endpoint have failed to completely replicate these findings, highlighting the difficulty of developing models that are sufficiently precise for routine use and the need for even larger, well-designed prospective studies [99, 112].

A recently introduced international prognostic index (CLL-IPI) performed multivariate analysis of 27 clinical and biological factors including 13q, 11q, 6q, and 17p loss; trisomy 12; and mutations of *TP53*, *SF3B1*, and *NOTCH1* on a large cohort of patients predominantly entered into first-line chemotherapy or chemo-immunotherapy trials. Five prognostic factors were identified: *TP53* status, *IGHV* mutational status, serum B2 microglobulin, clinical stage, and age, from which a prognostic index was derived identifying four risk groups with different overall survivals [158]. The CLL-IPI has subsequently been shown to predict TTFT in early-stage CLL [159].

Predicting Outcome Following Treatment

TP53 abnormalities. As outlined earlier in this chapter, copy number abnormalities such as del(11q) and deletion of *SETD2* and genomic mutations of *SF3B2, NOTCH1, BIRC3, SAMHD1, RPS15*, and *EGR2* appear to influence the outcome of patients receiving chemotherapy or chemo-immunotherapy. However the effect is either modest or has not been evaluated in multivariate analyses of large clinical trials. As a consequence the only genomic abnormalities that determine the choice of therapy in routine clinical practice are deletion and/or mutation of *TP53*, and current guidelines recommend screening for TP53 abnormalities prior to first-line and relapse therapy. Their presence is unequivocally linked to a dismal response to standard chemo-immunotherapy and is an indication for novel agents such as signaling inhibitors or pro-apoptotic BH3 mimetics acting through TP53-independant mechanisms. Conversely the absence of del(17p) or del(11q) in patients with mutated *IGHV* genes identifies patients with long overall survival following standard chemo-immunotherapy for fit patients (FCR) [160].

Although evidence for the predictive value of *TP53* abnormalities is overwhelming, the outcome of patients with these abnormalities is not uniform and is influenced by coexisting genomic abnormalities, immunogenetic status, and treatment type. As previously mentioned, it is well recognized that a small subset of early-stage patients with TP53 abnormalities may pursue a stable clinical course [161]. A more recent study of 69 patients with >10% TP53 loss using WES and SNP arrays to detect genomic mutations and CNAs, respectively, showed that the poorest outcomes were associated with bi-allelic TP53 abnormalities; clonal TP53 mutations; deletions of 3p, 4p, or 8p; and genomic complexity. Conversely cases that remained untreated for 5 years were enriched for mutated IGHV genes, subclonal or no TP53 mutations, and fewer CNAs [59]. Similarly, Guieze et al. noted that the poorest outcome of patients who received salvage therapy, having failed to respond to or relapsing after chemo-immunotherapy, had mutations of *TP53, ATM*, and *SF3B1* [162].

The impact of *TP53* abnormalities on treatments that act through *TP53*-independent mechanisms is mixed. *TP53* status does not influence the outcome of patients receiving an allogeneic stem cell transplant whereas the efficacy of ibrutinib in patients with a *TP53* abnormality is much greater than chemo-immunotherapy but inferior to *TP53* wild-type cases. This implies that *TP53* abnormalities may have an indirect effect on facilitating ibrutinib resistance possibly related to increased genomic instability.

NOTCH1 mutations. An interesting observation that emerged from genomic analysis of the German Study Group CLL8 trial was that the outcome of patients in the chemo-immunotherapy arm (FCR) was superior to those in the chemotherapy arm (FC) apart from those with *NOTCH1* mutations [153]. A similar phenomenon was observed in a trial of chlorambucil with or without the anti-CD20 antibody, ofatumumab, suggesting that NOTCH1 mutations may be a predictive factor for reduced benefit from chemotherapy and anti-CD20 antibody combinations [163].

Identifying Resistance Mechanisms

TP53 abnormalities account for primary or acquired resistance to chemotherapy-containing regimens in at least 50% of cases, reflecting the importance of an intact DNA damage response pathway for the activity of these agents. Unsurprisingly acquired resistance is encountered in a variety of hematological malignancies treated with signaling inhibitors or BH3 mimetics, and in CLL the mechanisms of resistance to ibrutinib have been partially elucidated. Whole exomic sequencing of tumor samples from six patients who relapsed during ibrutinib therapy identified a cysteine-to-serine mutation (C451S) in Bruton's tyrosine kinase (BTK). This reduced the binding affinity of ibrutinib for BTK, resulting in only transient, rather than the usual irreversible, inhibition of *BTK*. In addition three distinct gain-of-function mutations in *PLCG2*, the kinase immediately downstream of BTK, were found in two patients [164, 165]. A subsequent study used whole exomic and deep sequencing in serial samples from five patients who relapsed after an initial partial response to ibrutinib. At relapse, one patient had a *BTK* C4815 mutation and one had multiple *PLCG2* mutations. The remaining three cases showed expansion of a preexisting clone harboring del(8p) with additional driver mutations. Deletion of 8p resulted in halpoinsufficiency of the TRAIL receptor and the authors provided functional data to suggest that this may be a resistance mechanism [166].

A key question is whether *BTK* and *PLCG2* mutations can also be detected either prior to BTK administration or during BTK therapy before clinical relapse and therefore act as a predictive marker. Although computational analysis indicates that very small *BTK* mutant clones are present pretreatment, these have not been identified in deep sequencing studies [166, 167].

Summary

Since the previous edition of this book, our understanding of the CLL genome has been transformed by modern technology. New driver mutations have been discovered and it can be safely predicted that all clonal and subclonal genomic abnormalities that impact the survival and proliferation of tumor cells in at least 1% of CLL cases will be identified. It can also be anticipated that single platforms that robustly and affordably identify all common drivers will become available. Furthermore, mechanisms underlying genomic instability and phenotypic consequences of both single and multiple genomic abnormalities and their interaction with environmental factors are becoming increasingly understood.

These advances coincide with a revolution in treatment of CLL brought about by the introduction of novel small molecules and immune therapies which are highly effective, frequently easier to administer, and better tolerated than previous chemotherapy regimens. Importantly, the treatments that target key signaling and apoptosis pathways retain activity in cases that acquire the common genomic abnormalities including those affecting DNA repair.

Given the trend towards precision medicine, it is pertinent to ask what impact genomic advances might have in an era of increasingly effective therapies. It is probable that the genomic basis of familial CLL will be sufficiently understood to justify screening of high-risk individuals. The presence of key genomic lesions may have utility for the differential diagnosis of mature B-cell malignancies in general. It is also highly likely that screening for genomic abnormalities will contribute further to the recognition of early-stage patients at risk of disease progression who might benefit from early therapy prior to clonal evolution and expansion. It remains to be seen whether combinations of highly active agents targeting different pathways will be curative regardless of the genomic landscape, but should resistant clones emerge, then next-generation sequencing will be instrumental in determining resistance mechanisms and the choice of alternative therapies.

Acknowledgments Jonathan Strefford, Renata Walewska, and David Oscier wrote the chapter. This work was funded by Bloodwise (11052, 12036), Cancer Research UK (C34999/A18087, ECMC C24563/A15581), and the Kay Kendall Leukaemia Fund (873).

References

1. Gahrton G, et al. Extra chromosome 12 in chronic lymphocytic leukaemia. Lancet. 1980;2(8160):146–7.
2. Fitchett M, et al. Chromosome abnormalities involving band 13q14 in hematologic malignancies. Cancer Genet Cytogenet. 1987;24(1):143–50.
3. Dicker F, et al. Immunostimulatory oligonucleotide-induced metaphase cytogenetics detect chromosomal aberrations in 80% of CLL patients: a study of 132 CLL cases with correlation to FISH, IgVH status, and CD38 expression. Blood. 2006;108(9):3152–60.
4. Put N, et al. Improved detection of chromosomal abnormalities in chronic lymphocytic leukemia by conventional cytogenetics using CpG oligonucleotide and interleukin-2 stimulation: a Belgian multicentric study. Genes Chromosom Cancer. 2009;48(10):843–53.
5. Haferlach C, et al. Comprehensive genetic characterization of CLL: a study on 506 cases analysed with chromosome banding analysis, interphase FISH, IgV(H) status and immunophenotyping. Leukemia. 2007;21(12):2442–51.
6. Döhner H, et al. p53 gene deletion predicts for poor survival and non-response to therapy with purine analogs in chronic B-cell leukemias. Blood. 1995;85(6):1580–9.
7. Bastard C, et al. Comparison of a quantitative PCR method with FISH for the assessment of the four aneuploidies commonly evaluated in CLL patients. Leukemia. 2007;21(7):1460–3.
8. Coll-Mulet L, et al. Multiplex ligation-dependent probe amplification for detection of genomic alterations in chronic lymphocytic leukaemia. Br J Haematol. 2008;142(5):793–801.
9. Buijs A, Krijtenburg PJ, Meijer E. Detection of risk-identifying chromosomal abnormalities and genomic profiling by multiplex ligation-dependent probe amplification in chronic lymphocytic leukemia. Haematologica. 2006;91(10):1434–5.
10. Fabris S, et al. Multiplex ligation-dependent probe amplification and fluorescence in situ hybridization to detect chromosomal abnormalities in chronic lymphocytic leukemia: a comparative study. Genes Chromosom Cancer. 2011;50(9):726–34.
11. Kallioniemi A, et al. Comparative genomic hybridisation for molecular genetic analysis of solid tumours. Science. 1992;258(5083):818–21.
12. Pinkel D, et al. High resolution analysis of DNA copy number variation using comparative genomic hybridization to microarrays. Nat Genet. 1998;20(2):207–11.
13. Gaidano G, et al. p53 mutations in human lymphoid malignancies: association with Burkitt lymphoma and chronic lymphocytic leukemia. Proc Natl Acad Sci U S A. 1991;88(12):5413–7.

14. Stankovic T, et al. Inactivation of ataxia telangiectasia mutated gene in B-cell chronic lymphocytic leukaemia. Lancet. 1999;353(9146):26–9.
15. Bentley DR, et al. Accurate whole human genome sequencing using reversible terminator chemistry. Nature. 2008;456(7218):53–9.
16. Rossi D, et al. Integrated mutational and cytogenetic analysis identifies new prognostic subgroups in chronic lymphocytic leukemia. Blood. 2013;121(8):1403–12.
17. Landau DA, et al. Mutations driving CLL and their evolution in progression and relapse. Nature. 2015;526(7574):525–30.
18. Landau DA, et al. Evolution and impact of subclonal mutations in chronic lymphocytic leukemia. Cell. 2013;152(4):714–26.
19. Oakes CC, et al. Evolution of DNA methylation is linked to genetic aberrations in chronic lymphocytic leukemia. Cancer Discov. 2014;4(3):348–61.
20. Oakes CC, et al. DNA methylation dynamics during B cell maturation underlie a continuum of disease phenotypes in chronic lymphocytic leukemia. Nat Genet. 2016;48(3):253–64.
21. Landau DA, et al. Evolution and impact of subclonal mutations in chronic lymphocytic leukemia. Cancer Cell. 2013;152(4):714–26.
22. Rendeiro AF, et al. Chromatin accessibility maps of chronic lymphocytic leukaemia identify subtype-specific epigenome signatures and transcription regulatory networks. Nat Commun. 2016;7:11938.
23. Parker H, et al. 13q deletion anatomy and disease progression in patients with chronic lymphocytic leukemia. Leukemia. 2011;25(3):489–97.
24. Ouillette P, et al. The prognostic significance of various 13q14 deletions in chronic lymphocytic leukemia. Clin Cancer Res. 2011;17(21):6778–90.
25. Döhner H, et al. 11q deletions identify a new subset of B-cell chronic lymphocytic leukemia characterized by extensive nodal involvement and inferior prognosis. Blood. 1997;89(7):2516–22.
26. Hurley JN, et al. Chromosome abnormalities of leukaemic B lymphocytes in chronic lymphocytic leukaemia. Nature. 1980;283(5742):76–8.
27. Stilgenbauer S, et al. Incidence and clinical significance of 6q deletions in B cell chronic lymphocytic leukemia. Leukemia. 1999;13(9):1331–4.
28. Schwaenen C, et al. Automated array-based genomic profiling in chronic lymphocytic leukemia: development of a clinical tool and discovery of recurrent genomic alterations. Proc Natl Acad Sci U S A. 2004;101(4):1039–44.
29. Chapiro E, et al. Gain of the short arm of chromosome 2 (2p) is a frequent recurring chromosome aberration in untreated chronic lymphocytic leukemia (CLL) at advanced stages. Leuk Res. 2010;34(1):63–8.
30. Edelmann J, et al. High-resolution genomic profiling of chronic lymphocytic leukemia reveals new recurrent genomic alterations. Blood. 2012;120(24):4783–94.
31. de Paoli L, et al. MGA, a suppressor of MYC, is recurrently inactivated in high risk chronic lymphocytic leukemia. Leuk Lymphoma. 2013;54(5):1987–90.
32. Parker H, et al. Genomic disruption of the histone methyltransferase SETD2 in chronic lymphocytic leukaemia. Leukemia. 2016;30(11):2179–86.
33. Fabbri G, et al. Analysis of the chronic lymphocytic leukemia coding genome: role of NOTCH1 mutational activation. J Exp Med. 2011;208(7):1389–401.
34. Quesada V, et al. Exome sequencing identifies recurrent mutations of the splicing factor SF3B1 gene in chronic lymphocytic leukemia. Nat Genet. 2011;44(1):47–52.
35. Di Ianni M, et al. A new genetic lesion in B-CLL: a NOTCH1 PEST domain mutation. Br J Haematol. 2009;146(6):689–91.
36. Wang L, et al. SF3B1 and other novel cancer genes in chronic lymphocytic leukemia. N Engl J Med. 2011;365(26):2497–506.
37. Damm F, et al. Acquired initiating mutations in early hematopoietic cells of CLL patients. Cancer Discov. 2014;4(9):1088–101.
38. Puente XS, et al. Non-coding recurrent mutations in chronic lymphocytic leukemia. Nature. 2015;526(7574):519–24.
39. Ljungström V, et al. Whole-exome sequencing in relapsing chronic lymphocytic leukemia: clinical impact of recurrent RPS15 mutations. Blood. 2016;127(8):1007–16.
40. Rossi D, et al. Alteration of BIRC3 and multiple other NF-κB pathway genes in splenic marginal zone lymphoma. Blood. 2011;118(18):4930–4.
41. Kämpjärvi K, et al. Somatic MED12 mutations are associated with poor prognosis markers in chronic lymphocytic leukemia. Oncotarget. 2015;6(3):1884–8.
42. Puente XS, et al. Whole-genome sequencing identifies recurrent mutations in chronic lymphocytic leukemia. Nature. 2011;475(7354):101–5.
43. Clifford R, et al. SAMHD1 is mutated recurrently in chronic lymphocytic leukemia and is involved in response to DNA damage. Blood. 2014;123(7):1021–31.
44. Rodríguez D, et al. Functional analysis of sucrase-isomaltase mutations from chronic lymphocytic leukemia patients. Hum Mol Genet. 2013;22(11):2273–82.
45. Zhang X, et al. Sequence analysis of 515 kinase genes in chronic lymphocytic leukemia. Leukemia. 2011;25(12):1908–10.
46. Herling CD, et al. Complex karyotypes and KRAS and POT1 mutations impact outcome in CLL after chlorambucil-based chemotherapy or chemoimmunotherapy. Blood. 2016;128(3):395–404.
47. Havelange V, et al. IRF4 mutations in chronic lymphocytic leukemia. Blood. 2011;118(10):2827–9.
48. Kasar S, et al. Whole-genome sequencing reveals activation-induced cytidine deaminase signatures during indolent chronic lymphocytic leukaemia evolution. Nat Commun. 2015;6:8866.
49. Baca SC, et al. Punctuated evolution of prostate cancer genomes. Cell. 2013;153(3):666–77.
50. Calin GA, et al. Frequent deletions and down-regulation of microRNA genes miR15 and miR16 at 13q14 in chronic lymphocytic leukemia. Proc Natl Acad Sci U S A. 2002;99(24):15524–9.
51. Klein U, et al. The DLEU2/miR-15a/16-1 cluster controls B cell proliferation and its deletion leads to chronic lymphocytic leukemia. Cancer Cell. 2010;17(1):28–40.
52. Cimmino A, et al. miR-15 and miR-16 induce apoptosis by targeting BCL2. Proc Natl Acad Sci U S A. 2005;102(39):13944–9.
53. Fulci V, et al. Quantitative technologies establish a novel microRNA profile of chronic lymphocytic leukemia. Blood. 2007;109(11):4944–51.
54. Lia M, et al. Functional dissection of the chromosome 13q14 tumor-suppressor locus using transgenic mouse lines. Blood. 2011;119(13):2981–90.
55. Ouillette P, et al. Integrated genomic profiling of chronic lymphocytic leukemia identifies subtypes of deletion 13q14. Cancer Res. 2008;68(4):1012–21.
56. Rossi D, et al. Disruption of BIRC3 associates with fludarabine chemorefractoriness in TP53 wild-type chronic lymphocytic leukemia. Blood. 2012;119(12):2854–62.
57. Rose-Zerilli MJJ, et al. ATM mutation rather than BIRC3 deletion and/or mutation predicts reduced survival in 11q-deleted chronic lymphocytic leukemia: data from the UK LRF CLL4 trial. Haematologica. 2014;99(4):736–42.
58. Deneberg S, et al. microRNA-34b/c on chromosome 11q23 is aberrantly methylated in chronic lymphocytic leukemia. Epigenetics. 2014;9(6):910–7.
59. Yu L, et al. Survival of Del17p CLL depends on genomic complexity and somatic mutation. Clin Cancer Res. 2017;23(3):735–45.
60. Lazarian G, et al. TP53 mutations are early events in chronic lymphocytic leukemia disease progression and precede evolution to complex karyotypes. Int J Cancer. 2016;139(8):1759–63.
61. Rossi D, et al. Clinical impact of small TP53 mutated subclones in chronic lymphocytic leukemia. Blood. 2014;123(14):2139–47.

62. Nadeu F, et al. Clinical impact of clonal and subclonal TP53, SF3B1, BIRC3, NOTCH1, and ATM mutations in chronic lymphocytic leukemia. Blood. 2016;127(17):2122–30.
63. Best OG, et al. A novel functional assay using etoposide plus nutlin-3a detects and distinguishes between ATM and TP53 mutations in CLL. Leukemia. 2008;22(7):1456–9.
64. Schliemann I, et al. The t(11;14)(q13;q32)/CCND1-IGH translocation is a recurrent secondary genetic aberration in relapsed chronic lymphocytic leukemia. Leuk Lymphoma. 2016;57(11):2672–6.
65. Ouillette P, et al. Acquired genomic copy number aberrations and survival in chronic lymphocytic leukemia. Blood. 2011;118(11):3051–61.
66. Delgado J, et al. Genomic complexity and IGHV mutational status are key predictors of outcome of chronic lymphocytic leukemia patients with TP53 disruption. Haematologica. 2014;99(11):e231–4.
67. Stephens PJ, et al. Massive genomic rearrangement acquired in a single catastrophic event during cancer development. Cell. 2011;144(1):27–40.
68. Thompson PA, et al. Complex karyotype is a stronger predictor than del(17p) for an inferior outcome in relapsed or refractory chronic lymphocytic leukemia patients treated with ibrutinib-based regimens. Cancer. 2015;121(20):3612–21.
69. Ouillette P, et al. Aggressive chronic lymphocytic leukemia with elevated genomic complexity is associated with multiple gene defects in the response to DNA double-strand breaks. Clin Cancer Res. 2010;16(3):835–47.
70. Roos G, et al. Short telomeres are associated with genetic complexity, high-risk genomic aberrations, and short survival in chronic lymphocytic leukemia. Blood. 2008;111(4):2246–52.
71. Britt-Compton B, et al. Extreme telomere erosion in ATM-mutated and 11q-deleted CLL patients is independent of disease stage. Leukemia. 2012;26(4):826–30.
72. Crasta K, et al. DNA breaks and chromosome pulverization from errors in mitosis. Nature. 2012;482(7383):53–8.
73. Zhang CZ, et al. Chromothripsis from DNA damage in micronuclei. Nature. 2015;522(7555):179–84.
74. Rausch T, et al. Genome sequencing of pediatric medulloblastoma links catastrophic DNA rearrangements with TP53 mutations. Cell. 2012;148(1–2):59–71.
75. Nik-Zainal S, et al. Mutational processes molding the genomes of 21 breast cancers. Cell. 2012;149(5):979–93.
76. Alexandrov LB, et al. Signatures of mutational processes in human cancer. Nature. 2013;500(7463):415–21.
77. Bechter OE, et al. Telomere length and telomerase activity predict survival in patients with B cell chronic lymphocytic leukemia. Cancer Res. 1998;58(21):4918–22.
78. Damle RN, et al. Telomere length and telomerase activity delineate distinctive replicative features of the B-CLL subgroups defined by immunoglobulin V gene mutations. Blood. 2004;103(2):375–82.
79. Grabowski P, et al. Telomere length as a prognostic parameter in chronic lymphocytic leukemia with special reference to VH gene mutation status. Blood. 2005;105(12):4807–12.
80. Rossi D, et al. Telomere length is an independent predictor of survival, treatment requirement and Richter's syndrome transformation in chronic lymphocytic leukemia. Leukemia. 2009;23(6):1062–72.
81. Strefford JC, et al. Telomere length predicts progression and overall survival in chronic lymphocytic leukemia: data from the UK LRF CLL4 trial. Leukemia. 2015;29(12):2411–4.
82. Lin TT, et al. Telomere dysfunction and fusion during the progression of chronic lymphocytic leukemia: evidence for a telomere crisis. Blood. 2010;116(11):1899–907.
83. Lin TT, et al. Telomere dysfunction accurately predicts clinical outcome in chronic lymphocytic leukaemia, even in patients with early stage disease. Br J Haematol. 2014;167(2):214–23.
84. Ramsay AJ, et al. POT1 mutations cause telomere dysfunction in chronic lymphocytic leukemia. Nat Genet. 2013;45(5):526–30.
85. Rossi D, et al. Mutations of the SF3B1 splicing factor in chronic lymphocytic leukemia: association with progression and fludarabine-refractoriness. Blood. 2011;118(26):6904–8.
86. Alexandrov LB, et al. Clock-like mutational processes in human somatic cells. Nat Genet. 2015;47(12):1402–7.
87. Forbes SA, et al. COSMIC: mining complete cancer genomes in the catalogue of somatic mutations in cancer. Nucleic Acids Res. 2011;39:D945–50.
88. Messina M, et al. Genetic lesions associated with chronic lymphocytic leukemia chemo-refractoriness. Blood. 2014;123(15):2378–88.
89. Worrillow L, et al. An ultra-deep sequencing strategy to detect sub-clonal TP53 mutations in presentation chronic lymphocytic leukaemia cases using multiple polymerases. Oncogene. 2016;35(40):5328–36.
90. Rosati E, et al. Constitutively activated Notch signaling is involved in survival and apoptosis resistance of B-CLL cells. Blood. 2009;113(4):856–65.
91. Rosati E, et al. γ-Secretase inhibitor I induces apoptosis in chronic lymphocytic leukemia cells by proteasome inhibition, endoplasmic reticulum stress increase and Notch down-regulation. Int J Cancer. 2013;132(8):1940–53.
92. Oscier DG, et al. The clinical significance of NOTCH1 and SF3B1 mutations in the UK LRF CLL4 trial. Blood. 2013;120(22):4441–3.
93. Oscier D, et al. The morphology of CLL revisited: the clinical significance of prolymphocytes and correlations with prognostic/molecular markers in the LRF CLL4 trial. Br J Haematol. 2016;174(5):767–75.
94. Rossi D, et al. Mutations of NOTCH1 are an independent predictor of survival in chronic lymphocytic leukemia. Blood. 2011;119(2):521–9.
95. Larrayoz M, et al. Non-coding NOTCH1 mutations in chronic ltphocytic leukemia; Their clinical impact in the UK CLL4 trial. Leukemia. 2016;31(2):510–4.
96. Onaindia A, et al. Chronic lymphocytic leukemia cells in lymph nodes show frequent NOTCH1 activation. Haematologica. 2015;100(11):e450–3.
97. Arruga F, et al. Functional impact of NOTCH1 mutations in chronic lymphocytic leukemia. Leukemia. 2014;28(5):1060–70.
98. López-Guerra M, et al. The γ-secretase inhibitor PF-03084014 combined with fludarabine antagonizes migration, invasion and angiogenesis in NOTCH1-mutated CLL cells. Leukemia. 2014;29(1):96–106.
99. Jeromin S, et al. SF3B1 mutations correlated to cytogenetics and mutations in NOTCH1, FBXW7, MYD88, XPO1 and TP53 in 1160 untreated CLL patients. Leukemia. 2014;28(1):108–17.
100. Strefford JC, et al. Distinct patterns of novel gene mutations in poor-prognostic stereotyped subsets of chronic lymphocytic leukemia: the case of SF3B1 and subset #2. Leukemia. 2013;27(11):2196–9.
101. Rossi D, et al. Association between molecular lesions and specific B-cell receptor subsets in chronic lymphocytic leukemia. Blood. 2013;121(24):4902–5.
102. Darman RB, et al. Cancer-associated SF3B1 hotspot mutations induce cryptic 3′ splice site selection through use of a different branch point. Cell Rep. 2015;13(5):1033–45.
103. Ferreira PG, et al. Transcriptome characterization by RNA sequencing identifies a major molecular and clinical subdivision in chronic lymphocytic leukemia. Genome Res. 2014;24(2):212–26.
104. Te Raa GD, et al. The impact of SF3B1 mutations in CLL on the DNA-damage response. Leukemia. 2015;29(5):1133–42.
105. Xargay-Torrent S, et al. The splicing modulator sudemycin induces a specific antitumor response and cooperates with ibrutinib in chronic lymphocytic leukemia. Oncotarget. 2016;6(26):22734–49.
106. Larrayoz M, et al. The SF3B1 inhibitor spliceostatin A (SSA) elicits apoptosis in chronic lymphocytic leukaemia cells through downregulation of Mcl-1. Leukemia. 2016;30(2):351–60.

107. Lapalombella R, et al. Selective inhibitors of nuclear export show that CRM1/XPO1 is a target in chronic lymphocytic leukemia. Blood. 2012;120(23):4621–34.
108. Hing ZA, et al. Next-generation XPO1 inhibitor shows improved efficacy and in vivo tolerability in hematological malignancies. Leukemia. 2016;30(12):2364–72.
109. Herishanu Y, et al. The lymph node microenvironment promotes B-cell receptor signaling, NF-kappaB activation, and tumor proliferation in chronic lymphocytic leukemia. Blood. 2011;117(2):563–74.
110. Mansouri L, et al. Functional loss of IKBE leads to NF-KB deregulation in aggressive chronic lymphocytic leukemia. J Exp Med. 2015;212(6):833–43.
111. Lin SC, Lo YC, Wu H. Helical assembly in the MyD88-IRAK4-IRAK2 complex in TLR/IL-1R signalling. Nature. 2010;465(7300):885–90.
112. Baliakas P, et al. Recurrent mutations refine prognosis in chronic lymphocytic leukemia. Leukemia. 2015;29(2):329–36.
113. Martínez-Trillos A, et al. Mutations in TLR/MYD88 pathway identify a subset of young chronic lymphocytic leukemia patients with favorable outcome. Blood. 2014;123(24):37909–6.
114. Pandzic T, et al. Transposon mutagenesis reveals fludarabine-resistance mechanisms in chronic lymphocytic leukemia. Clin Cancer Res. 2016;22(24):6217–27.
115. Winkelmann N, et al. Low frequency mutations independently predict poor treatment free survival in early stage chronic lymphocytic leukemia and monoclonal B-cell lymphocytosis. Haematologica. 2015;100(6):e237–9.
116. Rodríguez D, et al. Mutations in CHD2 cause defective association with active chromatin in chronic lymphocytic leukemia. Blood. 2015;126(2):195–202.
117. Ouillette P, et al. Clonal evolution, genomic drivers, and effects of therapy in chronic lymphocytic leukemia. Clin Cancer Res. 2013;19(11):2893–904.
118. Stilgenbauer S, et al. Clonal evolution in chronic lymphocytic leukemia: acquisition of high-risk genomic aberrations associated with unmutated VH, resistance to therapy, and short survival. Haematologica. 2007;92(9):1242–5.
119. Shanafelt TD, et al. Prospective evaluation of clonal evolution during long-term follow-up of patients with untreated early-stage chronic lymphocytic leukemia. J Clin Oncol. 2006;24(28):4634–41.
120. Knight SJ, et al. Quantification of subclonal distributions of recurrent genomic aberrations in paired pre-treatment and relapse samples from patients with B-cell chronic lymphocytic leukemia. Leukemia. 2012;26(7):1564–75.
121. Greaves M, Maley CC. Clonal evolution in cancer. Nature. 2012;481(7381):306–13.
122. Schuh A, et al. Monitoring chronic lymphocytic leukemia progression by whole genome sequencing reveals heterogeneous clonal evolution patterns. Blood. 2012;120(20):4191–6.
123. Ojha J, et al. Deep sequencing identifies genetic heterogeneity and recurrent convergent evolution in chronic lymphocytic leukemia. Blood. 2015;125(3):492–8.
124. Rose-Zerilli MJ, et al. Longitudinal copy number, whole exome and targeted deep sequencing of 'good risk' IGHV-mutated CLL patients with progressive disease. Leukemia. 2016;30(6):1301–10.
125. Del Giudice I, et al. Inter- and intra-patient clonal and subclonal heterogeneity of chronic lymphocytic leukaemia: evidences from circulating and lymph nodal compartments. Br J Haematol. 2016;172(3):371–83.
126. Kulis M, et al. Epigenomic analysis detects widespread gene-body DNA hypomethylation in chronic lymphocytic leukemia. Nat Genet. 2012;44(11):1236–42.
127. Queirós AC, et al. A B-cell epigenetic signature defines three biologic subgroups of chronic lymphocytic leukemia with clinical impact. Leukemia. 2015;29(3):598–605.
128. Kopparapu PK, et al. Epigenetic silencing of miR-26A1 in chronic lymphocytic leukemia and mantle cell lymphoma: impact on EZH2 expression. Epigenetics. 2016;11(5):335–43.
129. Baer C, et al. Extensive promoter DNA hypermethylation and hypomethylation is associated with aberrant microRNA expression in chronic lymphocytic leukemia. Cancer Res. 2012;72(15):3775–85.
130. Claus R, et al. Quantitative DNA methylation analysis identifies a single CpG dinucleotide important for ZAP-70 expression and predictive of prognosis in chronic lymphocytic leukemia. J Clin Oncol. 2012;30(20):2483–91.
131. Claus R, et al. Validation of ZAP-70 methylation and its relative significance in predicting outcome in chronic lymphocytic leukemia. Blood. 2014;124(1):42–8.
132. Kulis M, et al. Whole-genome fingerprint of the DNA methylome during human B cell differentiation. Nat Genet. 2015;47(7):746–56.
133. Cahill N, et al. 450K-array analysis of chronic lymphocytic leukemia cells reveals global DNA methylation to be relatively stable over time and similar in resting and proliferative compartments. Leukemia. 2012;27(1):150–8.
134. Goldin LR, et al. Elevated risk of chronic lymphocytic leukemia and other indolent non-Hodgkin's lymphomas among relatives of patients with chronic lymphocytic leukemia. Haematologica. 2009;94(5):647–53.
135. Cerhan JR, Slager SL. Familial predisposition and genetic risk factors for lymphoma. Blood. 2015;126(20):2265–73.
136. Crowther-Swanepoel D, et al. Common variants at 2q37.3, 8q24.21, 15q21.3 and 16q24.1 influence chronic lymphocytic leukemia risk. Nat Genet. 2010;42(2):132–6.
137. Di Bernardo MC, et al. A genome-wide association study identifies six susceptibility loci for chronic lymphocytic leukemia. Nat Genet. 2008;40(10):1204–10.
138. Speedy HE, et al. A genome-wide association study identifies multiple susceptibility loci for chronic lymphocytic leukemia. Nat Genet. 2014;46(1):56–60.
139. Berndt SI, et al. Meta-analysis of genome-wide association studies discovers multiple loci for chronic lymphocytic leukemia. Nat Commun. 2016;7:10933.
140. Berndt SI, et al. Genome-wide association study identifies multiple risk loci for chronic lymphocytic leukemia. Nat Genet. 2013;45(8):868–76.
141. Kandaswamy R, et al. Genetic predisposition to chronic lymphocytic leukemia is mediated by a BMF super-enhancer polymorphism. Cell Rep. 2016;16(8):2061–7.
142. Speedy HE. et al. Germline mutations in shelterin complex genes are associated with familial chronic lymphocytic leukemia. Blood. 2016. doi: https://doi.org/10.1182/blood-2016-01-695692.
143. Chigrinova E, et al. Two main genetic pathways lead to the transformation of chronic lymphocytic leukemia to Richter syndrome. Blood. 2013;122(15):2673–82.
144. Fabbri G, et al. Genetic lesions associated with chronic lymphocytic leukemia transformation to Richter syndrome. J Exp Med. 2013;210(11):2273–88.
145. Rossi D, et al. Stereotyped B-cell receptor is an independent risk factor of chronic lymphocytic leukemia transformation to Richter syndrome. Clin Cancer Res. 2009;15(13):4415–22.
146. Rossi D, et al. Different impact of NOTCH1 and SF3B1 mutations on the risk of chronic lymphocytic leukemia transformation to Richter syndrome. Br J Haematol. 2012;158(3):426–9.
147. Rossi D, et al. The genetics of Richter syndrome reveals disease heterogeneity and predicts survival after transformation. Blood. 2011;117(12):3391–401.
148. Baliakas P, et al. Chromosomal translocations and karyotype complexity in chronic lymphocytic leukemia: a systematic reappraisal of classic cytogenetic data. Am J Hematol. 2014;89(3):249–55.

149. Kujawski L, et al. Genomic complexity identifies patients with aggressive chronic lymphocytic leukemia. Blood. 2008;112(5):1993–2003.
150. Oscier D, et al. Prognostic factors identified three risk groups in the LRF CLL4 trial, independent of treatment allocation. Haematologica. 2010;95(10):1705–12.
151. Zenz T, et al. TP53 mutation and survival in chronic lymphocytic leukemia. J Clin Oncol. 2010;28(29):4473–9.
152. Gonzalez D, et al. Mutational status of the TP53 gene as a predictor of response and survival in patients with chronic lymphocytic leukemia: results from the LRF CLL4 trial. J Clin Oncol. 2011;29(16):2223–9.
153. Stilgenbauer S, et al. Gene mutations and treatment outcome in chronic lymphocytic leukemia: results from the CLL8 trial. Blood. 2014;123(21):3247–54.
154. Schnaiter A, et al. NOTCH1, SF3B1, and TP53 mutations in fludarabine-refractory CLL patients treated with alemtuzumab: results from the CLL2H trial of the GCLLSG. Blood. 2013;122(7):1266–70.
155. Woyach JA, Johnson AJ. Targeted therapies in CLL: mechanisms of resistance and strategies for management. Blood. 2015;126(4):471–7.
156. Baliakas P, et al. Recurrent mutations refine prognosis in chronic lymphocytic leukemia. Leukemia. 2014;29(2):329–36.
157. Döhner H, et al. Genomic aberrations and survival in chronic lymphocytic leukemia. N Engl J Med. 2000;343(26):1910–6.
158. International CLL-IPI working group. An international prognostic index for patients with chronic lymphocytic leukaemia (CLL-IPI): a meta-analysis of individual patient data. Lancet Oncol. 2016;17(6):779–90.
159. Molica S, et al. The chronic lymphocytic leukemia international prognostic index predicts time to first treatment in early CLL: independent validation in a prospective cohort of early stage patients. Am J Hematol. 2016;91(11):1090–5.
160. Rossi D, et al. Molecular prediction of durable remission after first-line fludarabine-cyclophosphamide-rituximab in chronic lymphocytic leukemia. Blood. 2015;126(16):1921–4.
161. Best OG, et al. A subset of Binet stage A CLL patients with TP53 abnormalities and mutated IGHV genes have stable disease. Leukemia. 2009;23(1):212–4.
162. Guièze R, et al. Presence of multiple recurrent mutations confers poor trial outcome of relapsed/refractory CLL. Blood. 2015;126(18):2110–7.
163. Tausch E, et al. Gene mutations and treatment outcome in cll patients treated with chlorambucil (Chl) or Ofatumumab-Chl (O-Chl): results from the phase III study complement1 (OMB110911). Blood. 2014;124:1992.
164. Woyach JA, et al. Resistance mechanisms for the Bruton's tyrosine kinase inhibitor ibrutinib. N Engl J Med. 2014;370:2286–94.
165. Liu TM, et al. Hypermorphic mutation of phospholipase C, γ2 acquired in ibrutinib-resistant CLL confers BTK independency upon B-cell receptor activation. Blood. 2015;126(1):61–8.
166. Burger JA, et al. Clonal evolution in patients with chronic lymphocytic leukaemia developing resistance to BTK inhibition. Nat Commun. 2016;7:11589.
167. Famà R, et al. Ibrutinib-naïve chronic lymphocytic leukemia lacks Bruton tyrosine kinase mutations associated with treatment resistance. Blood. 2014;124(25):3831–3.

Treatment of Chronic Lymphocytic Leukemia and Related Disorders

9

Deepa Jeyakumar and Susan O'Brien

Burden of CLL

According to 2016 SEER data, there will be 18,960 new cases of CLL diagnosed and more than 100,000 people with CLL living in the USA [1]. The median age at diagnosis for chronic lymphocytic leukemia was 71 years and age-adjusted incidence rate was 4.6 per 100,000 men and women per year.

Diagnosis of CLL

The diagnosis requires peripheral blood clonal B lymphocytosis of $\geq 5 \times 10^9$/L persisting for at least 3 months [2]. The clonality of the cells needs to be confirmed by flow cytometry-based immunophenotyping demonstrating aberrant expression of the T-cell antigen CD5 along with B-cell antigens CD19, CD20, and CD23, and also by restriction of light-chain expression to either kappa or lambda (Table 9.1). The percentage of prolymphocytes in the peripheral blood may be up to 55%. Any excess of prolymphocytes will favor the diagnosis of B-cell prolymphocytic leukemia (B-PLL). Demonstration of cytopenias along with marrow infiltration by typical CLL cells is adequate for the diagnosis of CLL irrespective of the degree of lymphocytosis.

Small lymphocytic lymphoma (SLL) is a disease restricted to lymph nodes and lymphocytosis of $<5 \times 10^9$/L.

"Monoclonal B lymphocytosis" (MBL) is a disease comprised of clonal B-cell lymphocytosis $<5 \times 10^9$/L in the absence of lymph node involvement, disease-related symptoms, and cytopenias. The prevalence of MBL can be 4–5% [3, 4] among the general population over the age of 40 years. In a prospective study [3], 15% of subjects with MBL and lymphocytosis developed CLL after a median follow-up of 6.7 years. The absolute lymphocyte count correlated with progression to CLL.

Table 9.1 Criteria for diagnosis of CLL

	Working groups: NCIWG/IWCLL [2]
Parameter	
Diagnosis	
Lymphocytes (×10^9/L)	>5; ≥1 B-cell marker (CD19, CD20, CD23) + CD5
Atypical cells (%) (e.g. prolymphocytes)	<55
Duration of lymphocytosis	At least 3 months

NCIWG National Cancer Institute Working Group; *IWCLL* International Workshop on CLL

Table 9.2 Immunophenotypic analysis in chronic B-cell disorders

Disease	Sig	CD5	CD23	FMC7	CD22	CD79b
CLL	Weak	++	++	−/+	Weak/−	Weak/−
B-PLL	Strong	−/+	−	++	+	++
HCL	Strong	−	−	++	++	+
SL VL	Strong	−/+	−/+	++	++	++
FL	Strong	−/+	−/+	++	++	++
MCL	Strong	++	−/+	++	++	++

CLL chronic lymphocytic leukemia, *B-PLL* B-cell prolymphocytic leukemia

Modified from Matutes E, Owusu-Ankomah K, Morilla R, et al. The immunological profile of B-cell disorders and proposal of a scoring system for the diagnosis of CLL. Leukemia. 1994;8:1640–5

The differential diagnosis of CLL includes several other B-cell disorders. Flow cytometric analysis is critical for differentiating between CLL and other B-cell disorders (Table 9.2). A flow cytometry-based scoring system has been useful in situations where the diagnosis is not straightforward [5].

Clinical Features

At diagnosis, most patients are older than 70 years, with more than 95% over 45 years. The diagnosis of CLL is often incidental; routine blood counts may reveal an elevated absolute

D. Jeyakumar, M.D. (✉) • S. O'Brien, M.D.
Chao Family Comprehensive Cancer Center, Division of Hematology Oncology, Department of Medicine, University of California, Irvine, 101 The City Drive South, Building 56, Orange, CA 92868, USA
e-mail: djeyakum@uci.edu

P.H. Wiernik et al. (eds.), *Neoplastic Diseases of the Blood*, DOI 10.1007/978-3-319-64263-5_9

lymphocyte count (ALC). In symptomatic patients, fatigue and infections may be presenting features; B symptoms are rare. A smaller percentage of patients may present with autoimmune hemolytic anemia (AIHA) or autoimmune thrombocytopenia (AIT). Physical examination may reveal cervical, axillary, and/or inguinal lymphadenopathy. Splenomegaly is not uncommon. The majority of patients with CLL will develop hypogammaglobulinemia in their disease course [6, 7]; impaired cellular immunity is evidenced by lack of response to skin testing with tuberculin, candida, and other antigens. These immune defects predispose patients to recurrent infections [8].

Staging

The well-described staging systems for CLL include those of Rai [9] and Binet [10] staging (Table 9.3). The original Rai staging defined five stages from 0 to 4; this has been modified [11] to three stages by defining Rai stage 0 as low-risk group, stage 1 and 2 together designated as an intermediate-risk group, and joining stage 3 and 4 to form a high-risk group with a median survival of >12.5, 7, and 1.5 years for each risk group, respectively. Similarly in Binet stages A, B, and C median survivals are >10, 6, and 2 years, respectively [10]. Both these clinical staging systems are based on physical examination and routine blood counts and do not require radiological imaging. The value of computed tomography (CT) in early-stage CLL is not established.

Workup at Diagnosis

A physical examination that includes examination of the lymph nodes, routine blood counts, and peripheral blood flow cytometry to establish clonal B-cell lymphocytosis is sufficient to establish the diagnosis of CLL. Though the type of bone marrow infiltration (diffuse vs. nondiffuse) may carry prognostic information, the need for a bone marrow aspiration and biopsy can be replaced by new prognostic markers. FISH is required prior to any line of therapy given that therapy in patients with CLL with del(17p) may differ from first-line therapy for patients with CLL without del(17p).

Prognostic Factors

Clinical Prognostic Factors

In a randomized trial of chlorambucil versus observation in Binet stage A patients [12, 13], a subgroup of patients (designated "A") with hemoglobin ≥12 g/dL, lymphocyte count <30 × 10^9/L, and fewer than 80% lymphocytes in the bone marrow aspirate was identified and had an overall survival (OS) comparable to an age-matched French population. Similarly, a lymphocyte doubling time of >12 months, Rai stage 0 disease, nondiffuse bone marrow pattern, hemoglobin ≥13 g/dL, and absolute lymphocyte count <30 × 10^9/L define a group of "smoldering CLL" with an excellent prognosis [14]. Age and response to treatment are also prognostic factors [15]. Women fare better than men and this is independent of stage and age.

Laboratory Parameters

Several serum factors have been identified as prognostic indicators in early-stage CLL. Among patients with early-stage CLL (Binet stage A, Rai stage 0–2) considered to have "smoldering disease" (blood hemoglobin greater than 13.0 g/dL, a low absolute lymphocyte count (<30,000/μL), a lymphocyte doubling time greater than 12 months, and a nondiffuse pattern of lymphoid bone marrow infiltration [14]), serum thymidine kinase (TK) level >7.0 U/L identifies a group with significantly shorter progression-free survival (PFS) compared to those with lower TK levels [16]. Elevated serum β2-microglobulin level is also an adverse prognostic feature [17]. Serum soluble CD23 segregates Binet stage B disease into more or less aggressive forms [18]. High serum LDH levels indicate a poor prognosis [19]. These parameters appear to be surrogate markers of disease burden or cellular turnover.

Table 9.3 Staging of CLL

Rai stage [9]	Modified Rai stage [11]	Description	Binet stage [10]	Description	Median survival
0	Low risk	Lymphocytosis	A	Two or fewer lymphoid bearing areas	>10 Years
1	Intermediate risk	Lymphocytosis and lymphadenopathy	B	Three or more lymphoid bearing areas	5–7 Years
2	Intermediate risk	Lymphocytosis and splenomegaly with/without lymphadenopathy			
3	High risk	Lymphocytosis and anemia (hemoglobin <11 g/dL)	C	Anemia (hemoglobin <10 g/dL) or thrombocytopenia (platelets 100 × 10^6/dL)	2–3 Years
4	High risk	Lymphocytosis and thrombocytopenia (platelets <100 × 10^6/dL)			

A series of new prognostic markers have been identified. Testing for these is not needed for the diagnosis of CLL but may help clinicians to have an informed discussion with patients regarding prognosis. As most patients with CLL are diagnosed with early-stage disease, these data aid in predicting the likelihood of disease progression. Also, some (although not all) of the prognostic markers are correlated with response to therapy.

Genetic Studies

Using conventional chromosome banding techniques, cytogenetic abnormalities can be detected in 40–50% of cases of CLL [20]. This technique is hampered by the low mitotic activity of CLL cells; B-cell mitogens may be used to enhance this activity. In addition, metaphases obtained for karyotyping after mitogen stimulation may arise from normal T cells in the sample [21].

Fluorescence in situ hybridization (FISH) using genomic DNA probes has greatly enhanced the ability to detect molecular abnormalities in malignant cells. This technique can detect aberrations in interphase cells. FISH has demonstrated that molecular abnormalities occur in up to 80% of cases of CLL [22].

13q deletion is the most common genetic aberration found in CLL by FISH (55%) followed by 11q deletion (18%), 12q trisomy (16%), and 17p deletion (7%) [22]. Prior to the use of FISH, trisomy 12 was the most frequently detected chromosomal abnormality in CLL by conventional cytogenetic methods. Structural abnormalities of 13q were often missed by Giemsa banding, presumably because of the small size of the deletion. The prognosis of CLL varies with the chromosomal abnormality. When divided into five prognostic categories, 17p deletion, 11q deletion, 12q trisomy, normal karyotype, and 13q deletion (as sole abnormality), the survival times were 32, 79, 114, 111, and 133 months [22], respectively. Patients with 17p or 11q deletion [23] had more advanced disease with frequent splenomegaly, mediastinal and abdominal lymphadenopathy, as well as more extensive peripheral lymphadenopathy. As part of clonal evolution, patients with CLL can acquire additional mutations. Therefore, at the time of relapse, it is advisable to repeat FISH prior to selection of therapy.

The search for tumor-suppressor genes in the commonly deleted region of 13q14 led to the discovery that two microRNA genes, mir-15a and mir-16, are located in this region [24] and in majority of patients with CLL (approximately 68%) these microRNAs are deleted or downregulated. These two microRNAs are inversely linked to the expression of the antiapoptotic Bcl-2 protein at a posttranslational level [25]. Thus loss of these two microRNAs can be linked to apoptosis resistance in CLL cells through upregulation of Bcl-2. Additional targets of mir-15 and -16 include proteins related to cell cycle progression [26]. The 11q22-q23 deletion is associated with loss of the ataxia telangiectasia mutated (ATM) [27], a gene that is responsible for repair of DNA double-stranded breaks (DNA DSB), activation of cell cycle check points, and inducing of apoptosis in response to DNA DSB. ATM also functions directly in the repair of chromosomal DNA DSBs by maintaining DNA ends in repair complexes generated during VDJ gene rearrangement in the lymphocyte receptor assembly [28]. This explains the occurrence of lymphoid malignancies in patients with ataxia telangiectasia as chromosomal instability in the lymphoid population arises at a time when lymphoid cell receptor diversity is established. The residual ATM allele is mutated in 36% of CLLs with an 11q deletion [29]. Deletion of 17p13 in CLL always includes loss of tumor suppressor TP53 [30]. Deletion of the TP53 gene is associated with poor overall survival (OS) and chemoresistance [30, 31]. In CLL cases with monoallelic loss of TP53, the other allele is mutated in the vast majority [32]. TP53 mutation even in the absence of 17p13 abnormality is associated with poor OS in CLL [33]. The frequency of TP53 mutations is higher among patients with relapsed/refractory disease.

Somatic Hypermutation of Immunoglobulin Heavy-Chain Variable Gene

Recombination of variable (V), diversity (D), and joining (J) genes and insertion of nontemplated nucleotides at the V–D and D–J junction occur in the pregerminal phase of B-cell development. In addition to the diversity brought about by such VDJ recombination, somatic hypermutations are introduced in the V(D)J rearrangement in normal B cells in the germinal center to increase the B-cell repertoire. Assessment for somatic hypermutation in the immunoglobulin heavy-chain variable gene (IgV_H) defines two "subsets" of CLL. Approximately 50% of CLL cases have somatic hypermutation of the IgV_H gene and thus appear to arise from post-germinal B cells while the subset of CLL lacking IgV_H gene hypermutation appears to arise from naive B cells [34]. The mutation status of CLL cells appears fixed and mutational status is not gained or lost during the course of disease. The prognosis of patients with unmutated IgV_H gene is worse than that of patients with IgV_H mutations; the unmutated population is more likely to have advanced-stage and progressive disease [34, 35], as well as markedly shorter PFS and OS after chemoimmunotherapy. The prognostic value of mutation status may be changing in the era of targeted inhibitors.

Stereotyped B-Cell Receptors

Study of VDJ rearrangement of immunoglobulin gene in CLL indicates that certain gene segments are overrepresented across different patients, indicating a stereotyped use of these gene segments (an event occurring more frequently than by chance). A higher proportion of unmutated CLL cases carry stereotyped VDJ rearrangements resulting in similar complementarity-determining regions (CDRs) [34]. More than 20% of CLL cases can carry stereotyped BCRs which suggests exposure to similar antigens which are related to the pathogenesis [36–40]. Use of stereotyped IgV_H genes also affects prognosis. The use of IgV_H 3–21 gene is associated with an aggressive clinical course independent of the IgV_H mutation status [41].

ZAP-70 and CD38 Expression

An attempt was made to identify surrogate markers for IgV_H mutation status. A gene expression analysis identified ZAP-70, a tyrosine kinase protein normally expressed in T and NK cells, to be differentially expressed between mutated and unmutated CLL cases [42]. Immunophenotypic analysis of CLL cases with known mutation status identified higher CD38 expression in cases with unmutated IgV_H [35]. Thus CLL cell expression of ZAP-70 [43–46] and CD38 [35] tends to correlate with unmutated IgV_H and predict poor prognosis. However, their correlation with unmutated IgV_H is not absolute [47, 48], and CD38 and IgV_H mutation status can be independent prognostic factors. Moreover, unlike IgV_H mutation status, CD38 expression can change with time.

Factors That Identify Patients More Likely to Need Treatment

The CLL Research Consortium evaluated the relative value of ZAP-70, CD38 expression, and IgV_H mutation status for predicting time to treatment in patients with newly diagnosed CLL [49]. Based on the analysis of these three parameters, patients can be divided into three risk groups: low, ZAP-70 negative and IgV_H mutated; intermediate, ZAP-70 negative and IgV_H unmutated; and high, ZAP-70 positive irrespective of mutation status. Though ZAP-70 expression can predict for need for treatment, there are concerns about standardization of the procedure to detect ZAP-70 including whether flow cytometry or immunohistochemistry should be used and appropriate gating methods to detect ZAP-70 by flow cytometry. Information about CD38 expression did not appear to add any further prognostic information.

Combining FISH and IgV_H mutation status, the group in Ulm divided patients with early-stage CLL into three risk groups [50]: high risk, del (17p13) irrespective of IgV_H mutation status; intermediate risk, del (11q22) and/or unmutated IgV_H; and low risk, IgV_H mutated in the absence of del (17p13) or del (11q22).

Factors That Impact Response to Therapy

Deletion 17p13 and TP53 mutations are associated with resistance to treatment with nucleoside analogs or alkylating agents and their combinations. IgV_H mutation status does not predict for response, but responses (to chemoimmunotherapy) in patients with IgV_H mutations last longer [51, 52]. Ibrutinib does have activity in CLL with del(17p) [53].

Factors That Impact Overall Survival

Based on clinical and laboratory characteristics of 1674 patients with previously untreated CLL presenting to MDACC, Wierda et al. [54] developed a nomogram comprised of easily available parameters that include age, β2-microglobulin, absolute lymphocyte count, sex, Rai stage, and number of involved lymph node groups. This nomogram predicts for survival probability at 5 and 10 years.

Indications for Treatment

Outside the auspices of a clinical trial, patients with asymptomatic early-stage CLL (Rai stage = 0, Binet stage = A) should be observed until there is evidence of disease progression [2]. Patients with advanced disease (modified Rai stage intermediate or high or Binet B and C) may benefit from therapy. In addition to advanced stage, evidence of active disease should be present to initiate therapy. Such indicators of active disease include (1) marrow failure indicated by cytopenia, (2) splenomegaly (>6 cm below the costal margin or symptomatic splenomegaly), (3) massive (>10 cm) or symptomatic lymphadenopathy, (4) lymphocyte doubling time of <6 months, (5) autoimmune hemolytic anemia or thrombocytopenia poorly responsive to corticosteroids, and (6) a minimum of one disease-related symptom: (a) unintentional weight loss of ≥10% within the previous 6 months, (b) significant fatigue, (c) fevers for ≥2 weeks without any evidence of infection, and (d) night sweats for more than 1 month.

Treatment of CLL

Use of single alkylating agents such as chlorambucil for frontline therapy of CLL is now of historical interest though such an approach may have a role in the treatment of elderly patients with CLL and/or patients with significant comorbidities. See Table 9.4 for commonly used regimens in CLL. Purine analogs have shown single-agent activity and combinations built around the use of purine analogs have become the standard of care for patients with CLL.

Table 9.4 Commonly used chemoimmunotherapy regimens in CLL

Regimen	Schedule	ORR/CR	MRD negative	Remission duration
Fludarabine + rituximab [63]	F 25 mg/m² day 1–5 R 375 mg/m² day 1 for 6 cycles followed by R 375 mg/m² weekly × 4	90/47	N/A	70% at 2 years
Fludarabine + cyclophosphamide + rituximab (FCR) [65, 66]	**F** 25 mg/m² days 1–3 **C** 250 mg/m² days 1–3 **R** 500 mg/m² day 1 For 6 cycles	95/70	78% of CRs	68% at 5 years
Pentostatin + cyclophosphamide + rituximab (PCR) [69]	**P** 2 mg/m² day 1 **C** 600 mg/m² day 1 **R** 375 mg/m² day 1 For 6 cycles	91/41	73% of CRs	48% at 26 months
Bendamustine + rituximab (BR) [71]	**B** 70 mg/m² day 1–2 **R** 375 mg/m² day 1 **For** 6 cycles	88/23	29.2% of CRs in bone marrow; 57.8% in peripheral blood only	

Fludarabine

Fludarabine is the most extensively tested nucleoside analog in CLL. Cellular pharmacology suggests that intracellular accumulation of fludarabine triphosphate is dependent on both drug concentration and duration of exposure [55]. Thus a low-dose repeated dosing schedule was adopted for treatment of CLL.

Pentostatin or Deoxycoformycin

Deoxycoformycin is an inhibitor of adenosine deaminase (ADA), and based on lymphopenias observed in patients with ADA deficiency, pentostatin has been tested as single agent in CLL, both in frontline and salvage settings, yielding modest activity [56, 57]. Pentostatin is perceived to be less myelosuppressive than fludarabine and that led to it being investigated as part of chemoimmunotherapy regimens that will be discussed later.

Bendamustine

Bendamustine is a potent alkylating agent with a low rate of cross-resistance with other alkylating agents. In a phase III randomized, open-label trial comparing bendamustine to chlorambucil in previously untreated patients with CLL, the ORR (68% vs. 31%), CR rate (31% vs. 2%), and PFS (median, 21.8 months vs. 8.0 months) were better in the bendamustine-treated patients [58].

Combination of Purine Analogs with Other Chemotherapeutic Agents

Alkylating agents have been tested in combination with purine analogs. The rationale for such combinations is based on the fact that alkylating agents induce base excision, nucleotide excision, and mismatch repair. This involves removal of damaged nucleotides followed by resynthesis. Exposure to alkylating agents results in more CLL cells requiring DNA resynthesis. At this resynthesis step purine analogs are incorporated in DNA strand repair patch, stop elongation of DNA strands, and induce apoptosis [59].

Fludarabine/Pentostatin and Cyclophosphamide

In a cohort of 128 patients with CLL that included untreated and previously treated (including fludarabine refractory) patients, the combination of fludarabine (30 mg/m² intravenously daily for 3 days) and cyclophosphamide (FC) showed an ORR of ≥80% [60]. The cyclophosphamide dose was decreased from 500 mg/m²/day for 3 days to 300 mg/m²/day for 3 days because of myelosuppression in the early part of the study. The response to FC was higher compared to historical responses to single-agent fludarabine among patients undergoing salvage therapy, with a 38% response rate among patients refractory to fludarabine. While the CR rate (35%) was comparable to fludarabine alone among previously untreated patients, minimal residual disease elimination at the end of therapy was achieved at a higher rate compared to fludarabine alone. The German CLL Study Group (GCLLSG) reported similar activity with FC [61]. Myelosuppression leading to infections was the most common side effect of therapy in both studies.

Chemoimmunotherapy

Fludarabine and Rituximab

The combination of fludarabine and rituximab has been shown to have a synergistic effect against lymphoma cell lines [62]. This led to clinical investigations involving this combination. CALBG 9712 study compared concomitant fludarabine and rituximab with sequential regimen of fludarabine followed by rituximab in patients with previously untreated CLL [63]. The ORR and CR rate was higher in the concomitant arm. A retrospective comparison of 104 patients treated with fludarabine and rituximab on CALB 9712 with 171 patients treated with fludarabine alone in CALBG 9011 study indicated better OS and PFS in patients enrolled on CALBG 9712 [64].

Fludarabine, Cyclophosphamide, and Rituximab

Based on single-agent activity of rituximab in other studies and its synergism with fludarabine, the group at MD Anderson Cancer Center pioneered the combination of rituximab with the most effective chemotherapy combination of fludarabine and cyclophosphamide (FCR) [65]. In their initial report, they noted an ORR of 95% (CR = 70%, nodular PR = 10%, PR = 15%) with the combination regimen of fludarabine, cyclophosphamide, and rituximab (FCR). The CR rate with this regimen was significantly higher than that reported with FC. Moreover, 78% of the patients achieving CR also achieved MRD-negative status as assessed by flow cytometry [defined as CD5- and CD19-coexpressing cells of less than 1%, with normalization of the kappa:lambda ratio (<3:1 in patients with monotypic kappa and >1:3 in patients with monotypic lambda)]. Cytopenias precluded completion of the planned six cycles of treatment in 13% of patients. Neutropenia (≥ grade 3) was encountered in 52% of courses administered to all patients, but only 2.6% of these courses were associated with serious infectious episodes.

Long-term follow-up (median follow-up 6 years) results of this chemoimmunotherapy regimen administered to 300 patients showed a 6-year overall survival of 77% and progression-free survival of 51% with a median time to progression of 80 months [66].

Though all response parameters are superior with the FCR regimen compared to historical data with the FC regimen, a demonstrated survival benefit in a randomized comparison was lacking. The German CLL Study Group performed a multicenter randomized phase III trial [67] involving 817 patients; they reported a better overall survival in patients with previously untreated CLL with the FCR regimen compared to the FC regimen [84.1% in the FCR arm versus 79.0% in the FC arm ($p = 0.01$)]. This improvement in survival was seen in patients with Binet stage A and B CLL. Though cytopenias were more common in the FCR arm, no increased serious infectious episodes were seen (compared to the rate with FC). A multivariate analysis confirmed the beneficial effect of FCR regimen on OS and PFS.

In patients with previously treated CLL, the MD Anderson group reported that the FCR regimen produced a 73% ORR and 25% CR rate [68].

Pentostatin, Cyclophosphamide, and Rituximab

Clinical activity of the combination of pentostatin and cyclophosphamide also encouraged the chemoimmunotherapy regimen of pentostatin, cyclophosphamide, and rituximab (PCR) (see discussion to come). In an initial report of 64 patients, the ORR was 91% and the CR rate was 41% with 23% of patients in CR achieving a MRD-negative status (≤1% positive $CD5^+/CD19^+$ cells) [69]. A total of five patients required transfusions; grade 3/4 cytopenias were encountered in 14.5% of cycles with grade 3/4 infectious complication in only 2% of the cycles.

The initial expectation with the PCR regimen was that the infectious complications would be less than those seen with FCR regimen. However, a randomized community-based trial in previously untreated or minimally pretreated patients comparing the PCR regimen to FCR reported a better CR rate with FCR with a comparable overall response rate, as well as a comparable rate of cytopenias and infectious complications [70].

Bendamustine Rituximab

In a phase II trial of the GCLLSG, bendamustine was combined with rituximab in previously untreated patients with chronic lymphocytic leukemia [71]. The overall response rate was 88% with complete response rate of 23% and partial response rate of 64.9%. At a median follow-up of 27 months, median event-free survival was 33.9 months. The rate of grade 3 or 4 severe infection was 7.7%. Response to therapy was associated with cytogenetics. While 90% of patients with del(11q) and 94.7% of patients with trisomy 12 responded, only 37.5% of patients with del(17p) responded.

The CLL 10 study of the GCLLSG was a phase III, open-label, randomized study comparing bendamustine and rituximab (BR) to FCR [72]. At a median follow-up of 37.1 months, the median progression-free survival was 41.7 months with bendamustine and rituxan and 55.2 months with FCR. However, severe neutropenia and infection were more frequent in the FCR group. The incidence of infectious complications in the FCR group was more pronounced in patients older than 65 years. However, there was a benefit seen in patients with CLL with del(11q) with FCR over bendamustine and rituximab. Of note, patients with del(17p) were not included in this study. Therefore, FCR remains a standard of care in fit patients. However, bendamustine and rituximab are associated with less infectious complications.

Antibodies

CD20 Antibodies

Rituximab, ofatumumab, and obinutuzumab are three anti-CD20 antibodies approved for the treatment of CLL. Ublituximab is being developed as a novel anti-CD20 antibody. CD20 is an antigen expressed on the surface of CLL cells (dim expression by flow cytometry) and is tightly bound to the cell surface. The mechanisms of action of anti-CD20 antibodies against CLL cells include antibody-dependent cellular cytotoxicity [73] (ADCC) and complement-mediated cytotoxicity [74]. In addition, exposure of CLL cells to anti-CD20 antibody has been shown to reduce levels of antiapoptotic proteins including XIAP and Mcl-1 and to induce caspase activation and PARP cleavage [75].

Rituximab

Rituximab is a chimeric monoclonal antibody approved for the treatment of low-grade B-cell lymphomas. The pivotal trial in patients with relapsed low-grade B-cell lymphomas using 375 mg/m^2 weekly for 4 weeks showed responses in 48% of patients, but the response rate among patients with SLL (tissue equivalent of CLL) was 12% [76]. This was attributed to the fact that expression of CD20 was low on SLL/CLL cells compared to cells of follicular lymphomas. O'Brien et al. [77] conducted a dose escalation study of rituximab (375 mg/m^2 dose 1 and dose 2–4 at an escalated rituximab dose). For each patient, the dose of rituximab was kept constant and escalation range was 500–2250 mg/m^2. The ORR among patients with CLL was 36%, all responses being PR.

While Fcgamma RIIA [78] and RIIIA [79] gene polymorphism has been linked to responses to rituximab in patients with non-Hodgkin's lymphoma, no such association has been convincingly established in CLL [80].

Ofatumumab

Ofatumumab is a CD20 monoclonal antibody that binds to a unique epitope that is distinct from the epitope recognized by rituximab. Ofatumumab produces more complement-dependent cytotoxicity (CDC) than is seen with rituximab. As a single agent in patients with relapsed/refractory CLL, the overall response rate was 45% with a median PFS of 5 months [81]. Based on these results, ofatumumab was approved for patients with CLL refractory to fludarabine and alemtuzumab. Ofatumumab has been combined with chlorambucil as first-line therapy (Complement-1) trial [82]. The chlorambucil and ofatumumab combination significantly improved ORR compared to that seen with chlorambucil monotherapy (82% vs. 69%, $p < 0.001$). The combination also improved PFS (median 22.4 months vs. 13.1 months, $p < 0.001$). While ofatumumab is generally well tolerated, the most common side effects are infusion reactions and neutropenia. Based on these results, chlorambucil and ofatumumab were approved for first-line treatment of patients with CLL for whom fludarabine-based therapy is considered inappropriate.

Obinutuzumab

Obinutuzumab is a CD20 monoclonal antibody with a glycoengineered Fc portion leading to enhanced antibody-dependent cellular cytotoxicity (ADCC), increased direct cell death, and lower complement-dependent cytotoxicity (CDC) compared to that seen with rituximab [83]. The CLL11 trial randomized 781 previously untreated patients with CLL with comorbidities to receive chlorambucil monotherapy, chlorambucil with rituxan, or chlorambucil with obinutuzumab. The combination of chlorambucil and obinutuzumab produced an improved PFS compared with that seen with chlorambucil alone (26.7 vs. 11.1 months, $p < 0.001$) [84]. The combination of chlorambucil and obinutuzumab also showed an improved PFS when compared with the PFS noted with the chlorambucil and rituximab combination (median 26.7 vs. 16.3 months, $p < 0.001$). Chlorambucil and obinutuzumab produced a higher ORR as compared to that seen with chlorambucil and rituximab (78.4% vs. 65.1%, $p < 0.001$). These results led to FDA approval of the combination of chlorambucil and obinutuzumab for patients with previously untreated CLL not suitable for more aggressive chemoimmunotherapy. In a recent update, chlorambucil and obinutuzumab showed an improved PFS compared with chlorambucil and rituximab (29.2 months vs. 15.4 months, $p < 0.001$) [85]. However, no overall survival difference was noted between the two antibody arms.

Ublituximab

Ublituximab (TG-1101) is a chimeric IgG1 monoclonal antibody that targets a unique epitope on CD20. In a phase I trial, ublituximab demonstrated a 67% ORR in patients with relapsed/refractory CLL [86]. The combination of ublituximab and ibrutinib is being investigated. In an initial report of 20 patients with high-risk CLL, the overall response rate was 95% [87]. Final results of this trial are yet not reported.

CD52 Antibody

Alemtuzumab, originally known as Campath 1G, is a human immunoglobulin G1 (IgG1) anti-CD52 monoclonal antibody (MAb) that binds to nearly all B- and T-cell lymphomas and leukemias. Early phase II study with an administration schedule of a 30-mg 2-h intravenous (IV) infusion thrice weekly for a maximum period of 12 weeks produced an ORR of 42% [88]. Most disease elimination was seen in blood, bone marrow, and spleen while lymph node response was less. Keating et al. [89] reported on an international study involving 93 patients with fludarabine-refractory CLL using alemtuzumab 30 mg IV three times a week for 12 weeks. In the first week, the initial dose was 3 mg, which was increased to 10 mg, and then to 30 mg as soon as infusion-related reactions were tolerated. Infection prophylaxis with trimethoprim/sulfamethoxazole and famciclovir was mandatory. The intent-to-treat analysis showed an ORR of 33% (CR = 2%, PR = 31%). Though there was reduction in lymphadenopathy and other organomegalies, response in lymph nodes >2 cm was modest. In this pivotal trial, 25 patients had grade 3/4 infectious complications. Viral reactivation (cytomegalovirus = seven patients and herpes simplex virus = six patients) was seen in 13 patients. Infectious complications were more frequent in nonresponders to alemtuzumab than in responders.

Alemtuzumab is no longer available commercially but can be provided through the company through a distribution program.

Targeting Antiapoptotic Proteins

Antiapoptotic members of the Bcl-2 family of proteins can render CLL cells resistant to chemotherapeutic agents; increased expression of Bcl-2 family members is frequently seen in primary CLL cells [90]. Drugs targeting antiapoptotic members of the Bcl-2 family of proteins can induce apoptosis in CLL cells [91] and have synergistic/additive effect with chemotherapeutic agents.

In addition to antisense oligonucleotides, small-molecule inhibitors of Bcl-2 family members have been developed. These agents mimic the BH3 domain of pro-apoptotic Bcl-2 family proteins and work by releasing BH3 only pro-apoptotic members (BAX and BAK) from sequestration by the antiapoptotic members.

Venetoclax

Antiapoptotic proteins such as BCL-2 are expressed at high levels which make the cells resistance to senescence and death. Venetoclax is an oral BCL-2 inhibitor. In the phase I trial, 56 patients with relapsed chronic lymphocytic leukemia were treated in the dose-escalation cohort [92]. Clinical tumor lysis was diagnosed in three patients in that cohort with one death. Adjustments were made in the dose-escalation schema, increased tumor lysis prophylaxis was employed, and initial hospitalization was required, and the subsequent 60 patients tolerated the drug well. There was a 79% overall response rate with 20% complete responses. The 15-month progression-free survival was 69% in the 400 mg cohort. Other side effects were mild diarrhea (52%), upper respiratory tract infection (48%), nausea (47%), and grade 3 or 4 neutropenia (41%). In a phase II trial, 107 patients with relapsed or refractory CLL with 17p deletion were treated with venetoclax [93]. At a median follow-up of 12 months, the overall response rate was 85%. Most common grade 3–4 adverse events were neutropenia (40%), infection (20%), anemia (18%), and thrombocytopenia (15%). Serious adverse events included pyrexia, autoimmune hemolytic anemia (7%), pneumonia (6%), and febrile neutropenia (5%). These results led to the recent FDA approval of venetoclax in relapsed or refractory patients with CLL and del 17p.

Inhibitors of the B-Cell Receptor

B-cell receptor activation is known to play a crucial role in the pathogenesis of CLL. There are many potential targets for inhibition of the B-cell receptor pathway. Kinases for which targeting agents are commercially available include BTK and PI3K [94].

"Redistribution Lymphocytosis"

As a class effect, all inhibitors of the B-cell receptor appear to cause "redistribution lymphocytosis." During the first few weeks of therapy, these agents can cause transient lymphocytosis due to redistribution of CLL cells from the tissue to peripheral blood [95]. Normally, CLL cells circulate in the peripheral blood where they are attracted to tissue stromal cells by a chemokine gradient. The CXCR4-CXCL12 axis is the predominant one for marrow homing. Inhibition of these homing mechanisms by ibrutinib, a BTK inhibitor, leads to the exit of tissue cells into the blood, resulting in an increased lymphocytosis. Lymphocytosis occurs concomitantly with reduction in lymph node size [95]. The transient lymphocytosis should not be confused with disease progression and should not lead to discontinuation of the drug (Fig. 9.1).

Since this class of drugs is known to cause lymphocytosis, many patients do not meet response criteria defined in the 2008 International Workshop on Chronic lymphocytic leukemia (IWCLL) guidelines [2] despite clear and substantial clinical benefit. Thus, the IWCLL guidelines have been adjusted to define an initial response category called partial response with lymphocytosis (PRL), thus ensuring that patients with a partial response who have persistent lymphocytosis are considered responders [96].

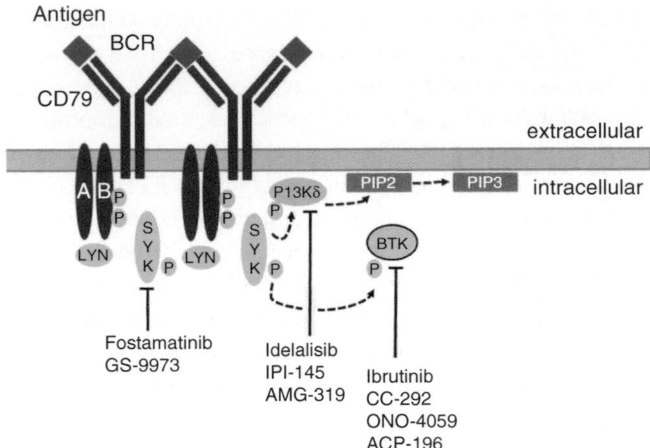

Fig. 9.1 BCR signaling and downstream pathways. The BCR consists of transmembrane receptors. Upon binding of antigen, BCR signaling induces LYN- and SYK-dependent phosphorylation of tyrosine motifs including PI3Kδ and BTK. Several small molecular inhibitors to this kinases are in development (adapted from Wiestner 2014 [94])

Bruton's Tyrosine Kinase (BTK)

BTK is a cytoplasmic tyrosine kinase which is essential to BCR signaling and couples BCR-induced calcium release to activation of the NK-κB pathway and cellular proliferation. X-linked agammaglobulinemia (or Bruton's agammaglobulinemia), which typically presents during childhood, is characterized by an absence of mature B cells and immunoglobulins and leads to recurrent bacterial infections. Loss-of-function mutations in BTK block B-cell maturation at the pre-B-cell stage [97].

Ibrutinib

Ibrutinib is the first BTK inhibitor studied in clinical trials; it inactivates BTK through the formation of an irreversible covalent bond with Cys-481 in the ATP-binding domain [98]. Ibrutinib is also known to inhibit other kinases including ITK (interleukin-2-inducible T-cell kinase), TEC, BMX, and EGFR, which may explain some of the toxicities seen with this agent. Ibrutinib is currently FDA approved for use as initial therapy as well as for the treatment of relapsed disease.

Byrd et al. reported the outcomes of 101 patients with relapsed/refractory CLL, who received ibrutinib [99, 100]. The median age was 64 years old (range, 37–82). Thirty-four percent of the patients had del(17p) and 78% had unmutated IGVH. The median number of prior regimens was four. The overall response rate was 90% with 7% with complete remission (CR). The estimated progression-free survival at 30 months in this heavily pretreated group was 69%. The median PFS in patients with del(17p) and del(11q) was 28 months and 38.7 months, respectively. While this median PFS is a significant improvement over prior experience with chemotherapy regimens in this high-risk group, there is clearly a shorter PFS in patients with del(17p). The most common toxicity was diarrhea which occurred in 55% of patients and was predominately grade 1–2. Notable toxicities >grade 3 included bleeding (8%) and atrial fibrillation (6%).

Ibrutinib was compared to ofatumumab in previously treated patients with CLL in a randomized trial, with results demonstrating improved progression-free and overall survival in the ibrutinib arm [101]. At 12 months, the overall survival was 90% in the ibrutinib arm versus 81% in the ofatumumab arm. The overall response rate was higher with ibrutinib at 43% versus 4% with ofatumumab.

Patients with CLL and a 17p deletion typically have aggressive disease and respond poorly to chemotherapy regimens [102]. A recent report described the outcome of 144 patients with CLL and a 17p deletion who had failed at least one therapy and received ibrutinib 420 mg daily until disease progression [53]. The median number of prior therapies was two with a range of 1 to 7 prior therapies. At a median follow-up of 13 months, the median PFS had not been reached. At 12 months, 79% were alive and progression free and 88% of the responders were progression free. Progressive disease was reported in 13% of patients; 7% of patients developed Richter's transformation and seven of those cases occurred within the first 24 weeks of therapy. The most frequent adverse events were diarrhea in 36% (grades 3–4 in 2%), fatigue in 30% (grades 3–4 in 1%), cough in 24% (grades 3–4 in 1%), and arthralgias in 22% (1% with grades 3–4). Another report described 51 patients with CLL and deletion 17p who were treated with ibrutinib [103]. At 24 weeks, 80% of patients had an objective response: 40% had a PR, 40% had a PRL, and the remaining 20% had stable disease. The adverse effects were similar to those seen in previous reports.

The frontline trial leading to approval of ibrutinib as initial therapy randomized 269 patients who were 65 years or older to receive either ibrutinib or chlorambucil [104]. With a median follow-up of 18.4 months, the median progression-free survival was not reached with ibrutinib versus 18.9 months with chlorambucil. The 24-month overall survival with ibrutinib was 98% versus 85% with chlorambucil.

Toxicity

The incidence of bleeding with ibrutinib was found to be increased. In the phase I/II studies, bruising was seen in 17% of patients: 2% had intracranial hemorrhage [105]. Subsequent trials with ibrutinib have excluded patients on warfarin therapy. In the phase III trial of ibrutinib versus ofatumumab, the bleeding rates were 44% with ibrutinib and

12% with ofatumumab but the rates of serious bleeding were low at 1% versus 2%, respectively [101]. An earlier analysis of the bleeding events with ibrutinib was attributed to effects on the collagen and von Willebrand-dependent platelet functions [106]. However, a more recent analysis attributes the bleeding to inhibition of collagen-dependent platelet aggregation by ibrutinib [107].

The incidence of atrial fibrillation is also increased with ibrutinib. In the phase III trial of ibrutinib versus ofatumumab, ten patients on the ibrutinib arm developed atrial fibrillation versus only one patient on the ofatumumab arm. This led to discontinuation of ibrutinib in one patient [101].

Finally, as with other BCR inhibitors, ibrutinib does cause lymphocytosis. This generally resolves after 6–9 months with continued treatment. Approximately 20% of patients have prolonged lymphocytosis (greater than 12 months) with ibrutinib therapy. Development of lymphocytosis does not appear to be detrimental to long-term clinical outcomes [108].

Ibrutinib Resistance

The outcome of heavily pretreated patients who fail ibrutinib is poor. A previous report described outcomes in 33 patients (26%) (of 127 patients) enrolled on clinical trials of ibrutinib at MD Anderson who discontinued the drug [109]. The majority of these patients had high-risk features including 94% with unmutated IgVH, 58% with 17p deletion by FISH, and 54% with complex karyotype. The reason for discontinuation of ibrutinib included disease transformation in 7%, progressive disease in 7%, and adverse events in 11%; 3% of patients underwent stem cell transplantation. Seventy-six percent of patients died after discontinuing ibrutinib, with a median overall survival after discontinuation of only 3 months. These patients who discontinued ibrutinib had aggressive disease and were heavily pretreated. Recent analysis of outcomes of patients with ibrutinib therapy demonstrated that this does not hold true for patients who receive ibrutinib earlier in their disease course [110]. Patients who were treatment naïve in the Resonate-2 trial and patients that had several lines of prior therapy prior to ibrutinib were compared. The median overall survival in patients post-ibrutinib therapy who had ibrutinib as either first- or second-line therapy was not reached. The median overall survival in patients who had ibrutinib as third-line (or beyond) therapy was only 7–9 months. Therefore, patients who receive ibrutinib in first or second line of therapy were less likely to progress and also experienced better post-ibrutinib survival.

Mutations in the BTK-binding site of ibrutinib have been described in patients who developed resistance while on ibrutinib therapy [111]. Mutations in the cysteine-to-serine in BTK at position 481 (C481S) were seen in five patients. The C481S mutation elicits BTK-independent activation after B-cell receptor activation [112]. Two patients had mutations in PLCγ2 (a downstream kinase from BTK), one at position 665 (R665W) and the other at L845F, leading to gain-of-function mutations that led to potential autonomous B-cell receptor activity. Proximal kinases of SYK and LYN would be critical for activation of mutant PLCG2 and targeting LYN and SYK may combat molecular resistance in cell line models as well as in primary CLL cells from ibrutinib-resistant patients. There has also been a report of clonal evolution leading to ibrutinib resistance. One patient acquired a new clonal mutation in SF3B1(K666 T) and two patients had clonal deletion in chromosome 8p [113]. Other proposed mechanisms for resistance to ibrutinib as well as the other BCR antagonists are reviewed elsewhere [114].

Clinical data are limited on how to proceed after a patient has disease progression on ibrutinib. These patients may be considered for stem cell transplantation, if they are eligible candidates for this intervention [115]. This group may benefit from development of other novel therapies. Because the current second-generation BTK inhibitors bind to the same binding site as ibrutinib, using them in this setting would likely not be productive. A phase I study of the dual-PI3K inhibitor IPI-145 included some patients previously treated with ibrutinib [116]. There was one PR and five patients had stable disease. For further details, refer to the section on IPI-145.

Based on ex vivo data supporting the use of selinexor in the setting of acquired resistance to ibrutinib, as well as in vitro synergy with ibrutinib in chronic lymphocytic leukemia [117], a clinical trial is investigating the combination of selinexor and ibrutinib in relapsed/refractory CLL [118].

Preliminary results from a phase II study of venetoclax in patients with CLL relapsed after ibrutinib or idelalisib are encouraging [119]. In this heavily pretreated group (median of 5 prior regimens) of 54 patients, 41 patients had had prior ibrutinib and 13 patients had prior idelalisib. In the group which had been pretreated with ibrutinib, 13% CR, 48% PR, and 13% SD at 24 weeks were seen. In the group who had been pretreated with idelalisib, the response rate was 50% PR and 25% SD at 24 weeks. At 36 weeks, the overall response rate was 61% in the ibrutinib-pretreated group and 50% in the idelalisib-pretreated group. The drug was well tolerated but serious adverse events were seen, 7% pneumonia and 7% neutropenia.

Second-Generation BTK Inhibitors

Other BTK inhibitors in earlier clinical development include GS-4059 (ONO-4059) [120, 121], acalabrutinib [122, 123], and BGB-3111 [124]. These inhibitors all covalently bind to Cys481 leading to irreversible inhibition. These second-generation inhibitors may have more selective binding to BTK and fewer off-target effects, such as diarrhea, bleeding, and atrial fibrillation.

GS-4059 (ONO-4059)

GS-4059 is a potent and selective BTK inhibitor with an IC50 in the sub-nmol/L range. In a phase I study, the oral inhibitor was given as monotherapy to patients with relapsed/refractory CLL [119]. Of the 16 patients evaluable, 38% of patients had a 17p deletion and 19% of patients had an 11q deletion. Twelve of 16 patients had an unmutated IgVH gene. Eight of 16 patients had a TP53 mutation. The median number of prior therapies was 3. This inhibitor was well tolerated; grade 3 toxicities included febrile neutropenia, as well as one grade 4 neutropenia. The best overall response was 70% as per IWCLL criteria. Two patients had a PR and five patients had a PRL, two had stable disease, and one progressed with Richter's transformation. The results in 60 patients with relapsed hematologic malignancies treated with GS-4059 were recently published [120]. Of 25 patients with relapsed CLL, 24 responded to and 21 patients remained on therapy. One patient had grade 3 bleeding but no diarrhea, cardiac events, or arthralgias were reported. There is an ongoing clinical trial evaluating GS-4057 in various combinations of other agents. There are five different arms comparing GS-4057 with idelalisib, GS-4057 with entospletinib, GS-4057 with idelalisib and obinutuzumab, GS-4057 with entospletinib and obinutuzumab, and just single agent GS-4057 [125]. There is an upcoming clinical trial comparing the combination of GS-4057 and idelalisib with or without obinutuzumab in patients with relapsed/refractory CLL [126].

ACP-196 (Acalabrutinib)

ACP-196 is a second-generation BTK inhibitor which binds covalently to Cys481 with improved selectivity and in vivo target coverage [121]. ACP-196 was able to inhibit 94% of BTK target occupancy after 7 days of dosing in patients with CLL. The results of a phase I–II multicenter study of ACP-196 in patients with relapsed CLL were recently published [122]. Sixty-one patients with relapsed CLL had received a median of three prior regimens and 31% had deletion 17p. No dose-limited toxicities were seen. At a median follow-up of 14.3 months, the overall response rate was 95%, including 85% with partial response and 10% with PRL. The remainder (5%) had stable disease. The response rate in the patients with deletion 17p was 100%. There is an ongoing registration trial randomizing patients with relapsed CLL and deletion 17p or 11q to ibrutinib or acalabrutinib [127]. The FDA registration phase III study for potential frontline approval randomizes patients to one of the three arms, acalabrutinib, acalabrutinib and obinutuzumab, or chlorambucil and obinutuzumab [126].

BGB-3111

BGB-3111 is another oral BTK inhibitor. Ibrutinib antagonizes rituximab-induced antigen-dependent cell-mediated cytotoxicity (ADCC) by inhibiting ITK kinase activity [128]. In murine models BGB-3111 resulted in a tenfold weaker inhibition of rituximab-induced ADCC and was threefold more potent than ibrutinib in target organs [129]. The results of a phase I study of BGB-3111 in patients with B-cell lymphoid malignancies were recently reported [130]. Of 25 patients enrolled, 8 patients had CLL. There were other patients including mantle cell lymphoma, Waldenstrom's, DLBCL, follicular lymphoma, marginal zone lymphoma, and hairy cell leukemia. There were no serious adverse events leading to drug discontinuation or adverse-related disease reported. Of 21 adverse events grade 3 or greater, only 3 were felt to potentially be related to the drug which were neutropenia. There were no grade 3 or 4 bleeding events or cases of atrial fibrillation. Of the CLL patients, two had stable disease and six had partial response. The results of 45 patients with CLL treated with BGB-3111 were recently presented [131]. The drug was well tolerated with 69% of patients without any AE greater than grade 1 within the first 12 weeks of therapy. The most frequent AEs were petechiae/bruising, upper respiratory infection, diarrhea, fatigue, and cough. Three serious adverse events were reported which possibly could have been related to the drug which were grade 2 cardiac failure, grade 2 pleural effusion, and grade 3 purpura. At a median follow-up of 7.5 months, the response rate was 90% with PR in 79% of patients and PR-L in 10%, and stable disease in 7%. These results are encouraging and further studies are planned.

PI3K Inhibitor

The PI3K pathway is a key component of survival in a variety of cancers including CLL. There are three classes of PI3K isoforms. Class I isoforms are made up of two subsets: 1A, which includes p110α, p110β, and p110δ bound by regulatory domains, and 1B, which is composed of p110-γ coupled with p101 [132]. The p110δ is abundantly expressed in CLL as the delta isoform is the most important isoform in hematologic cells. Idelalisib is the first PI3K inhibitor in combination with rituximab approved by the FDA in patients with relapsed CLL. PI3K inhibitors in clinical development include duvelisib, and TGR-1202.

Idelalisib

Idelalisib is a selective oral reversible inhibitor of the p110δ isoform of PI3Kδ. In the phase I study of idelalisib, 72% of patients had an objective response with a median progression-free survival of 16 months [133]. Overall, the patients on this trial had less functional reserve than the patients on ibrutinib trials, with decreased renal function, therapy-induced myelosuppression, or major coexisting illness. Furthermore, at the optimal doses, progression-free survival was 32 months. Median overall survival was not reached, with a 36-month overall survival of 75%. The most common >grade 3 adverse events were pneumonia in 20%, neutropenic fever in 11%, and diarrhea in 6% of patients. At the second interim analysis, the phase III randomized clinical trial of idelalisib with rituximab versus placebo with rituximab reported that the addition of idelalisib led to an overall response rate of 77% versus 15% with rituximab plus placebo [133]. Furthermore, in the idelalisib and rituximab arm, there was a 12-month progression-free survival of 66% [134, 135]. Serious adverse events occurred in 40% of patients in the idelalisib arm. The most common adverse events were pneumonia, pyrexia, and febrile neutropenia. Grade 3 or higher transaminitis occurred in 5% of patients in the idelalisib arm with onset at 8–16 weeks. The study drug was withheld and four of six patients were successfully rechallenged. Furthermore, in the idelalisib arm, gastrointestinal and skin toxicities led to discontinuation of the drug in six patients. Because PI3kδ influences clonal expansion and differentiation of suppressor T cells, diarrhea and colitis may be an expected autoimmune toxicity. A phase II trial evaluated the combination of idelalisib and rituximab in previously untreated patients with CLL/SLL who were 65 years or older [136]. This combination produced a high ORR of 97%. However, the adverse side effect profile was higher in this previously untreated cohort compared to that seen in relapsed/refractory patients treated with idelalisib The incidence of transaminitis was 67% with 23% of patients having grade 3 or higher toxicity. Diarrhea or colitis was reported in 64% of patients; 42% was grade 3 or higher. On the colonoscopic biopsies, T-cell infiltration was present in the patients with colitis. The authors noted that T-cell levels are typically normal in previously untreated patients with CLL but are quite low in patients with relapsed/refractory disease. This is one possible reason for the increased toxicity noted in the previously untreated group compared with the relapsed/refractory group.

These findings were confirmed in another phase II trial evaluating idelalisib in the frontline setting [137]. This trial enrolled 24 patients with newly diagnosed CLL who were treated with 2 months of idelalisib followed by 6 months of the combination of idelalisib and ofatumumab. Hepatotoxicity was reported in 79% of patients with 54% being grade 3 or higher. The median time to development of transaminitis was 28 days which was prior to the administration of ofatumumab. The transaminitis did resolve with holding the drug and, in some cases, addition of immunosuppressants. This study showed that the toxicity was increased in the younger frontline patients, presumably because they have better functioning immune systems. Clinical trials with idelalisib in the frontline setting have been discontinued because of a higher rate of infections and death than was seen in the control arm.

IPI-145 (Duvelisib)

IPI-145 is another inhibitor of PI3K. It inhibits both the p110δ and the p110γ isoforms. Duvelisib antagonizes BCR cross-linking activated pro-survival signals in primary CLL cells [138] and causes direct killing of primary CLL cells in a dose-dependent fashion while it spares normal B cells. Furthermore, based on ex vivo models, duvelisib could possibly overcome ibrutinib resistance resulting from the BTK C481S mutation [116].

In a phase I/II study of monotherapy with IPI-145, 54 patients with relapsed/refractory CLL were enrolled [139]. The patients were heavily pretreated with 82% having received more than three prior lines of therapy. The median time from prior therapy was 3.5 months. Cytogenetics were poor risk with 49% having TP53 mutations or a 17p deletion and 89% having an unmutated IgVH. The expansion cohort enrolled patients at either 25 or 75 mg twice daily. The best overall response rate was 55% in 49 evaluable patients including 1 CR and 26 partial responses (PR). There were 21 patients with stable disease (in this study PRL was counted as stable disease) and 1 patient with progressive disease. The overall response rate was independent of dose or the presence of TP53/17p deletion. There was early resolution in the lymphocytosis. Overall, the drug was well tolerated with transient cytopenias, with 31% neutropenia, 11% thrombocytopenia, 15% febrile neutropenia, and 11% pneumonia. Treatment was discontinued in 31% of patients due to adverse events, and in another 24% of patients because of disease progression. DUO is a phase III study in relapsed/refractory CLL randomizing 300 patients to either duvelisib 25 mg twice daily or ofatumumab for up to 18 cycles [140].

In the phase I study a cohort of patients with CLL resistant to ibrutinib were treated with duvelisib [116]. This included six patients with relapsed/refractory CLL and six patients with aggressive B-cell NHL (aNHL, including two with DBLCL and four with Richter's transformation). Two patients received duvelisib at 25 mg twice daily and ten patients received duvelisib at 75 mg twice daily. All patients had received more than three prior therapies. The median time from prior therapy to duvelisib was 0.3 months and 67% of patients received it within 2 weeks of ibrutinib. The patients with CLL had received a median of four cycles of duvelisib. The best response in patients with relapsed/refractory CLL was one PR; five patients had stable disease. Of these six patients, two patients remained on the drug for 8 and 9 months and four patients discontinued the drug due to disease progression or physician decision.

TGR-1202

TGR-1202 is a second-generation PI3Kδ inhibitor. In a phase I study, patients with relapsed/refractory hematologic malignancies were administered monotherapy with TGR-1202 orally once daily following a 3 + 3 dose escalation design [141]. Preliminary results from this phase I study were notable for PR in four of the six patients with CLL treated at doses above 800 mg daily. The nodal reduction occurred rapidly and was accompanied by lymphocytosis. Subsequent reporting revealed that of nine evaluable patients with CLL, eight (89%) achieved a PR in the nodes with a median nodal reduction of 71%, of whom five achieved a PR [142]. Notably, in comparison to other PI3kδ inhibitors, there were no cases of hepatotoxicity or colitis observed. Rates of infection and pneumonia were low at 12% and 6%, respectively, with no cases of febrile neutropenia.

Based on the encouraging phase I data, the combination of TGR-1202 and ublituximab (a glycoengineered anti-CD20 mAb) was studied in a phase I trial following a 3 + 3 dose escalation design [143]. Ublituximab was administered weekly for the first two cycles and then on day 1 of cycle numbers 4, 6, 9, and 12 while TGR-1202 was administered daily. There were 12 patients with CLL included in the trial. Reported toxicities were 44% day 1 infusion reactions, 41% neutropenia, 34% diarrhea, and 28% nausea; no grade 3 or 4 toxicities were seen. There were no cases of hepatotoxicity. In the ten patients with CLL, there was a median progression-free survival of 8 months. Enrollment continues in the higher dose cohort.

The combination of ublituximab with TGR-1202 and ibrutinib has also been administered to patients with B-cell malignancies [144]. Ublituximab was dosed at 900 mg weekly for the first two cycles and then on day 1 of cycles 4, 6, 9, and 12. TGR-1202 was dose escalated at 400, 600, 800, and 1200 mg while the ibrutinib dose was held stable at 420 mg for patients with CLL and 560 mg for patients with NHL. There were three patients with CLL and SLL included. Of the adverse events, 20% of patients experienced day 1 infusion reactions with no grade 3 or 4 reactions noted, while 20% of patients experienced neutropenia which was grade 3 or 4, and 30% experienced diarrhea, constipation, or fatigue with no grade 3 or 4 events. The overall response rate was 86% with two of three patients with CLL/SLL responding. Based on these findings, phase II studies are planned.

Adoptive Cellular Therapy

New cellular therapies including CAR-T cells are being developed for patients with B-cell malignancies including patients with CLL [145]. CAR-T cells can be associated with adverse events including neurotoxicity and cytokine release syndrome. Experience with managing the toxicities of these therapies is critical for safe delivery of these therapies.

Targeting Minimal Residual Disease in CLL

In patients achieving complete remission after therapy for CLL, those who achieve MRD-negative CR tend to have responses that last longer and also have better OS. Four-color flow cytometry or allele-specific oligonucleotide PCR (ASO-PCR) with a sensitivity of detecting 1 CLL cell in 10,000 leukocytes is recommended for use in clinical trials reporting on MRD eradication.

Disease-Related Complications of CLL

Immune-Mediated Cytopenias in CLL

Autoimmune hemolytic anemia (AIHA), autoimmune thrombocytopenia (AIT), and pure red cell aplasia (PRCA) develop in some patients with CLL. The incidence of AIHA is 4–11% [6, 146, 147] and that of AIT 2–3%. PRCA is least common. Fludarabine has been associated with AIT and AIHA [148]. Prednisone is the usual treatment for AIHA and AIT, with a high likelihood of response initially. However, more than 60% of patients relapse when treatment is stopped. Intravenous immunoglobulin produces response in 40% of patients, but these responses tend to be transient. Cyclosporine A is another option for treatment of immune-mediated cytopenias and can produce responses even in patients with steroid refractory immune cytopenias [149]. Rituximab, alemtuzumab, and the combination of rituximab, cyclophosphamide, and dexamethasone [150–152] have also been used to treat autoimmune complications of CLL.

Hypogammaglobulinemia

Hypogammaglobulinemia is a frequent complication of CLL. Because of the high cost of therapy and its limited activity in preventing serious infections, monthly intravenous gammaglobulin replacement therapy is usually limited to hypogammaglobulinemic patients who experience repeated sino-pulmonary bacterial infections.

Transformations

Richter's Syndrome

The term Richter's syndrome (RS) refers to the development of large-cell lymphoma (LCL) during the course of CLL. RS is usually associated with worsening systemic symptoms including B symptoms, elevated LDH, rapid tumor growth, and/or extranodal involvement. Diagnosis requires tissue biopsy. PET scanning helps in identifying sites to direct tissue biopsy. Gene rearrangement studies and isotype analysis suggest that the CLL and LCL cells frequently share identical clonal origins. The LCL is usually resistant to therapy, and the median survival of patients who develop RS is approximately 6–9 months [153, 154]. If the gene rearrangement studies do not show the identical clonal origin, then the LCL should be treated as independent of the history of CLL and the prognosis can be excellent [155]. The presence of NOTCH mutations increases the risk of transformation. The presence of NOTCH mutation was associated with a risk of development of DLBCL in 30% of patients at 10 years [156].

Prolymphocytic Transformation

The NCIWG criteria allow a diagnosis of CLL to be made in the presence of ≤55% prolymphocytes. The presence of prolymphocytes >55% indicates prolymphocytic transformation.

Prolymphocytic Leukemia

Prolymphocytic leukemia (PLL) is characterized by splenomegaly, a high number of circulating prolymphocytes, minimal lymphadenopathy, and a median survival of less than 3 years. Prolymphocytes are larger and less homogenous than CLL cells, and have abundant clear cytoplasm, clumped chromatin, and a prominent nucleolus. Prolymphocytes can be of either B- or T-cell type. B-PLL cells usually do not express CD5 but stain strongly for surface immunoglobulin and FMC-7. TP53 mutations and 11q23 or 13q14 deletions are common in B-PLL [157–159]. Approximately 20% of cases of PLL are of T-cell phenotype. Over 70% of T-PLL shows overexpression of the oncoprotein TCL-1 [160, 161].

Splenectomy and lymphoma-like regimens have been used to treat PLL without much success. In a study at MDACC, a 38% ORR (18% CR) was seen with a 5-day schedule of fludarabine administered every 4 weeks. Dearden et al. reported an ORR of 48% with pentostatin (2′ deoxycoformycin) [162]. Alemtuzumab (Campath-1H) also has shown promising activity in T- and B-PLL [163–165] with an ORR of 51%, CR rates of up to 39.5%, and median survival of 7.5 months. In a study from Royal Marsden Hospital, alemtuzumab (Campath-1H) was administered intravenously three times weekly to patients with previously treated T-PLL until maximal response [166]. The ORR was 76% with 60% CR. However, responses with alemtuzumab are short-lasting and disease progression is the norm. Ibrutinib and idelalisib may have a role in this disease.

Conclusion

Based on the advances made in our understanding of the biology of CLL, there are now many avenues for investigation for novel therapies. Given that these newer therapies are generally better tolerated than chemoimmunotherapy, many more patients are eligible for therapy than in the past. This will hopefully lead to a prolongation in remissions in these patients while maintaining a good quality of life.

References

1. http://seer.cancer.gov/statfacts/html/clyl.html.
2. Hallek M, Cheson BD, Catovsky D, et al. Guidelines for the diagnosis and treatment of chronic lymphocytic leukemia: a report from the International Workshop on Chronic Lymphocytic Leukemia updating the National Cancer Institute-Working Group 1996 guidelines. Blood. 2008;111:5446–56.
3. Rawstron AC, Bennett FL, O'Connor SJ, et al. Monoclonal B-cell lymphocytosis and chronic lymphocytic leukemia. N Engl J Med. 2008;359:575–83.
4. Shanafelt TD, Ghia P, Lanasa MC, Landgren O, Rawstron AC. Monoclonal B-cell lymphocytosis (MBL): biology, natural history and clinical management. Leukemia. 2010;24(3):512–20.
5. Matutes E, Owusu-Ankomah K, Morilla R, et al. The immunological profile of B-cell disorders and proposal of a scoring system for the diagnosis of CLL. Leukemia. 1994;8:1640–5.
6. Dearden C. Disease-specific complications of chronic lymphocytic leukemia. Hematology Am Soc Hematol Educ Program. 2008:450–6.
7. Ben-Bassat I, Many A, Modan M, Peretz C, Ramot B. Serum immunoglobulins in chronic lymphocytic leukemia. Am J Med Sci. 1979;278:4–9.
8. Morrison VA. Management of infectious complications in patients with chronic lymphocytic leukemia. Hematology Am Soc Hematol Educ Program. 2007:332–8.
9. Rai KR, Sawitsky A, Cronkite EP, Chanana AD, Levy RN, Pasternack BS. Clinical staging of chronic lymphocytic leukemia. Blood. 1975;46:219–34.
10. Binet JL, Auquier A, Dighiero G, et al. A new prognostic classification of chronic lymphocytic leukemia derived from a multivariate survival analysis. Cancer. 1981;48:198–206.
11. Rai KR, Han T. Prognostic factors and clinical staging in chronic lymphocytic leukemia. Hematol Oncol Clin North Am. 1990;4:447–56.
12. Effects of chlorambucil and therapeutic decision in initial forms of chronic lymphocytic leukemia (stage A): results of a randomized clinical trial on 612 patients. The French Cooperative Group on Chronic Lymphocytic Leukemia. Blood. 1990;75:1414–21.
13. Dighiero G, Maloum K, Desablens B, et al. Chlorambucil in indolent chronic lymphocytic leukemia. French Cooperative Group on Chronic Lymphocytic Leukemia. N Engl J Med. 1998;338:1506–14.
14. Montserrat E, Vinolas N, Reverter JC, Rozman C. Natural history of chronic lymphocytic leukemia: on the progression and progres-

sion and prognosis of early clinical stages. Nouv Rev Fr Hematol. 1988;30:359–61.
15. Catovsky D, Fooks J, Richards S. Prognostic factors in chronic lymphocytic leukaemia: the importance of age, sex and response to treatment in survival. A report from the MRC CLL 1 trial. MRC Working Party on Leukaemia in Adults. Br J Haematol. 1989;72:141–9.
16. Hallek M, Langenmayer I, Nerl C, et al. Elevated serum thymidine kinase levels identify a subgroup at high risk of disease progression in early, nonsmoldering chronic lymphocytic leukemia. Blood. 1999;93:1732–7.
17. Ibrahim S, Keating M, Do KA, et al. CD38 expression as an important prognostic factor in B-cell chronic lymphocytic leukemia. Blood. 2001;98:181–6.
18. Molica S, Levato D, Dell'Olio M, et al. Cellular expression and serum circulating levels of CD23 in B-cell chronic lymphocytic leukemia. Implications for prognosis. Haematologica. 1996;81:428–33.
19. Lee JS, Dixon DO, Kantarjian HM, Keating MJ, Talpaz M. Prognosis of chronic lymphocytic leukemia: a multivariate regression analysis of 325 untreated patients. Blood. 1987;69:929–36.
20. Dohner H, Stilgenbauer S, Fischer K, Bentz M, Lichter P. Cytogenetic and molecular cytogenetic analysis of B cell chronic lymphocytic leukemia: specific chromosome aberrations identify prognostic subgroups of patients and point to loci of candidate genes. Leukemia. 1997;11(Suppl 2):S19–24.
21. Autio K, Elonen E, Teerenhovi L, Knuutila S. Cytogenetic and immunologic characterization of mitotic cells in chronic lymphocytic leukaemia. Eur J Haematol. 1987;39:289–98.
22. Dohner H, Stilgenbauer S, Benner A, et al. Genomic aberrations and survival in chronic lymphocytic leukemia. N Engl J Med. 2000;343:1910–6.
23. Dohner H, Stilgenbauer S, James MR, et al. 11q deletions identify a new subset of B-cell chronic lymphocytic leukemia characterized by extensive nodal involvement and inferior prognosis. Blood. 1997;89:2516–22.
24. Calin GA, Dumitru CD, Shimizu M, et al. Frequent deletions and down-regulation of micro-RNA genes miR15 and miR16 at 13q14 in chronic lymphocytic leukemia. Proc Natl Acad Sci U S A. 2002;99:15524–9.
25. Cimmino A, Calin GA, Fabbri M, et al. miR-15 and miR-16 induce apoptosis by targeting BCL2. Proc Natl Acad Sci U S A. 2005;102:13944–9.
26. Calin GA, Cimmino A, Fabbri M, et al. MiR-15a and miR-16-1 cluster functions in human leukemia. Proc Natl Acad Sci U S A. 2008;105:5166–71.
27. Stilgenbauer S, Liebisch P, James MR, et al. Molecular cytogenetic delineation of a novel critical genomic region in chromosome bands 11q22.3-923.1 in lymphoproliferative disorders. Proc Natl Acad Sci U S A. 1996;93:11837–41.
28. Bredemeyer AL, Sharma GG, Huang CY, et al. ATM stabilizes DNA double-strand-break complexes during V(D)J recombination. Nature. 2006;442:466–70.
29. Austen B, Skowronska A, Baker C, et al. Mutation status of the residual ATM allele is an important determinant of the cellular response to chemotherapy and survival in patients with chronic lymphocytic leukemia containing an 11q deletion. J Clin Oncol. 2007;25:5448–57.
30. Dohner H, Fischer K, Bentz M, et al. p53 gene deletion predicts for poor survival and non-response to therapy with purine analogs in chronic B-cell leukemias. Blood. 1995;85:1580–9.
31. el Rouby S, Thomas A, Costin D, et al. p53 gene mutation in B-cell chronic lymphocytic leukemia is associated with drug resistance and is independent of MDR1/MDR3 gene expression. Blood. 1993;82:3452–9.
32. Zenz T, Krober A, Scherer K, et al. Monoallelic TP53 inactivation is associated with poor prognosis in chronic lymphocytic leukemia: results from a detailed genetic characterization with long-term follow-up. Blood. 2008;112:3322–9.
33. Rossi D, Cerri M, Deambrogi C, et al. The prognostic value of TP53 mutations in chronic lymphocytic leukemia is independent of Del17p13: implications for overall survival and chemorefractoriness. Clin Cancer Res. 2009;15:995–1004.
34. Hamblin TJ, Davis Z, Gardiner A, Oscier DG, Stevenson FK. Unmutated Ig V(H) genes are associated with a more aggressive form of chronic lymphocytic leukemia. Blood. 1999;94:1848–54.
35. Damle RN, Wasil T, Fais F, et al. Ig V gene mutation status and CD38 expression as novel prognostic indicators in chronic lymphocytic leukemia. Blood. 1999;94:1840–7.
36. Ghia P, Stamatopoulos K, Belessi C, et al. Geographic patterns and pathogenetic implications of IGHV gene usage in chronic lymphocytic leukemia: the lesson of the IGHV3-21 gene. Blood. 2005;105:1678–85.
37. Murray F, Darzentas N, Hadzidimitriou A, et al. Stereotyped patterns of somatic hypermutation in subsets of patients with chronic lymphocytic leukemia: implications for the role of antigen selection in leukemogenesis. Blood. 2008;111:1524–33.
38. Stamatopoulos K, Belessi C, Moreno C, et al. Over 20% of patients with chronic lymphocytic leukemia carry stereotyped receptors: Pathogenetic implications and clinical correlations. Blood. 2007;109:259–70.
39. Fais F, Ghiotto F, Hashimoto S, et al. Chronic lymphocytic leukemia B cells express restricted sets of mutated and unmutated antigen receptors. J Clin Invest. 1998;102:1515–25.
40. Mauerer K, Zahrieh D, Gorgun G, et al. Immunoglobulin gene segment usage, location and immunogenicity in mutated and unmutated chronic lymphocytic leukaemia. Br J Haematol. 2005;129:499–510.
41. Tobin G, Thunberg U, Johnson A, et al. Chronic lymphocytic leukemias utilizing the VH3-21 gene display highly restricted Vlambda2-14 gene use and homologous CDR3s: implicating recognition of a common antigen epitope. Blood. 2003;101:4952–7.
42. Rosenwald A, Alizadeh AA, Widhopf G, et al. Relation of gene expression phenotype to immunoglobulin mutation genotype in B cell chronic lymphocytic leukemia. J Exp Med. 2001;194:1639–47.
43. Crespo M, Bosch F, Villamor N, et al. ZAP-70 expression as a surrogate for immunoglobulin-variable-region mutations in chronic lymphocytic leukemia. N Engl J Med. 2003;348:1764–75.
44. Orchard JA, Ibbotson RE, Davis Z, et al. ZAP-70 expression and prognosis in chronic lymphocytic leukaemia. Lancet. 2004;363:105–11.
45. Rassenti LZ, Huynh L, Toy TL, et al. ZAP-70 compared with immunoglobulin heavy-chain gene mutation status as a predictor of disease progression in chronic lymphocytic leukemia. N Engl J Med. 2004;351:893–901.
46. Wiestner A, Rosenwald A, Barry TS, et al. ZAP-70 expression identifies a chronic lymphocytic leukemia subtype with unmutated immunoglobulin genes, inferior clinical outcome, and distinct gene expression profile. Blood. 2003;101:4944–51.
47. Hamblin TJ, Orchard JA, Gardiner A, Oscier DG, Davis Z, Stevenson FK. Immunoglobulin V genes and CD38 expression in CLL. Blood. 2000;95:2455–7.
48. Hamblin TJ, Orchard JA, Ibbotson RE, et al. CD38 expression and immunoglobulin variable region mutations are independent prognostic variables in chronic lymphocytic leukemia, but CD38 expression may vary during the course of the disease. Blood. 2002;99:1023–9.
49. Rassenti LZ, Jain S, Keating MJ, et al. Relative value of ZAP-70, CD38, and immunoglobulin mutation status in predicting aggressive disease in chronic lymphocytic leukemia. Blood. 2008;112:1923–30.
50. Krober A, Seiler T, Benner A, et al. V(H) mutation status, CD38 expression level, genomic aberrations, and survival in chronic lymphocytic leukemia. Blood. 2002;100:1410–6.

51. Byrd JC, Gribben JG, Peterson BL, et al. Select high-risk genetic features predict earlier progression following chemoimmunotherapy with fludarabine and rituximab in chronic lymphocytic leukemia: justification for risk-adapted therapy. J Clin Oncol. 2006;24:437–43.
52. Lin KI, Tam CS, Keating MJ, et al. Relevance of the immunoglobulin VH somatic mutation status in patients with chronic lymphocytic leukemia treated with fludarabine, cyclophosphamide, and rituximab (FCR) or related chemoimmunotherapy regimens. Blood. 2009;113:3168–71.
53. O'Brien SM, Jones JA, Coutre S, et al. Efficacy and Safety of ibrutinib in patients with relapsed or refractory chronic lymphocytic leukemia or small lymphocytic leukemia with 17p deletion: results from the Phase II Resonate-17 Trial. Blood. 2014;124(21):327.
54. Wierda WG, O'Brien S, Wang X, et al. Prognostic nomogram and index for overall survival in previously untreated patients with chronic lymphocytic leukemia. Blood. 2007;109:4679–85.
55. Gandhi V, Kemena A, Keating MJ, Plunkett W. Cellular pharmacology of fludarabine triphosphate in chronic lymphocytic leukemia cells during fludarabine therapy. Leuk Lymphoma. 1993;10:49–56.
56. Dillman RO, Mick R, McIntyre OR. Pentostatin in chronic lymphocytic leukemia: a phase II trial of cancer and leukemia group B. J Clin Oncol. 1989;7:433–8.
57. Johnson SA, Catovsky D, Child JA, Newland AC, Milligan DW, Janmohamed R. Phase I/II evaluation of pentostatin (2′-deoxycoformycin) in a five day schedule for the treatment of relapsed/refractory B-cell chronic lymphocytic leukaemia. Investig New Drugs. 1998;16:155–60.
58. Knauf WU, Lissichkov T, Aldaoud A, et al. Phase III randomized study of bendamustine compared with chlorambucil in previously untreated patients with chronic lymphocytic leukemia. J Clin Oncol. 2009;27:4378–84.
59. Carson DA, Carrera CJ, Wasson DB, Yamanaka H. Programmed cell death and adenine deoxynucleotide metabolism in human lymphocytes. Adv Enzym Regul. 1988;27:395–404.
60. O'Brien SM, Kantarjian HM, Cortes J, et al. Results of the fludarabine and cyclophosphamide combination regimen in chronic lymphocytic leukemia. J Clin Oncol. 2001;19:1414–20.
61. Hallek M, Schmitt B, Wilhelm M, et al. Fludarabine plus cyclophosphamide is an efficient treatment for advanced chronic lymphocytic leukaemia (CLL): results of a phase II study of the German CLL Study Group. Br J Haematol. 2001;114:342–8.
62. Di Gaetano N, Xiao Y, Erba E, et al. Synergism between fludarabine and rituximab revealed in a follicular lymphoma cell line resistant to cytoxic activity of either drug alone. Br J Hematol. 2001;114:800–9.
63. Byrd JC, Peterson BL, Morrison VA, et al. Randomized phase 2 study of fludarabine with concurrent or sequential rituximab in symptomatic untreated patients with B cell chronic lymphocytic leukemia: results from Cancer and Leukemia Group B 9712 (CALBG 9712). Blood. 2003;101:6–14.
64. Byrd JC, Rai K, Peterson BL, et al. Addition of rituximab to fludarabine may prolong progression free survival and overall survival in patients with previously untreated chronic lymphocytic leukemia: an updated retrospective comparative analysis of CALBG 9712 and CALBG 9011. Blood. 2005;23:4070–8.
65. Keating MJ, O'Brien S, Albitar M, et al. Early results of a chemoimmunotherapy regimen of fludarabine, cyclophosphamide, and rituximab as initial therapy for chronic lymphocytic leukemia. J Clin Oncol. 2005;23:4079–88.
66. Tam CS, O'Brien S, Wierda W, et al. Long-term results of the fludarabine, cyclophosphamide, and rituximab regimen as initial therapy of chronic lymphocytic leukemia. Blood. 2008;112:975–80.
67. Hallek M, Fingerle-Rowson G, Fink A-M, et al. First-line treatment with fludarabine (F), cyclophosphamide (C), and rituximab (R) (FCR) improves overall survival (OS) in previously untreated patients (pts) with advanced chronic lymphocytic leukemia (CLL): results of a randomized phase III trial on behalf of an international group of investigators and the German CLL Study Group. Blood (ASH Annual Meeting Abstracts). 2009;114:535.
68. Wierda W, O'Brien S, Wen S, et al. Chemoimmunotherapy with fludarabine, cyclophosphamide, and rituximab for relapsed and refractory chronic lymphocytic leukemia. J Clin Oncol. 2005;23:4070–8.
69. Kay NE, Geyer SM, Call TG, et al. Combination chemoimmunotherapy with pentostatin, cyclophosphamide, and rituximab shows significant clinical activity with low accompanying toxicity in previously untreated B chronic lymphocytic leukemia. Blood. 2007;109:405–11.
70. Reynolds C, Di Bella N, Lyons RM, et al. Phase III trial of fludarabine, cyclophosphamide, and rituximab vs. pentostatin, cyclophosphamide, and rituximab in B-cell chronic lymphocytic leukemia. Blood (ASH Annual Meeting Abstracts). 2008;112:327.
71. Fischer K, Cramer P, Busch R, et al. Bendamustine in combination with rituximab for previously untreated patients with chronic lymphocytic leukemia: a multicenter phase II trial of the German Chronic lymphocytic leukemia study group. J Clin Oncol. 2012;30:3209–16.
72. Eichhorst B, Fink AM, Bahlo J, et al. First-line chemoimmunotherapy with bendamustine and rituximab versus fludarabine, cyclophosphamide and rituximab in patients with advanced chronic lymphocytic leukemia (CLL10): an international, open-label, randomized, phase 3, non-inferiorty trial. Lancet Oncol. 2016;17:928–42.
73. Lefebvre ML, Krause SW, Salcedo M, Nardin A. Ex vivo-activated human macrophages kill chronic lymphocytic leukemia cells in the presence of rituximab: mechanism of antibody-dependent cellular cytotoxicity and impact of human serum. J Immunother. 2006;29:388–97.
74. Di Gaetano N, Cittera E, Nota R, et al. Complement activation determines the therapeutic activity of rituximab in vivo. J Immunol. 2003;171:1581–7.
75. Byrd JC, Kitada S, Flinn IW, et al. The mechanism of tumor cell clearance by rituximab in vivo in patients with B-cell chronic lymphocytic leukemia: evidence of caspase activation and apoptosis induction. Blood. 2002;99:1038–43.
76. McLaughlin P, Grillo-Lopez AJ, Link BK, et al. Rituximab chimeric anti-CD20 monoclonal antibody therapy for relapsed indolent lymphoma: half of patients respond to a four-dose treatment program. J Clin Oncol. 1998;16:2825–33.
77. O'Brien SM, Kantarjian H, Thomas DA, et al. Rituximab dose-escalation trial in chronic lymphocytic leukemia. J Clin Oncol. 2001;19:2165–70.
78. Paiva M, Marques H, Martins A, Ferreira P, Catarino R, Medeiros R. FcgammaRIIa polymorphism and clinical response to rituximab in non-Hodgkin lymphoma patients. Cancer Genet Cytogenet. 2008;183:35–40.
79. Weng WK, Levy R. Two immunoglobulin G fragment C receptor polymorphisms independently predict response to rituximab in patients with follicular lymphoma. J Clin Oncol. 2003;21:3940–7.
80. Farag SS, Flinn IW, Modali R, Lehman TA, Young D, Byrd JC. Fc gamma RIIIa and Fc gamma RIIa polymorphisms do not predict response to rituximab in B-cell chronic lymphocytic leukemia. Blood. 2004;103:1472–4.
81. Osterborg A, Jewell RC, Padmanabhan-Iyer S, et al. Ofatumumab monotherapy in fludarabine-refractory chronic lymphocytic leukemia: final results from a pivotal study. Haematologica. 2015;100:e311–4.
82. Hillmen P, Robak T, Janssens A, et al. Chlorambucil plus ofatumumab versus chlorambucil alone in previously untreated patients with chronic lymphocytic leukemia (complement 1): a randomized multicenter, open-label phase 3 trial. Lancet. 2015;385:1873–83.

83. Herter S, Herting F, Mundigl O, et al. Preclinical activity of the type II CD20 antibody GA101 (obinutuzumab) compared with rituximab and ofatumumab in vitro and in xenograft models. Mol Cancer Ther. 2013;12:2031–42.
84. Goede V, Fischer K, Busch R, et al. Obinutuzumab plus chlorambucil in patients with CLL and coexisting conditions. N Engl J Med. 2014;370:1101–10.
85. Goede V, Fischer K, Engelke A, et al. Obinutuzumab as frontline treatment of chronic lymphocytic leukemia: updated results of the CLL 1 study. Leukemia. 2015;29:1602–4.
86. O'Connor OA, Schreeder MT, Deng C, et al. Ublituximab (TG-1101), a novel anti-CD20 monoclonal antibody for rituximab relapsed/refractory B cell malignancies. Milan, Italy: European Hematology Association (EHA); 2014.
87. Sharman J, Farber CM, Mahadevan D, et al. Ublituximab (TG-1101), a novel glycoengineered anti-CD20 mAb, in combination with ibrutinib achieves 95% ORR in patients with high-risk relapsed/refractory CLL. Presented at: 13th International Congress on Malignant Lymphoma; June 17–20, 2015; Lugano, Switzerland. Abstract 105.
88. Lundin J, Kimby E, Bjorkholm M, et al. Phase II trial of subcutaneous anti-CD52 monoclonal antibody alemtuzumab (Campath-1H) as first-line treatment for patients with B-cell chronic lymphocytic leukemia (B-CLL). Blood. 2002;100:768–73.
89. Keating MJ, Flinn I, Jain V, et al. Therapeutic role of alemtuzumab (Campath-1H) in patients who have failed fludarabine: results of a large international study. Blood. 2002;99:3554–61.
90. McConkey DJ, Chandra J, Wright S, et al. Apoptosis sensitivity in chronic lymphocytic leukemia is determined by endogenous endonuclease content and relative expression of BCL-2 and BAX. J Immunol. 1996;156:2624–30.
91. Robertson LE, Plunkett W, McConnell K, Keating MJ, McDonnell TJ. Bcl-2 expression in chronic lymphocytic leukemia and its correlation with the induction of apoptosis and clinical outcome. Leukemia. 1996;10:456–9.
92. Roberts AW, Davids MS, Pagel JM, et al. Targeting BCL2 with venetoclax in relapsed chronic lymphocytic leukemia. N Engl J Med. 2016;374:311–22.
93. Stilgenbauer S, Eichhorst B, Schetelig J, et al. Venetoclax in relapsed or refractory chronic lymphocytic leukemia with 17p deletion: a multicenter, open-label, phase 2 study. Lancet Oncol. 2016;17:768–78.
94. Wiestner A. BCR pathway inhibition as therapy for chronic lymphocytic leukemia and lymphoplasmacytic lymphoma. ASH Education Book. 2014;2014:125–34.
95. Woyach JA, Smucker K, Smith LL, et al. Prolonged lymphocytosis during ibrutinib therapy is associated with distinct molecular characteristics and does not indicate a suboptimal response to therapy. Blood. 2014;123(12):1810–7.
96. Cheson BD, Byrd JC, Rai KR, et al. Novel targeted agents and the need to refine clinical end points in chronic lymphocytic leukemia. J Clin Onc. 2012;30:2820–2.
97. Singh J, Petter RC, Kluge AF. Targeting covalent drugs of the kinase family. Curr Opin Chem Biol. 2010;14(4):475–80.
98. Dubovsky JA, Beckwith KA, Natarajan G, et al. Ibrutinib is an irreversible molecular inhibitor of ITK driving a Th-1-selective pressure in T lymphocytes. Blood. 2013;122(15):2539–49.
99. Byrd JC, Furman RR, Coutre SE, et al. Targeting BTK with ibrutinib in relapsed chronic lymphocytic leukemia. N Engl J Med. 2013;369(1):32–42.
100. Byrd JC, Furman RR, Coutre SE, et al. Three-year follow-up in treatment-naïve and previously treated patients with CLL and SLL receiving single-agent ibrutinib. Blood. 2015;125(16):2497–506.
101. Byrd JC, Brown JR, O'Brien S, et al. Ibrutinib versus ofatumumab in previously treated chronic lymphoid leukemia. N Engl J Med. 2014;371(3):213–23.
102. Stephens DM, Byrd JC. Chronic lymphocytic leukemia with del(17p13.1): a distinct clinical subtype requiring novel treatment approaches. Oncology. 2012;11:1044–54.
103. Farooqui MZ, Valdez J, Martyr S, et al. Ibrutinib for previously untreated and relapsed or refractory chronic lymphocytic leukemia with TP53 aberrations: a phase 2 single arm trial. Lancet Oncol. 2015;16:169–76.
104. Burger JA, Tedeschi A, Barr PM, et al. Ibrutinib as initial therapy for patients with chronic lymphocytic leukemia. NEJM. 2015;373:2425–37.
105. Advani RH, Buggy JJ, Sharman JP, et al. Bruton tyrosine kinase inhibitor ibrutinib (PCI-32765) has significant activity in patients with relapsed/refractory B-cell malignancies. J Clin Onc. 2013;31(1):88–94.
106. Levade M, David E, Garcia C, et al. Ibrutinib treatment affects collagen and von Willebrand factor-dependent platelet functions. Blood. 2014;124(26):3991–5.
107. Kamel S, Horton L, Ysebaert L, et al. Ibrutinib inhibits collagen-mediated but not ADP-mediated platelet aggregration. Leukemia. 2015;29:783–7.
108. Herman SE, Niemann CU, Farooqui M, et al. Ibrutinib-induced lymphocytosis in patients with chronic lymphocytic leukemia: correlative analysis from phase II study. Leukemia. 2014;28:2188–96.
109. Jain P, Keating M, Wierda W, et al. Outcomes of patients with chronic lymphocytic leukemia after discontinuing ibrutinib. Blood. 2015;125(13):2062–7.
110. O'Brien SM, Byrd JC, Hillmen P, et al. Outcomes with ibrutinib by line of therapy in patients with CLL: analyses from phase III data. J Clin Oncol. 2016;34(suppl):abstr 7520.
111. Woyach JA, Furmann RR, Liu TM, et al. Resistance mechanisms for the Bruton's tyrosine kinase inhibitor ibrutinib. N Engl J Med. 2014;270(24):2286–94.
112. Liu TM, Woyach JA, Zhong Y, et al. Hypermorphic mutation of phospholipase C, γ2 acquired in ibrutinib-resistant CLL confer BTK independency upon B cell receptor activation. Blood. 2015;126(1):61–8.
113. Landau D, Hoellenriegel J, Sougnez C, et al. Clonal evolution in patients with chronic lymphocytic leukemia (CLL) developing resistance to BTK inhibition. Blood. 2013;122(21):866.
114. Woyach JA, Johnson AJ. Targeted therapies in CLL: mechanisms of resistance and strategies for management. Blood. Prepublished online June 11, 2015.
115. Daver N, Cortes J, Ravandi F, et al. Secondary mutations as mediators of resistance to targeted therapy in leukemia. Blood. 2015;125(21):3236–45.
116. Porcu P, Flinn I, Kahl BS, et al. Clinical activity of Duvelisib (IPI-145), a phosphoinositide-3-kinsase-∂/γ inhibitor in patients previously treated with ibrutinib. Blood. 2014;123(21):3335.
117. Hing ZA, Mantle R, Beckwith KA, et al. Selinexor is effective in acquired resistance to ibrutinib and synergizes with ibrutinib in chronic lymphocytic leukemia. Blood. 2015;125(20):3128–32.
118. https://clinicaltrials.gov/ct2/show/NCT02303392.
119. Jones J, Mato AR, Coutre S, et al. Preliminary results of phase 2 open-label study of venetoclax (ABT-199/GDC-0199) monotherapy in patients with CLL relapsed after or refractory to ibrutinib or idealisib therapy. Oral presentation abstract 715.
120. Sales G, Karlin L, Rule S, Shah N, et al. A phase I study of oral BTK inhibitor ONO-4059 in patients with relapsed/refractory or high-risk chronic lymphocytic leukemia (CLL). ASH Annual Meeting Abstracts. 2013;122(21):676.
121. Walters HS, Rule SA, Dyer MJ, et al. A phase 1 clinical trial of the selective BTK inhibitor ONO/GS-4059 in relapsed and refractory mature B-cell malignancies. Blood. 2016;127:411–9.
122. Covey T, Barf T, Gulrajani M, et al. ACP-196: a novel covalent Bruton's tyrosine kinase (BTK) inhibitor with improved selectivity and in vivo target coverage in chronic lymphocytic leukemia.

123. Byrd JC, Harrington B, O'Brien S, et al. Acalabrutinib (ACP-196) in relapsed chronic lymphocytic leukemia. NEJM. 2016;374:323–32.
124. Li Na SZ, Ye L, et al. BGB-311 is a novel and highly selective Bruton's tyrosine kinase (BTK) inhibitor. Cancer Res. 2015;75:Abstract nr 2597.
125. https://clinicaltrials.gov/ct2/show/NCT02457598.
126. https://clinicaltrials.gov/ct2/show/NCT02968563.
127. https://clinicaltrials.gov/ct2/show/NCT02477696.
128. https://clinicaltrials.gov/ct2/show/NCT02337829.
129. Kohrt HE, Sagiv-Barfi I, Rafiq S, Herman SE, Butchar JP, Cheney C, et al. Ibrutinib antagonizes rituximab-dependent NK cell-mediated cytotoxicity. Blood. 2014;123:1957–60.
130. Tam C, Grigg AP, Opat S, et al. The BTK inhibitor, BGB 3111, is safe, tolerable and highly active in patients with relapsed/refractory B-cell malignancies: initial report of a phase 1 first-in-human trial. Blood. 2015;126:832.
131. Tam C, Opat S, Cull G, et al. Twice daily dosing with the highly specific BTK inhibitor, BGB-3111, achieved complete and continuous BTK occupancy in lymph nodes and is associated with durable responses in patients with chronic lymphocytic leukemia (CLL)/Small lymphocytic leukemia (SLL). Blood 2016. Oral session 642.
132. Herman SE, Gordon AL, Wagner AJ, et al. Phosphatidylinositol 3-kinase-δ inhibitor shows promising preclinical activity in chronic lymphocytic leukemia by antagonizing intrinsic and extrinsic cellular survival signals. Blood. 2010;116(12):2078–88.
133. Brown JR, Byrd JC, Coutre SE, et al. Idelalisib, an inhibitor of phosphatidylinositol 3-kinase p110delta, for relapsed/refractory chronic lymphocytic leukemia. Blood. 2014;123(22):3390–7.
134. Furman RR, Sharman JP, Coutre SE, et al. Idelalisib and rituxan in relapsed chronic lymphocytic leukemia. N Engl J Med. 2014;370(11):997–1007.
135. Sharman JP, Coutre SE, Furman RR, et al. Second interim analysis of a phase 3 study of idelalisib (Zydelig) plus Rituximab for relapsed chronic lymphocytic leukemia: Efficacy analysis in patient subpopulations with del(17p) and other adverse prognostic factors. Blood (ASH Annual Meeting Abstracts) 2014; Abstract 330.
136. O'Brien S, Lamanna N, Kipps TJ, et al. A phase 2 study of idelalisib plus rituximab in treatment-naïve older patients with chronic lymphocytic leukemia. Blood. 2015;126(25):2686–94.
137. Lampson BL, Kasar SN, Matos TR, et al. Idelalisib given front-line for treatment of chronic lymphocytic leukemia causes frequent immune-mediated hepatotoxicity. Blood. 2016;128(2):195–203.
138. Dong S, Guinn D, Dubovsky, et al. IPI-145 antagonizes intrinsic and extrinsic survival signals in chronic lymphocytic leukemia cells. Blood. 2014;124(24):3583–6.
139. O'Brien S, Patel M, Kahl BS, et al. Duvelisib (IPI-145), a PI3K-∂/γ inhibitor, is clinically active in patients with relapsed/refractory chronic lymphocytic leukemia. Blood. 2014;124(21):3334.
140. https://clinicaltrials.gov/ct2/show/NCT02004522.
141. Burris HA, Patel MA, Lanasa MC, et al. Activity of TGR-1202, a novel once-daily PI3k**δ** inhibitor in patients with relapsed and refractory hematologic malignancies. J Clin Onc. 2014;32(suppl 5s):abstr 2513.
142. Burris HA, Patel MR, Brander DM, et al. TGR-1202, a novel once daily PI3kδ inhibitor, demonstrates clinical activity with a favorable safety profile, lacking hepatotoxicity, in patients with chronic lymphocytic leukemia and B cell lymphoma. Blood. 2014;124(21):1984.
143. Lunning MA, Vose J, Fowler NH, et al. Ublituximab plus TGR-1202 activity and safety profile in relapsed/refractory B-cell NHL and high risk CLL. J Clin Onc. 2015;33(suppl):abstr 8548.
144. Flower NH, Nastoupil LJ, Lunning MA, et al. Safety and activity of the chemotherapy-free triplet of ublituximab, TGR-1202 and ibrutinib in relapsed B cell malignancies. J Clin Onc. 2015;33(suppl):abstr 8501.
145. Castro JE, Kipps TJ. Adoptive cellular therapy for chronic lymphocytic leukemia and B cell malignancies. CARs and more. Best Pract Res Clin Haematol. 2016;29:15–29.
146. Diehl LF, Ketchum LH. Autoimmune disease and chronic lymphocytic leukemia: autoimmune hemolytic anemia, pure red cell aplasia, and autoimmune thrombocytopenia. Semin Oncol. 1998;25:80–97.
147. Weiss RB, Freiman J, Kweder SL, Diehl LF, Byrd JC. Hemolytic anemia after fludarabine therapy for chronic lymphocytic leukemia. J Clin Oncol. 1998;16:1885–9.
148. Kyasa MJ, Parrish RS, Schichman SA, Zent CS. Autoimmune cytopenia does not predict poor prognosis in chronic lymphocytic leukemia/small lymphocytic lymphoma. Am J Hematol. 2003;74:1–8.
149. Cortes J, O'Brien S, Loscertales J, et al. Cyclosporin a for the treatment of cytopenia associated with chronic lymphocytic leukemia. Cancer. 2001;92:2016–22.
150. Hegde UP, Wilson WH, White T, Cheson BD. Rituximab treatment of refractory fludarabine-associated immune thrombocytopenia in chronic lymphocytic leukemia. Blood. 2002;100:2260–2.
151. Lundin J, Karlsson C, Celsing F. Alemtuzumab therapy for severe autoimmune hemolysis in a patient with B-cell chronic lymphocytic leukemia. Med Oncol. 2006;23:137–9.
152. Kaufman M, Limaye SA, Driscoll N, et al. A combination of rituximab, cyclophosphamide and dexamethasone effectively treats immune cytopenias of chronic lymphocytic leukemia. Leuk Lymphoma. 2009;50:892–9.
153. Robertson LE, Pugh W, O'Brien S, et al. Richter's syndrome: a report on 39 patients. J Clin Oncol. 1993;11:1985–9.
154. Tsimberidou AM, Keating MJ. Richter syndrome: biology, incidence, and therapeutic strategies. Cancer. 2005;103:216–28.
155. Rossi D. Richter's syndrome: novel and promising therapeutic alternatives. Best Pract Res Clin Hematol. 2016;29:30–9.
156. Vollamor N, Conde L, Martinez-Trillos A, et al. NOTCH1 mutations identify a genetic subgroup of chronic lymphocytic leukemia patients with high risk of transformation and poor outcome. Leukemia. 2013;27:1100–6.
157. Lens D, De Schouwer PJ, Hamoudi RA, et al. p53 abnormalities in B-cell prolymphocytic leukemia. Blood. 1997;89:2015–23.
158. Lens D, Coignet LJ, Brito-Babapulle V, et al. B cell prolymphocytic leukaemia (B-PLL) with complex karyotype and concurrent abnormalities of the p53 and c-MYC gene. Leukemia. 1999;13:873–6.
159. Lens D, Matutes E, Catovsky D, Coignet LJ. Frequent deletions at 11q23 and 13q14 in B cell prolymphocytic leukemia (B-PLL). Leukemia. 2000;14:427–30.
160. Herling M, Khoury JD, Washington LT, Duvic M, Keating MJ, Jones D. A systematic approach to diagnosis of mature T-cell leukemias reveals heterogeneity among WHO categories. Blood. 2004;104:328–35.
161. Herling M, Patel KA, Teitell MA, et al. High TCL1 expression and intact T-cell receptor signaling define a hyperproliferative subset of T-cell prolymphocytic leukemia. Blood. 2008;111:328–37.
162. Dearden C, Matutes E, Catovsky D. Deoxycoformycin in the treatment of mature T-cell leukaemias. Br J Cancer. 1991;64:903–6.
163. Ferrajoli A, O'Brien SM, Cortes JE, et al. Phase II study of alemtuzumab in chronic lymphoproliferative disorders. Cancer. 2003;98:773–8.
164. Keating MJ, Cazin B, Coutre S, et al. Campath-1H treatment of T-cell prolymphocytic leukemia in patients for whom at least one prior chemotherapy regimen has failed. J Clin Oncol. 2002;20:205–13.
165. Pawson R, Dyer MJ, Barge R, et al. Treatment of T-cell prolymphocytic leukemia with human CD52 antibody. J Clin Oncol. 1997;15:2667–72.
166. Dearden CE, Matutes E, Cazin B, et al. High remission rate in T-cell prolymphocytic leukemia with CAMPATH-1H. Blood. 2001;98:1721–6.

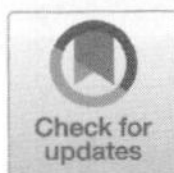

Hairy Cell Leukemia

10

Sonia Ali and Alan Saven

Introduction

The WHO categorizes hairy cell leukemia (HCL) as a mature B-cell neoplasm. HCL is characterized by lymphocytes with prominent cytoplasmic projections (hairy cells) infiltrating the bone marrow and spleen, leading to pancytopenia, bone marrow fibrosis, and splenic enlargement. Hairy cells have a unique immunophenotypic profile—CD11c+, CD20+, CD25+, and CD103+—that confirms its diagnosis. The course of HCL is usually chronic, but can often be progressive, and most patients require treatment at some point. The purine nucleoside analogues, pentostatin and cladribine, are highly active, but cladribine is the preferred first-line choice due to its efficacy, brief treatment duration, and favorable toxicity profile. Other therapeutic options include rituximab, interferon-alpha, vemurafenib, and splenectomy. With current therapy, an overall survival of 87% at 12 years has been reported.

History

HCL was originally recognized in the 1920s but was not identified as a unique entity with distinct pathological and clinical characteristics until 1958 when Bouroncle and colleagues characterized it as *leukemic reticuloendotheliosis* [1] and described the first 26 cases. In their landmark article, the authors provided a comprehensive description of the clinical course, pathology, and limited treatment at the time with alkylating agents and splenectomy. The term "hairy cell leukemia" was first coined by Schreck and Donnelly in 1966 when they noted hairlike cytoplasmic projections on phase-contrast microscopy [2]. The last 50 years, and especially the last two decades, have been spent defining HCL as a B-cell neoplasm [3, 4] and have heralded dramatic therapeutic advances with the purine nucleoside analogues.

Epidemiology and Etiology

HCL is uncommon and accounts for 2–3% of all adult leukemias in the USA [5]. According to the Surveillance Epidemiology and End Results (SEER) database, 2856 cases were diagnosed between 1978 and 2004 [6]. There is a 4:1 male predominance and the median age at presentation is 50 years [5]. New data suggest a bimodal incidence pattern, with an early peak around age 40 years and a later peak at 80 years [6]. The disease is more common in Caucasians, with an increased incidence in Ashkenazi Jewish men.

No well-defined etiology for HCL has been reported. Case reports have suggested an association with farming, woodworking, and exposure to organic solvents [7]. A recent hospital-based case-control study in France noted significant associations between HCL and organochlorine insecticides, and phenoxyacetic and triazine herbicides, though the numbers in the study were small [8]. Infectious etiologies such as EBV and HTLV-1 have also been postulated as causes [9, 10]. Familial cases of HCL have been rarely reported. Makower et al. described two cases of familial HCL. In one case, a 50-year-old man developed HCL and a year later his mother was diagnosed with the same entity. In the other family, an aunt of a patient with HCL was diagnosed with Hodgkin's disease. Interestingly, in both families, the younger generation developed the hematologic malignancy at an earlier age. This phenomenon, known as anticipation, has been noted in other malignancies [11]. Cases of familial HCL have also identified HLA haplotypes specific to each family. Each family's HLA haplotype was unique and there has been no identification of a common HLA haplotype among unrelated cases of HCL [11, 12].

S. Ali, M.D. (✉) • A. Saven, M.D.
Division of Hematology/Oncology, Scripps Clinic, 10666 North Torrey Pines Road, La Jolla, CA 92037, USA
e-mail: ali.sonia@scrippshealth.org; saven.alan@scrippshealth.org

P.H. Wiernik et al. (eds.), *Neoplastic Diseases of the Blood*, DOI 10.1007/978-3-319-64263-5_10

Pathogenesis

Ontogeny

With the advances in molecular techniques, the ontogeny of HCL is becoming clearer. The hairy cell phenotype is that of a late B-cell precursor, likely an activated memory B cell, with aberrant gene expression [13]. The post-germinal center origin is supported by the presence of Bcl-6 mutations and somatic point mutations in the immunoglobulin variable region of the heavy chain [14, 15]. Furthermore, hairy cells express several pan B-cell markers including CD19, CD20, and CD37, but are devoid of the early markers of B-cell development, including CD21 and CD 24 [16]. Hairy cells express the plasma cell antigen-1 (PCA-1) but lack expression of PC-1 which appears later in B-cell ontogeny. This observation suggests that hairy cells do not differentiate into terminal B cells, i.e., plasma cells [3]. DNA microarray analysis illustrates a homogeneous phenotype distinct from other B-cell malignancies. When compared to normal B cells, hairy cells share many genes with memory B cells involved in proliferation and apoptosis [4].

Adhesion/Homing

Hairy cells are highly adherent and can spontaneously bind to several matrices, including fibronectin, vitronectin, and hyaluronan [17, 18]. This binding is facilitated by specific adhesive proteins on hairy cells, including the integrins $\alpha 4\beta$ 1, $\alpha 5\beta 1$, and $\alpha v\beta 3$ [18]. Hairy cells characteristically disseminate into the red pulp of the spleen and hepatic sinusoids and portal tracts, but spare lymph nodes [19]. Not only do hairy cells infiltrate many different types of tissues, but they also modify the tissues they infiltrate. Thus, they cause bone marrow fibrosis and form vascular lakes (pseudosinuses) in the spleen [20]. This modification is inherent to the tissue matrix and is enhanced by hairy cell interactions [18]. For example, fibronectin is important in the development of bone marrow fibrosis and it is thought that hairy cells themselves are intricately involved in its production and assembly [17]. Recently, gene analysis has provided more insights into hairy cell adhesion and targeting. For instance, the lack of hairy cell lymph node infiltration can be explained by downregulation of CCR7, a chemokine receptor that allows B cells to enter lymph nodes. Also, hairy cells remain confined to blood-related compartments due to upregulation of genes that prevent their extravasation [4].

Cytogenetics

No karyotypic abnormality is pathognomonic for HCL. Clonal karyotypic abnormalities are variable and range from 20 to 67% of patients [21]. Unlike most other B-cell malignancies, HCL lack balanced chromosomal translocations which occur with immunoglobulin gene rearrangements that are switched off in memory B cells [13]. Instead, chromosomal gains, deletions, and inversions have been identified. In one study, 40% of karyotypic abnormalities involved chromosome 5, with aberrations in band 5q13 being most common [21]. Other chromosomal abnormalities include deletion of 14q and losses of the long arm of chromosome 7 [22, 23]. Evaluation by FISH has revealed that p53 deletions, a marker found in aggressive disease, occur in HCL. The clinical significance of this finding in an indolent disease is currently under investigation [24].

Diagnosis

Histopathologic and morphologic evaluation of the bone marrow is key to establishing the diagnosis of HCL [25]. Classical cytochemical stainings such as tartrate-resistant acid phosphatase (TRAP) have generally been supplanted by modern diagnostic techniques of flow cytometry and immunohistochemical (IHC) staining.

Cytology

Hairy cells are uniform and monotonous in their appearance [25]. A typical hairy cell is slightly larger than a mature lymphocyte with a distinct nucleus that is usually ovoid, but can also be slightly indented [25]. Unlike other B-cell malignancies, the chromatin is uniformly granular without clumping [26]. Morphologically, hairy cells display features suggestive of a metabolically active cell [27]. They have variable amounts of blue-gray cytoplasm and abundant mitochondria and ribosomes. Hairy cells exhibit thin cytoplasmic "hair-like" projections often appearing as serrated borders (Fig. 10.1). Phase-contrast microscopic studies of live cells show that the surface of these cells is in a constant state of change, reflecting ongoing cytoskeletal and signaling activity [13, 28].

Rarely, ribosomal lamellar complexes, or broad-shaped inclusions, can be seen in the cytoplasm on electron microscopy. These organelles are thought to originate from the endoplasmic reticulum and are characterized by alternating layers of ribosome-like granules and fibrous lamellae [29, 30]. Present in half of the cases, the ultrastructural inclusions are not unique to HCL and have been noted in other lymphoid malignancies [30]. They are of unclear clinical significance [31].

Hairy cell cytoplasm stains strongly for TRAP [32]. Isoenzyme 5 acid phosphatase present in hairy cell cytoplasm resists decoloration with tartrate [33]. Most other lymphoid cells, monocytes, and myeloid cells stain variably for

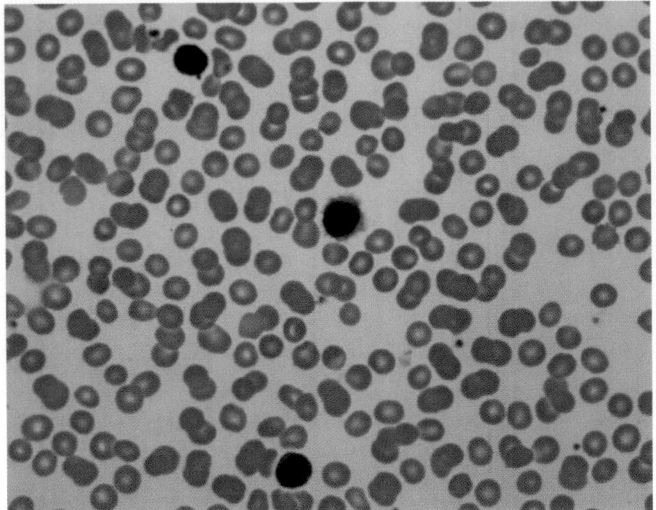

Fig. 10.1 Peripheral blood smear from a patient with HCL. The hairy cell is slightly larger than a mature lymphocyte with ovoid nuclei. Hairy cells characteristically have abundant, *gray-blue* cytoplasm with thin "hairlike" projections (×1000) (corresponds to figure pb 1000×)

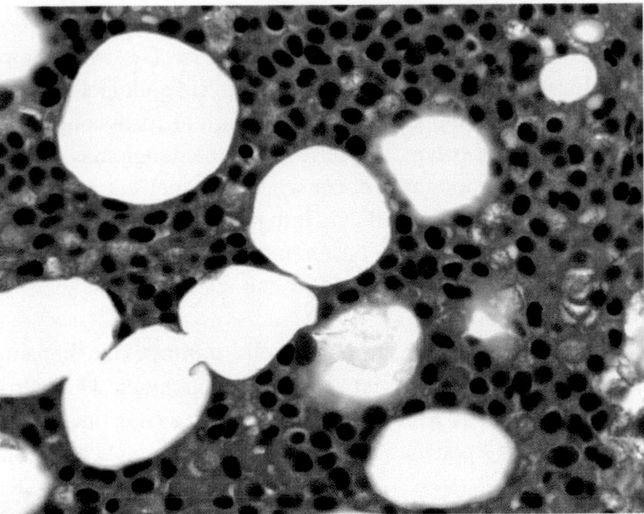

Fig. 10.2 Hairy cell leukemia in the bone marrow, characterized by well-spaced lymphocytes with a "fried-egg" appearance due to the distinct round to oval nuclei, which are centrally placed within a pale staining cytoplasmic domain (×1000) (corresponds to figure bm 1000×)

acid phosphatase activity in the absence of tartrate [16]. TRAP staining is labor intensive and difficult to perform in paraffin-embedded tissues and it is rarely used in the era of immunophenotyping.

Histopathology

Blood and Bone Marrow

Abnormalities in the hemogram are classically seen at presentation in HCL patients [26]. Pancytopenia is common and reported in 80% of patients. Leukopenia is frequently noted [5]. Circulating monocytes are usually absent from the peripheral blood. Despite findings of marrow fibrosis, leukoerythroblastosis is not seen. Circulating hairy cells are variable and oftentimes very difficult to identify [26].

Bone marrow involvement is seen in nearly all patients with HCL [34]. It is often difficult or impossible to obtain an aspirate [25]. The biopsy can show a hypercellular picture. Hairy cells demonstrate patchy or diffuse infiltration of the marrow. A closer examination of the infiltrate reveals a distinctive wide-spaced separation of cells with a surrounding halo, often referred to as a "fried-egg" appearance (Fig. 10.2) [34]. This loose packing of cells results from hairy cells adhering to the reticulin–fibronectin network. Few fibroblasts are seen and trichrome staining does not show deposition of mature collagen [26]. The residual hematopoietic tissues exhibit nonspecific changes [34]. Other collection of cells including small lymphocytes, plasma cells, and mast cells is often identified. Not uncommonly, HCL produces a hypocellular marrow which can be difficult to distinguish from aplastic anemia. Immunostains with CD20 may be helpful (see Fig. 10.3) [35].

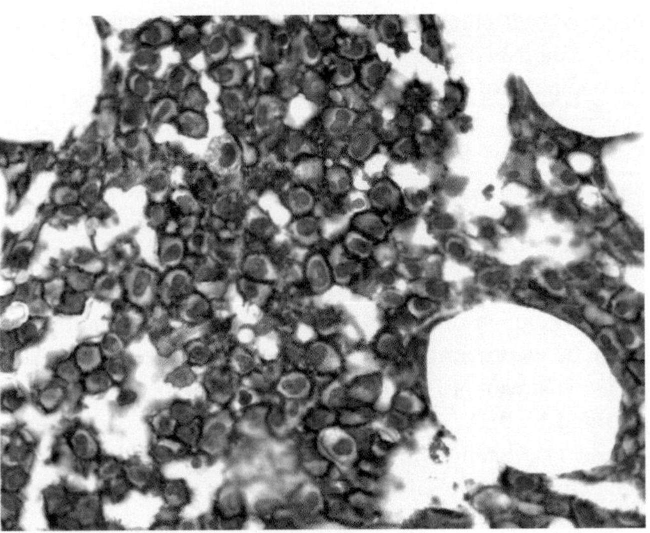

Fig. 10.3 Immunoperoxidase staining with anti-CD20 (B-cell marker), demonstrating strong membrane positivity (×1000). This stain is very useful in evaluating MRD in bone marrow specimens (corresponds to figure bm cd20 1000×)

Spleen and Liver

Splenic sequestration of hematopoietic elements is a characteristic feature of HCL [36]. HCL mostly affects the red pulp. On microscopy, there is a heavy infiltration of monotonous cells in the expanded red pulp, sometimes making the individual cords and sinuses indistinguishable. The white pulp atrophies overtime [36]. Hairy cells replace endothelial cells that line the splenic sinusoids and merge to form congested splenic lakes, often appearing as hemangiomas [20]. Remodeling is thought to occur when hairy cells directly network with endothelial cells via integrin receptors and the vitronectin matrix of the basement membrane [13]. Such splenic findings are striking and can sometimes be seen in the bone marrow.

Similarly in the liver, hairy cells infiltrate the hepatic sinuses and portal tracts but spare the parenchyma. They also form characteristic lesions but appear more as angiomas than pseudosinuses since they lack circumferential ring fibers [20].

Genetic Features

With the use of whole-exome sequencing, Tacci et al. recently detected the BRAF V600E mutation in an entire cohort of 48 HCL patients. The absence of this variant in 195 patients with other peripheral B-cell lymphomas or leukemias established it as a key genetic lesion in HCL [37]. The oncogenicity of this mutation results from constitutive activation of the RAF-MEK-ERK mitogen-activated protein kinase pathway. Subsequent studies have confirmed the presence of the BRAF V600E mutation in HCL, with two exceptions [38, 39]; the molecular variants HCL-variant [38] and HCL with IGHV4–34 immunoglobulin rearrangement [39] lack this mutation. Thus, while distinct in the indolent lymphoproliferative disorders, the BRAF V600E mutation has yet to be incorporated into the diagnostic criteria for HCL.

Downstream of BRAF is MEK1, a dual-specificity kinase encoded by MAP 2 K1 (mitogen-activated protein kinase kinase 1). Mutations of the MAP 2 K1 gene have recently been identified in classical, variant, and IGHV-34-expressing HCL patients and appear to be mutually exclusive of the BRAF V600E mutation [40]. Aside from isolated reports [41, 42], MAP 2 K1 mutations in other hematologic malignancies have not been reported. This seemingly unique mutation makes it an attractive target for therapeutic manipulation and warrants further investigation.

Immunophenotyping: Flow Cytometry

Hairy cells can be identified by multicolor flow cytometry to a high degree of certainty even when they compose less than 1% of circulating lymphocytes [43, 44]. They display a mature B-cell phenotype and express pan B-cell markers including CD19, CD20, CD22, and CD 79A [16]. One or more heavy chains and a single light chain are displayed on the cell surface [45, 46]. Frequently, hairy cells demonstrate the presence of surface IgG, specifically the IgG3 isotype, and do not undergo normal B-cell differentiation with class switching [47]. Three markers of importance in the characterization of HCL include CD11c (common in myelomonocytic cells), CD25 (the IL-2 receptor), and CD103 (the alpha subunit of the alpha-beta integrin in intraepithelial T cells) [48–50]. Though these markers are not limited to HCL and can be seen in other lymphoproliferative disorders, such as splenic marginal zone lymphoma (SMZL), their co-expression is unique. For instance, CD11c is distinguished from other disorders by its nearly 30-fold higher intensity of expression in HCL [47, 49]. Moreover, CD103 has the greatest sensitivity and specificity for HCL [26, 51]. Researchers have evaluated the predictive value of the composite phenotype of these antigens. A scoring system was developed by the Royal Marsden Group using the markers: CD11c, CD25, CD103, and HC2 (HCL-associated antigen involved in cell differentiation). Ninety-eight percent of the evaluated cases of HCL had a score of 3 or 4 [52]. Also of note, primarily due to its potential therapeutic implications, is CD52, a marker that has recently been identified in both variant and classical HCL [53].

Further distinctions between variant and classical HCL can be made via flow cytometry. CD123, which is the alpha chain of the IL-3 receptor, is positive in the majority of classical HCL and dim or negative in variant HCL [54–56]. Additionally, CD25 has been shown to be commonly absent in HCL variant [56].

Immunophenotyping: Immunostains

Monoclonal antibodies with specificity for HCL are useful diagnostic tools. They can be performed easily in peripheral blood and paraffin-embedded tissues, and are thus valuable in the evaluation of minimal residual disease (MRD) in treated patients [16]. In addition to the routine B-cell markers like CD20 and PAX5, specific markers for HCL include TRAP, DBA.44, and cyclin D1 [27, 57, 58]. DBA.44 recognizes an unknown fixation-resistant B-cell antigen that is expressed in mantle zone lymphocytes, reactive immunoblasts, and monocytoid B cells [57]. It reacts strongly with HCL (Fig. 10.4) [59]. Although DBA.44 is expressed in other low-grade B-cell lymphoproliferative disorders, a recent study suggests that the combination of DBA.44/TRAP staining has a 97% specificity for HCL [60]. Moreover, CD20 immunostaining is a useful marker in quantifying disease, as it often highlights HCL infiltrates not detected on routine hematoxylin and eosin staining [61].

Annexin A1 (ANXA1) has been identified as a gene that is upregulated in HCL. One study evaluated samples of 500 B-cell tumors for the anti-ANXA-1 monoclonal antibody and found the assay to be both highly sensitive and specific

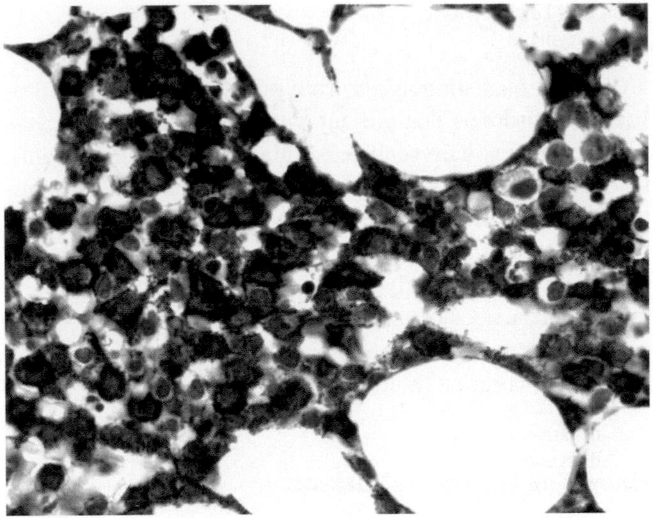

Fig. 10.4 Immunoperoxidase staining with DBA.44. in bone marrow of HCL patient. DBA.44 reacts strongly with HCL. A combination of DBA.44/TRAP staining has a 97% specificity for HCL (corresponds to figure dba-44 1000×)

for HCL (100%) [62]. This precision was not reproduced in a subsequent study, in which only 74% of HCL cases stained positive for ANXA1. Interestingly, none of the HCL variant or BRAF V600E-mutated HCL cases stained for ANXA1 [56].

Clinical Features

General

The onset of HCL may be insidious and its course chronic. It is characterized by pancytopenia and in particular monocytopenia, splenomegaly, and impaired immunity without significant lymphadenopathy [36]. This unique clinical presentation reflects the leukemic infiltration of hairy cells in the bone marrow, spleen, and liver.

In the original description of HCL, fatigue and weakness were the most common symptoms on initial presentation [1]. Also, frequently noted are symptoms of an opportunistic infection and abdominal fullness from splenomegaly. Some patients are incidentally found on physical examination or laboratory workup [5].

On physical examination, splenomegaly is the most prominent finding seen in 80–90% of patients. Spleen size may be variable, but sometimes can be massive [34]. Older studies have suggested that massive splenomegaly, along with patient age and hemoglobin concentration, is associated with a worse prognosis [63]. When present, hepatomegaly usually accompanies splenomegaly, and is seen in 50% of patients [5]. Palpable peripheral lymphadenopathy, unlike other chronic lymphoproliferative disorders, is not common [64]. Internal adenopathy is recognized in one-third of patients with HCL and is thought to be related to disease duration and may correlate with overall survival [64, 65].

Infectious Complications

Infections are a common complication in HCL and a cause of death throughout its course [36, 45]. Among multiple case series, the incidence of serious infections has ranged from 20 to 47%, which includes pneumonia and septicemia [36, 66, 67]. Pyogenic organisms consist of *Pseudomonas aeruginosa*, *Escherichia coli*, and *Enterococcus* species [68]. A higher frequency of intracellular organisms such as *Legionella pneumophila* and *Mycobacterium kansasii* has also been noted and thought to arise from defects in monocytes and decreased dendritic cells [45, 69]. Multiple studies have chronicled neutropenia and monocytopenia as contributing causes of the immunodeficiency in HCL [5]. A study of 73 long-term patients found that baseline lymphopenia may be a prognostic factor of increased risk of infectious complications [67].

Secondary Malignancies

Patients with HCL are at increased risk of secondary malignancies [70–72]. Secondary cancers have been attributed to decreased T-cell function from treatment as well as immunologic aberrations from the underlying disease itself [70, 73, 74]. In their 20-year experience with HCL, Wing et al. noted that 22% of their 117 patients developed second malignancies. Cancer risk peaked at 2 years after the diagnosis of HCL and then steadily declined [73]. The authors in this study conclude that HCL patients may be prone to secondary malignancies from the HCL tumor burden rather than genetic predisposition or the immunosuppressive effects of treatment.

Long-term data suggest that secondary cancers are only moderately increased with exposure to purine nucleoside analogues. In their extended follow-up of HCL patients treated with cladribine at Scripps Clinic, Goodman et al. noted 58 second malignancies in 379 treated patients [75]. A subsequent study at the same institution evaluated 83 patients ≤40 years with HCL treated with cladribine; though the excess frequency of developing a second primary malignancy was 1.60 (95% confidence interval, 0.80–2.89), it was not statistically significant [76]. In a retrospective analysis of 487 patients with HCL treated with purine nucleoside analogs, Cornet et al. reported an increased incidence of second malignancies, especially hematological malignancies (standardized incidence ratio 1.86, CI 1.34–2.51 for all malignancies; 5.32, CI 2.90–8.92 for hematological malignancies) [74]. The National Cancer

Institute (NCI) quantified second cancer incidence and cause-specific mortality among 3104 survivors of HCL between 1973 and 2002. They found that the rate of second cancers was 32% compared to the expected 23% in the general population [70].

Other

Extremely rare manifestations of HCL include cutaneous, bone, serosal, and meningeal involvement [77]. Hypocholesterolemia and elevated liver function tests are disease-related findings in HCL [78, 79]. Polyclonal and monoclonal gammopathies have also been noted in 3–20% of patients and can be associated with plasma cell disorders, lymphoma, or autoimmune processes. Autoimmune-associated disorders include polyarthritis nodosa and leukocytoclastic vasculitis [78, 80].

Differential Diagnosis

HCL must be distinguished from other chronic lymphoproliferative disorders that present with splenomegaly and cytopenias, such as hairy cell leukemia variant (HCL variant), splenic lymphoma with villous lymphocytes, and prolymphocytic leukemia. This distinction is critical since these different disorders have unique management approaches and respond quite differently to treatment with interferon-alpha and purine nucleoside analogues.

The differential diagnosis is based on morphologic and phenotypic criteria (Table 10.1).

Hairy Cell Leukemia Variant

HCL variant is a very rare B-cell lymphoproliferative disorder with features distinct from HCL. Patients with HCL variant

Table 10.1 HCL differential diagnosis

Lymphoid malignancy	Clinical characteristics (age/sex)	Morphology	Peripheral blood count	Immunophenotype	Genetics	Spleen	Survival
HCL	Median age: 50 years	Cytoplasm: Irregular	Neutropenia and lymphopenia	CD11c:+++	BRAF V600E mutation ++/–	Red pulp	87% at 12 years
	Male predominance: 4:1	Nucleus: Reniform	Monocytopenia:+	CD25: ++			
		Nucleolus: Not present		CD 103:+++			
				TRAP: ++			
				CD 123 ++			
				ANXA1 +/–			
HCL-variant	Median age: 80 years	Cytoplasm: Irregular	Lymphocytosis	CD11c:++	BRAF V600E mutation ––/––	Red pulp	Median: 9 years
	Male predominance: <2:1	Nucleus: Round	Monocytopenia:–	CD25: ––/–			
		Nucleolus: Present		CD 103:++			
				TRAP: +/–			
				CD 123 +/––			
				ANXA1 –/–			
SMZL	Median age: 65 year	Cytoplasm: Irregular	Lymphocytosis	CD11c:+		White pulp	80% at 5 years
	No gender predominance	Nucleus: Round	Monocytopenia:–	CD25: +/–			
		Nucleolus: Often present		CD 103:+/–			
				TRAP: +/–			
				CD123 +/–			
				ANXA1 –/–			
CLL	Median age: 70 years	Cytoplasm: Smooth	Lymphocytosis	CD11c:+/–			Median: 3 years
	Male predominance: <2:1	Nucleus: Round	Monocytopenia:–	CD25: –			
		Nucleolus: Present		CD 103: –			
				TRAP: –			

+ present, – absent
HCL hairy cell leukemia, *SMZL* splenic marginal zone lymphoma, *CLL* chronic lymphocytic leukemia

are often diagnosed in their seventh or eighth decades and unlike HCL lack a strong male predominance. They typically present with splenomegaly and high leukocyte counts. Though cytopenias may be noted, neither monocytopenia nor neutropenia is a feature of HCL variant [81, 82]. The bone marrow and splenic histologies are similar to those of HCL [81]. Morphologically, cells of HCL variant are intermediate between HCL and B-cell prolymphocytic leukemia [83]. The cells lack monotony and are more varied in appearance. The nucleus is well circumscribed with a prominent nucleolus similar to that of prolymphocytes, while the cytoplasm is more basophilic [81]. Akin to the morphology, the diagnostic profile for HCL variant can be quite distinct. TRAP staining is variable and often negative. Considering the three markers that are characteristically expressed in HCL, CD11c is strongly positive, CD103 is positive in 60% of cases, and CD25 is negative [83, 84].

Examination of the immunoglobulin heavy-chain (IGH) rearrangements and somatic hypermutation patterns has noted significant differences between HCL and HCL variant. In fact, the mutation status of HCL variant mirrored splenic marginal zone lymphoma (SMZL) more than HCL. Specifically, IGHV4–34 was overrepresented in patients with HCL variant and SMZL [85]. Exploration of IGHV4–34 overexpression has established it as a distinct and separate entity from HVL variant, predicting an even worse prognosis [86, 87].

With an aggressive clinical course and refractoriness to traditional therapy, the median survival of patients with HCL variant is 9 years [84]. In addition, approximately 5–10% of patients have transformation to a large-cell process, characterized by significant leukocytosis, B symptoms, and an overall poor prognosis [88]. Moreover, a Japanese variant of HCL has also been described with large granular lymphocytosis [89].

Splenic Marginal Zone Lymphoma

SMZL is a chronic B-cell lymphoproliferative disorder characterized by splenomegaly and lymphocytosis with more polar villous projections. These cells are smaller than hairy cells and have more condensed chromatin [90]. When the hairy cell scoring system is applied to SMZL, the score is usually low [52]. CD103 is rarely positive in SMZL, and in most studies, CD25 and CD11c were positive in 25–47% of cases [91]. The immunologic profile of SMZL is very similar to that of HCL variant and can present a diagnostic challenge. Histologically, SMZL can be distinguished from HCL and HCL variant by splenic expansion of the white pulp and appearance of nodularity in the bone marrow [26].

SMZL usually has a more indolent clinical course with reported 5-year overall survivals of 80% [90].

B-Cell Prolymphocytic Leukemia

B-cell prolymphocytic leukemia is frequently noted in elderly males with prominent splenomegaly without significant lymphadenopathy [92]. The presenting WBC is elevated and often greater than 100 × 10^9/L with predominant prolymphocytes [93]. Like SMZL, B-cell prolymphocytic leukemia shares many similarities with HCL variant. B-prolymphocytes are larger lymphocytes with a condensed chromatin and a prominent central nucleolus. Immunophenotypically, they are CD25, CD103, and CD11c negative. Overall, they have a poor prognosis and their median survival is 3 years [94].

Treatment

General

Though HCL is an indolent disease, most patients ultimately require treatment [66]. Generally, patients are treated for worsening cytopenias (hemoglobin <10 g/dL, platelet count <100 × 10^9/L, or absolute neutrophil count <1.0 × 10^9/L), infectious complications, and symptomatic splenomegaly. Other less common reasons include bulky lymphadenopathy, progressive visceral or bony disease, or significant autoimmune processes.

Purine Nucleoside Analogues

For many years, splenectomy and interferon-alpha were the standard therapeutic approaches to HCL. The purine nucleoside analogues, cladribine [2-chlorodeoxyadenosine (2-CdA)] and pentostatin (2′-deoxycoformycin), came into clinical use in the mid-1980s and are considered to be the cornerstone of HCL therapy. The discovery that adenosine deaminase (ADA) deficiency produced lymphopenia in children with combined immunodeficiency syndrome led to the development of purine nucleoside analogues [95]. ADA is the major pathway for deoxypurine nucleoside degradation. Resistance to or inhibition of ADA can lead to a buildup of intracellular purine nucleotides which are very toxic to lymphocytes [96–98]. Cladribine (substrate analogue) and pentostatin (direct inhibitor) were developed to oppose the action of ADA.

Cladribine (2-CdA)

Cladribine is commonly chosen as the initial therapy because of its brief treatment administration and high, durable response rates. As a purine nucleoside analogue, it is resistant to ADA. Cladribine accumulates in lymphoid cells because they have high levels of deoxycytidine kinase [98]. This enzyme phosphorylates cladribine, creating a deoxynucleotide which is then incorporated into DNA, thereby inducing DNA strand breaks and inhibiting repair. Cladribine's potency in indolent lymphomas is a function of its cytotoxicity to both dividing and nondividing lymphocytes [99].

Cladribine was first reported to be effective for HCL in 1990. Under the leadership of Ernest Beutler, investigators at Scripps Clinic first reported on 12 HCL patients treated with a single 7-day course of cladribine at 0.1 mg/kg/day by continuous intravenous infusion. Of those 12 patients, 11 achieved a complete response and the responses were maintained for 16 months [100].

The largest single-institution series was at Scripps Clinic and evaluated 349 previously treated and untreated HCL patients [71]. After a median follow-up of 52 months, 91% of patients achieved a complete response and 7% a partial response. Ninety patients (26%) had relapsed at a median of 29 months. The median survival rate at 48 months was 96%. Rosenberg et al. subsequently reported on 83 patients aged 40 years or less [76]. After a median follow-up of 251 months, 88% of patients achieved a complete response and 12% a partial response. Forty-five (54%) of patients who achieved a response ultimately relapsed at a median of 54 months. Median overall survival for all patients following the first cladribine course was 231 months. The authors hypothesized that the variation in survival data may be attributable to the intrinsic biologic differences between young and old HCL patients.

In the 25-year interval since the introduction of cladribine, many studies have acquired long-term patient data (Table 10.2). Among the assessable patients with HCL treated with cladribine as a single 7-day continuous infusion, complete responses have ranged between 76 and 100%. The majority of these patients have enjoyed long-term remissions with relapse rates of 14% at 24 months and 36% at 9.7 years [101, 102]. In one of the longest follow-up studies, 85% of the patients were alive at 20.9 years [76].

Standard cladribine dosing is a 7-day continuous infusion at a dose of 0.1 mg/kg/day. Alternative treatment schemes have been developed in the hopes of ameliorating prolonged myelosuppression and obviating the need for a pump. Alternative schedules have included a 5-day 2-h infusion at a dose of 0.14 mg/kg/day, weekly 2-h intravenous infusion, subcutaneous administration, and oral administration. Several studies have shown that the 2-h 5-day infusion is equally efficacious with a similar toxicity profile [111]. Robak et al. conducted a prospective study of 132 patients, comparing cladribine administered in a weekly versus daily schedule. Patients were randomized to receive either cladribine 0.12 mg/kg as a 2-h intravenous infusion daily for 5 days or 0.12 mg/kg in a 2-h intravenous infusion once a week for 6 weeks. Results of the trial showed similar complete remission rates, progression-free survival, and overall survival between the two groups. Despite prior reports showing improvement in infectious complications with the weekly dosing, there was no significant difference in grade 3 or 4 infections [112]. Similar results were noted in a Swiss study that compared subcutaneous daily 2-CdA with weekly treatment [113]. Though treatments with these alternative schedules appear promising, they lack the support of long-term follow-up, and the 7-day continuous infusion and 2-h 5-day infusion of cladribine are both considered standard.

Neutropenic fever is the principal acute toxicity of cladribine therapy in HCL, occurring in 42% of treated patients [71]. Infectious complications include bacterial and opportunistic infections. Immunosuppressive effects of

Table 10.2 Long-term follow-up studies with cladribine

Study	Patients (no.)	Median F/U (years)	Initial complete remission rate (%)	Relapse rate (%)	Median time to relapse (months)	Overall survival
Seymour et al. [103]	46	2.5	78	20	16	NA
Hoffman et al. [104]	49	4.6	76	20	NA	95% at 4.6 years
Goodman et al. [75]	209	7	95	37	42	97% at 9 years
Jehn et al. [105]	44	8.5	98	39	48	79% at 12 years
Chadha et al. [106]	86	9.7	79	36	35	87% at 12 years
Else et al. [101]	45	16	76	38	NA	100% at 15 years
Rosenberg et al. [76]	83	20.9	88	54	54	85% at 20.9 years
Lopez et al. [107]	80	5.2	88*	25	NA	NA
Cornet et al. [74]	281	4.4	83	18	NA	NA
Hacioglu et al. [108]	78	2.3	81	17	24	96% at 2.1 years
Somasundaram et al. [109]	27	2.2	100	18	48	96% at 2.2 years
Ruiz-Delgado et al. [110]	11	2.1	100	27	NA	91% at 11 years

NA data not available
aafter a second course of cladribine in some patients

cladribine can persist for extended periods with decreases in CD4+ lymphocytes [103]. Herpes zoster is the most frequently reported late infection [75]. Granulocyte colony-stimulating factor (G-CSF) was evaluated in patients treated with cladribine therapy. Although G-CSF ameliorated neutropenia, it did not improve rates of neutropenic fever or hospital admissions for antibiotics and is thus not routinely recommended [114].

Pentostatin (2′-Deoxycoformycin)

Pentostatin is a natural product that is derived from *Streptomyces antibioticus*. Unlike cladribine, it irreversibly inhibits ADA and leads to the accumulation of cytotoxic metabolites. Pentostatin was first described to be an effective agent against HCL in the mid-1980s [115].

One of the largest studies evaluating its efficacy randomized 313 patients to pentostatin or interferon-alpha-2a for 6–12 months. This study used a crossover design where patients in the interferon arm could cross over to pentostatin upon progression. In the initial results, 76% of pentostatin patients achieved a complete remission compared to only 11% treated with interferon-alpha. In patients who crossed over from initial interferon to pentostatin, the complete response rate was 66% [63]. This study underscores the benefits of pentostatin both in treated and untreated patients. Flinn et al. reported on the long-term data from this trial with a median follow-up duration of 9.3 years. The relapse rate was 18% and included both patients initially treated with pentostatin and those who crossed over from the interferon arm. The estimated 5- and 10-year relapse-free survival rates were 85% and 67%, respectively. The 5-year survival was 81%. Acknowledging that this was a crossover design, the survival outcomes were similar between the two groups [116]. The findings in this study have mirrored other long-term follow-up trials with pentostatin (Table 10.3).

Currently, pentostatin is given every 2 weeks usually at a dose of 4 mg/m^2 for 3–6 months until maximum response is achieved. Previous experience with high-dose pentostatin (twice the standard dose) was associated with serious infectious complications [118]. With this interrupted dosing schedule, febrile neutropenia is significantly reduced, especially in comparison to cladribine [63, 71]. Other common side effects of pentostatin include nausea, vomiting, photosensitivity, and keratoconjunctivitis [119].

Cladribine and pentostatin have amassed significant long-term data with many years of follow-up. Else et al. reported on outcomes of 233 patients with a median follow-up of 16 years. In this retrospective review, treatment with single cycle of cladribine or multiple cycles of pentostatin showed equal efficacy: complete remissions (76% vs. 82%) and overall survival (100% vs. 95%) [101]. Lopez et al. described a median treatment-free interval of 95 months with first-line pentostatin and 144 months with first-line cladribine; the difference was not statistically different (p = 0.476) [107]. Despite similar effectiveness, a single course of cladribine is generally considered the preferred first-line treatment because of its brief treatment duration and paucity of adverse effects.

Other Treatments

Splenectomy

Historically, splenectomy was the first effective therapy for HCL. Splenectomy did not affect bone marrow infiltration, but did remove a major site of hairy cell proliferation and alleviated the symptoms of hypersplenism [120]. Most studies noted 60–80% improvement of blood counts with rapid improvements in thrombocytopenia [121, 122]. These responses were not consistent. The degree of splenomegaly was not predictive of hematological improvement or duration of response [123] and most patients ultimately relapsed. The median time to failure with splenectomy was variable, ranging from 5.4 to 56.5 months [124]. No randomized trial has shown a survival benefit with splenectomy [121, 125]. The present indications for splenectomy are active and uncontrolled infection, the resolution of which can be rapid and reflects the improvement of peripheral blood counts. Splenectomy is used in the rare event of a splenic rupture and is beneficial in patients with splenomegaly and severe

Table 10.3 Long-term follow-up studies with pentostatin

Study	Patients (no.)	Patients (no.) with prior therapy	Median F/U (years)	Initial complete remission rate (%)	Relapse rate (%)	Overall survival
Cassileth et al. [117]	50	31	3.25	64	20	NA
Malosiel et al. [65]	238	154	5.3	79	15	89% at 5 years
Flinn et al. [116]	241	87	9.3	71	18	81% at 10 years
Else et al. [101]	188	108	16	82	44	95% at 15 years
Lopez et al. [107]	27	0	12.1	92	51	NA
Cornet [74]	99	0	4.8	82	23	NA

NA data not available

thrombocytopenia who are bleeding. Splenectomy can also be considered in the refractory setting as well as in the second trimester of pregnancy [121, 126].

Interferon

Interferon-alpha is an active agent in HCL and had a significant impact on treatment prior to purine nucleoside analogues. The exact mechanism of action is unknown, but it is thought that interferon-alpha acts as a cytostatic agent in HCL, inducing hairy cell differentiation and making these cells less responsive to growth stimuli [127].

In 1984, Quesada and colleagues first reported the successful use of partially purified alpha human interferon in seven patients with HCL. All seven had normalization of their blood counts with the responses maintained for 6–10 months [128]. Two recombinant interferon-alpha drugs were subsequently developed and approved by the FDA: interferon-alpha-2a and interferon-alpha-2b. Differing by only an amino acid, the recombinant forms showed equal efficacy [129].

Quesada's landmark trial has paved the way to many national and international trials. Treatment with interferon-alpha results mostly in partial remissions ranging from 69 to 87%. Few complete responses are noted and the duration of response is 18–25 months [129–131]. Long-term studies have reported improved survivals of 85–90% at 5 years [132, 133]. Interferon-alpha has activity even in previously treated patients and response rates are robust in patients with splenomegaly [131, 134]. The standard treatment for interferon-alpha-2b is 2×10^6 U/m^2 subcutaneously three times per week for 6–12 months and for interferon-alpha-2a is 3×10^6 U/m^2 three times per week for 12 months. The most common side effects of interferon-alpha are a flu-like syndrome consisting of fever, myalgias, and malaise. Rarely, central and peripheral nervous system complaints have been documented [128, 129].

Although interferon-alpha is an active agent in HCL, it does not induce the same complete responses seen with purine nucleoside analogues and thus is no longer utilized as initial therapy. Treatment with interferon-alpha should be reserved for patients with active infection who cannot receive a purine nucleoside analogue because of its associated immunosuppression.

Evaluation and Follow-Up of Treatment

Patients with HCL should be followed closely for months after treatment to evaluate for cytopenias, possible infectious complications, and ultimately treatment responses [113]. Recovery of blood counts may take weeks to several months following treatment with purine nucleoside analogues. In one study, the median recovery time to normalization of peripheral blood counts after the first cladribine course was 49 days (range 9–379 days) [71]. In addition to evaluating bone marrows for treatment response, translational studies have shown that soluble serum IL-2 secreted by hairy cells correlates closely with disease course and can be used as a noninvasive parameter for disease response [135]. Resolution of hepatosplenomegaly, adenopathy, cytopenias, and eradication of hairy cells from the peripheral blood and bone marrow by non-immunologic studies currently constitutes a complete response [136].

Despite robust responses to treatment with purine nucleoside analogues, long-term studies continue to show late relapses [76, 101]. With this in mind, researchers turned their attention to evaluating minimal residual disease (MRD) in posttreatment bone marrows, in the hopes of more completely eradicating hairy cell infiltrates. MRD can be identified by several techniques: immunohistochemistry using CD20, DBA.44, and CD45RO immunostains; immunophenotyping by flow cytometry; or polymerase chain reaction (PCR) [137–139]. Immunohistochemistry was initially thought to be more sensitive for detecting MRD [43]; however, upon direct comparison, PCR was found to be the most sensitive and specific test [138]. With increased diagnostic sensitivity, these studies have identified residual disease in 10–50% of patients previously thought to be in a complete remission [137, 140] (Table 10.4). This MRD usually represents <1% of the total cell population [137, 141].

Using a strategy of initial cladribine therapy followed by rituximab, researchers have shown that they can successfully eradicate MRD [144, 145]; however, it is not clear if this preemptive treatment strategy translates into improved clinical outcomes. Studies evaluating this question have shown mixed results. Sigal et al. reported on 19 patients who were

Table 10.4 Evaluation of minimal residual disease (MRD)

Study	Method of evaluation	Treatment	Patient (no.)	MRD (%)
Ellison et al. [137]	IHC with anti-CD20 and DBA.44	Cladribine	154	50
Hakimian et al. [140]	IHC with anti-CD20, anti-MB2, anti-UCHL-1	Cladribine	34	21
Wheaton et al. [141]	IHC with anti-CD20 DBA.44, anti-CD45RO	Cladribine	39	13
Matutes et al. [142]	IHC with anti-CD11c, anti-CD25, anti-CD103, and anti-HC2	Pentostatin	31	43
Filleul et al. [143]	PCR, IGH genes	Cladribine	10	100

in complete hematologic remission following initial treatment with cladribine with a median follow-up of 16 years [146]. Using flow cytometry and immunohistochemical staining (CD20, DBA.44, TRAP, and annexin positive), these investigators were able to determine that 47% of patients had no MRD. They also found that in patients with MRD or even gross bone marrow involvement, normal blood counts are possible. The study concluded that HCL is potentially curable and that patients with MRD can have long periods of complete remission [146]. More recently, Lopez et al. reported on a group of 82 patients initially treated with purine analogs and found a shorter treatment-free interval in patients with MRD compared to those without MRD (97 months vs. not reached, $p < 0.049$) [107]. Long-term follow-up with greater number of patients will be needed to fully appreciate the clinical significance of MRD.

Treatment for Relapsed and Resistant Disease

Purine nucleoside analogues elicit noteworthy responses in HCL. Despite this, there are a minority of patients who are refractory to treatment, and their prognosis is inferior. Researchers in Italy investigated biologic parameters in patients who did not respond to cladribine therapy. They found that the unmutated status of IGH variable region paralleled treatment failure and rapid progression of disease. Moreover, they identified defects in TP53 gene as a possible mechanism for resistance. These authors suggested that in such patients, a rituximab-based regimen may be more appropriate [147].

In addition to patients who are resistant to purine nucleoside therapy, long-term follow-up studies suggest that 20–40% of patients who initially had a response will eventually relapse. These patients have several options for therapy when treatment is indicated.

Re-treatment with Purine Nucleoside Analogue

Multiple studies have shown good efficacy when patients are re-treated with purine nucleosides. In the Scripps Clinic series, 62% of patients treated with a second course of cladribine on first relapse achieved a complete remission [71]. Similarly, in the Northwestern experience 83% of relapsed patients responded to a second cycle of cladribine therapy [106]. Even though cladribine and pentostatin have similar chemical structures, there is little clinical cross-resistance between the two drugs [148]. Else et al. showed that relapsed patients had a high rate of remission when treated with the other purine nucleoside analogue. On multivariate analysis, a shorter median duration of first remission was the only variable associated with a failure to attain a complete response [101]. Other studies have noted responses with purine nucleosides in the third- and fourth-line setting, but responses decline with each successive course [149]. No randomized trial exists to determine the optimal duration before re-treatment. Balancing efficacy with immunosuppressive effects of therapy, most experts recommend a 1-year interval before reconsidering purine nucleoside therapy [113].

Immunoconjugates and Targeted Therapies

Rituximab

Because hairy cells express CD20 brightly, rituximab, a chimeric monoclonal antibody against CD20, has become an important agent in salvage therapy. Hagberg first described rituximab as an effective therapy in a patient relapsing from HCL in 1999 [150]. Since then, multiple studies with rituximab have been conducted. Use of single-agent rituximab in the relapsed setting have shown response rates ranging from 25 to 80%, with complete response rates as high at 53% [151, 152]. Given these robust response rates, attention then turned to combination regimens with purine nucleoside analogs. Else and colleagues recently updated their results from a series of 26 patients treated with rituximab and either pentostatin ($n = 15$) or cladribine ($n = 11$) following purine analog treatment failure. Rituximab was administered at a dose of 375 mg/m^2 for 4–8 intravenous infusions (median 6.5). Twenty patients received rituximab concurrently and the remainder received sequential therapy. The overall response rate was 96%, and the complete response rate was 88%. At a median follow-up of 78 months, relapse-free survival following combination therapy was markedly improved compared to the RFS of the same patients following their prior first-line treatment (hazard ratio: 0.10; 95% CI: 0.03–0.32; log-rank $p < 0.0001$). Relapse-free survival at 10 years was 87% (95% CI: 75–100%) following combination therapy, versus 12% (95% CI: 0–24%) following the patient's same first-line treatment [153]. The authors did note certain discrepancies: some patients may have had a heavier baseline disease burden at the time of initial therapy compared to relapse, and 8 of the 26 patients received purine analog in combination therapy that they had not been previously exposed to. Though additional studies of rituximab combination therapy with purine analogs have also shown high response rates for classical [154–156] and variant HCL [157], true randomized trials are lacking.

BRAF Inhibitors

Building on the Italian group's discovery of the BRAF V600E mutation in a very high percentage of classical HCL patients, studies exploring the role of BRAF inhibitors have

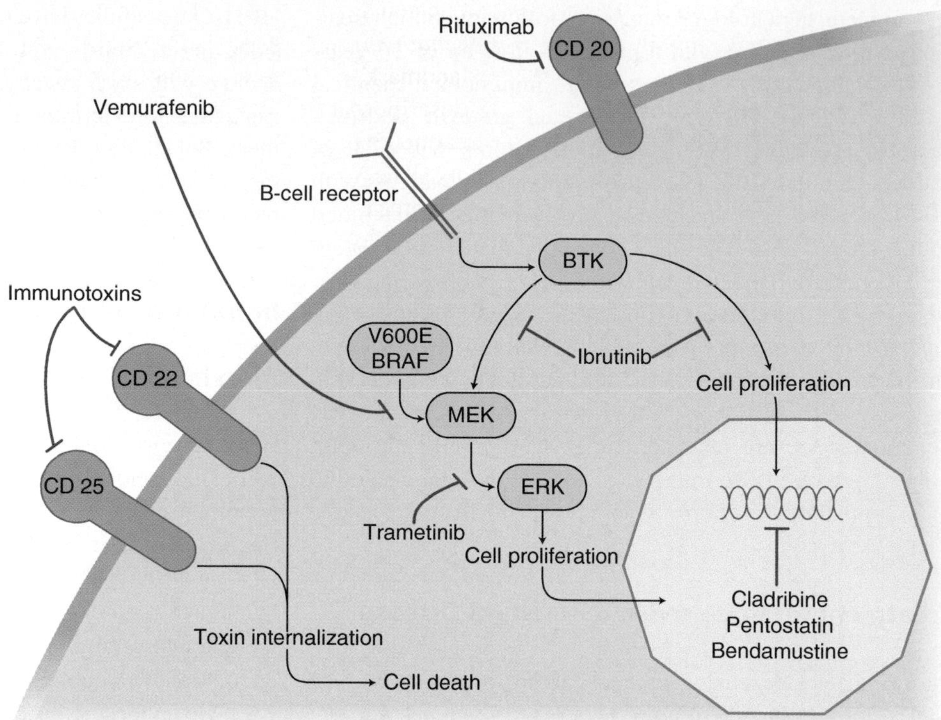

Fig. 10.5 Hairy Cell leukemia therapeutic pathways. *MEK* indicates mitogen-activated protein kinase, *ERK* extracellular signal-regulated kinase, *BTK* Bruton's tyrosine kinase

yielded encouraging results. Early case reports revealed rapid responses, including complete responses, in multiply treated relapsed and refractory classical HCL patients treated with the oral BRAF inhibitor, vemurafenib [158–161] (Fig. 10.5). More recently, results from two phase 2, single-group, multicenter studies of vemurafenib at a dose of 960 mg twice daily were published [162]. The studies were conducted in Italy and the United States. In the Italian study, treatment was administered for a minimum of 8 weeks and, if patients did not have a complete response, for a maximum of 16 weeks. At a median follow-up of 23 months, relapse-free survival was 19 months among patients with a CR. In the US study, patients received treatment on a continuous schedule for 12 weeks; however, patients with residual disease were allowed to receive vemurafenib for up to 12 additional weeks. Median treatment duration was 18 weeks and resulted in an overall survival rate of 91% after a median follow-up of 12 weeks. Therapy was generally well tolerated; drug-related adverse events were mostly grade 1 or 2. Toxicities included rash, arthralgias, and arthritis, among others. However, despite the high response rates, MRD was noted in all patients with complete responses at the end of treatment. In both trials, re-treatment with vemurafenib at relapse elicited some responses.

In the Italian study, bone marrow specimens from 13 of 26 patients were evaluated for phosphorylated ERK and PAX5 double immunostaining. Residual hairy cells expressing ERK were seen in 6 of the 13 patients. All 6 of these patients had a partial response to vemurafenib. Conversely, two patients with complete responses did not express phosphorylated ERK. Post hoc analysis revealed a prolonged median progression-free survival for patients with phosphorylated ERK compared to those lacking this (8 months vs. 13 months, respectively). In addition, residual disease (assessed by the Hairy Cell Index) was greater in patients with persistent phosphorylated ERK than those without measurable ERK. These investigators proposed that circumvention of BRAF inhibition may be explained by alternative mechanisms for reactivating MEK and ERK. The persistence of HCL cells and potential identification of resistance mechanisms indicate the need for additional therapy to improve response rates. One potential method may be to combine a BRAF inhibitor with another drug that targets the pathway, like an MEK inhibitor, as has been done in melanoma patients [163].

MEK Inhibition

The activity of the MEK inhibitor, trametinib, was recently supported by both in vivo and in vitro studies [164]. Pettirossi et al. isolated HCL cells from 26 patients and exposed them in vitro to active BRAF inhibitors (vemurafenib or dabrafenib) or trametinib. The in vitro results were subsequently validated in vivo in the phase 2 study of refractory and relapsed HCL patients treated with oral vemurafenib as detailed above. Vemurafenib, dabrafenib, and trametinib incubation resulted in dose-dependent MEK and ERK dephosphorylation as well as considerable loss of the hairy morphology. Moreover, the ERK dephosphorylation and apoptosis appeared to be potentiated by the combination of BRAF and MEK blockade with dabrafenib and trametinib. These findings highlight feasible approaches for new treatment options and warrant investigation.

Recombinant Immunotoxins (CD22, CD25)

Recombinant immunotoxins are antibody-toxin chimeric proteins. By engineering the antibody moiety to target antigens expressed preferentially in HCL cells, the toxin moiety is able to exert lethal effects selectively. Recombinant immunotoxin research in HCL has focused on CD25 and CD22.

Kreitman et al. have extensively reported on the efficacy of BL22, a recombinant immunotoxin comprised of a pseudomonas exotoxin fused to a single-chain variable fragment of anti-CD22 [165–168]. Initial results revealed complete remissions in patients with HCL resistant to purine analog therapy [165]. Phase 2 testing of 36 patients with relapsed and refractory HCL, including three patients with variant HCL, was completed [167]. In this study, the complete response rate was 25% after one cycle. Twenty patients were then re-treated, and 47% achieved a complete response. Interestingly, response rates were higher in non-splenectomized patients without massive splenomegaly. Two patients experienced reversible grade 3 hemolytic uremic syndrome, which did not require plasmapheresis. Subsequently, moxetumomab pasudotox, a new recombinant immunotoxin with a 14-fold increased binding affinity for CD22, was developed. Phase 1 testing results are encouraging; the overall response rate was 86% and complete remissions were seen in 46% (13 patients). At 26 months, the median disease-free survival had not been reached. No dose-limiting toxicities were observed [169].

LMB-2 is a recombinant immunotoxin formed from the fusion of a CD25 antibody to the PE38 toxin. Phase 1 testing of this agent in 35 patients with chemotherapy-refractory CD25-expressing hematologic malignancies revealed measurable responses [170]. The most dramatic activity was seen in the HCL cohort. In this group of four patients, one had a complete response, two had partial responses, and the remaining patient had stable disease. Dose-limiting toxicities included reversible cardiomyopathy and transaminitis.

Alemtuzumab

Though it has not been extensively studied, there have been case reports suggesting the activity of alemtuzumab, a humanized monoclonal antibody against CD52, in HCL [171, 172]. Sasaki et al. treated a patient with variant HCL with splenic irradiation followed by alemtuzumab [171]. Splenomegaly resolved, and leukemic cells were eliminated from the peripheral blood by day 12. These reports warrant further investigation into the role of CD52 targeting in the treatment of HCL.

Bendamustine

Bendamustine is a chemotherapeutic agent with features of both alkylators and purine analogs. Following its initial report [173], bendamustine was further studied in relapsed and refractory HCL patients [174]. The results were encouraging; the overall response rate was 100%. At a dose of 90 mg/m^2 on days 1 and 2, for 6 cycles at 4-week intervals, 67% achieved CR, 100% of which were without MRD. At a median follow-up of 31 months, all complete responders with absent MRD remained in CR. Phase 2 trials are currently under way [175].

Ibrutinib

Ibrutinib, a selective and irreversible inhibitor of Bruton's tyrosine kinase (BTK), has activity in multiple low-grade lymphoproliferative disorders including chronic lymphocytic leukemia, mantle cell lymphoma, and Waldenstrom's macroglobulinemia. Recently, Sivina et al. reported their findings showing that BTK protein is expressed in HCL cells, and ibrutinib significantly inhibited HCL cell proliferation, cycling, and survival [176]. Preliminary safety and efficacy data was recently presented [177], and a phase 2 clinical trial is currently under way [178].

Conclusion

Since its initial description more than 50 years ago, the natural history of HCL has been dramatically altered. In the era of Bouroncle, treatment options were few, including splenectomy, and the median survival was only 4 years. Now with purine nucleoside therapies, many patients enjoy long-term remissions frequently surpassing 10 years with good quality of life. The final chapter in this remarkable tale, however, has not been written. Despite excellent responses to the purine nucleoside analogues, cladribine and pentostatin, a small minority of patients will not respond and a proportion who do will eventually relapse. Though these patients respond upon re-treatment, the responses are less rigorous and there is a concern that further therapy will cause long-term immunosuppression. Moreover, disease-free survival curves have failed to show a plateau after 10 years [149]. A few long-term studies, however, have suggested that some patients may be cured. Focusing attention on identifying refractory patients with HCL through biologic parameters and employing treatment strategies with targeted agents, monoclonal antibodies, and recombinant immunotoxins are currently under investigation. Introduction of BRAF targeting agents represents a major therapeutic advance and addition to the therapeutic armamentarium for patients with refractory or relapsed disease. More research is still needed in understanding the fundamental biology of this disease. Filling in the gaps in our knowledge of the pathophysiology will aid in the development of better treatments with the prospect of more patients enjoying long-term disease-free survival and perhaps even a curative strategy. Also, delving into the biology of HCL will provide insights and potential treatment directions for more common indolent lymphoproliferative diseases.

References

1. Bouroncle BA, Wiseman BK, Doan CA. Leukemic reticuloendotheliosis. Blood. 1958;13:609–30.
2. Schreck R, Donnelly WJ. Hairy cells in blood in lymphoreticular neoplastic disease and flagellated cells of normal lymph nodes. Blood. 1966;27:199–211.
3. Anderson KC, Boyd AW, Fisher DC, et al. Hairy cell leukemia: a tumor of pre-plasma cells. Blood. 1986;65:620–9.
4. Basso K, Liso A, Tiacci E, et al. Gene expression profiling of hairy cell leukemia reveals a phenotype related to memory B cells with altered expression of chemokine and adhesion receptors. J Exp Med. 2003;199:59–68.
5. Flandrin G, Sigaux F, Sebahoun G, et al. Hairy cell leukemia: clinical presentation and follow-up of 211 patients. Semin Oncol. 1984;11:458–71.
6. Dores GM, Matsuno RK, Weisenburger DD, et al. Hairy cell leukaemia: a heterogeneous disease. Br J Haematol. 2008;142:45–51.
7. Oleske D, Golomb HM, Farber MD, et al. A case control inquiry into the etiology of hairy cell leukemia. Am J Epidemiol. 1985;121:675–83.
8. Orsi L, Delabre L, Monnereau A, et al. Occupational exposure to pesticides and lymphoid neoplasms among men: results of a French case-control study. Occup Environ Med. 2009;66:291–8.
9. Wolf BC, Martin AW, Neiman RS. The detection of Epstein-Barr virus in hairy cell leukemia cells by in situ hybridization. Am J Pathol. 1990;136:717–23.
10. Wachsman W, Golde DW, Chen IS. Hairy cell leukemia and human T cell leukemia virus. Semin Oncol. 1984;11:446–50.
11. Makower D, Marino P, Frank M, et al. Familial hairy cell leukemia. Leuk Lymphoma. 1998;29:193–7.
12. Colovic MD, Jankovic GM, Wiernik PH. Hairy cell leukemia in first cousins and review of the literature. Eur J Haematol. 2001;67:185–8.
13. Cawley JC. The pathophysiology of the hairy cell. Hematol Oncol Clin North Am. 2006;20:1011–21.
14. Capello D, Vitolo U, Pasqualucci L, et al. Distribution and pattern of BCL-6 mutations throughout the spectrum of B-cell neoplasms. Blood. 2000;95:651–9.
15. Forconi F, Sahota S, Raspadori D, et al. Tumor cells of hairy cell leukemia expresses multiple clonally related immunoglobulin isotypes via RNA splicing. Blood. 2001;98:1174–81.
16. Matutes E. Immunophenotyping and differential diagnosis of hairy cell leukemia. Hematol Oncol Clin North Am. 2006;20:1051–63.
17. Burthem J, Cawley JC. The bone marrow fibrosis of hairy-cell leukemia is caused by the synthesis and assembly of a fibronectin matrix by the hairy cells. Blood. 1994;83:497–504.
18. Burthem J, Baker PK, Hunt JA, et al. Hairy cell interactions with extracellular matrix:expression of specific integrin receptors and their role in the cell's response to specific adhesive proteins. Blood. 1994;84:873–82.
19. Aziz KA, Till KJ, Zuzel M, et al. Involvement of CD 44-hyaluronan interaction in malignant cell homing and fibronectin synthesis in hairy cell leukemia. Blood. 2000;96:3161–7.
20. Nanba K, Soban E, Bowling M. Splenic pseudosinuses and hepatic angiomatous lesions. Am J Clin Pathol. 1977;67:415–26.
21. Haglund U, Juliusson G, Birgitta S, et al. Hairy cell leukemia is characterized by clonal chromosome abnormalities clustered to specific regions. Blood. 1994;83:2637–45.
22. Sambani C, Trafalis DT, Mitsoulis-Mentzikoff C, et al. Clonal chromosome rearrangements in hairy cell leukemia: personal experience and review of literature. Cancer Genet Cytogenet. 2001;129:138–44.
23. Anderson CL, Gruszka-Westwood A, Ostergaard M, et al. A marrow deletion of 7q is common to HCL and SMZL, but not CLL. Eur J Haematol. 2004;72:390–402.
24. Vallianatou K, Brito-Babapulle V, Matutes E, et al. P53 gene deletion and trisomy 12 in hairy cell leukemia and its variant. Leuk Res. 1999;23:1041–5.
25. Burke JS. The value of the bone marrow biopsy in the diagnosis of hairy cell leukemia. Am J Clin Pathol. 1978;70:876–84.
26. Sharpe RW, Bethel KJ. Hairy cell leukemia: diagnostic pathology. Hematol Oncol Clin North Am. 1996;20:1023–49.
27. Zuzel M, Cawley JC. The biology of hairy cells. Best Pract Res Clin Haematol. 2003;16:1–13.
28. Cawley JC. What is the nature of the hairy cell and why should we be interested? Br J Haematol. 1997;97:511–4.
29. Rosner MC, Golomb HM. Ribosome-lamella complex in hairy cell leukemia: ultrastructure and distribution. Lab Investig. 1980;42:236–47.
30. Brunning RD, Parkin J. Ribosome-lamella complexes in neoplastic hematopoietic cells. Am J Pathol. 1975;79:565–78.
31. Katayama I, Li Y, Tam LT. Ultrastructural characteristics of the "hairy cells" of leukemic reticuloendotheliosis. Am J Pathol. 1972;67:361–70.
32. Yam LT, Li CY, Lam KW. Tartrate-resistant acid phosphatase isoenzyme in the reticulum cells of leukemic reticuloendotheliosis. N Engl J Med. 1971;284:357–60.
33. Li CY, Yam LT, Lam KW. Studies of acid phosphatase isoenzymes in human leukocytes demonstration of isoenzyme cell specificity. J Histochem Cytochem. 1970;19:901–10.
34. Bartl R, Frisch B, Hill W, et al. Bone marrow histology in hairy cell leukemia. Identification of subtype and their prognosis. Am J Clin Pathol. 1983;79:531–45.
35. Krause JR. Aplastic anemia terminating in hairy cell leukemia. A report of two cases. Cancer. 1984;53:1533–7.
36. Turner A, Kjeldsberg CR. Hairy cell leukemia: a review. Medicine. 1978;57:477–99.
37. Tiacci E, Trionov V, Shiavoni G, et al. BRAF mutations in hairy-cell leukemia. N Engl J Med. 2011;364:2305–15.
38. Jain P, Ok CY, Konoplev S, et al. Relapsed refractory BRAF-negative, IGHV4-34-positive variant of hairy cell leukemia: a distinct entity? J Clin Oncol. 2016;34(7):e57–60.
39. Xi L, Arons E, Navarro W, et al. Both variant and IGHV4-34-expressing hairy cell leukemia lack the BRAF V600E mutation. Blood. 2012;119:3330.
40. Waterfall JJ, Arons E, Walker RL, et al. High prevalence of MAP 2K1 mutations in variant and IGHV4-34-expressing hairy-cell leukemias. Nat Genet. 2014;46:8.

41. Rossi D, et al. The coding genome of splenic marginal zone lymphoma: activation of NOTCH2 and other pathways regulating marginal zone development. J Exp Med. 2012;209:1537–51.
42. Brown NA, Furtado LV, Betz BL, et al. High prevalence of somatic MAP 2K1 mutations in BRAF V600E-negative Langerhans cell histiocytosis. Blood. 2014;124(10):1655–8.
43. Sausville JE, Salloum RG, Sorbara L, et al. Minimal residual disease detection in hairy cell leukemia. Comparison of flow cytometric immunophenotyping with clonal analysis using consensus primer polymerase chain reaction for the heavy chain gene. Am J Clin Pathol. 2003;119:213–7.
44. Robbins BA, Ellison DJ, Spinosa JC, et al. Diagnostic application of two-color flow cytometry in 161 cases of hairy cell leukemia. Blood. 1993;82:1277–87.
45. Golomb HM, Hadad LJ. Infectious complications in 127 patients with hairy cell leukemia. Am J Hematol. 1984;16:393–401.
46. Burns GF, Cawley JC, Karpas WA, et al. Multiple heavy chain isotypes on the surface of the cells of hairy cell leukemia. Blood. 1978;52:1132–47.
47. Kluin-Nelemans HC, Krouwels MM, Jansen JH, et al. Hairy cell leukemia preferentially expresses the IgG3-subclass. Blood. 1990;75:972–5.
48. Hanson CA, Gribbon TE, Schnitzer B, et al. CD11c (LEU-M5) expression characterizes a B-cell chronic lymphoproliferative disorder with features of both chronic lymphocytic leukemia and hairy cell leukemia. Blood. 1990;76:2360–7.
49. Visser L, Shaw A, Slupsky J, et al. Monoclonal antibodies reactive with hairy cell leukemia. Blood. 1989;74:320–5.
50. Flenghi L, Spinozzi F, Stein H, et al. LF61: a new monoclonal antibody directed against a trimeric molecule (150 kDa, 125 kDa, 105 kDa) associated with hairy cell leukemia. Br J Haematol. 1990;76:451–9.
51. Dong HY, Weisberger J, Liu Z, et al. Immunophenotypic analysis of CD103+ B-lymphoproliferative disorders: hairy cell leukemia and its mimics. Am J Clin Pathol. 2009;131:586–95.
52. Matutes E, Morilla R, Owusu-Ankomah K, et al. The immunophenotype of hairy cell leukemia (HCL). Proposal for a scoring system to distinguish HCL from B-cell disorders with hairy or villous lymphocytes. Leuk Lymphoma. 1994, 14(Suppl 1):57–61.
53. Quigley MM, Bethel KJ, Sharpe RW, et al. CD52 expression in hairy cell leukemia. Am J Hematol. 2003;74(4):227–30.
54. Del Giudice I, Matutes E, Morilla R, et al. The diagnostic value of CD 123 in B cell disorders with hairy or villous lymphocytes. Haematologica. 2004;89:303–8.
55. Munoz L, Nomededeu JF, Lopez O, et al. Interleukin-3 receptor alpha chain (CD 123) is widely expressed in hematologic malignancies. Haematologica. 2001;86:1261–9.
56. Shao H, Calvo KR, Grönborg M, et al. Distinguishing hairy cell leukemia variant from hairy cell leukemia: development and validation of diagnostic criteria. Leuk Res. 2013;37:401.
57. Hounieu H, Chittal SM, Saati TA, et al. Hairy cell leukemia. Diagnosis of bone marrow involvement in paraffin-embedded sections with monoclonal antibody DBA.44. Am J Clin Pathol. 1992;98:26–33.
58. Janckila AJ, Cardwell EM, Yam LT, et al. Hairy cell identification by immunohistochemistry of tartrate-resistant acid phosphatase. Blood. 1995;85:2939–44.
59. Saati TA, Caspar S, Brousset P, et al. Production of anti-B monoclonal antibodies (DBB.44, DBA.44, DNA.7, and DND.53) reactive on paraffin-embedded tissues with a new B-lymphoma cell line grafted into athymic nude mice. Blood. 1989;74:2476–85.
60. Went PT, Zimpfer A, Pehrs AC, et al. High specificity of combined TRAP and DBA.44 expression for hairy cell leukemia. Am J Surg Pathol. 2005;29:474–8.
61. Lauria F, Raspadori L, Benfenati D, et al. Biological markers and minimal residual disease in hairy cell leukemia. Leukemia. 1992;6(Suppl 4):149–51.
62. Falini B, Tiacci E, Liso A, et al. Simple diagnostic assay for hairy cell leukemia by immunocytochemical detection of annexin a (ANXA 1). Lancet. 2004;363:1869–70.
63. Grever M, Kopecky K, Foucar MK, et al. Randomized comparison of pentostatin versus interferon alfa-2a in previously untreated patients with hairy cell leukemia: an intergroup study. J Clin Oncol. 1995;13:974–82.
64. Hakimian D, Tallman MS, Hogan DK, et al. Prospective evaluation of internal adenopathy in a cohort of 43 patients with hairy cell leukemia. J Clin Oncol. 1994;12:268–72.
65. Maloisel F, Benboubker L, Gardembas M, et al. Long-term outcome with pentostatin treatment in hairy cell leukemia patients. A French retrospective study of 238 patients. Leukemia. 2003;17:45–51.
66. Golomb HM, Catovsky D, Golde DW. Hairy cell leukemia: a clinical review based on 71 cases. Ann Intern Med. 1978;89:677–83.
67. Damaj G, Kuhnowski F, Marolleau JP, et al. Risk factors for severe infection in patients with hairy cell leukemia: a long term study of 73 patients. Eur J Haematol. 2009;83:246–50.
68. Vardiman JW, Golomb HM. Autopsy findings in hairy cell leukemia. Semin Oncol. 1984;11:370–80.
69. Bourguin-Plonquet A, Rourad H, Roudot-Thoraval F, et al. Severe decrease in peripheral blood dendritic cell in hairy cell leukemia. Br J Haematol. 2002;116:595–7.
70. Hisada M, Chen BE, Jaffe ES, et al. Second cancer incidence and cause-specific mortality among 3104 patients with hairy cell leukemia: a population based study. J Natl Cancer Inst. 2007;99:215–22.
71. Saven A, Burian C, Koziol J, et al. Long term follow-up of patients with hairy cell leukemia after cladribine treatment. Blood. 1998;92:1918–26.
72. Kampmeier P, Spielberger R, Dickstein J, et al. Increased incidence of second neoplasms in patients treated with interferon alpha 2b for hairy cell leukemia: a clinicopathologic assessment. Blood. 1994;83:2931–8.
73. Wing YA, Klasa RJ, Gallagher R, et al. Second malignancies in patients with hairy cell leukemia in British Columbia: a 20 year experience. Blood. 1998;92:1160–4.
74. Cornet E, Tomowiak C, Tanguy-Schmidt A, et al. Long-term follow-up and second malignancies in 487 patients with hairy cell leukemia. Br J Haematol. 2014;166(3):390–400.
75. Goodman GR, Burian C, Koziol JA, et al. Extended follow-up of patients with hairy cell leukemia after treatment with cladribine. J Clin Oncol. 2003;21:891–6.
76. Rosenberg JD, Burian C, Waalen J, et al. Clinical characteristics and long-term outcome of young hairy cell leukemia patients treated with cladribine: a single-institution series. Blood. 2014;123(2):177–83.
77. Wolfe DW, Scopelliti JA, Boselli BD. Leukemic meningitis in a patient with hairy cell leukemia. A case report. Cancer. 1984;54:1085–7.
78. Dorsey JK, Penick GD. The association of hairy cell leukemia with unusual immunologic disorders. Arch Intern Med. 1982;142:902–3.
79. Juliusson G, Vitols S, Lilemark J, et al. Disease-related hypocholesterolemia in patients with hairy cell leukemia. Cancer. 1995;76:423–8.
80. Eklon KB, Hughes GR, Catovsky D. Hairy cell leukemia with polyarteritis nodosa. Lancet. 1979;2:280–2.
81. Matutes E, Wotherspoon A, Catovsky D. The variant form of hairy-cell leukemia. Best Pract Res Clin Haematol. 2003;16:41–56.
82. Cawley JC, Burns GF, Hayhoe FG, et al. A chronic lymphoproliferative disorder with distinctive features: a distinct variant of hairy-cell leukemia. Leuk Res. 1980;4:547–59.
83. Sainati L, Matutes E, Mulligan S, et al. A variant form of hairy cell leukemia resistant to alpha-interferon: clinical and phenotypic characteristics of 17 patients. Blood. 1990;76:157–62.

84. Matutes E, Wotherspoon A, Brito-Babapulle V, et al. The natural history and clinico-pathological features of the variant form of hairy cell leukemia. Leukemia. 2001;15:184–6.
85. Hockley SL, Giannouli S, Morrilla A, et al. Insights into the molecular pathogenesis of hairy cell leukemia, hairy cell leukemia variant and splenic marginal zone lymphoma, provided by the analysis of their IGH rearrangements and somatic hypermutation patterns. Br J Haematol. 2010;148(4):666–9.
86. Arons E, Kreitman RJ. Molecular variant of hairy cell leukemia with poor prognosis. Leuk Lymphoma. 2011;52(Suppl 2):99–102.
87. Arons E, Suntum T, Stetler-Stevenson M, Kreitman RJ. VH4-34+ hairy cell leukemia, a new variant with poor prognosis despite standard therapy. Blood. 2009;114:4687–95.
88. Martin JL, Li C, Banks P, et al. Blastic variant of hairy-cell leukemia. Am J Clin Pathol. 1987;87:576–83.
89. Machii T, Tokumine Y, Inoue R, et al. Predominance of a distinct subtype of hairy cell leukemia in Japan. Leukemia. 1983;7:181–6.
90. Troussard X, Valensi F, Duchayne E, et al. Splenic lymphoma with villous lymphocytes: clinical presentation, biology and prognostic factors in a series of 100 patients. Br J Haematol. 1996;93:731–6.
91. Matutes E, Morilla R, Owusu-Ankomah K, et al. The immunophenotype of splenic lymphoma with villous lymphocytes and its relevance to the differential diagnosis with other B-cell disorders. Blood. 1994;83:1558–62.
92. Pollack A. Hairy cell leukemia: biology, clinical diagnosis, unusual manifestations and associated disorders. Rev Clin Exp Hematol. 2002;6:366–88.
93. Galton DA, Wiltshaw GE, Catovsky D, et al. Prolymphocytic leukemia. Br J Haematol. 1974;27:7–23.
94. Dungarawalla M, Matutes E, Dearden E. Prolymphocytic leukemia of B- and T-cell subtype: a state-of-the-art paper. Eur J Haematol. 2008;80:469–76.
95. Giblet ER, Anderson JE, Cohen F, et al. Adenosine deaminase deficiency in two patients with severely impaired cellular immunity. Lancet. 1972;2:1067–9.
96. Cohen A, Hirschhorn R, Horowitz SD, et al. Deoxyadenosine triphosphate as a potentially toxic metabolite in adenosine deaminase deficiency. Proc Natl Acad Sci U S A. 1978;75:472–6.
97. Carson DA, Kaye J, Seegmiller JE. Lymphospecific toxicity in adenosine deaminase deficiency and purine nucleoside phosphorylase deficiency: possible role of nucleoside kinase(s). Proc Natl Acad Sci U S A. 1977;74:5677–88.
98. Carson DA, Wasson DB, Kaye J, et al. Deoxycytidine kinase-mediated toxicity of deoxyadenosine analogs toward malignant human lymphoblasts in vitro and toward murine L1210 leukemia in vivo. Proc Natl Acad Sci U S A. 1980;77:6865–9.
99. Carson DA, Wasson DB, Taetle R, et al. Specific toxicity of 2-chlorodeoxyadenosine toward resting and proliferating human lymphocytes. Blood. 1983;62:737–43.
100. Piro LD, Carrerra CJ, Carson DA, et al. Lasting remissions in hairy-cell leukemia induced by a single infusion of 2-chlorodeoxyadenosine. N Engl J Med. 1990;322:1117–21.
101. Else M, Dearden CE, Matutes E, et al. Long term follow-up of 233 patients with hairy cell leukaemia, treated initially with pentostatin or cladribine, at a median of 16 years from diagnosis. Br J Haematol. 2009;145:733–40.
102. Tallman MS, Hakimian D, Rademaker AW, et al. Relapse of hairy cell leukemia after 2-chlorodeoxyadenosine: long term follow-up of the northwestern experience. Blood. 1996;88:1954–9.
103. Seymour J, Kurzrock R, Freireich EJ, et al. 2-Chlorodeoxyadenosine induces durable remissions and prolonged suppression of CD4+ lymphocyte counts in patients with hairy cell leukemia. Blood. 1994;83:2906–11.
104. Hoffman MA, Janson D, Rose E, et al. Treatment with hairy cell leukemia with cladribine: response, toxicity and long term follow-up. J Clin Oncol. 1997;15:1131–42.
105. Jehn U, Bartl R, Dietzfelbinger H, et al. An update: 12 year follow up of patients with hairy cell leukemia following treatment with 2-chlorodeoxyadenosine. Leukemia. 2004;18:1476–81.
106. Chadha P, Rademaker AW, Mendiratta P, et al. Treatment of hairy cell leukemia with 2-chlorodeoxyadenosine (2-CdA): long-term follow-up of the Northwestern University experience. Blood. 2005;106:241–6.
107. Lopez RM, Da Silva C, Loscertales J, et al. Hairy cell leukemia treated initially with purine analogs: a retrospective study of 107 patients from the Spanish Cooperative Group on Chronic Lymphocytic Leukemia (CELLC). Leuk Lymphoma. 2014;55(5):1007–12.
108. Hacioglu S, Bilen Y, Eser A, et al. Multicenter retrospective analysis regarding the clinical manifestations and treatment results in patients with hairy cell leukemia: twenty-four year Turkish experience in cladribine therapy. Hematol Oncol. 2015;33(4):192–8.
109. Somasundaram V, Purohit A, Aggarwal M, et al. Hairy cell leukemia: a decade long experience of North Indian Hematology Center. Indian J Med Paediatr Oncol. 2013;35(4):271–5.
110. Ruiz-Delgado GJ, Tarin-Arzaga LC, Alarcon-Urdaneta C, et al. Treatment of hairy cell leukemia: long-term results in a developing country. Hematology. 2012;17(3):140–3.
111. Golomb HM. Hairy cell leukemia: treatment successes in the past 25 years. J Clin Oncol. 2008;26:2607–9.
112. Robak T, Jamroziak K, Gora-Tybor J, et al. Cladribine in a weekly versus daily schedule for untreated active hairy cell leukemia: final report, from the Polish Adult Leukemia Group (PALG) of a prospective randomized, multicenter trial. Blood. 2007;109:3672–5.
113. Grever MR. How I treat hairy cell leukemia. Blood. 2010;115:21–8.
114. Saven A, Burian C, Adusumali J, et al. Filgrastim for cladribine-induced neutropenic fever in patients with hairy cell leukemia. Blood. 1999;93:2471–7.
115. Spiers ASD, Parek SK. Complete remission in hairy cell leukemia achieved with pentostatin. Lancet. 1984;1:1080–1.
116. Flinn IW, Kopecky KJ, Foucar MK, et al. Long term follow-up of remission, duration, mortality, and second malignancies in hairy cell leukemia patients treated with pentostatin. Blood. 2000;96:2981–6.
117. Cassileth PA, Cheuvart B, Spiers ASD, et al. Pentostatin induces durable remissions in hairy cell leukemia. J Clin Oncol. 1991;9:243–6.
118. O'Dwyer PJ, Spiers ASD, Marsoni S. Association of severe and fatal infections and treatment with pentostatin. Cancer Treat Rep. 1986;70:1117–20.
119. Johnston JB, Glazer RI, Pugh L, et al. The treatment of hairy-cell leukaemia with 2′-deoxycoformycin. Br J Haematol. 1986;63:525–34.
120. Smalley RV, Connors J, Tuttle RL, et al. Splenectomy vs. alpha interferon: a randomized study in patients with previously untreated hairy cell leukemia. Am J Hematol. 1992;41:13–8.
121. Zakarija A, Peterson LC, Tallman M, et al. Splenectomy and treatments of historical interest. Best Pract Res Clin Haematol. 2003;16:57–68.
122. Mintz U, Golomb HM. Splenectomy as initial therapy in twenty six patients with leukemic reticuloendotheliosis (hairy cell leukemia). Cancer Res. 1979;39:2366–70.
123. Golomb HM, Vardiman JW. Response to splenectomy in 65 patients with hairy cell leukemia: an evaluation of spleen weight and bone marrow involvement. Blood. 1983;61:349–52.
124. Ratain MJ, Vardiman JW, Barker CM. Prognostic variables in hairy cell leukemia after splenectomy as initial therapy. Cancer. 1988;62:2420–4.
125. Frassoldati A, Lamparelli T, Federico M, et al. Hairy cell leukemia: a clinical review based on 725 cases of the Italian Cooperative Group (ICGHCL). Italian Cooperative Group for Hairy Cell Leukemia. Leuk Lymphoma. 1995;13:307–16.
126. Stiles GM, Stanco LM, Saven A, et al. Splenectomy for hairy cell leukemia in pregnancy. J Perinatol. 1998;18:200.

127. Vendantham S, Gamliel H, Golomb HM. Mechanisms of interferon action in hairy cell leukemia: a model of effective cancer biotherapy. Cancer Res. 1992;52:1056–66.
128. Quesada JR, Reuben J, Manning JT, et al. Alpha-interferon for induction of remission in hairy cell leukemia. N Engl J Med. 1984;310:15–8.
129. Quesada JR, Hersh EM, Manning J, et al. Treatment of hairy cell leukemia with recombinant alpha-interferon. Blood. 1986;68:493–7.
130. Golomb HM, Jacobs A, Fefer A, et al. Alpha-2 interferon therapy for hairy cell leukemia: a multicenter study of 64 patients. J Clin Oncol. 1986;4:900–5.
131. Ratain MJ, Golomb HM, Vardiman JW, et al. Relapse after interferon-alpha-2b for hairy cell leukemia: analysis of prognostic variables. J Clin Oncol. 1988;6:1714–21.
132. Damasio EE, Masoudi CM, Spriano IA, et al. Alpha-interferon as induction and maintenance therapy in hairy cell leukemia: a long term follow-up analysis. Eur J Haematol. 2000;64:47–52.
133. Capnist G, Federico M, Chisesi T, et al. Long term results of interferon treatment in hairy cell leukemia. Italian Cooperative Group of Hairy Cell Leukemia. Leuk Lymphoma. 1994;14:457–64.
134. Hoffmen MA. Interferon-alpha is a very effective salvage therapy for patients with hairy cell leukemia relapsing after cladribine: a report of three cases. Med Oncol. 2011;28:1537.
135. Steis RG, Marcon L, Clark J, et al. Serum soluble IL-2 receptor as a tumor marker in patients with hairy cell leukemia. Blood. 1988;71:1304–9.
136. Naik R, Saven A. My treatment approach to hairy cell leukemia. Mayo Clin Proc. 2012;87(1):67–76.
137. Ellison DJ, Sharp RW, Robbins BA, et al. Immunomorphologic analysis of bone marrow biopsies after treatment with 2-chlorodeoxyadenosine for hairy cell leukemia. Blood. 1994;84:4310–5.
138. Arons E, Margulies I, Sorbara L, et al. Minimal residual disease in hairy cell leukemia patients assessed by clone-specific polymerase chain reaction. Clin Cancer Res. 2006;12:2804–11.
139. Bengio R, Narbaitz MI, Sarmiento MA, et al. Comparative analysis of immunophenotypic methods for the assessment of minimal residual disease in hairy cell leukemia. Haematologica. 2000;85:1227–9.
140. Hakimian D, Tallman MS, Kiley C, et al. Detection of minimal residual disease by immunostaining of bone marrow biopsies after 2-chlorodeoxyadenosine for hairy cell leukemia. Blood. 1993;82:1798–802.
141. Wheaton S, Tallman MS, Hakimian D. Minimal residual disease may predict bone marrow relapse in patients with hairy cell leukemia treated with 2-chlorodeoxyadenosine. Blood. 1996;87:1556–60.
142. Matutes E, Meeus P, McLennan K, et al. The significance of minimal residual disease in hairy cell leukaemia treated with deoxycoformycin: a long-term follow-up study. Br J Haematol. 1997;98:375–83.
143. Filleul B, Delannoy A, Ferrant A, et al. A single course of 2-chloro-deoxyadenosine does not eradicate leukemic cells in hairy cell leukemia patients in complete remission. Leukemia. 1994;8:1153–6.
144. Ravandi F, Jorgensen JL, O'Brien SM, et al. Eradication of minimal residual disease in hairy cell leukemia. Blood. 2006;107:4658–62.
145. Cervetti G, Galimberti S, Andreazzoli F, et al. Rituximab as treatment for minimal residual disease in hairy cell leukemia. Eur J Haematol. 2004;73:412–7.
146. Sigal DS, Sharpe R, Burian C, et al. Very long term eradication of minimal residual disease in patients with hairy cell leukemia following a single course of cladribine. Blood. 2010;115:1893–6.
147. Forconi F, Sozzi E, Cencini E, et al. Hairy cell leukemias with unmutated IGHV genes define the minor subset refractory to single-agent cladribine with more aggressive behavior. Blood. 2009;114:4696–702.
148. Saven A, Piro LD. Complete remissions in hairy cell leukemia with 2-chlorodeoxyadenosine after failure with 2-deoxycoformycin. Ann Intern Med. 1993;119(4):278–83.
149. Kreitman RJ, Fitzgerald DJP, Pastan I, et al. Approach to the patient after relapse of hairy cell leukemia. Leuk Lymphoma. 2009;50(Suppl 1):32–7.
150. Hagberg H. Chimeric monoclonal anti-CD20 antibody (rituximab)—an effective treatment for a patient with relapsing hairy cell leukemia. Med Oncol. 1999;14:221–2.
151. Nieva J, Bethel K, Saven A. Phase II study of rituximab in the treatment of cladribine-failed patients with hairy cell leukemia. Blood. 2003;102:810–3.
152. Thomas DA, O'Brien S, Bueso-Ramos C, et al. Rituximab in relapsed or refractory hairy cell leukemia. Blood. 2003;102:3906–11.
153. Else M, Dearden CE, Catovsky D. Long-term follow-up after purine analogue therapy in hairy cell leukaemia. Best Pract Res Clin Haematol. 2015;28(4):217–29.
154. Ravandi F, O'Brien S, Jorgensen J, et al. Phase 2 study of cladribine followed by rituximab in patients with hairy cell leukemia. Blood. 2011;118(14):3818–23.
155. Leclerc M, Suarez F, Noel MP, et al. Rituximab therapy for hairy cell leukemia: a restrospective study of 41 cases. Ann Hematol. 2015;94(1):89–95.
156. Gerrie AS, Zypchen LN, Connors JM. Fludarabine and rituximab for relapsed or refractory hairy cell leukemia. Blood. 2012;119(9):1988–91.
157. Kreitmaan RJ, Wilson W, Calvo KR, et al. Cladribine with immediate rituximab for the treatment of patients with variant hairy cell leukemia. Clin Cancer Res. 2013;19(24):6873–81.
158. Munoz J, Schlette E, Kurzrock R. Rapid response to vemurafenib in a heavily pretreated patient with hairy cell leukemia and a BRAF mutation. J Clin Oncol. 2013;31(20):e351–2.
159. Peyrade F, Re D, Ginet C, et al. Low-dose vemurafenib induces complete remission in a case of hairy-cell leukemia with a V600E mutation. Haematologica. 2013;98(2):e20–2.
160. Samuel J, Macip S, Dyer MJ. Efficacy of vemurafenib in hairy-cell leukemia. N Engl J Med. 2014;370(3):286–8.
161. Dietrich S, Hullein J, Hundemer M, et al. Continued response off treatment after BRAF inhibition in refractory hairy cell leukemia. J Clin Oncol. 2013;31(19):e300–3.
162. Tiacci E, Park JH, De Carolis SS, et al. Targeting mutant BRAF in relapsed or refractory hairy-cell leukemia. N Engl J Med. 2015;373:1733–47.
163. Long GV, Stroyakovskiy D, Gogas H, et al. Combined BRAF and MEK inhibition versus BRAF inhibition alone in melanoma. N Engl J Med. 2014;371:1877–88.
164. Pettirossi V, Santi A, Imperi E, et al. BRAF inhibitors reverse the unique molecular signature and phenotype of hairy cell leukemia and exert potent antileukemic activity. Blood. 2015;125(8):1207–16.
165. Kreitman RJ, Wilson WH, Bergeron K, et al. Efficacy of the anti-CD22 recombinant immunotoxin BL22 in chemotherapy-resistant hairy-cell leukemia. N Engl J Med. 2001;345(4):241–7.
166. Kreitman RJ, Squires DR, Stetler-Stevenson M, et al. Phase 1 trial of recombinant immunotoxin RFB4(dsFv)-PE38 (BL22) in patients with B-cell malignancies. J Clin Oncol. 2005;23(27):6719–29.
167. Kreitman RJ, Stetler-Stevenson M, Margulies I, et al. Phase II trial of recombinant immunotoxin RFB4(dsFv)-PE38 (BL22) in patients with hairy cell leukemia. J Clin Oncol. 2009;27(18):2983–90.
168. Kreitman RJ, Pastan I. Antibody fusion proteins: anti-CD22 recombinant immunotoxin moxetumomab pasudotox. Clin Cancer Res. 2011;17(20):6398–405.
169. Kreitman RJ, Tallman MS, Robak T, et al. Phase 1 trial of anti-CD22 recombinant immunotoxin moxetumomab pasudotox (CAT-8015 or HA22) in patients with hairy cell leukemia. J Clin Oncol. 2012;30(15):1822–8.

170. Kreitmen RJ, Wilson WH, White JD, et al. Phase 1 trial of recombinant immunotoxin anti-Tac(Fv)-PE38 (LMB-2) in patients with hematologic malignancies. J Clin Oncol. 2000;18(8):1622–36.
171. Sasaki M, Sugimoto K, Mori T, et al. Effective treatment of a refractory hairy cell leukemia variant with splenic pre-irradiation and alemtuzumab. Acta Haematol. 2008;119(1):48–53.
172. Fietz T, Rieger K, Schmittel A, Thiel E, Knauf W. Alemtuzumab (Campath 1H) in hairy cell leukaemia relapsing after rituximab treatment. Hematol J. 2004;5(5):451–2.
173. Kreitman RJ, Arons E, Stetler-Stevenson M, et al. Response of hairy cell leukemia to bendamustine. Leuk Lymphoma. 2011;52(6):1153–6.
174. Burotto M, Stetler-Stevenson M, Arons E, et al. Bendamustine and rituximab in relapsed and refractory hairy cell leukemia. Clin Cancer Res. 2013;19(22):6313–21.
175. Randomized Phase II trial of rituximab with either pentostatin or bendamustine for multiply relapsed or refractory hairy cell leukemia. https://clinicaltrials.gov/ct2/show/NCT01059786.
176. Sivina M, Kreitman RJ, Arons E, et al. The bruton tyrosine kinase inhibitor ibrutinib (PCI-32765) blocks hairy cell leukaemia survival, proliferation and B cell receptor signalling: a new therapeutic approach. Br J Haematol. 2014;166(2):177–88.
177. Jones JA, Andritsos LA, Lucas DM, et al. Preliminary safety and efficacy of the Bruton's tyrosine kinase (BTK) inhibitor ibrutinib (IBR) in patients (pts) with hairy cell leukemia (HCL). J Clin Oncol. 2014;32(5 Suppl):abstract 7063.
178. Ibrutinib in treating patients with relapsed hairy cell leukemia. https://clinicaltrials.gov/ct2/show/NCT01841723.

Part II

Acute Leukemias

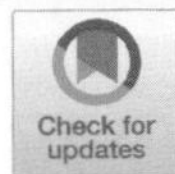

History of Acute Leukemia

11

Emil J Freireich

Introduction

In 1953, the United States Public Health Service opened the 500-bed clinical center on the Bethesda campus of the National Institutes of Health. James Holland, who had trained at the Francis Delafield Hospital of the Columbia University School of Medicine, was among the first clinicians to join the faculty of the National Cancer Institute's clinical center and he began to utilize these agents for the treatment of children with acute leukemia. In 1954, Charles Gordon Zubrod was recruited to the clinical center to become the head of the medicine branch in the Cancer Institute and he recruited Emil Frei III, who was his chief resident, to come with him to the Cancer Institute. Early in 1955, Emil J. Freireich joined the Cancer Institute with a background in hematology.

Dr. Holland left the Cancer Institute in 1954 to move to Buffalo, the Roswell Park Memorial Institute, and when Freireich arrived in Bethesda there were three patients in the hospital with acute lymphoblastic leukemia. What the new group decided to do was to utilize the newly described technique of the prospective randomized controlled clinical trial which was so successful in developing the antimalarial drugs during the war, and secondly, to test the hypothesis that combination chemotherapy would provide synergistic effects—this had been demonstrated in the treatment of infectious diseases, particularly tuberculosis. In reviewing what was published up to that date on the chemotherapy of acute leukemia, these young investigators discovered that the agents that were described to induce temporary remissions when used singularly [1–8] did not significantly affect the natural history of acute leukemia [9]. They initiated a collaborative study between the group at the Cancer Institute in Bethesda and Dr. Holland and his group at Roswell Park in Buffalo. The goal of the first study was to evaluate the effectiveness of a combination of 6-mercaptopurine and methotrexate. They first reviewed the world's literature on the normal values for blood and bone marrow, physical findings, and symptoms, and published objective criteria for defining complete remission, partial remission, and hematological improvement which were to be used in this cooperative group study [10].

Secondly, a detailed research protocol was constructed and agreed to by the investigators at both institutions, and they devised data collecting flow sheets which mandated the measurement of bone marrow, blood, physical findings, and symptoms at regular intervals. This first study was a landmark study in that it established the feasibility of doing formal clinical trials, and it provided objective quantitative information of the frequency and duration of response and survival for a group of 63 consecutive patients [11].

Because the results of the combination study looked promising, the second protocol, Protocol 2, systematically compared the combination to each of the two drugs used as single agents followed, on failure, by a crossover to the other agent. These studies were designed based on mouse leukemia studies conducted by Lloyd Law and Abe Golden which suggested not only the concept of combination chemotherapy, but also the possibility that there was collateral sensitivity, i.e., the disease resistant to one agent would have enhanced sensitivity to the other. Protocol 2 had three arms—the combination of methotrexate and 6-mercaptopurine which was given at 60% of their maximum tolerated dose that was worked out in mouse toxicology studies because these two drugs were both myelosuppressive agents; and 60% of each combined to a maximum tolerated dose for the two drugs, which was compared with the full therapeutic dose of methotrexate, followed by 6-mercaptopurine upon failure; and the third arm was 6-mercaptopurine followed by methotrexate upon failure. While this study was being prepared, the results of Protocol 1 were publicized through scientific meetings and a number of institutions, specifically ten institutions, elected to join in the study; so Protocol 2 was

E. J Freireich, M.D.
Department of Leukemia, University of Texas MD Anderson Cancer Center, SMEP Y7.5338, Unit 55, 1515 Holcombe Blvd, Houston, TX 77030, USA
e-mail: efreirei@mdanderson.org

P.H. Wiernik et al. (eds.), *Neoplastic Diseases of the Blood*, DOI 10.1007/978-3-319-64263-5_11

able to accrue a much larger sample size in a reasonable period of time. The results of that study were positive in the sense that the combination of the two agents was more effective—in terms of frequency and duration of response, and survival—than the two agents used in either sequence, but no collateral sensitivity was demonstrated [12].

It was clear that one strategy for the control of acute leukemia was to discover new agents with unique mechanisms of action. In the first such study undertaken by the National Cancer Institute group—the study of 6-azauracil which was shown by Arnold Welch in experimental animals to have a high degree of activity—the results of the Phase 2 study revealed some hematological improvements in the patients, suggesting that this was a potential drug for using in newly diagnosed patients [13]. But, before that was undertaken, they recognized that they had little information on patients who had been extensively treated previously with the three active drugs. So, they undertook the first prospective randomized controlled trial in cancer research comparing 6-azauracil to a placebo in these terminal advanced refractory leukemia and found that there was no significant difference between those treated with placebo or the active drug [14]. This was an important study because it demonstrated the importance of concurrent controls and quantitative assessment of response—because the disease was not inevitably progressive and quantitative information to build new hypotheses was essential.

For Protocol 3 [15], they hypothesized that the patients would be in better physical and clinical condition in remission, and therefore, they would have a better opportunity to assess the activity of new agent. The clinical trial was designed to expose all children to the most active remission-inducing drug which, at that time, was hydrocortisone, resulting in approximately 60% of the children achieving complete clinical and hematological remission. The children were then randomized to receive either placebo or 6-mercaptopurine, which was known to be active in inducing complete clinical and hematological remission in approximately 30% of the patients with active leukemia. The study was designed in an innovative way using a sequential design, so that when the probability that one was better than the other was greater than 95% the study stopped automatically. The results of this study were impressive because it first demonstrated a substantial prolongation of remission with 6-mercaptopurine, and it established that corticosteroid-induced remissions had a median remission of only 8 weeks and all patients had recurrence at approximately 10 months. In contrast, the patients who received mercaptopurine, all patients, not just 30%, had significant prolongation of remission and approximately 10–15% of the patients remained in remission for more than a year, which was an unheard of result with any prior therapy. Moreover, those who received placebo and were subsequently treated with 6-mercaptopurine and methotrexate had overall survival which was comparable to the patients who received 6MP during remission, indicating that their survival was not significantly compromised. The results of this study demonstrated, for the first time, the principle of adjuvant chemotherapy, i.e., chemotherapy given to patients free of clinical disease was substantially more effective than the same therapy given to patients with active disease. That was the major outcome of this study, even though that was not the initial plan.

The next major development was the discovery of the vinca alkaloids by Irving Johnson working at Eli Lilly Laboratories. In an effort to develop new antidiabetic drugs, Eli Lilly screened many natural products and the extract from the periwinkle plant contained alkaloids that had little effect on glucose metabolism, but did cause substantial myelosuppression in mice. Dr. Johnson had the impressive thought that this drug might be active in leukemia. To that end, Eli Lilly, at great expense, extracted this alkaloid from very large quantities of the periwinkle plant and initiated clinical trials in Children's Hospital in Boston and with the group at the National Cancer Institute. The Phase 2 trial with this drug gave dramatic responses. Over 50% of the children with far advanced disease refractory to the three known agents developed rapid, complete clinical and hematological remissions [16]. Like steroids, these remissions were short, approximately 8 weeks on average, but the results were impressive and the limiting dose toxicity for this drug was not myelosuppression, but central nervous system and peripheral nervous system toxicity. The group had learned that one could add the full therapeutic dose of adrenocortical steroids, which is not myelosuppressive, to the myelosuppressive drugs methotrexate or 6-mercaptopurine, and in both instances, frequency of complete response to the combination was higher than that predicted from the results of each individual drug used in previously untreated patients. This led the NCI group to consider the possibility of combining all four known active agents into a single therapy because they recognized that vincristine and prednisone did not have additive toxicity, nor were they myelosuppressive. They knew the maximum tolerated dose of the combination mercaptopurine methotrexate, so they created the first multi-agent four-drug chemotherapy regimen, and even more importantly created the first eponym for this combination (VAMP): vincristine, amethopterin, mercaptopurine, and prednisone. The results of the VAMP study were impressive—over 90% of the children entered remission rapidly and with minimal side effects. Since they had recognized the importance of adjuvant chemotherapy from Protocol 3, the NCI investigators used early intensification of the remission induced by VAMP and gave three induction courses to the children in remission. What they observed was that the duration of remission was as long as that achieved with adjuvant 6-mercaptopurine. Then they introduced the concept of continuous intermittent re-induction therapy specifically; they gave the same four agents for induction, consolidation, and continued intermittent therapy at monthly intervals for 1 year (POMP). By 1964, with over 3 years of follow-up, they reported that one-third of the patients were still alive and disease free, and they suggested that these patients were "cured" of their childhood lymphoblastic leukemia—a prediction which has proven to be correct [17–19].

Treatment of childhood ALL progressively improved over the next 40 years with the addition of new agents, such as asparaginase. The recognition of the importance of meningeal leukemia and the role of prophylaxis for central nervous system involvement is such that at present at least 80–90% of such patients are literally cured of their disease with chemotherapy alone [20].

When the activity of 6-mercaptopurine, methotrexate, and prednisone was described, it was early recognized that the cytological details of the morphology of these leukemia cells were suddenly extremely important. Those leukemia patients who had a lymphoid phenotype responded dramatically, whereas those who had myeloid characteristics had the same natural history as in the untreated state and were found to be quite resistant to chemotherapy [21]. The other prognostic factor that was identified was that the optimal responses occurred in patients under 10, and in patients over 20, the frequency of response and survival was significantly lower.

In addition, they recognized the importance of the degree of leukocytosis as an important prognostic factor.

VAMP was primarily active in children with acute lymphoblastic leukemia. The investigators attempted the same four-drug combination (POMP) therapy in children with myeloid phenotype and in young adults. Although the effects were much less dramatic and quantitatively less effective, they nonetheless reported that approximately 25% of adults in this case (median age well below median age of approximately 40) could achieve complete hematological remission, and with intermittent maintenance, these remissions could last for approximately 1 year. These data were assembled and submitted to the journal, *Blood*, for publication. The manuscript was rejected and Dr. Dameshek, founder of the journal and the editor-in-chief, was inclined to write editorials on the progress in hematology and he wrote an editorial in 1965 which said, "However, not only was this method unscientific, but the initial toxic reaction may be lethal, particularly in adults. Furthermore, it has not yet been clearly shown that this treatment program offers a significant advantage over more conservative approaches. In general, however, they may be thought to represent 'gropings' which engender little enthusiasm for long-term advantages" [22].

The situation for adults in 1965 was still poor—prednisone and 6MP gave 10% responses, and POMP reported to give 25% responses; these were largely ignored by the medical community as being too toxic for adult patients. The breakthrough occurred with the description of the activity of arabinosyl cytosine in 1963 [23].

In 1968, Ellison and Holland described the induction of remission in adults with acute myeloblastic leukemia [24]. Based on the animal experiments which were conducted by Skipper and Schabel at Southern Research Institute [25], it was demonstrated that Ara-C was schedule dependent.

M.D. Anderson reported that a group of patients in 1967 were treated by continuous infusion over 120 h or 5 days [26]. The Southwest Oncology Group conducted a dose schedule study which demonstrated that single injection of Ara-C as high as 3 g/m^2 did not cause myelosuppression, but infusion of 48 h or longer had dose-responsive myelosuppression [27]. The Southwest Oncology Group then compared 48- and 120-h infusions which showed higher frequency and longer duration of response with 120-h infusions [28].

In 1964, an Italian group discovered the natural product, daunorubicin, an anthracycline, antibiotic [29]. And in 1969, adriamycin, another anthracycline antibiotic, was discovered [30]. Both of these drugs had substantial single-agent activity in patients refractory to Ara-C. What followed was a series of studies combining the anthracycline antibiotics with Ara-C in its best schedule. Many of these combinations were studied in cooperative groups, but the one that proved to be best tolerated and most effective for the highest number of patients was the famous 3 and 7 regimen—3 days of daunorubicin and 7 days of continuous infusion of arabinosyl cytosine [31].

The academic hematology community received these reports with skepticism. As late as 1974, one of the giants of hematology, William Crosby, published "chemotherapy should be used only sparing in related cases of leukemia, since the treatment may be killing more patients than proponents of aggressive therapy realize" [32].

In 1976, the editors of the Archives of Internal Medicine published a series of papers in rebuttal of Crosby's comments supporting the use of chemotherapy for adults with AML [33–35].

In 1981, it was clear that the natural history of AML had changed substantially at least for a fraction of these patients [36]. For the first time, completed 5-year survival was observed in approximately 15% of the patients diagnosed with AML before 1976. Shortly thereafter, a major review of the treatment of acute leukemia in many centers and in the cooperative groups was conducted and it was clear that these results from a single institution were confirmed not only in many institutions but also in multi-institution studies. And an analysis of long-term survival was published in 1983 [37].

With the advent of techniques to study the human chromosomes, including banding to identify the individual chromosomes, many investigators reported that acute leukemia patients had a number of abnormalities in the chromosomes which were apparently random. However, in 1979 Trujillo recognized the first nonrandom chromosome abnormality—the translocation between chromosomes 8 and 21 [38]. Over the following years, many nonrandom chromosome abnormalities were identified which allowed a systematic classification of acute leukemia into groups [39]. Favorable was the inversion 16, the translocation 8:21, and the translocation 15:17, which constituted approximately 20% of all the acute myeloid leukemias. For these diseases, chemotherapy provided long-term (3 years or longer) survival for the majority of the patients. About one-third of the patients had complex cytogenetic and these were clearly unfavorable, where long-term survival occurred rarely. Then the remaining 50% were intermediate: mostly diploid patients who had an intermediate outcome of approximately 20% long-term survival. The most dramatically distinctive group of AML patients was the group which had the translocation between chromosomes 15 and 17 which created a neo-gene (the RARA/PML gene) which was susceptible to remission induction by all-trans-retinoic acid. With the addition of arsenic trioxide it became possible for this small subset of AML patients (approximately 6–10%) to enter complete remission with long-term survival and without any cytotoxic chemotherapy [40]. The discovery of the cytogenetic classifications of patients formed the basis for the new molecular oncology so that now specific genetic traits are used not only for diagnosis and choice of therapy, but also for the detection of residual disease and for guiding the courses of therapy [41].

Another important advance was the development of myeloablative allogeneic stem cell transplantations [42, 43]. This was shown to result in long-term survival for a significant fraction of patients with acute leukemia. This therapy has become a significant therapy, particularly for patients in remission. The transplant techniques have also improved rapidly with the use of peripheral blood stem cells, reduced intensity conditioning and improved tissue typing, matched unrelated donor pools, and improved control of complications such as infection and graft-versus-host diseases [44].

Conclusion

Considering the transformation of AML from a universally fatal untreatable disease in the mid-1960s to one with a significant portion of cured patients and a very high proportion of patients who respond to therapy in a half century, this rapid progress suggests strongly that knowledge about the biology and therapy of acute leukemia will increase at an accelerating pace and hopefully lead to control of this disease in the near future. Recent authoritative reviews of progress in acute leukemia treatment have appeared [45, 46].

References

1. Freireich EJ, Lemak NA. Milestones in leukemia research and therapy. London: The John Hopkins University Press; 1991.
2. Virchow R. Weisses Blut. Neue Notizen Gebiete Natur-Heilkunde. 1845;36:151–7.
3. Farber S, Daimond LK, Mercer RD, et al. Temporary remission in acute leukemia in children prolonged by folic acid antagonist, 4-aminopteroylglutamic acid (aminopterin). N Engl J Med. 1948;238:787–93.
4. Pearson OH, Eliel LP, Rawson RW, et al. ACTH- and cortisoneinduced regression of lymphoid tumors in man. Cancer. 1949;2:943–5.
5. Farber S, Shwachman H, Toch R, et al. The effect of ACTH in acute leukemia in childhood. In: Mote JR, editor. Proceedings of the first clinical ACTH conference. Philadelphia: Blakiston; 1950. p. 328–30.
6. Hitchings GH, Elion GB. The chemistry and biochemistry of purine analogs. Ann N Y Acad Sci. 1954;60:195–9.
7. Burchenal JH, Murphy ML, Ellison RR, et al. Clinical evaluation of a new antimetabolite, 6-mercaptopurine, in the treatment of leukemia and allied diseases. Blood. 1953;8:965–99.
8. MacMahon B, Forman D. Variation and duration of survival of patients with acute leukemia. Blood. 1957;12:683–93.
9. Haut A, Altman SJ, Cartwright GE, Wintrobe MM. The influence of chemotherapy on survival in actute leukemia. Blood. 1955;10:875–95.
10. Holland JF, Frei E III, Burchenal JH. Criteria for the evaluation of response to therapy of acute leukemia. In: Proceedings of the fourth congress of the International Society for Hematology, Boston; 1956. p. 213.
11. Frei E III, Holland JF, Schneiderman MA, Pinkel D, Selkirk G, Freireich EJ, Silver RT, Gold GL, Regelson W. A comparative study of two regimens of combination chemotherapy in acute leukemia. Blood. 1958;13:1126–48.
12. Frei IIIE, Freireich EJ, Gehan E, Pinkel D, Holland JF, Selawry O, Haurani F, Spurr CL, Hayes DM, James GW, Rothberg H, Sodee DB, Rundles RW, Schroeder LR, Hoogstraten B, Wolman IJ, Traggis DG, Cooper T, Gendel BR, Ebaugh F, Taylor R. Studies of sequential and combination antimetabolite therapy in acute leukemia: 6-mercaptopurine and methotrexate. Blood. 1961;18:431–54.
13. Shnider BI, Frei IIIE, Tuohy JH, Gorman J, Freireich EJ, Brindley Jr CO, Clements J. Clinical studies of 6-azauracil. Cancer Res. 1960;20:28–33.
14. Freireich EJ, Frei IIIE, Holland JF, Pinkel D, Selawry O, Rothberg H, Haurani F, Taylor R, Gehan EA. Evaluation of a new chemotherapeutic agent in patients with "advanced refractory" acute leukemia. Studies of 6-azauracil. Blood. 1960;16:1268–78.
15. Freireich EJ, Gehan EA, Frei IIIE, Schroeder LR, Wolman IJ, Anbari R, Burgert EO, Mills SD, Pinkel D, Selawry OS, Moon JH, Gendel BR, Spurr CL, Storrs R, Haurani F, Hoogstraten B, Lee S. The effect of 6-mercaptopurine on the duration of steroid-induced remissions in acute leukemia: a model for evaluation of other potentially useful therapy. Blood. 1963;21:699–716.
16. Karon MR, Freireich EJ, Frei E III. A Preliminary report of vincristine sulphate—a new active agent for the treatment of acute leukemia. Pediatrics. 1962;30:791–6.
17. Freireich EJ, Frei E III. Recent advances in acute leukemia. In: Moore CV, Brown EB, editors. Progress in hematology. New York: Grune and Stratton; 1964. p. 189–202.
18. Frei E III, Freireich EJ. Progress and perspectives in the chemotherapy of acute leukemia. In: Goldin A, Hawking F, Schnitzer RJ, editors. Advances in chemotherapy, vol. 2. New York: Academic; 1965. p. 269–98.
19. Freireich EJ, Henderson ES, Karon M, Frei III E. The treatment of acute leukemia considered with respect to cell population kinetics. In: Proliferation and spread of neoplastic cells, The University of Texas MD Anderson Cancer Center, 21st Annual Symposium on Fundamental Cancer Research. Baltimore: The Williams and Wilkins Co; 1968. p. 441–53.
20. Pui CH, Pei D, et al. Long term results of St. Jude. Total therapy studies for childhood ALL. Leukemia. 2010;24:371–82.
21. Freireich EJ, Gehan EA, Sulman D, Boggs DR, Frei E III. The effect of chemotherapy on acute leukemia in the human. J Chronic Dis. 1961;14:593–608.
22. Dameshek W, Necheles TF, Finkel HE, Allen DM. Therapy of acute leukemia, 1965. Blood. 1965;26:220–5.
23. Talley RW, Viatkevicius VK. Megaloblastosis produced by a cytosine antagonist 1-B-D-arabinofuranosylcytosine. Blood. 1963;21:352–62.

24. Ellison RR, Holland JF, Weil M, et al. Arabinosyl cytosine: useful agent in the treatment of acute leukemia in adults. Blood. 1968;32:507–23.
25. Skipper HE, Schabel Jr FM, Wilcox WS. Experimental evaluation of potential anticancer agents: XXI. Scheduling of arabinosylcytosine to take advantage of its S-phase specificity against leukemic cells. Cancer Chemother Rep. 1967;51:125–65.
26. Freireich EJ, Bodey GP, Harris JE, Hart JS. Therapy for acute granulocytic leukemia. Cancer Res. 1967;27:2573–7.
27. Frei IIIE, Bickers JN, Hewlett JS, et al. Dose schedule and antitumor studies or arabinosyl cytosine. Cancer Res. 1969;29:1325–32.
28. Bickers JN, Gehan EA, Freireich EJ, Coltman CA, Wilson HE, Hewlett JS, Stuckey JW, Van Slyck EJ. Cytarabine for acute leukemia in adults. Effect of schedule on therapeutic response. Arch Intern Med. 1974;133:251–9.
29. DiMarco A, Gaetani M, Orezzi P, et al. Antitumor activity of a new antibiotic: Daunomycin. In: Proceedings of the third international congress of chemotherapy, vol. 2, Stuttgart, 1963. New York: Hafner; 1964. p. 1023–31.
30. DiMarco A, Gaetani M, Scarpinato B. Adriamycin: a new antibiotic with antitumor activity. Cancer Chemother Rep. 1969;53:33–7.
31. Yates JW, Wallace Jr J, Ellison RR, Holland JF. Cytosine arabinosyl and daunorubicin in acute non-lymphocytic leukemia. Cancer Chemother Rep. 1973;57:485.
32. Crosby WH. Grounds for optimism in treating actue granulocytic luekemia. Arch Intern Med. 1974;184:177.
33. Freireich EJ. Grounds for optimism in treating acute granulocytic leukemia (adult acute leukemia). Symposium on leukemia. Arch Intern Med. 1976;136:1375–6.
34. Bodey GP, Coltman CA, Hewlett JS, Freireich EJ. Progress in the treatment of adults with acute leukemia. Symposium on leukemia. Arch Intern Med. 1976;136:1383–8.
35. Freireich EJ, Bodey GP, McCredie KB, Hersh EM, Gehan EA, Hart JS, Gutterman JU, Rodriguez V, Smith T, Hester JP. Developmental therapy in adult acute leukemia. Symposium on Leukemia. Arch Intern Med. 1976;136:1417–21.
36. Keating MJ, Smith TL, McCredie KB, Bodey GP, Hersh EM, Gutterman JU, Gehan E, Freireich EJ. A four-year experience with anthracycline, cytosine arabinoside, vincristine and prednisone combination chemotherapy in 325 adults with acute leukemia. Cancer. 1981;47:2779–88.
37. Keating MJ, McCredie KB, Bodey GP, Smith TL, Gehan E, Freireich EJ. Improved prospects for long-term survival in adults with acute myelogenous leukemia. J Am Med Assoc. 1982;248:2481–6.
38. Trujillo JM, Cork A, Ahearn MJ, Youness EL, McCredie KB. Hematologic and cytologic characterization of 8:21 translocation acute granulocytic leukemia. Blood. 1979;53:659.
39. Keating MJ, Cork A, Broach Y, Smith T, Walters RS, McCredie KB, Trujillo J, Freireich EJ. Toward a clinically relevant cytogenetic classification of acute myelogenous leukemia. Leukemia Res. 1987;11:119–33.
40. Ravandi F, Estey E, Jones D, Faderl S, et al. Effective treatment of acute promyelocytic leukemia with a trans-retinoic acid, arsenic trioxide, and gemtuzumab ozoga. J Clin Oncol. 2009;27(4):504–10.
41. Kantarjian H. Acute myeloid leukemia—major progress over four decades and glimpses into the future. Am J Hematol. 2016;91(1):131–45.
42. Thomas ED, Storb R, Clift RA, et al. Bone marrow transplantation: Part I. N Engl J Med. 1975;292:832–43.
43. Mathé G, Jammet H, Pendic B, et al. Transfusions et greffes de moelle osseuse homologue chez des humains irradiés à haute dos accidentellement. Rev Fr Etud Clin Biol. 1959;4:226–38.
44. Freireich E. Commentary on Thomas and Epstein: "Bone marrow transplantation in acute leukemia". Cancer Res. 2016;76(6):1301–2.
45. Freireich EJ, Wiernik PH, Steensma DP. The leukemias: a half-century of discovery. J Clin Oncol. 2014;32:3463–9.
46. Wiernik PH. Inching toward cure of acute myeloid leukemia: a summary of the progress made in the last 50 years. Med Oncol. 2014;8(136):31.

The Etiology of Acute Leukemia

12

J.N. Nichol, M. Kinal, and W.H. Miller Jr.

Introduction

Leukemia is a clonal disorder of deranged and disordered hematopoiesis that results from the acquisition of mutations in hematopoietic progenitors that confer a proliferative and/or survival advantage, and impair hematopoietic differentiation. In the case of acute myeloid leukemia (AML), these progenitors are from the myeloid lineage and for acute lymphocytic leukemia (ALL), these progenitors are from the lymphoid lineage (Fig. 12.1). Specifics concerning the clinical features and treatment of acute leukemia can be found elsewhere in this textbook. This chapter focuses on the molecular pathogenesis of acute leukemia.

Over a decade ago, Kelly and Gilliland [1] proposed a two-hit model for the development of AML, which is also applicable to the development of acute lymphoblastic leukemia ALL, whereby they hypothesize that these diseases emerge as a consequence of an association between at least two broad classes of mutations (Fig. 12.2). Class I, or activating, mutations typically result in the aberrant activation of signal transduction pathways and provide a proliferative and/or survival advantage to hematopoietic progenitors. Class II mutations arrest differentiation because of loss-of-function (LOF) mutations in key transcription factors or cofactors that are important for normal hematopoietic differentiation.

Cumulative evidence from different murine models of leukemia provides support for the necessity of cooperative transforming events for leukemogenesis. Induced mutations in these models result in increased self-renewal capacity and reduced differentiation, but are not sufficient to induce malignant transformation, and acute leukemia was not observed in mice until the mutations were combined with a dose of the chemical mutagenic agent, *N*-ethyl-*N*-nitrourea (ENU) [2–4].

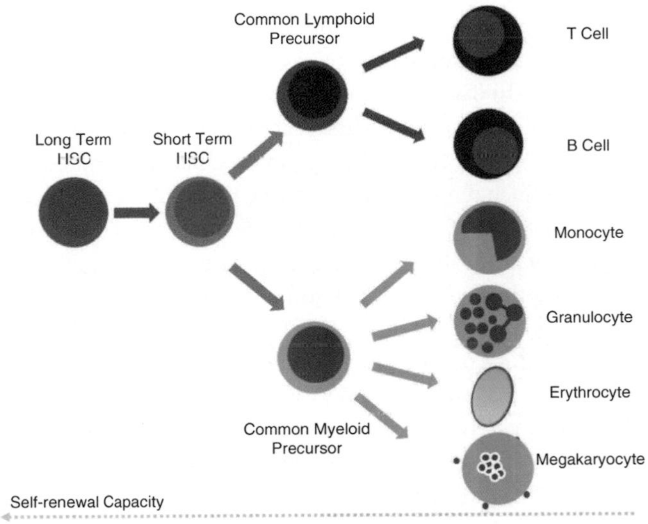

Fig. 12.1 *The hierarchy of hematopoietic development.* Long-term stem cells (HSCs) develop into different precursor cells, whose self-renewal capacity and developmental potential become progressively more restricted

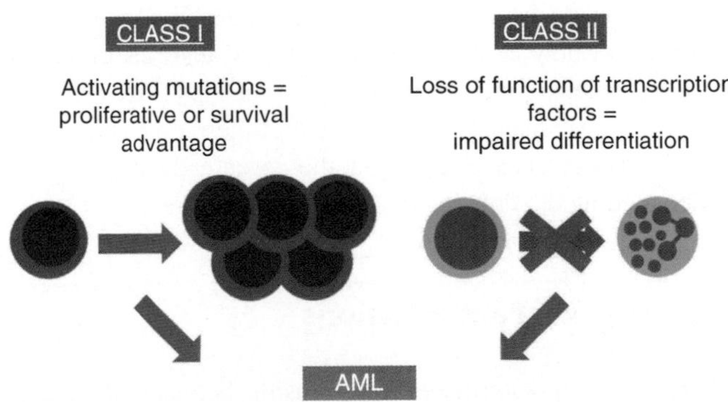

Fig. 12.2 *The two-hit model of acute leukemogenesis.* This model hypothesizes that AML and ALL are the consequence of a combination of at least two broad classes of mutations. Class I mutations involve an activating lesion in signaling pathways and confer a proliferative and/or survival advantage to hematopoietic cells. Class II mutations lead to an arrest of lymphoid or myeloid differentiation as a result of loss of function of transcription factors or cofactors that are important for normal hematopoietic differentiation

J.N. Nichol, Ph.D. (✉) • M. Kinal, M.Sc. • W.H. Miller Jr., M.D., Ph.D.
Segal Cancer Centre and Lady Davis Institute, Jewish General Hospital, Department of Oncology, McGill University, Montréal, QC, Canada, H3T 1E2
e-mail: jessica.nichol@mail.mcgill.ca; menakinal@gmail.com; wmiller@jgh.mcgill.ca

P.H. Wiernik et al. (eds.), *Neoplastic Diseases of the Blood*, DOI 10.1007/978-3-319-64263-5_12

A study of monozygotic twins who both developed ETV6/RUNX1-positive ALL [5] with identical chromosome breakpoints, but with different timelines, provides further support for the requirement of secondary genetic insults. Additionally, common leukemia- and lymphoma-associated genetic rearrangements are found in the peripheral blood of individuals with no history of either disease [6] and there are rare familial leukemia syndromes, involving germline *CEBPA* [7] and *RUNX1* mutations [8], where affected individuals exhibit an enhanced, but not guaranteed, risk of developing leukemia.

Over the past decade, technological advances have revolutionized our ability to interrogate cancer genomes, culminating in whole-genome sequencing (WGS), which provides genome-wide coverage at a single base-pair resolution. The information provided by these more sophisticated methods reveals that class I and II mutations are only one part of a more intricate framework. To date, the tumor genome has been sequenced in hundreds of cases of acute leukemia [9–14], and the latest numbers suggest that each AML genome contains hundreds of mutations, including anywhere between 5 and 23 coding mutations [14]. Most of these mutations are "background," or passenger mutations that were acquired during normal aging of hematopoietic stem cells, but some novel "driver" mutations have been discovered through WGS analysis [11]. Many of these mutations do not fit into either Class I or Class II, suggesting that the "two-hit model" is perhaps oversimplified [9]. Moreover, there is evidence that the sequence and timing of the aberrations during development may be important, suggesting that the cellular milieu in which the transcripts are expressed is relevant. This has been reported, for example, in acute promyelocytic leukemia (APL). The PML/RARA fusion protein in APL may occur at any point in the development of the myeloid cell, but is associated only with leukemia if the translocation occurs at an early stage, while expression of the fusion in late myeloid cells has little effect [15].

Based on the discoveries made by next-generation sequencing, we can now expand the initial two categories of genes relevant for leukemic pathogenesis into nine [9] (Fig. 12.3). In this review, we discuss in detail some of these nine categories and, in particular, we highlight the recent advances in the understanding of acute leukemia in the WGS era.

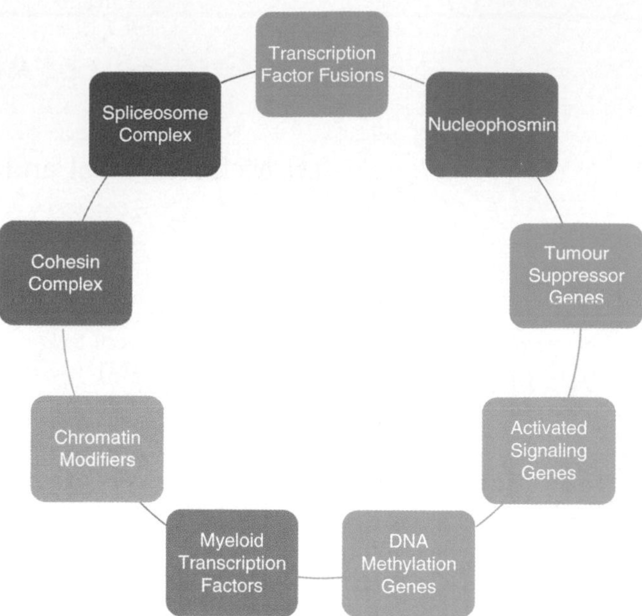

Fig. 12.3 *Functional categories of gene mutations in acute leukemia.* Genes found to be mutated via whole-genome sequencing of patient samples can be organized into nine categories based on related biological function

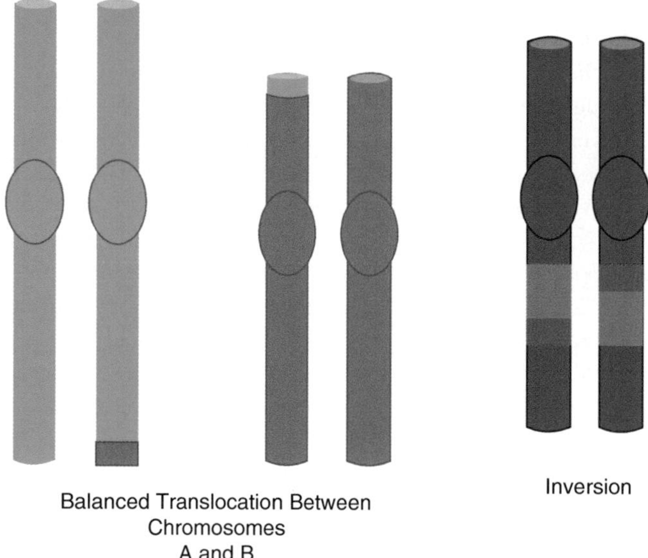

Fig. 12.4 *Structural chromosomal abnormalities.* A translocation arises when an exchange of chromosomal material takes place between two different chromosomes. If the translocation is balanced, the pieces of the chromosomes are rearranged but there is no loss or gain of genetic material (*left*). An inversion occurs when a segment of the chromosome is excised, rotated 180 degrees, and then reinserted into the same chromosome (*right*)

Transcription Factor Fusions

There is a long-established relationship between structural genomic aberrations, especially chromosome translocations and inversions, and acute leukemia. Specific cytogenetic abnormalities are often uniquely associated with clinically distinct subsets of the disease. Identifying the DNA sequences surrounding the chromosomal breakpoints has had an enormous impact on our understanding of leukemogenesis, carcinogenesis in general, and normal cellular functions of the protein products of the involved genes.

A chromosome translocation is a structural abnormality resulting from the exchange of pieces between two nonhomologous chromosomes. Reciprocal translocations are those in which there is no obvious overall loss of chromosomal material, and they probably result from a failure to properly repair DNA double-strand breaks (Fig. 12.4).

Several recurrent reciprocal translocations are frequently found in acute leukemia. Specific translocations are often consistently associated with specific subtypes of leukemia, providing strong support that they represent causal events during leukemogenesis in developing hematopoietic cells. For example, the t(15;17) is found only in patients with APL and not other forms of leukemia, while the t(1;19) is found only in the leukemic cells of patients with B-cell precursor acute lymphoblastic leukemia (ALL). However, there are exceptions to this phenomenon. For instance, the t(4;11) translocation occurs in patients with both AML and ALL. Chromosomal inversions are also seen in acute leukemia. An inversion occurs when a single chromosome undergoes breakage and rearrangement within itself (Fig. 12.4).

Identifying the genes disrupted by breakpoints in translocations and inversions provided the first mechanistic insights into understanding why chromosome abnormalities can be leukemogenic.

X/RARA

Acute promyelocytic leukemia (APL) is a subtype of acute myelogenous leukemia, representing 5–8% of AML cases in adults. At the genetic level, APL is characterized by a specific chromosomal rearrangement between the retinoic acid receptor alpha (*RARA*) on chromosome 17, and a number of partners. The majority of patients (98%) present with the 15;17 translocation, t(15;17), which results in a fusion of *RARA* with the promyelocytic leukemia (*PML*) gene on chromosome 15 [16, 17]. In normal cells, the retinoic acid receptors (RARs) heterodimerize with the retinoid X receptors (RXRs) to form a transcriptional complex. In the absence of ligand, all-trans retinoic acid (RA), a vitamin A derivative, the heterodimers are found bound, along with inhibitory co-repressor molecules, to the retinoic acid response elements (RAREs) of target genes. Treatment with ligand causes a release of the co-repressors and a concurrent recruitment of co-activators, leading to initiation of transcription of genes important for stimulating myeloid differentiation and regulating the cell cycle.

In APL cells, the prevailing view is that the leukemic effects of the resulting chimeric protein, X/RARA, are due to its function as a dominant negative inhibitor of normal retinoid receptor function. The chimera locates to promoters normally regulated by RARA, aberrantly recruits co-repressor proteins, and thereby inhibits the RARA-mediated gene expression. Therapeutic doses of RA can circumvent the differentiation block [18].

To date, eight different chromosomal translocation partners have been identified in patients with APL [19–26] (Fig. 12.5), and, as mentioned above, all involve the *RARA* gene on chromosome 17q21. The N-terminal fractions contributed by the fusion partners donate additional dimerization domains. These acquired dimerization domains, together with the DNA-binding domain of RARA, are required for the oncogenic effect of the fusion proteins and promote formation of chimeric receptor homodimers and provide additional co-repressor binding domains. The resulting X/RARA fusion proteins have been shown to recruit the HDAC, NCOR1 and NCOR2 (NCoR) complex, DNMT1, DNMT3A, repressive histone methyl-transferases, and polycomb group proteins.

However, disruption of the normal RARA signaling pathway does not solely account for the pathogenesis of APL. As mentioned previously, the differentiation block mediated by the X/RARAs is necessary, but not sufficient to cause APL. This suggests that a second transformative event is required for full neoplastic development. Mutations in oncogenes such as *FLT3* can cooperate with the fusions to provide the second hit necessary to generate leukemia. The presence of these second mutations might also explain why APL cannot be cured by differentiation therapy with ATRA alone, but is highly curable by combinations of ATRA and cytotoxic chemotherapy. Additionally, some translocations generate the reciprocal *RARA/X* fusion genes which can result in the co-expression of their transcripts in leukemic blasts [27–29]. Important roles in oncogenesis are now being identified for the co-expressed RARA/X reciprocal fusion proteins [27, 28, 30, 31]. Additionally, the partner proteins in APL have important growth-regulatory roles in normal myeloid cells. It may

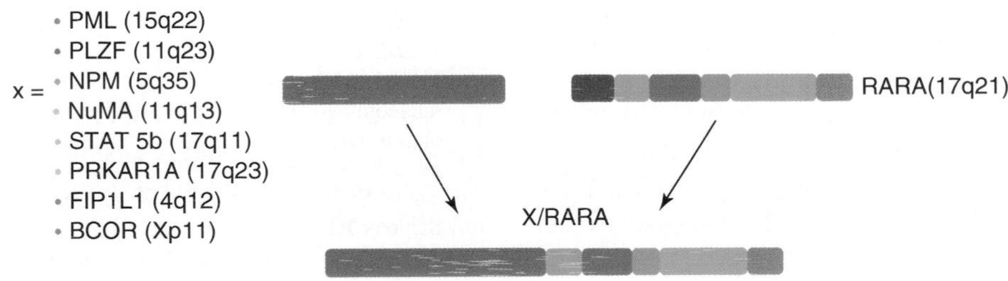

Fig. 12.5 *Identified chromosomal translocations associated with APL.* Acute promyelocytic leukemia (APL) is the result of chromosomal rearrangements in which part of the retinoic acid receptor alpha (*RARA*) gene is linked to the amino-terminal domains of eight genes (*X*) that encode different nuclear proteins. All of the translocations produce a chimeric protein (X/RARA) that disrupts the normal function of RARA and arrests the maturation of myeloid cells at the promyelocyte stage. The most common translocation, t(15;17), involves a break in chromosome 15 and disrupts the promyelocytic leukemia (*PML*) gene, producing the *PML/RARA* fusion

be that the loss of one allele of the partner protein combined with the effects of the X/RARA or reciprocal RARA/X fusion protein, which compromises normal partner protein function, contributes to the development of leukemia.

Core Binding Factor Rearrangements

Core binding factor (CBF) leukemias refer to a subset of AML bearing t(8;21)(q22;q22), which generates the RUNX1/CBFA2T1 fusion protein (previously known as AML1/ETO) and inv.(16)(p13q22), which generates the CBFB/MYH11 fusion protein. These genomic rearrangements are characterized by disruption of the *RUNX1* gene at 21q22 and the *CBFbeta (CBFB)* gene at 16q22, respectively. These are two of the most prevalent cytogenetic subtypes of AML.

Native RUNX1 and CBFB form a heterodimeric transcription factor [32] which regulates the transcription of genes required for the development of definitive hematopoiesis, including macrophage colony-stimulating factor (CSF) receptor [33], granulocyte-macrophage CSF [34], myeloperoxidase [35], and interleukin-3 [36].

RUNX1/CBFA2T1

The chromosomal translocation t(8;21) fuses the DNA-binding runt domain from RUNX1 (previously known as AML1) to almost the entirety of the CBFA2T1 (previously known as ETO) repressor protein [37]. The t(8;21)(q22;q22) translocation is present in 10–15% of AML cases and is associated with the M2 subtype of AML. Expression of the resulting fusion protein, RUNX1/CBFA2T1, in mouse models induces a pre-leukemic state, but requires cooperating mutations for full leukemogenesis [38–41]. An early hypothesis for the pathogenic role of RUNX1/CBFA2T1, postulating that it functions as a transcriptional repressor, was dervied from models based on the archetypal leukemiaassociated transcription factor, PML/RARA, and are supposrted by several lines of evidence:

1. Repression by RUNX1/CBFA2T1 is mediated by the CBFA2T1 moiety, which recruits co-repressors, such as HDACs 1–3, NCoR, SMRT, and mSin3A [42–44], and produces the secondary effect of altering the chromatin structure of target promoters.
2. RUNX1/CBFA2T1 binds to the promoters of tumor-suppressor genes which are normally activated by RUNX1, such as $p14^{ARF}$ [45] and CCAAT/enhancer-binding protein alpha (C/EBPA) [46], and represses their transcriptional activation.
3. Treatment of t(8;21)-positive AML cell lines with HDACis [47] and DNMT inhibitors relieves the repressive effects of RUNX1/CBFA2T1 on chromatin, gene expression, and cell differentiation [48].

However, evidence has suggested that the model of RUNX1/CBFA2T1's leukemogenic effect through repressive transcriptional activity needs to be broadened. Microarray data shows that RUNX1/CBFA2T1 activates as many genes as it represses, including genes not normally under the control of wild-type RUNX1. Many of the genes upregulated by RUNX1/CBFA2T1, for example *JAG1* [49], play a role in promoting stem cell renewal. Furthermore, RUNX1/CBFA2T1 is a potent transcriptional activator of the anti-apoptotic *BCL2* gene [50]. Thus RUNX1/CBFA2T1 expression may result in leukemia by two opposing effects on transcription: by simultaneously repressing tumor-suppressor genes while upregulating genes that drive expansion or prolong the survival of t(8;21) early multipotent progenitors.

Furthermore, researchers have identified, in patients, a spliced isoform of the RUNX1/CBFA2T1 fusion protein, called AE9a, which is coexpressed with the full-length fusion and is capable of inducing leukemia in a murine transduction/transplantation model [51]. High levels of AE9a in patients are associated with poor disease outcome [52] and it was recently demonstrated that binding of AE9a to CBFB, leading to dysregulation of Notch target genes, is necessary for AML initiation [53].

Finally, an alternative explanation for the pathogenesis of t(8,21) acute myeloid leukemia is the loss of function of lineage-program-transcription factors [54]. These transcription factors strictly control gene expression during hematopoiesis, and instruct a precursor cell to commit to a certain differentiation program by initiating expression of a characteristic set of lineage-specific target genes in response to diverse signals [55]. There are four central hematopoietic transcription factors that are functionally repressed by RUNX1/CBFA2T1 through protein-protein interactions: PU.1 [56], CEBPA [57], GATA-1 [58], and the E proteins [59]. These inhibitory interactions with RUNX1/CBF2AT1 may expand stem cell pools by promoting stem cell renewal and blocking commitment to the various lineages. The expanded stem cell pool may then be primed for leukemic transformation through acquisition of additional mutations. The development of these secondary mutations is again facilitated by RUNX1/CBFA2T1 expression through the fusion protein's ability to repress DNA repair genes [49].

CBFB/MYH11

Inversion of chromosome 16, inv.(16), or the related t(16;16) is associated with the M4Eo subtype of AML, and results in the fusion of *CBFB* with *MYH11*, the gene encoding smooth-muscle myosin heavy chain. The resulting fusion protein CBFB/MYH11 is composed of the heterodimerization domain of CBFB fused to the C-terminal coiled-coil domain from MYH11. Studies suggest that CBFB/MYH11 has a higher affinity for RUNX1 than wild-type CBFB [60], and at the molecular level, CBFB/MYH11 has been suggested to alter the normal transcription program by several mechanisms. These include the tethering of RUNX1 outside the nucleus [61, 62], recruitment of HDACs/co-repressors [63, 64], and inhibiting RUNX1 activity [65]. However, most of these studies were based on in vitro and overexpression experiments.

Furthermore, there are data suggesting that CBFB/MYH11 has activities independent of RUNX1/CBFB repression. CBFB/MYH11 expression has been shown to reduce levels of CEBPA protein, which is crucial for normal granulopoiesis, without affecting mRNA levels, but rather by the translational inhibition of CEBPA [66]. Additionally, microarray analyses have determined that CBFB/MYH11 expression results in a significant upregulation of many genes, including those involved in DNA replication, cell cycle regulation, and proliferation [67], again indicating that CBFB/MYH11 has RUNX1/CBFB repression-independent activities that may contribute to leukemogenesis.

CBFB/MYH11 rearrangements co-occur with RAS gene, or RAS-regulating gene mutations that lead to RAS pathway activation, in more than 90% of CBFB/MYH11 patients, indicating that changes to this pathway play an important role in AML pathogenesis [68]. In addition to RAS genes, whole-genome and whole-exome sequencing analysis of adult and pediatric leukemia samples identified recurrent stabilizing mutations in *CCND2* [69], the gene encoding cyclin D2. All the mutations surrounded the codon for a conserved phosphorylation site (Thr280) that regulates ubiquitination of Lys270 and degradation by the proteasome [70]. The mutations led to increased stability of the CCND2 protein [69] and suggest that stabilization of CCND2 is a previously unidentified and potentially targetable mutation in CBF-AML.

BCR/ABL

The BCR/ABL gene fusion is the result of the t(9;22), and although present in approximately 20% of B-ALL cases is most often associated with chronic myelogenous leukemia (CML). The translocation generates the BCR-ABL fusion protein, in which the N-terminal domains of BCR are combined with almost the entirety of ABL, a nonreceptor tyrosine kinase, whose activity is tightly regulated in normal cells. The oligomerization domain contributed by BCR constitutively activates ABL tyrosine kinase activity and is essential for BCR-ABL transformation.

Depending on the site of the breakpoint in the *BCR* gene, the fusion protein can vary in size from 190 to 230 kDa. Each fusion protein contains the same portion of the ABL protein but differs in the length of the BCR portion. In two-thirds of ALL cases with BCR/ABL, the breakpoint in *BCR* occurs in the region known as the minor-breakpoint cluster region (m-bcr), resulting in a fusion protein of 190 kDa (p190). In CML, however, the *BCR* breakpoint occurs further upstream, in a region referred to as the major breakpoint cluster region (M-bcr), resulting in a protein of 210 kDa (p210). A constitutively active ABL is produced by both the p190 and p210 fusion. Due to the well-characterized mechanisms of BCR/ABL oncogenicity in CML, this fusion will not be discussed further in this chapter and readers are instead directed to other chapters within this textbook which deal specifically with CML.

ETV6/RUNX1

The t(12;21) translocation is the most common genetic lesion in pediatric ALL [71], occurring in 17% of patients. The translocation generates a fusion between *ETV6* and *RUNX1* and occurs prior to the onset of immunoglobulin gene rearrangement, giving rise to leukemic blasts that appear to be blocked at the pre-B stage [72]. As noted in the introduction to this chapter, evidence from twin studies has demonstrated that the *ETV6/RUNX1* fusion is most likely an initiating event in ALL, but expression of the fusion alone is insufficient to cause leukemia. Most cases of ETV6/RUNX1 also have deletions in the wild-type *ETV6* allele [73], and mutations in *PAX5* [74, 75].

The fusion gene encodes a chimeric protein that contains the helix–loop–helix domain of the ETV6 transcription factor fused to nearly all RUNX1. The molecular mechanisms underlying ETV6/RUNX1-induced leukemogenesis remain poorly understood; however, there are some commonalities with the other fusions previously discussed, with ETV6/RUNX1 seemingly to inhibit wild-type RUNX1 transcriptional activity through the aberrant recruitment of HDACs and other transcriptional co-repressors [76, 77].

E2A Fusions

B-cell commitment and development require the sequential action of transcription factors positioned within a hierarchical network and which activate or repress genes to specify the B-cell-specific transcriptome. The *TCF3* gene encodes two basic helix–loop–helix (bHLH) transcription factors, E12 and E47, through alternative splicing and both of these proteins play an indispensable role in the earliest defined stages of B lineage development [78, 79]. Known collectively as the E2A proteins, E12 and E47 form heterodimers with other bHLH proteins and bind to the regulatory regions of many genes expressed in early- and late-stage B cells [80–82]. In common lymphoid progenitors, E2A lies in the middle of the transcription factor hierarchy. E2A expression is induced by the macrophage and B-cell-specific transcription factor and E2A itself then stimulates expression of *EBF1* [83]. EBF1, in turn, remodels the promoter region and thereby activates the expression of *PAX5* [84], which definitively commits lymphoid progenitors to the B-cell pathway. Data from E2A-deficient cells substantiate the pivotal role of E2A in B-cell commitment; E2A$^{-/-}$ cells possess stem-cell-like properties, including promiscuous expression of genes that are normally associated with non-B-cell lineages.

Approximately 5% of all B-lineage ALLs and 25% of cases with a pre-B phenotype possess the E2A-PBX1 chimera. This translocation fuses the transactivation domain of E2A to the majority of the homeobox protein, PBX1, including its DNA-binding domain. While it is speculated that the E2A/PBX1 chimera blocks differentiation of B cells, no leukemic property of E2A/PBX1 has been identified in pre-B cells. It is possible, considering the central role of E2A in the B-cell transcription cascade, that the E2A/PBX1 oncoproteins may act via a dominant-negative mechanism in which they sequester coactivators, thereby disrupting the function of endogenous E2A proteins. Additionally, the fact that the E2A/PBX1 fusions found in human pre-B acute lymphoblastic leukemia all contain the PBX1 DNA-binding domain suggests that direct gene targeting by E2A-PBX1 is critical for the development of ALL.

Nucleophosmin

Mutations in *NPM1* represent the most common genetic change in adult patients with cytogenetically normal AML, and are seen in approximately 35% of cases [85, 86]. The latest WHO classification of AML recognizes AML with *NPM1* mutations as its own separate category [biological and clinical consequences of NPM1 mutations in AML (2017), 2]. *NPM1* mutation, when present alone, is associated with a more favorable outcome, and when co-expressed with *FLT3-ITD*, it is associated with an improved clinical outcome over *FLT3-ITD* mutations alone [87]. Interestingly, *FLT3-ITD* is about twice as frequent in *NPM1*-mutated AML compared to *NPM1* wild-type AML, which may suggest a mechanistic link between these two mutations [85, 86, 88–92]. Recently, whole-genome or whole-exome sequencing of the genomes of 200 adult cases of de novo AML revealed that the most prominent co-occurring mutations in AML are *NPM1, FLT3*, and *DNMT3A* and the combination of the three mutations is associated with extensive loss of DNA methylation, occurring mostly in coding regions. This observation, along with the fact that this co-occurrence occurs at higher frequency than expected by chance, suggests that harboring mutations in all three genes represents a novel subtype of AML [9]. In AML where all three mutations are present, evidence has shown that the *DNMT3A* mutation occurs first, then *NPM1*, and lastly *FLT3* [93, 94]. *NPM1* mutations are usually stable throughout disease and disappear with remission; therefore these could potentially be used to monitor residual disease, or to detect relapse [88, 91, 95].

The protein product of *NPM1*, nucleophosmin (NPM), is normally an abundant, ubiquitous, and highly conserved phosphoprotein that resides primarily in the nucleolus, although it shuttles rapidly between the nucleus and cytoplasm. By shuttling between these subcellular compartments, NPM plays a role in diverse processes including the regulation of centrosome duplication, transport of preribosomal particles and ribosome biogenesis, maintenance of genomic stability, participation in DNA repair processes, and regulation of DNA transcription (reviewed in [92]). In addition, within the nucleolus, NPM has been demonstrated to bind the important tumor suppressor, p53, and to its regulatory proteins, including ARF [96, 97]. The numerous functional domains of NPM (Fig. 12.6) account for its diverse biochemical functions in both cellular proliferation and growth suppression.

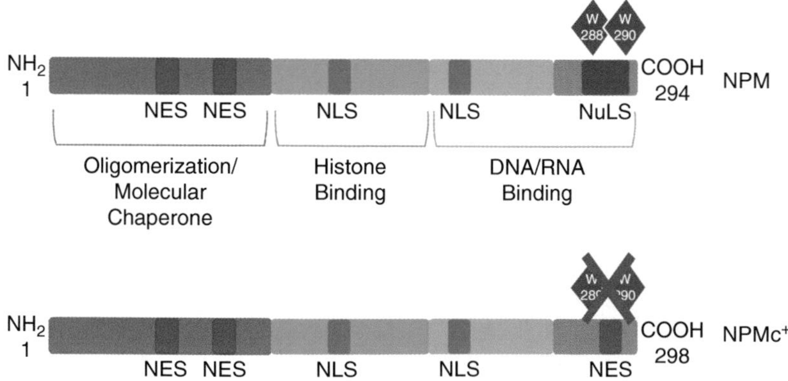

Fig. 12.6 *The functional domains and motifs of wild-type and mutant nucleophosmin.* Wild-type nucleophosmin (NPM, top panel) consists of 294 amino acids that can be subdivided into various functional domains. The cellular localization of NPM1 is dictated by three functional motifs: (1) two leucine-rich nuclear export signals (NES) located in the N-terminal domain (oligomerization domain), (2) a classic bipartite nuclear localization signal (NLS, residues 152–157 and 190–197), and (3) a C-terminal nucleolar localization signal (NuLS) containing two tryptophan residues (W288, W290) which are critical for its nucleolar localization. The mutated NPM1 protein (NPMc$^+$, bottom panel) in AML acquires a new NES at the C-terminus and loses at least one of the two tryptophans in the NuLS. Both alterations are responsible for the exclusion of NPMc$^+$ from the nucleus and its aberrant accumulation in the cytoplasm

In AML, the most common mutations of *NPM1* involve the insertion of four base pairs at the C-terminal portion of the protein. These mutations are unique to AML, and are not seen in other cancers where NPM is usually upregulated through genetic translocations [98]. The C-terminal mutations are usually heterozygous and result in an inability of the protein to perform its usual nuclear-cytoplasmic shuttling function. The cytoplasmic mutant (NPM^{c+}) has been isolated from leukemic blasts [85].

It has been shown that NPM^{c+} relocalizes ARF to the cytoplasm, thus inhibiting its functional interaction with the p53-negative regulator, MDM2, and blunting ARF-induced activation of the p53 transcriptional program. Despite this, the inactivation of ARF by NPM^{c+} is insufficient to cause oncogenesis [97]. This may be because of its dual role as an inactivator of ARF, and an inducer of cellular senescence, as discovered in experiments where NPM^{c+} is overexpressed in fibroblasts [99]. A transgenic mouse model of AML with NPM^{c+} has been generated by placing NPM^{c+} under the human myeloid-specific *MRP8* promoter. In this experimental setting, the cytoplasmic mutation of NPM induces myeloproliferation of mature monocytes and granulocytes but does not induce a maturation arrest [100]. Finally, data from in vitro, cell-free experiments using recombinant NPM^{c+}, patient NPM^{c+}, and leukemia cell lines show that NPM^{c+} reduces apoptosis through an inhibition of caspase-6 and -8 signaling, and inhibits myeloid differentiation also through a caspase-mediated process. Identifying this myeloid-specific function for NPM^{c+} may explain why this mutant is uniquely found in AML [101].

Similar to the model of cytoplasmic ARF sequestration, the NPM1^{c+} mutation causes delocalization of the F-box protein, Fbw7γ, to the cytoplasm, which accelerates this protein's degradation. As Fbw7γ regulates the turnover of MYC, expression of NPM^{c+} ultimately leads to MYC stabilization [102]. MYC overexpression favors myeloid leukemogenesis in mouse models [103]; therefore the resulting elevated MYC expression might also contribute to leukemogenesis in the NPM^{c+} AMLs.

Finally, in the context of wild-type *NPM1* in acute leukemia, a novel function for NPM as a negative regulator of retinoic acid (RA)-induced gene regulation and differentiation toward granulocytes was recently uncovered. In stable RA-resistant acute leukemia cells, NPM is highly overexpressed and resistance is driven by an aberrant association with a putative co-repressor complex containing wild-type NPM and topoisomerase II beta (TOP2B) leading to recruitment of the chromatin remodeler BRG1 to RA-target genes [104].

Activated Signaling

Mutations in proteins involved in cell signaling transduction pathways typically result in the aberrant activation of these pathways, and provide a proliferative and/or survival advantage to hematopoietic progenitors.

FLT3

FLT3 (FMS-like tyrosine kinase 3) is a transmembrane receptor tyrosine kinase that belongs to the same family, the type III receptor tyrosine kinases (RTKs), as FMS, KIT, and platelet-derived growth factor receptors (PDGFRs) [105–108]. The structure of type III RTKs consists of five extracellular immunoglobulin-like domains, a transmembrane and juxtamembrane domain, and an intracellular kinase domain [109].

FLT3 has been found to be mutated in 25% of all AML, and to be overexpressed in some cases of B- and T-cell precursor ALL [110]. In AML, the recurrent mutations include in-frame internal tandem duplication (ITD) of the transmembrane domain in 95% of cases, and a tyrosine kinase domain (TKD) mutation at aspartic acid residue 835 in the remainder [111]. Other transmembrane and kinase domain mutations have been reported at a much lower frequency. For patients with AML with normal cytogenetics, the presence of an FLT3-ITD mutation is associated with a poorer response to therapy and poorer overall survival [87]. It is less clear whether TKD mutations are associated with a poor outcome (reviewed in [111]).

In normal hematopoiesis, binding of FLT3 ligand to FLT3 results in dimerization of the receptor and its activation. In combination with other growth factors, activation of FLT3 results in expansion of the hematopoietic stem/progenitor cells in vitro. For all but dendritic cells, once hematopoietic cells differentiate, the expression of FLT3 is lost [112, 113]. The proliferative role of FLT3 is further supported by knockout mouse models of FLT3 or FLT3 ligand. These mice have a normal life expectancy but show subtle deficits in hematopoietic cells, including a reduction in the number of B progenitor cells, NK cells, and dendritic cells, and reconstitute lethally irradiated mice with only 25% of the efficiency of bone marrow from wild-type mice [114, 115]. Thus, although FLT3 contributes to hematopoietic proliferation, its function is not essential.

In AML, there is constitutive activation of FLT3 due to either interference with the negative regulatory function of the juxtamembrane region with ITD mutations or changes in the activation loop with TKD mutations [116]. As a result, there is autophosphorylation and direct or indirect phosphorylation of several proteins that in turn activate the PI-3-kinase/AKT, RAS/MAPK, and STAT5 pathways, ultimately inducing cellular proliferation, and inhibiting apoptosis (reviewed in [117]).

It is postulated that FLT3 mutations allow for unrestricted growth of the leukemia stem cells. In support of this hypothesis, it has been shown that retroviral transfection of primary murine bone marrow cells with human AML *FLT3* mutation does not cause leukemia, but rather results in an oligoclonal myeloproliferative disease manifested by splenomegaly and leukocytosis [118]. Full development of leukemia occurs when *FLT3-ITD* mutations are combined with other genetic alterations known to inhibit hematopoietic differentiation, including PML/RARA, NUP98/HOX, RUNX1/CBFA2, MLL/ENL, and MLL/SEPT6 (reviewed in [117]).

Finally, isolation of a stem cell-enriched fraction from patients with FLT3-ITD AML and subsequent injection of these primary cells into NOD/SCID mice resulted in leukemogenesis with identical FLT3-ITD mutations [119]. These data imply that FLT3-ITD mutations occur at the level of the leukemia stem cell (LSC). However, other clinical evidence suggests that the *FLT3* mutation may occur in a subclone of the LSC, including the finding that in the context of relapsed AML, there is loss of the ITD mutation 16% of the time and loss of the TKD mutation 50% of the time [120, 121].

KIT

Human KIT is located on chromosome 4 and encodes a 145 kD transmembrane glycoprotein. Like FLT3, KIT is a member of the type III RTK family [122]. The kinase activity of KIT is tightly regulated by its ligand, stem cell factor (SCF) [123–125]. SCF binding promotes KIT dimerization and transphosphorylation of KIT at specific tyrosine residues that can serve as docking sites for src-homology-2 (SH2) domain-containing signaling and adaptor proteins [108]. KIT signal transduction plays an important role in the proliferation, differentiation, migration, and survival of hematopoietic stem cells, as well as mast cells, neural crest-derived melanocytes, and germ cells [126].

Point mutations in KIT have been identified in AML. Some of the mutations localize within exon 8 [127] and result in hyperactivation of the receptor in response to SCF [128]. Other KIT mutations cluster within exon 17, which encodes the KIT activation loop in the kinase domain [129]. These mutations lead to ligand-independent activation of the kinase domain. KIT mutations are also found in other human malignancies, such as gastrointestinal stromal tumors [130], mastocytosis [131], and germ cell tumors [132].

KIT mutations are observed mostly in association with CBF-AML [133, 134]. It may be that the KIT mutations in this subset of AML provide the myeloid blasts with the necessary extra hit by conferring a proliferative and/or survival advantage, because, as discussed previously, the chimeric transcription factor blocks differentiation, but has a limited effect on cellular proliferation [38–41].

The prognostic significance of KIT mutations in CBF-AML is uncertain [135–138]. A recent meta-analysis evaluating the impact of *KIT* mutations on the prognosis of CBF-AML found that *KIT* mutations had no effect on complete remission (CR) rates, but they resulted in a significantly increased relapse risk [139].

Myeloid Transcription Factors

Hematopoietic stem cells (HSCs) are pluripotent stem cells that give rise to all the circulating blood cell types. They are defined by their ability to self-renew while generating differentiated daughter cells [140]. The maturation of HSCs into blood cells has been suggested to follow a hierarchical model, in which the stem cells undergo a reduction in self-renewal potential while simultaneously gaining functional specialization [141]. Several key transcription factors (TFs) maintain HSC self-renewal, whereas others specify differentiated hematopoietic lineages. As discussed earlier, chromosomal translocations that disrupt the normal functioning of these essential TFs are one way that hematopoiesis becomes deregulated. However, beyond fusions involving these transcription factors, mutations altering their functions have also been uncovered with new sequencing technologies [9, 75].

CCAAT-Enhancer-Binding Protein Alpha (CEBPA)

CEBPA is a tumor-suppressor gene that encodes a transcription factor associated with inhibiting cell proliferation. Mutations in this gene have been reported in 7–16% of AML patients, with a close to equal distribution of patients with either a single- or a double-*CEBPA* mutation. AML patients with a *CEBPA* mutation have improved prognosis versus wild-type patients, and those with a double mutation have better overall survival compared to those with a single mutation. Of note, this improvement in survival is lost if there is a co-occurring FLT3-ITD mutation [87, 142–148].

Mutations in *CEBPA* can occur across the whole coding region; however, two clusterings of mutation hot spots have been identified. The more common N-terminal mutations increase the use of an alternative initiation codon that then leads to the formation of a short p30 isoform, which inhibits the function of the full-length protein by a dominant negative mechanism [145]. C-terminal mutations are generally in-frame insertions/deletions in the DNA-binding or basic leucine zipper domains that disrupt binding to DNA or dimerization. The less frequent C-terminal mutations are generally in-frame insertions/deletions that prevent CEBPA DNA binding via alteration of the protein's basic-leucine zipper (bZIP) domain [149].

Recently, whole-exome sequencing detected a high frequency of *CEBPA* mutations in a subtype of AML, acute erythroid leukemia (AEL) [150]. Significantly, the biallelic *CEBPA* mutations co-occur with *GATA2* mutations. GATA2 is a transcription factor that is crucial for hematopoietic development. Considering the prominent expression of GATA2 and CEBPA in early hematopoietic progenitor cells and the direct protein-protein interaction between GATA2 and CEBPA proteins, further studies are needed to clarify whether and how mutations of both genes contribute to the pathogenesis of AEL [151].

Paired Box Protein 5 (PAX5)

B-progenitor acute lymphoblastic leukemia (B-ALL) is a common pediatric malignancy. A genome-wide analysis of leukemic cells from B-ALL patients using high-resolution single-nucleotide polymorphism arrays and DNA sequencing was performed to identify cooperating oncogenic lesions in this disease. *PAX5* was found to be the most frequent target of somatic mutations, with lesions found in ~30% of the cases analyzed [75]. PAX5 is the essential regulator of B-cell identity and function. Consistent with this view, *PAX5*-deficient pro-B cells, unlike their wild-type counterparts, exhibit promiscuous gene expression and a lack of lineage commitment [152]. Additionally, *PAX5*$^{-/-}$ pro-B cells have the capacity to differentiate into a variety of non-B-cell lineages, including functional macrophages, osteoclasts, dendritic cells, granulocytes, and natural killer cells, when stimulated with the appropriate cytokines [152]. Similarly, in mice, the absence of PAX5 results in the arrest of B-cell development at a pro-B-cell-like stage [153].

The *PAX5* gene encodes a 52 kDa transcription factor, expressed within the hematopoietic system exclusively in the B-lymphoid lineage. By recognizing DNA through the highly conserved paired domain characteristic of the PAX family of transcription factors [154], PAX5 functions both as a transcriptional activator and a repressor. PAX5 activates expression of B-lineage-specific genes such as *CD19* [155], *BLK* [156], and *CD72* [157] while concurrently repressing lineage-inappropriate genes such as *NOTCH1* [158], *M-CSFR* [152], and *FLT3* [159].

The overall effect of the *PAX5* alterations seen in B-ALL is to reduce or inhibit the level of normal PAX5 functional activity, either because of monoallelic deletions or the generation of altered forms of the PAX5 protein [75]. In the context of leukemogenesis, it is important to note that during the normal development of B cells, *PAX5* is subjected to allele-specific regulation, being predominantly transcribed from only one allele in early progenitors and then switched to a biallelic transcription mode as B cells begin to differentiate [160]. It is tempting to speculate that this allelic type of regulation has been imposed because the levels of PAX5 need to be finely tuned, as subtle decreases or increases may dramatically modify B-cell development. Therefore, the loss of wild-type *PAX5* allele due to the identified mutations would eliminate the possibility to turn on normal biallelic transcription, which may directly contribute to the arrest in differentiation arrest seen in ALL [75].

Chromatin Modifiers

Epigenetic information is deposited by "writer" proteins, such as histone methyl lysine and arginine transferases; removed by "eraser" proteins, such as histone deacetylases and demethylases; and decoded by "reader" proteins adapted to bind to chromatin marks using specific structures such as chromo, bromo, and PHD domains [161]. Together, these "chromatin modifiers" help to integrate signals that lead to meaningful changes in gene expression. Several alterations in chromatin modifiers, such as the "readers" ASXL1 [162–164]; the "writers" NSD1 [165, 166], MLL [167, 168], and EZH2 [169, 170]; and the "eraser" KDM6A [171], repeatedly occur in acute leukemia.

MLL Fusions and MLL-PTD

The MLL (mixed-lineage leukemia) gene is located on chromosome 11q23, and fusions involving this gene are seen in both de novo and therapy-related acute myeloid and lymphoid leukemia. MLL is a large DNA-binding protein ubiquitously expressed in hematopoietic cells, including stem and progenitor populations. Using chromatin immunoprecipitation (ChIP) analysis, MLL has been found to be associated with a subset of transcriptionally active human promoters [172, 173] and with RNA polymerase II, suggesting that MLL has a specific role in the regulation of transcription. A SET domain is located at the carboxy-terminal of MLL, and this domain mediates methylation of histone H3 lysine 4 (H3K4), a histone modification which is associated with transcription at active gene loci [174]. Importantly, in mammals, MLL positively regulates the expression of the homeobox (*HOX*) genes. *HOX* genes are transcription factors that participate in the development of multiple tissues, including the hematopoietic system.

Some of the roughly 50 characterized MLL fusion partners (FPs) can be grouped into families based on cellular localization and function (Table 12.1) [175, 176]. All identified MLL fusions contain the first 8–13 exons of *MLL* and a variable number of exons from the FP gene. Furthermore, another type of *MLL* rearrangement, *MLL-PTD* (partial tandem duplication), is a result of internal tandem duplication of select exons. MLL mutant proteins are always in-frame chimeras that reside in the nucleus, regardless of whether the fusion partner is normally nuclear or cytoplasmic in origin. Despite the large number and functional diversity of the fusion partners, there are some common principles that can be applied to all MLL fusions [175]. First, all MLL fusions retain its amino-terminal domains required for the association of MLL with chromatin, so the fusion proteins are still able to bind DNA. Second, expression of the amino-terminal region of MLL (the region retained in MLL fusions) alone

Table 12.1 Classification of MLL fusion partners

Group	MLL fusion partner	Location	Function
1	**AF4**, **AF9**, **AF10**, **ENL**, **ell**	Nuclear	Putative DNA-binding proteins
2	CBP, p300	Nuclear	Histone acetyltransferases
3	AF1P, **AF6**, AFX, EEN, EPS15, GAS7, LARG	Cytoplasm	Presence of coiled-coil oligomerization domain
4	SEPT2, SEPT5, SEPT6, SEPT9, SEPT11	Cytoplasm	Septin family, interact with cytoskeletal filaments, have a role in mitosis
5	N/A	N/A	MLL partial tandem duplication of exons 5–11 (MLL/PTD)

There are more than 50 known MLL partners; therefore this table is not an exhaustive compilation. The six most common fusion partners are highlighted in bold. *N/A* not applicable

does not lead to myeloid transformation [177], indicating that the fusion partners make critical contributions to the oncogenicity of MLL fusions [178]. Third, MLL fusion proteins enforce continuous expression of the *HOX* genes, *HOXA9* and *MEIS1*, which are normally downregulated during hematopoietic differentiation. This sustained induction appears to be critical for leukemogenesis, since forced expression of *HOXA9* and *MEIS1*, in the absence of an MLL fusion, immortalizes hematopoietic progenitors in vitro and results in AML development in transplanted mice [179, 180].

MLL fusions are hypothesized to disrupt normal gene expression patterns, especially those of the *HOX* genes, maintained by wild-type MLL. However, discerning one unifying mechanism of leukemogenesis by MLL fusion proteins is difficult due to the heterogeneity of the MLL fusion partners. The putative mechanisms of MLL fusion-induced transformation may be more easily characterized by dividing the fusion partners into two broad classes based on their normal cellular localization (either nuclear or cytoplasmic). The fusion partners that are nuclear have been associated with various aspects of transcriptional regulation. Therefore, the fusions involving these proteins may lead to transcriptional deregulation of the *HOX* genes through alterations in the histone modification pattern and chromatin structure. An early insight into this possibility was provided by the characterization of the nuclear MLL/CREBBP fusion [181]. CREBBP (also known as CBP) is a well-characterized global transcriptional activator with intrinsic histone acetyltransferase (HAT) activity. Structure–function analysis demonstrated that inclusion of the portion of CREBBP that contains its HAT domain in the fusion is required for full in vitro transformation and is sufficient to induce the leukemic phenotype in vivo [182]. These data suggest that the leukemic effect of MLL/CREBBP results from the combination of the chromatin association and modifying activities of CREBBP with the DNA-binding activities of MLL. Additionally, although the SET domain, which mediates MLL's H3K4 methyltransferase activity, is consistently lost in all the MLL fusions, several MLL fusion partners, for example AF4, AF9, AF10, and ENL [183], associate with the DOT1L histone methyltransferase that methylates lysine 79 residues in histone H3 (H3K79). Methylation of H3K79 is also associated with positive transcriptional regulation [184]. As different methylation marks may positively control transcription in unique ways [185], the replacement of H3K4 activity in wild-type MLL with H3K79 activity in the MLL fusion complex could perturb transcriptional control. In the case of the MLL-PTD, where the SET domain is maintained, the characterization of a mouse model of *MLL-PTD* demonstrated that MLL-PTD facilitates histone H3K4 trimethylation as well as H3/H4 acetylation within target *HOX* gene promoters [186]. This provides further evidence for an epigenetic mechanism as the underlying cause of *HOX* overexpression.

Some MLL fusion partners are normally localized to the cytoplasm and do not display inherent transactivation properties. However, they do possess structural domains responsible for protein-protein interactions. Therefore dimerization/oligomerization mediated by these domains may create a transcriptional activator complex capable of stimulating gene expression. Experiments have been performed where fusion of the first eight exons of *MLL* to β-galactosidase (a bacterial enzyme) resulted in the development of AML in mice [187]. β-Galactosidase is known to oligomerize but has not known leukemogenic potential suggesting that the mere oligomerization of MLL is sufficient to achieve transforming potential. Examples of translocations that produce fusions where the fusion partner probably imparts oligomerization include MLL/GAS7, MLL/AF1P [188], and MLL/LARG [189]. However, when tested in animal models these fusions develop leukemia after a longer latency when compared with the nuclear fusion partners, which suggests a further specific biological contribution, beyond oligomerization, of the fusion partners in dynamics and penetrance of tumorigenesis.

EZH2

A broad class of protein complexes, known as the polycomb group (PcG), are responsible for writing the histone methylation marks that suppress gene expression. PcG is correlated with transcriptional silencing and trimethylation of lysine 27 of histone H3 (H3K27me^3) [190]. In mammals, there are two distinct PcG complexes, PRC1 and PRC2 (Fig. 12.1). PRC2 is the primary writer of di- and tri-methylation of H3K27 [191]. PRC2 is composed of four core components (Fig. 12.7), enhancer of zeste homologue 2 (EZH2), suppressor of zeste 12 (SUZ12), and two WD40 domain proteins, EED and RBBP4 [192, 193]. The catalytic domain of EZH2 is its SET domain, and this has

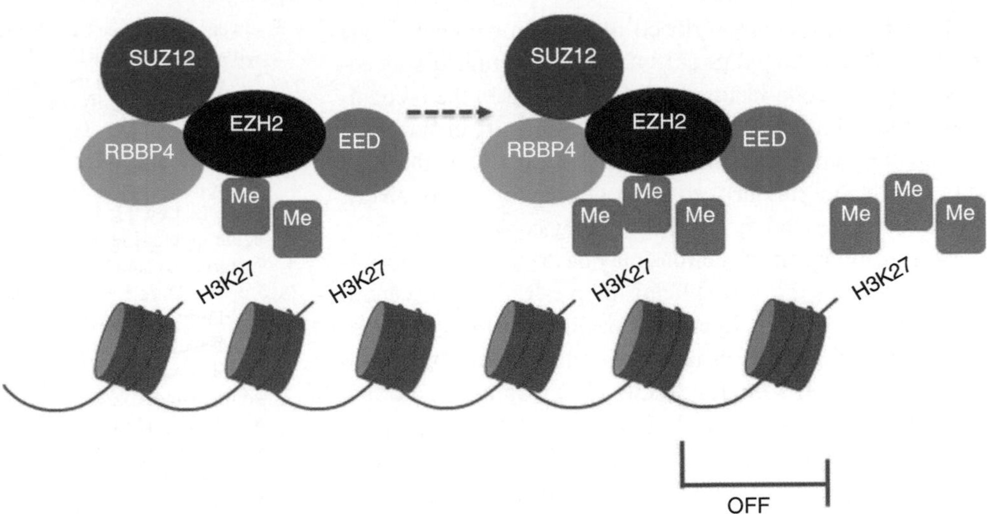

Fig. 12.7 *EZH2 is a histone methyltransferase*. PRC2 is composed of the core subunits, EZH2, SUZ12, RBBP4, and EED. EZH2 catalyzes the addition of methyl groups to histone H3 lysine 27 (H3K27me), ultimately resulting in histone H3 lysine 27 tri-methylation (H3K27me^3), a mark associated with transcriptional repression

methyltransferase activity not only toward H3K27, but also weakly toward lysine 26 of histone H1 [194].

EZH2 has a complex role in cancer pathogenesis, acting as an oncogene or as a tumor suppressor, depending on the type of cancer. Evidence in leukemia suggests that it is the loss of EZH2 that contributes to tumor development. In T-cell acute lymphoblastic leukemia (T-ALL), myeloproliferative disorders, and myeloid malignancies, a range of missense, nonsense, and frameshift mutations of *EZH2* occur [169, 170, 195]. These lesions can be heterozygous or homozygous, are found throughout the gene body, and generally are predicted to ablate histone methyltransferase activity via truncation of the SET domain. Loss of EZH2 potentiates oncogenic NOTCH1 and RUNX1 signaling in T-ALL and myelodysplastic syndromes (MDS), respectively [195, 196]. Loss of EZH2 is an indicator of poor prognosis in MDS [169, 170], but the same association with de novo AML cannot be drawn, as EZH2 mutations remain comparatively rare in this setting [197]. While MDS may often progress to AML, this is not to be the case for MDS with EZH2 loss, and genetic deletion of EZH2 in a syngeneic mouse model was shown to prevent the transformation of MDS to AML [196]. Additionally, loss of EZH2 protein occurs in about 45% of relapsed AML samples due to posttranslational deregulation of EZH2 protein [198], and this loss is associated with chemoresistance toward multiple drugs. These findings indicate that inhibition of EZH2 degradation in combination with chemotherapy, and/or targeted inhibitors, may be a novel therapeutic approach in drug-resistant AML.

Cohesin

The cohesin complex is composed of four core components that hold chromatin strands in a ringlike structure that regulates sister chromatid alignment during mitosis (16). The complex has also been shown to play a role in double-stranded DNA damage repair and regulation of transcription (17). Cohesin complex mutations in all four components, STAG1/2, RAD21, SMC1A, and SMC3, have been found in AML and other myeloid malignancies [199–202]. Mutations of cohesin complex components occur in approximately 13% of AML patients [9]. The mutations are almost always mutually exclusive, and occur early in leukemogenesis, at the stage of pre-leukemic hematopoietic stem cells [199].

In most AML cases, cohesion mutations are not associated with genomic instability [9, 203], suggesting that defects in chromatid cohesion do not contribute to leukemogenesis. What, then, are the mechanistic implications of cohesion mutations in leukemia? One hypothesis put forward is that reduced cohesion function alters chromatin structure, disrupting *cis*-regulatory architecture of hematopoietic progenitors and impairing hematopoietic differentiation [204–206]. In agreement with this, using an assay for transposable-accessible chromatin combined with high-throughput sequencing (ATAC-Seq), it was shown that there was a global loss of open chromatin in cohesin-mutant-expressing cells, with a concomitant increase in accessibility at specific motifs for key hematopoietic transcription factors [205], including ERG [207], GATA2 [208], and RUNX1 [209], and enforcing stem cell transcriptional programs.

Spliceosome

The spliceosome is a large and complex cellular machine comprised of multiple protein subunits and small nuclear RNAs (snRNAs) used to remove introns from pre-mRNA during constitutive and alternative splicing [210–212]. Mutations in the spliceosome genes *SF3B1, SRSF2*, and *U2AF1* have been found in myelodysplastic syndromes (MDS) and myeloid malignancies, including 10–25% of

AML patients, and are enriched in patients who developed AML secondary to MDS [213–215]. The mutated spliceosome genes encode factors that are involved in the recognition of the 3′-end of the intron, and are mutually exclusive of one another in patient samples [214–217], implying that they may contribute similarly to pathogenesis or, alternatively, may not be tolerated by a cell when they co-occur.

Spliceosome gene mutations may be driving leukemogenesis by causing the mis-splicing of pre-RNA from central hematopoietic drivers. In support of this hypothesis, expression of all three mutations in human cell line models, murine cells, and patient samples results in disruption of normal splicing patterns [218–220]. Furthermore, modulation of splicing catalysis via a spliceosome inhibitor reduced leukemic burden in mouse models, indicating that targeting the spliceosome may represent a novel therapeutic strategy in genetically defined subsets of leukemia [221].

Conclusions and Perspectives

Acute leukemia represents a heterogeneous collection of diseases harboring numerous molecular abnormalities. Earlier research identified recurrent fusion proteins directly linked to the pathogenesis of acute leukemia, while more recent work has focused on the role of an ever-increasing number of specific genetic and epigenetic alterations. However, as whole-genome sequencing becomes increasingly accessible for scientists, clinicians, and patients, there is a need for clarification of the prognostic and therapeutic implications of these alterations.

References

1. Kelly LM, Gilliland DG. Genetics of myeloid leukemias. Annu Rev Genomics Hum Genet. 2002;3:179–98.
2. Higuchi M, O'Brien D, Kumaravelu P, Lenny N, Yeoh EJ, Downing JR. Expression of a conditional AML1-ETO oncogene bypasses embryonic lethality and establishes a murine model of human t(8;21) acute myeloid leukemia. Cancer Cell. 2002;1(1):63–74.
3. Castilla LH, Garrett L, Adya N, et al. The fusion gene Cbfb-MYH11 blocks myeloid differentiation and predisposes mice to acute myelomonocytic leukaemia. Nat Genet. 1999;23(2):144–6.
4. Wang J, Iwasaki H, Krivtsov A, et al. Conditional MLL-CBP targets GMP and models therapy-related myeloproliferative disease. EMBO J. 2005;24(2):368–81.
5. Ford AM, Bennett CA, Price CM, Bruin MC, Van Wering ER, Greaves M. Fetal origins of the TEL-AML1 fusion gene in identical twins with leukemia. Proc Natl Acad Sci U S A. 1998;95(8):4584–8.
6. Song J, Mercer D, Hu X, Liu H, Li MM. Common leukemia- and lymphoma-associated genetic aberrations in healthy individuals. J Mol Diagn. 2011;13(2):213–9.
7. Pabst T, Eyholzer M, Haefliger S, Schardt J, Mueller BU. Somatic CEBPA mutations are a frequent second event in families with germline CEBPA mutations and familial acute myeloid leukemia. J Clin Oncol. 2008;26(31):5088–93.
8. Owen CJ, Toze CL, Koochin A, et al. Five new pedigrees with inherited RUNX1 mutations causing familial platelet disorder with propensity to myeloid malignancy. Blood. 2008;112(12):4639–45.
9. Cancer Genome Atlas Research N, Ley TJ, Miller C, et al. Genomic and epigenomic landscapes of adult de novo acute myeloid leukemia. N Engl J Med. 2013;368(22):2059–74.
10. Ding L, Ley TJ, Larson DE, et al. Clonal evolution in relapsed acute myeloid leukaemia revealed by whole-genome sequencing. Nature. 2012;481(7382):506–10.
11. Ley TJ, Ding L, Walter MJ, et al. DNMT3A mutations in acute myeloid leukemia. N Engl J Med. 2010;363(25):2424–33.
12. Li M, Collins R, Jiao Y, et al. Somatic mutations in the transcriptional corepressor gene BCORL1 in adult acute myelogenous leukemia. Blood. 2011;118(22):5914–7.
13. Mardis ER, Ding L, Dooling DJ, et al. Recurring mutations found by sequencing an acute myeloid leukemia genome. N Engl J Med. 2009;361(11):1058–66.
14. Welch JS, Ley TJ, Link DC, et al. The origin and evolution of mutations in acute myeloid leukemia. Cell. 2012;150(2):264–78.
15. Lane AA, Ley TJ. Neutrophil elastase cleaves PML-RARalpha and is important for the development of acute promyelocytic leukemia in mice. Cell. 2003;115(3):305–18.
16. de The H, Lavau C, Marchio A, Chomienne C, Degos L, Dejean A. The PML-RAR alpha fusion mRNA generated by the t(15;17) translocation in acute promyelocytic leukemia encodes a functionally altered RAR. Cell. 1991;66(4):675–84.
17. Kakizuka A, Miller WH Jr, Umesono K, et al. Chromosomal translocation t(15;17) in human acute promyelocytic leukemia fuses RAR alpha with a novel putative transcription factor, PML. Cell. 1991;66(4):663–74.
18. Fenaux P, Le Deley MC, Castaigne S, et al. Effect of all transretinoic acid in newly diagnosed acute promyelocytic leukemia. Results of a multicenter randomized trial. European APL 91 group. Blood. 1993;82(11):3241–9.
19. Arnould C, Philippe C, Bourdon V, Gr goire MJ, Berger R, Jonveaux P. The signal transducer and activator of transcription STAT5b gene is a new partner of retinoic acid receptor alpha in acute promyelocytic-like leukaemia. Hum Mol Genet. 1999;8(9):1741–9.
20. Catalano A, Dawson MA, Somana K, et al. The PRKAR1A gene is fused to RARA in a new variant acute promyelocytic leukemia. Blood. 2007;110(12):4073–6.
21. Chen SJ, Zelent A, Tong JH, et al. Rearrangements of the retinoic acid receptor alpha and promyelocytic leukemia zinc finger genes resulting from t(11;17)(q23;q21) in a patient with acute promyelocytic leukemia. J Clin Invest. 1993;91(5):2260–7.
22. de The H, Chomienne C, Lanotte M, Degos L, Dejean A. The t(15;17) translocation of acute promyelocytic leukaemia fuses the retinoic acid receptor alpha gene to a novel transcribed locus. Nature. 1990;347(6293):558–61.
23. Kondo T, Mori A, Darmanin S, Hashino S, Tanaka J, Asaka M. The seventh pathogenic fusion gene FIP1L1-RARA was isolated from a t(4;17)-positive acute promyelocytic leukemia. Haematologica. 2008;93(9):1414–6.
24. Redner RL, Rush EA, Faas S, Rudert WA, Corey SJ. The t(5;17) variant of acute promyelocytic leukemia expresses a nucleophosmin-retinoic acid receptor fusion. Blood. 1996;87(3):882–6.
25. Wells RA, Catzavelos C, Kamel-Reid S. Fusion of retinoic acid receptor alpha to NuMA, the nuclear mitotic apparatus protein, by a variant translocation in acute promyelocytic leukaemia. Nat Genet. 1997;17(1):109–13.
26. Yamamoto Y, Tsuzuki S, Tsuzuki M, Handa K, Inaguma Y, Emi N. BCOR as a novel fusion partner of retinoic acid receptor alpha in a t(X;17)(p11;q12) variant of acute promyelocytic leukemia. Blood. 2010;116(20):4274–83.
27. Pollock JL, Westervelt P, Kurichety AK, Pelicci PG, Grisolano JL, Ley TJ. A bcr-3 isoform of RARalpha-PML potentiates the

development of PML-RARalpha-driven acute promyelocytic leukemia. Proc Natl Acad Sci U S A. 1999;96(26):15103–8.
28. He LZ, Bhaumik M, Tribioli C, et al. Two critical hits for promyelocytic leukemia. Mol Cell. 2000;6(5):1131–41.
29. Sitterlin D, Tiollais P, Transy C. The RAR alpha-PLZF chimera associated with acute promyelocytic leukemia has retained a sequence-specific DNA-binding domain. Oncogene. 1997;14(9):1067–74.
30. Mozziconacci MJ, Liberatore C, Brunel V, et al. In vitro response to all-trans retinoic acid of acute promyelocytic leukemias with nonreciprocal PML/RARA or RARA/PML fusion genes. Genes Chromosomes Cancer. 1998;22(3):241–50.
31. Guidez F, Parks S, Wong H, et al. RARalpha-PLZF overcomes PLZF-mediated repression of CRABPI, contributing to retinoid resistance in t(11;17) acute promyelocytic leukemia. Proc Natl Acad Sci U S A. 2007;104(47):18694–9.
32. Ogawa E, Inuzuka M, Maruyama M, et al. Molecular cloning and characterization of PEBP2 beta, the heterodimeric partner of a novel drosophila runt-related DNA binding protein PEBP2 alpha. Virology. 1993;194(1):314–31.
33. Zhang DE, Fujioka K, Hetherington CJ, et al. Identification of a region which directs the monocytic activity of the colony-stimulating factor 1 (macrophage colony-stimulating factor) receptor promoter and binds PEBP2/CBF (AML1). Mol Cell Biol. 1994;14(12):8085–95.
34. Takahashi A, Satake M, Yamaguchi-Iwai Y, et al. Positive and negative regulation of granulocyte-macrophage colony-stimulating factor promoter activity by AML1-related transcription factor, PEBP2. Blood. 1995;86(2):607–16.
35. Nuchprayoon I, Meyers S, Scott LM, Suzow J, Hiebert S, Friedman AD. PEBP2/CBF, the murine homolog of the human myeloid AML1 and PEBP2 beta/CBF beta proto-oncoproteins, regulates the murine myeloperoxidase and neutrophil elastase genes in immature myeloid cells. Mol Cell Biol. 1994;14(8):5558–68.
36. Cameron S, Taylor DS, TePas EC, Speck NA, Mathey-Prevot B. Identification of a critical regulatory site in the human interleukin-3 promoter by in vivo footprinting. Blood. 1994;83(10):2851–9.
37. Erickson P, Gao J, Chang KS, et al. Identification of breakpoints in t(8;21) acute myelogenous leukemia and isolation of a fusion transcript, AML1/ETO, with similarity to drosophila segmentation gene, runt. Blood. 1992;80(7):1825–31.
38. Okuda T, Cai Z, Yang S, et al. Expression of a knocked-in AML1-ETO leukemia gene inhibits the establishment of normal definitive hematopoiesis and directly generates dysplastic hematopoietic progenitors. Blood. 1998;91(9):3134–43.
39. Rhoades KL, Hetherington CJ, Harakawa N, et al. Analysis of the role of AML1-ETO in leukemogenesis, using an inducible transgenic mouse model. Blood. 2000;96(6):2108–15.
40. Yergeau DA, Hetherington CJ, Wang Q, et al. Embryonic lethality and impairment of haematopoiesis in mice heterozygous for an AML1-ETO fusion gene. Nat Genet. 1997;15(3):303–6.
41. Yuan Y, Zhou L, Miyamoto T, et al. AML1-ETO expression is directly involved in the development of acute myeloid leukemia in the presence of additional mutations. Proc Natl Acad Sci U S A. 2001;98(18):10398–403.
42. Wang J, Hoshino T, Redner RL, Kajigaya S, Liu JM. ETO, fusion partner in t(8;21) acute myeloid leukemia, represses transcription by interaction with the human N-CoR/mSin3/HDAC1 complex. Proc Natl Acad Sci U S A. 1998;95(18):10860–5.
43. Lutterbach B, Westendorf JJ, Linggi B, et al. ETO, a target of t(8;21) in acute leukemia, interacts with the N-CoR and mSin3 corepressors. Mol Cell Biol. 1998;18(12):7176–84.
44. Gelmetti V, Zhang J, Fanelli M, Minucci S, Pelicci PG, Lazar MA. Aberrant recruitment of the nuclear receptor corepressor-histone deacetylase complex by the acute myeloid leukemia fusion partner ETO. Mol Cell Biol. 1998;18(12):7185–91.
45. Linggi B, Muller-Tidow C, van de Locht L, et al. The t(8;21) fusion protein, AML1 ETO, specifically represses the transcription of the p14(ARF) tumor suppressor in acute myeloid leukemia. Nat Med. 2002;8(7):743–50.
46. Pabst T, Mueller BU, Harakawa N, et al. AML1-ETO downregulates the granulocytic differentiation factor C/EBPalpha in t(8;21) myeloid leukemia. Nat Med. 2001;7(4):444–51.
47. Wang J, Saunthararajah Y, Redner RL, Liu JM. Inhibitors of histone deacetylase relieve ETO-mediated repression and induce differentiation of AML1-ETO leukemia cells. Cancer Res. 1999;59(12):2766–9.
48. Liu S, Shen T, Huynh L, et al. Interplay of RUNX1/MTG8 and DNA methyltransferase 1 in acute myeloid leukemia. Cancer Res. 2005;65(4):1277–84.
49. Alcalay M, Meani N, Gelmetti V, et al. Acute myeloid leukemia fusion proteins deregulate genes involved in stem cell maintenance and DNA repair. J Clin Invest. 2003;112(11):1751–61.
50. Klampfer L, Zhang J, Zelenetz AO, Uchida H, Nimer SD. The AML1/ETO fusion protein activates transcription of BCL-2. Proc Natl Acad Sci U S A. 1996;93(24):14059–64.
51. Yan M, Kanbe E, Peterson LF, et al. A previously unidentified alternatively spliced isoform of t(8;21) transcript promotes leukemogenesis. Nat Med. 2006;12(8):945–9.
52. Jiao B, Wu CF, Liang Y, et al. AML1-ETO9a is correlated with C-KIT overexpression/mutations and indicates poor disease outcome in t(8;21) acute myeloid leukemia-M2. Leukemia. 2009;23(9):1598–604.
53. Thiel VN, Giaimo BD, Schwarz P, et al. Heterodimerization of AML1/ETO with CBFbeta is required for leukemogenesis but not for myeloproliferation. Leukemia. 2017. https://doi.org/10.1038/leu.2017.105.
54. Elagib KE, Goldfarb AN. Oncogenic pathways of AML1-ETO in acute myeloid leukemia: multifaceted manipulation of marrow maturation. Cancer Lett. 2007;251(2):179–86.
55. Lessard J, Faubert A, Sauvageau G. Genetic programs regulating HSC specification, maintenance and expansion. Oncogene. 2004;23(43):7199–209.
56. Vangala RK, Heiss-Neumann MS, Rangatia JS, et al. The myeloid master regulator transcription factor PU.1 is inactivated by AML1-ETO in t(8;21) myeloid leukemia. Blood. 2003;101(1):270–7.
57. Westendorf JJ, Yamamoto CM, Lenny N, Downing JR, Selsted ME, Hiebert SW. The t(8;21) fusion product, AML-1-ETO, associates with C/EBP-alpha, inhibits C/EBP-alpha-dependent transcription, and blocks granulocytic differentiation. Mol Cell Biol. 1998;18(1):322–33.
58. Choi Y, Elagib KE, Delehanty LL, Goldfarb AN. Erythroid inhibition by the leukemic fusion AML1-ETO is associated with impaired acetylation of the major erythroid transcription factor GATA-1. Cancer Res. 2006;66(6):2990–6.
59. Zhang J, Kalkum M, Yamamura S, Chait BT, Roeder RG. E protein silencing by the leukemogenic AML1-ETO fusion protein. Science. 2004;305(5688):1286–9.
60. Lukasik SM, Zhang L, Corpora T, et al. Altered affinity of CBF beta-SMMHC for Runx1 explains its role in leukemogenesis. Nat Struct Biol. 2002;9(9):674–9.
61. Adya N, Stacy T, Speck NA, Liu PP. The leukemic protein core binding factor beta (CBFbeta)-smooth-muscle myosin heavy chain sequesters CBFalpha2 into cytoskeletal filaments and aggregates. Mol Cell Biol. 1998;18(12):7432–43.
62. Lu J, Maruyama M, Satake M, et al. Subcellular localization of the alpha and beta subunits of the acute myeloid leukemia-linked transcription factor PEBP2/CBF. Mol Cell Biol. 1995;15(3):1651–61.
63. Durst KL, Lutterbach B, Kummalue T, Friedman AD, Hiebert SW. The inv(16) fusion protein associates with corepressors via a smooth muscle myosin heavy-chain domain. Mol Cell Biol. 2003;23(2):607–19.

64. Lutterbach B, Hou Y, Durst KL, Hiebert SW. The inv(16) encodes an acute myeloid leukemia 1 transcriptional corepressor. Proc Natl Acad Sci U S A. 1999;96(22):12822–7.
65. Wee HJ, Voon DC, Bae SC, Ito Y. PEBP2-beta/CBF-beta-dependent phosphorylation of RUNX1 and p300 by HIPK2: implications for leukemogenesis. Blood. 2008;112(9):3777–87.
66. Helbling D, Mueller BU, Timchenko NA, et al. CBFB-SMMHC is correlated with increased calreticulin expression and suppresses the granulocytic differentiation factor CEBPA in AML with inv(16). Blood. 2005;106(4):1369–75.
67. Hyde RK, Kamikubo Y, Anderson S, et al. Cbfb/Runx1 repression-independent blockage of differentiation and accumulation of Csf2rb-expressing cells by Cbfb-MYH11. Blood. 2010;115(7):1433–43.
68. Haferlach C, Dicker F, Kohlmann A, et al. AML with CBFB-MYH11 rearrangement demonstrate RAS pathway alterations in 92% of all cases including a high frequency of NF1 deletions. Leukemia. 2010;24(5):1065–9.
69. Faber ZJ, Chen X, Gedman AL, et al. The genomic landscape of core-binding factor acute myeloid leukemias. Nat Genet. 2016;48(12):1551–6.
70. Kida A, Kakihana K, Kotani S, Kurosu T, Miura O. Glycogen synthase kinase-3beta and p38 phosphorylate cyclin D2 on Thr280 to trigger its ubiquitin/proteasome-dependent degradation in hematopoietic cells. Oncogene. 2007;26(46):6630–40.
71. Jamil A, Theil KS, Kahwash S, Ruymann FB, Klopfenstein KJ. TEL/AML-1 fusion gene. Its frequency and prognostic significance in childhood acute lymphoblastic leukemia. Cancer Genet Cytogenet. 2000;122(2):73–8.
72. Romana SP, Mauchauffe M, Le Coniat M, et al. The t(12;21) of acute lymphoblastic leukemia results in a tel-AML1 gene fusion. Blood. 1995;85(12):3662–70.
73. Patel N, Goff LK, Clark T, et al. Expression profile of wild-type ETV6 in childhood acute leukaemia. Br J Haematol. 2003;122(1):94–8.
74. Lilljebjorn H, Soneson C, Andersson A, et al. The correlation pattern of acquired copy number changes in 164 ETV6/RUNX1-positive childhood acute lymphoblastic leukemias. Hum Mol Genet. 2010;19(16):3150–8.
75. Mullighan CG, Goorha S, Radtke I, et al. Genome-wide analysis of genetic alterations in acute lymphoblastic leukaemia. Nature. 2007;446(7137):758–64.
76. Hiebert SW, Sun W, Davis JN, et al. The t(12;21) translocation converts AML-1B from an activator to a repressor of transcription. Mol Cell Biol. 1996;16(4):1349–55.
77. Fuka G, Kauer M, Kofler R, Haas OA, Panzer-Grumayer R. The leukemia-specific fusion gene ETV6/RUNX1 perturbs distinct key biological functions primarily by gene repression. PLoS One. 2011;6(10):e26348.
78. Zhuang Y, Soriano P, Weintraub H. The helix-loop-helix gene E2A is required for B cell formation. Cell. 1994;79(5):875–84.
79. Bain G, Maandag EC, Izon DJ, et al. E2A proteins are required for proper B cell development and initiation of immunoglobulin gene rearrangements. Cell. 1994;79(5):885–92.
80. Murre C, McCaw PS, Vaessin H, et al. Interactions between heterologous helix-loop-helix proteins generate complexes that bind specifically to a common DNA sequence. Cell. 1989;58(3):537–44.
81. Sigvardsson M, Clark DR, Fitzsimmons D, et al. Early B-cell factor, E2A, and Pax-5 cooperate to activate the early B cell-specific mb-1 promoter. Mol Cell Biol. 2002;22(24):8539–51.
82. Sayegh CE, Quong MW, Agata Y, Murre C. E-proteins directly regulate expression of activation-induced deaminase in mature B cells. Nat Immunol. 2003;4(6):586–93.
83. Kee BL, Murre C. Induction of early B cell factor (EBF) and multiple B lineage genes by the basic helix-loop-helix transcription factor E12. J Exp Med. 1998;188(4):699–713.
84. Decker T, Pasca di Magliano M, Mc Manus S, et al. Stepwise activation of enhancer and promoter regions of the B cell commitment gene Pax5 in early lymphopoiesis. Immunity. 2009;30(4):508–20.
85. Falini B, Mecucci C, Tiacci E, et al. Cytoplasmic nucleophosmin in acute myelogenous leukemia with a normal karyotype. N Engl J Med. 2005;352(3):254–66.
86. Verhaak RG, Goudswaard CS, van Putten W, et al. Mutations in nucleophosmin (NPM1) in acute myeloid leukemia (AML): association with other gene abnormalities and previously established gene expression signatures and their favorable prognostic significance. Blood. 2005;106(12):3747–54.
87. Schlenk RF, Dohner K, Krauter J, et al. Mutations and treatment outcome in cytogenetically normal acute myeloid leukemia. N Engl J Med. 2008;358(18):1909–18.
88. Chou WC, Tang JL, Lin LI, et al. Nucleophosmin mutations in de novo acute myeloid leukemia: the age-dependent incidences and the stability during disease evolution. Cancer Res. 2006;66(6):3310–6.
89. Dohner K, Schlenk RF, Habdank M, et al. Mutant nucleophosmin (NPM1) predicts favorable prognosis in younger adults with acute myeloid leukemia and normal cytogenetics: interaction with other gene mutations. Blood. 2005;106(12):3740–6.
90. Schnittger S, Schoch C, Kern W, et al. Nucleophosmin gene mutations are predictors of favorable prognosis in acute myelogenous leukemia with a normal karyotype. Blood. 2005;106(12):3733–9.
91. Suzuki T, Kiyoi H, Ozeki K, et al. Clinical characteristics and prognostic implications of NPM1 mutations in acute myeloid leukemia. Blood. 2005;106(8):2854–61.
92. Thiede C, Koch S, Creutzig E, et al. Prevalence and prognostic impact of NPM1 mutations in 1485 adult patients with acute myeloid leukemia (AML). Blood. 2006;107(10):4011–20.
93. Papaemmanuil E, Gerstung M, Bullinger L, et al. Genomic classification and prognosis in acute myeloid leukemia. N Engl J Med. 2016;374(23):2209–21.
94. Shlush LI, Zandi S, Mitchell A, et al. Identification of pre-leukaemic haematopoietic stem cells in acute leukaemia. Nature. 2014;506(7488):328–33.
95. Schnittger S, Kern W, Tschulik C, et al. Minimal residual disease levels assessed by NPM1 mutation-specific RQ-PCR provide important prognostic information in AML. Blood. 2009;114(11):2220–31.
96. Colombo E, Marine JC, Danovi D, Falini B, Pelicci PG. Nucleophosmin regulates the stability and transcriptional activity of p53. Nat Cell Biol. 2002;4(7):529–33.
97. den Besten W, Kuo ML, Williams RT, Sherr CJ. Myeloid leukemia-associated nucleophosmin mutants perturb p53-dependent and independent activities of the Arf tumor suppressor protein. Cell Cycle. 2005;4(11):1593–8.
98. Grisendi S, Mecucci C, Falini B, Pandolfi PP. Nucleophosmin and cancer. Nat Rev Cancer. 2006;6(7):493–505.
99. Cheng K, Grisendi S, Clohessy JG, et al. The leukemia-associated cytoplasmic nucleophosmin mutant is an oncogene with paradoxical functions: Arf inactivation and induction of cellular senescence. Oncogene. 2007;26(53):7391–400.
100. Cheng K, Sportoletti P, Ito K, et al. The cytoplasmic NPM mutant induces myeloproliferation in a transgenic mouse model. Blood. 2010;115(16):3341–5.
101. Leong SM, Tan BX, Bte Ahmad B, et al. Mutant nucleophosmin deregulates cell death and myeloid differentiation through excessive caspase-6 and -8 inhibition. Blood. 2010;116(17):3286–96.
102. Bonetti P, Davoli T, Sironi C, Amati B, Pelicci PG, Colombo E. Nucleophosmin and its AML-associated mutant regulate c-Myc turnover through Fbw7 gamma. J Cell Biol. 2008;182(1):19–26.
103. Luo H, Li Q, O'Neal J, Kreisel F, Le Beau MM, Tomasson MH. C-Myc rapidly induces acute myeloid leukemia in mice without evidence of lymphoma-associated antiapoptotic mutations. Blood. 2005;106(7):2452–61.

104. Nichol JN, Galbraith MD, Kleinman CL, Espinosa JM, Miller WH Jr. NPM and BRG1 mediate transcriptional resistance to retinoic acid in acute promyelocytic leukemia. Cell Rep. 2016;14(12):2938–49.
105. Besmer P, Murphy JE, George PC, et al. A new acute transforming feline retrovirus and relationship of its oncogene v-kit with the protein kinase gene family. Nature. 1986;320(6061):415–21.
106. Qiu FH, Ray P, Brown K, et al. Primary structure of c-kit: relationship with the CSF-1/PDGF receptor kinase family--oncogenic activation of v-kit involves deletion of extracellular domain and C terminus. EMBO J. 1988;7(4):1003–11.
107. Rosnet O, Schiff C, Pebusque MJ, et al. Human FLT3/FLK2 gene: cDNA cloning and expression in hematopoietic cells. Blood. 1993;82(4):1110–9.
108. Ullrich A, Schlessinger J. Signal transduction by receptors with tyrosine kinase activity. Cell. 1990;61(2):203–12.
109. Roskoski R Jr. Structure and regulation of kit protein-tyrosine kinase--the stem cell factor receptor. Biochem Biophys Res Commun. 2005;338(3):1307–15.
110. Carow CE, Levenstein M, Kaufmann SH, et al. Expression of the hematopoietic growth factor receptor FLT3 (STK-1/Flk2) in human leukemias. Blood. 1996;87(3):1089–96.
111. Renneville A, Roumier C, Biggio V, et al. Cooperating gene mutations in acute myeloid leukemia: a review of the literature. Leukemia. 2008;22(5):915–31.
112. Gilliland DG, Griffin JD. The roles of FLT3 in hematopoiesis and leukemia. Blood. 2002;100(5):1532–42.
113. Stirewalt DL, Radich JP. The role of FLT3 in haematopoietic malignancies. Nat Rev Cancer. 2003;3(9):650–65.
114. Mackarehtschian K, Hardin JD, Moore KA, Boast S, Goff SP, Lemischka IR. Targeted disruption of the flk2/flt3 gene leads to deficiencies in primitive hematopoietic progenitors. Immunity. 1995;3(1):147–61.
115. McKenna HJ, Stocking KL, Miller RE, et al. Mice lacking flt3 ligand have deficient hematopoiesis affecting hematopoietic progenitor cells, dendritic cells, and natural killer cells. Blood. 2000;95(11):3489–97.
116. Griffith J, Black J, Faerman C, et al. The structural basis for autoinhibition of FLT3 by the juxtamembrane domain. Mol Cell. 2004;13(2):169–78.
117. Small D. FLT3 mutations: biology and treatment. Hematology Am Soc Hematol Educ Program. 2006:178–84.
118. Kelly LM, Liu Q, Kutok JL, Williams IR, Boulton CL, Gilliland DG. FLT3 internal tandem duplication mutations associated with human acute myeloid leukemias induce myeloproliferative disease in a murine bone marrow transplant model. Blood. 2002;99(1):310–8.
119. Levis M, Murphy KM, Pham R, et al. Internal tandem duplications of the FLT3 gene are present in leukemia stem cells. Blood. 2005;106(2):673–80.
120. Shih LY, Huang CF, Wu JH, et al. Internal tandem duplication of FLT3 in relapsed acute myeloid leukemia: a comparative analysis of bone marrow samples from 108 adult patients at diagnosis and relapse. Blood. 2002;100(7):2387–92.
121. Shih LY, Huang CF, Wu JH, et al. Heterogeneous patterns of FLT3 asp(835) mutations in relapsed de novo acute myeloid leukemia: a comparative analysis of 120 paired diagnostic and relapse bone marrow samples. Clin Cancer Res. 2004;10(4):1326–32.
122. Yarden Y, Kuang WJ, Yang-Feng T, et al. Human proto-oncogene c-kit: a new cell surface receptor tyrosine kinase for an unidentified ligand. EMBO J. 1987;6(11):3341–51.
123. Flanagan JG, Leder P. The kit ligand: a cell surface molecule altered in steel mutant fibroblasts. Cell. 1990;63(1):185–94.
124. Williams DE, Eisenman J, Baird A, et al. Identification of a ligand for the c-kit proto-oncogene. Cell. 1990;63(1):167–74.
125. Zsebo KM, Williams DA, Geissler EN, et al. Stem cell factor is encoded at the Sl locus of the mouse and is the ligand for the c-kit tyrosine kinase receptor. Cell. 1990;63(1):213–24.
126. Furitsu T, Tsujimura T, Tono T, et al. Identification of mutations in the coding sequence of the proto-oncogene c-kit in a human mast cell leukemia cell line causing ligand-independent activation of c-kit product. J Clin Invest. 1993;92(4):1736–44.
127. Gari M, Goodeve A, Wilson G, et al. C-kit proto-oncogene exon 8 in-frame deletion plus insertion mutations in acute myeloid leukaemia. Br J Haematol. 1999;105(4):894–900.
128. Kohl TM, Schnittger S, Ellwart JW, Hiddemann W, Spiekermann K. KIT exon 8 mutations associated with core-binding factor (CBF)-acute myeloid leukemia (AML) cause hyperactivation of the receptor in response to stem cell factor. Blood. 2005;105(8):3319–21.
129. Beghini A, Larizza L, Cairoli R, Morra E. C-kit activating mutations and mast cell proliferation in human leukemia. Blood. 1998;92(2):701–2.
130. Hirota S, Isozaki K, Moriyama Y, et al. Gain-of-function mutations of c-kit in human gastrointestinal stromal tumors. Science. 1998;279(5350):577–80.
131. Longley BJ Jr, Metcalfe DD, Tharp M, et al. Activating and dominant inactivating c-KIT catalytic domain mutations in distinct clinical forms of human mastocytosis. Proc Natl Acad Sci U S A. 1999;96(4):1609–14.
132. Kemmer K, Corless CL, Fletcher JA, et al. KIT mutations are common in testicular seminomas. Am J Pathol. 2004;164(1):305–13.
133. Care RS, Valk PJ, Goodeve AC, et al. Incidence and prognosis of c-KIT and FLT3 mutations in core binding factor (CBF) acute myeloid leukaemias. Br J Haematol. 2003;121(5):775–7.
134. Park SH, Chi HS, Min SK, Park BG, Jang S, Park CJ. Prognostic impact of c-KIT mutations in core binding factor acute myeloid leukemia. Leuk Res. 2011;35(10):1376–83.
135. Cairoli R, Beghini A, Grillo G, et al. Prognostic impact of c-KIT mutations in core binding factor leukemias: an Italian retrospective study. Blood. 2006;107(9):3463–8.
136. Pollard JA, Alonzo TA, Gerbing RB, et al. Prevalence and prognostic significance of KIT mutations in pediatric patients with core binding factor AML enrolled on serial pediatric cooperative trials for de novo AML. Blood. 2010;115(12):2372–9.
137. Shih LY, Liang DC, Huang CF, et al. Cooperating mutations of receptor tyrosine kinases and Ras genes in childhood core-binding factor acute myeloid leukemia and a comparative analysis on paired diagnosis and relapse samples. Leukemia. 2008;22(2):303–7.
138. Shimada A, Taki T, Tabuchi K, et al. KIT mutations, and not FLT3 internal tandem duplication, are strongly associated with a poor prognosis in pediatric acute myeloid leukemia with t(8;21): a study of the Japanese childhood AML cooperative study group. Blood. 2006;107(5):1806–9.
139. Chen W, Xie H, Wang H, et al. Prognostic significance of KIT mutations in core-binding factor acute myeloid leukemia: a systematic review and meta-analysis. PLoS One. 2016;11(1):e0146614.
140. Orlic D, Bodine DM. What defines a pluripotent hematopoietic stem cell (PHSC): will the real PHSC please stand up! Blood. 1994;84(12):3991–4.
141. Orkin SH. Diversification of haematopoietic stem cells to specific lineages. Nat Rev Genet. 2000;1(1):57–64.
142. Barjesteh van Waalwijk van Doorn-Khosrovani S, Erpelinck C, Meijer J, et al. Biallelic mutations in the CEBPA gene and low CEBPA expression levels as prognostic markers in intermediate-risk AML. Hematol J. 2003;4(1):31–40.
143. Frohling S, Schlenk RF, Stolze I, et al. CEBPA mutations in younger adults with acute myeloid leukemia and normal cytogenetics: prognostic relevance and analysis of cooperating mutations. J Clin Oncol. 2004;22(4):624–33.
144. Green CL, Koo KK, Hills RK, Burnett AK, Linch DC, Gale RE. Prognostic significance of CEBPA mutations in a large cohort of younger adult patients with acute myeloid leukemia: impact of double CEBPA mutations and the interaction with FLT3 and NPM1 mutations. J Clin Oncol. 2010;28(16):2739–47.

145. Pabst T, Mueller BU, Zhang P, et al. Dominant-negative mutations of CEBPA, encoding CCAAT/enhancer binding protein-alpha (C/EBPalpha), in acute myeloid leukemia. Nat Genet. 2001;27(3):263–70.
146. Patel JP, Gonen M, Figueroa ME, et al. Prognostic relevance of integrated genetic profiling in acute myeloid leukemia. N Engl J Med. 2012;366(12):1079–89.
147. Preudhomme C, Sagot C, Boissel N, et al. Favorable prognostic significance of CEBPA mutations in patients with de novo acute myeloid leukemia: a study from the acute leukemia French association (ALFA). Blood. 2002;100(8):2717–23.
148. Fasan A, Haferlach C, Alpermann T, et al. The role of different genetic subtypes of CEBPA mutated AML. Leukemia. 2014;28(4):794–803.
149. Gombart AF, Hofmann WK, Kawano S, et al. Mutations in the gene encoding the transcription factor CCAAT/enhancer binding protein alpha in myelodysplastic syndromes and acute myeloid leukemias. Blood. 2002;99(4):1332–40.
150. Ping N, Sun A, Song Y, et al. Exome sequencing identifies highly recurrent somatic GATA2 and CEBPA mutations in acute erythroid leukemia. Leukemia. 2017;31(1):195–202.
151. Tong Q, Tsai J, Tan G, Dalgin G, Hotamisligil GS. Interaction between GATA and the C/EBP family of transcription factors is critical in GATA-mediated suppression of adipocyte differentiation. Mol Cell Biol. 2005;25(2):706–15.
152. Nutt SL, Heavey B, Rolink AG, Busslinger M. Commitment to the B-lymphoid lineage depends on the transcription factor Pax5. Nature. 1999;401(6753):556–62.
153. Urbanek P, Wang ZQ, Fetka I, Wagner EF, Busslinger M. Complete block of early B cell differentiation and altered patterning of the posterior midbrain in mice lacking Pax5/BSAP. Cell. 1994;79(5):901–12.
154. Czerny T, Schaffner G, Busslinger M. DNA sequence recognition by Pax proteins: bipartite structure of the paired domain and its binding site. Genes Dev. 1993;7(10):2048–61.
155. Kozmik Z, Wang S, Dorfler P, Adams B, Busslinger M. The promoter of the CD19 gene is a target for the B-cell-specific transcription factor BSAP. Mol Cell Biol. 1992;12(6):2662–72.
156. Zwollo P, Desiderio S. Specific recognition of the blk promoter by the B-lymphoid transcription factor B-cell-specific activator protein. J Biol Chem. 1994;269(21):15310–7.
157. Ying H, Healy JI, Goodnow CC, Parnes JR. Regulation of mouse CD72 gene expression during B lymphocyte development. J Immunol. 1998;161(9):4760–7.
158. Souabni A, Cobaleda C, Schebesta M, Busslinger M. Pax5 promotes B lymphopoiesis and blocks T cell development by repressing Notch1. Immunity. 2002;17(6):781–93.
159. Holmes ML, Carotta S, Corcoran LM, Nutt SL. Repression of Flt3 by Pax5 is crucial for B-cell lineage commitment. Genes Dev. 2006;20(8):933–8.
160. Nutt SL, Vambrie S, Steinlein P, et al. Independent regulation of the two Pax5 alleles during B-cell development. Nat Genet. 1999;21(4):390–5.
161. Falkenberg KJ, Johnstone RW. Histone deacetylases and their inhibitors in cancer, neurological diseases and immune disorders. Nat Rev Drug Discov. 2014;13(9):673–91.
162. Schnittger S, Eder C, Jeromin S, et al. ASXL1 exon 12 mutations are frequent in AML with intermediate risk karyotype and are independently associated with an adverse outcome. Leukemia. 2013;27(1):82–91.
163. Boultwood J, Perry J, Pellagatti A, et al. Frequent mutation of the polycomb-associated gene ASXL1 in the myelodysplastic syndromes and in acute myeloid leukemia. Leukemia. 2010;24(5):1062–5.
164. Carbuccia N, Trouplin V, Gelsi-Boyer V, et al. Mutual exclusion of ASXL1 and NPM1 mutations in a series of acute myeloid leukemias. Leukemia. 2010;24(2):469–73.
165. Cerveira N, Correia C, Doria S, et al. Frequency of NUP98-NSD1 fusion transcript in childhood acute myeloid leukaemia. Leukemia. 2003;17(11):2244–7.
166. Wang GG, Cai L, Pasillas MP, Kamps MP. NUP98-NSD1 links H3K36 methylation to Hox-a gene activation and leukaemogenesis. Nat Cell Biol. 2007;9(7):804–12.
167. Gu Y, Nakamura T, Alder H, et al. The t(4;11) chromosome translocation of human acute leukemias fuses the ALL-1 gene, related to drosophila trithorax, to the AF-4 gene. Cell. 1992;71(4):701–8.
168. Tkachuk DC, Kohler S, Cleary ML. Involvement of a homolog of drosophila trithorax by 11q23 chromosomal translocations in acute leukemias. Cell. 1992;71(4):691–700.
169. Ernst T, Chase AJ, Score J, et al. Inactivating mutations of the histone methyltransferase gene EZH2 in myeloid disorders. Nat Genet. 2010;42(8):722–6.
170. Nikoloski G, Langemeijer SM, Kuiper RP, et al. Somatic mutations of the histone methyltransferase gene EZH2 in myelodysplastic syndromes. Nat Genet. 2010;42(8):665–7.
171. van Haaften G, Dalgliesh GL, Davies H, et al. Somatic mutations of the histone H3K27 demethylase gene UTX in human cancer. Nat Genet. 2009;41(5):521–3.
172. Guenther MG, Jenner RG, Chevalier B, et al. Global and Hox-specific roles for the MLL1 methyltransferase. Proc Natl Acad Sci U S A. 2005;102(24):8603–8.
173. Milne TA, Dou Y, Martin ME, Brock HW, Roeder RG, Hess JL. MLL associates specifically with a subset of transcriptionally active target genes. Proc Natl Acad Sci U S A. 2005;102(41):14765–70.
174. Milne TA, Briggs SD, Brock HW, et al. MLL targets SET domain methyltransferase activity to Hox gene promoters. Mol Cell. 2002;10(5):1107–17.
175. Dou Y, Hess JL. Mechanisms of transcriptional regulation by MLL and its disruption in acute leukemia. Int J Hematol. 2008;87(1):10–8.
176. Krivtsov AV, Armstrong SA. MLL translocations, histone modifications and leukaemia stem-cell development. Nat Rev Cancer. 2007;7(11):823–33.
177. Lavau C, Szilvassy SJ, Slany R, Cleary ML. Immortalization and leukemic transformation of a myelomonocytic precursor by retrovirally transduced HRX-ENL. EMBO J. 1997;16(14):4226–37.
178. Slany RK, Lavau C, Cleary ML. The oncogenic capacity of HRX-ENL requires the transcriptional transactivation activity of ENL and the DNA binding motifs of HRX. Mol Cell Biol. 1998;18(1):122–9.
179. Zeisig BB, Milne T, Garcia-Cuellar MP, et al. Hoxa9 and Meis1 are key targets for MLL-ENL-mediated cellular immortalization. Mol Cell Biol. 2004;24(2):617–28.
180. Kroon E, Krosl J, Thorsteinsdottir U, Baban S, Buchberg AM, Sauvageau G. Hoxa9 transforms primary bone marrow cells through specific collaboration with Meis1a but not Pbx1b. EMBO J. 1998;17(13):3714–25.
181. Sobulo OM, Borrow J, Tomek R, et al. MLL is fused to CBP, a histone acetyltransferase, in therapy-related acute myeloid leukemia with a t(11;16)(q23;p13.3). Proc Natl Acad Sci U S A. 1997;94(16):8732–7.
182. Lavau C, Du C, Thirman M, Zeleznik-Le N. Chromatin-related properties of CBP fused to MLL generate a myelodysplastic-like syndrome that evolves into myeloid leukemia. EMBO J. 2000;19(17):4655–64.
183. Bitoun E, Oliver PL, Davies KE. The mixed-lineage leukemia fusion partner AF4 stimulates RNA polymerase II transcriptional elongation and mediates coordinated chromatin remodeling. Hum Mol Genet. 2007;16(1):92–106.
184. Schubeler D, MacAlpine DM, Scalzo D, et al. The histone modification pattern of active genes revealed through genome-wide chromatin analysis of a higher eukaryote. Genes Dev. 2004;18(11):1263–71.

185. Shilatifard A. Chromatin modifications by methylation and ubiquitination: implications in the regulation of gene expression. Annu Rev Biochem. 2006;75:243–69.
186. Dorrance AM, Liu S, Yuan W, et al. Mll partial tandem duplication induces aberrant Hox expression in vivo via specific epigenetic alterations. J Clin Invest. 2006;116(10):2707–16.
187. Dobson CL, Warren AJ, Pannell R, Forster A, Rabbitts TH. Tumorigenesis in mice with a fusion of the leukaemia oncogene Mll and the bacterial lacZ gene. EMBO J. 2000;19(5):843–51.
188. So CW, Lin M, Ayton PM, Chen EH, Cleary ML. Dimerization contributes to oncogenic activation of MLL chimeras in acute leukemias. Cancer Cell. 2003;4(2):99–110.
189. Grabocka E, Wedegaertner PB. Disruption of oligomerization induces nucleocytoplasmic shuttling of leukemia-associated rho guanine-nucleotide exchange factor. Mol Pharmacol. 2007;72(4):993–1002.
190. Schuettengruber B, Martinez AM, Iovino N, Cavalli G. Trithorax group proteins: switching genes on and keeping them active. Nat Rev Mol Cell Biol. 2011;12(12):799–814.
191. Margueron R, Reinberg D. The Polycomb complex PRC2 and its mark in life. Nature. 2011;469(7330):343–9.
192. Cao R, Wang L, Wang H, et al. Role of histone H3 lysine 27 methylation in Polycomb-group silencing. Science. 2002;298(5595):1039–43.
193. Muller J, Hart CM, Francis NJ, et al. Histone methyltransferase activity of a drosophila Polycomb group repressor complex. Cell. 2002;111(2):197–208.
194. Kuzmichev A, Nishioka K, Erdjument-Bromage H, Tempst P, Reinberg D. Histone methyltransferase activity associated with a human multiprotein complex containing the enhancer of Zeste protein. Genes Dev. 2002;16(22):2893–905.
195. Ntziachristos P, Tsirigos A, Van Vlierberghe P, et al. Genetic inactivation of the polycomb repressive complex 2 in T cell acute lymphoblastic leukemia. Nat Med. 2012;18(2):298–301.
196. Sashida G, Harada H, Matsui H, et al. Ezh2 loss promotes development of myelodysplastic syndrome but attenuates its predisposition to leukaemic transformation. Nat Commun. 2014;5:4177.
197. Wang X, Dai H, Wang Q, et al. EZH2 mutations are related to low blast percentage in bone marrow and −7/del(7q) in de novo acute myeloid leukemia. PLoS One. 2013;8(4):e61341.
198. Gollner S, Oellerich T, Agrawal-Singh S, et al. Loss of the histone methyltransferase EZH2 induces resistance to multiple drugs in acute myeloid leukemia. Nat Med. 2017;23(1):69–78.
199. Corces-Zimmerman MR, Hong WJ, Weissman IL, Medeiros BC, Majeti R. Preleukemic mutations in human acute myeloid leukemia affect epigenetic regulators and persist in remission. Proc Natl Acad Sci U S A. 2014;111(7):2548–53.
200. Diaz-Martinez LA, Clarke DJ. Chromosome cohesion and the spindle checkpoint. Cell Cycle. 2009;8(17):2733–40.
201. Panigrahi AK, Pati D. Higher-order orchestration of hematopoiesis: is cohesin a new player? Exp Hematol. 2012;40(12):967–73.
202. Yan J, Enge M, Whitington T, et al. Transcription factor binding in human cells occurs in dense clusters formed around cohesin anchor sites. Cell. 2013;154(4):801–13.
203. Thol F, Bollin R, Gehlhaar M, et al. Mutations in the cohesin complex in acute myeloid leukemia: clinical and prognostic implications. Blood. 2014;123(6):914–20.
204. Kagey MH, Newman JJ, Bilodeau S, et al. Mediator and cohesin connect gene expression and chromatin architecture. Nature. 2010;467(7314):430–5.
205. Mazumdar C, Shen Y, Xavy S, et al. Leukemia-associated cohesin mutants dominantly enforce stem cell programs and impair human hematopoietic progenitor differentiation. Cell Stem Cell. 2015;17(6):675–88.
206. Viny AD, Ott CJ, Spitzer B, et al. Dose-dependent role of the cohesin complex in normal and malignant hematopoiesis. J Exp Med. 2015;212(11):1819–32.
207. Chen Y, Chi P, Rockowitz S, et al. ETS factors reprogram the androgen receptor cistrome and prime prostate tumorigenesis in response to PTEN loss. Nat Med. 2013;19(8):1023–9.
208. Wang Q, Li W, Liu XS, et al. A hierarchical network of transcription factors governs androgen receptor-dependent prostate cancer growth. Mol Cell. 2007;27(3):380–92.
209. Lichtinger M, Ingram R, Hannah R, et al. RUNX1 reshapes the epigenetic landscape at the onset of haematopoiesis. EMBO J. 2012;31(22):4318–33.
210. Berget SM, Moore C, Sharp PA. Spliced segments at the 5′ terminus of adenovirus 2 late mRNA. Proc Natl Acad Sci U S A. 1977;74(8):3171–5.
211. Chow LT, Gelinas RE, Broker TR, Roberts RJ. An amazing sequence arrangement at the 5′ ends of adenovirus 2 messenger RNA. Cell. 1977;12(1):1–8.
212. Lerner MR, Boyle JA, Mount SM, Wolin SL, Steitz JA. Are snRNPs involved in splicing? Nature. 1980;283(5743):220–4.
213. Graubert TA, Shen D, Ding L, et al. Recurrent mutations in the U2AF1 splicing factor in myelodysplastic syndromes. Nat Genet. 2011;44(1):53–7.
214. Papaemmanuil E, Cazzola M, Boultwood J, et al. Somatic SF3B1 mutation in myelodysplasia with ring sideroblasts. N Engl J Med. 2011;365(15):1384–95.
215. Yoshida K, Sanada M, Shiraishi Y, et al. Frequent pathway mutations of splicing machinery in myelodysplasia. Nature. 2011;478(7367):64–9.
216. Haferlach T, Nagata Y, Grossmann V, et al. Landscape of genetic lesions in 944 patients with myelodysplastic syndromes. Leukemia. 2014;28(2):241–7.
217. Walter MJ, Shen D, Shao J, et al. Clonal diversity of recurrently mutated genes in myelodysplastic syndromes. Leukemia. 2013;27(6):1275–82.
218. Kim E, Ilagan JO, Liang Y, et al. SRSF2 mutations contribute to myelodysplasia by mutant-specific effects on exon recognition. Cancer Cell. 2015;27(5):617–30.
219. Obeng EA, Chappell RJ, Seiler M, et al. Physiologic expression of Sf3b1(K700E) causes impaired erythropoiesis, aberrant splicing, and sensitivity to therapeutic spliceosome modulation. Cancer Cell. 2016;30(3):404–17.
220. Shirai CL, Ley JN, White BS, et al. Mutant U2AF1 expression alters hematopoiesis and pre-mRNA splicing in vivo. Cancer Cell. 2015;27(5):631–43.
221. Lee SC, Dvinge H, Kim E, et al. Modulation of splicing catalysis for therapeutic targeting of leukemia with mutations in genes encoding spliceosomal proteins. Nat Med. 2016;22(6):672–8.

Epidemiology and Hereditary Aspects of Acute Leukemia

13

Logan G. Spector, Erin L. Marcotte, Rebecca Kehm, and Jenny N. Poynter

Introduction

Recent projections for the USA estimate that 6590 patients are diagnosed annually with acute lymphocytic leukemia (ALL) and 19,950 with acute myeloid leukemia (AML), while approximately 1430 patients die from ALL and 10,430 from AML [1]. Together these forms of acute leukemia represent about 1.6% of all newly diagnosed cancers and 2.0% of all cancer deaths in the USA [1]. Advances in the understanding of immunology and molecular/genetic features of the acute leukemias along with laboratory improvements in immunophenotyping and cytogenetic characterization have led to the recognition of molecularly defined subtypes of ALL and AML, targeted therapeutics, and recognition of distinct prognostic groups. The most recent World Health Organization (WHO) classification of hematopoietic malignancies considers three major categories of acute leukemia: AML and related myeloid precursor neoplasms, precursor lymphoid neoplasms (encompassing the entities previously known as ALL), and acute leukemias of ambiguous lineage [2]. Consistent with classifications used in cancer registries, to date most epidemiologic investigations have considered all acute leukemias combined or the broad categories of ALL and AML, although an increasing number of studies, especially those of genetic risk factors, examine cases by molecular subtype. Traditionally pediatric acute leukemias, defined either as those diagnosed at 0–14 or 0–19 years of age, have been studied separately from that in adults.

ALL and AML demonstrate substantial differences in incidence patterns by age and risk factors, although some risk factors overlap (e.g., ionizing radiation). Childhood forms of ALL and AML are distinct from those occurring in adulthood with respect to certain molecular (e.g., cytogenetic) features, demographic characteristics (e.g., incidence according to racial/ethnic group), risk factors, leukemogenic susceptibility associated with certain exposures, and prognosis. There also appear to be important differences in the critical time windows for specific leukemogenic exposures [3] and in the relevant contributions of genetic and environmental factors to the etiology of childhood- versus adult-onset acute leukemias. This chapter reviews acute leukemias in terms of their descriptive epidemiology, risk factors for childhood- and adult-onset disease, and hereditary and genetic aspects. Quantitative measures of risk, described as estimated relative risks (RRs), are defined as estimates of the ratios of risks in exposed versus unexposed populations. For the purposes of this chapter, high RRs are considered to be those ≥4, moderate RRs are 2 to <4, and modest RRs are <2.

Descriptive Characteristics of Acute Leukemias Occurring at All Ages

Age-adjusted incidence of leukemia varies internationally by a factor of about six- to eightfold in women and men, respectively, with the lowest rates in Middle and Western Africa and the highest rates in Northern American and Australia/New Zealand [4]. The International Agency for Research on Cancer (IACR), the primary reporting source for international cancer trends, does not subclassify leukemias into acute and chronic, and myeloid or lymphoid, preventing international comparisons of leukemia subclassifications. Rates also vary across racial and ethnic populations within countries. In the USA, for example, rates of ALL are highest among Hispanics [5].

In the USA, the incidence of AML is 2.6 times that of ALL, with age-adjusted incidence rates of 3.6 versus 1.4 cases per 100,000 person-years, based on data from the nine long-standing cancer registry areas of the Surveillance, Epidemiology and End Results Program (SEER-9), 1975–2013 [5]. Incidence is higher among males than females—by

L.G. Spector, Ph.D. (✉) • E.L. Marcotte, M.P.H., Ph.D.
R. Kehm, M.P.H. • J.N. Poynter, Ph.D.
Division of Epidemiology and Clinical Research, Department of Pediatrics, University of Minnesota Medical School, Minneapolis, MN 55455, USA
e-mail: spector@umn.edu; marcotte@umn.edu; kehmx003@umn.edu; poynt006@umn.edu

P.H. Wiernik et al. (eds.), *Neoplastic Diseases of the Blood*, DOI 10.1007/978-3-319-64263-5_13

nearly 40% for ALL and 50% for AML—and lower among blacks than whites—by 36% for ALL and 11% for AML. Despite differences in incidence by sex and race, age-specific rate patterns are similar within each acute leukemia subtype among all sex and race groups (Fig. 13.1a). Leukemia subtypes differ notably in incidence by age: the age-specific curve for ALL is bimodal, with peaks at the youngest and oldest ages, whereas rates for AML rise consistently over the entire age range. Prior to age 20 years, ALL incidence is four times that of AML, but this pattern reverses with age, with AML incidence 11 times that of ALL among individuals ≥60 years of age. Over the past three decades in the USA, age-adjusted rates of ALL and AML have gradually increased among all sex and race groups (Fig. 13.1b).

Relative survival (RS) rates for individuals diagnosed in SEER-9 during 1975–2012 and followed through 2013 are considerably more favorable for patients with ALL than AML, with approximately 81% and 62% 1- and 5-year overall RS, respectively, for ALL, and 39% and 20%, respectively, for AML. Overall RS for ALL and AML is somewhat more favorable for females than males; overall ALL survival is slightly more favorable for whites than blacks, whereas the reverse is true for AML. Over the past three decades, overall ALL and AML survival has improved, with the greatest strides apparent among the youngest age groups. During 1975–1982, 5-year RS for ALL was 61%, 22%, 11%, and 8% for those <20, 20–39, 40–59, and ≥60 years, respectively, and this increased to 88, 47, 32, and 18% in the corresponding age groups during 2005–2012. During these same two time periods, AML 5-year RS increased prominently from 22 to 65% among those <20 years, 13–55% among those 20–39 years, and 10–40% among those 40–59 years, with a less striking improvement of 3–9% among those ≥60 years.

Risk Factors for Acute Leukemia in Children

Chromosomal translocations have been demonstrated to initiate pediatric leukemia in utero based on studies of leukemia arising in identical twins, investigations in newborn blood spots, and the short latency period characterizing pediatric leukemia [6]. Agents causing such translocations have not been identified, and it is suspected that additional molecular

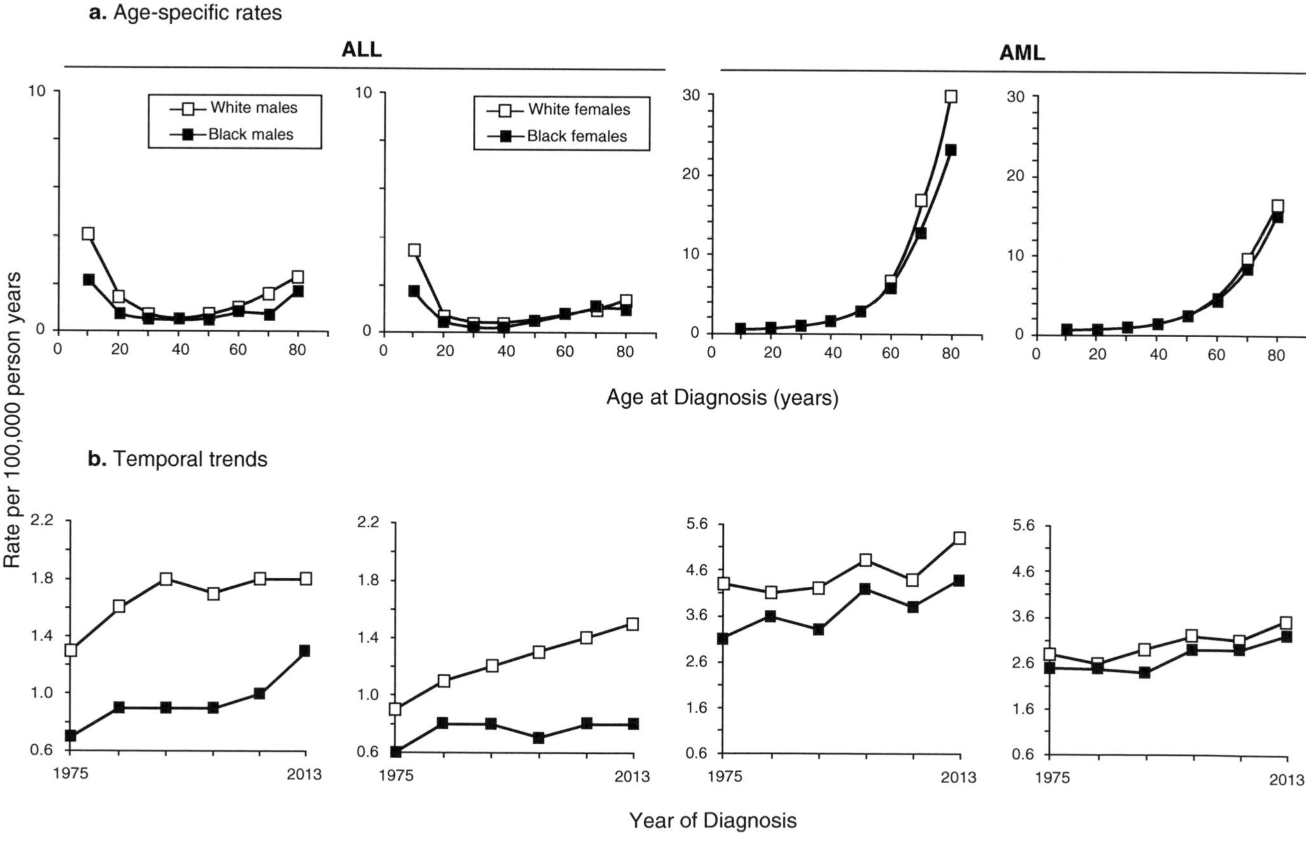

Fig. 13.1 US acute lymphocytic leukemia (ALL) and acute myeloid leukemia (AML) incidence rates (age-adjusted, 2000 US standard) by race and sex, diagnosed among residents of nine cancer registry areas of the Surveillance, Epidemiology and End Results Program, 1975–2013. (**a**) Age-specific rates (<15, 15–24, 25–34, 35–44, 45–54, 55–64, 65–74, 75+); (**b**) temporal trends (1975–1981, 1982–1988, 1989–1995, 1996–2001, 2002–2007, 2008–2013)

changes are required for pediatric leukemia to develop. Data supporting the requirement for additional events in pediatric leukemogenesis include twin concordance rates and results from animal studies. Notably, there is ongoing debate on the frequency at which these translocations occur in healthy newborns [7–9]. Next, we summarize the epidemiologic findings on preconception and prenatal risk factors followed by results for postnatal leukemogenic factors.

Prenatal and Preconception Factors

Reproductive History

Long-standing efforts to identify reproductive factors associated with risk of pediatric ALL and AML have not yielded clearly established etiologic factors. Associations of prior maternal fetal loss with increased risk of acute pediatric leukemias [10–12] were not confirmed in subsequent studies of pediatric [13, 14] or infant [15] leukemia. Although results from individual studies have been inconsistent, a recent meta-analysis reported increased risk of both ALL and AML for older maternal age and increased risk of AML for offspring of young mothers [16]. In the same analysis, older paternal age was associated with ALL while younger paternal age was associated with AML. Inconsistent findings also have been reported for birth order, although two recent large, independent pooled analyses showed slight reductions in risk for ALL with increasing birth order [17, 18].

Medical Conditions and Treatments

Decades of efforts to identify infectious agents causing pediatric ALL have been unsuccessful, and more recent studies of maternal medical conditions and/or treatments generally have not been replicated. It has long been postulated that a viral agent infecting a susceptible mother during pregnancy may play an etiologic role in pediatric leukemias [19]. However, reports linking in utero influenza infection [20] and Epstein–Barr virus [21] with pediatric leukemia and ALL, respectively, were not subsequently confirmed [22–24], and specific leukemogenic infectious agents have not been identified [24–27].

Inconsistent findings have been reported for both maternal hypertension [28–31] and diabetes [11, 28–30]. Observations requiring replication include findings of excess risks of pediatric common B-cell precursor leukemia in offspring of women with a previous molar pregnancy [14] and those receiving antibiotics [32] or mind-altering drugs during pregnancy [33], pediatric AML in offspring of mothers with polyhydramnios or anemia [14], and pediatric hematopoietic malignancies in offspring of mothers who had undergone fertility treatment [13, 34, 35]. An excess of pediatric leukemia in mothers using marijuana before or during pregnancy [36] was not confirmed [37].

Medical Radiation Exposures

Diagnostic X-ray exposures from the late 1940s through the mid-1970s have been associated consistently with modest elevation in the risk of pediatric leukemia, although risks have declined over time as radiation doses have decreased [38, 39]. Increased risk of pediatric leukemia was first linked with fetal exposure to abdominal or pelvic diagnostic X-ray of the pregnant mother nearly 60 years ago [40]. Subsequently, additional data from the large Oxford Survey of Childhood Cancers, a medical record-based study in hospitals in the northeast UK, and close to 30 other case–control studies support an overall RR of 1.4 (i.e., 40% increased risk) for pediatric leukemia associated with diagnostic ionizing radiation exposure in utero, but the interpretation of the statistical association has been debated [39]. Data are insufficient to determine risks of pediatric leukemia in offspring of women undergoing radiotherapy for cancer, and there is no evidence linking ultrasonography during pregnancy with risk of pediatric leukemia [38].

Environmental Ionizing Radiation Exposures

Data evaluating leukemia risk with in utero exposure to environmental sources of ionizing radiation are limited. The cohort study of survivors who were in utero at the time of the atomic bombings of Hiroshima and Nagasaki "… cannot provide information on the effect of radiation on the incidence of childhood cancers" in the absence of complete information for the first 5 years of follow-up and insufficient size to assess such rare outcomes [41]. Similar limitations characterize a cohort of persons who were in utero at the time of the Chernobyl accident [42]. Existing data are not informative about pediatric leukemia risks in offspring of female airline crew or women living in proximity to nuclear testing or nuclear installations [43]. However recent population-based studies have reported elevated risk of childhood leukemia associated with residential gamma radiation [44, 45], but not radon [44, 46].

Parental Occupational Radiation Exposures

A small study linking paternal preconception occupational exposure of nuclear industry workers with excess leukemia risks in offspring [47] was not confirmed in a study of 39,557 children of male nuclear workers [48]. Furthermore, there was no excess of pediatric leukemia in offspring of female or male medical radiation workers in the UK [49] or the USA [50]. A meta-analysis of all studies of parental occupational exposure to extremely low-frequency magnetic fields (ELF-MF) revealed no association with the risk of childhood leukemia for either maternal or paternal exposure [51].

Parental Pesticide Exposures

Risks of leukemia in offspring of parents occupationally exposed to pesticides have been extensively investigated, but few investigations have identified the specific pesticides to which the fetus has been exposed. Meta-analysis of more than 30 case–control and 5 cohort studies revealed similarly increased risks for both ALL and AML (RR = 2.64, 95% CI = 1.00–5.00; RR = 2.64, 95% CI = 1.48–4.71, respectively) with maternal occupational exposure, with higher risks in studies of farm-related exposures compared with studies of mixed or unknown place of exposure [52–55]. No consistent association was observed for childhood leukemia with paternal occupational exposure to pesticides [54]. A subsequent pooled analysis of 13 case–control studies reported elevated risk of ALL following paternal occupation exposure (OR = 1.20, 95% CI = 1.06, 1.38) and increased risk of AML following maternal occupational exposure (OR = 1.94, 95% CI = 1.19, 3.18) [56]. A recent pooled analysis of home pesticide exposure found 40–55% increased risk for ALL and AML for the preconception and pregnancy time periods [57].

Parental Chemical Exposures

Findings from epidemiological studies of pediatric leukemia in offspring of parents exposed to heavy metals (including arsenic), polychlorinated biphenyls, dioxin, indices for outdoor air pollution, traffic density, drinking water disinfection by-products, and specified and unspecified solvents are generally limited by a scarcity of data available. However some pooled studies and meta-analyses have recently become available for these exposures. A meta-analysis of benzene exposure, and established risk factor for adult leukemia, revealed an association between maternal and paternal exposure and both ALL and AML, with a particularly strong effect for AML (OR = 2.34, 95% CI = 1.72, 3.18) [58]. Pooled analyses from the Childhood Leukemia International Consortium (CLIC) examining occupational [59] and home [60] paint exposure reported null associations for occupation exposures and modest positive associations for home exposure (OR = 1.54, 95% CI = 1.28, 1.85 and OR = 1.14, 95% CI = 1.04, 1.25 for exposure preconception and during pregnancy, respectively). Limited evidence has linked pediatric leukemia in offspring with parental exposure to motor vehicle emissions [61, 62], driving or inhaled particulate hydrocarbons [63], or maternal exposure to unspecified solvents [64]. Maternal exposure to petroleum products during pregnancy has also been linked to infant AML [65].

Parental Cigarette Smoking

The role of maternal smoking in the development of pediatric leukemia has been evaluated for several decades, with a few studies reporting an increased risk. However, a meta-analysis [66] and subsequent studies concluded that maternal smoking during pregnancy is not a major risk factor for childhood acute leukemia [67–69]. Paternal preconception smoking has been investigated less extensively, but a recent meta-analysis of 20 studies showed a modest association with childhood ALL (RR = 1.25, 95% CI = 1.08–1.46) [70].

Parental Alcohol Consumption

A comprehensive assessment of pediatric leukemia risk and parental alcohol consumption in 33 case–control studies did not strongly support an association [71]. Paternal preconception consumption of alcohol has also not been linked with elevated risk [72]. However, a meta-analysis of 21 case–control studies concluded that maternal consumption of alcohol during pregnancy was associated with increased risk of pediatric AML (RR = 1.56, 95% CI = 1.13–2.15), but not ALL [73]. The association between maternal alcohol consumption and AML has also been reported in a subsequent study [69]. Reasons why in utero exposure to alcohol increases AML but not ALL risk are unknown.

Maternal Diet and Vitamin Supplements

The possible role of maternal diet or vitamin supplements in risk of acute leukemia has been investigated by several studies, although heterogeneity between dietary components studied and exposure categories used makes drawing conclusions difficult. Four investigations found reduced risks of pediatric leukemia in offspring of mothers who consumed higher levels of fruits and vegetables during pregnancy [74–77]. A recent pooled analysis reported reduced risk of ALL associated with prenatal vitamin supplementation and weak evidence for a reduced risk of AML associated with maternal vitamin use [78], and a subsequent study reported similar results for both ALL and AML [79]. Other studies also found reduced risk with maternal use of iron supplements [33, 80]. Spector et al. found that maternal consumption of foods that inhibit DNA topoisomerase II was linked with increased risk of infant AML [74]. Finally, a meta-analysis linked maternal coffee consumption to increased risk of both ALL and AML and cola consumption to increased risk of ALL, whereas tea consumption was associated with decreased risk of overall leukemia in offspring [81].

Mode of Birth

Mode of birth has recently become an exposure of interest for several long-term outcomes in offspring. Support for a role of mode of birth in immune system development includes observations that cesarean delivery alters both the composition [82] and diversity [83] of intestinal microbiota, and these differences can persist through the first 12 months of life [84]; reported associations between cesarean delivery and immune-related disorders, including type I diabetes mellitus [85], asthma [86], and allergies [87]; and evidence that infants born by cesarean delivery experience a markedly diminished stress response before birth, including reduced levels of cortisol and catecholamines [88–90]. A recent pooled analysis of 13 studies found an association between pre-labor cesarean delivery and risk of ALL (OR = 1.23 95% CI = 1.04, 1.47) but not AML [91].

Postnatal Factors

Birth Weight

High birth weight has been linked consistently with increased risk of ALL, and recent studies suggest a similar relationship for AML. A meta-analysis of 31 studies demonstrated significantly increased risks of ALL (RR = 1.23, 95% CI = 1.15–1.32) associated with birth weight of ≥4 kg, and seven of these studies showed a similar relationship for AML (RR = 1.40, 95% CI = 1.11–1.76) [92]. It has been suggested that accelerated growth rather than high birth weight per se is etiologically linked with ALL, and a recent pooled analysis of 12 case–control studies found evidence of moderate increased risk of ALL for large-for-gestational-age infants and those with a higher proportion of optimal birth weight [93]. Low birth weight (<1.5 kg) has been associated with increased risk of AML (RR = 1.49, 95% CI = 1.03–2.15) but not ALL [92].

Breast-Feeding

Large case–control studies examining the association of breast-feeding and risk of childhood acute leukemias have reported 9–20% decreased risk for ALL, but a less consistent picture for AML, ranging from no reduction to 23% reduction in risk [94, 95]. A meta-analysis found that any breast-feeding for 6 months or more was associated with an 18% reduced risk of ALL based on 11 studies and no reduction in risk of AML based on 6 studies [96]. A subsequent pooled analysis of 11 studies found a similar reduction in the risk of ALL for children who were breast-fed for 6 months or more (OR = 0.86, 95% CI = 0.79, 0.94) [17]. Although few studies have examined risks for combined breast-feeding and milk supplementation, one reported a moderately increased risk of childhood leukemia among those infants who received milk supplementation with breast-feeding more than 50% of the time [97].

Medical Conditions and Treatments: Infections, Vaccinations, Allergy, and Atopy

Clusters (a group of cases representing an excess intensity within the population at risk which is unlikely to be due to chance) of pediatric leukemia have been described for decades, but no infectious or other causal agent(s) have been linked with these clusters [98, 99]. A comprehensive, broad-based epidemiologic and laboratory investigation of the largest pediatric acute leukemia cluster to date, diagnosed in residents of Churchill County, Nevada, was unable to identify a causal agent [100].

Two mechanisms have been suggested by which infectious agents might be associated with the age peak from 2 to 5 years in the common form of pediatric ALL. Greaves postulated a two-hit model of leukemogenesis, with the first event or mutation occurring in rapidly dividing immature B cells in utero and the second event arising in early childhood as a result of delayed exposure to infectious agents [101]. Epidemiologic studies of proxy measures of early-life exposure to infections, including daycare attendance [17, 102], birth order [18], and timing of birth [103], generally support a reduced risk of ALL associated with early exposure to infectious agents. However, studies of clinically diagnosed infectious episodes during infancy are not consistent [17, 104].

Kinlen proposed that childhood ALL occurs as a rare response to a specific, albeit currently unknown, viral agent(s), particularly when there is mixing of rural (or other low-density) populations with urban (or other high-density) populations [105]. Summarizing multiple extreme examples of population mixing in Britain, Kinlen observed significant short-term excesses of pediatric leukemia [106], although others reviewing the population mixing studies have disagreed with the conclusions drawn by Kinlen [107].

A limited number of studies investigating an infectious etiology for pediatric acute leukemia have reported a protective effect from vaccination in infancy or early childhood, with risks varying according to the type of vaccine and age at immunization [108]. A meta-analysis of epidemiologic studies examining atopy and risk of childhood leukemia revealed a 31% significantly reduced risk of ALL based on six studies and no significant association for AML based on two studies [109]. Inverse associations were seen for ALL with asthma, eczema, and hay fever, but the authors caution about overinterpretation of the results in light of the limited number of studies, substantial heterogeneity, and potential misclassification. Finally, a meta-analysis based on eight studies of allergies and ALL reported a 33% reduction in risk [110].

Medical Radiation and Chemotherapy

In general, studies of low-dose postnatal diagnostic radiographic exposures (estimated organ doses range from 0.01 to 6 mGy) have not observed increased risks of pediatric leukemia; the results were based on questionnaire responses and estimated doses were not evaluated [111]. Two reports assessing pediatric cancer risks in children who have undergone computed tomographic (CT) examinations, which are higher dose diagnostic imaging procedures (estimated organ doses from CT scans of the chest, abdomen, brain, spine, and face range from 10 to 80 mGy), reported excess risk of leukemia among children following postnatal CT, with one study reporting a threefold increase in risk (RR = 3.18, 95% CI 1.46, 6.94) for doses of 30 mGy or more [112, 113].

Earlier cohort studies of infants or children irradiated for benign conditions were generally too small to estimate the risk of pediatric leukemia accurately [114], but radiotherapy during childhood for tinea capitis was associated with a subsequent moderately increased risk of leukemia mortality (RR mortality = 2.3, estimated bone marrow dose = 30 mGy) [115]. Two of three earlier small studies found a dose–response relationship between estimated radiation dose to the bone marrow from radiotherapy for treatment of pediatric cancer and subsequent risk of secondary leukemia. A larger more recent investigation did not confirm this relationship; however, excess secondary leukemia was evident—likely due to chemotherapy treatment [116], a strong and well-established risk factor for acute leukemia. More information on the relationship between chemotherapeutic agents and acute leukemia risk is provided in the section of this chapter on adult leukemia.

Environmental Exposures: Ionizing Radiation

Environmental ionizing radiation has been examined as a potential risk factor for childhood leukemia since the establishment of the cohort of Hiroshima and Nagasaki atomic bomb survivors. Investigation of this cohort has demonstrated that survivors who were less than 10 years old at exposure had moderate-to-high relative risks for both ALL and AML [86] [117]. Relative and absolute risks were higher among children than adults, and these risks peaked within 10 years. The absolute risk for incidence was estimated to decrease by about 5% for each year's increase in age, and risk for ALL among females was about 40% of that among males. A recent analysis of this population confirmed excess risk of leukemia among children within the cohort [118].

Results from other studies of postnatal environmental ionizing radiation and risk of pediatric acute leukemias are less clear. Leukemia and lymphoma risks were found to be increased in persons under age 25 among populations living near nuclear fuel reprocessing or weapon production plants in the UK, but not among populations residing close to nuclear plants generating electricity; however, environmental radiation levels measured in proximity to these facilities were considered too low to ascribe to the radiation exposures from these plants [119]. Residential exposure to radon was linked with elevated risk of pediatric ALL in an ecological study but was not associated with an increased risk in studies in the USA [120], Germany [121], France [122], or the UK [123]. Although there was no overall association of residential radon with pediatric AML, a borderline increase was observed in children aged 2 or older [124]. The study from France also revealed no association between childhood leukemia and any type of natural background radiation, including gamma radiation [122].

Environmental Exposures: Nonionizing Radiation

Initial reports of two- to threefold excess risks of pediatric leukemia in children residing in homes with high levels of 60-Hz magnetic field exposures from residentially proximate power lines were assessed further in large studies with more extensive and direct measurements. Results from pooled analyses of these high-quality studies revealed that pediatric leukemia risks were not increased among children residing in homes with power frequency magnetic field exposures under 0.4 μT (which included more than 99% of residences internationally), but were twofold increased among the <1% of children living in homes with exposures ≥0.4 μT [125]. A recent study found that there may be some selection bias in a study of EMF, although no association was found between childhood leukemia and residential exposure to EMF even when accounting for potential biases [126]. Reasons for the suggested increased risk among children with the highest exposure levels are unclear, particularly since experimental studies have not linked power frequency magnetic fields with carcinogenesis [127].

Environmental Exposures: Chemicals

Residential use of pesticides demonstrated a relationship with total childhood leukemia [94] and ALL in two studies, including a large pooled analysis [57, 95, 128], although another study found no association between organochlorine pesticides and leukemia [129]. Exposures to insecticides in agricultural settings were not associated with risk, nor was use of herbicides or fungicides in any setting [64]. There is some evidence that supports a relationship of pediatric leukemia with childhood residential exposure to nearby high traffic density, car repair garages, or gasoline stations [64, 130, 131], and with household use of petroleum products, solvents, and paint [60, 64, 132–134]. No clear association was observed with pediatric leukemia risk and exposure to drinking water disinfection by-products, drinking water nitrate, residence near hazardous waste disposal sites, or exposure to environmental tobacco smoke [64].

Diet and Vitamin Supplements

Only a few small studies have assessed the risk of pediatric leukemia with dietary components, and replication of the results is needed. Findings were mixed for consumption of cured meats [135, 136], and reduced risks were associated with intake of bean, curd, and vegetables in a study in Taiwan [136] and with consumption of foods containing vitamin C and/or potassium in a study in California, particularly during the earliest years of life [135]. Postnatal consumption of cola has not been associated with leukemia [81]. Concern about a report linking intramuscular vitamin K with risk of pediatric leukemia [137] was dispelled following a pooled analysis showing no association [138].

Risk Factors for Acute Leukemia in Adults

Chemotherapy

The development of therapy-related myeloid neoplasms, typically AML (t-AML), is a rare but highly fatal complication of cytotoxic treatments for both malignant and nonmalignant diseases [139–143]. Exposure to such treatments is associated with RRs ≥ 3 and incidence ranging from <1 to 7% for t-AML following conventional therapy, with even higher rates following hematopoietic cell transplantation (HCT) [144].

Therapy-related myeloid neoplasms are classified as a distinct entity in the World Health Organization (WHO) classification system [145], with two types of therapy-related myelodysplastic syndromes (t-MDS) and t-AML differentiated by previous therapeutic exposure. Patients treated with alkylating agents are more prone to t-AML that is preceded by MDS, develops 5–7 years after exposure, and is characterized by loss or deletion of chromosome 5 and/or 7 [−5/del(5q), −7/del(7q)] and presence of somatically acquired loss-of-function mutations in p53 [146]. In contrast, patients treated with topoisomerase II inhibitors, including the epipodophyllotoxins, are more prone to t-AML that is rarely preceded by MDS, arises after a latency of 2–5 years, and is characterized by balanced translocations involving the *MLL* gene at 11q23 [147, 148].

Antimetabolites used for treatment of malignancies (e.g., fludarabine) and for immunosuppressive therapy for autoimmune diseases and transplantation (e.g., azathioprine) have also been shown to increase the risk of t-AML. Abnormalities in chromosomes 5 and/or 7, similar to t-AML associated with alkylating agents, have been described [149, 150]. Population-based studies showing an increased risk of MDS/AML in patients with autoimmune disease have also been published in recent years [151, 152], with evidence suggesting that the association may be attributed to immunosuppressive therapy [153]. Further, solid organ transplant recipients who received azathioprine for initial maintenance immunosuppression had increased risk for both MDS and AML [154].

Although the vast majority of therapy-related leukemias are of myeloid lineage, increased risk of ALL following exposure to chemotherapy has been reported in the literature [155–158]. Several common abnormalities are observed in these cases of t-ALL, including 11q23 abnormalities and t(9;22)(q34;q11) (Ph chromosome) [156–158]. With the introduction and increasing use of a number of new chemotherapeutic agents in recent years, future studies are needed to evaluate the acute leukemia risks and identify cytogenetic abnormalities associated with current treatments.

Medical Radiation

Most epidemiologic studies have not reported a significant association between radiation exposure from diagnostic imaging procedures and AML [159–163]. Use of the radiographic contrast medium, Thorotrast (an alpha-emitting contrast medium with a half-life of 400 years that was used in earlier time periods for cerebral angiography), has been consistently linked with an increased risk of MDS/AML [164–166]. Increased risk of AML has also been associated with radiation treatment for benign conditions, including ankylosing spondylitis [167], benign gynecologic disorders [168, 169], tinea capitis [115], and peptic ulcer disease [170]. Individuals treated with radiotherapy for non-Hodgkin lymphoma, Ewing sarcoma, or cancer of the breast, uterine cervix, or uterine corpus also have moderately increased risks of secondary AML, although the absolute risk is small [114]. Similar to the pattern for primary AML occurring among the

Japanese atomic bomb survivors, initial cases of secondary AML following radiotherapy for another primary cancer often appear within 5 years of treatment (with most cases occurring within 10–15 years) and are associated with estimated bone marrow doses ranging from 1 to 15 Gy [169].

Environmental Exposures: Ionizing Radiation

Compared with Japanese atomic bomb survivors exposed during childhood and adolescence, those exposed in adulthood had lower estimated relative risks of ALL, but the pattern was similar to that following childhood exposure, with risk peaking at less than 10 years since exposure, a declining risk for each year's increase in age at exposure, and risks for women about half the level of risks for men [117, 171]. For AML, relative risks were similar for males and females, but males had twofold higher absolute risks. A recent analysis suggests that excess risk of acute leukemia mortality continues to persist decades after the bombings [172]. The population living on the banks of the Techa River in the Southern Urals region in Russia, who received chronic low-dose-rate internal and external radiation exposures from releases of radionuclides into the river from the Mayak nuclear weapon plant plutonium production facility, experienced excess risk of leukemias other than chronic lymphocytic leukemia (i.e., non-CLL leukemias) with an excess relative risk estimate of 0.22 per 100 mGy [173, 174].

Occupational Exposures: Radiation

Studies of radiation-exposed workers are important for clarifying the effects of protracted radiation doses, since animal studies suggest that protracted low doses may allow for DNA repair and thus lower risks of leukemia or other cancers compared with risks associated with an acute, single radiation dose [114]. Medical radiation workers were the first population observed to develop radiation-related leukemia within a few years of the discovery of X-rays due to the very high radiation exposures of early workers [175]. This increased risk was largely confined to those working prior to 1960 due to implementation of radiation protection methods in the late 1950s [176, 177]. A meta-analysis of epidemiologic studies in workers who experience low, protracted radiation exposures has shown modest increases in risk for non-CLL leukemias [178]. The International Nuclear WORKers Study (INWORKS), a large international cohort study designed to evaluate cancer risk in radiation-monitored workers, quantified this excess relative risk at 2.96 per Gy for non-CLL leukemia [179]. Leukemia mortality risks were significantly elevated and risk rose significantly with increasing external radiation dose among workers at the Mayak nuclear complex in Russia where effects of plutonium exposures have been under investigation for years [180].

Occupational Exposures: Benzene

For more than 100 years, there has been recognition that occupational benzene exposure is related to risk of leukemia. IARC has determined that benzene exposure is carcinogenic to the bone marrow and causes both AML and MDS, with several potential mechanistic explanations for this association [181]. Currently, the major occupational uses of benzene are in the manufacture of organic chemicals and chemical intermediates [181]. Benzene also occurs naturally in petroleum products and is added to unleaded gasoline [181]. Nonoccupational sources of exposure also exist, with the majority of exposure due to cigarette smoking and emissions from automobiles and industry [182]. A literature review identified 9 cohort and 13 case–control studies that included estimates of benzene exposure, excluded ecologic or proportionate mortality methods, included a comparison group, and assessed risks for one or more subtypes of leukemia [183]. High RRs and a positive dose–response relationship were seen across study designs for AML, especially in more highly exposed workers in the rubber, shoe, and paint industries. Data on ALL were judged to be sparse and inconclusive. A subsequent systematic review and meta-analysis of four studies focusing on cumulative exposure to benzene and AML found a clear dose–response pattern, with RRs of 1.94 (95% CI = 0.95–3.95), 2.32 (95% CI = 0.90–5.94), and 3.20 (95% CI = 1.09–9.45) for low, medium, and high benzene exposure, respectively [184]. A long-standing cohort study of occupational benzene exposure in China has also documented increased risks of MDS/AML in benzene-exposed workers [185–187], with the most recent report showing similar elevated risks in males and females and across different occupations after 28 years of follow-up [188].

Occupational Exposures: Farming and Pesticide Exposure

Increased risks of leukemias and lymphomas have been linked with farming, but relatively few studies have focused on risks of ALL or AML. Some data link occupation as a farmer with increased risk of ALL, but the data are not conclusive [189]. A few studies have examined risks of AML, and results have been mixed. Data from the Iowa Women's Health Study linked residence on a farm or rural area with a small but significant excess of AML, but data were not available to determine if the women worked as farmers or to assess their exposures [190]. In contrast, data from the Women's Health Initiative did not find an association between living on a farm and myeloid leukemia [191].

Exposure to a variety of agricultural chemicals has been evaluated as a risk factor for AML incidence and/or mortality [192–196]. For AML, a significant association was reported in a meta-analysis of cohort studies evaluating pesticide exposure (OR = 1.55, 95% CI 1.02, 2.34), with evidence that this association was significant for pesticide manufacturers or pesticide applicators but not for agricultural/farm workers [194]. Data from the Agricultural Health Study suggest that the risk of leukemia overall may differ for individual agricultural chemicals, with significant associations detected between leukemia and organochlorine insecticides, fonofos, diazinon, and EPTC [197–200] while no associations being detected for other chemicals [201–203].

Cigarette Smoking

Cigarette smoking was first associated with the risk of adult leukemia in the mid-1980s. Several studies have suggested a small but consistent increased risk of acute leukemia among smokers. In a meta-analysis of studies published through 1992, the estimated relative risks for all leukemia were 1.1 (95% CI 1.0–1.2) and 1.3 (95% CI = 1.2–1.6) for case–control and cohort studies, respectively [204]. A more recent meta-analysis of smoking and AML including studies published through 2013 reported that current smokers (RR = 1.40, 95% CI 1.22–1.60) and ever smokers (1.15, 95% CI 1.15–1.36) have increased risk of developing AML when compared with nonsmokers [205]. Few studies have looked specifically at the risk of adult ALL and smoking; however, studies that have evaluated associations by subtype have typically reported stronger associations for myeloid leukemia [206].

BMI and Diet

The majority of studies have shown a modest, but statistically significant, association between obesity and leukemia, with a recent meta-analysis of 16 prospective studies yielding an adjusted relative risk (RR) for AML of 1.53 (95% confidence interval (CI) 1.26–1.85) and for ALL of 1.62 (95% CI 1.12–2.32) for individuals with a BMI > 30.0 kg/m^2 compared to individuals with a BMI < 24.9 kg/m^2 [207]. A limited number of studies have investigated dietary factors and AML [206, 208–213]. A large prospective cohort study identified higher meat intake with increased risk of AML [212], and this finding was supported by a recent case–control study [211]. Mixed evidence has been reported for associations between AML and fruit and vegetable consumption [206, 208, 211–213]. Alcohol intake has not been shown to be an important risk factor for adult acute leukemia [214–216]. The few studies conducted to date along with methodologic issues related to dietary assessment, particularly in case–control studies, suggest that additional epidemiologic research is needed.

Physical Activity

A recent pooled analysis of 12 prospective cohorts reported a significant reduction in the risk of myeloid leukemia associated with high levels of leisure-time physical activity (HR, 0.80; 95% CI 0.70–0.92) while no significant association was observed for lymphocytic leukemia (HR, 0.98; 95% CI 0.88–1.12) [217]. In contrast, a previous meta-analysis including eight published studies reported no significant association between leukemia overall and physical activity (RR, 0.97; 95% CI 0.84–1.13); however, this analysis did not stratify by subtype of leukemia [218]. Data from the prospective VITamins And Lifestyle (VITAL) study which were not included in either the pooled or meta-analysis also support an association with myeloid neoplasms [219]. Additional studies of AML and ALL will be required to clarify this association.

Nonsteroidal Anti-inflammatory Drug and Acetaminophen Use

Studies of a wide range of malignancies have demonstrated a potential chemopreventive role for frequent nonsteroidal anti-inflammatory drug (NSAID) use. Further, there is evidence that these effects may be specific to certain classes of NSAIDs. Recent evidence from case–control and cohort studies suggests that aspirin use may be associated with reduced risk of AML [220–224]. In contrast, acetaminophen use may be associated with increased risk of AML [221–224]. Given the limited number of studies conducted to date and the small sample size in some studies, further research on the topic is warranted.

Hereditary and Genetic Aspects of Acute Leukemias

Familial Aggregation and Genetic Syndromes

Familial aggregation of acute leukemias is rare. Studies of the few pure familial AML pedigrees have identified germline mutations in *RUNX1* and *CEBPA* [225]. Few studies have described familial aggregation of ALL, although novel familial syndromes involving germline mutation genes frequently somatically mutated in the disease (e.g., PAX5, ETV6) have recently been described [226–228]. Individuals having a twin with ALL have substantially elevated risk for ALL, particularly among monozygotic twins [229], although this risk is due to transplacental migration of preleukemic cells rather than genetic predisposition [230].

A much larger body of evidence regarding the hereditary component of acute leukemia derives from the study of patients with rare genetic syndromes, but these patients also account for only a small proportion of the total population burden of acute leukemia. Among children with rare inherited bone marrow failure syndromes, including Fanconi anemia, dyskeratosis congenita, congenital neutropenia, and Shwachman-Diamond syndrome, risk of AML is strikingly elevated—often more than 100-fold [231, 232]. The molecular events that predispose to AML among these individuals are not completely understood but are thought to differ by syndrome and involve defective DNA repair, shortened telomere length, and abnormal hematopoietic differentiation and proliferation [233]. Other hereditary conditions associated with increased risk of acute leukemia include Li-Fraumeni syndrome, ataxia–telangiectasia, Bloom syndrome, Noonan syndrome, and neurofibromatosis 1 [234–238].

Myeloid proliferations related to Down syndrome (trisomy 21) have unique morphologic, immunophenotypic, clinical, and molecular features [2]. Children with Down syndrome have a 100-fold risk of AML, as well as approximately 15-fold risk of ALL [239]. Individuals with Down syndrome are disproportionately found to have somatic mutations in the hematopoietic transcription factor *GATA1*, which results in impaired hematopoietic cell differentiation [240].

Genetic Susceptibility

Numerous studies have investigated common genetic variation in germline DNA in relation to leukemia risk. Candidate gene studies of acute leukemias have frequently focused on carcinogen metabolism, folate metabolism, and DNA repair in the past, and have shown some consistency of findings [241]. However, the same genes have not been identified by agnostic methods such as genome-wide association studies (GWAS), which casts doubt on previous findings.

Rather than implicating previously hypothesized pathways or mechanisms, GWAS of childhood ALL have identified risk loci in or near several genes that regulate the transcription and differentiation of B-cell progenitors (*IKZF1*, *ARID5B*, *CEBPE, and GATA3*) and the tumor-suppressor genes *CDKN2A* and *CDK2NB*, which is also frequently somatically altered in hematologic malignancies [242–253]. Although the leukemia risks associated with these loci are low, these inherited genetic susceptibilities can be common in the general population, and it is estimated that common variants identified to date account for about 25% of pediatric ALL [254]. These common variants appear to cause ALL in children with non-European ancestries to a similar degree, but differences in allele frequency may explain a portion of interethnic differences in the disease rate [255, 256]. It is also notable that some variants discovered by GWAS are particularly associated with cytogenetically defined subtypes of ALL, for instance *GATA3* with Ph+-like disease [249]. Additional research is needed to understand the biological basis of these findings, identify other genetic loci that confer acute leukemia risk, and investigate the potential interaction of genetic susceptibility with environmental and individual risk factors.

Summary

Causes of the acute leukemias in children and adults have not been fully identified, but recent progress has provided new etiologic insights. The most well-established risk factors for acute leukemias include ionizing radiation, benzene, and cytotoxic chemotherapy, with increasing risks associated with increasing doses. Among children, risks of pediatric leukemia (ALL and AML) are modestly increased with maternal in utero exposures to diagnostic X-rays in earlier decades, moderately increased with radiotherapy treatments, and moderate-to-highly increased with childhood exposure to the atomic bombings. Among persons exposed as adults, acute leukemia risks are moderately increased among atomic bomb survivors, individuals living near the Mayak nuclear weapon plant, and patients receiving radiotherapy treatments, and AML risks are moderate-to-highly increased with occupational benzene exposure. High risks of AML occur among children and adults receiving cytotoxic treatments (e.g., alkylating agent and epipodophyllotoxin chemotherapy) for benign and malignant disease.

Although pediatric ALL has long been thought to have an infectious etiology, no infectious agent has been isolated. However, recent research has identified modest associations with other environmental, lifestyle, and medical factors for all acute leukemias. Pediatric leukemia has been linked with prenatal maternal occupational pesticide exposure (ALL and AML) and postnatal residential use of insecticides (ALL only). Modest associations have been reported for pediatric AML with maternal prenatal alcohol consumption, pediatric ALL with paternal preconception smoking, and adult AML with cigarette smoking. Anthropometric measures have also been associated with both ALL and AML in children (high birth weight) and adults (high body mass index). Dietary factors may play a role in both pediatric and adult leukemia, but more studies are needed to clarify associations. Interestingly, pediatric ALL risk appears modestly reduced among children who were breast-fed or have a history of atopy.

Recent progress has been made in understanding the germline mutations underlying familial AML, the molecular events by which rare genetic syndromes predispose to the acute leukemias, common genetic variants that confer increased susceptibility to the acute leukemias, and agents causing recurrent chromosomal and genetic abnormalities associated with acute leukemia molecular subtypes.

Although insights into etiology to date have facilitated some prevention efforts for the acute leukemias, additional epidemiologic work is needed to further impact the disease burden worldwide.

References

1. Siegel RL, Miller KD, Jemal A. Cancer statistics, 2016. CA Cancer J Clin. 2016;66(1):7–30.
2. Swerdlow SHCE, Harris NL, et al., editors. World Health Organization classification of tumours of haematopoietic and lymphoid tissues. 4th ed. Lyon: International Agency for Research on Cancer; 2008.
3. Anderson LM, Diwan BA, Fear NT, Roman E. Critical windows of exposure for children's health: cancer in human epidemiological studies and neoplasms in experimental animal models. Environ Health Perspect. 2000;108(Suppl 3):573–94.
4. Ferlay J, Soerjomataram I, Dikshit R, et al. Cancer incidence and mortality worldwide: sources, methods and major patterns in GLOBOCAN 2012. Int J Cancer. 2015;136(5):E359–E86.
5. National Cancer Institute S, Epidemiology, and End Results (SEER) Program. SEER*Stat Database: Incidence—SEER-9 Regs Research Data (1975–2013). In: DCCPS SRP, Cancer Statistics Branch, editor. National Cancer Institute, DCCPS, Surveillance Research Program, Cancer Statistics Branch, released April 2010, based on the November 2009 submission: National Cancer Institute; 2016.
6. Greaves MF. Biological models for leukaemia and lymphoma. IARC Sci Publ. 2004;157:351–72.
7. Mori H, Colman SM, Xiao Z, et al. Chromosome translocations and covert leukemic clones are generated during normal fetal development. Proc Natl Acad Sci U S A. 2002;99(12):8242–7.
8. Lausten-Thomsen U, Madsen HO, Vestergaard TR, et al. Prevalence of t(12;21)[ETV6-RUNX1]-positive cells in healthy neonates. Blood. 2011;117(1):186–9.
9. Brown P. TEL-AML1 in cord blood: 1% or 0.01%? Blood. 2011;117(1):2–4.
10. Ma X, Metayer C, Does MB, Buffler PA. Maternal pregnancy loss, birth characteristics, and childhood leukemia (United States). Cancer Causes Control. 2005;16(9):1075–83.
11. Podvin D, Kuehn CM, Mueller BA, Williams M. Maternal and birth characteristics in relation to childhood leukaemia. Paediatr Perinat Epidemiol. 2006;20(4):312–22.
12. van Steensel-Moll HA, Valkenburg HA, Vandenbroucke JP, van Zanen GE. Are maternal fertility problems related to childhood leukaemia? Int J Epidemiol. 1985;14(4):555–9.
13. Schuz J, Kaatsch P, Kaletsch U, Meinert R, Michaelis J. Association of childhood cancer with factors related to pregnancy and birth. Int J Epidemiol. 1999;28(4):631–9.
14. Roman E, Simpson J, Ansell P, et al. Perinatal and reproductive factors: a report on haematological malignancies from the UKCCS. Eur J Cancer. 2005;41(5):749–59.
15. Ross JA, Potter JD, Shu XO, et al. Evaluating the relationships among maternal reproductive history, birth characteristics, and infant leukemia: a report from the Children's cancer group. Ann Epidemiol. 1997;7(3):172–9.
16. Sergentanis TN, Thomopoulos TP, Gialamas SP, et al. Risk for childhood leukemia associated with maternal and paternal age. Eur J Epidemiol. 2015;30(12):1229–61.
17. Rudant J, Lightfoot T, Urayama KY, et al. Childhood acute lymphoblastic leukemia and indicators of early immune stimulation: a childhood leukemia international consortium study. Am J Epidemiol. 2015;181(8):549–62.
18. Von Behren J, Spector LG, Mueller BA, et al. Birth order and risk of childhood cancer: a pooled analysis from five US states. Int J Cancer. 2011;128(11):2709–16.
19. Smith M. Considerations on a possible viral etiology for B-precursor acute lymphoblastic leukemia of childhood. J Immunother. 1997;20(2):89–100.
20. Hakulinen T, Hovi L, Karkinen J, Penttinen K, Saxen L. Association between influenza during pregnancy and childhood leukaemia. Br Med J. 1973;4(5887):265–7.
21. Lehtinen M, Koskela P, Ogmundsdottir HM, et al. Maternal herpesvirus infections and risk of acute lymphoblastic leukemia in the offspring. Am J Epidemiol. 2003;158(3):207–13.
22. Randolph VL, Heath CW Jr. Influenza during pregnancy in relation to subsequent childhood leukemia and lymphoma. Am J Epidemiol. 1974;100(5):399–409.
23. Tedeschi R, Luostarinen T, Marus A, et al. No risk of maternal EBV infection for childhood leukemia. Cancer Epidemiol Biomark Prev. 2009;18(10):2790–2.
24. Bzhalava D, Hultin E, Arroyo Muhr LS, et al. Viremia during pregnancy and risk of childhood leukemia and lymphomas in the offspring: nested case-control study. Int J Cancer. 2016;138(9):2212–20.
25. Smith MA, Strickler HD, Granovsky M, et al. Investigation of leukemia cells from children with common acute lymphoblastic leukemia for genomic sequences of the primate polyomaviruses JC virus, BK virus, and simian virus 40. Med Pediatr Oncol. 1999;33(5):441–3.
26. MacKenzie J, Gallagher A, Clayton RA, et al. Screening for herpesvirus genomes in common acute lymphoblastic leukemia. Leukemia. 2001;15(3):415–21.
27. Isa A, Priftakis P, Broliden K, Gustafsson B. Human parvovirus B19 DNA is not detected in Guthrie cards from children who have developed acute lymphoblastic leukemia. Pediatr Blood Cancer. 2004;42(4):357–60.
28. Cnattingius S, Zack M, Ekbom A, et al. Prenatal and neonatal risk factors for childhood myeloid leukemia. Cancer Epidemiol Biomark Prev. 1995;4(5):441–5.
29. Cnattingius S, Zack MM, Ekbom A, et al. Prenatal and neonatal risk factors for childhood lymphatic leukemia. J Natl Cancer Inst. 1995;87(12):908–14.
30. Johnson KJ, Soler JT, Puumala SE, Ross JA, Spector LG. Parental and infant characteristics and childhood leukemia in Minnesota. BMC Pediatr. 2008;8:7.
31. Oksuzyan S, Crespi CM, Cockburn M, Mezei G, Kheifets L. Birth weight and other perinatal characteristics and childhood leukemia in California. Cancer Epidemiol. 2012;36(6):e359–65.
32. Kaatsch P, Scheidemann-Wesp U, Schuz J. Maternal use of antibiotics and cancer in the offspring: results of a case-control study in Germany. Cancer Causes Control. 2010;21(8):1335–45.
33. Wen W, Shu XO, Potter JD, et al. Parental medication use and risk of childhood acute lymphoblastic leukemia. Cancer. 2002;95(8):1786–94.
34. Rudant J, Amigou A, Orsi L, et al. Fertility treatments, congenital malformations, fetal loss, and childhood acute leukemia: the ESCALE study (SFCE). Pediatr Blood Cancer. 2013;60(2):301–8.
35. Brinton LA, Kruger Kjaer S, Thomsen BL, et al. Childhood tumor risk after treatment with ovulation-stimulating drugs. Fertil Steril. 2004;81(4):1083–91.
36. Robison LL, Buckley JD, Daigle AE, et al. Maternal drug use and risk of childhood nonlymphoblastic leukemia among offspring. An epidemiologic investigation implicating marijuana (a report from the Childrens cancer study group). Cancer. 1989;63(10):1904–11.
37. Trivers KF, Mertens AC, Ross JA, et al. Parental marijuana use and risk of childhood acute myeloid leukaemia: a report from the Children's cancer group (United States and Canada). Paediatr Perinat Epidemiol. 2006;20(2):110–8.

38. Shu XO, Potter JD, Linet MS, et al. Diagnostic X-rays and ultrasound exposure and risk of childhood acute lymphoblastic leukemia by immunophenotype. Cancer Epidemiol Biomark Prev. 2002;11(2):177–85.
39. Wakeford R. Childhood leukaemia following medical diagnostic exposure to ionizing radiation in utero or after birth. Radiat Prot Dosim. 2008;132(2):166–74.
40. Stewart A, Webb J, Hewitt D. A survey of childhood malignancies. Br Med J. 1958;1(5086):1495–508.
41. Preston DL, Cullings H, Suyama A, et al. Solid cancer incidence in atomic bomb survivors exposed in utero or as young children. J Natl Cancer Inst. 2008;100(6):428–36.
42. Hatch M, Brenner A, Bogdanova T, et al. A screening study of thyroid cancer and other thyroid diseases among individuals exposed in utero to iodine-131 from Chernobyl fallout. J Clin Endocrinol Metab. 2009;94(3):899–906.
43. United Nations. Scientific committee on the effects of atomic radiation. Sources and effects of ionizing radiation: United Nations scientific committee on the effects of atomic radiation : UNSCEAR 2008 report to the general assembly, with scientific annexes. New York: United Nations; 2010.
44. Kendall GM, Little MP, Wakeford R, et al. A record-based case-control study of natural background radiation and the incidence of childhood leukaemia and other cancers in great Britain during 1980–2006. Leukemia. 2013;27(1):3–9.
45. Spycher BD, Lupatsch JE, Zwahlen M, et al. Background ionizing radiation and the risk of childhood cancer: a census-based nationwide cohort study. Environ Health Perspect. 2015;123(6):622–8.
46. Del Risco KR, Blaasaas KG, Claussen B. Risk of leukaemia or cancer in the central nervous system among children living in an area with high indoor radon concentrations: results from a cohort study in Norway. Br J Cancer. 2014;111(7):1413–20.
47. Gardner MJ, Snee MP, Hall AJ, et al. Results of case-control study of leukaemia and lymphoma among young people near Sellafield nuclear plant in west Cumbria. BMJ. 1990;300(6722):423–9.
48. Roman E, Doyle P, Maconochie N, et al. Cancer in children of nuclear industry employees: report on children aged under 25 years from nuclear industry family study. BMJ. 1999;318(7196):1443–50.
49. Roman E, Doyle P, Ansell P, Bull D, Beral V. Health of children born to medical radiographers. Occup Environ Med. 1996;53(2):73–9.
50. Johnson KJ, Alexander BH, Doody MM, et al. Childhood cancer in the offspring born in 1921–1984 to US radiologic technologists. Br J Cancer. 2008;99(3):545–50.
51. Su L, Fei Y, Wei X, et al. Associations of parental occupational exposure to extremely low-frequency magnetic fields with childhood leukemia risk. Leuk Lymphoma. 2016;57(12):2855–62.
52. Zahm SH, Ward MH. Pesticides and childhood cancer. Environ Health Perspect. 1998;106(Suppl 3):893–908.
53. Infante-Rivard C, Weichenthal S. Pesticides and childhood cancer: an update of Zahm and Ward's 1998 review. J Toxicol Environ Health B Crit Rev. 2007;10(1–2):81–99.
54. Wigle DT, Turner MC, Krewski D. A systematic review and meta-analysis of childhood leukemia and parental occupational pesticide exposure. Environ Health Perspect. 2009;117(10):1505–13.
55. Van Maele-Fabry G, Lantin AC, Hoet P, Lison D. Childhood leukaemia and parental occupational exposure to pesticides: a systematic review and meta-analysis. Cancer Causes Control. 2010;21(6):787–809.
56. Bailey HD, Fritschi L, Infante-Rivard C, et al. Parental occupational pesticide exposure and the risk of childhood leukemia in the offspring: findings from the childhood leukemia international consortium. Int J Cancer. 2014;135(9):2157–72.
57. Bailey HD, Infante-Rivard C, Metayer C, et al. Home pesticide exposures and risk of childhood leukemia: findings from the childhood leukemia international consortium. Int J Cancer. 2015;137(11):2644–63.
58. Carlos-Wallace FM, Zhang L, Smith MT, Rader G, Steinmaus C. Parental, in utero, and early-life exposure to benzene and the risk of childhood leukemia: a meta-analysis. Am J Epidemiol. 2016;183(1):1–14.
59. Bailey HD, Fritschi L, Metayer C, et al. Parental occupational paint exposure and risk of childhood leukemia in the offspring: findings from the childhood leukemia international consortium. Cancer Causes Control. 2014;25(10):1351–67.
60. Bailey HD, Metayer C, Milne E, et al. Home paint exposures and risk of childhood acute lymphoblastic leukemia: findings from the childhood leukemia international consortium. Cancer Causes Control. 2015;26(9):1257–70.
61. Ghosh JK, Heck JE, Cockburn M, et al. Prenatal exposure to traffic-related air pollution and risk of early childhood cancers. Am J Epidemiol. 2013;178(8):1233–9.
62. Heck JE, Wu J, Lombardi C, et al. Childhood cancer and traffic-related air pollution exposure in pregnancy and early life. Environ Health Perspect. 2013;121(11–12):1385–91.
63. McKinney PA, Fear NT, Stockton D, Investigators UKCCS. Parental occupation at periconception: findings from the United Kingdom childhood cancer study. Occup Environ Med. 2003;60(12):901–9.
64. Wigle DT, Arbuckle TE, Turner MC, et al. Epidemiologic evidence of relationships between reproductive and child health outcomes and environmental chemical contaminants. J Toxicol Environ Health B Crit Rev. 2008;11(5–6):373–517.
65. Slater ME, Linabery AM, Spector LG, et al. Maternal exposure to household chemicals and risk of infant leukemia: a report from the Children's oncology group. Cancer Causes Control. 2011;22(8):1197–204.
66. Klimentopoulou A, Antonopoulos CN, Papadopoulou C, et al. Maternal smoking during pregnancy and risk for childhood leukemia: a nationwide case-control study in Greece and meta-analysis. Pediatr Blood Cancer. 2012;58(3):344–51.
67. Bonaventure A, Goujon-Bellec S, Rudant J, et al. Maternal smoking during pregnancy, genetic polymorphisms of metabolic enzymes, and childhood acute leukemia: the ESCALE study (SFCE). Cancer Causes Control. 2012;23(2):329–45.
68. Milne E, Greenop KR, Scott RJ, et al. Parental prenatal smoking and risk of childhood acute lymphoblastic leukemia. Am J Epidemiol. 2012;175(1):43–53.
69. Orsi L, Rudant J, Ajrouche R, et al. Parental smoking, maternal alcohol, coffee and tea consumption during pregnancy, and childhood acute leukemia: the ESTELLE study. Cancer Causes Control. 2015;26(7):1003–17.
70. Liu R, Zhang L, McHale CM, Hammond SK. Paternal smoking and risk of childhood acute lymphoblastic leukemia: systematic review and meta-analysis. J Oncol. 2011;2011:854584.
71. Infante-Rivard C, El-Zein M. Parental alcohol consumption and childhood cancers: a review. J Toxicol Environ Health B Crit Rev. 2007;10(1–2):101–29.
72. MacArthur AC, McBride ML, Spinelli JJ, et al. Risk of childhood leukemia associated with parental smoking and alcohol consumption prior to conception and during pregnancy: the cross-Canada childhood leukemia study. Cancer Causes Control. 2008;19(3):283–95.
73. Latino-Martel P, Chan DS, Druesne-Pecollo N, et al. Maternal alcohol consumption during pregnancy and risk of childhood leukemia: systematic review and meta-analysis. Cancer Epidemiol Biomark Prev. 2010;19(5):1238–60.
74. Spector LG, Xie Y, Robison LL, et al. Maternal diet and infant leukemia: the DNA topoisomerase II inhibitor hypothesis: a report from the children's oncology group. Cancer Epidemiol Biomark Prev. 2005;14(3):651–5.

75. Jensen CD, Block G, Buffler P, et al. Maternal dietary risk factors in childhood acute lymphoblastic leukemia (United States). Cancer Causes Control. 2004;15(6):559–70.
76. Petridou E, Ntouvelis E, Dessypris N, et al. Maternal diet and acute lymphoblastic leukemia in young children. Cancer Epidemiol Biomark Prev. 2005;14(8):1935–9.
77. Kwan ML, Jensen CD, Block G, et al. Maternal diet and risk of childhood acute lymphoblastic leukemia. Public Health Rep. 2009;124(4):503–14.
78. Metayer C, Milne E, Dockerty JD, et al. Maternal supplementation with folic acid and other vitamins and risk of leukemia in offspring: a childhood leukemia international consortium study. Epidemiology. 2014;25(6):811–22.
79. Singer AW, Selvin S, Block G, et al. Maternal prenatal intake of one-carbon metabolism nutrients and risk of childhood leukemia. Cancer Causes Control. 2016;27(7):929–40.
80. Kwan ML, Metayer C, Crouse V, Buffler PA. Maternal illness and drug/medication use during the period surrounding pregnancy and risk of childhood leukemia among offspring. Am J Epidemiol. 2007;165(1):27–35.
81. Thomopoulos TP, Ntouvelis E, Diamantaras AA, et al. Maternal and childhood consumption of coffee, tea and cola beverages in association with childhood leukemia: a meta-analysis. Cancer Epidemiol. 2015;39(6):1047–59.
82. Dominguez-Bello MG, Costello EK, Contreras M, et al. Delivery mode shapes the acquisition and structure of the initial microbiota across multiple body habitats in newborns. Proc Natl Acad Sci U S A. 2010;107(26):11971–5.
83. Jakobsson HE, Abrahamsson TR, Jenmalm MC, et al. Decreased gut microbiota diversity, delayed Bacteroidetes colonisation and reduced Th1 responses in infants delivered by caesarean section. Gut. 2014;63(4):559–66.
84. Gronlund MM, Lehtonen OP, Eerola E, Kero P. Fecal microflora in healthy infants born by different methods of delivery: permanent changes in intestinal Flora after cesarean delivery. J Pediatr Gastroenterol Nutr. 1999;28(1):19–25.
85. Cardwell CR, Stene LC, Joner G, et al. Caesarean section is associated with an increased risk of childhood-onset type 1 diabetes mellitus: a meta-analysis of observational studies. Diabetologia. 2008;51(5):726–35.
86. Thavagnanam S, Fleming J, Bromley A, Shields MD, Cardwell CR. A meta-analysis of the association between caesarean section and childhood asthma. Clin Exp Allergy. 2008;38(4):629–33.
87. Bager P, Wohlfahrt J, Westergaard T. Caesarean delivery and risk of atopy and allergic disease: meta-analyses. Clin Exp Allergy. 2008;38(4):634–42.
88. Mears K, McAuliffe F, Grimes H, Morrison JJ. Fetal cortisol in relation to labour, intrapartum events and mode of delivery. J Obstet Gynaecol. 2004;24(2):129–32.
89. Lagercrantz H. Stress, arousal, and gene activation at birth. News Physiol Sci. 1996;11:214–8.
90. Zanardo V, Solda G, Trevisanuto D. Elective cesarean section and fetal immune-endocrine response. Int J Gynaecol Obstet. 2006;95(1):52–3.
91. Marcotte EL, Thomopoulos TP, Infante-Rivard C, et al. Caesarean delivery and risk of childhood leukaemia: a pooled analysis from the childhood leukemia international consortium (CLIC). Lancet Haematol. 2016;3(4):e176–85.
92. Caughey RW, Michels KB. Birth weight and childhood leukemia: a meta-analysis and review of the current evidence. Int J Cancer. 2009;124(11):2658–70.
93. Milne E, Greenop KR, Metayer C, et al. Fetal growth and childhood acute lymphoblastic leukemia: findings from the childhood leukemia international consortium. Int J Cancer. 2013;133(12):2968–79.
94. Shu XO, Linet MS, Steinbuch M, et al. Breast-feeding and risk of childhood acute leukemia. J Natl Cancer Inst. 1999;91(20):1765–72.
95. Investigators UKCCS. Breastfeeding and childhood cancer. Br J Cancer. 2001;85(11):1685–94.
96. Amitay EL, Keinan-Boker L. Breastfeeding and childhood leukemia incidence: a meta-analysis and systematic review. JAMA Pediatr. 2015;169(6):e151025.
97. MacArthur AC, McBride ML, Spinelli JJ, et al. Risk of childhood leukemia associated with vaccination, infection, and medication use in childhood: the cross-Canada childhood leukemia study. Am J Epidemiol. 2008;167(5):598–606.
98. Alexander FE. Clusters and clustering of childhood cancer: a review. Eur J Epidemiol. 1999;15(9):847–52.
99. Heath CW Jr. Community clusters of childhood leukemia and lymphoma: evidence of infection? Am J Epidemiol. 2005;162(9):817–22.
100. Rubin CS, Holmes AK, Belson MG, et al. Investigating childhood leukemia in Churchill County, Nevada. Environ Health Perspect. 2007;115(1):151–7.
101. Greaves M. Infection, immune responses and the aetiology of childhood leukaemia. Nat Rev Cancer. 2006;6(3):193–203.
102. Urayama KY, Buffler PA, Gallagher ER, Ayoob JM, Ma X. A meta-analysis of the association between day-care attendance and childhood acute lymphoblastic leukaemia. Int J Epidemiol. 2010;39(3):718–32.
103. Marcotte EL, Ritz B, Cockburn M, Yu F, Heck JE. Exposure to infections and risk of leukemia in young children. Cancer Epidemiol Biomark Prev. 2014;23(7):1195–203.
104. Roman E, Simpson J, Ansell P, et al. Childhood acute lymphoblastic leukemia and infections in the first year of life: a report from the United Kingdom childhood cancer study. Am J Epidemiol. 2007;165(5):496–504.
105. Kinlen L. Evidence for an infective cause of childhood leukaemia: comparison of a Scottish new town with nuclear reprocessing sites in Britain. Lancet. 1988;2(8624):1323–7.
106. Kinlen LJ. Epidemiological evidence for an infective basis in childhood leukaemia. Br J Cancer. 1995;71(1):1–5.
107. Law GR, Parslow RC, Roman E. United Kingdom childhood cancer study I. Childhood cancer and population mixing. Am J Epidemiol. 2003;158(4):328–36.
108. Pagaoa MA, Okcu MF, Bondy ML, Scheurer ME. Associations between vaccination and childhood cancers in Texas regions. J Pediatr. 2011;158(6):996–1002.
109. Linabery AM, Jurek AM, Duval S, Ross JA. The association between atopy and childhood/adolescent leukemia: a meta-analysis. Am J Epidemiol. 2010;171(7):749–64.
110. Dahl S, Schmidt LS, Vestergaard T, Schuz J, Schmiegelow K. Allergy and the risk of childhood leukemia: a meta-analysis. Leukemia. 2009;23(12):2300–4.
111. Linet MS, Kim KP, Rajaraman P. Children's exposure to diagnostic medical radiation and cancer risk: epidemiologic and dosimetric considerations. Pediatr Radiol. 2009;39(Suppl 1):S4–26.
112. Pearce MS, Salotti JA, Little MP, et al. Radiation exposure from CT scans in childhood and subsequent risk of leukaemia and brain tumours: a retrospective cohort study. Lancet. 2012;380(9840):499–505.
113. Krille L, Dreger S, Schindel R, et al. Risk of cancer incidence before the age of 15 years after exposure to ionising radiation from computed tomography: results from a German cohort study. Radiat Environ Biophys. 2015;54(1):1–12.
114. BJ J. Ionizing radiation. In: Schottenfeld D, Fraumeni JF, editors. Cancer epidemiology and prevention. New York: Oxford University Press; 2006. p. 259–935.
115. Ron E, Modan B, Boice JD Jr. Mortality after radiotherapy for ringworm of the scalp. Am J Epidemiol. 1988;127(4):713–25.
116. Allard A, Haddy N, Le Deley MC, et al. Role of radiation dose in the risk of secondary leukemia after a solid tumor in childhood treated between 1980 and 1999. Int J Radiat Oncol Biol Phys. 2010;78(5):1474–82.

117. Preston DL, Kusumi S, Tomonaga M, et al. Cancer incidence in atomic bomb survivors. Part III. Leukemia, lymphoma and multiple myeloma, 1950–1987. Radiat Res. 1994;137(2 Suppl):S68–97.
118. Hsu WL, Preston DL, Soda M, et al. The incidence of leukemia, lymphoma and multiple myeloma among atomic bomb survivors: 1950–2001. Radiat Res. 2013;179(3):361–82.
119. Darby SC, Doll R. Fallout, radiation doses near Dounreay, and childhood leukaemia. Br Med J (Clin Res Ed). 1987;294(6572):603–7.
120. Lubin JH, Linet MS, Boice JD Jr, et al. Case-control study of childhood acute lymphoblastic leukemia and residential radon exposure. J Natl Cancer Inst. 1998;90(4):294–300.
121. Kaletsch U, Kaatsch P, Meinert R, et al. Childhood cancer and residential radon exposure—results of a population-based case-control study in lower Saxony (Germany). Radiat Environ Biophys. 1999;38(3):211–5.
122. Demoury C, Marquant F, Ielsch G, et al. Residential exposure to natural background radiation and risk of childhood acute leukemia in France, 1990–2009. Environ Health Perspect. 2017;125(4):714–20.
123. Investigators UKCCS. The United Kingdom childhood cancer study of exposure to domestic sources of ionising radiation: 1: radon gas. Br J Cancer. 2002;86(11):1721–6.
124. Steinbuch M, Weinberg CR, Buckley JD, Robison LL, Sandler DP. Indoor residential radon exposure and risk of childhood acute myeloid leukaemia. Br J Cancer. 1999;81(5):900–6.
125. Ahlbom A, Day N, Feychting M, et al. A pooled analysis of magnetic fields and childhood leukaemia. Br J Cancer. 2000;83(5):692–8.
126. Slusky DA, Does M, Metayer C, et al. Potential role of selection bias in the association between childhood leukemia and residential magnetic fields exposure: a population-based assessment. Cancer Epidemiol. 2014;38(3):307–13.
127. Boorman GA, Rafferty CN, Ward JM, Sills RC. Leukemia and lymphoma incidence in rodents exposed to low-frequency magnetic fields. Radiat Res. 2000;153(5 Pt 2):627–36.
128. Infante-Rivard C, Labuda D, Krajinovic M, Sinnett D. Risk of childhood leukemia associated with exposure to pesticides and with gene polymorphisms. Epidemiology. 1999;10(5):481–7.
129. Ward MH, Colt JS, Metayer C, et al. Residential exposure to polychlorinated biphenyls and organochlorine pesticides and risk of childhood leukemia. Environ Health Perspect. 2009;117(6):1007–13.
130. Janitz AE, Campbell JE, Magzamen S, et al. Traffic-related air pollution and childhood acute leukemia in Oklahoma. Environ Res. 2016;148:102–11.
131. Spycher BD, Feller M, Roosli M, et al. Childhood cancer and residential exposure to highways: a nationwide cohort study. Eur J Epidemiol. 2015;30(12):1263–75.
132. Buckley JD, Robison LL, Swotinsky R, et al. Occupational exposures of parents of children with acute nonlymphocytic leukemia: a report from the Childrens cancer study group. Cancer Res. 1989;49(14):4030–7.
133. Freedman DM, Stewart P, Kleinerman RA, et al. Household solvent exposures and childhood acute lymphoblastic leukemia. Am J Public Health. 2001;91(4):564–7.
134. Scelo G, Metayer C, Zhang L, et al. Household exposure to paint and petroleum solvents, chromosomal translocations, and the risk of childhood leukemia. Environ Health Perspect. 2009;117(1):133–9.
135. Kwan ML, Block G, Selvin S, Month S, Buffler PA. Food consumption by children and the risk of childhood acute leukemia. Am J Epidemiol. 2004;160(11):1098–107.
136. Liu CY, Hsu YH, Wu MT, et al. Cured meat, vegetables, and bean-curd foods in relation to childhood acute leukemia risk: a population based case-control study. BMC Cancer. 2009;9:15.
137. Golding J, Greenwood R, Birmingham K, Mott M. Childhood cancer, intramuscular vitamin K, and pethidine given during labour. BMJ. 1992;305(6849):341–6.
138. Roman E, Fear NT, Ansell P, et al. Vitamin K and childhood cancer: analysis of individual patient data from six case-control studies. Br J Cancer. 2002;86(1):63–9.
139. Pedersen-Bjergaard J, Andersen MK, Christiansen DH. Therapy-related acute myeloid leukemia and myelodysplasia after high-dose chemotherapy and autologous stem cell transplantation. Blood. 2000;95(11):3273–9.
140. Boice JD Jr, Greene MH, Killen JY Jr, et al. Leukemia and preleukemia after adjuvant treatment of gastrointestinal cancer with semustine (methyl-CCNU). N Engl J Med. 1983;309(18):1079–84.
141. Pedersen-Bjergaard J, Daugaard G, Hansen SW, et al. Increased risk of myelodysplasia and leukaemia after etoposide, cisplatin, and bleomycin for germ-cell tumours. Lancet. 1991;338(8763):359–63.
142. McLaughlin P, Estey E, Glassman A, et al. Myelodysplasia and acute myeloid leukemia following therapy for indolent lymphoma with fludarabine, mitoxantrone, and dexamethasone (FND) plus rituximab and interferon alpha. Blood. 2005;105(12):4573–5.
143. Hershman D, Neugut AI, Jacobson JS, et al. Acute myeloid leukemia or myelodysplastic syndrome following use of granulocyte colony-stimulating factors during breast cancer adjuvant chemotherapy. J Natl Cancer Inst. 2007;99(3):196–205.
144. Bhatia S. Therapy-related myelodysplasia and acute myeloid leukemia. Semin Oncol. 2013;40(6):666–75.
145. Vardiman JW. The World Health Organization (WHO) classification of tumors of the hematopoietic and lymphoid tissues: an overview with emphasis on the myeloid neoplasms. Chem Biol Interact. 2010;184(1–2):16–20.
146. Godley LA, Larson RA. Therapy-related myeloid leukemia. Semin Oncol. 2008;35(4):418–29.
147. Pedersen-Bjergaard J, Philip P. Balanced translocations involving chromosome bands 11q23 and 21q22 are highly characteristic of myelodysplasia and leukemia following therapy with cytostatic agents targeting at DNA-topoisomerase II. Blood. 1991;78(4):1147–8.
148. Pedersen-Bjergaard J, Andersen MK, Christiansen DH, Nerlov C. Genetic pathways in therapy-related myelodysplasia and acute myeloid leukemia. Blood. 2002;99(6):1909–12.
149. Leone G, Fianchi L, Pagano L, Voso MT. Incidence and susceptibility to therapy-related myeloid neoplasms. Chem Biol Interact. 2010;184(1–2):39–45.
150. Kwong YL. Azathioprine: association with therapy-related myelodysplastic syndrome and acute myeloid leukemia. J Rheumatol. 2010;37(3):485–90.
151. Anderson LA, Gadalla S, Morton LM, et al. Population-based study of autoimmune conditions and the risk of specific lymphoid malignancies. Int J Cancer. 2009;125(2):398–405.
152. Johnson KJ, Blair CM, Fink JM, et al. Medical conditions and risk of adult myeloid leukemia. Cancer Causes Control. 2012;23(7):1083–9.
153. Lopez A, Mounier M, Bouvier AM, et al. Increased risk of acute myeloid leukemias and myelodysplastic syndromes in patients who received thiopurine treatment for inflammatory bowel disease. Clin Gastroenterol Hepatol. 2014;12(8):1324–9.
154. Morton LM, Gibson TM, Clarke CA, et al. Risk of myeloid neoplasms after solid organ transplantation. Leukemia. 2014;28(12):2317–23.
155. Pagano L, Pulsoni A, Tosti ME, et al. Acute lymphoblastic leukaemia occurring as second malignancy: report of the GIMEMA archive of adult acute leukaemia. Gruppo Italiano Malattie Ematologiche Maligne dell'Adulto. Br J Haematol. 1999;106(4):1037–40.
156. Shivakumar R, Tan W, Wilding GE, Wang ES, Wetzler M. Biologic features and treatment outcome of secondary acute lymphoblastic leukemia—a review of 101 cases. Ann Oncol. 2008;19(9):1634–8.
157. Tang G, Zuo Z, Thomas DA, et al. Precursor B-acute lymphoblastic leukemia occurring in patients with a history of prior malignancies: is it therapy-related? Haematologica. 2012;97(6):919–25.

158. Aldoss I, Dagis A, Palmer J, Forman S, Pullarkat V. Therapy-related ALL: cytogenetic features and hematopoietic cell transplantation outcome. Bone Marrow Transplant. 2015;50(5):746–8.
159. Linos A, Gray JE, Orvis AL, et al. Low-dose radiation and leukemia. N Engl J Med. 1980;302(20):1101–5.
160. Boice JD Jr, Morin MM, Glass AG, et al. Diagnostic x-ray procedures and risk of leukemia, lymphoma, and multiple myeloma. JAMA. 1991;265(10):1290–4.
161. Zheng W, Linet MS, Shu XO, et al. Prior medical conditions and the risk of adult leukemia in shanghai, People's republic of China. Cancer Causes Control. 1993;4(4):361–8.
162. Yuasa H, Hamajima N, Ueda R, et al. Case-control study of leukemia and diagnostic radiation exposure. Int J Hematol. 1997;65(3):251–61.
163. Pogoda JM, Nichols PW, Ross RK, et al. Diagnostic radiography and adult acute myeloid leukaemia: an interview and medical chart review study. Br J Cancer. 2011;104(9):1482–6.
164. Martling U, Mattsson A, Travis LB, Holm LE, Hall P. Mortality after long-term exposure to radioactive thorotrast: a forty-year follow-up survey in Sweden. Radiat Res. 1999;151(3):293–9.
165. Andersson M, Carstensen B, Visfeldt J. Leukemia and other related hematological disorders among Danish patients exposed to Thorotrast. Radiat Res. 1993;134(2):224–33.
166. Travis LB, Hauptmann M, Gaul LK, et al. Site-specific cancer incidence and mortality after cerebral angiography with radioactive thorotrast. Radiat Res. 2003;160(6):691–706.
167. Weiss HA, Darby SC, Fearn T, Doll R. Leukemia mortality after X-ray treatment for ankylosing spondylitis. Radiat Res. 1995;142(1):1–11.
168. Sakata R, Kleinerman RA, Mabuchi K, et al. Cancer mortality following radiotherapy for benign gynecologic disorders. Radiat Res. 2012;178(4):266–79.
169. Inskip PD, Kleinerman RA, Stovall M, et al. Leukemia, lymphoma, and multiple myeloma after pelvic radiotherapy for benign disease. Radiat Res. 1993;135(1):108–24.
170. Griem ML, Kleinerman RA, Boice JD Jr, et al. Cancer following radiotherapy for peptic ulcer. J Natl Cancer Inst. 1994;86(11):842–9.
171. Ozasa K. Epidemiological research on radiation-induced cancer in atomic bomb survivors. J Radiat Res. 2016;57(Suppl 1):i112–7.
172. Richardson D, Sugiyama H, Nishi N, et al. Ionizing radiation and leukemia mortality among Japanese atomic bomb survivors, 1950–2000. Radiat Res. 2009;172(3):368–82.
173. Krestinina L, Preston DL, Davis FG, et al. Leukemia incidence among people exposed to chronic radiation from the contaminated Techa River, 1953–2005. Radiat Environ Biophys. 2010;49(2):195–201.
174. Krestinina LY, Davis FG, Schonfeld S, et al. Leukaemia incidence in the Techa River cohort: 1953-2007. Br J Cancer. 2013;109(11):2886–93.
175. Yoshinaga S, Mabuchi K, Sigurdson AJ, Doody MM, Ron E. Cancer risks among radiologists and radiologic technologists: review of epidemiologic studies. Radiology. 2004;233(2):313–21.
176. Berrington de Gonzalez A, Ntowe E, Kitahara CM, et al. Long-term mortality in 43 763 U.S. radiologists compared with 64 990 U.S. Psychiatrists. Radiology. 2016;281(3):847–57.
177. Liu JJ, Freedman DM, Little MP, et al. Work history and mortality risks in 90,268 US radiological technologists. Occup Environ Med. 2014;71(12):819–35.
178. Daniels RD, Schubauer-Berigan MK. A meta-analysis of leukaemia risk from protracted exposure to low-dose gamma radiation. Occup Environ Med. 2011;68(6):457–64.
179. Leuraud K, Richardson DB, Cardis E, et al. Ionising radiation and risk of death from leukaemia and lymphoma in radiation-monitored workers (INWORKS): an international cohort study. Lancet Haematol. 2015;2(7):e276–81.
180. Shilnikova NS, Preston DL, Ron E, et al. Cancer mortality risk among workers at the Mayak nuclear complex. Radiat Res. 2003;159(6):787–98.
181. International Agency for Research on Cancer. IARC Monographs on the Evaluation of Carcinogenic Risks to Humans. Volume 100F: A Review of Human Carcinogens: Chemical Agents and Related Occupations. 2012. http://monographs.Iarc.Fr/ENG/monographs/vol100F/mono100F-24.Pdf. Accessed Mar 29 2016.
182. Wallace LA. Major sources of benzene exposure. Environ Health Perspect. 1989;82:165–9.
183. Schnatter AR, Rosamilia K, Wojcik NC. Review of the literature on benzene exposure and leukemia subtypes. Chem Biol Interact. 2005;153–154:9–21.
184. Khalade A, Jaakkola MS, Pukkala E, Jaakkola JJ. Exposure to benzene at work and the risk of leukemia: a systematic review and meta-analysis. Environ Health. 2010;9:31.
185. Yin SN, Hayes RB, Linet MS, et al. A cohort study of cancer among benzene-exposed workers in China: overall results. Am J Ind Med. 1996;29(3):227–35.
186. Linet MS, Yin SN, Travis LB, et al. Clinical features of hematopoietic malignancies and related disorders among benzene-exposed workers in China. Benzene study group. Environ Health Perspect. 1996;104(Suppl 6):1353–64.
187. Hayes RB, Yin SN, Dosemeci M, et al. Benzene and the dose-related incidence of hematologic neoplasms in China. Chinese academy of preventive medicine—National Cancer Institute benzene study group. J Natl Cancer Inst. 1997;89(14):1065–71.
188. Linet MS, Yin SN, Gilbert ES, et al. A retrospective cohort study of cause-specific mortality and incidence of hematopoietic malignancies in Chinese benzene-exposed workers. Int J Cancer. 2015;137(9):2184–97.
189. Linet MS, Devesa SS, Morgan GJ. The leukemias. In: Schottenfeld D, Fraumeni JF, editors. Cancer epidemiology and prevention. 3rd ed. New York: Oxford University Press; 2006. p. 841–71.
190. Jones RR, Yu CL, Nuckols JR, et al. Farm residence and lymphohematopoietic cancers in the Iowa Women's health study. Environ Res. 2014;133:353–61.
191. Schinasi LH, De Roos AJ, Ray RM, et al. Insecticide exposure and farm history in relation to risk of lymphomas and leukemias in the Women's health initiative observational study cohort. Ann Epidemiol. 2015;25(11):803–10.
192. Descatha A, Jenabian A, Conso F, Ameille J. Occupational exposures and haematological malignancies: overview on human recent data. Cancer Causes Control. 2005;16(8):939–53.
193. Travis LB, Li CY, Zhang ZN, et al. Hematopoietic malignancies and related disorders among benzene-exposed workers in China. Leuk Lymphoma. 1994;14(1–2):91–102.
194. Van Maele-Fabry G, Duhayon S, Lison D. A systematic review of myeloid leukemias and occupational pesticide exposure. Cancer Causes Control. 2007;18(5):457–78.
195. Waggoner JK, Kullman GJ, Henneberger PK, et al. Mortality in the agricultural health study, 1993–2007. Am J Epidemiol. 2011;173(1):71–83.
196. Frost G, Brown T, Harding AH. Mortality and cancer incidence among British agricultural pesticide users. Occup Med (Lond). 2011;61(5):303–10.
197. Beane Freeman LE, Bonner MR, Blair A, et al. Cancer incidence among male pesticide applicators in the agricultural health study cohort exposed to diazinon. Am J Epidemiol. 2005;162(11):1070–9.
198. van Bemmel DM, Visvanathan K, Beane Freeman LE, et al. S-ethyl-N,N-dipropylthiocarbamate exposure and cancer incidence among male pesticide applicators in the agricultural health study: a prospective cohort. Environ Health Perspect. 2008;116(11):1541–6.
199. Mahajan R, Blair A, Lynch CF, et al. Fonofos exposure and cancer incidence in the agricultural health study. Environ Health Perspect. 2006;114(12):1838–42.
200. Purdue MP, Hoppin JA, Blair A, Dosemeci M, Alavanja MC. Occupational exposure to organochlorine insecticides and

cancer incidence in the agricultural health study. Int J Cancer. 2007;120(3):642–9.
201. Lerro CC, Koutros S, Andreotti G, et al. Use of acetochlor and cancer incidence in the agricultural health study. Int J Cancer. 2015;137(5):1167–75.
202. Silver SR, Bertke SJ, Hines CJ, et al. Cancer incidence and metolachlor use in the agricultural health study: an update. Int J Cancer. 2015;137(11):2630–43.
203. Freeman LE, Rusiecki JA, Hoppin JA, et al. Atrazine and cancer incidence among pesticide applicators in the agricultural health study (1994-2007). Environ Health Perspect. 2011;119(9):1253 9.
204. Brownson RC, Novotny TE, Perry MC. Cigarette smoking and adult leukemia. A meta-analysis. Arch Intern Med. 1993;153(4):469–75.
205. Fircanis S, Merriam P, Khan N, Castillo JJ. The relation between cigarette smoking and risk of acute myeloid leukemia: an updated meta-analysis of epidemiological studies. Am J Hematol. 2014;89(8):E125–32.
206. Kasim K, Levallois P, Abdous B, Auger P, Johnson KC. Lifestyle factors and the risk of adult leukemia in Canada. Cancer Causes Control. 2005;16(5):489–500.
207. Castillo JJ, Reagan JL, Ingham RR, et al. Obesity but not overweight increases the incidence and mortality of leukemia in adults: a meta-analysis of prospective cohort studies. Leuk Res. 2012;36(7):868–75.
208. Ross JA, Kasum CM, Davies SM, et al. Diet and risk of leukemia in the Iowa Women's health study. Cancer Epidemiol Biomark Prev. 2002;11(8):777–81.
209. Li Y, Moysich KB, Baer MR, et al. Intakes of selected food groups and beverages and adult acute myeloid leukemia. Leuk Res. 2006;30(12):1507–15.
210. Zhang M, Zhao X, Zhang X, Holman CD. Possible protective effect of green tea intake on risk of adult leukaemia. Br J Cancer. 2008;98(1):168–70.
211. Yamamura Y, Oum R, Gbito KY, Garcia-Manero G, Strom SS. Dietary intake of vegetables, fruits, and meats/beans as potential risk factors of acute myeloid leukemia: a Texas case-control study. Nutr Cancer. 2013;65(8):1132–40.
212. Ma X, Park Y, Mayne ST, et al. Diet, lifestyle, and acute myeloid leukemia in the NIH-AARP cohort. Am J Epidemiol. 2010;171(3):312–22.
213. Saberi Hosnijeh F, Peeters P, Romieu I, et al. Dietary intakes and risk of lymphoid and myeloid leukemia in the European prospective investigation into cancer and nutrition (EPIC). Nutr Cancer. 2014;66(1):14–28.
214. Gorini G, Stagnaro E, Fontana V, et al. Alcohol consumption and risk of leukemia: a multicenter case-control study. Leuk Res. 2007;31(3):379–86.
215. Klatsky AL, Li Y, Baer D, et al. Alcohol consumption and risk of hematologic malignancies. Ann Epidemiol. 2009;19(10):746–53.
216. Kroll ME, Murphy F, Pirie K, et al. Alcohol drinking, tobacco smoking and subtypes of haematological malignancy in the UK million women study. Br J Cancer. 2012;107(5):879–87.
217. Moore SC, Lee IM, Weiderpass E, et al. Association of leisure-time physical activity with risk of 26 types of cancer in 1.44 million adults. JAMA Intern Med. 2016;176(6):816–25.
218. Jochem C, Leitzmann MF, Keimling M, Schmid D, Behrens G. Physical activity in relation to risk of hematologic cancers: a systematic review and meta-analysis. Cancer Epidemiol Biomark Prev. 2014;23(5):833–46.
219. Walter RB, Buckley SA, White E. Regular recreational physical activity and risk of hematologic malignancies: results from the prospective VITamins and lifestyle (VITAL) study. Ann Oncol. 2013;24(5):1370–7.
220. Traversa G, Menniti-Ippolito F, Da Cas R, et al. Drug use and acute leukemia. Pharmacoepidemiol Drug Saf. 1998;7(2):113–23.
221. Kasum CM, Blair CK, Folsom AR, Ross JA. Non-steroidal anti-inflammatory drug use and risk of adult leukemia. Cancer Epidemiol Biomark Prev. 2003;12(6):534–7.
222. Weiss JR, Baker JA, Baer MR, et al. Opposing effects of aspirin and acetaminophen use on risk of adult acute leukemia. Leuk Res. 2006;30(2):164–9.
223. Ross JA, Blair CK, Cerhan JR, et al. Nonsteroidal anti-inflammatory drug and acetaminophen use and risk of adult myeloid leukemia. Cancer Epidemiol Biomark Prev. 2011;20(8):1741–50.
224. Walter RB, Milano F, Brasky TM, White E. Long-term use of acetaminophen, aspirin, and other nonsteroidal anti-inflammatory drugs and risk of hematologic malignancies: results from the prospective vitamins and lifestyle (VITAL) study. J Clin Oncol. 2011;29(17):2424–31.
225. Owen C, Barnett M, Fitzgibbon J. Familial myelodysplasia and acute myeloid leukaemia--a review. Br J Haematol. 2008;140(2):123–32.
226. Noetzli L, Lo RW, Lee-Sherick AB, et al. Germline mutations in ETV6 are associated with thrombocytopenia, red cell macrocytosis and predisposition to lymphoblastic leukemia. Nat Genet. 2015;47(5):535–8.
227. Topka S, Vijai J, Walsh MF, et al. Germline ETV6 mutations confer susceptibility to acute lymphoblastic leukemia and thrombocytopenia. PLoS Genet. 2015;11(6):e1005262.
228. Shah S, Schrader KA, Waanders E, et al. A recurrent germline PAX5 mutation confers susceptibility to pre-B cell acute lymphoblastic leukemia. Nat Genet. 2013;45(10):1226–31.
229. Couto E, Chen B, Hemminki K. Association of childhood acute lymphoblastic leukaemia with cancers in family members. Br J Cancer. 2005;93(11):1307–9.
230. Greaves MF, Maia AT, Wiemels JL, Ford AM. Leukemia in twins: lessons in natural history. Blood. 2003;102(7):2321–33.
231. Alter BP, Giri N, Savage SA, et al. Malignancies and survival patterns in the National Cancer Institute inherited bone marrow failure syndromes cohort study. Br J Haematol. 2010;150(2):179–88.
232. Rommens J, Durie P. Shwachman-diamond syndrome. In: Pagon R, Bird T, Dolan C, Stephens K, editors. Gene reviews [internet]. Seattle, WA: University of Washington; 2008.
233. Federman N, Sakamoto KM. The genetic basis of bone marrow failure syndromes in children. Mol Genet Metab. 2005;86(1–2):100–9.
234. Gelb BD, Tartaglia M. Noonan syndrome and related disorders: dysregulated RAS-mitogen activated protein kinase signal transduction. Hum Mol Genet. 2006;15 Spec No 2:R220–6.
235. German J. Bloom's syndrome. XX. The first 100 cancers. Cancer Genet Cytogenet. 1997;93(1):100–6.
236. Olsen JH, Hahnemann JM, Borresen-Dale AL, et al. Cancer in patients with ataxia-telangiectasia and in their relatives in the Nordic countries. J Natl Cancer Inst. 2001;93(2):121–7.
237. Varley JM, Evans DG, Birch JM. Li-Fraumeni syndrome--a molecular and clinical review. Br J Cancer. 1997;76(1):1–14.
238. Yohay K. Neurofibromatosis type 1 and associated malignancies. Curr Neurol Neurosci Rep. 2009;9(3):247–53.
239. Ross JA, Spector LG, Robison LL, Olshan AF. Epidemiology of leukemia in children with down syndrome. Pediatr Blood Cancer. 2005;44(1):8–12.
240. Xavier AC, Taub JW. Acute leukemia in children with down syndrome. Haematologica. 2010;95(7):1043–5.
241. Vijayakrishnan J, Houlston RS. Candidate gene association studies and risk of childhood acute lymphoblastic leukemia: a systematic review and meta-analysis. Haematologica. 2010;95(8):1405–14.
242. Migliorini G, Fiege B, Hosking FJ, et al. Variation at 10p12.2 and 10p14 influences risk of childhood B-cell acute lymphoblastic leukemia and phenotype. Blood. 2013;122(19):3298–307.
243. Papaemmanuil E, Hosking FJ, Vijayakrishnan J, et al. Loci on 7p12.2, 10q21.2 and 14q11.2 are associated with risk of childhood acute lymphoblastic leukemia. Nat Genet. 2009;41(9):1006–10.

244. Prasad RB, Hosking FJ, Vijayakrishnan J, et al. Verification of the susceptibility loci on 7p12.2, 10q21.2, and 14q11.2 in precursor B-cell acute lymphoblastic leukemia of childhood. Blood. 2010;115(9):1765–7.
245. Sherborne AL, Hosking FJ, Prasad RB, et al. Variation in CDKN2A at 9p21.3 influences childhood acute lymphoblastic leukemia risk. Nat Genet. 2010;42(6):492–4.
246. Vijayakrishnan J, Kumar R, Henrion MY, et al. A genome-wide association study identifies risk loci for childhood acute lymphoblastic leukemia at 10q26.13 and 12q23.1. Leukemia. 2017;31(3):573–9.
247. Vijayakrishnan J, Sherborne AL, Sawangpanich R, et al. Variation at 7p12.2 and 10q21.2 influences childhood acute lymphoblastic leukemia risk in the Thai population and may contribute to racial differences in leukemia incidence. Leuk Lymphoma. 2010;51(10):1870–4.
248. Hungate EA, Vora SR, Gamazon ER, et al. A variant at 9p21.3 functionally implicates CDKN2B in paediatric B-cell precursor acute lymphoblastic leukaemia aetiology. Nat Commun. 2016;7:10635.
249. Perez-Andreu V, Roberts KG, Harvey RC, et al. Inherited GATA3 variants are associated with Ph-like childhood acute lymphoblastic leukemia and risk of relapse. Nat Genet. 2013;45(12):1494–8.
250. Trevino LR, Yang W, French D, et al. Germline genomic variants associated with childhood acute lymphoblastic leukemia. Nat Genet. 2009;41(9):1001–5.
251. Xu H, Yang W, Perez-Andreu V, et al. Novel susceptibility variants at 10p12.31-12.2 for childhood acute lymphoblastic leukemia in ethnically diverse populations. J Natl Cancer Inst. 2013;105(10):733–42.
252. Yang JJ, Cheng C, Devidas M, et al. Genome-wide association study identifies germline polymorphisms associated with relapse of childhood acute lymphoblastic leukemia. Blood. 2012;120(20):4197–204.
253. Yang W, Trevino LR, Yang JJ, et al. ARID5B SNP rs10821936 is associated with risk of childhood acute lymphoblastic leukemia in blacks and contributes to racial differences in leukemia incidence. Leukemia. 2010;24(4):894–6.
254. Enciso-Mora V, Hosking FJ, Sheridan E, et al. Common genetic variation contributes significantly to the risk of childhood B-cell precursor acute lymphoblastic leukemia. Leukemia. 2012;26(10):2212–5.
255. Lim JY, Bhatia S, Robison LL, Yang JJ. Genomics of racial and ethnic disparities in childhood acute lymphoblastic leukemia. Cancer. 2014;120(7):955–62.
256. Moriyama T, Relling MV, Yang JJ. Inherited genetic variation in childhood acute lymphoblastic leukemia. Blood. 2015;125(26):3988–95.

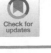

Classification of the Acute Leukemias: Cytochemical and Morphologic Considerations

14

N. Nukhet Tuzuner and John M. Bennett

Definition and Classification

The acute leukemias are a heterogeneous group of neoplasms affecting uncommitted or partially committed hematopoietic stem cells. The origin of the malignant neoplasm is almost invariably within the marrow. Replacement of the marrow pulp or repression of normal hematopoietic cells results in variable degrees of anemia, neutropenia, and thrombocytopenia.

Historically, the term acute implied not only a poorly differentiated blast population, but also a clinical syndrome that led to a rapid fatal outcome. Since it is apparent that, with modern chemotherapy, including bone marrow transplantation (BMT), patients with acute leukemia of several morphologic types can enjoy complete remission (CR), and indeed cure, the term acute can be maintained for nosologic reasons only.

Traditionally, morphology and cytochemistry identified the different involved lineages. During the past 25 years, major advances in our knowledge of the nature of acute leukemia consequent to the application of the techniques of immunology, cytogenetics, and molecular studies have taken place. The demonstration of membrane and cytoplasmic antigen or enzyme by immunologic or immunocytochemical methods and detection of the recurring chromosomal abnormalities either conventional cytogenetic or molecular methods, studies utilizing microarray analysis of gene expression, DNA copy number alterations, and next-generation sequencing provides supplementary arguments for accurate classification.

Identification of subclasses of acute leukemia is important for three reasons. First, some leukemias have clinical features that influence the therapeutic approaches; that is, central nervous system (CNS) is more frequently involved in acute lymphocytic leukemia (ALL) than in acute myelocytic leukemia (AML). Acute promyelocytic leukemia (APL) is associated with intravascular coagulation [1] and acute monocytic leukemia (AMoL) with skin and gum infiltration [2]. Second, differences in response rate and survival are observed in the treatment of acute leukemias; that is, the percentage of CR rate is higher in childhood ALL than in adult ALL. Third, classification greatly facilitates communication and cooperation around the world, and comparisons of results are possible only through reproducible definitions of the acute leukemias.

Examination of both peripheral blood and bone marrow smears is necessary for the diagnosis and the classification of acute leukemias. The most useful cytochemical stains are myeloperoxidase (MPO); Sudan Black B (SBB); specific and nonspecific esterase, such as chloroacetate esterase, naphthol ASD acetate esterase with and without sodium fluoride (NAF), α-naphthyl acetate esterase (ANAE), or butyrate esterase; periodic acid-Schiff (PAS); and acid phosphatase (Figs. 14.1, 14.2, and 14.3).

There are two instances in which the diagnosis of acute leukemia can be made on the basis of histologic material. The first occurs when there is an abundance of reticulin in the bone marrow, resulting in a so-called dry tap [3]. This can be present in any of acute leukemias and is recognized most commonly associated with acute megakaryoblastic leukemia and acute panmyelosis with myelofibrosis. Although touch preparation smears may be of help in such cases, well-prepared hematoxylin and eosin (H&E) stains of paraffin-embedded

One of the coauthors of this chapter (JMB) participated in the WHO Clinical Advisory committee on hematologic neoplasms and coauthored several of the upcoming chapters on MDS and MDS/MPN. The review article by Arber and Hasserjian (Reclassifying Myelodysplastic Syndromes: what's where in the new WHO and why. Hematol. Am. Soc. Hematol. Educ. Program. 2015:294–298) discusses many but not all of the proposed changes. Availability of the chapters was made possible by the WHO to facilitate the writing and revisions necessary.
We anticipate that the entire fascicle will be available in hard copy and via the Internet late in 2017. "We are indebted to the many authors who wrote the revised chapters and have incorporated the changes in this chapter."

N.N. Tuzuner, M.D.
Department of Pathology/Hematopathology, Cerrahpasa Medical Faculty, Istanbul University, Istanbul 34303, Turkey
e-mail: tuzunern@yahoo.com; tuzunern@istanbul.edu.tr

J.M. Bennett, M.D. (✉)
Department of Pathology, University of Rochester, 601 Elmwood Ave, Rochester, NY 14642, USA
e-mail: John_Bennett@URMC.rochester.edu

P.H. Wiernik et al. (eds.), *Neoplastic Diseases of the Blood*, DOI 10.1007/978-3-319-64263-5_14

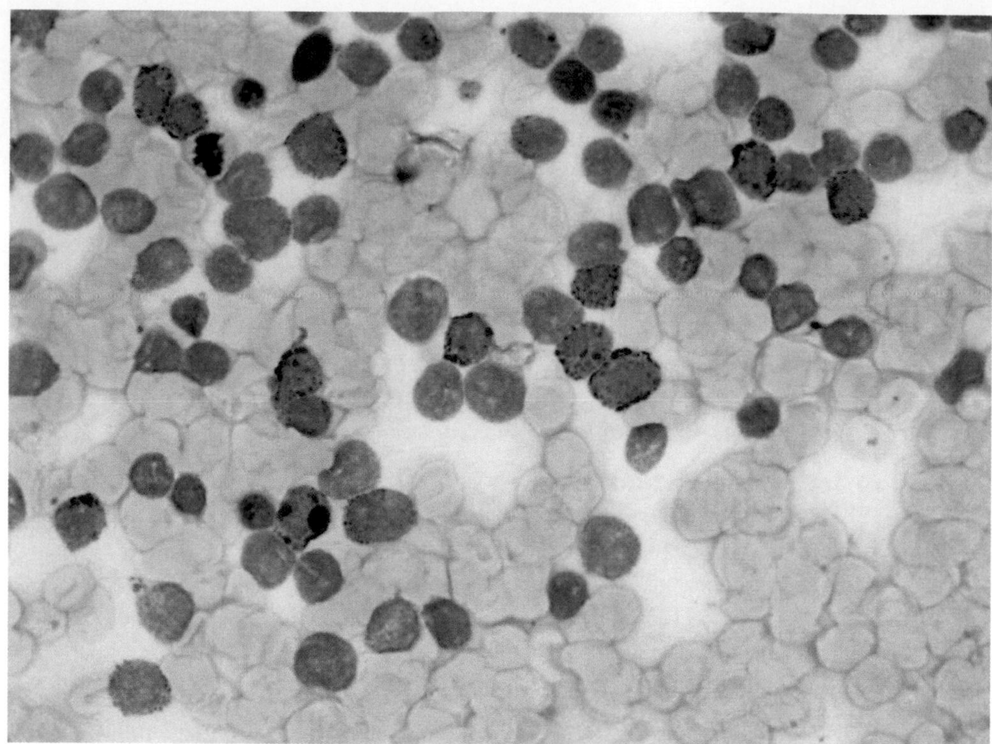

Fig. 14.1 ALL: PAS reaction. Note the blocklike reaction product

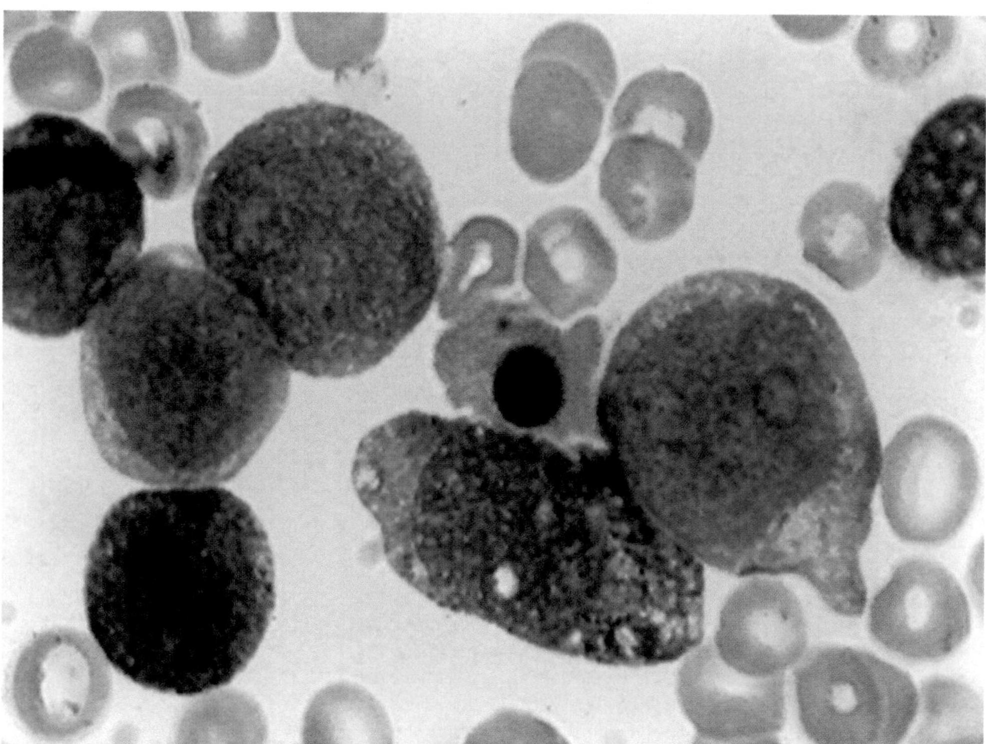

Fig. 14.2 AML (FABM0). Blasts with no differentiation. Peroxidase negative but with positive myeloid antigens by flow cytometry

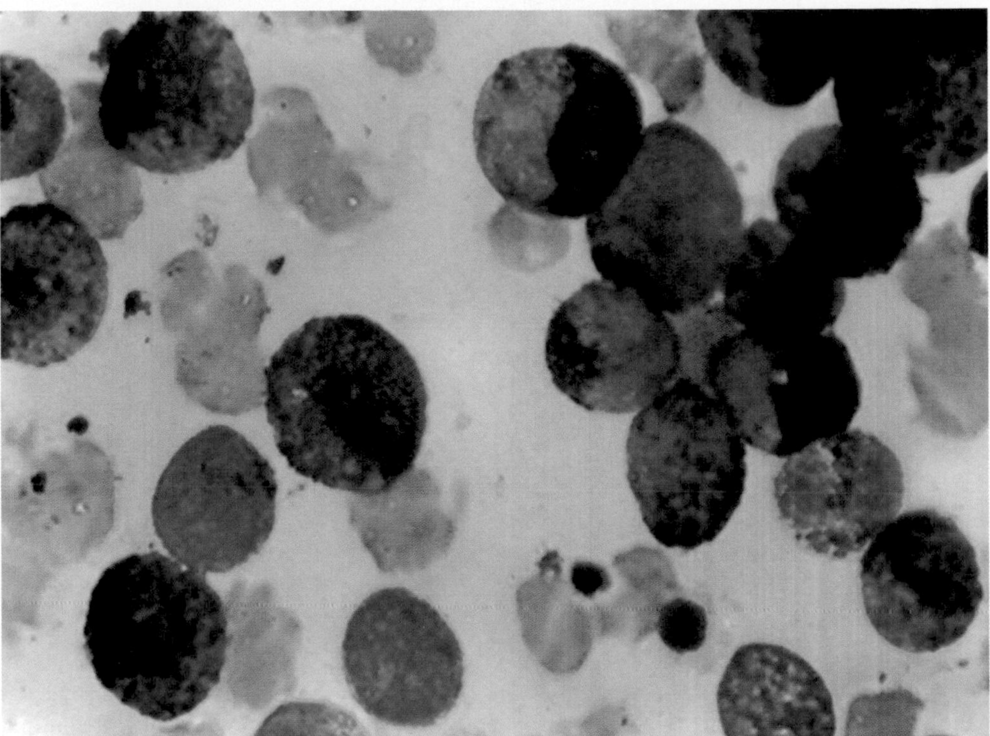

Fig. 14.3 AML (myeloperoxidase stain). *Black* reaction product with Auer rods

material, PAS, chloroacetate esterase stains, and immunologic methods identifying antigens on cell surface (CD41, CD61 or factor VIII) may establish the diagnosis. However, the distinction between acute megakaryoblastic leukemia with myelofibrosis and acute panmyelosis with myelofibrosis may be difficult, particularly if no specimen suitable for cytogenetic analysis can be obtained [4].

The second example is hypocellular (hypoplastic) acute myeloid leukemia in which bone marrow aspirations from several sites and biopsy from one site are necessary for diagnosis [5]. The correct diagnosis depends on a representative biopsy specimen. The third example is that of an uncommon localized extramedullary mass of cells of the granulocytic–monocytic series (myeloid sarcomas) [6]. These tumors can be seen in an established diagnosis of AML, either at presentation or as the first manifestation of relapse.

Diagnosis of Acute Leukemias

The diagnosis of acute leukemia is based exclusively on the morphology of the bone marrow and peripheral blood leukemic cells in the Romanowsky-stained smears. The initial intent was to separate ALL and AML into easily identifiable cell types. In attempting to define boundaries between overlapping groups, major attention is given to the predominant cell type present. An essential cytochemical stain is one that demonstrates MPO, an enzyme restricted to the primary granules of granulocytes and monocytes [7]. Morphologic classification of acute leukemia was that proposed by the French–American–British (FAB) Cooperative group [8], widely used for over two decades. In the meantime, genetic features (cytogenetic, molecular genetic, and gene expression) as well as history of myelodysplasia and prior therapy have been shown to have a significant impact on the clinical behavior of acute leukemias. In 2001 World Health Organization (WHO) proposed a classification in which genetic information was incorporated with morphologic, cytochemical, immunophenotypic, and clinical information into diagnostic algorithms for the acute leukemias [9]. WHO 2008 classification and upcoming revised edition (expected in late 2016) expanded the number of entities with recurrent chromosomal translocations and gene mutations and included new provisional entities [10].

Acute Lymphoblastic Leukemia/Lymphoma (ALL/LBL)

ALL/LBL is one of the most common malignancies observed in the pediatric age group. It derives from the clonal proliferation of lymphoid progenitors in the bone marrow. ALL represents about 80% of cases of acute leukemia in children but only 20% in adults. The consequence of bone marrow infiltration is various cytopenias in the peripheral blood and is associated with the appearance of peripheral blast cells. In some instances, leukemic cells are not seen in the peripheral blood. Thus examination of bone marrow is usually necessary to confirm the diagnosis. Since the CNS is infiltrated at diagnosis in 5% of patients, examination of the cerebrospinal fluid (CSF) by cytocentrifuge is also necessary.

Morphologic Features

Morphologic classification of ALL was proposed by the FAB group in 1976 [8] and widely used for over two decades. However, the WHO 2008 no longer emphasizes the morphologic classification and separation of the morphologic subtypes. The morphologic features of B- and T-ALL/LBLs are indistinguishable. The lymphoblasts in ALL/LBL vary from small blasts with high nuclear/cytoplasmic (N/C) ratio, scant cytoplasm, condensed nuclear chromatin, a small inconspicuous nucleolus, and a regular nucleus (Fig. 14.4) to larger cell with irregular nuclear membranes, one or more nucleoli, more cytoplasm, and lower N/C ratio (Fig. 14.5). A rare type of leukemia seen in approximately equal percentages in children and adults (about 3–5%) is morphologically identical to the cell characteristics of Burkitt lymphoma. The cells are large and homogeneous with round-to-oval nuclei. The chromatin is finely dispersed with prominent nucleoli. The cytoplasm is intensely basophilic with or without vacuoles (Fig. 14.6). The term B-ALL/LBL should not be used to indicate Burkitt lymphoma/leukemia since it is constantly associated with surface immunoglobulin (sIg) (mature B-ALL) [11]. In addition, an identical nonrandom chromosomal abnormality t(8;14) translocation has been described in both Burkitt lymphoma and leukemia [12]. In rare instances, terminal deoxynucleotidyl transferase-positive (TdT+) B-cell lymphoma/leukemias with BCL2 and/or MYC alterations have been reported [13–15]. These cases do not have the typical morphologic features and chromosomal translocation.

Cytochemistry

By standard definition, the peroxidase reaction is totally negative in leukemic lymphoblasts. SBB stain is also negative. However, it has been suggested that SBB is less specific than MPO because positive reactions have been reported in ALL [16]. It should be remembered that in case of negative MPO or SBB reaction, megakaryocytic, erythroid, some monocytic, and AML with minimal differentiation subtype as well as lymphoid lineage may be involved.

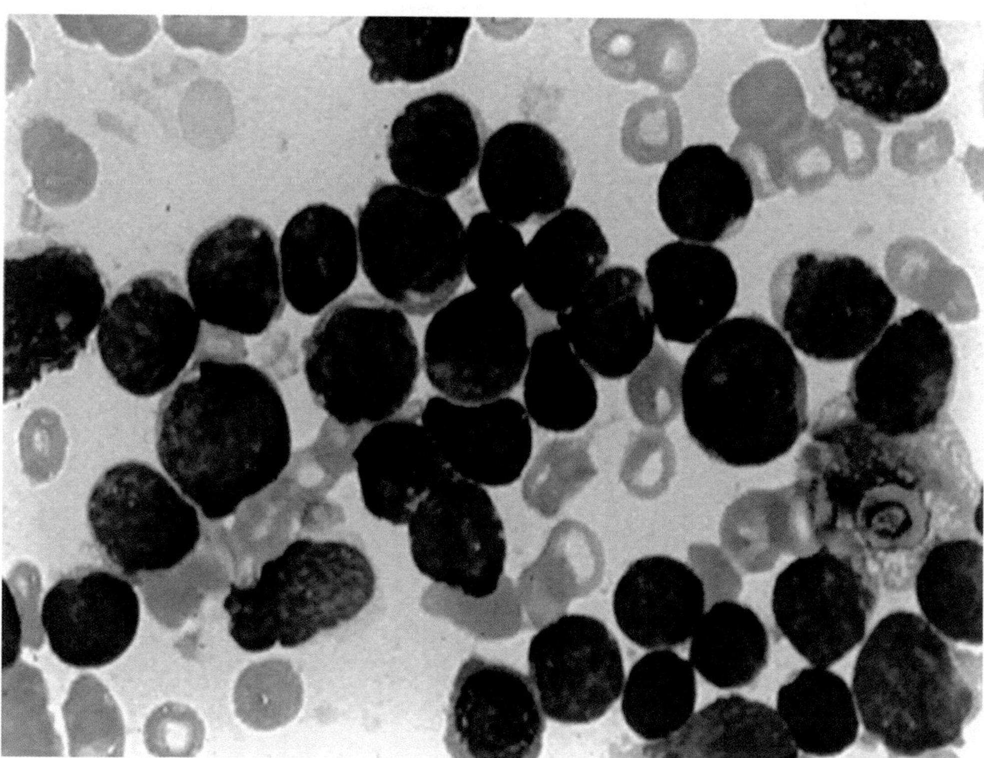

Fig. 14.4 Acute lymphocytic leukemia (ALL): agranular blasts with high nuclear/cytoplasmic ratio; smooth nuclear membrane; rare nucleoli. WG stain

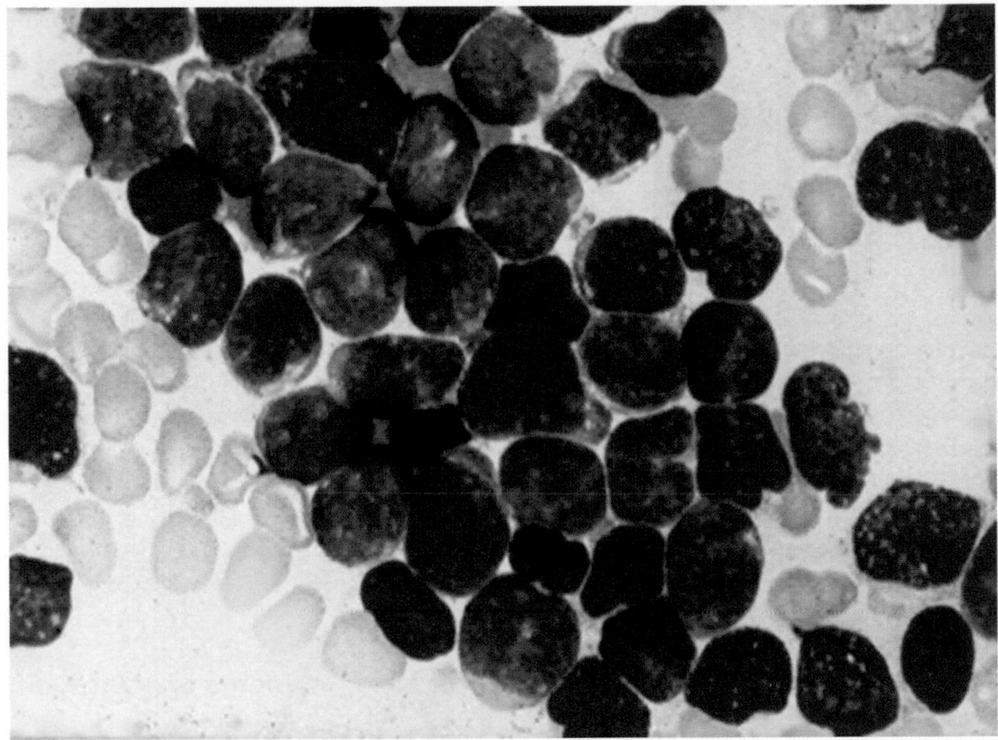

Fig. 14.5 ALL: More cytoplasm than L1 with prominent nucleoli. WG stain

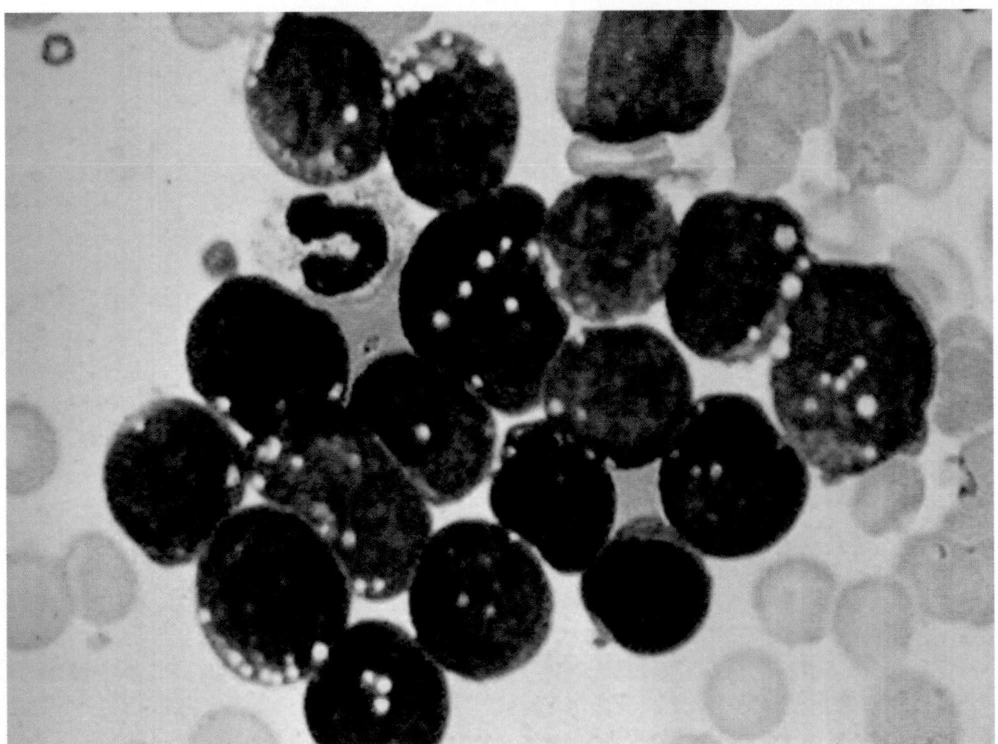

Fig. 14.6 Burkitt lymphoma/leukemia (mature B-ALL): blasts with oval nuclei, finely dispersed chromatin, basophilic cytoplasm with vacuoles. WG stain

The PAS reaction is useful in supporting the diagnosis of ALL (Table 14.1), but its importance has declined, as immunophenotyping has become more important for this purpose. Although blocklike PAS positivity is considered characteristic of ALL, only 15% of cases have this type of PAS reaction (Fig. 14.1) [17]. This pattern of PAS positivity correlates with the immunologic phenotype which is more common in B-lineage cases. The presence of both vacuolated blasts and PAS positivity correlates with reactivity of CD10 antigen [18]. It should be noted that blocklike PAS positivity can be seen in monoblasts in acute monoblastic leukemia and in erythroblasts in acute erythroleukemia [19]. Moreover, fine granular activity in blocks of PAS material can be identified in all AML cell types (Fig. 14.7). PAS stain is therefore a poor discriminator of various cell types, but it may be useful as a part of battery of stains, particularly when many of the reactions are negative or nonspecific. A strong focal (paranuclear) acid phosphatase (ACP) activity or a strong focal ANAE activity greater than 75% of blasts is characteristic of T-ALL [20]. However, it should be remembered that a localized ACP and ANAE reaction is also a feature of rare forms of acute megakaryoblastic and erythroleukemia [21].

Table 14.1 Reaction of acute leukemic cells to cytochemical stains

Stain	AML (M1–M3)	AMML (M4)	AMoL (M5)	ALL (L1–L2)
PAS	±	+	++	++
Acid phosphatase	–	±	++	+++
Peroxidase	+	+	±	–
Chloroacetate esterase	+	+	–	–
α-Naphthyl acetate esterase	±	+	++	++++

PAS Periodic acid-Schiff, – absent, ± occasional activity, + moderate activity, ++ strong activity, +++ focally strong activity in T cells, ++++ focally strong activity at acid pH in T cells

Immunohistochemistry

Indirect immunoperoxidase and indirect alkaline phosphatase anti-alkaline phosphatase (APAAP) techniques are applied to fixed cells in blood and bone marrow smears, cytospin preparations [22], or paraffin-embedded material. These methods permit the detection of surface antigens (i.e., CD19, CD20, CD3, CD1a, and CD10), cytoplasmic antigens (CD79a, MPO, or cytoplasmic μ chain), and nuclear antigens (e.g., TdT and PAX5) [23].

Genetics of Acute Lymphoblastic Leukemia/Lymphoma

Acute lymphoblastic leukemia/lymphoma is relatively homogeneous at morphologic level. However, significant heterogeneity is seen at the genetic level. These genetic lesions define disease subsets with distinct biology and response to treatment and are used in the risk stratification schemas for current protocols [10, 24]. In the last decade,

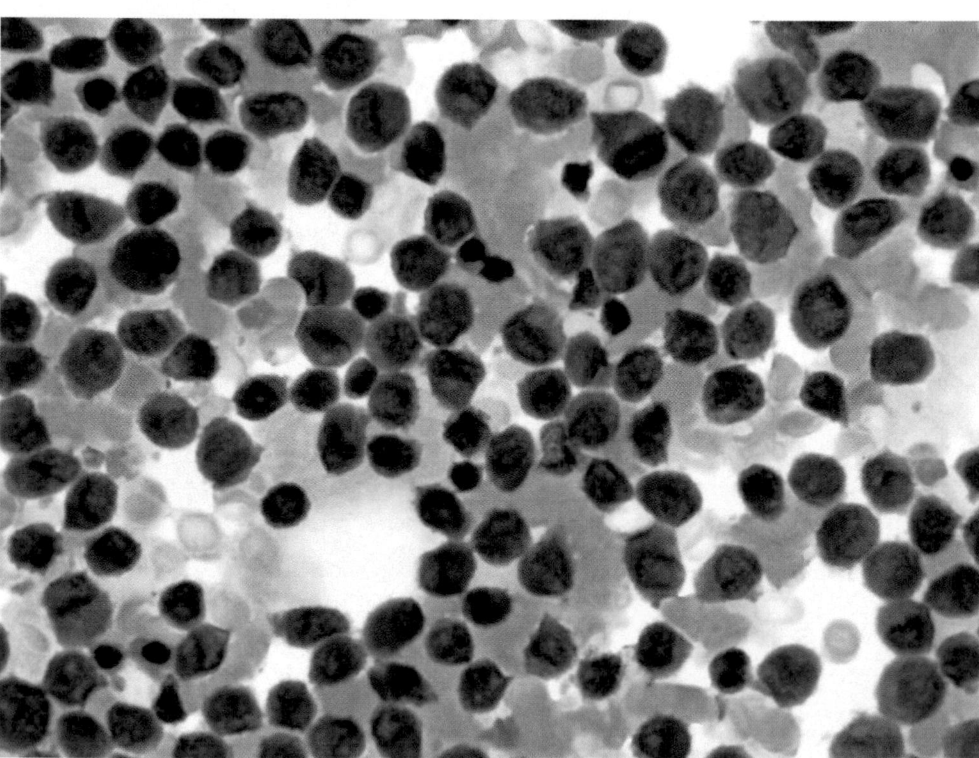

Fig. 14.7 AML: PAS reaction. Note the blush background

studies utilizing microarray analysis and next-generation sequencing have provided major insights into the pathogenesis and clinical behavior of ALL. These studies have identified new ALL subtypes. High hyperdiploidy (>50 chromosomes) occurs in 25–30% of childhood B-ALL and is associated with favorable outcome. Hypodiploidy with 44 chromosomes is uncommon (2–3% of cases) and is associated with poor outcome [25, 26]. Chromosomal rearrangements commonly involve hematopoietic transcription factors, cytokine receptors, epigenetic modifiers, and tyrosine kinases [27]. Common rearrangements in acute B lymphoblastic leukemia are as follows: the t(12;21)(p13;q22) (TEL-AML1) occurs in 15–25% of pediatric cases and is associated with excellent prognosis; t(1;19)(q23;p13) (E2A-PBX1) is seen in 2–6% of pediatric cases, associated with excellent prognosis and CNS relapse; t(9;22)(q34;q11.2) resulting in formation of the "Philadelphia" chromosome (Ph) encoding BCR-ABL1 is associated with 2–4% of pediatric and 25% of adult cases and with poor prognosis; rearrangements of MLL at 11q23 to a range of fusion partners are common in infant ALL (1–2%) with poor prognosis; rearrangement of the cytokine receptor gene CRLF2 is common in Down syndrome-associated and Ph-like ALL and with poor prognosis in non-Down syndrome-associated ALL; t(8;14)(q24;q32), t(2;8)(q12;q24), and t(2;8) (q12;q24) encoding; and MYC rearrangement is associated with Burkitt lymphoma/leukemia which is a neoplasm of mature B cells (2% of cases) and associated with favorable prognosis with short-term high-dose chemotherapy [28, 29]. Approximately 20% of childhood B-ALL cases lack one of these alterations and have alternative sentinel genetic lesions, including deregulation of the ETS family transcription factor ERG, or one of a diverse range of alterations that drive kinase signaling in Ph-like ALL.

T-ALL is also characterized by translocations that deregulate transcription factors, commonly by rearrangement to T-cell antigen receptor loci, and recurring sequence mutations and DNA copy number alterations that disrupt developmental, signaling, and tumor-suppressor pathways, including activating mutations of NOTCH1 and rearrangements of transcription factors TLX1 , TLX3, LYL1, TAL1, and MLL [9, 30, 31].

The finding of prominent eosinophilia either T or B lymphoblastic leukemia/lymphoma must be considered for a rearrangement involving PDGFRA, PDGFRB, or FGFR1. It is important to identify these cases with PDGFRA or PDGFRB abnormalities because these patients are often responsive to TKI therapy [32].

If none of the particular cytogenetic abnormalities (listed previously) are found in a case of B or T lymphoblastic leukemia/lymphoma, the designation of "B or T lymphoblastic leukemia/lymphoma not otherwise specified" is recommended.

Philadelphia-Positive (Ph) ALL and Ph-Like ALL

Cytogenetic studies suggest that Ph chromosome occurs in 2–4% of children with ALL [33], but it is as high as 30% in adults [34]. Thus, this chromosome appears to be the single most common genetic finding in adult ALL. Moreover, the presence of the Philadelphia chromosome identifies a subgroup of ALL with a poor prognosis [35]. Most BCR-ABL1-positive childhood cases express p190 fusion protein, whereas in adults, approximately 50% of the cases express p210 kDa fusion protein (more likely in chronic granulocytic leukemia). It has been suggested that Philadelphia-positive-BCR-positive ALL cases expressing p210 may be CML in lymphoid blast crisis; BCR-negative cases expressing variant p190 may be true de novo ALL [36]. However, no clinical data have been reported to substantiate this claim. One characteristic of Philadelphia-positive ALL is the expression of both myeloid and lymphoid antigens [37]. This feature supports that the cell origin is more immature than the other B-ALL cases [38]. There are no unique morphologic or cytochemical features that distinguish Philadelphia chromosome-positive ALL from other types of ALL.

Recently in about 20% of patients with B lymphoblastic acute leukemia/lymphoma that lack the BCR-ABL1 translocation but that show similar pattern of gene expression profile to B-ALL with BCR-ABL1 which are called as B lymphoblastic leukemia/lymphoma, BCR-ABL1-like or B lymphoblastic leukemia/lymphoma, Ph-like [39]. Leukemias with these properties have poor outcome and frequently have translocations involving other receptor tyrosine kinases, or alternatively have translocations involving either the cytokine receptor-like factor 2 (CRLF2) or less commonly rearrangements of the erythropoietin receptor (EPOR) [40]. Identification of these cases has clinical importance since they are potentially amenable to thyrosine kinase inhibitor (TKI) therapy [41].

There are no unique morphologic or cytochemical features that distinguish Ph-like ALL from other types of ALL. Blasts typically have a CD19+,CD10+ phenotype. The subset of cases with CRLF2 translocations shows very high levels of surface expression of this protein by flow cytometry.

Myeloid Leukemias

AMLs result from a neoplastic transformation of a single pluripotential hematopoietic stem cell. Evidence to support this statement is morphologic [42], immunologic [43], and chromosomal [44] as well as from in vitro cell culture studies. These studies have demonstrated trilineage dysplastic features or lymphoid antigen expressions in AML, monocytic, and erythroid precursors in cultures and elaboration of colony-stimulating factors (CSFs) from monocytes.

Four major types of AML have long been recognized: acute myeloid, acute myelomonocytic, acute monocytic, and acute erythroid leukemia. Despite these subtype definitions, Auer rods are the only consistent neoplastic marker demonstrating that a blast is myeloid and of leukemic origin. Auer rods are abnormal azurophilic crystalline-like granules that represent the coalescence of primary lysosomal granules of myeloid precursors as documented by cytochemical and ultrastructural studies [45, 46]. We have demonstrated that the addition of a peroxidase or another specific stain for primary granules increases the percentage of positive blast cells that contain Auer rods from 21 to 60%. The clinical relevance of these observations is uncertain at the present time.

Classification

The minimal requirements for morphologic specification of each case of AML are well-prepared peripheral blood and bone marrow smears prepared with a Romanowsky stain such as a Wright-Giemsa stain. To prove lineage, some routine cytochemical stains can be applied. These techniques are discussed next.

A uniform reproducible subtype classification in AML is necessary for several reasons; first, it permits comparison among various therapeutic regimens from different groups and from program to program within the same institution or cooperative group. Second, it allows for the potential identification of different clinical features and laboratory aspects that may be unique to certain subtypes. Finally with the increasing sophistication of chromosomal abnormalities and gene mutations in the AML, accurate description of myeloid subsets may permit a meaningful association of nonrandom rearrangements and translocations.

Morphologic classification of AML was proposed by the FAB Cooperative Group in 1976 [8] based on the morphologic and cytochemical features of the blast cells. The original proposal was revised and expanded in 1985 [47]. In the 2008 World Health Organization (WHO) classification, and in the upcoming revision, most of the morphologic FAB subgroups are retained in the AML, NOS category because they define criteria for the diagnosis of AML across a diverse morphological spectrum [48].

Morphologic classification accepts two types of blasts: type I (agranular) blasts are myeloblasts with open chromatin, distinct nucleoli, and immature cytoplasm without granules; type II (granular) blasts are similar to type I, except that they contain up to 20 delicate cytoplasmic azurophilic granules or Auer rods, or both (Fig. 14.8). Goasguen et al. [49] distinguished another type of blasts from promyelocytes, referred to as type III blasts; these lack major characteristics of the promyelocyte, especially the Golgi zone and eccentric

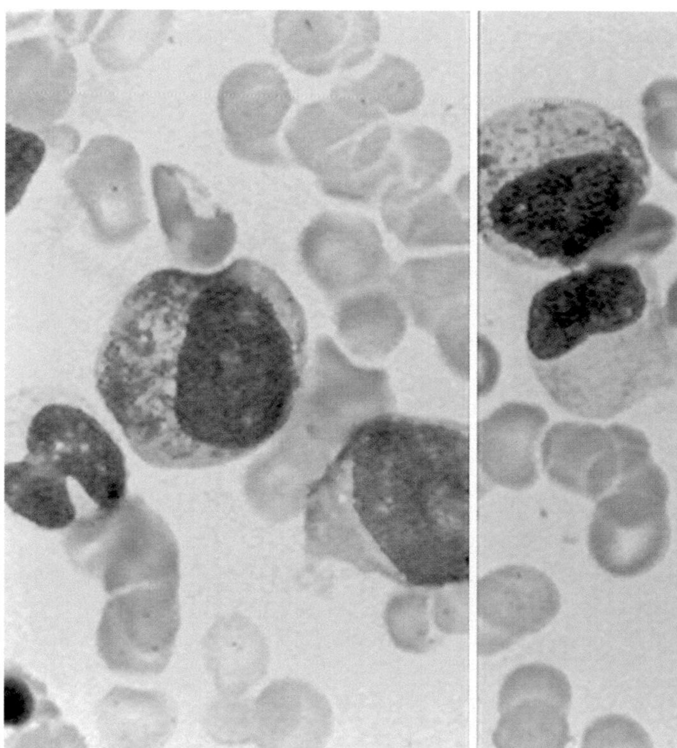
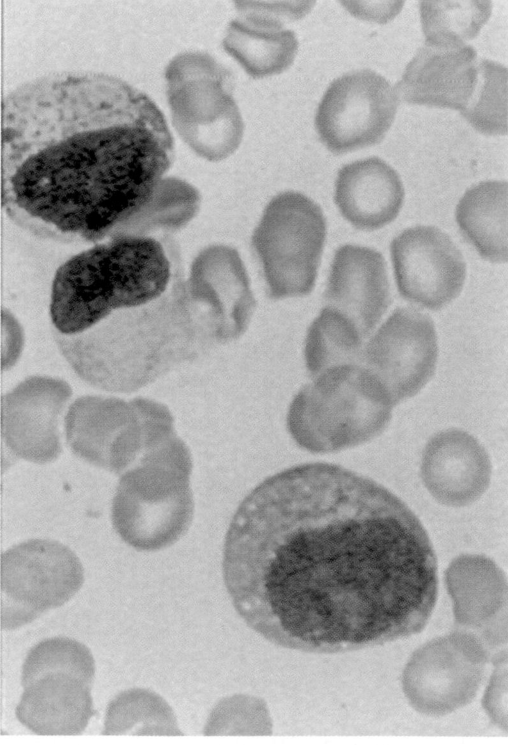

Fig. 14.8 Myeloblast morphology. *Left panel*: agranular blast and promyelocytes (note: Golgi zone); *right panel*: granular blast

nuclear location, but they have many azurophilic granules. Type III blasts are characteristically identified in AML M2 associated with t(8;21), in secondary AML and AML developing from MDS [50]. In practice, although FAB type I and type II blasts can generally be distinguished from each other it has proved difficult to distinguish FAB type II blasts from type III blasts. In addition, the enumeration of abnormal promyelocytes in MDS or AML with multilineage dysplasia remains problematic and their separation from type II and type III blasts has remained imprecise. A group of international experts in morphology has provided guidelines to assist in this regard [51].

FAB criteria identify one clinically significant type of AML, acute promyelocytic leukemia (M3); however, the remaining AML subtypes appear to be cytogenetically and immunologically heterogeneous group of diseases. AML is now classified according to the World Health Organization (WHO) Classification of Tumours of Haematopoietic and Lymphoid Tissues, which was last updated in 2008 [52]. The major categories of the current classification include AML with recurrent genetic abnormalities, AML with myelodysplasia-related changes, therapy-related AML, and AML not otherwise specified. Myeloid proliferations of Down syndrome and blastic plasmacytoid dendritic cell neoplasm are separately classified [53].

A revision of the WHO classification is under way. Changes to the section on AML with recurrent genetic abnormalities are being discussed. First, the molecular basis of inv(3)(q21q26.2) or t(3;3)(q21;q26.2) has been revisited [54]. Second, the provisional entities "AML with NPM1 mutation" and "AML with CEBPA mutation" will become entities; "AML with CEBPA mutation" will be restricted to patients with AML in whom there is a biallelic (and not a monoallelic) mutation, and third, "AML with RUNX1 mutation" [55, 56] and "AMLwith BCR-ABL1" gene [57] are being considered as provisional entities. Finally, a section on familial myeloid neoplasms, which reflects the increasing recognition of familial syndromes, is also under development [58] (Table 14.2).

In the WHO scheme, a myeloid neoplasm with 20% or more blasts in the peripheral blood or bone marrow is considered to be AML [9]. The blast count should be obtained from at least a 200-cell count of all nucleated cells in the peripheral blood and a 500-cell count of all nucleated cells in the bone marrow. In certain cases associated with specific genetic abnormalities inv (16), t(8;21), t(16;16), or t(15;17), the diagnosis of AML is made regardless of the blast count in the peripheral blood or bone marrow. Similarly, the presence of granulocytic sarcoma is diagnostic of AML even if the blast count is less than 20% in the blood or bone marrow [59].

Table 14.2 Proposed WHO revised classification of acute myeloid leukemias (AML)—2016

AML with recurrent genetic abnormalities
Acute myeloid leukemia with t(8;21)(q22;q22.1); *RUNX1-RUNX1T1*
Acute myeloid leukemia with inv(16)(p13.1q22) or t(16;16)(p13.1;q22); *CBFB-MYH11*
Acute promyelocytic leukemia with *PML-RARA*
Acute myeloid leukemia with t(9;11)(p21.3;q23.3); *KMT2A/MLL-MLLT3*
Acute myeloid leukemia with t(6;9)(p23;q34.1); *DEK-NUP214* 9869/3
Acute myeloid leukemia with inv.(3)(q21.3q26.2) or t(3;3)(q21.3;q26.2); GATA2, MECOM (EVI1)
AML (megakaryoblastic) with t(1;22)(p13.3;q13.1); RBM15-MKL1
AML with *BCR-ABL1*
AML with gene mutations
AML with mutated *NPM1*
AML with mutated *CEBPA*
AML with mutated *RUNX1*
Acute myeloid leukemia (AML) with myelodysplasia-related changes
Therapy-related myeloid neoplasms
Acute myeloid leukemia, NOS
Acute myeloid leukemia with minimal differentiation
Acute myeloid leukemia without maturation
Acute myeloid leukemia with maturation
Acute myelomonocytic leukemia
Acute monoblastic and monocytic leukemia
Acute erythroid leukemia
Acute megakaryoblastic leukemia
Acute basophilic leukemia
Acute panmyelosis with myelofibrosis
Myeloid sarcoma
Myeloid proliferations related to Down syndrome
Transient abnormal myelopoiesis associated with Down syndrome
Myeloid leukemia associated with Down syndrome
Blastic plasmacytoid dendritic cell neoplasm

Cytochemistry

Myeloperoxidase and Sudan Black B

An essential cytochemical stain is one that demonstrates the presence of MPO, an enzyme restricted to the primary granules of granulocytes and monocytes [7]. This enzyme can be identified by performing a benzidine-based peroxidase reaction or SBB staining or by diaminobenzidine reaction. The benzidine method is the best available method against which other methods should be compared. However, because of the concern for its potential carcinogenicity, it should not be adopted as the reference method [60].

The SBB reaction, a general stain for intracellular lipids, can be used in the same way. This stain is present in both primary and secondary granules. Sudanophilia and MPO activity are closely parallel [61].

Specific and Nonspecific Esterases

The chloroacetate esterase reaction can also be used to identify myeloid lineage. Although it is less sensitive than either MPO or SBB in detecting myeloid differentiation, it can be useful, when combined with ANAE in double-esterase stain, in confirming a monocytic component. Because ANAE is positive both in neutrophils and in monocytes, inhibition by NAF in monocytes should be used to identify these cells [62, 63].

Periodic Acid-Schiff Reaction

All glycogen-containing cells as well as neutrophils and granulocytes at all stages of maturation stain with this reaction. Our experience in more than 200 patients has shown that fine granular PAS reaction can be identified in all AML subtypes, ranging from 60% in AML (M1–M3) to 80% in AML M5. Moreover, the latter often demonstrates a blocklike reaction pattern characteristic of ALL (Bennett J.M., unpublished observation). The blocklike pattern of PAS reactivity is seen in erythroid precursors of acute erythroid leukemia.

Electron Microscopy

Electron microscopy (EM) is used to demonstrate either MPO or platelet peroxidase (PPO). These ultrastructural studies are useful in the confirmation of myeloid (MO) or megakaryocytic (M7) origin of blasts. MPO can be demonstrated by electron microscopy in blast cells that previously had negative results (less than 3% positive blasts) by conventional criteria. It is also useful to define the myeloid component in biphenotypic leukemias [62, 63]. In megakaryoblasts, the PPO reaction is localized exclusively on the nuclear membrane and the endoplasmic reticulum, whereas in myeloblasts it occurs in the Golgi area and cytoplasmic granules.

Immunohistochemistry

Cytospin preparations or direct marrow or peripheral blood smears as well as bone marrow paraffin sections are used to demonstrate the presence of specific lineage antigens using a secondary technique (e.g., PAP, APAAP) to show antibody fixation [22]. Its advantage includes confirmation of morphologic features, the possibility of performing retrospective studies, and in situations where peripheral blood and bone marrow smears are inadequate for study such as bone marrow fibrosis or hypocellular acute myeloid leukemia. Paraffin-reactive antibodies, i.e., CD34, MPO, CD68, CD117, CD41, CD61, glycophorin A, and factor VIII-related antigen, can successfully be used to subclassify AML [64].

Acute Myeloid Leukemias with Recurrent Cytogenetic Abnormalities

All patients morphologically diagnosed with AML must have bone marrow cytogenetic studies performed. WHO 2008 classification is recommended to incorporate recently described genetic aberrations into classification and define, biologically relevant, homogeneous entities based on not only the prognostic value of a genetic abnormality but also morphologic, clinical, and phenotypic properties [59, 65]. The contribution of cytogenetics to the classification of AML and acute myeloid leukemias with recurrent cytogenetic abnormalities are briefly discussed as follows.

Acute Myeloid Leukemia with t(8;21)(q22;q22);RUNX1-RUNX1T1

AML with t(8;21) is common in children and adults accounting for approximately 7–12% of AML overall and 20–25% of AML M2. Myeloid sarcomas may be present at presentation. Cases with t(8;21) should be diagnosed as AML regardless of a blast percentage in the bone marrow. The translocation results in a fusion product involving the RUNX1 gene (also known as core-binding factor alpha or AML1) on chromosome 21 and the RUNX1T1 (also known as ETO) gene on chromosome 8 [66]. Cases of AML with t(8;21) are associated with characteristic morphologic features [67]. Blasts are large cells with a distinctive nucleolus. The cytoplasm contains abnormal heavy azurophilic granulations (type III blasts) with tiny needlelike Auer rods (Fig. 14.9). The maturing neutrophils are commonly dysplastic. However, dysplasia of other cell lines is uncommon. Background eosinophilia is variably present. Blasts may express B-lineage antigens such as CD19, CD79a, PAX5, and TdT. These findings do not indicate the presence of mixed-phenotype leukemia in the presence of t(8;21) [68]. Acute myeloid leukemia with t(8;21) is usually associated with favorable prognosis in children and adults [69]. Mutations of KIT occur in 20–30% of cases [70]. Most published reports indicate a higher relapse rate and lower overall survival when mutated KIT is present [70, 71]. Additional mutations in ASXL2 and ASXL1 were also recently described in t(8;21) AML [72]. The presence of monosomy 7 as an additional cytogenetic abnormality may adversely impact prognosis [73]. Quantitative PCR measuring of RUNX1-RUNX1T1 transcripts is useful for monitoring minimal residual disease [74].

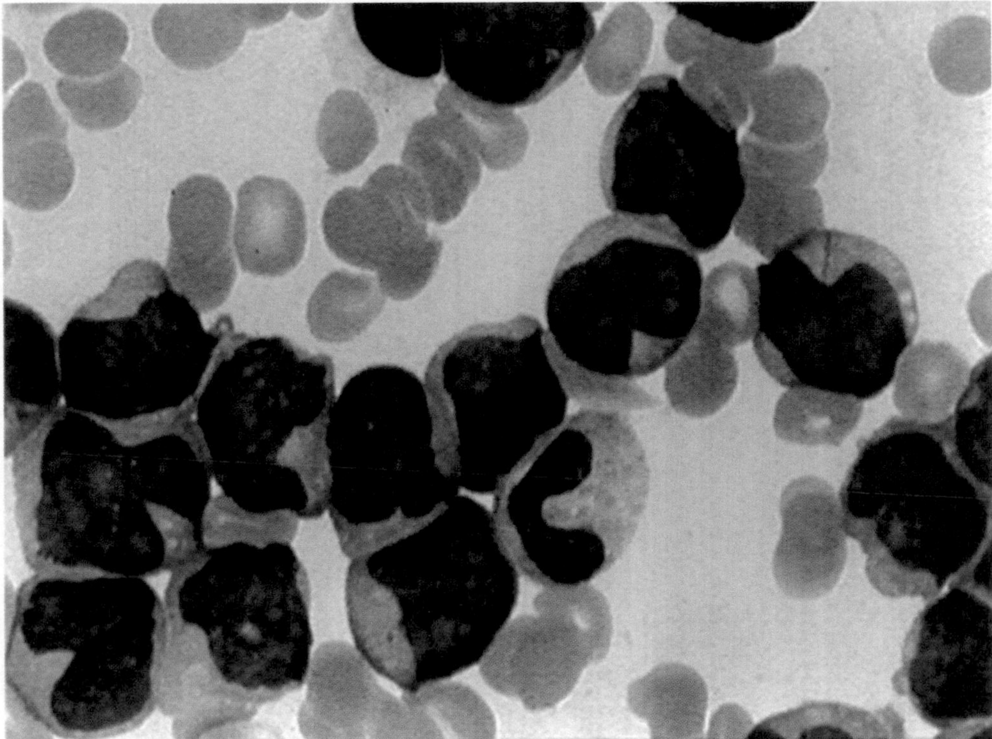

Fig. 14.9 AML –t(8;21). Note thin Auer rod in a myeloblast

Acute Promyelocytic Leukemia with t(15;17)/q22;q12, PML–RARA

APL is a distinct class of AML characterized by specific morphologic, cytogenetic, and clinical features. In most series, M3 accounts for about 10% of cases in adults and for 4–8% in children [75].

The highly specific t(15;17) translocation is present in at least 90% of all APL cases. Using molecular techniques, virtually 100% of APL cases have t(15;17). This translocation fuses the PML gene of the chromosome 15 to the retinoic acid receptor-α (RARA) gene, producing chimeric PML–RARA gene [76–78]. Cytogenetic analysis, FISH, or RT-PCR is necessary for genetic confirmation of the PML–RARA fusion. Detection of this abnormality is diagnostic of APL regardless of the blast count. The involvement of RARA at the translocation breakpoints may explain the clinical response to all-trans retinoic acid (ATRA) [79, 80].

Morphology is still highly relevant in APL diagnosis and is a very rapid modality [81]. Typical APL is characterized by the presence of hypergranular blast cells, which have the appearance of abnormal promyelocytes. The cytoplasm is dense with coarse dark-staining granules that often obscure the nucleus. The nuclear border is generally irregular and has a folded or reniform appearance (Fig. 14.10). Cells contain bundles of delicate needlelike Auer rods, giving a meshwork appearance (so-called Faggots), found in some of the leukemic blasts. These abnormal promyelocytes are strongly positive for the MPO or SBB reactions. In contrast to other AML subtypes, dysplastic features of the myeloid series associated with leukemic proliferation are not seen. In adult patients with typical APL that achieve a CR, the prognosis is better than for any category of AML.

The FAB classification recognizes a variant of APL (FAB M3v) [82], characterized by bilobate cells or by cells with reniform nucleus and cytoplasm with minimal or no granulations (Fig. 14.11). Typical M3 cells are infrequent in the bone marrow. Hypogranular promyelocytes are strongly positive for the MPO or SBB, as in typical APL. The immunophenotype of M3v is identical to that described for the typical APL (expressing of myeloid antigens in the absence of HLA-DR reactivity) [83, 84]. Special attention should be given to differentiate these cases from M4 and M5b subtypes. The distinction is important because of the well-known association of M3 with disseminated intravascular coagulation (DIC) [1]. The DIC syndrome is present equally in the M3v. In adults, the hypogranular or "microgranular" variant constitutes 25% of APL cases [85]. It may also occur in children [86]. The hematological characteristic of M3v at onset, in addition to DIC, is hyperleukocytosis (>20,000/mm^3). M3v has been associated with shorter CR and poorer overall survival, reflecting early hemorrhagic deaths [85, 86].

FLT3 mutations are common in APL with the majority being internal tandem duplication (ITD) mutations. These mutations are strongly associated with the hypogranular subtype with hyperleukocytosis [87].

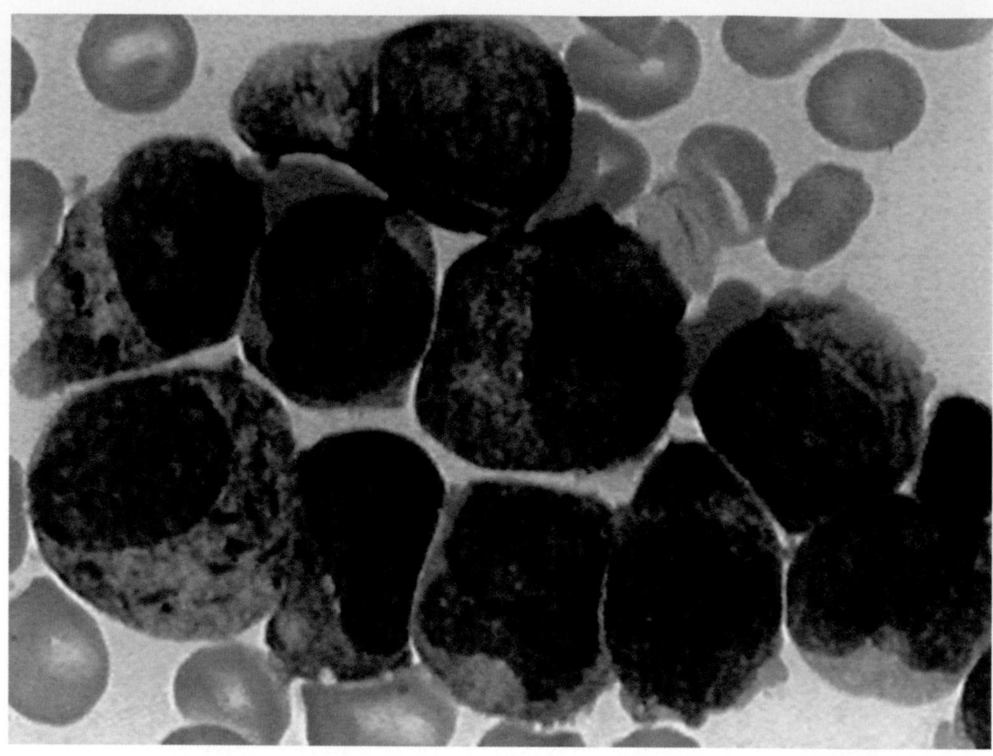

Fig. 14.10 APL (FABM3). Hypergranular promyelocytes with bundles of Auer rods

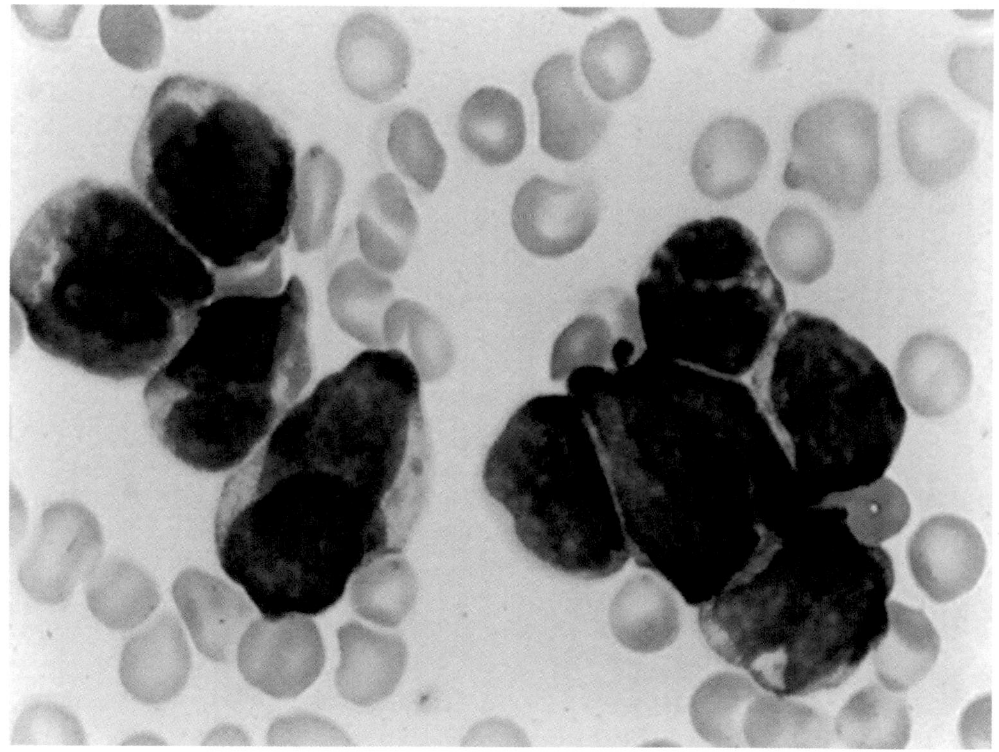

Fig. 14.11 APL variant (FABM3v). Only occasional cells have granules but prominent bilobed and reniform nuclei. WG stain

A small numbers of cases, often with morphologic features resembling APL, show variant translocations involving RARA gene on chromosome 17, but not the PML gene on chromosome 15, such as t(11;17) (ZBTB16-RARA), t(5;17)(NPM-1-RARA), and t(17;17)(STAT5B-RARA) [88]. Patients with variant RARA translocations often experience DIC. Cases with t(11;17) show morphologic differences in which Auer rods are usually absent and pelgeroid neutrophils may be seen. Importantly, some of these variant PML–RARA transcripts are associated with ATRA resistance, and some are not detected by current PCR techniques [89, 90].

Acute Myeloid Leukemia with inv(16)(p13.1q22) or t(16;16)p13.1;q22;CBFB-MYH11

AML with chromosome 16 abnormalities comprises 10% of adult and 6% of childhood AML. The inv(16) and the t(16;16) both result in the fusion of the beta-subunit of core-binding factor (CBFB) gene at 16q22 to the gene encoding smooth muscle myosin heavy chain (MYH11) at 16p13.1 [91]. The presence of this genetic abnormality is diagnostic of AML regardless of the blast count [52]. In these cases, in addition to characteristic morphologic features of acute myelomonocytic leukemia, the bone marrow shows a variable number of abnormal eosinophil components (AML-M4Eo) (Fig. 14.12). Eosinophils account for 5% or more of nonerythroid cells. The eosinophils are abnormal; in addition to the specific eosinophilic granules, they have large basophilic granules and demonstrate chloroacetate esterase and PAS (coarse granules) positivity. Often the nuclei have pseudo-Pelger features. At least 3% of the blasts show myeloperoxidase (MPO) or Sudan Black B reactivity. The monoblasts and promonocytes usually show NSE or ANAE reactivity [92]. The incidence of extramedullary disease is higher than for most types of AML, with a high incidence of CNS relapse. Patients with chromosome 16 abnormalities tend to respond to chemotherapy better, experience relatively long remissions, and have a better prognosis [69, 93]. KIT mutations are present in 30% of cases and negatively impact prognosis in older patients [70]. AML with t(8;21) or inv(16) and mutated KIT are considered as intermediate-risk AML, not favorable-risk AML [94].

Acute Myeloid Leukemia with t(9;11)(p22-q23); MLLT3-MLL

Translocations involving the MLL gene on chromosome 11q23 are seen in approximately 6% of cases of AML and secondary leukemias that occur in patients treated with topoisomerase II inhibitors [95], in patients with acute lymphoblastic leukemia, and rarely in patients with MDS [96]. However, with regard to copy number alterations (CNAs), no differences were found in the number or type of lesions between de novo and therapy-related AML with t(9;11) [97]. A number of different partners for the balanced 11q23 translocations have been identified. However, the WHO 2008 classification only recognizes t(9;11) (MLLT3-MLL) as a specific entity. This type of AML occurs at any age but is more common in children [98, 99]. Leukemic blasts containing 11q23 translocations generally have monocytic features and are subclassified as FAB M4 or M5 [100]. However, it is also detected in AML with or without maturation. Monoblasts and promonocytes show strong positive NSE reactions and often lack MPO reactivity. Extramedullary disease of the skin and gingiva and presentation with DIC have also been described.

Although pediatric cases with t(9;11) have an intermediate prognosis, leukemias associated with a different chromosome 11q23 translocations have poor prognosis [101]. Recently, within all t(11q23) AMLs, EVI1 positivity was found to be sole prognostic factor, predicting for inferior overall survival [102]. KIT or FLT3-ITD mutations are rare in AML with 11q23 translocations [59].

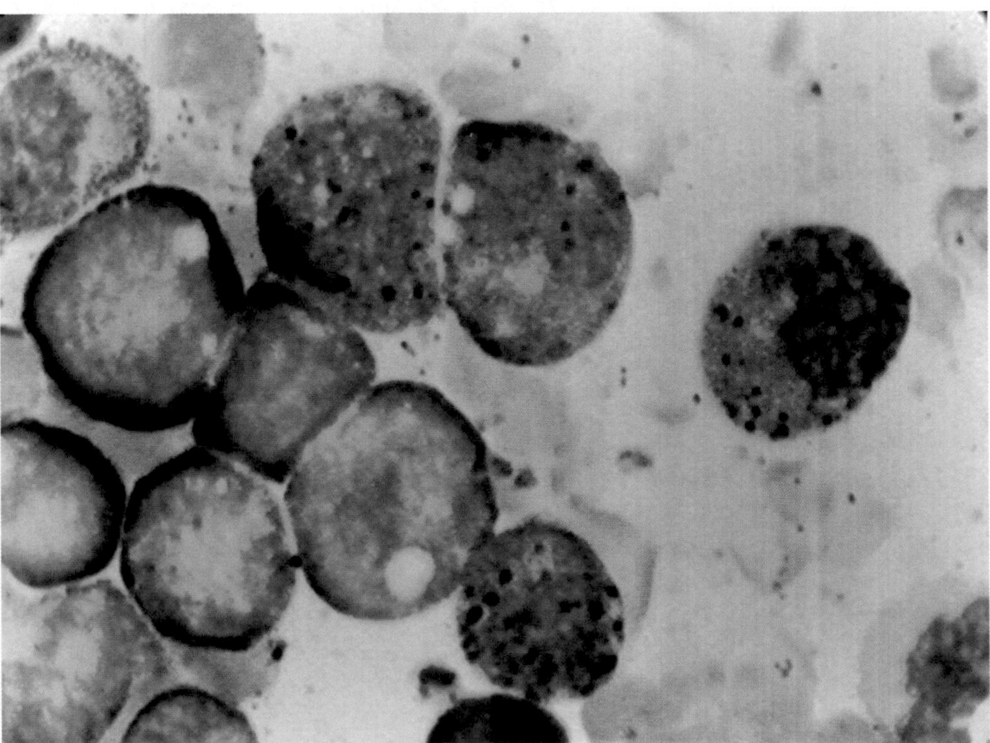

Fig. 14.12 AMML with eosinophils (FAB M4Eos). Note the magenta staining granules in the myelocyte. WG stain

Acute Myeloid Leukemia with t(6;9)(p23;q34);DEK-NUP214

The t(6;9) is detected in 0.7–1.8% of AML that occurs in both children and adults.

In this entity there are no features specific to blast cells. The blasts may show occasional Auer rods and may exhibit monocytic features. Marrow and peripheral blood basophilia defined as more than 2% is seen in half of the reported cases. Multilineage dysplasia may be evident in most of the cases [103, 104]. Blasts are MPO positive. TdT may be positive in some cases. FLT3-ITD mutations are common in this type of AML occurring in 69% of childhood and 78% of adult cases [103, 104]. AML with t(6;9)(p23;q34) represents a unique subtype of acute myeloid leukemia with a high risk of relapse, high frequency of FLT3-ITD mutations, and a specific gene expression signature including several upregulated genes involved in histone modification, and a typical HOXA/B profile, which may be a target for future therapy [105]. AML with t(6;9)(p23;q34) has poor outcome in both adults and children. However, recent smaller studies, including both adult and pediatric patients, have shown that treatment with early allogeneic hematopoietic stem cell transplantation in first complete remission may improve the outcome [106, 107].

Acute Myeloid Leukemia with inv (3)(q21q26.2) or t(3;3)(q21;q26.2);RPN1-EVI1

Various categories of 3q abnormalities in AML can be distinguished according to their genetic features. But 2008 WHO classification of hematopoietic tumors only recognizes AML with inv(3)(q21q26.2) or t(3;3)(q21;q26.2);RPN1-EVI1 as an independent clinicopathological entity, with an extremely poor prognosis. In the upcoming revised WHO classification, the molecular basis of inv(3)(q21q26.2) or t(3;3)(q21;q26.2) shows rearrangement of a GATA2 oncogenic enhancer element, rather than of the RPN1 gene, in band 3q21 with the EVI gene in band 3q26.2 [54]. High expression of the oncogene EVI1 at 3q26.2 is a poor prognostic indicator independent of 3q26 rearrangement. Deregulated expression of EVI1 is the molecular hallmark of this disease; however, when the genome-wide spectrum of cooperating mutations is elucidated it has been shown that 98% of inv(3)/t(3;3) myeloid malignancies harbor mutations in genes activating RAS/receptor tyrosine kinase (RTK) signaling pathways which may provide a target for a rational treatment strategy [108].

Acute myeloid leukemia with inv (3) or t(3;3) may represent de novo or may arise from MDS. It accounts for about 1–2% of all AML cases and occurs most commonly in adults [98, 109]. Patients typically present with anemia and sometimes thrombocytosis [110, 111]. Dysplastic hypogranular neutrophils, pseudo-Pelger cells, dysplastic thrombocytes, and naked megakaryocyte nuclei associated with or without blast cells are noted as peripheral blood changes. Bone marrow blasts may show all morphological FAB diagnoses from M0 to M7 (except M3) subtypes. MPO reactivity is often low. Multilineage dysplasia of bone marrow elements other than blast cells is a common finding. Dyserithropoesis and/or dysgranulopoiesis are frequent. Megakaryocytes may be normal or increased in number and usually have dysplastic features [111–113]. Bone marrow cellularity and fibrosis are variable.

Secondary karyotypic abnormalities including monosomy 7, 5q deletions, and complex karyotypes are present in most of the cases and associated with poor prognosis [112]. Some patients having these translocations may present less than 20% blasts in the bone marrow and should be closely monitored for development of AML.

Acute Myeloid Leukemia (Megakaryoblastic) with t(1;22)(p13;q13); RBM15-MKL1

Acute megakaryoblastic leukemia (AMKL) with t(1;22) is a rare form of AML and restricted to infants and children younger than 3 years. It commonly occurs in infants without Down syndrome (DS) [52, 114]. Non-DS AMKL is characterized by chimeric oncogenes consisting of genes known to play a role in normal hematopoiesis [115, 116]. The median age at diagnosis is 4 months. Majority of cases present with marked hepatosplenomegaly and/or osteolytic skeletal lesions with or without bone marrow involvement [117]. Patients also have anemia and thrombocytopenia with a moderately elevated white blood cell count. The morphology of the blast cells reveals that cells are very pleomorphic that may vary from very small with dense chromatin to somewhat larger with a fine reticulated nuclear chromatin and prominent nucleoli. Cytoplasmic blebs or actual platelet shedding may be found surrounding some blasts. The blasts are MPO or SBB negative. Micromegakaryocytes are common, but dysplastic features of erythroid and granulocytic cells are not present. Bone marrow biopsy may show many clusters of micromegakaryoblasts, as well as more mature megakaryoblasts (Fig. 14.13). This is associated with an increase in reticulin formation and a corresponding decrease in normal hematopoietic precursors. Patients with t(1;22) and less than 20% blasts on bone marrow aspiration should be correlated with the bone marrow biopsy. The presence of myeloid sarcoma is diagnostic of AML regardless of the marrow blast count. Megakaryoblasts express one or more of the platelet glycoproteins (CD41 and CD61). Cytoplasmic expression of these markers is more specific and sensitive than surface staining. The myeloid-associated markers CD13 and CD33 may be positive. CD36 is characteristically positive. CD34,

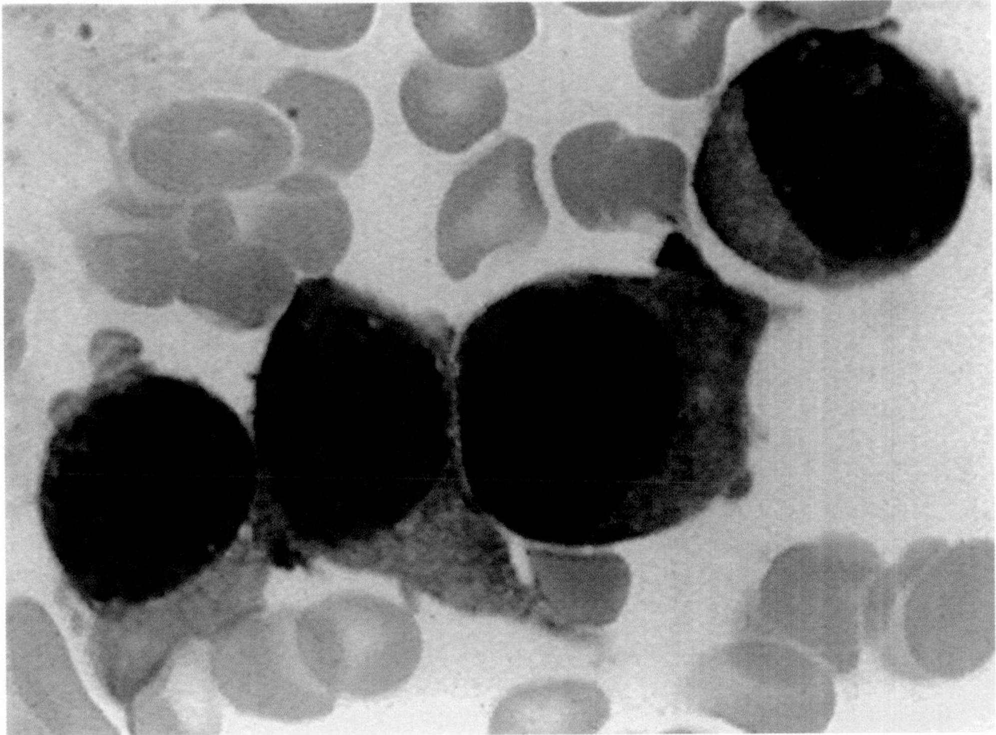

Fig. 14.13 Acute megakaryocytic leukemia. (FABM7). Large blasts with cytoplasmic projections. Immunostain for CD41 was positive. WG stain

MPO, HLA-DR, and TdT are negative [49]. The outcome of non-DS AMKL is generally poor, with lower event-free survival even in the face of intensified treatment [118]. Monitoring of MRD using RBM15-MKL1 fusion transcript would be useful in the treatment of AMKL with t(1 ; 22)(p13; q13) [119].

AML with Gene Mutations

In addition to translocation and inversions, specific gene mutations also occur in AML. Alone or in combination NPM1, FLT3-ITD, CEBPA, and KIT mutations have been reported in AML patients with a normal karyotype. However, they may also be seen in patients with translocation and inversions as well [119]. Recent studies have also shown that the mutations of ASXL1 and TP53 as well as RUNX1 have consistently been associated with an inferior outcome and they will be included in these recommendations [65, 120]. In the 2008 WHO classification [52], mutations of NPM1, FLT3-ITD, and CEBPA are listed among the most common recurrently mutated genes, and those with the NPM1 or CEBPA mutation are designated as provisional entities; in revised upcoming edition they will become entities. On the other hand, AML with CEBPA mutation will be restricted to patients with AML in whom there is a biallelic (and not a monoallelic) mutation, because only that form of AML defines a clinicopathologic entity that is associated with a favorable prognosis [121]. Finally, "AML with RUNX1 mutation" [56] is being considered as provisional entity on the basis of their characteristic clinicopathologic features. FLT3-ITD gene mutations may occur with any type of AML and MDS (20–40% of cases) but is more common in AML with t(15;17) and AML with a normal karyotype and their presence is associated with an adverse outcome [122, 123]. KIT mutations have prognostic significance in cases of AML with t(8;21), inv(16), and t(16;16) (core-binding factor leukemias), in which they are associated with a poor prognosis [70]. AML with mutated NPM1 is found in 50% of adult and 20% of pediatric AML patients with a normal karyotype [124, 125]. AML with mutated NPM1 in the absence of a FLT1-ITD mutation has a favorable prognosis [124, 126]. In adults, most of the NPM1-mutated cases show monocytic differentiation. Along with molecular techniques, paraffin sections are also used to show aberrant cytoplasmic expression of NPM by immunohistochemistry [125]. Around 10% of AML cases with normal karyotype carry the CEBPA mutation. Most CEBPA-mutated cases are double mutated (biallelic); only a few cases of AML cases with normal karyotype carry a singly mutated CEBPA [127]. There are no distinctive morphologic features of AML with biallelic mutations of CEBPA, but the vast majority of cases have features of either AML without or with maturation [127, 128]. Multilineage dysplasia is reported in 26% of cases with no adverse prognostic significance [129]. *RUNX1* mutations have been identified in a substantial proportion of AML patients with normal karyotype [55, 56] as well as in myelodysplastic syndromes [130]. AML with RUNX1 mutations are often associated with undifferentiated morphology (M0). RUNX1 mutations are frequently associated with ASXL1 mutations; however they never coexisted with NPM1 and CEBPA mutations [56]. Since RUNX1 mutations are associated with poor clinical outcome in both younger and older patients treated with intensive induction chemotherapy [55] patients harboring RUNX1 mutations warrant novel therapies and/or early alloSCT.

Acute Myeloid Leukemia with Myelodysplastic Related Changes

Patients are assigned to "AML with myelodysplasia-related changes" if they have 20% or more blasts in the blood or marrow and (1) arise from previous myelodysplastic syndrome (MDS) or a myelodysplastic/myeloproliferative (MDS/MPN) neoplasm, (2) have specific MDS-related cytogenetic abnormalities, and/or (3) exhibit multilineage dysplasia (50% or more of the cells in two or more myeloid lineages) [49]. Patients should not have a history of prior cytotoxic or radiation therapy for an unrelated disease. The specific genetic abnormalities of AML with recurrent genetic abnormalities are absent.

This category of AML occurs mainly in elderly patients and is rare in children [131]. Although the definition of multilineage dysplasia is variable in the literature, this category appears to represent 24–35% of all cases of AML [132, 133]. Myeloid sarcomas may be present at presentation and should be diagnosed as AML regardless of the bone marrow blast percentage [52].

To classify an AML as having myelodysplasia-related changes based on morphology, dysplasia must be present in at least 50% of the cells in at least two myeloid cell lines. Morphologic dysplasias are characterized by neutrophils with hypogranular cytoplasm or hyposegmented nuclei; erythroblasts with megaloblastoid changes, nuclear irregularity, multinuclearity, and ringed sideroblasts; megakaryocytes with nonlobated or multiple nuclei; and micromegakaryocytes. Dysmegakaryopoiesis may be more easily recognized in paraffin sections [132, 134]. Some cases do not meet the criteria for a morphologic diagnosis. However, they are diagnosed as AML with myelodysplastic related changes by the detection of MDS-related cytogenetic abnormalities and/or by a prior history of MDS or MDS/MPN. Chromosome abnormalities are similar to those found in MDS and often involve gain or loss of major segments of certain chromosomes with complex karyotypes, −7/del(7q) and del(5q), and unbalanced translocations involving 5q being most common [93, 135]. Cases of AML with multilineage dysplasia may carry NPM1 and/or FLT3 mutations, or biallelic mutations of CEBPA [136]. Most NPM1-mutated or CEBPA double-mutated cases would be expected to have a normal karyotype and no history of prior MDS [137]. Prognosis of these cases is similar to cases without multilineage dysplasia [129]. Therefore, such cases are now considered as part of the respective entities of AML with mutated NPM1 or AML with double-mutated CEBPA and not as AML with myelodysplasia-related changes. Other gene mutations, such as U2AF1, ASXL1, and TP53, are fairly common in AML with myelodysplasia-related changes [9, 138]. Blasts often express panmyeloid markers (CD13, CD33), but aberrantly high or low expression is common. There is frequent aberrant expression of CD56 and/or CD7 [139].

The principal differential diagnoses are MDS with excess blasts (MD-EB), acute erythroid leukemia, acute megakaryoblastic leukemia, and other categories of AML, not otherwise specified (NOS). Careful blast cell counts, adherence to the diagnostic criteria for morphological dysplasia, and evaluation for MDS-related cytogenetic abnormalities should resolve most cases, with this category having priority over the purely morphological categories of AML, NOS. For example, a case with ≥20% total BM myeloblasts, multilineage dysplasia, ≥50% BM erythroid precursors, and monosomy 7 should be considered as AML with myelodysplasia-related changes rather than acute erythroid leukemia. Similarly, a case with 20% or more BM megakaryoblasts and multilineage dysplasia would be considered AML with myelodysplasia-related changes if AML with t(1;22)(p13.3;q13.1) and myeloid neoplasms of Down syndrome are excluded.

Although AML with multilineage dysplasia is generally associated with a poor prognosis, several studies have not found morphology to be a significant parameter when using multivariate analysis that also incorporates the results of cytogenetic analysis, high-risk cytogenetic abnormalities being more significantly associated with prognosis [136]; however, the presence of multilineage dysplasia in the absence of prior MDS or an MDS-related cytogenetic abnormality appears to remain to be a significantly poor prognostic indicator in adults [140, 141].

Therapy-Related Myeloid Neoplasms

This category includes therapy-related AML, MDS, and MDS/MPN occurring as late complication of cytotoxic and/or radiation therapy administered for a neoplastic or non-neoplastic disorder [142]. Therapy-related myeloid neoplasms account for 10–20% of all cases of AML, MDS, and MDS/MPN [143].

Two subsets of therapy-related neoplasms are recognized. The longer latency cases (5–10 years after therapy) are associated with alkylating agents and ionizing radiation. This category is commonly associated with chromosomal losses, often of −5,−7 in a setting of complex karyotype and mutations or loss of TP53 [144, 145]. Shorter latency cases may arise 1–5 years after therapy and comprise 20–30% of patients. These cases are usually associated with topoisomerase II inhibitor therapy and majority of these cases are associated with recurrent balanced chromosomal translocations that frequently involve 11q23 (MLL orKMT2A) or 21q22.1 (RUNX1) and have morphology resembling de novo acute leukemia associated with these same chromosomal abnormalities [146]. On the other hand, division of patients according to the type of the therapy is not practical since most patients have received polychemotherapy that includes both classes of drugs [147]. The bone marrow may be hypercellular, normocellular, or hypocellular and may have been associated with fibrosis. Blast counts are variable; approximately half of the t-MDS patients will have less than 5% blasts but often exhibit poor-risk cytogenetics [148, 149]. Dysgranulopoiesis and dyserythropoiesis are present in most cases. Megakaryocytes vary in number but the majority of cases show dysplastic megakaryocytes with mono- or hypolobated nuclei. In 20–30% of cases the first manifestation of a therapy-related myeloid neoplasm is overt acute leukemia without a preceding myelodysplastic phase [146–148]. Many of these cases have monoblastic or myelomonocytic morphology. Some cases may have karyotypic and morphologic changes identical to de novo AML with recurring cytogenetic abnormalities, including t-APL with RARA-PML. Such cases should be designated as t-AML with the appropriate cytogenetic abnormality indicated [150]. The prognosis of t-MN is generally poor although it is strongly influenced by the associated karyotypic abnormality as well as the comorbidity of the underlying malignancy or illness for which the cytotoxic therapy was given [151].

Acute Myeloid Leukemia, Not Otherwise Specified

Acute myeloid leukemia, not otherwise specified (AML, NOS), encompasses those cases that do not fulfill the criteria for any of the other previously described AML categories. AML, NOS accounts for 25–30% of all cases. The subgroups of AML, NOS are not prognostically significant [132, 152] when AML with mutated *NPM1* and double-mutated *CEBPA* are removed [48]. Mutation analysis and cytogenetic studies are essential before a case can be placed into this category.

The primary basis for subclassification within AML, NOS category is the morphological and cytochemical/immunophenotypic features of the leukemic cells that indicate the major lineages involved and their degree of maturation. The defining criterion for AML is the presence of 20% or more myeloblasts in the peripheral blood (PB) or bone marrow (BM); the promonocytes in AML with monocytic differentiation are considered blast equivalents. The classification of pure erythroid leukemia is unique and is based on the percentage of abnormal, immature erythroblasts. The previous category of erythroid/myeloid type of erythroleukemia has been eliminated from AML, NOS; cases with a myeloblast count of less than 20% of total BM and PB cells are considered as myelodysplastic syndrome, while cases with greater than 20% myeloblasts will continue to be classified according to standard AML criteria.

Acute Myeloid Leukemia with Minimal Differentiation (M0)

AML M0 is a rare form of acute myeloid leukemia consisting approximately less than 5% of AMLs and may occur at any age. Morphologically, blasts are large with open chromatin and prominent single or multiple nucleoli. The N/C ratio is low. Cytoplasm is moderately basophilic. Azurophilic granules or Auer rods are not seen (Fig. 14.2). MPO- or SBB-positive blasts are less than 3% by light microscopy. Without immunophenotyping, AML M0 may be misdiagnosed as ALL based on the negative cytochemical reactions. So, it is important to stress that a diagnosis of AML M0 cannot be made on morphologic grounds alone and that always requires confirmation by immunologic techniques. Blast cells usually expressed CD13 and CD117 as well as early, hematopoietic associated antigens (CD34, HLA-DR, CD38), while expression of CD33 is found in approximately 60% of cases. Since CD13 antigen is expressed in the cytoplasm of myeloblasts earlier than on the surface, CD13 should be tested by immunohistochemistry whenever the flow cytometry on the cell suspensions is negative. Moreover lymphoid differentiation antigens should be absent, except for CD7 and TdT. TdT is positive in approximately 50% of cases and has been suggested to be of favorable prognostic significance [153]. Patients with the AML M0 subtype have a poorer response to combination therapy.

Acute Myeloblastic Leukemia with Minimal Differentiation (M1)

Poorly differentiated myeloblasts are the predominant non-erythroid cell type (type I and type II). Auer rods may be present and consistent with the diagnosis (Fig. 14.14). More than 3% of these blast cells are MPO or SBB positive by conventional cytochemistry (Fig. 14.3). The low percentage of MPO-positive (3–10%) M1 cases may constitute up to 25% of all M1 cases [154]. In such cases, M1 should be differentiated from ALL L2, acute megakaryoblastic leukemia, and acute monoblastic leukemia without differentiation (M5a). Cytochemical stains and immunophenotyping using a classic panel (MPO, CD13, CD33, CD15, CD34, CD117) to confirm the myeloid nature of blasts are necessary for the differential diagnosis. Blasts are negative for B- and T-associated

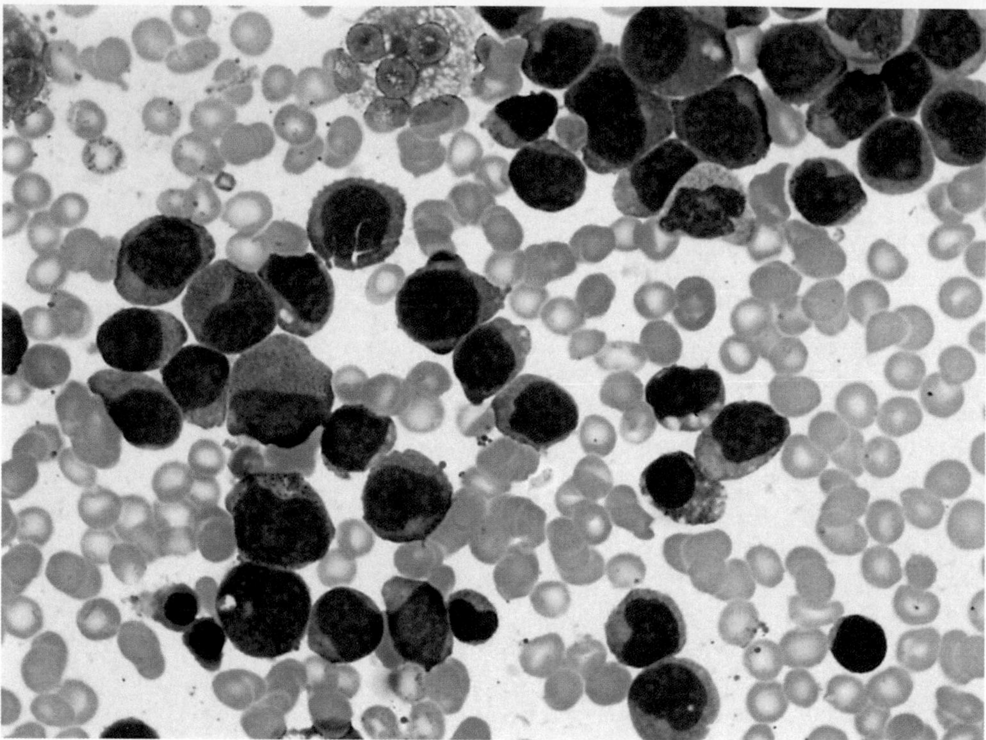

Fig. 14.14 AML (FABM1). Myeloblasts with <10% maturation of granulocytes. WG stain

cytoplasmic lymphoid markers: cCD3, cCD79a, and cCD22. CD7 is found in ~30% of cases, while expression of other lymphoid-associated membrane markers such as CD2, CD4, CD19, and CD56 has been described in 10–20% of cases.

Acute Myeloblastic Leukemia with Maturation (M2)

Acute myeloid leukemia with maturation is characterized by the presence of ≥20% blasts in the BM or PB and evidence of significant differentiation in all cells beyond the promyelocyte state (Fig. 14.15). Granular and agranular blasts are present. Auer rods are frequently seen. Monocytic precursors cannot exceed 20%. Increased numbers of eosinophilic precursors may be seen but they do not exhibit the cytological or cytochemical abnormalities characteristic of the abnormal eosinophils in acute myelomonocytic leukemia associated with inv(16)(p13.1q22) or t(16;16)(p13.1;q22). Variable degrees of dysplasia as pseudo-Pelger-Hüet cells and hypogranular neutrophils are frequently present, but no more than 50% of cells in two lineages are dysplastic. The MPO and SBB reactions are strongly positive. However, cases with a partial MPO deficiency in the granulocytic precursors and mature granulocytes have been reported [155]. Basophils are sometimes increased in this rare form and, therefore, this type of leukemia must be separated from CML in blast crisis by appropriate cytogenetic studies [156].

Leukemic blasts in AML with maturation usually express one or more of the myeloid-associated antigens, CD13, CD33, CD65, CD11b, and CD15. Early stem cell antigens like HLA-DR, CD34, and/or CD117 are also expressed. CD7 is expressed in 20–30% of cases.

Acute Myelomonocytic Leukemia (M4)

Acute myelomonocytic leukemia comprises 5–10% of cases of AML. It occurs in all age groups but is more common in older individuals; the median age is 50 years. Acute myelomonocytic leukemia is morphologically characterized by the proliferation of both neutrophil and monocyte precursors (Fig. 14.16). The PB or BM has ≥20% blasts including promonocytes; neutrophils, monocytes, and their precursors each comprise at least 20% of BM cells. This arbitrary minimal limit of 20% monocytes and their precursors distinguishes acute myelomonocytic leukemia from cases of AML with or without maturation in which some monocytes may be present. The PB typically shows an increase in monocytes, which are often more mature than those in the BM.

The monoblasts are large cells, with abundant cytoplasm basophilic cytoplasm, and have round nuclei with delicate lacy chromatin and one or more large prominent nucleoli. Promonocytes have a more irregular and delicately convoluted nuclear configuration; the cytoplasm is usually less basophilic and sometimes more obviously granulated. Monocytes and promonocytes may not always be readily distinguishable from maturing myeloid cells in routinely stained BM smears. In this regard cytochemical stains are necessary

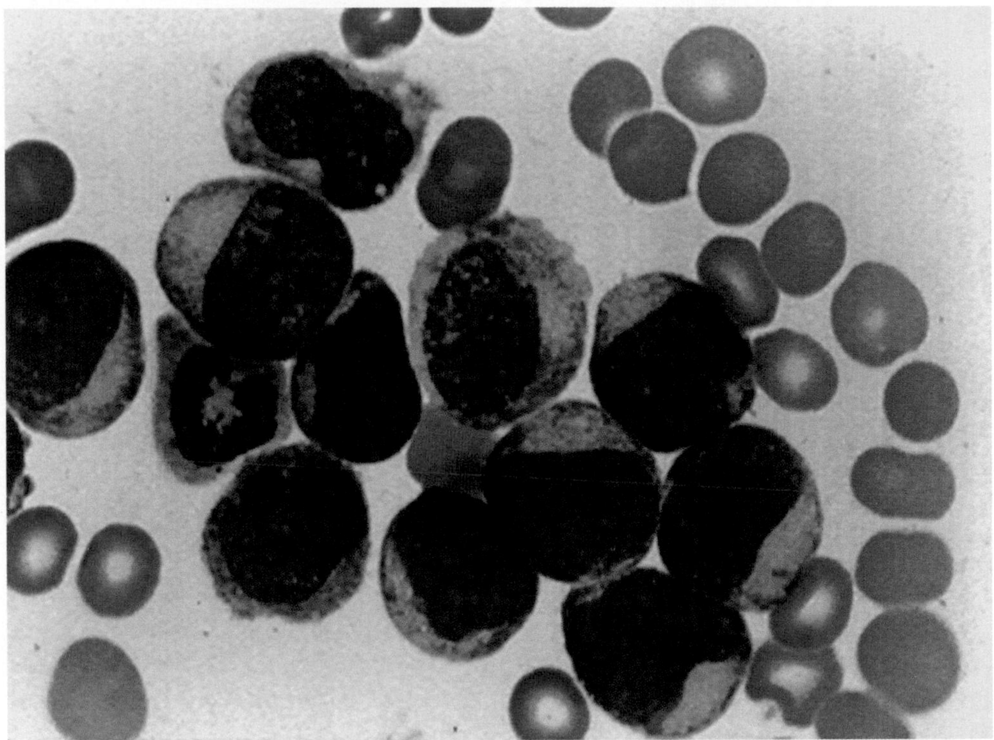

Fig. 14.15 AML (FABM2). Blasts with significant maturation of granulocytes at the promyelocyte and beyond. A single cell has an Auer rod. WG stain

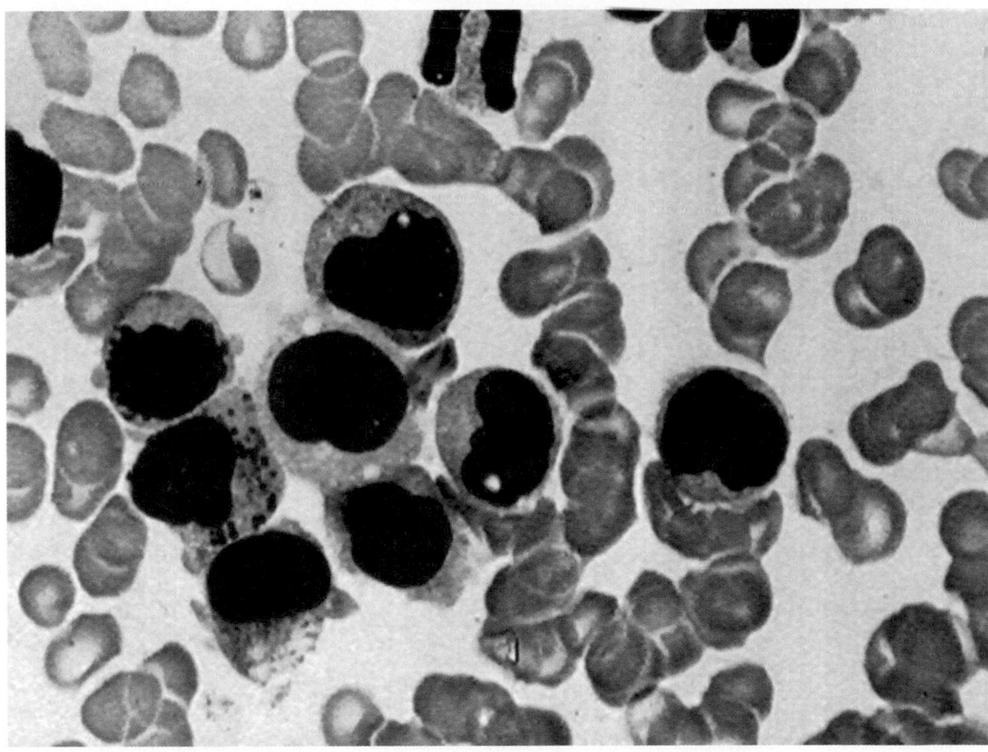

Fig. 14.16 AMML (FAB M4). Both myeloblasts and monocytic precursors are present. WG stain

for confirming the diagnosis. The monoblasts, promonocytes, and monocytes are typically nonspecific esterase (NSE) positive, although in some cases reactivity may be weak or absent. If the cells meet morphologic criteria for monocytes, absence of NSE does not exclude the diagnosis. Double staining for NSE and CAE or MPO may show dual-positive cells (Fig. 14.17). At least 3% of the blasts should show MPO positivity. Monocytic component can be identified by immunophenotyping using CD14, CD11c, CD11b, and CD68 in conjunction with other granulocyte-restricted antibodies.

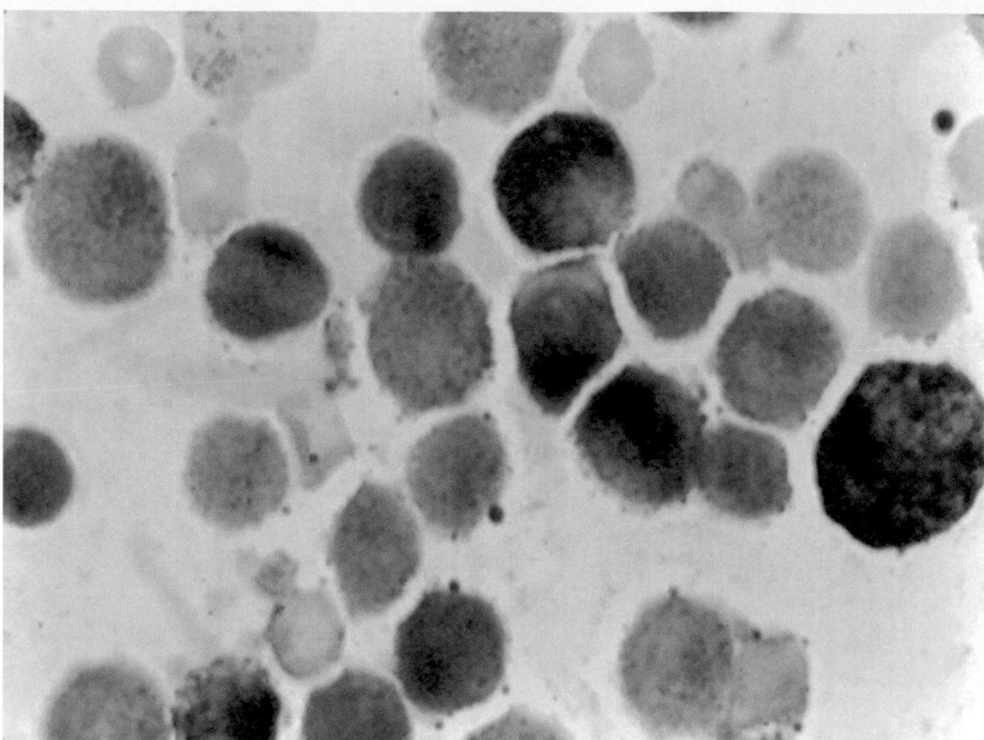

Fig. 14.17 Double-esterase reaction. *Black* product in monocytes and *brick red* color in granulocytes

Dysplastic features involving granulocytic, erythroid, and megakaryocytic lineages can be identified in approximately 20% of patients. The major differential diagnoses include AML with maturation, acute monocytic leukemia, and chronic myelomonocytic leukemia. The differential diagnosis with chronic myelomonocytic leukemia is critical and relies on the proper identification of promonocytes.

Acute Monoblastic and Monocytic Leukemia (M5a and M5b)

Acute monoblastic and acute monocytic leukemias both account for about 10% of the AML. They are clonally expressed in cells committed to differentiation to monocytic pathway [157]. The PB or BM has ≥20% blasts (including promonocytes) and in which 80% or more of the leukemic cells are of monocytic lineage including monoblasts, promonocytes, and monocytes; a minor neutrophil component, <20%, may be present.

Acute monoblastic leukemia is frequently observed in children; it can be confused with the Burkitt lymphoma/leukemia. In the bone marrow, 80% or more of all monocytic cells are monoblasts. Blast cells display abundant deep basophilic cytoplasm, which is often vacuolated and has no or few azurophilic granules and no Auer rods. The nuclei are round to oval, with one or more prominent nucleoli (Fig. 14.18). Since the peroxidase reaction may be negative in 40–50% of such cases and the PAS reaction is often strongly positive with a blocklike pattern, it is very useful to use nonspecific esterase (NSE) staining differential diagnosis. This stain will be strongly positive in more than 90% of cases. Occasionally, the SBB reaction will be positive in the absence of a peroxidase reaction. Cells with monocytic differentiation can express at least two markers characteristic of monocyte differentiation such as CD14, CD4, CD11B, CD64, CD68, and CD36 on the cell surface.

Acute monocytic leukemia is defined by the presence of 20% or more of abnormal cells being (promonocytes) with twisted or folded nuclei, gray-blue cytoplasm, and scattered azurophilic granules (Fig. 14.19). Rarely, a few cells will contain Auer rods. The percentage of mature monocytes is often much higher in the blood than in the bone marrow.

Extramedullary masses (monocytic sarcomas), cutaneous or gingival infiltration, and CNS involvement are common. MPO and CEA are typically negative, but CD68 and CD168 are often positive in extramedullary myeloid (monoblastic) sarcomas. Hemophagocytosis may be observed and is often associated with myeloid-associated, nonspecific cytogenetic abnormalities such as t(8;16)(p11.2;p13.3) [158].

The differential diagnosis of acute monoblastic leukemia includes AML without maturation, AML with minimal differentiation, and acute megakaryoblastic leukemia. Extramedullary myeloid (monoblastic) sarcoma may be confused with malignant lymphoma or soft-tissue sarcomas. However, they are readily distinguished by immunophenotypic analysis and cytochemistry. The differential

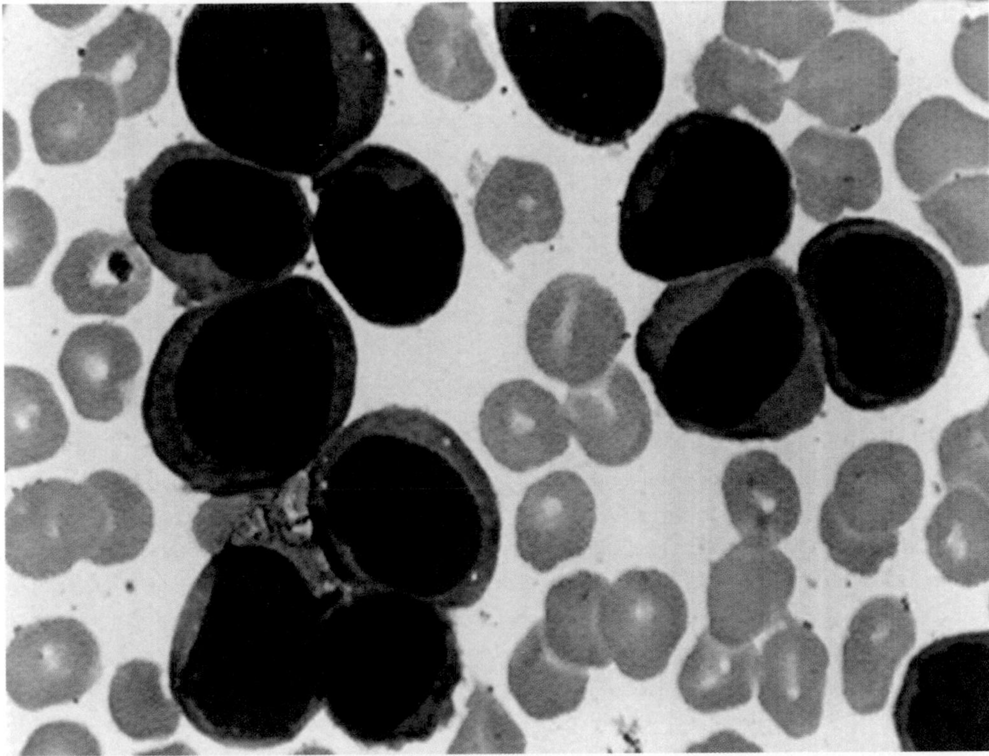

Fig. 14.18 AMOL (acute monocytic leukemia) (FABM5A). Large blasts with nuclear indentation without granules. WG stain

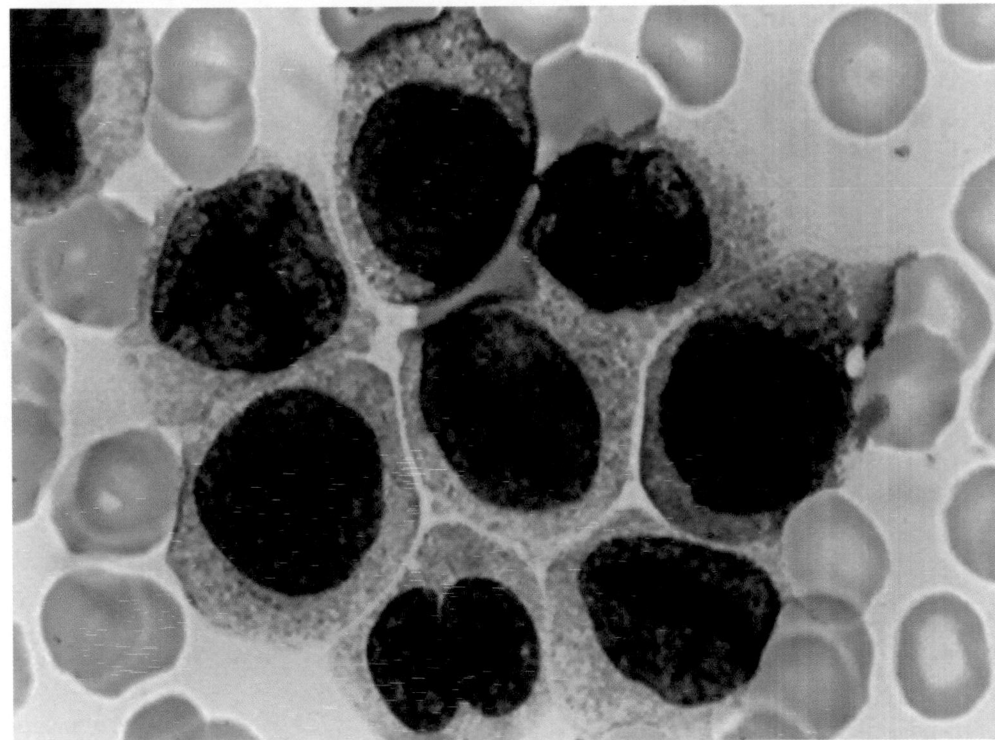

Fig. 14.19 AMOL (FABM5B). Promonocytes are apparent with occ. Azurophil granules. WG stain

diagnosis of acute monocytic leukemia includes chronic myelomonocytic leukemia, acute myelomonocytic leukemia, and microgranular acute promyelocytic leukemia (APL). These can be distinguished by careful examination of well-stained smears and by cytochemistry. The differential diagnosis with chronic myelomonocytic leukemia is critical and relies on the proper identification of promonocytes and their inclusion as blast equivalents.

Acute Erythroid Leukemia (M6)

Pure erythroid leukemia is extremely rare and defined as a neoplastic proliferation of immature (or more mature) cells committed exclusively to the erythroid lineage (80% of total nucleated cells) with no evidence of a significant myeloblastic component [159, 160]. It can occur at any age, including in childhood.

Cases previously classified as the erythroid/myeloid subtype of erythroleukemia (Fig. 14.20), based on counting myeloblasts as a percentage of nonerythroid cells when erythroid cells comprised ≥50% of marrow cells, are now classified based on the total bone marrow or peripheral blood blast cell count. Such cases are classified as myelodysplastic syndromes (usually MDS with excess blasts) when the blast count is <20% of all cells and usually as AML with myelodysplasia-related changes when blasts are ≥20% of marrow or blood cells, irrespective of the erythroid precursor cell count.

Pure erythroid leukemia may occur as a de novo disease, but more frequently occurs as progression of a prior myelodysplastic syndrome or as therapy-related disease [161, 162]. In the latter setting, the case should be diagnosed as a therapy-related myeloid neoplasm.

Morphologically, pure erythroid leukemia is characterized by the presence of medium-sized to large proerythroblasts, with round nuclei, fine chromatin, and one or more nucleoli; the cytoplasm is deeply basophilic and agranular and frequently contains PAS-positive vacuoles (Fig. 14.21). Occasionally the blasts are smaller with scanty cytoplasm and can resemble the lymphoblasts of ALL. The cells are negative for MPO and SBB; they show reactivity with α-naphthyl acetate esterase, acid phosphatase, and blocklike PAS positivity. Pure erythroid leukemia without morphologic evidence of erythroid maturation is difficult to distinguish from megakaryoblastic leukemia and ALL. Moreover, differentiation of the more differentiated forms of pure erythroid leukemia from megaloblastic anemia is difficult.

Acute Megakaryoblastic Leukemia (M7)

Acute megakaryoblastic leukemia (AMkL) in this category is probably an uncommon disease since it would not include cases with t(1;22), AML with inv(3) or t(3;3), AML of Down syndrome, and cases meeting the criteria for AML with myelodysplasia-related changes. The WHO defines AMkL as 20% or more blasts of which at least 50% are of megakaryocyte lineage. The morphologic and immunophenotypic features are those of the megakaryoblasts (Fig. 14.13) described in the aforementioned entities. Cytochemical stains for SBB, CAE, and MPO are consistently negative in the megakaryoblasts; the blasts may show reactivity with PAS and for acid phosphatase and punctate or focal nonspecific esterase reactivity. The megakaryoblasts express one or more of the platelet glycoproteins such as CD41, and/or CD61. In some cases, because of marked fibrosis resulting in a "dry tap" the percent of blasts is estimated from the biopsy.

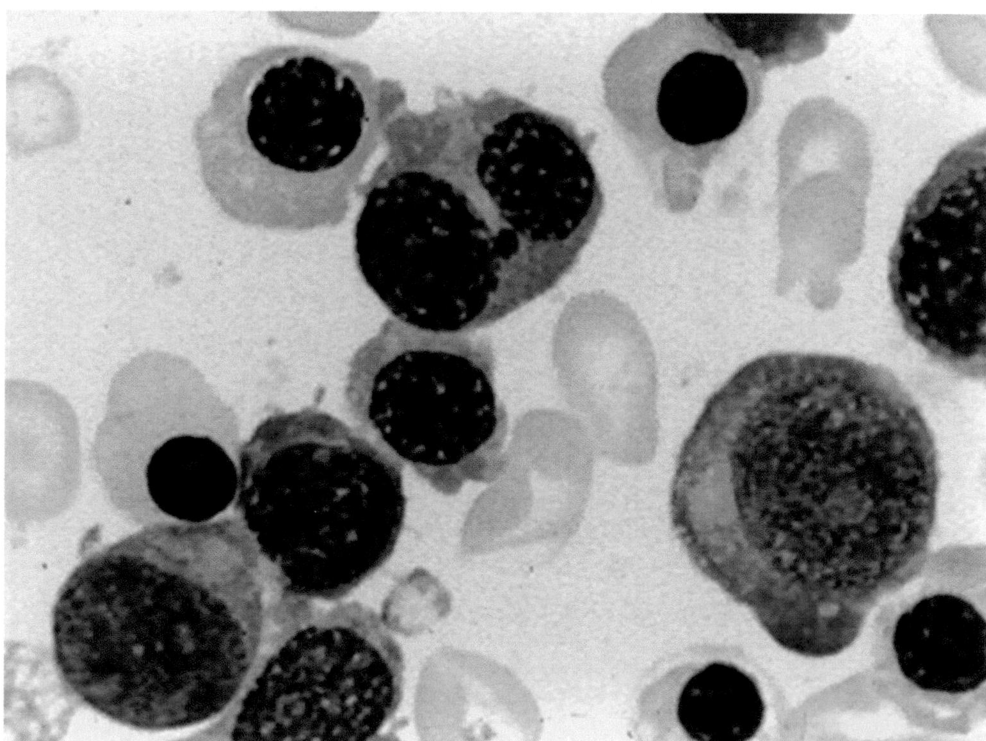

Fig. 14.20 Basophilic erythroid precursors and maturing erythroid cells. Megaloblastic changes. One myeloblast with an Auer rod (previously classified as the erythroid/myeloid subtype of erythroleukemia) WG stain

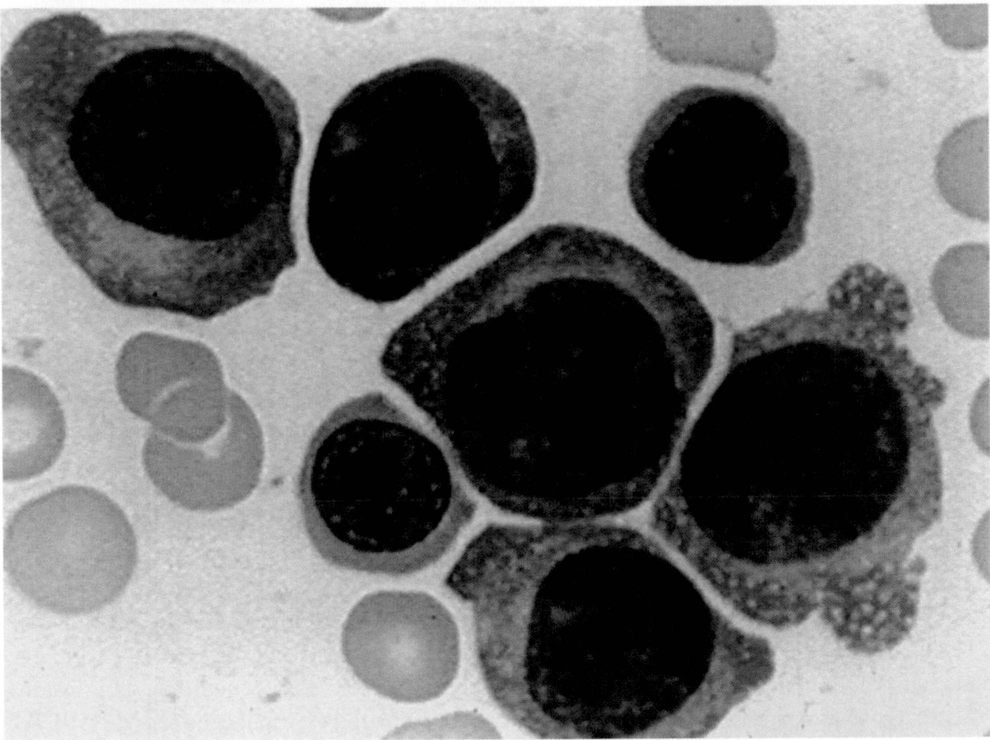

Fig. 14.21 Acute erythroleukemia (FAB M6B). No myeloblasts and many basophilic megaloblasts. WG stain

Acute Basophilic Leukemia

This is a very rare disease comprising <1% of all cases of AML. The circulating PB and BM blasts are of medium size with a high nuclear-cytoplasmic ratio; an oval, round, or bilobed nucleus characterized by dispersed chromatin; and one to three prominent nucleoli. The cytoplasm is moderately basophilic and contains a variable number of coarse basophilic granules which are positive with metachromatic stains such as toluidine blue. The differential diagnosis includes blast phase of CML, other AML subtypes with basophilia such as acute myeloid leukemia with t(6;9), AML with BCR-ABL1, and mast cell leukemia [163, 164].

Acute Panmyelosis with Myelofibrosis

Acute panmyelosis with myelofibrosis (APMF) is a very rare form of de novo AML. APMF is characterized by an acute panmyeloid proliferation with increased blasts and accompanying bone marrow fibrosis that does not meet the criteria for AML with myelodysplasia-related changes [165, 166].

The term APMF is intended to denote involvement of all three hematopoietic cell lineages. Similar features are seen in cases of MDS associated with an excess blasts and fibrosis; AML with myelodysplasia-related changes with multilineage dysplasia and fibrosis; and acute megakaryoblastic leukemia with myelofibrosis and in fibrotic phases of myeloproliferative neoplasms. The distinction between these entities and APMF may be difficult, particularly if no specimen suitable for cytogenetic analysis can be obtained.. Bone marrow biopsy supplemented with immunohistochemistry is required for diagnosis [4, 167]. Immunohistochemistry used by myeloid (MPO, CD13), megakaryocytic (CD61, CD41, factor VIII), and erythroid (glycophorin) markers confirms the presence of panmyelosis. Blasts usually express the progenitor (CD34) or more myeloid-associated (CD13, CD117) markers [4, 167, 168]. The distinction between APMF and MDS with excess blasts (MDS-EB) and myelofibrosis is very difficult since the latter cases can share most of the morphological findings seen in APMF. Cases of MDS-EB and fibrosis, except for their usually less acute clinical presentation, may be otherwise indistinguishable from APMF [4].

Myeloid Sarcoma

Myeloid sarcomas are solid myelogeneous tumors that can occur in 3–7% of AML [169], most frequently observed in children. These tumors either appear green or may become green in diluted acid because of their high MPC content (chloroma). Myeloid sarcomas can be localized in a number of locations including the skin, breast, gastrointestinal tract, lymph nodes, soft tissues, ovaries, and brain. However, most of these tumors arise adjacent to bony or neural structures [170, 171]. Myeloid sarcomas can be recognized in three types of clinical setting [6]: (1) de novo presentation without generalized bone marrow involvement (these cases should be considered as synonymous with AML); (2) in an established diagnosis of AML either at presentation or as the first manifestation of relapse; and (3) may represent acute blastic transformation of myelodysplastic syndromes (MDS), myelodysplastic/myeloproliferative neoplasm (MDS/MPN), or myeloproliferative neoplasms (MPN) [170, 171].Myeloid sarcomas display myeloblastic, myelomonocytic, or pure monoblastic morphology [170]. The morphologic features are highly variable, ranging from little to no differentiation, where the differential diagnosis includes large-cell lymphomas and blastic plasmacytoid dendritic cell neoplasm. The histological diagnosis should be validated by immunohistochemistry (MPO, CD117, CD68, CD34, TdT, CD45, CD56 CD123, BDCA/2) [75, 172]. A more traditional stain is the specific granulocyte esterase reaction, naphthol ASD chloroacetate esterase stain on air-dried touch preparations, or non-Zenker fixed solutions. Moreover, correlation with cytogenetic and molecular genetic status is necessary to provide the correct diagnosis. AML with t(8;21), inv(16), t(1;22), and some 11q23 translocations are frequently associated with extramedullary presentations [5]. About 16% of cases carry evidence of *NPM1* mutations as shown by aberrant cytoplasmic NPM expression [173]. Inv(16) or amplification of *CBFB* has been related to breast, uterus, or intestinal involvement and possible foci of plasmacytoid dendritic cell differentiation [174].

Myeloid Proliferations Related to Down Syndrome

Patients with Down syndrome (DS) have an increased risk of leukemia. There is an approximately 50-fold increase of AML in children with DS younger than 5 years, and 70% of these neoplasms are AMKL. In contrast, AMKL comprises only 3–6% of AML in children without DS. The acute myeloblastic leukemia which occurs in children with DS has unique morphologic, immunophenotypic clinical, and molecular features [175–177] that distinguish it from other forms of AML. It commonly occurs in the first 3 years of life. Morphology of the leukemic blasts shows particular features with round nuclei and moderate amount of basophilic cytoplasm with or without blebs. Some blast contains MPO-negative coarse granules. Bone marrow core biopsy may show dense reticulin network. In these cases, antibodies to CD41 and CD61 may be particularly useful in identifying cells of megakaryocytic lineage in immunohistologic preparations. Leukemic blasts in acute megakaryocytic leukemia of DS display a similar immunophenotype to blasts in transient abnormal myelopoiesis (TAM) [178] (*positive for CD117, CD13, CD33, CD7, CD4, CD42, TPO-R, IL-3R, CD36, CD41, CD61, CD71, and are negative for myeloperoxidase, CD15, CD14, and glycophorin A*). On the other hand, TAM is a unique disorder of DS newborns in which morphologic and clinical features are indistinguishable from AML with DS [177]. The process in the majority of patients undergoes spontaneous remission within the first 3 months of life.

In addition to trisomy 21, acquired GATA-1 mutations are considered pathognomonic of TAM or AML of DS and are associated with a better response to chemotherapy and favorable prognosis compared to children with AML without DS [175]. While gene array studies have suggested differences in expression between AML of DS and TAM, however, these findings have not yet been confirmed [179].

Blastic Plasmacytoid Dendritic Cell Neoplasm

Blastic plasmacytoid dendritic cell neoplasm (BPDCN) is a clinically aggressive neoplasm derived from the precursors of plasmacytoid dendritic cells that is characterized by solitary or multiple skin lesions, often associated with regional lymphadenopathy [180]. Many cases tend to involve bone marrow and peripheral blood as well. Morphology is characterized by a diffuse monomorphous infiltrate of medium-sized blasts with scant cytoplasm, irregular nuclei, fine chromatin, and several small nucleoli. The blasts express CD4, CD56, CD43, as well as plasmacytoid dendritic cell-associated antigens (CD123, BDCA-2/CD303, TCL-1, and CLA). CD68 is expressed in 50% and TdT in 30% of cases [180–182]. In about 8% of cases CD4 or CD56 can be negative, which does not rule out the diagnosis if other PDC-associated antigens (especially CD123, TCL1, or CD303) are expressed [183, 184]. Other hematologic neoplasms especially AML with monocytic differentiation may share morphological and immunophenotypical features with BPDCN [185, 186]; an extensive immunohistochemical and/or genetic analysis is mandatory before a definitive diagnosis of BPDCN is made. On the other hand, BPDCN must be distinguished from mature plasmacytoid dendritic cell proliferation (MPDCP) in which plasmacytoid dendritic cells are morphologically mature and CD56 negative. MPDCP is invariably associated with a myeloid disorder most commonly with chronic myelomonocytic leukemia [186, 187].

Two-thirds of patients with BPDCN have an abnormal karyotype; specific chromosomal aberrations are lacking, but complex karyotypes are common [188]. Genomic abnormalities mainly involve tumor-suppressor genes [189].

The clinical course is aggressive, with a median survival ranging from 10.0 to 19.8 months, irrespective of the initial pattern of disease. Most cases (80–90%) show an initial response to multiagent chemotherapy, but relapses with subsequent resistance to drugs are regularly observed [190, 191].

Acute Leukemias of Ambiguous Lineage

Acute leukemias of ambiguous lineage show no clear evidence of differentiation along a single lineage. Cases with no lineage-specific antigens are designated as acute undifferentiated leukemia (AUL). They often express CD34, HLA-DR, and/or CD38 and TdT but lack specific myeloid and/or lymphoid antigens [192]. Leukemias that coexpress antigens of more than one lineage on the same cells or that have separate populations of blasts that are of different lineages are referred to as mixed-phenotype acute leukemia (MPAL). Some examples of MPAL blasts reveal B lineage and myeloid differentiation (MPAL, B/Myeloid) whereas other cases have both T lineage and myeloid markers (MPAL, T/Myeloid) [193, 194]. On the basis of associated cytogenetic anomalies, MPAL can be subdivided into three subgroups according to the presence of chromosome abnormalities: t(9;22)/BCR-ABL1, t(v;11q23)/MLL, or not otherwise specified (NOS) [195]. Therefore, mixed blast phase of CML must be excluded. All other unusual immunophenotypes, including early natural killer (NK) leukemias, constitute the remainder of leukemias of ambiguous origin. There may be cases that cannot be adequately classified due to insufficient immunophenotyping data or discordant expression of various markers, rendering definitive classification impossible. These cases should be designated as acute unclassifiable leukemia, which is different from AUL [196].

Central Nervous System Leukemia

Without CNS prophylaxis against CNS leukemia in ALL, isolated CNS relapse occurs in 50% of patients and is associated with subsequent systemic relapse. Therefore, CNS prophylaxis is routinely used in ALL. Although testicular and other extramedullary relapses have become exceedingly rare in ALL, in contemporary clinical trials [197] central nervous system (CNS) relapse remains a major obstacle to cure, accounting for 30–40% of initial relapses [198]. The incidence of CNS leukemia is lower in AML, and CNS prophylaxis is not usually used [199]. It should be remembered that CNS leukemia occurs frequently in patients with a prominent monocytic component (i.e., acute monocytic leukemia or acute myelomonocytic leukemia), acute promyelocytic leukemia (APL) in systemic relapse, AML with inversion or deletion of chromosome 16 (16) or chromosome 11 abnormality, hyperleukocytosis, or an elevated lactate dehydrogenase [200, 201].

The most likely explanation of CNS leukemia is direct extension from bone marrow in the skull, extending along the dura mater. Additional venules provide a direct route for leukemic infiltration of brain parenchyma [202].

Diagnostic lumbar puncture is recommended for all patients with ALL and for patients with AML who have WBC counts higher than 40,000 mm^3 [203]. Careful cytologic investigation of CNS fluid is essential to establish a diagnosis of involvement.

A CSF leukocyte count greater than 5 leukocytes/mL with the presence of unequivocal blasts on cytocentrifuge preparation is accepted as minimum cytologic criteria for CNS leukemia [204]. The two most common techniques include a cytocentrifuge preparation and a Wright-Giemsa stain or Millipore filtration technique and the Papanicolaou method. It is important to distinguish atypical but reactive cells secondary to drug-related arachnoiditis from leukemia blasts.

Evaluation of Remission

In a patient treated with acute leukemia, CR is considered when peripheral blood cell counts approach the normal range, and the bone marrow is normocellular, and shows orderly maturation of hematopoietic cells with less than 5% blast cells. The criteria for morphologic remission of less than 5% bone marrow blasts are arbitrary. The leukemic blasts in AML M3 or ALL L3, or blasts containing Auer rods, can be readily identified, even when present in small numbers. In other types of leukemia, a definitive diagnosis of residual leukemia may not be possible by morphologic examination. Persistence of dysplastic hematopoiesis in a patient who might otherwise fulfill the criteria for CR results in a much higher relapse rate. It should be remembered that the bone marrow regeneration occurs more quickly in pediatric patients (3 or 4 weeks). Therefore, one can observe a modest increase in myeloblasts and promyelocytes during recovery that may persist for 1–2 weeks. This should not be over-interpreted as a regrowth of leukemic cells.

The definition of partial remission is accepted when less than 25% leukemic cells are counted in the bone marrow smears. Relapse is defined by the presence of more than 25% leukemic cells in the bone marrow aspirate and is usually associated with peripheral cytopenias and sometimes presence of blasts.

Myelodysplastic Syndrome

Myelodysplastic syndromes (MDS) are a clonal proliferation of multipotential hematopoietic stem cells. Clinically, MDS represents a condition of bone marrow failure, usually of the elderly (primary MDS), or of patients previously exposed to prior chemotherapy or radiation or both (secondary MDS). The correlation of the biology of this clonal disorder with its clinical presentation of cytopenias is varied ranging from an incidental mild anemia stable for years to a rapidly evolving leukemia [205].

MDS is a disease of elderly, with the annual incidence of 4 cases per 100,000 in the general population.

The underlying causes in the pathogenesis of MDS remain elusive. Analyses of G6PD isoenzymes, restriction-linked polymorphisms, X-linked DNA polymorphisms of the androgen receptor (HUMARA), cytogenetic abnormalities, gene mutations, and recently targeted gene sequencing and SNP array analysis can identify somatic events in the majority of MDS patients, and have shown that MDS is a clonal abnormality of the hematopoietic stem cell characterized by defective maturation and in advanced stages uncontrolled proliferation [206–209].

Chromosomal anomalies are detected in approximately 50% of patients with de novo MDS and in up to 80% of patients with MDS secondary to chemotherapy or other toxic agent [210–212]. Balanced cytogenetic abnormalities, including reciprocal translocations, inversions, and insertions, are uncommon in MDS, in which unbalanced chromosomal abnormalities reflecting a gain or loss of chromosomal material are more prevalent [210–212]. Upcoming WHO 2008 revision recognized the importance of recent discoveries regarding the clinical significance of specific gene mutations in MDS. However, most mutations do not appear to correlate with specific disease entities with the exception for SF3B1 mutations [213, 214].

The examination of an appropriately prepared and stained bone marrow and peripheral blood smear remains the most important diagnostic approach in morphologic diagnosis [215–217]. Well-prepared thin smears with an excellent Romanowsky stains should be utilized. Iron stains are essential to address the percentage of ring sideroblasts. For an accurate differential count, at least 500 nucleated cells should be counted.

Reticulin stains prepared from bone marrow biopsy cores are recommended, since some cases will demonstrate an increased score that is viewed as impacting adversely on prognosis.

Finally, cytogenetics are critical to obtain because prognostic information is provided and is an important component of several scoring systems. Conventional cytogenetics obtained from bone marrow aspirate could be complemented by interphase FISH (with probes, i.e., 5q–,7–,8+,20q–) tests.

Morphologic Characteristics

The following discussion highlights the morphologic features used to define MDS [218–222]. In general, these features should be present in at least 10% or greater of cells of the respective lineage under consideration. The upcoming proposal is to retain the 10% threshold but provide more detailed morphologic definitions of dysplasia [217, 222–224].

Dyserythropoiesis

Morphologic bone marrow dyserythropoiesis (DysE) may include the presence of ringed sideroblasts, multinuclear fragments, bizarre nuclear shapes, internuclear bridging, mitosis, abnormal intensity of the chromatin or fine chromatin with asynchronous cytoplasm, and abnormal cytoplasmic features (intense basophilia, Howell-Jolly bodies, and ghosted cytoplasm). Marked macrocytosis (at least 100 fmol/L), basophilic stippling, anisocytosis, and poikilocytosis may be observed in the peripheral blood. Quantitative changes include the presence of ringed sideroblasts (exceeding 15% of all nucleated erythroid cells) and a number of megaloblastic erythroid precursors. However, the evaluation of dysplastic features in erythroid lineage such as megaloblastoid and cytoplasmic changes is poorly reproducible [222].

The MDS working group [51] defines three types of sideroblast: type 1 sideroblasts: fewer than five siderotic granules in the cytoplasm; type 2 sideroblasts: five or more siderotic granules but not in preinuclear distribution; and type 3 or ring sideroblasts: five or more granules in a perinuclear position, surrounding the nucleus or encompassing at least one-third of the nuclear circumference (Fig. 14.22). This definition of ring sideroblasts has been incorporated into WHO 2008 and revised WHO classification. For the definition of MDS-RS, the required number of ring sideroblasts remains at 15%.

Dysgranulopoiesis

In dysgranulopoiesis (DysG), the peripheral blood can be notable for hypogranulation and hyposegmentation of the polymorphonuclear leukocytes (PMLs) with excessive chromatin condensation (pseudo-Pelger-Hüet anomaly) (Fig. 14.23). Hypogranulation is most commonly noted and can be associated with a negative MPO reaction. The cells can be devoid of all granules, often in the more immature forms. Nuclear sticks can be seen, particularly in cases of secondary MDS or therapy-related MDS. These morphologic features may explain in part the frequency of infection in these patients (i.e., phagocytic adhesion, chemotaxis, and microbiocidal capacities may be impaired), but no correlation has been found between the loss of granules and impaired function.

Dysmegakaryopoiesis

Qualitative changes are more common in dysmegakaryopoiesis (DysM) as the number of megakaryocytes is usually normal, although hypoplasia or hyperplasia can

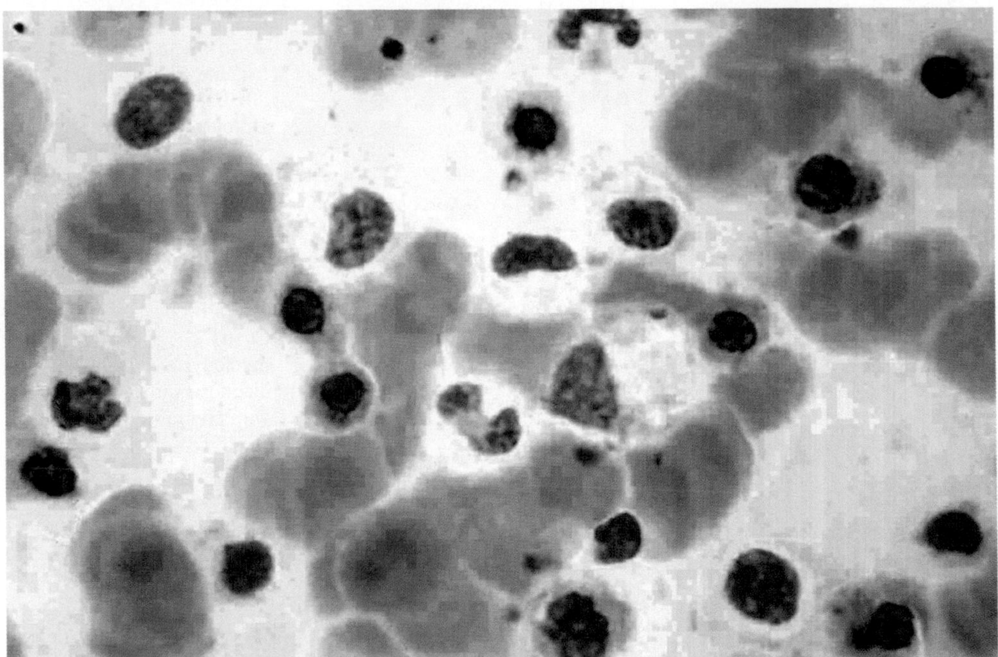

Fig. 14.22 Myelodysplastic syndrome (MDS). RARS with ring sideroblasts. Prussian *blue* reaction

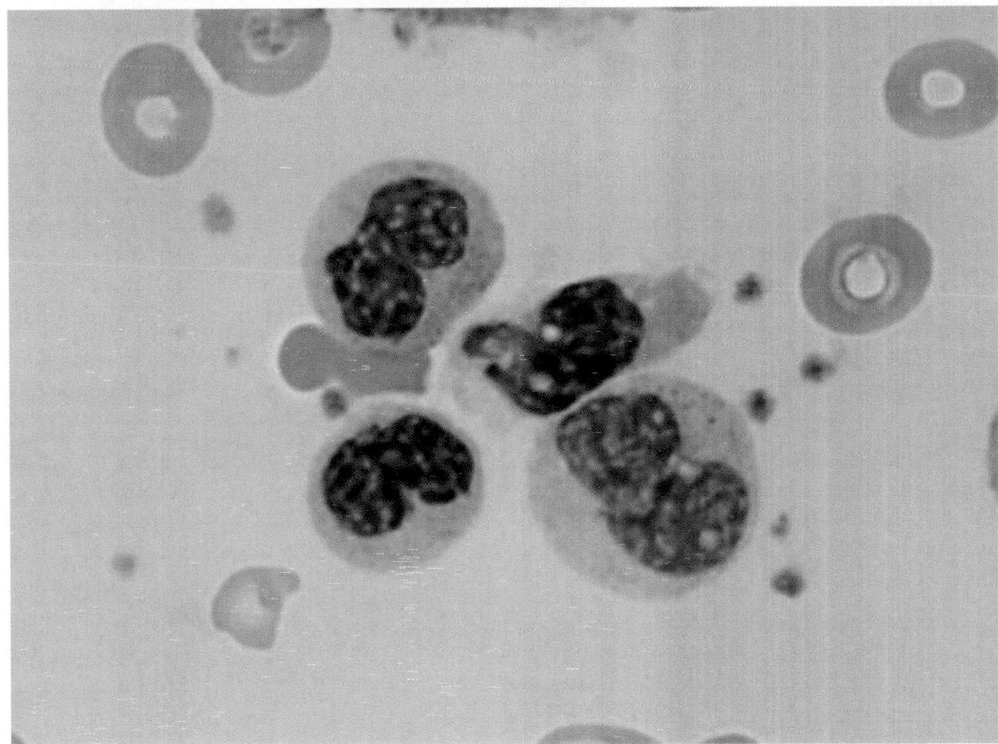

Fig. 14.23 MDS. Dysplastic granulocytes with clumped chromatin and hypogranular cytoplasm. WG stain

occasionally be seen. In the peripheral blood, large hypo- or hypergranular platelets can be found. In the bone marrow, morphologic abnormalities of the megakaryocytic precursors can be seen in half of the patients. Commonly there are micromegakaryocytes (dwarf forms) (Fig. 14.24), megakaryocytes with multiple small round, and separate nuclei and large mononuclear forms. Micromegakaryocytes can be further recognized by using CD41 and antifactor VIII antibodies on bone marrow smears with the APAAP technique. Small mononuclear megakaryocytes with a single eccentric nucleus are strongly correlated with 5q– syndrome [225].

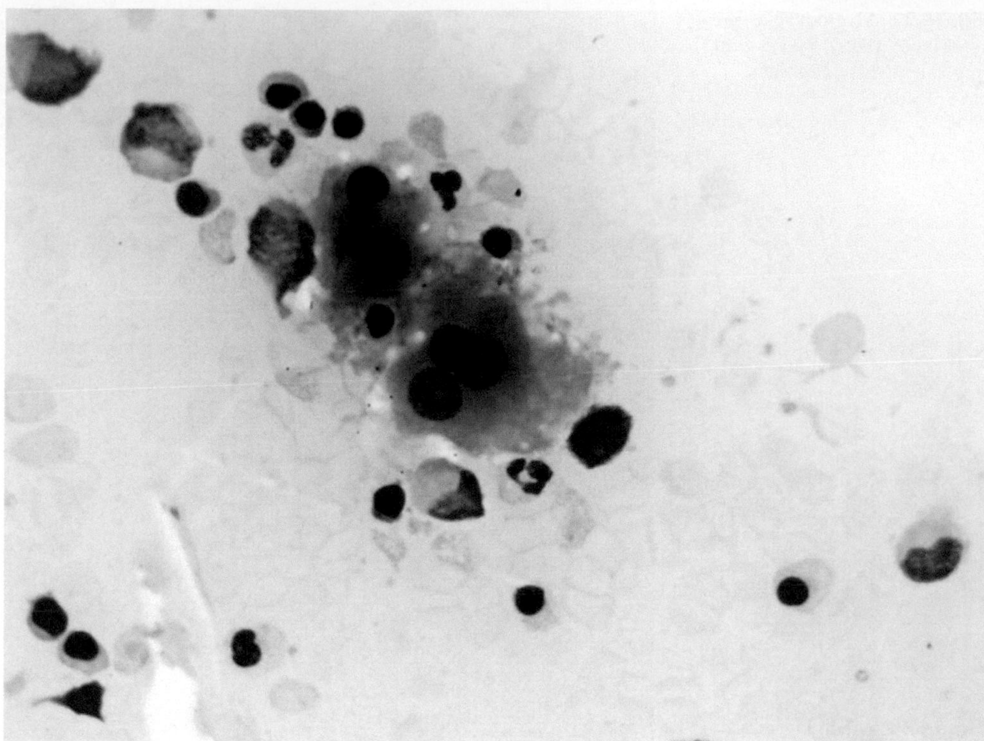

Fig. 14.24 MDS. Dysplastic megakaryocytes with separated nuclei. WG stain

Dysmonocytopoiesis

Identification of the monocyte precursors in the bone marrow is sometimes difficult, and the use of double-esterase staining may be necessary. CD14 and CD68 antibodies can also be used to identify monocytic population.

Blast Cell Characteristics

One of the most important criteria for MDS subclassification is the number (quantity) of blast cells. An area of confusion has been the identification of blasts in MDS. Recently, the international working group of morphology (IWGM) [51] recommended that myeloblasts in MDS should be classified as agranular or granular. The agranular blasts correspond to the type I blasts of the FAB classification. Granular blasts are cells that have not only the nuclear features of blast cells but also cytoplasmic granules. These cells will thus include type II blasts as defined by FAB as well as type III blasts as defined by Goasguen and coworkers [49]. Granular blasts must be distinguished from promyelocytes.

Bone Marrow Histology

The value of bone marrow biopsy in MDS is well established [64]. Bone marrow histology provides useful information on cellularity, relative proportions of three hematopoietic cell lines, architectural disorganization, and increase in the reticulin fibers.

The bone marrow cellularity should be determined as percentage of bone marrow section area according to the standard proposed by our group [226, 227]. We recommended that the bone marrow cellularity should be determined as "normocellular," "hypercellular," or "hypocellular" based on an age-adapted estimate.

Reticulin stain provides additional information about the degree of reticulin fibrosis which can add prognostic information.

Aggressive types of MDS (MD-EB) characterized by clusters of blast in bone marrow biopsies localized in the central part of the bone marrow away from the vascular structures and endosteal surfaces of the trabecule (Figs. 14.25 and 14.26). The blast can also be identified by immunohistochemistry using anti-CD34 antibody. Detection of blasts by anti-CD34 is especially useful in cases with fibrosis and hypocellular MDS to assess blast percentage. Previous studies have reported on the diagnostic and prognostic value of an atypical localization of immature progenitor cells (ALIP) in MDS [228]. These studies have been confirmed using anti-CD34 antibodies. In contrast to other bone marrow cells, it is possible to assess cytologic atypia of megakaryocytes in an adequately processed bone marrow sections. Megakaryocyte markers such as CD41 and CD61 are also helpful for the detection of atypical grouping or clustering and morphologic atypia of megakaryocytes. Tryptase immunohistochemistry is useful to detect coexisting occult mastocytosis [229].

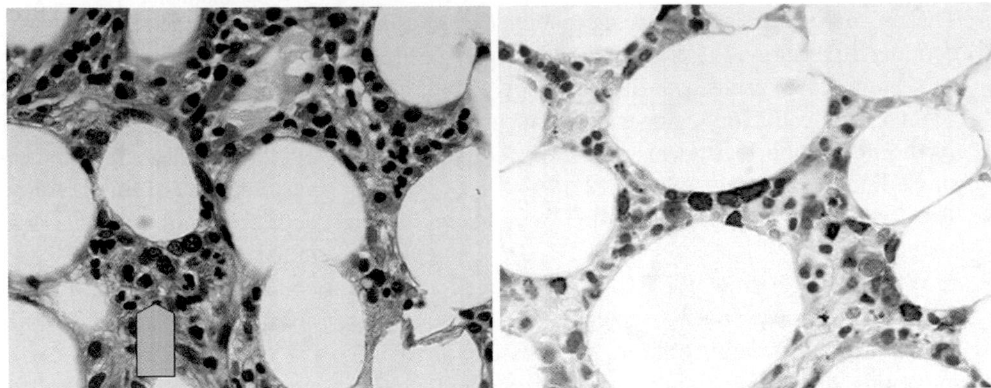

Fig. 14.25 MDS. Abnormal localization of immature precursors (ALIP). *Arrow points* to cluster and right panel shows CD34+ blasts. H&E stain

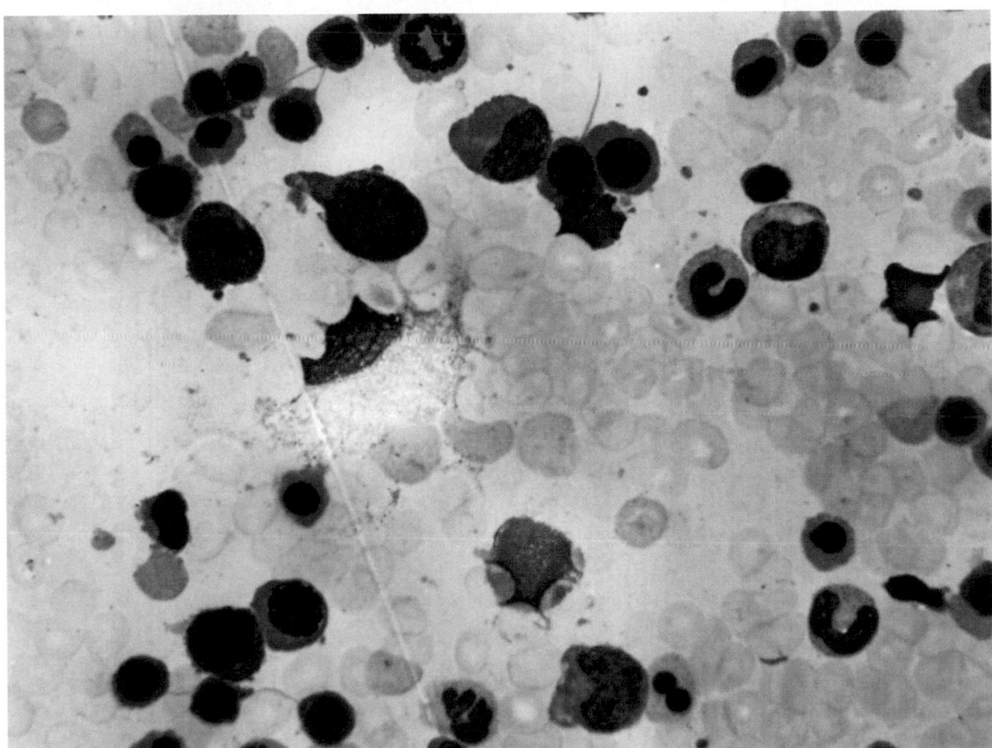

Fig. 14.26 MD-EB2. Note: increased number of blasts and megaloblastic erythroid precursors. MGG stain

Classification of MDS

In 1982, the FAB group introduced a classification system for patients with MDS [230]. The main discriminators were peripheral and medullary blast count, the percentage of ring sideroblasts, and the absolute monocyte count. This classification provided standard diagnostic procedures and became a gold standard for more than two decades.

The World Health Organization (WHO) revised and updated the MDS classification in 1997 and a revised version of the WHO classification is published in 2008 [231]. However, after 7 years, it needs to be updated. The summary of the proposed major changes to the classification related to the myelodysplastic syndromes in revised upcoming 5th edition can be summarized as follows [232]:

1- Significant changes to the morphologic criteria are not proposed. Although the current threshold of 10% to define a lineage as dysplastic may result in overcalling of dysplasia in non-MDS cases, the current proposal is to retain the 10% threshold but provide more detailed morphologic definitions of dysplasia and emphasize the importance of carefully considering non-MDS causes of dysplasia [217–224].

2. Blast cell counts resulted in no change so the classification will continue to recommend that blast cell counts should ideally be performed on well-stained, cellular bone marrow aspirate smears; although the utility of CD34 staining on a trephine biopsy may be helpful for blast cell estimates in the absence of cellular aspirate smears, such as in the setting of marrow fibrosis.

3. The use of cytopenias versus morphologic dysplasia in defining MDS subtypes is sometimes leading to confusion. It is proposed to replace the terminology of "refractory anemia" and "refractory cytopenia" with "myelodysplastic syndrome" in the revised classification [i.e., MDS with single-lineage dysplasia (MDS-SLD)].
4. The cytogenetic criteria for MDS will likely remain unchanged.
5. In WHO 2008 classification RCMD-RS was incorporated in RCMD; however this category is reinstated as RCMD-RS in upcoming edition. MDS cases with SF3B1 mutations have a distinctive gene expression pattern [233], with a large number of differentially expressed genes [234]. This combination of shared morphology (ring sideroblasts) and a shared underlying driver mutation (SF3B1) now favors separating MDS with ring sideroblasts as distinct entities, which may have single or multilineage dysplasias. Thus, MDS cases with SF3B1 mutation can be classified as RARS or RCMD-RS if any ring sideroblasts are present. Ring sideroblasts and SF3B1 mutations also occur in high-grade MDS with excess blasts and even in AML. It should be remembered that RARS or RCMD-RS only defines a specific MDS entity in cases with <5% bone marrow blasts.
6. Recent studies have shown that the del(5q) abnormality in MDS is prognostically similar whether it is isolated or occurs with one additional low-risk cytogenetic aberration [235]. Based on this finding, the category of MDS with isolated del(5q) will be expanded to encompass cases with one additional non-high-risk cytogenetic abnormality. Blasts are <5% in bone marrow, and <1% in blood; dysplasia is uni- or multilineage but cases with significant myeloid dysplasia are excluded [236].
7. The category of MDS unclassified in the revised 2008 classification is retained and includes patients with pancytopenia and unilineage dysplasia, and patients with no overt dysplasia but cytogenetic evidence of cytogenetics. Unilineage dysplasia cases with 1% blood blasts are detected on at least two separate occasions.
8. In upcoming revision erythroid/myeloid type of erythroleukemia with >50% erythroid precursors and 5–19% blasts are now considered as MDS-EB rather than AML. Acute erythroid/myeloid leukemia is linked with MDS, since they share both morphologic and genetic features [237, 238]. Cases with ≥20% blasts and >50% erythroid precursors will still be classified as AML with myelodysplastic changes. Pure erythroleukemia will remain in AML.
9. A provisional entity, refractory cytopenia of childhood (RCC), has been added in 2008 classification to include children with cytopenia(s) with less than 2% peripheral blood and less than 5% bone marrow blasts and evidence of dysplasia in two or more lineages. It remains as a provisional entity in the updated classification.

Morphologic Subtypes

MDS with Single-Lineage Dysplasia (MDS-SLD)

MDS with single-lineage dysplasia (MDS-SLD) comprises 10–20% of all cases. It is primarily disease of elderly. The vast majority of MDS-SLD cases are associated with unilineage erythroid dysplasia (RA). Anemia is the main manifestation (hemoglobin below 11 g/dL with a low reticulocyte count) with variable dyserythropoiesis. Blast cells usually are not present in the peripheral blood (<1%) and fewer than 5% in the bone marrow. Dyserythropoiesis varies from slight to moderate. The bone marrow biopsy is generally hypercellular but may be normocellular or even hypocellular. In general, RA can be considered as a "low-grade" MDS with median survival in the range of 6–7 years and only 5–10% of cases progressing to overt acute leukemia [239, 240]. Other forms of MDS-SLD are rare.

MDS with Single-Lineage Dysplasia and Ring Sideroblasts (MDS-RSSLD)

The morphologic features of MDS with ring sideroblast single-lineage dysplasia (MDS-RSSLD) are similar to those of MDS with single-lineage dysplasia (MDS-SLD) except that there are more than 15% ringed sideroblasts in the bone marrow. However, patients with ring sideroblasts but not meeting the 15% threshold used to define MDS-RSSLD will still be diagnosed if an SF3B1 mutation is detected. Macrocytosis and dysmorphic red cells are present in the peripheral blood (Fig. 14.27). MDS-RSSLD accounts for 3–11% of all MDS cases. It is primarily disease of elderly with a median age of 60–73 years [232, 239]. Ring sideroblasts represent erythroid precursors with abnormal accumulation of iron within mitochondria [51]. It should be remembered that ring sideroblasts are frequently observed in other types of MDS (i.e., MD-EB). If the platelet count is 450 × 103/μL (450 × 109/L) or greater and the megakaryocytes have features of those described in the myeloproliferative neoplasms (MPNs), an analysis for JAK2 and SF3B1 mutations is indicated. Most of these cases may be assigned to the provisional entity of RA with ring sideroblasts and thrombocytosis [241] which is considered within the MDS/MPN group.

MDS with Multilineage Dysplasia (MDS-MLD)

MDS-MLD accounts for approximately 30% of all MDS cases. It is a disease of elderly. The median age is 70 years [232]. Bone marrow aspiration and/or biopsy are usually hypercellular and characterized by erythroid, granulocytic, and megakaryocytic dysplasias. Bone marrow blasts are less than 5%. Auer rods are not seen. If present those cases should be classified as MDS-EB2. The clinical course varies. Patients with RCMD have a worse outcome (reported median survival of 17–33 months) than patients with RA [240]. The frequency of AML evaluation at 2 years is approximately 10%.

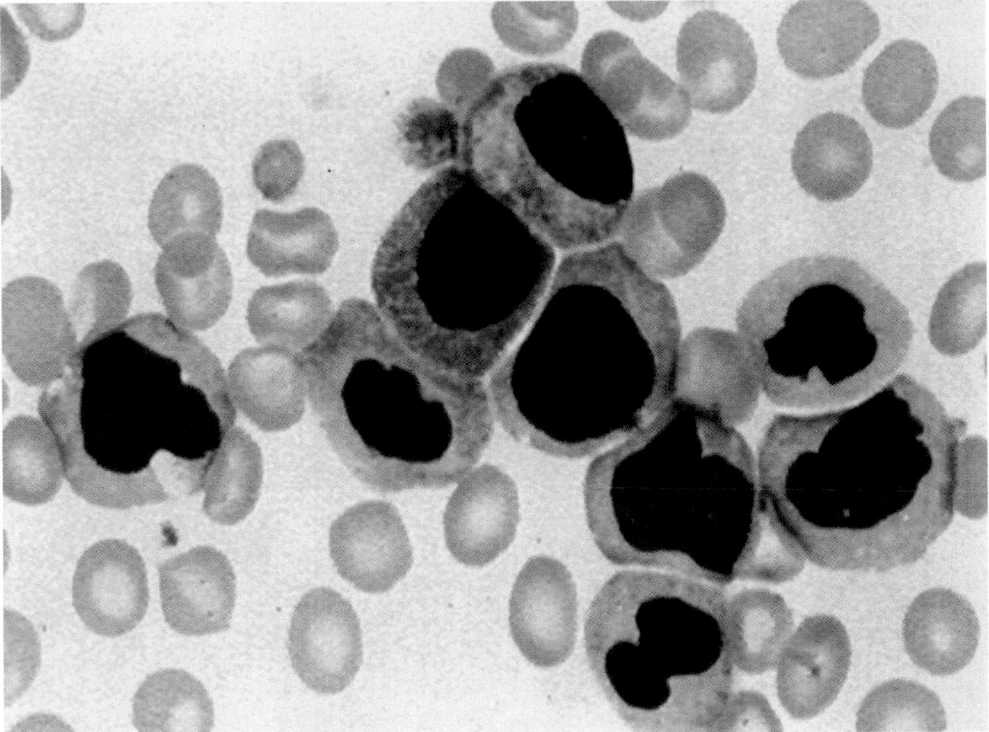

Fig. 14.27 MDS. CMML. Monocytic precursors and myeloblasts. WG stain

MDS with Multilineage Dysplasia and Ring Sideroblasts (MDS-RSMLD)

The category of RCMD-RS was originally eliminated in the 2008 WHO Classification and merged with RCMD because it was shown to be prognostically similar to RCMD lacking ring sideroblasts [242]. Although this still appears to be the case, the recent discovery of mutations in the spliceosome gene SF3B1 that are associated with ring sideroblasts provided a link between morphology and genetics in MDS [243]. Other morphologic features, except ringed sideroblasts, are similar as MDS with multilineage dysplasia.

MDS with Excess of Blasts (MDS-EB)

Conspicuous changes in all three lineages are present associated with variable cytopenia affecting two or more of the hematopoietic lines. Blasts (granular and agranular) range from greater than 5% but less than 20% in the bone marrow or 2–19% in peripheral blood. Two categories of MDS with excess of blasts (MDS-EB) are recognized: MDS-EB1, defined by 5–9% blasts in the bone marrow or 2–4% blasts in peripheral blood, and MDS-EB2, defined by 10–19% blasts in the bone marrow or 5–19% blasts in the peripheral blood [240]. The presence of Auer rods in blasts qualifies a case as MDS-EB2 regardless of the blast percentage. The bone marrow biopsy is very useful in documenting the presence of blast clusters particularly in cases with extensive fibrosis or hypocellularity. Blasts in MDS-EB tend to form cell aggregates that are usually located away from the trabecule and vascular structures. CD34 staining is helpful in their identification. Patients with MDS-EB2 have worse survival and a higher rate of disease transformation to AML. Median survival time for MDS-EB1 is approximately 18 months vs. 10 months for MDS-EB2 [240].

MDS with Fibrosis

Moderate-to-severe (Grades 2–3) bone marrow fibrosis is observed in 10–15% of patients with MDS. These cases have been referred to as MDS with fibrosis [244]. Most of these cases belong to the MDS-EB category. These cases may morphologically overlap acute panmyelosis with fibrosis (APMF). It has been shown that bone marrow fibrosis represents an independent prognostic parameter and identifies a distinct group of MDS with multilineage dysplasia, high transfusion requirement, poor-risk cytogenetics, and poor prognosis. Furthermore, the presence of CD34+ cell clusters is an independent risk factor for progression to AML [245].

Myelodysplastic Syndrome with Isolated del (5q)

Myelodysplastic syndrome with isolated del (5q) is characterized by severe anemia, absence of or mild neutrophenia, and/or thrombocytosis. Blast cells usually are not present in the peripheral blood (<1%) and fewer than 5% in the bone marrow. There is marked female predominance. Bone marrow hypercellular or normocellular frequently exhibits erythroid hypoplasia. Megakaryocytes increase in number. Small mononuclear hypolobated megakaryocytes with single eccentric nucleus and many granulations are strongly correlated with isolated del(5)q [225]. Recent studies have shown that the del(5q) abnormality in MDS is prognostically similar whether it is isolated or occurs with one additional low-risk cytogenetic aberration [246]. Based on this finding, the category of MDS with isolated del(5q) will be expanded to encompass cases with one additional cytogenetic abnormality (excluding monosomy 7).

MDS in Children

Primary MDS is very rare in pediatric population and accounts to less than 5% of all malignant hematopoietic neoplasms among children under the age of 14 years [247]. Although many morphologic and genetic features are common in adult and pediatric cases, there are some significant differences present, particularly in patients with low-grade MDS (RA, RARS, del.5q) categories. Unlike adults, children with MDS present with thrombocytopenia in approximately 75% of cases [248]. Moreover, hypocellularity of the bone marrow is more commonly observed in children than in adults [249]. For these reasons, a provisional entity, refractory cytopenia of childhood (RCC), has been added to include children with cytopenia(s) with less than 2% blasts in the peripheral blood and less than 5% in the bone marrow and evidence of dysplasia in two or more lineages. It remains as a provisional entity in the updated classification for children with 2–19% blasts in the blood and/or 5–19% in the bone marrow; the MDS subclassification should be made using the same criteria used for adults.

Hypocellular Myeloid Neoplasms

Hypocellular AML and hypocellular MDS represent small (10–15%) but significant number of patients diagnosed with myeloid malignancies [250, 251]. Hypocellular AML affects elderly and accounts for 5–12% of de novo AML. In a recent study although the outcome of hypocellular acute myeloid leukemia does not differ from that of non-hypocellular acute myeloid leukemia, hypocellular AML is characterized by prominent cytopenias, older age, a high percentage of antecedent hematologic disorders or prior chemotherapy/radiotherapy, and a low frequency of proliferative mutations [252]. Hypocellular MDS is more frequent in women and occurs with an age-related frequency which is similar to that seen in primary MDS. Bone marrow cellularity is the critical determinant to recognize hypocellular myeloid neoplasm and a bone marrow biopsy is necessary to diagnose these variants in all patients including children. According to our experience [228], by using anatomic comparisons, 13% of AML and 29% of MDS patients had hypocellular marrows. Correcting for age lowered the percentage of hypocellular marrows 2.2% and 7%, respectively. Therefore, age correction is necessary and should be considered as one of the defining criteria for such diagnoses. Bone marrow cellularity may be an important prognostic factor in hypocellular MDS. There is some controversy on survival differences between hypocellular MDS and normo/hypercellular MDS, but patients appear to do at least as well or better [251, 253, 254]. The separation between hypocellular AML, hypocellular MDS, and aplastic anemia (AA) can be problematic. Most hypocellular MDS cases fall into the categories of MD-SLD and MD-EB. The presence of easily identifiable megakaryocytes and patchy erythropoiesis with defective maturation within an architecturally disorganized marrow and the presence of reticulin fibrosis favor MDS over aplastic anemia [249, 250, 253, 255]. An important feature provided by the bone marrow biopsy is to identify blasts. In patients with myeloid neoplasia, blasts often form clusters in central marrow cavity location in contrast to paratrabecular location in reactive marrows. The presence of such clusters is mainly seen in the aggressive MDS subtypes. Immunohistochemical stains, mainly CD34, have provided additional assistance for counting blast in tissue sections. Increase in the percentage of CD34/CD117-positive blast cells and a tendency to form aggregates are useful in distinguishing hypoplastic myeloid neoplasms from aplastic anemia [256]. Although cytogenetic studies may be of particular value in this group of disorders, cytogenetic failures are frequently observed due to severe hypocellularity. FISH studies on paraffin sections or from peripheral blood may be useful for the detection of particular chromosome abnormalities (i.e., 7–, 5–). A recent study revealed that single-nucleotide polymorphisms-array (SNP-A) karyotyping in aplastic anemia and hypocellular MDS can complement metaphase cytogenetics and lead to the identification of cryptic clonal genomic aberrations in both disorders leading to improved distinction of these disease entities [257].

Myelodysplastic/Myeloproliferative Diseases

The WHO classification [9] recommends that a separate category to be formed to include disorders that have both myelodysplastic and myeloproliferative features including CMML, JMML, and aCML. These disorders have many common features including abnormalities of both granulocytic and monocytic lines and a relatively aggressive course.

Chronic Myelomonocytic Leukemia

The criterion for the diagnosis of CMML is the presence of peripheral absolute monocytosis higher than 1×10^9/L, associated with a marrow proliferation of monocytes. For most cases, the peripheral blood and bone marrow smears of patients fulfill all of the classical criteria for MDS (variable degrees of trilineage dysplasia) and show identical chromosome abnormalities. In the WHO classification [258], CMML is further divided into two subcategories, depending on the number of blasts and promonocytes found in the bone marrow and peripheral blood: CMML1, blasts and promonocytes less than 5% in the peripheral blood and less than 10% in the bone marrow, and CMML2, blasts and promonocytes 5–19% in peripheral blood and 10–19% in the bone marrow. Presence of Auer rods qualify as CMML2 regardless of the blast percentage. The value of this approach has been validated [259].

A subset of patients with eosinophilia, which are formerly included in the CMML category associated with genetic abnormalities including PDGFR, are classified as myeloid neoplasms with eosinophilia.

The percentage of bone marrow and peripheral blasts and the presence of cytogenetic aberrations have been associated with shorter survival and a higher risk of AML evolution [260]. Moreover, the presence of EZH2 implies an unfavorable prognosis [261] while mutation of ASXL1 correlates with evolution to AML and a shorter overall survival [262]. The median survival time varies from 20 to 40 months in most reported series. Progression to AML occurs in 15–30% of cases.

Atypical Chronic Myeloid Leukemia, BCR-ABL1 Negative

This disease predominantly involves the neutrophilic series as CML but lacked Ph1 chromosome or BCR/ABL translocation. Therefore, it is renamed as atypical CML. BCR/ABL negative emphasizes importance of obtaining these tests. aCML has dysplastic and proliferative features. Dysgranulopoiesis is a constant finding. Leukocyte alkaline phosphatase score (LAP) is not useful for diagnosis. Specific and nonspecific esterase stains are useful to detect monocytic component and exclude CMML. aCML is a disease of elderly but has also been reported in young patients. Its prognosis is significantly worse than Ph1+ CML and other MDS/MPNs with a median survival of 14–30 months, and an acute myeloid leukemia (AML) progression rate of approximately 40% [263]. MPN-related mutations are either absent or very infrequent in aCML, and the detection of CSF3R T618I, MPL, CALR, or JAK2V617F mutations should prompt a differential diagnosis of chronic neutrophilic leukemia (CNL), primary myelofibrosis (PMF), or myeloproliferative neoplasm-unclassifiable (MPN-U), which can share overlapping features with aCML [264].

Juvenile Myelomonocytic Leukemia

This is a separate disorder seen in children and adolescents and distinct from adult CMML. Blasts and promonocytes account for less than 20% of cells in both bone marrow and peripheral blood. Erythroid and megakaryocytic dysplasias are frequently seen [265]. Young patient age (median 1.8 years), predominant hepatosplenomegaly, frequent skin involvement, leukocytosis, monocytosis, and presence of immature precursors in peripheral blood characterize juvenile myelomonocytic leukemia (JMML). Ten percent of patients are known to have neurofibromatosis type I by clinical criteria [266]. It is a rapidly fatal disorder; however it rarely transforms into AML. Approximately 90% of patients carry either somatic or germline mutations of PTPN-11, K-RAS, N-RAS, CBL, *or* NF1 in their leukemic cells. These genetic aberrations are largely mutually exclusive and activate the Ras/mitogen-activated protein kinase pathway [267, 268].

References

1. Gralnick HR, Sultan C. Acute promyelocytic leukemia, hemorrhagic manifestations and morphologic criteria. Br J Haematol. 1975;29:373.
2. Sultan C, Deregnaucourt J, Ko YW, et al. Distribution of 250 cases of acute myeloid leukemia(AML) according to FAB classification and response to therapy. Br J Haematol. 1981;47:545.
3. Manohoran A, Horsley R, Ptiney WR. The reticulin content of bone marrow in acute leukemia in adults. Br J Haematol. 1979;43:185.
4. Orazi A, O'Malley DP, Jiang J, Vance GH, Thomas J, Czader M, Fang W, An C, Banks PM. Acute panmyelosis with myelofibrosis: an entity distinct from acute megakaryoblastic leukemia. Mod Pathol. 2005;18:603.
5. Islam A. Proposal for a classification of acute myeloid leukemia based on plastic embedded bone marrow biopsy section. Leuk Res. 1993;17:421.
6. Neiman RS, Barcos M, Berard C, et al. Granulocytic sarcoma. Cancer. 1981;48:1426.
7. Bennet JM, Reed CE. Acute leukemia cytochemical implications. Blood Cells. 1975;1:101.
8. Bennett JM, Catovsky D, Daniel MT, et al. Proposal for classification of acute leukemias. Br J Haematol. 1976;33:451.
9. Jaffe ES, Harris NL, Stein H, Vardiman JW, editors. World Health Organization classification of tumors. In: Pathology and genetics of tumors of haematopoietic and lymphoid tissues. Lyon: IARC; 2001.
10. Schrappe M, Reiter A, Ludwig WD, et al. Improved outcome in childhood acute lymphoblastic leukemia despite reduced use of anthracyclines and cranial radiotherapy: result of trial ALL BFM 90.German-Austrian-Swiss ALL-BFM Study Group. Blood. 2000;95:3310.
11. Flandrin G, Brouet JC, Daniel MT, et al. Acute leukemia with Burkitt's tumor cell. Blood. 1975;45:183.
12. Berger R, Bernheim A, Brouet JC, et al. t(8;14) translocation in a Burkitt's type of lymphoblastic leukemia(L3). Br J Haematol. 1979;43:81.
13. Michiels JJ, Adriiaansen HJ, Hagemeijer A, et al. TdT positive B cell acute lymphoblastic leukemia(B-ALL). Br J Haematol. 1988;68:423.
14. Chapiro E, Radford-Weiss I, Cung HA, et al. Chromosomal translocations involving the IGH@ locus in B-cell precursor acute lymphoblastic leukemia: 29 new cases and a review of the literature. Cancer Genet. 2013;206:162.
15. Seo JY, Lee SH, Kim HJ, et al. MYC rearrangement involving a novel non-immunoglobulin chromosomal locus in precursor B-cell acute lymphoblastic leukemia. Ann Lab Med. 2012;32:289.
16. Tricot G, Broeckaert-Van Orshoren A, Van Hoof A, et al. Sudan Black B positivity in acute lymphoblastic leukemia. Br J Haematol. 1982;51:615.
17. Bennett JM, Catovsky D, Daniel MT, et al. The morphologic classification of acute lymphoblastic leukemia: the morphologic classification of acute lymphoblastic leukemia: concordance among observers and clinical correlations. Br J Haematol. 1981;47:553.
18. Lillyman JS, Hann IM, Stevens RF, et al. Blast vacuoles in childhood acute lymphoblastic leukemia. Br J Haematol. 1988;70:183.
19. Bain B, Catovsky D. Current concerns in hematology. 2. Classification of acute leukemia. J Clin Pathol. 1990;43:882.

20. Catovsky D, Cherchi M, Graves MF, et al. Acid phosphatase reaction in acute lymphoblastic leukemia. Lancet. 1978;1:749.
21. De Olivera MP, Matutes E, Catovsky D. The cytochemistry, membrane markers and ultrastructure of megakaryoblastic (M7) and erythro (M6) leukemias. In: Scott CS, Harwood E, editors. Leukemia cytochemistry: principles and practice. Chichester: Wiley; 1989. p. 137.
22. Cordell JL, Fallini B, Erber WN, et al. Immunoenzymatic labeling of monoclonal antibodies using immunocomplexes of alkaline phosphatase and monoclonal alkaline phosphatase(APAAP complex). J Histochem Cytochem. 1984;32:219.
23. Olsen RJ, Chang CC, Herrick JL, et al. Acute leukemia immunohistochemistry: a systemic diagnostic approach. Arch Pathol Lab. 2008;132:462.
24. Pui CH, Yang JJ, Hunger SP, et al. Childhood acute lymphoblastic leukemia: progress through collaboration. J Clin Oncol. 2015;33(27):2938–48.
25. Nachman JB, Heerema NA, Sather H, et al. Outcome of treatment in children with hypodiploid acute lymphoblastic leukemia. Blood. 2007;110(4):1112.
26. Hunger PS, Mullighan CG. Redefining ALL classification: toward detecting high-risk ALL and implementing precision medicine. Blood. 2015;125:3977.
27. Harrison CJ. Cytogenetics of paediatric and adolescent acute lymphoblastic leukaemia. Br J Haematol. 2009;144(2):147.
28. Mullighan CG, Collins-Underwood JR, Phillips LA, et al. Rearrangement of CRLF2 in B-progenitor- and Down syndrome-associated acute lymphoblastic leukemia. Nat Genet. 2009;41:1243.
29. Russell LJ, Capasso M, Vater I, et al. Deregulated expression of cytokine receptor gene, CRLF2, is involved in lymphoid transformation in B-cell precursor acutelymphoblastic leukemia. Blood. 2009;114:2688.
30. Cazzaniga G, van Delft FW, Lo Nigro L, et al. Developmental origins and impact of BCR-ABL1 fusion and IKZF1 deletions in monozygotic twins with Ph1 acute lymphoblastic leukemia. Blood. 2011;118:5559.
31. Safavi S, Forestier E, Golovleva I, et al. Loss of chromosomes is the primary event in nearhaploid and low-hypodiploid acute lymphoblastic leukemia. Leukemia. 2013;27:248.
32. von Bubnoff N, Gorantla SP, Thone S, et al. The FIP1L1-PDGFRA T674I mutation can be inhibited by the tyrosine kinase inhibitor AMN107 (nilotinib). Blood. 2006;107:4970.
33. Crist W, Caroll A, Shuster J, et al. Philadelphia chromosome positive childhood acute lymphoblastic leukemia: clinical and cytogenetic characteristics and treatment outcome. A Pediatric Oncology Group Study. Blood. 1990;76:489.
34. Hoberman AL, Westbrook CA, Davey FR, et al. Molecular detection of Philadelphia (Ph1) chromosome in acute lymphoblastic leukemia (ALL): clinical, cytogenetic and immunologic correlations in a CALGB Study. Blood. 1989;74:52a.
35. Bloomfield CD, Goldman AI, Alimena G, et al. Chromosomal abnormalities identify high risk and low risk patients with acute lymphoblastic leukemia. Blood. 1986;67:415.
36. Champlin G, Gale RP. Acute lymphoblastic leukemia: recent advances in biology and therapy. Blood. 1989;73:2051.
37. Altman AJ. Clinical features and biological implications of acute mixed lineage (Hybrid) leukemias. Am J Pediatr Hematol Oncol. 1990;12:123.
38. Cobaleda C, Gutierez-Cianca N, Perez-Losada J, et al. A primitive hematopietic cell is the target for the leukemic transformation in human Philadelphia positive acute lymphoblastic leukemia. Blood. 2000;95:1007.
39. Roberts KG, Li Y, Payne-Turner D, et al. Targetable kinase-activating lesions in Ph-likeacute lymphoblastic leukemia. N Engl J Med. 2014;371:1005.
40. Boer JM, Marchante JR, Evans WE, et al. BCR-ABL1-like cases in pediatric acute lymphoblastic leukemia: a comparison between DCOG/Erasmus MC and COG/St. Jude signatures. Haematologica. 2015;100:e354–7.
41. Weston BW, Hayden MA, Roberts KG, et al. Tyrosine kinase inhibitor therapy induces remission in a patient with refractory EBF1-PDGFRB-positive acute lymphoblastic leukemia. J ClinOncol. 2013;31:e413–6.
42. Morley A, Higgs D. Abnormal differentiation of leukemic cells in-vitro. Cancer. 1974;33:716.
43. Drexler HG, Thiel E, Ludwig WD. Acute myeloid leukemias expressing lymphoid associated antigens: diagnostic incidence and prognostic significance. Leukemia. 1993;7:489.
44. Jensen MK, Killman SA. Additional incidence for chromosomal abnormalities in the erythroid precursors in acute leukemia. Acta Med Scand. 1971;189:97.
45. Ackerman GA. Microscopic and histochemical studies on the Auer bodies in leukemic cells. Blood. 1950;7:1230.
46. Bainon DF, Friedlander LM, Shohet SB. Abnormalites in granule formation in acute myelogeneous leukemia. Blood. 1977;49:639.
47. Bennett JM, Catovsky D, Daniel MT, et al. Proposed revised criteria for classification of acute myeloid leukemia. Ann Intern Med. 1985;103:626.
48. Walter RB, Othus M, Burnett AK, et al. Significance of FAB subclassification of "acute myeloid leukemia, NOS" in the 2008 WHO classification: analysis of 5848 newly diagnosed patients. Blood. 2013;121:2424.
49. Goasguen JE, Bennett JM, Cox C, et al. Prognostic implication and characterization of blast cell population in myelodysplastic syndrome. Leuk Res. 1991;15:1159.
50. Cheson BD, Cassileth A, Head DR, et al. Report of National Cancer Institute Sponsored Workshop on definitions of diagnosis and response in acute myeloid leukemia. J Clin Oncol. 1950;8:813.
51. Mufti JG, Bennett JM, Goasguen JE, et al. Diagnosis and classification of myelodysplastic syndrome: international working group on morphology of myelodysplastic syndrome (IWGM.MDS) consensus proposals for the definition and enumeration of myeloblasts and ring sideroblasts. Hematologica. 2008;93:1712.
52. Arber DA, Brunning RD, LeBeau MM, et al. Acute myeloid leukemia with recurrent genetic abnormalities. In: Swerdlow SH, Compo E, Harris NL, et al., editors. WHO classification of tumors of haematopoietic and lymphoid tissues. Lyon: IARC; 2008. p. 110–23.
53. Baumann I, Neimeyer CM, Brunning RD, et al. Myeloid proliferations related to Down syndrome. In: Swerdlow SH, Compo E, Harris NL, et al., editors. WHO classification of tumors of haematopoietic and lymphoid tissues. Lyon: IARC; 2008. p. 142–4.
54. Gröschel S, Sanders MA, Hoogenboezem R, et al. A single oncogenic enhancer rearrangement causes concomitant *EVI1*and *GATA2* deregulation in leukemia. Cell. 2014;157:369.
55. Gaidzik VI, Bullinger L, Schlenk RF, et al. *RUNX1* mutations in acute myeloid leukemia: results from a comprehensive genetic and clinical analysis from the AML study group. J Clin Oncol. 2011;29:1364–72.
56. Mendler JH, Maharry K, Radmacher MD, et al. *RUNX1* mutations are associated with poor outcome in younger and older patients with cytogenetically normal acute myeloid leukemia and with distinctgene and microRNA expression signatures. J Clin Oncol. 2012;30:3109–18.
57. Nacheva EP, Grace CD, Brazma D, et al. Does *BCR/ABL1* positive acute myeloid leukaemia exist? Br J Haematol. 2013;161:541–50.
58. Godley LA. Inherited predisposition to acute myeloid leukemia. Semin Hematol. 2014;51:306–21.
59. Wardiman JW, Thiele J, Arber DA, et al. The 2008 revision of the World Health Organization (WHO) classification of myeloid neoplasms and acute leukemia: rationale and important changes. Blood. 2009;114:937.

60. Bennett JM, Castoldi D, Catovsky D, et al. Recommended methods for cytological procedures in hematology. Clin Lab Hematol. 1985;7:55.
61. Goasguen JE, Bennett JM. Classification of acute leukemia. Clin Lab Med. 1990;10:661.
62. Van Wering ER, Brederoo P, Staalduien GJ, et al. Contribution of electron microscopy to the classification of minimally differentiated acute leukemia in children. Recent Results Cancer Res. 1993;13:177.
63. Van Wering ER, Brederoo P, Van Dijk-de-Leeuw JHS. Electron microscopy: a contribution to further classification of acute unclassifiable childhood leukemia. Blut. 1990;60:291.
64. Orazi A. Histopathology in the diagnosis and classification ao acute myeloid leukemia, myelodysplastic syndrome and myelodysplastic/myeloproliferative diseases. Pathobiology. 2007;74:97.
65. Döhner H, Weisdorf DJ, Bloomfield CD. Acute myeloid leukemia. N Engl J Med. 2015;373:1136–52.
66. Downing JR. The AML1-ETO chimeric transcription in acute myeloid leukemia biology and clinical significance. Br J Haematol. 1999;106:296.
67. Second International Workshop on Chromosomes in Leukemia. Cytogenetic, morphologic and clinical correlations in acute nonlymphocytic leukemia with t(8;21). Cancer Genet Cytogenet. 1980;2:99.
68. Kita K, Nakase K, et al. Phenotypical characteristics of acute myelocytic leukemi associated with the t(8;21)(q22;q22) chromosomal abnormality frequent expression of immature B cell antigen CD19 together with stem cell antign CD34. Blood. 1992;80:470.
69. Grimwade D, Walker H, Oliver F, et al. The importance of diagnostic cytogenetics on outcome in AML: analysis of 1612 patients entered into the MRC-AML10 trial. The Medical Research Council Adult and Children's Leukemia Working Parties. Blood. 1998;92:2322.
70. Paschka P, Marrucci G, Ruppert AS, et al. Adverse prognostic signifcance of KIT mutations in adult acute myeloid leukemia with inv(16) and t(8;21): a Cancer and Leukemia Group B Study. J Clin Oncol. 2006;24:3904.
71. Boissel N, Leroy H, Brethon B, et al. Incidence and prognostic inpact of c-KIT, FLR3 and Ras gene mutations in core binding factor acute myeloid leukemia (CBF-AML). Leukemia. 2006;20:965.
72. Micol J-B, Duployez N, Boissel N, et al. Frequent ASXL2 mutations in acute myeloid leukemia patients with t(8;21)/RUNX1-RUNX1T1 chromosomal translocations. Blood. 2014;124(9):1445.
73. Paschka P. Core binding factor acute myeloid leukemia. Semin Oncol. 2008;35:410.
74. Duployez N, Nibourel O, Marceau-Renaut A, et al. Minimal residual disease monitoring in *t*(8;21) acute myeloid leukemia based on RUNX1-RUNX1T1 fusion quantification on genomic DNA. Am J Hematol. 2014;89:610.
75. Cartrer M, Kalwinsky DR, Dahl GV, et al. Childhood acute promyelocytic leukemia: a rare variant of nonlymphoid leukemia with distinctive clinical and biologic features. Leukemia. 1989;4:298.
76. Chang KS, Stass SA, Chu DT, et al. Characterization of a fusion cDNA(RARA/myl) transcribed from the t(15;17) translocation breakpoint in acute promyelocytic leukemia. Mol Cell Biol. 1992;12:800.
77. Chang KS, Lu J, Wang G, et al. The t(15;15) breakpoint in acute promyelocytic leukemia cluster within two different sites on the myl gene. Targets for the detection of minimal residual disease by the polymerase chain reaction. Blood. 1992;79:554.
78. De The H, Lavau C, Marchio A, et al. The PML-RAR fusion mRNA generated by the t(15;17) translocation in acute promyelocytic leukemia encodes a functionally altered RAR. Cell. 1991;66:675.
79. Castaigne S, Chomienne C, Daniel MT, et al. All trans retinoic acid as a differentiating therapy for acute promyelocytic leukemia. Blood. 1990;76:1704.
80. Warrell RP, Frankel SR, Miller WH Jr, et al. Differentiation therapy of acute promyelocytic leukemia with tretinoin (all-trans-retinoic acid). N Engl J Med. 1991;324:1385.
81. Fouchar K, Anastasi J. Acute myeloid leukemia with recurrent cytogenetic abnormalities. Am J Clin Pathol. 2015;144:6.
82. Bennett JM, Catovsky D, Daniel MT, et al. A variant form of hypergranular acute promyelocytic leukemia(M3) French-American-British (FAB) classification. Br J Haematol. 1980;44:169.
83. San Miguel JF, Gonzales M, Canizo MC, et al. Surface marker analysis in acute myeloid leukemia and correlation with FAB classification. Br J Haematol. 1986;64:547.
84. Dong HY, Kung JX, Bhardwaj V, et al. Flow cytometry rapidly identifies all acute promyelocytic leukemias with high specificity independent of underlying cytogenetic abnormalities. Am J Clin Pathol. 2011;135:76.
85. Scott RM, Mayer RJ. The unique aspects of acute promyelocytic leukemia. J Clin Oncol. 1990;8:1913.
86. Roveli A, Biondi A, Rajnoldi AC, et al. Microgranular variant of acute promyelocytic leukemia in children. J Clin Oncol. 1992;10:1413.
87. Kussick SJ, Stirewalt DL, Yi HS, et al. A distinctive nuclear morphology in acute myeloid leukemia is strongly associated with loss of HLA-DR expression and FLT3 internal tandem duplication. Leukemia. 2004;18:1591.
88. Zelent A, Guidez F, Melnick A, et al. Translocation of the RAR-alpha gene in acute promyelocytic leukemia. Oncogene. 2001;20:7186.
89. Melnick A, Licht JD. Deconstructing a disease: RARalpha, its fusion partners and their roles in the pathogenesis of acute promyelocytic leukemia. Blood. 1999;93:3167.
90. Yi Y, Pei M, Xiao L, et al. Acute promyelocytic leukemia with insertion of PML exon 7c: a novel variant transcript related to good prognosis that is not detected with real-time polymerase chain reaction. Leuk Lymphoma. 2013;54:2294.
91. Shigesada K, van de Sluis B, Liu PP. Mechanism of leukomogenesis by the inv (16) chimeric gene CBFB/PEBP2B-MHY11. Oncogene. 2004;23:4297.
92. Mariton P, Keating M, Kantarjian H, et al. Cytogenetic and clinical correlates in AML patients with abnormalities of chromosome 16. Leukemia. 1995;9:965.
93. Mrozek K, Heinonen K, de la Chapelle A, et al. Clinical significance of cytogenetics in acute myeloid leukemia. Semin Oncol. 1997;24:17.
94. O'Donnell MR, Abboud CN, Altman J, et al. Acute myeloid leukemia. J Natl Compr Canc Netw. 2012;10(8):984.
95. Pui CH, Relling MV. Topoisomerase II inhibitor-related acute myeloid leukemia. Br J Heamatol. 2000;109:13.
96. Bain BJ, Moorman AV, Johansson B, et al. Myelodysplastic syndromes associated with 11q23 abnormalities. Leukemia. 1998;12:834.
97. Kühn WM, Bullinger L, Gröschel S, et al. Genome-wide genotyping of acute myeloid leukemia with translocation t(9;11)(p22;q23) reveals novel recurrent genomic alterations. Hematologica. 2014;99(8):e133–5.
98. Byrd JC, Mrozek K, Dodge RK, et al. Pretreatment cytogenetic abnormalities are predictive of induction success, cumulative incidence of relapse and overal survival in adult patients with de novo acute myeloid leukemia results from Cancer and Leukemia Group B (CALGB 8461). Blood. 2002;100:4325.
99. Forestier E, Heim S, Blennow E, et al. Cytogenetic abnormalities in childhood acute myeloid leukemia: a Nordic series comprising a children enrolled in the NOPHO-93-AML trial between 1993 and 2001. Br J Haematol. 2003;121:566.

100. Sorensen PH, Chen CS, Smith FO, et al. Molecular rearrangements of the MLL gene are present in most cases of infant acute myeloid leukemia and are strongly correlated with monocytic or myelomonocytic phenotypes. J Clin Invest. 1994;93:429.
101. Lugthart S, van Drunen E, van Norden Y, et al. High EVI1 levels predict adverse outcome in acute myeloid leukemia: prevalence of EVI1 overexpression and chromosome 3q26 abnormalities underestimated. Blood. 2008;111:4329.
102. Gröschel S, Schlenk RF, Engelmann J, et al. Deregulated expression of EVI1 defines a poor prognostic subset of MLL-rearranged acute myeloid leukemias: a study of the German-Austrian Acute Myeloid Leukemia Study Group and the Dutch-Belgian-Swiss HOVON/SAKK Cooperative Group. J Clin Oncol. 2013;31:95.
103. Slovak ML, Gundacker H, Bloomfield CD, et al. A retrospective study of 69 patients with t(6;9)(p23;q34) AML emphasized the need for a prospective multicenter initiative for rare poor prognosis myeloid malignancies. Leukemia. 2006;20:1295.
104. Oyarzo MP, Lin P, Glassman A, et al. Acute myeloid leukemia with t(6;9)(p23;q34) is associated with dysplasia and high frequency of FLT3 gene mutations. Am J Clin Pathol. 2004;122:348.
105. Sandahl JD, , Coenen EA , Forestier E, et al. t(6;9)(p22;q34)/*DEK-NUP214*-rearranged pediatric myeloid leukemia: an international study of 62 patients. Hematologica. 2014;90:865.
106. Ishiyama K, Takami A, Kanda Y, et al. Allogeneic hematopoietic stem cell transplantation for acute myeloid leukemia with t(6;9)(p23;q34) dramatically improves the patient prognosis: a matched-pair analysis. Leukemia. 2012;26:461.
107. Ishiyama K, Takami A, Kanda Y, et al. Prognostic factorsfor acute myeloid leukemia patients with t(6;9)(p23;q34) who underwent an allogeneichematopoietic stem cell transplant. Leukemia. 2012;26:1416.
108. Gröschel S, Sanders MA, Hoogenboezem R, et al. Mutational spectrum of myeloid malignancies with inv(3)/t(3;3) reveals a predominant involvement of RAS/RTK signaling pathways. Blood. 2015;125:133.
109. Slovak ML, Kopecky KJ, Cassileth PA, et al. Karyotypic analysis predicts outcome of preremission and postremission therapy in adult acute myeloid leukemia: a southwest oncology group/eastern cooperative oncology group study. Blood. 2000;96:4075.
110. Grigg AP, Gascoyne RD, Phillips GL, et al. Clinical, haematological and cytogenetic features in 24 patients with structural rearrangements of the Q arm of chromosome 3. Br J Haematol. 1993;83:158.
111. Jenkins RB, Tefferi A, Solberg LA, et al. Acute leukemia with abnormal thrombopoiesis and invertions of chromosome 3. Cancer Genet Cytogenet. 1989;39:167.
112. Secker-Walker LM, Mehta A, Bain B. Abnormalities of 3q21 and 3q26 in myeloid malignancy. A United Kingdom Cancer Cytogenetic Group study. Br J Haematol. 1995;91:490.
113. Raya HM, Martín-Santos T, Luño E, et al. Acute myeloid leukemia with inv(3)(q21q26.2) or t(3;3)(q21;q26.2): clinical and biological features and comparison with other acute myeloid leukemias with cytogeneticaberrations involving long arm of chromosome 3. Hematology. 2015;20:435.
114. Hama A, Yagasaki H, Takahashi Y, et al. Acute megakaryoblastic leukemia (AMKL) in children in comparison of AKML with and without Down syndrome. Br J Haematol. 2008;140:552.
115. Gruber TA, Larson Gedman A, Zhang J, et al. An Inv(16)(p13.3q24.3)-encoded CBFA2T3-GLIS2 fusion protein defines an aggressive subtype of pediatric acute megakaryoblastic leukemia. Cancer Cell. 2012;22:683.
116. de Rooij JD, Hollink IH, Arentsen-Peters ST, et al. NUP98/JARID1A is a novel recurrent abnormality in pediatric acute megakaryoblastic leukemia with a distinct HOX gene expression pattern. Leukemia. 2013;27:2280.
117. Athale UH, Kaste SC, Razzouk BL, et al. Skeletal manifestations of pediatric acute magakaryoblastic leukemia. J Pediatr Heamatol Oncol. 2002;24:561.
118. Reinhardt D, Diekamp S, Langebrake C, et al. Acute megakaryoblastic leukemia in children and adolescents, excluding Down's syndrome: improved outcome with intensified induction treatment. Leukemia. 2005;19:1495.
119. Ballerini P, Blaise A, Mercher T, et al. A novel real-time RT-PCR assay for quantification of OTT-MAL fusion transcript reliable for diagnosis of t(1 ; 22) and minimal residual disease (MRD) detection. Leukemia. 2003;17:1193.
120. Döhner H, Estey EH, Amadori S, et al. Diagnosis and management of acute myeloid leukemia in adults: recommendationsfrom an international expert panel, on behalf of the European Leukemia Net. Blood. 2010;115:453.
121. Taskesen E, Bullinger L, Corbacioglu A, et al. Prognostic impact, concurrent genetic mutations, and gene expression features of AML with CEBPA mutations in a cohort of 1182 cytogenetically normal AML patients: further evidence for CEBPA double mutant AML as a distinctive disease entity. Blood. 2011;117:2469.
122. Whitman SP, Ruppert AS, Radmacher MD, et al. FLT3 D835/I836 mutations are associated with poor disease free survival and a distinct gene expression signature among younger adults with de novo cytogenetically normal acute myeloid leukemia lackinf FLT3 internal tandem duplications. Blood. 2008;111:1552.
123. Ofran Y, Rowe JM. Genetic profiling in acute myeloid leukaemia—where are we and what is its role in patient management. Br J Haematol. 2013;160:303.
124. Brown P, McIntyre E, Rau R, et al. The incidence and clinical significance of nucleophosmin mutations in childhood AML. Blood. 2007;110:979.
125. Fallini B, Mecucci C, Saglio G, et al. NPM1 mutations and cytoplasmic nucleophosmin are mutually exclusive of recurrent genetic abnormalities: a comparative analysis of 2562 patients with acute myeloid leukemia. Hematologica. 2008;93:439.
126. Dohner K, Schlenk RF, Habdank M, et al. Mutant nucleophosmin(MPM1) predicts favurable prognosis in younger adults with acute myeloid leukemia and normal cytogenetics: interaction with other gene mutations. Blood. 2005;106:3740.
127. Green CL, Koo KK, Hills RK, et al. Prognostic significance of CEBPA mutations in a large cohort of younger adult patients with acute myeloid leukemia: impact of double CEBPA mutations and the interaction with FLT3 and NPM1 mutations. J Clin Oncol. 2010;28:2739.
128. Dufour A, Schneider F, Metzeler KH, et al. Acute myeloid leukemia with biallelic CEBPA gene mutations and normal karyotype represents a distinct genetic entity associated with a favorable clinical outcome. J Clin Oncol. 2010;28:570.
129. Bacher U, Schnittger S, Macijewski K, et al. Multilineage dysplasia does not influence prognosis in CEBPA-mutated AML, supporting the WHO proposal to classify these patients as a unique entity. Blood. 2012;119:4719.
130. Chen CY, Lin LI, Tang JL, et al. RUNX1 gene mutation in primary myelodysplastic syndrome: the mutation can be detected early at diagnosis or acquired during disease progression and is associated with poor outcome. Br J Haematol. 2007;139:405–14.
131. Head DR. Revised classification of acute myeloid leukemia. Leukemia. 1996;10:1826.
132. Arber DA, Stein AS, Carter NH, Ikle D, Forman SJ, Slovak ML. Prognostic impact of acute myeloid leukemia classification. Importance of detection of recurring cytogenetic abnormalities and multilineage dysplasia on survival. Am J ClinPathol. 2003;119:672.
133. Davis KL, Marina N, Arber DA, Ma L, Cherry A, Dahl GV, Heerema-McKenney A. Pediatric acute myeloid leukemia as clas-

sified using 2008 WHO criteria: a single-center experience. Am J ClinPathol. 2013;139:818.
134. Gahn B, Haase D, Unterhalt M, et al. De novo AML with dysplastic hematopoiesis: cytogenetic and prognostic significance. Leukemia. 1996;10:946.
135. Odenike O, Anastasi J, Le Beau MM. Myelodysplastic syndromes. Clin Lab Med. 2011;31:763.
136. Wandt H, Schäkel U, Kroschinsky F, et al. MLD according to the WHO classification in AML has no correlation with age and no independent prognostic relevance as analyzed in 1766 patients. Blood. 2008;111:1855.
137. Shiseki M, Kitagawa Y, Wang YH, et al. Lack of nucleophosmin mutation in patients with myelodysplastic syndrome and acute myeloid leukemia with chromosome 5 abnormalities. Leuk Lymphoma. 2007;48:2141.
138. Devillier R, Mansat-De Mas V, Gelsi-Boyer V, et al. Role of ASXL1 and TP53 mutations in the molecular classification and prognosis of acute myeloid leukemias with myelodysplasia-related changes. Oncotarget. 2015;6:8388.
139. Ogata K, Kakumoto K, Matsuda A, et al. Differences in blast immunophenotypes among disease types in myelodysplastic syndromes: a multicenter validation study. Leuk Res. 2012;36:1229.
140. Díaz-Beyá M, Rozman M, Pratcorona M, et al. The prognostic value of multilineage dysplasia in de novo acute myeloid leukemia patients with intermediate-risk cytogenetics is dependent on NPM1 mutational status. Blood. 2010;116:6147.
141. Rozman M, Navarro JT, Arenillas L, et al. Multilineage dysplasia is associated with a poorer prognosis in patients with de novo acute myeloid leukemia with intermediate-risk cytogenetics and wild-type NPM1. Ann Hematol. 2014;93:1695.
142. Wardiman JW, Arber DA, Brunning D, et al. Therapy related myeloid neoplasms. In: Swerdlow SH, Compo E, Harris NL, et al., editors. WHO classification of tumors of haematopoietic and lymphoid tissues. Lyon: IARC; 2008. p. 127–9.
143. Granfeldt Østgård LS, Medeiros BC, Sengeløv H, et al. Epidemiology and clinical significance of secondary and therapy-related acute myeloid leukemia: a national population-based cohort study. J Clin Oncol. 2015;33:3641.
144. Shih AH, Chung SS, Dolezal EK, et al. Mutational analysis of therapy-related myelodysplastic syndromes and acute myelogenous leukemia. Haematologica. 2013;98:908.
145. Wong TN, Ramsingh G, Young AL, et al. Role of TP53 mutations in the origin and evolution of therapy-related acute myeloid leukaemia. Nature. 2015;518:552.
146. Rowley JD, Olney HJ. International workshop on the relationship of prior therapy to balanced chromosome aberrations in therapy-related myelodysplatic syndromes and acute leukemia: overview report. Genes Chromosomes Cancer. 2002;33:331.
147. Smith SM, Le Beau MM, Hou D. Clinical cytogenetic associations in 306 patients with therapy related myelodysplasia and myeloid leukemia: the university of Chicago series. Blood. 2003;102:43.
148. Michels SD, McKenna RW, Arthur DC, et al. Therapy-related acute myeloid leukemia and myelodysplastic syndrome: a clinical and morphologic study of 65 cases. Blood. 1985;65:1364.
149. Singh ZN, Huo D, Anastasi J, et al. Therapy-related myelodysplastic syndrome: morphologic subclassification may not be clinically relevant. Am J Clin Pathol. 2007;127:197.
150. Andersen MK, Larson RA, Mauritzson N, et al. Balanced chromosome abnormalities inv(16) and t(15;17) in therapy-related myelodysplastic syndromes and acute leukemia: report from an international workshop. Genes Chromosomes Cancer. 2002;33:395–400.
151. Fianchi L, Pagano L, Piciocchi A, et al. Characteristics and outcome of therapy-related myeloid neoplasms: Report from the Italian network on secondary leukemias. Am J Hematol. 2015;90:E80.
152. Tallman MS, Kim HT, Paietta E, et al. Acute monocytic leukemia (French-American-British classification M5) does not have a worse prognosis than other subtypes of acute myeloid leukemia: a report from the Eastern Cooperative Oncology Group. J ClinOncol. 2004;22:1276.
153. Patel KP, Khokhar FA, Muzzafar T, et al. TdT expression in acute myeloid leukemia with minimal differentiation is associated with distinctive clinicopathological features and better overall survival following stem cell transplantation. Mod Pathol. 2013;26:195.
154. Matsuo T, Cox C, Bennett JM. Prognostic significance of myeloperoxidase positivity of blast cells in acute myeloid leukemia without maturation (FAB M1). Hematol Pathol. 1989;3:153.
155. Loeffler H. Morphologic basis for the MIC classification in acute myeloid leukemia. Recent Results Cancer Res. 1993;131:339.
156. Catovsky D, Matutes E, Buccheri V, et al. Classification of acute leukemia for the 1990s. Ann Hematol. 1991;62:16.
157. Ferraris AM, Broccia G, Meloni T, et al. Clonal origin of cells restricted to monocytic differentiation in acute nonlymphocytic leukemia. Blood. 1984;64:817.
158. Diab A, Zickl L, Abdel-Wahab O, et al. Acute myeloid leukemia with translocation t(8;16) presents with features which mimic acute promyelocytic leukemia and is associated with poor prognosis. Leuk Res. 2013;37:32.
159. Garand R, Duchayne E, Blanchard D, Robillard N, et al. Minimally differentiated erythroleukaemia(AML M6 'variant'): a rare subset of AML distinct from AML M6. Groupe Francais d'Hematologie Cellulaire. Br J Haematol. 1995;90:868.
160. Lessard M, Struski S, Leymarie V, et al. Cytogenetic study of 75 erythroleukemias. Cancer Genet Cytogenet. 2005;163:113.
161. Wang SA, Hasserjian RP. Acute erythroleukemias, acute megakaryoblastic leukemias, and reactive mimics: a guide to a number of perplexing entities. Am J Clin Pathol. 2015;144:44.
162. Liu W, Hasserjian RP, Hu Y, Zhang L, Miranda RN, Medeiros LJ, Wang SA. Pure erythroid leukemia: a reassessment of the entity using the 2008 World Health Organization classification. Mod Pathol. 2011;24:375.
163. Lichtman MA, Segel GB. Uncommon phenotypes of acute myelogenous leukemia: basophilic, mast cell, eosinophilic, and myeloid dendritic cell subtypes: a review. Blood Cells Mol Dis. 2005;35:370.
164. Staal-Viliare A, Latger-Cannard V, Rault JP, Didion J, et al. A case of de novo acute basophilic leukaemia: diagnostic criteria and review of the literature. Ann BiolClin (Paris). 2006;64:361.
165. Bearman RM, Pangalis GA, Rappaport H. Acute (malignant) myelosclerosis. Cancer. 1979;43:279.
166. Sultan C, Sigaux F, Imbert M, Reyes F. Acute myelodysplasia with myelofibrosis: a report of eight cases. Br J Haematol. 1981;49:11.
167. Thiele J, Kvasnicka HM, Zerhusen G, et al. Acute panmyelosis with myelofibrosis: a clinicopathological study on 46 patients including histochemistry of bone marrow biopsies and follow-up. Ann Hematol. 2004;83:513.
168. Suvajdzic N, Marisavljevic D, Kraguljac N, Pantic M, Djordjevic V, Jankovic G, Cemerikic-Martinovic V, Colovic M. Acute panmyelosis with myelofibrosis: clinical, immunophenotypic and cytogenetic study of twelve cases. Leuk Lymphoma. 2004;45:1873–9.
169. Muss HB, Moleney WC. Chloroma and other myeloblastic tumors. Blood. 1973;42:721.
170. Pileri SA, Asacni S, Cox MC, et al. Myeloid sarcoma: clinicopathologic, phenotypic and cytogenetic analysis of 92 adult patients. Leukemia. 2007;21:340.
171. Movassaghian M, Brunner AM, Blonquist TM, et al. Presentation and outcomes among patients with isolated myeloid sarcoma: a Surveillance, Epidemiology, and End Results database analysis. Leuk Lymphoma. 2015;56:1698.

172. Alexiev BA, Wang W, Ning Y, et al. Myeloid sarcomas,a histologic, immunohistochemical and cytogenetic study. Diagn Pathol. 2007;2:42.
173. Falini B, Lenze D, Hasserjian R, et al. Cytoplasmic mutated nucleophosmin (NPM) defines the molecular status of a significant fraction of myeloid sarcomas. Leukemia. 2007;21:1566.
174. Mallo M, Espinet B, Salido M, et al. Gain of multiple copies of the CBFB gene: a new genetic aberration in a case of granulocytic sarcoma. Cancer Genet Cytogenet. 2007;179:62.
175. Greene ME, Mundschau G, Wechsler J, et al. Mutations in GATA1 in both transient myeloproliferative disorder and acute megakaryoblastic leukemia of Down syndrome. Blood Cells Mol Dis. 2003;31:351.
176. Gurbuxani S, Vyas P, Crispino JD. Recent insights into the mechanisms of myeloid leukemogenesis in Down syndrome. Blood. 2004;103:399.
177. Massey GV, Zipursky A, Chang MN, et al. A prospective study of the natural history of transient leukemia (TL) in neonates with Down syndrome (DS): Children's Oncology Group (COG) study POG-9481. Blood. 2006;107:4606.
178. Langebrake C, Creutzig U, Reinhardt D. Immunophenotype of Down syndrome acute myeloid leukemia and transient myeloproliferative disease differs significantly from other diseases with morphologically identical or similar blasts. KlinPadiatr. 2005;217:126–34.
179. McElwaine S, Mulligan C, Groet J, et al. Microarray transcript profiling distinguishes the transient from the acute type of megakaryoblasticleukaemia (M7) in Down's syndrome, revealing PRAME as a specific discriminating marker. Br J Haematol. 2004;125:729.
180. Herling M, Jones D. CD4+/CD56+ hematodermic tumor: the features of an evolving entity and its reletionship to dendritic cells. Am J Clin Pathol. 2007;127:687.
181. Herling M, Teitell MA, Shen PR, et al. TCL1 expression in plasmacytoid dendritic cells (DC2c) and the related CD4+, CD56+ blastic tumors of skin. Blood. 2003;101:5007.
182. Pilicowska ME, Fleming MD, Pinkus JL, Pinkus GS. CD4+/ CD56+ hematodermicneoplasm (blastic natural killer lymphoma): neoplastic cells express the immature dendritic cell marker BDCA-2 and produce interferon. Am J Clin Pathol. 2007;128:445.
183. Boiocchi L, Lonardi S, Vermi W, Fisogni S, Facchetti F. BDCA-2 (CD303): a highly specific marker for normal and neoplastic plasmacytoid dendritic cells. Blood. 2013;122:296.
184. Julia F, Dalle S, Duru G, et al. Blastic plasmacytoid dendritic cell neoplasms: clinico-immunohistochemical correlations in a series of 91 patients. Am J Surg Pathol. 2014;38:673.
185. Assaf C, Gellrich S, Whittaker S, et al. CD56-positive haematological neoplasms of the skin: a multicentre study of the Cutaneous Lymphoma Project Group of the European Organisation for Research and Treatment of Cancer. J Clin Pathol. 2007;60:981.
186. Vitte F, Fabiani B, Bénet C, et al. Specific skin lesions in chronic myelomonocytic leukemia: a spectrum of myelomonocytic and dendritic cell proliferations: a study of 42 cases. Am J Surg Pathol. 2012;36:1302.
187. Dargent JL, Delannoy A, Pieron P, et al. Cutaneous accumulation of plasmacytoid dendritic cells associated with acute myeloid leukemia: a rare condition distinct from blastic plasmacytoid dendritic cell neoplasm. J Cutan Pathol. 2011;38:893.
188. Leroux D, Mugneret F, Callanan M, et al. CD4(+), CD56(+) DC2 acute leukemia is characterized by recurrent clonal chromosomal changes affecting 6 major targets: a study of 21 cases by the Groupe Français de Cytogénétique Hématologique. Blood. 2002;99:4154.
189. Jardin F, Ruminy P. Parmentier F, et al TET2 and TP53 mutations are frequently observed in blastic plasmacytoid dendritic cell neoplasm. Br J Haematol. 2011;153:413.
190. Rauh MJ, Rahman F, Good D, et al. Blastic plasmacytoid dendritic cell neoplasm with leukemic presentation, lacking cutaneous involvement: case series and literature review. Leuk Res. 2012;36:81.
191. Pagano L, Valentini CG, Pulsoni A, et al. Blastic plasmacytoid dendritic cell neoplasm with leukemic presentation: an Italian multicenter study. Haematologica. 2013;98:239.
192. Borowitz M, Bene MC, Harris NL, et al. In: Swerdlow S, Campo E, Harris NL, et al., editors. WHO classification of tumours of haematopoietic and lymphoid tissues. 4th ed. Lyon: IARC; 2008. p. 149.
193. Porwit A, Béné MC. Acute leukemias of ambiguous origin. Am J Clin Pathol. 2015;144:361.
194. Béné MC, Nebe T, Bettelheim P, et al. Immunophenotyping of acute leukemia and lymphoproliferative disorders: a consensus proposal of the European Leukemia Net Work Package 10. Leukemia. 2011;25:567.
195. Manola KN. Cytogenetic abnormalities in acute leukaemia of ambiguous lineage: an overview. Br J Haematol. 2013;163:24.
196. Merzianu M, Wallace PK. Case study interpretation—Portland: Case 4: acute leukemia of ambiguous lineage, unclassifiable. Cytometry B Clin Cytom. 2012;82:186.
197. Pui C-H, Evans WE. Treatment of acute lymphoblastic leukemia. N Engl J Med. 2006;354:166–78.
198. Bostrom BC, Sensel MR, Sather HN, et al. Dexamethasone versus prednisone and daily oral versus weekly intravenous mercaptopurine for patients with standard-risk acute lymphoblastic leukemia: a report from the Children's Cancer Group. Blood. 2003;101:3809.
199. Martínez-Cuadrón D, Montesinos P, Pérez-Sirvent M, et al. Central nervous system involvement at first relapse in patients with acute myeloid leukemia. Haematologica. 2011;96:1375.
200. Montesinos P, Díaz-Mediavilla J, Debén G, et al. Central nervous system involvement at first relapse in patients with acute promyelocytic leukemia treated with all-trans retinoic acid and anthracycline monochemotherapy without intrathecal prophylaxis. Haematologica. 2009;94:1242.
201. Shihadeh F, Reed V, Faderl S, et al. Cytogenetic profile of patients with acute myeloid leukemia and central nervous system disease. Cancer. 2012;118:112.
202. Thomas LB. Pathology of leukemia in the brain and meninges: postmortem studies of patients with acute and of mice given L1210 leukemia. Cancer Res. 1965;25:155.
203. Cassileth PA, Sylvester LS, Bennett JM, Begg CB. High peripheral blast count in acute myelogeneous leukemia is a primary risk factor for CNS leukemia. J Clin Oncol. 1988;6:495.
204. Mastrangelo R, Roplack D, Bleyer A, et al. Report on recommendations of the Rome workshop concerning poor prognosis acute lymphoblastic leukemia in children: biologic basis for staging, stratification and treatment. Med Pediatr Oncol. 1986;14:191.
205. Anastasi J, Freg J, Le Beau MM, et al. Cytogenetic clonality in myelodysplastic syndromes studied with fluorescent insitu hybridization: lineage, response to growth factor therapy and clone expression. Blood. 1993;81:1580.
206. Jansen JWG, Bushle M, Drexler HG, et al. Clonal analysis of myelodysplastic syndromes: evidence of multipotent stem cell origin. Blood. 1984;73:24.
207. Turhan AG, Humpheries RK, Phillips GL, et al. Clonal hematopoiesis demonstratred by X-linked DNA polymorphism after allogeneic bone marrow transplantation. N Engl J Med. 1989;320:1655.
208. Haferlach T, Nagata Y, Grossmann V, et al. Landscape of genetic lesions in 944 patients with myelodysplastic syndromes. Leukemia. 2014;28:241.
209. Naqvi K, Jabbour E, Bueso-Ramos C, et al. Implications of discrepancy in morphologic diagnosis of myelodysplastic syndrome between referral and tertiary care centers. Blood. 2011;118:4690.

210. Toyama K, Ohyashiki K, Yoshida Y, et al. Clinical implications of chromosomal abnormalities in 401 patients with myelodysplastic syndromes: a multicentric study in Japan. Leukemia. 1993;7:499.
211. Haase D, Germing U, Schanz J, et al. New insights into the prognostic impact of the karyotype in MDS and correlation with subtypes: evidence from a core dataset of 2124 patients. Blood. 2007;110:4385.
212. Pozdnyakova O, Miron PM, Tang G, et al. Cytogenetic abnormalities in a series of 1,029 patients with primary myelodysplastic syndromes: a report from the US with a focus on some undefined single chromosomal abnormalities. Cancer. 2008;113:3331.
213. Papaemmanuil E, Gerstung M, Malcovati L, et al. Clinical and biological implications of driver mutations in myelodysplastic syndromes. Blood. 2013;122:3616. quiz 3699
214. Bejar R, Stevenson K, Abdel-Wahab O, et al. Clinical effect of point mutations in myelodysplastic syndromes. N Engl J Med. 2011;364:2496.
215. Mauritzson N, Albin M, Rylander L, et al. Pooled analysis of clinical and cytogenetic features intreatment-related and de novo adult acute myeloid leukemia and myelodysplastic syndromes based on a consecutive series of 761 patients analyzed 1976–1993 and on 5098 unselected cases reported in the literature 1974–2001. Leukemia. 2002;16:2366.
216. Bennett JM. A comparative review of classification systems in myelodysplastic syndromes (MDS). Semin Oncol. 2005;32:3.
217. Della Porta MG, Travaglino E, Boveri E, et al. Minimal morphological criteria for defining bone marrow dysplasia: a basis for clinical implementation of WHO classification of myelodysplastic syndromes. Leukemia. 2015;29:66.
218. Valent P, Horny HP, Bennett JM, et al. Definitions and standarts in the diagnosis and treatment of the myelodysplastic syndromes: consensus statements and report from a working conference. Leuk Res. 2007;31:227.
219. Bennett JM. The classification and management of the myelodysplastic syndromes: areas of controversy. Hematol Rev. 1993;7:189.
220. Goasguen JE, Bennett JM. Classification and morphologic features of myelodysplastic syndromes. Semin Oncol. 1992;19:4.
221. Kouides PA, Bennett JM. Morphology and classification of myelodysplastic syndromes. Hematol Oncol Clin N Am. 1992;6:485.
222. Bennett JM. Morphological classification of the myelodysplastic syndromes: how much more education of diagnosticians is necessary? Haematologica. 2013;98:490.
223. Senent L, Arenillas L, Luno E, Ruiz JC, Sanz G, Florensa L. Reproducibility of the World Health Organization 2008 criteria formyelodysplastic syndromes. Haematologica. 2013;98:568.
224. Matsuda A, Germing U, Jinnai I, et al. Improvement of criteria for refractory cytopenia with multilineage dysplasia according to the WHO classification based on prognostic significance of morphological features in patients with refractory anemia according to the FAB classification. Leukemia. 2007;21:678.
225. Thide T, Engquist L, Billstrom R. Application of megakaryocyte morphology in diagnosis of –5q syndrome. Eur J Hematol. 1988;41:434.
226. Tuzuner N, Bennett JM. Reference standards for bone marrow cellularity. Leuk Res. 1994;18:645.
227. Tuzuner N, Cox C, Rowe JM, Bennett JM. Bone marrow cellularity in myeloid stem cell disorders: impact of age correction. Leuk Res. 1994;18:559.
228. Tricot G, De Wolf-Peeters C, Vlietinck R, Verwilghen RL. Bone marrow histology in myelodysplastic syndromes. II. Prognostic value of abnormal localization of immature precursors in MDS. Br J Haematol. 1984;58:217.
229. Horny HP, Greschniok A, Jordan JH, Menke DM, Valent P. Chymase expressing bone marrow mast cells in mastocytosis and myelodysplastic syndromes: an immunohistochemical and morphometric study. J Clin Pathol. 2003;56:103.
230. Bennett JM, Catovsky D, Daniel MT, et al. Proposals for the classification of myelodysplastic syndrome. Br J Haematol. 1982;51:189.
231. Brunning RD, Orazi A, Germing U, et al. Myelodysplastic syndromes/neoplasms, overview. In: Swerdlow SH, Campo E, Harris NL, editors. World Health Organization classification of tumours of haematopoietic and lymphoid tissues. Lyon: IARC; 2008. p. 92–3.
232. Arber DA, Hasserjian R. Reclassifying myelodysplastic syndromes: what's where in the new WHO and why. Am Soc Hematology. 2015;2015:294–8.
233. Pellagatti A, Cazzola M, Giagounidis AA, et al. Gene expression profiles of CD34_ cells in myelodysplastic syndromes: involvement of interferon-stimulated genes and correlation to FAB subtype and karyotype. Blood. 2006;108:337.
234. Gerstung M, Pellagatti A, Malcovati L, et al. Combining gene mutation with gene expression data improves outcome prediction in myelodysplastic syndromes. Nat Commun. 2015;6:590.
235. Germing U, Lauseker M, Hildebrandt B, et al. Survival, prognostic factors and rates of leukemic transformation in 381 untreated patients with MDS and del(5q): a multicenter study. Leukemia. 2012;26:1286.
236. Geyer JT, Verma S, Mathew S, et al. Bone marrow morphology predicts additional chromosomal abnormalities in patients with myelodysplastic syndrome with del(5q). Hum Pathol. 2013;44:346.
237. Zuo Z, Medeiros LJ, Chen Z, et al. Acute myeloid leukemia (AML) witherythroid predominance exhibits clinical and molecular characteristics that differ from other types of AML. PLoS One. 2012;7:e41485.
238. Grossmann V, Bacher U, Haferlach C, et al. Acute erythroid leukemia (AEL) can be separated into distinct prognostic subsets based on cytogenetic and molecular genetic characteristics. Leukemia. 2013;27:1940.
239. Maassen A, Strupp C, Giagoinidis A, Germing U. Validation and proposals for a refinement of the WHO 2008 classification of myelodysplastic syndromes without excess of blasts. Leuk Res. 2012;37:64.
240. Orazi A, Czader MB. Myelodysplastic syndromes. Am J Clin Pathol. 2009;132:290.
241. Szpurka H, Tiu R, Murugesan G, et al. Refractory anemia with ringed sideroblasts associated with marked thrombocytosis (RARS-T), another myeloproliferative condition characterized by JAK2 V617F mutation. Blood. 2006;108:2173.
242. Malcovati L, Germing U, Kuendgen A, et al. Time-dependent prognostic scoring system for predicting survival and leukemic evolution in myelodysplastic syndromes. J Clin Oncol. 2007;25:3503.
243. Patnaik MM, Hanson CA, Sulai NH, et al. Prognostic irrelevance of ring sideroblast percentage in World Health Organization-defined myelodysplastic syndromes without excess blasts. Blood. 2012;119:5674.
244. Maschek H, Georgii A, Kaloutsi V, et al. Myelofibrosis in primary myelodysplastic syndromes: a retrospective study of 352 patients. Eur J Haematol. 1992;48:208.
245. Della Porta MG, Malcovati L, Boveri E, et al. Clinical relevance of bone marrow fibrosis and CD 34 positive cell clusters in primary myelodysplastic syndrome. J Clin Oncol. 2009;27:754.
246. Schanz J, Tuchler H, Sole F, et al. New comprehensive cytogenetic scoring system for primary myelodysplastic syndromes (MDS) andoligoblastic acute myeloid leukemia after MDS derived from an international database merge. J Clin Oncol. 2012;30:820.
247. Bauman I, Niemeyer CM, Bennett JM, Shannon K. Childhood myelodysplastic syndrome. In: Swerdlow SH, Campo E, Harris NL, editors. World Health Organization classification of tumours of haematopoietic and lymphoid tissues. Lyon: IARC; 2008. p. 104–7.

248. Kardos G, Baumann I, Passmore SJ, et al. Refractory anemia in childhood: a retrospective analysis of 67 patients with particular reference to monosomy 7. Blood. 2003;102:1997.
249. Baumann I, Führer M, Behrendt S, et al. Morphological differentiation of severe aplastic anaemia from hypocellular refractory cytopenia of childhood: reproducibility of histopathological diagnostic criteria. Histopathology. 2012;61:10.
250. Tuzuner N, Cox C, Rowe JM, Bennett JM. Hypocellular acute myeloid leukemia: the Rochester (New York) experience. Hematol Pathol. 1995;9:195.
251. Tuzuner N, Cox C, Rowe JM, Watrous D, Bennett JM. Hypocellular myelodysplastic syndrome: new proposals. Br J Haematol. 1995;91:612.
252. Al-Kali A, Konoplev S, Lin E, et al. Hypocellular acute myeloid leukemia in adults: analysis of the clinicaloutcome of 123 patients. Haematologica. 2012;97:235.
253. Bennet JM, Orazi A. Diagnostic criteria to distinguish hypocellular acute myeloid leukemia from hypocellular myelodysplastic syndromes and aplastic anemia: recomendations for a standardized approach. Hematologica. 2009;94:264.
254. Yue G, Hao S, Fadare O, et al. Hypocellularity in myelodysplastic syndrome is an independent factorwhich predicts a favorable outcome. Leuk Res. 2008;32:553.
255. Fohlmeister I, Fischer R, Mödder B, et al. Aplastic anemia and the hypocellular myelodysplastic syndrome: histomorphological, diagnostic and prognostic features. J Clin Pathol. 1985;38:1218.
256. Orazi A, Albitar M, Heerema NA, et al. Hypocellular myelodtsplastic syndromes can be distinguished from acquired aplastic anemia by CD34 and PCNA immunostaining of bone marrow biopsy specimens. Am J Clin Pathol. 1997;107:268.
257. Afable MG, Wlodarski M, Makishima H, et al. SNP array–based karyotyping: differences and similarities between aplastic anemia and hypocellular myelodysplastic syndromes. Blood. 2011;117:6876.
258. Orazi A, Bennett JM, Germing U, et al. Chronic myelomonocytic leukemia. In: Swerdlow SH, Campo E, Harris NL, editors. World Health Organization classification of tumours of haematopoietic and lymphoid tissues. Lyon: IARC; 2008. p. 76–9.
259. Germing U, Strupp C, Knipp S, et al. Chronic myelomonocytic leukemia in the light of the WHO proposals. Hematologica. 2007;92:974.
260. Such E, Cervera J, Costa D, et al. Cytogenetic risk stratification in chronic myelomonocytic leukemia. Haematologica. 2011;96:375.
261. Grossmann V, Kohlmann A, Eder C, et al. Molecular profiling of chronic myelomonocytic leukemia reveals diverse mutations in >80% of patients with TET2 and EZH2 being of high prognostic relevance. Leukemia. 2011;25:877.
262. Gelsi-Boyer V, Trouplin V, Adélaïde J, et al. Mutations of polycomb-associated gene ASXL1 in myelodysplastic syndromes and chronic myelomonocytic leukaemia. Br J Haematol. 2009;145:788.
263. Breccia M, Biondo F, Latagliata R, Carmosino I, Mandelli F, Alimena G. Identification of risk factors in atypical chronic myeloid leukemia. Haematologica. 2006;91:1566.
264. Wang AS, Hasserjian RP, Fox SP. et al.Atypical chronic myeloid leukemia is clinically distinct from unclasifiable myelodysplastic/ myeloproliferative neoplasms. Blood. 2014;123:2645.
265. Baumann I, Bennett JM, Niemeyer CM, Thiele J, Shannon K. Juvenile myelomonocytic leukemia. In: Swerdlow SH, Campo E, Harris NL, editors. World Health Organization classification of tumours of haematopoietic and lymphoid tissues. Lyon: IARC; 2008. p. 82.
266. Neimeyer CM, Arico M, Basso B, et al. Chronic myelomonocytic leukemia in childhood: a retrospective analysis of 110 cases. European Working Group on Myelodysplastic Syndromes of Childhood (EWOG-MDS). Blood. 1997;89:3534.
267. de Vries AC, Zwaan CM, van den Heuvel-Eibrink MM. Molecular basis of juvenile myelomonocytic leukemia. Haematologica. 2010;95:179.
268. Chang TY, Dvorak CC, Loh ML. Bedside to bench in juvenile myelomonocytic leukemia: insights into leukemogenesis from a rare pediatric leukemia. Blood. 2014;124:2487.

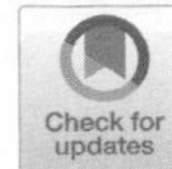

Immunobiology of Acute Leukemia

15

Elisabeth Paietta

Introduction

Acute leukemias are commonly defined as the expansion of immature cells that are derived from rare transformed hematopoietic progenitor cells, termed the leukemic stem cells (LSC) or leukemia-initiating cells (LIC), which have the capacity of self-renewal, a defining characteristic also of normal hematopoietic stem cells [1]. As an alternative to originating in a primitive stem cell, leukemias may be derived from transformation of a committed progenitor cell, as is the case with the PML/RARα fusion gene which confers self-renewal to the promyelocyte compartment [2]. The specific cell surface phenotype of LSCs is CD34$^+$, CD38$^-$ [3]. To distinguish between normal and malignant CD34$^+$, CD38$^-$ cells, additional markers are required, such as the C-type lectin-like molecule (CLL-1) [4], CD123 [5], and CD47 [6]. Remarkably, however, even this basic LSC phenotype may vary among patients, such as in truly CD34$^-$, often *NPM1* (nucleophosmin 1)-mutated AML [7], or in leukemias with rearrangement of the *MLL* (mixed-lineage leukemia) gene, in which surface antigen expression of LSCs depends on gene fusion partners [8]. Together with the loss of long-term repopulating potential, the phenotypic features of the LSC blast cell progeny that invade the bone marrow and the peripheral blood of leukemia patients are different from those of the LSC and typically characterized by different morphology and antigen profiles. Despite limited morphologic variability, which forms the basis of the FAB classification, the genetic heterogeneity of both acute myeloid (AML) and lymphoid leukemias (ALL) is vast. With very few exceptions, namely hypergranular *PML/RARα^{POS}* acute promyelocytic leukemia (APL) associated with FAB M3, the t(8;21) and inv(16) core-binding factor (CBF) leukemias associated with M2 and M4Eo, respectively [9], and *RUNX1* mutations, which are associated with the M0 FAB type [10], the morphologic appearance of leukemic cells lacks predictive power with respect to their genetic makeup. While FAB classes may still be collected as part of the biologic characterization of study cohorts, they are no longer part of multivariate analyses establishing the prognostic significance of mutational landscapes [9–15].

For some of the cytogenetic/genetic aberrations, specific antigen profiles have been established, termed surrogate marker profiles, which, in itself, are independent of the underlying genetic lesion, e.g., for APL, for *AML1/ETO* (now termed *RUNX1/RUNX1T1*), and for *BCR/ABL^{POS}* ALL [16, 17]. For other genotypic subtypes, such as BCR/ABL1-like or Ph-like ALL, overexpression of the cytokine receptor-like factor 2 (CRLF2), found in approximately 50% of cases [18], can be reliably detected with an antibody to surface expression of CRLF2 by the leukemic B-lymphoblasts when compared to CRLF2 analysis by fluorescence in situ hybridization [19]. The 2016 revision to the World Health Organization (WHO) classification of myeloid neoplasms and acute leukemia [13] illustrates clearly the increased impact of genetic aberrations in the standardized classification of the acute leukemias. The newly defined concept of pre-leukemic cell clones which carry recurrent mutations, particularly of epigenetic regulator genes (*DNMT3A, TET2*), has revealed novel insights into the intricacies of hematopoiesis and the development of acute leukemia [20–22]. These pre-leukemic stem cells are resistant to standard chemotherapy, persist during remission, and may correspond to a patient's risk of relapse. The fact that these somatic mutations are found with astonishing high frequency in clonally expanded hematopoetic stem cells of healthy subjects [23–26], however, may challenge the notion that pre-leukemic stem cells are the most important target for minimal residual disease (MRD) monitoring.

Antigens expressed by leukemic cells are identical to those expressed by normal hematopoietic cells. To date,

E. Paietta, Ph.D.
Department of Oncology, Albert Einstein College of Medicine, Montefiore Medical Center, 111 East 210th Street, Bronx, NY 10467, USA
e-mail: epaietta@montefiore.org

P.H. Wiernik et al. (eds.), *Neoplastic Diseases of the Blood*, DOI 10.1007/978-3-319-64263-5_15

there is no evidence for the existence of leukemia-specific antigens, with the exception of proteins that are encoded by novel fusion genes as a result of leukemia-specific chromosomal aberrations [27] or by mutated genes, e.g., *NPM1* [28]. The value of these antibodies to leukemia-specific proteins lies in their ability to detect genetic aberrations by alternative techniques.

The concept of surrogate marker profiles for genetic lesions [16, 17] follows the basic hypothesis that molecular features determine the cellular phenotype. For leukemic clones, this notion implies that the expression of (altered) genes associated with leukemogenesis will cause characteristic distortions of the cellular phenotype with some predictable consistency that can be exploited by sophisticated immunophenotyping. This explains the occurrence of unique antigens or antigen patterns in leukemia subtypes characterized by particular cytogenetic and/or molecular abnormalities. Examples are the typical antigen profile of AML with t(8;21) *(RUNX1/RUNX1T1)*, the classical marker composition of *PML/RARα*^{POS} APL, and the association of CD25, the α-chain of the interleukin-2 receptor, with BCR/ABL^{POS} ALL, all of which will be discussed in detail.

Unfortunately, reliable surrogate marker profiles for genetic lesions are rare and even the finding of a CD34^{-}, HLA-DR^{-}, CD11a^{-}, CD18^{-} phenotype, which is strongly indicative of APL [29], is only that, indicative of APL, and must be confirmed by the molecular presence of the *PML/RARα*-fusion gene by the polymerase chain reaction (PCR) assay. On the other hand, elevated surface expression of CRLF2 by B-lymphoblasts is almost invariably associated with the Ph-like CRLF2 phenotype [18, 30]. It does not, however, distinguish between *IGH@-CRLF2*, *P2RY8-CRLF2*, and other kinase fusions.

The characterization of universal markers for poor treatment response with current treatment strategies is another aspect of antigen expression worth mentioning. Besides CRLF2, CD25 is one such antigen both in B-lineage ALL [31] and AML [32]. Other antigens exhibit their unfavorable prognostic significance only in association with a certain maturation stage of acute leukemia, such as the poor outcome associated with expression of the myeloid antigen CD13 in cortical, mature but not in immature T-ALL [33].

The finding that particular combinations of antigens expressed by leukemic cells may be rarely or never be seen in normal hematopoietic tissues has important implications for the detection of MRD, whether the different-from-normal approach or the concept of leukemia-associated immunophenotypes (LAIP) is used [34]. The best example is the differentiation between hematogones, normal B-cell precursor cells, and leukemic B-lymphoblasts while monitoring MRD in B-lineage ALL, which requires extensive knowledge of the intricate antigen expression by hematogones and their various differentiation stages [35, 36]. With more sophisticated immunophenotypic analyses, it has become apparent that leukemic cells differ from normal hematopoietic cells and that leukemia categorization cannot be based solely on presumed normal counterparts [37]. Of course, it is still valid to group the acute leukemias according to the major hematopoietic cell lineages (T-lymphoid, B-lymphoid, myeloid), based on the expression of lineage-specific antigens, and to distinguish between precursor and more mature subtypes based on the hierarchy of antigen expression observed in normal hematopoiesis. However, refined, clinically relevant subgrouping focuses increasingly on prognostically significant and/or therapy-determining features, which may cross lineage borders, as seen, for instance, with the CD25 antigen, mentioned above. The 2008 WHO classification of neoplastic diseases of the hematopoietic and lymphoid tissues [9] and its recent revision [13] clearly reflect this tendency by increasingly recognizing cytogenetic/molecular categories in the new nomenclature of the acute leukemias, thereby reducing those disease entities which rely on morphology and/or immunophenotype alone and invariably suffer from reduced prognostic significance. Comprehensive genomic profiling can now be performed in the clinical setting to improve the diagnosis of hematologic malignancies [38, 39] and more precisely match patients with targeted therapies [40]. The emphasis on marker compositions and single antigens which are associated with genetic features and/or carry prognostic significance irrespective of lineage affiliation should be viewed as a new role for immunophenotyping that deviates from mere lineage identification.

Clinical flow cytometrists today most commonly are still charged solely with determining the lineage affiliation of a given leukemia population to provide an immunodiagnosis which is then routinely compared with the morphologic evaluation of the same tissue under the microscope and, hopefully, with cytogenetic data, to provide the diagnostic basis for therapy. There remains the challenge of accurately interpreting the rare true bilineal (BLL) or mixed-phenotype acute leukemia (MPAL), though any controversies as to whether T/MPALs or B/MPALs [9, 13] should be treated as lymphoid or myeloid leukemias are determined by their genetic makeup rather than their presumed lineage affiliation. I am saying presumed lineage affiliation, because recognizing true lineage affiliation depends on the detection of lineage-specific, predominantly intracellular antigens, which remain to present a challenge to many. Genomic characterization of immunophenotypically distinct subpopulations from two patients with T/myeloid BLL failed to demonstrate genetic diversity, suggesting that the cells with T-, myeloid-, or T/myeloid features all derived from a common LSC with multilineage differentiation capacity [41]. This concept of inherent leukemic plasticity [37, 42, 43] emphasizes that treating BLL or MPAL leukemias according to the dominant phenotype seen at the time of testing is ill advised; genotypic features should guide the treatment decision.

Inevitably, routine clinical flow cytometry laboratories are limited in their efforts due to costs and time restraints. Even if involved in clinical trials with protocol-derived correlative studies, the laboratory must strike a balance between routine immunophenotyping for diagnostic purposes and science-driven, prognostically pertinent testing, if only limited material is available and more sophisticated correlatives, such as genomic studies, must be performed on the same tissue. Ideally, the number of cells required for mere diagnosis-confirming flow cytometry is reduced to a minimum by using multiple fluorochromes in combination and a selection of most informative antibodies. This chapter discusses the various roles of immunophenotyping and the relation between antigen expression and other biologic or clinical aspects in the acute leukemias. In particular, it emphasizes on novel developments, such as the exciting developments in immunotherapy, MRD detection, and novel genotype-driven leukemia subsets. The discussion of lineage-affiliated antigen expression and immunophenotypic classification systems, areas which have been introduced extensively in the previous editions [44, 45], this time will be touched on only peripherally, as far as they relate to the other topics.

Immunophenotyping Versus Morphology

The classification of the acute leukemias has relied on the evaluation of cell size, granularity, nuclear shape, cytoplasmic appearance, cytochemical reactions, and dysplastic features of cells surrounding the "leukemic blasts" since the introduction of the French-American-British (FAB) classification system first in 1976, followed by more recent modifications [46]. Twenty years later, when the WHO published its first proposed classification for hematopoietic tumors [47], FAB terms for ALL were no longer found relevant. For AML, the new classification encompassed four major categories: (1) AML with recurrent genetic abnormalities; (2) AML with multilineage dysplasia; (3) AML and myelodysplastic syndromes, therapy related; and (4) AML not otherwise categorized. In the 2008 WHO edition [9], category 1 was significantly expanded by incorporating more balanced chromosomal translocations and inversions as well as a list of gene mutations that had been found to be of prognostic significance and/or associated with a normal karyotype in the years between the two publications. Despite these additions, which to some extent reduced the number of cases previously left uncategorized, particularly in elderly AML [48], a large group of patients still remained in category 4, not otherwise categorized molecularly and therefore still classified by FAB criteria. Proteomic profiling confirmed the ability of the FAB classification to distinguish between the major lineages by aligning protein signatures with myeloid (M0, M1, M2), monocytic (M4, M5), or M6/M7, though without discriminating the degree of maturation [49]. This may explain why FAB classes are usually not good predictors of prognosis, with the exception of FAB M3 or hypergranular APL. Critics of the WHO classification blame it for emphasizing simplicity of classification at the expense of prognostic significance [50].

An excellent example for underappreciated discordance between information provided by FAB criteria and the actual level of maturation arrest indicated by antigen expression in a recurrent cytogenetic aberration is t(8;21) or *RUNX1/RUNX1T1*^{POS} AML. Incredible effort has gone into accurately identifying this AML subtype based on morphology. Nucifora et al. [51] proposed a scoring system for the identification of t(8;21) AML based on a list of morphologic characteristics—a total score of 6 or 7 would be suggestive of t(8;21). This scoring system was subsequently adjusted to capture more t(8;21) positive cases while simultaneously decreasing the false-positive rate from 12% with the Nucifera score to 7% with the weighted score [52]. This better recognition rate was accomplished simply by altering the scores assigned to the various morphologic features, reflecting the randomness of such scoring systems. Although predominantly associated with FAB M2 (AML with maturation) [9], 20% of t(8;21) AML cases presented with M1 features (AML without maturation) upon central morphology review (Bennett JM, personal communication) of a recently completed phase III trial of the Eastern Cooperative Oncology Group (ECOG) in >600 younger AML patients [53]. A characteristic feature of the t(8;21) AML immunophenotype is a striking myeloid immaturity, such as weak or absent expression of CD33 [52] and/or the more mature myeloid antigen, $CD65_{(S)}$ (Paietta E, personal observation), and failure to detect myeloperoxidase by antibody binding [54], and consistent with the suggestion that the *RUNX1/RUNX1T1* fusion event occurs at an early stem/(progenitor cell stage [55]). This lack of myeloid maturation has mostly gone unnoticed due to the continuing tendency of pathologists to place more weight on morphology rather than immunophenotype, particularly in AML. The unique B-lymphoid antigenic features of t(8;21) AML, with expression of PAX5, CD19, and CD79a [56], are a further indication for focusing on refined immunophenotyping, especially since immunostaining for PAX5 is a valuable diagnostic tool for t(8;21) AML presenting with extramedullary masses, which occur frequently in this disease [9]. The absence of expression of the T-lymphoid antigen, CD7, in t(8;21) AML was reported many years ago [52, 57]. More recently, however, we described a subtype of AML which resembles closely the phenotype of t(8;21) AML but expresses CD7 together with CD19 [58]. Strikingly, this novel AML presents with a normal karyotype, lacks *RUNX1/RUNXT1* transcripts, but instead contains internal tandem duplications of the *FLT3* gene (*FLT3ITD*^{POS}) and mutated *NPM1* (*NPM1MUT*^{POS}).

An intriguing observation is the application of immunophenotyping in the discovery of the genetic diversity of morphologically defined APL. Flow cytometry recognizes the characteristic cellular structures of hypergranular (FAB M3) APL by producing a scattergram that reflects cells of large size (high forward-angle light scatter, FSC) with a high degree of granularity (high 90° angle scatter or side scatter, SSC). However, for variant hypogranular APL cells (FAB M3v), the scatter signal can be quite variable and misleading [59]. In a report from the Europena Working Party [60], the majority of cases with FAB M3 or M3v morphology contained t(15;17)(q22;q12)/PML/RARα or other cytogenetic aberrations involving the RARα gene. To account for a small subgroup of morphologic APL patients apparently lacking a RARα rearrangement, a new morphological subclass was introduced and termed "M3r," which also covered APL presenting with PLZF/RARα transcripts. Although the immunophenotype of M3r cases shared the negativity for CD34 and HLA-DR, which is part of the surrogate marker profile for t(15;17) APL [29], M3r patients lacked response to all-trans retinoic acid (ATRA) in vivo. In other words, the main rationale for classifying APL, namely to recognize ATRA-responsive disease, was invalid in this morphologic subtype. The other lesson that should have been learned from these data was that the standard CD34- and HLA-DR-negative marker profile, still widely accepted as sufficient for the diagnosis of APL, is unreliable in predicting the disease. Contrary to this overzealous attempt to define APL by morphology, t(15;17) leukemia without M3/M3v features is often ignored. Among larger studies [59, 61], the incidence of such APL cases ranges between 1 and 2%. For these as well as patients with cryptic t(15;17) [59], the improved surrogate antigen profile for PML/RARα^{POS} APL applies, consisting of negativity for HLA-DR, CD11a, and CD18 [29]. While this antigen combination pertains to both M3 and M3v morphologies, there are immunophenotypic peculiarities that are limited to M3v and/or leukemic promyelocytes containing the S-isoform of PML/RARα transcripts; these are expression of CD34 and of the T-cell-affiliated antigen, CD2 [29]. In fact, CD2^{POS} leukemic promyelocytes frequently lack all of the antigenic properties associated with APL. In such cases, expression of CD2 by myeloid blasts per se is the strongest indication that one is dealing with an APL. It is important to remember that CD2 expression in AML is rare and if present most commonly suggests APL or AML FAB M4Eo with inv(16)(p13q22) resulting in the *CBFβ/MYH11* fusion transcript [62]. In confirmation of a biologic heterogeneity within the APL phenotype, results from gene expression profiling demonstrated that M3 and M3v APL were clearly separable [63]. Furthermore, the origin of CD2^{POS} APL has been localized to a progenitor cell more immature than that of CD2^{NEG} APL [64].

The role of morphology in the diagnosis of "acute leukaemias of ambiguous lineage" [9] is difficult to assess, since this leukemia subtype is frequently erroneously diagnosed. Occasionally, two morphologically distinct blast populations are readily distinguishable in individual patients; still, even in such cases, the demonstration of lineage-specific antigens is essential for the differential diagnosis of "mixed" (distinct expression of lineage-specific antigens in the two morphologically different populations) versus "biphenotypic" leukemia (expression of lineage-specific antigens by one and the same blast cell irrespective of morphology). More common is the finding of antigens specific for more than one cell lineage in a morphologically homogenous blast cell population, e.g., myeloperoxidase and cytoplasmic CD22 (cCD22) or myeloperoxidase and cytoplasmic CD3 (cCD3), the antigens specific for the myeloid, B-lymphoid, and T-lymphoid lineage, respectively. An instructive example for such a true biphenotype is that of CD117^{POS}, FLT3-gene mutated T-lineage ALL [65]. This rare leukemia subtype simultaneously expresses cCD3 and, in a subset of blast cells (5–10%), myeloperoxidase. Despite the presence of the myeloid-specific antigen in only a minor portion of the blasts, the morphology of these cases varied between FAB M2 (occasionally with Auer rods) and FAB L2, independent of the percentage of myeloperoxidase^{pos} blasts.

Minimally differentiated AML is considered to be equivalent to FAB M0, with no evidence of myeloid differentiation by morphology or cytochemistry [9]. Based on a retrospective analysis of >700 adult AML patients across all ages, ECOG defined this undifferentiated phenotype based on lack of expression of the more mature myeloid antigen, CD65(s), a carbohydrate antigen that can be expressed in an asialostate (CD65) or with a sialic acid residue in terminal position of the carbohydrate chain (CD65s) [66]. Morphologically, the majority of these patients belonged to the FAB M0/M1 classes. Important hints in the correct interpretation of this AML subtype are the following: (a) blasts must be negative for lymphoid-specific antigens, cCD22 and cCD3; (b) although blasts do not show an enzymatic reaction for myeloperoxidase, they frequently stain for the myeloperoxidase protein by antibody staining; (c) even if blasts are negative with antimyeloperoxidase antibody, they are considered myeloid given that they lack lymphoid-specific antigens; (d) in most cases, the blasts will stain for CD33 and/or CD13, the pan-myeloid antigens; (e) immature antigens, such as CD34, CD117, HLA-DR, CD133, and CD123, are common; (f) frequently, the T-lymphoid-affiliated antigen CD7 is found; (g) expression of the B-lymphoid antigen CD19 by these undifferentiated blasts suggests t(8;21)/AML1/ETO^{POS}AML. Minimally differentiated AML more often occurs in older patients and carries inferior prognosis [66].

In summary, diagnoses based on morphology cannot be easily correlated with immunophenotypic findings. With the exception of FAB-M3, morphologic subclasses rarely relate to specific immunophenotypes. The presence of monocytes and/or monocytic features in a leukemia population, however, requires special discussion. Invariably, when CD14, the prototype mature monocytic antigen, is detected on an abnormally large fraction of white blood cells (WBC) or on blasts cells defined by the expression of immature markers, such as CD34 or CD117, the morphologic evaluation will yield FAB M4 (myelomonocytic) or M5 (monocytic), respectively. It should be emphasized here that CD123 (α-chain of the IL-3 receptor), an antigen associated with the hematopoietic stem cell [67] and expressed by >99% of AML [68], cannot be used to diagnose leukemic monocytes, because normal monocytes show weak, though persistent, CD123 expression. The strong association of CD14 with monocytic morphology stands in contrast to CD11b (Mac-1), an integrin α-subunit (adhesion molecule) [69], which in monocytic development appears earlier than CD14 [70] and which is also expressed by myeloid cells starting at the myelocyte stage [71]. Given its appearance late in myeloid maturation, one would expect CD11b expression by nonlymphoid leukemic cells to reflect monocytic features. However, in a retrospective evaluation of 382 patients with $CD11b^{POS}CD14^{NEG/LOW}$ AML, ECOG found that less than half of those patients belonged to FAB classes M4/M5, whereas the other half demonstrated FAB M1/M2 features [72].

An instructive tale relates to the "cuplike" nuclei which have been published as a distinct morphologic feature in AML with FLT3-gene internal tandem duplication (FLT3-ITD) [73]. According to Kussick et al. [73], non-APL AML-cuplike was more likely to lack HLA-DR and CD34, to express CD123 without CD133, and to have a normal karyotype. A few years later, Chen et al. [74] associated the same prominent nuclear invaginations with NPM1-mutated AML, which is characterized by negativity for CD34 and CD133, normal cytogenetics, and a high incidence of FLT3 gene mutations. These structural nuclear features prevail in NPM1-mutated AML irrespective of FAB categories, which typically span a wide spectrum in this genetic subtype. Furthermore, NPM1 mutations involve all but lymphoid hematopoietic cell lineages and, as FAB criteria, also this feature is independent of the presence of FLT3-ITD [75]. While previously [47] included in the class of "AML not otherwise characterized" and subjected to diagnosis based on FAB criteria, the newest WHO classification [13] recognizes NPM1-mutated AML as a distinct disease category rather than mere prognostic factor.

Immunophenotypes Versus Genetic Lesions

Chromosome translocations can have two distinct effects at the molecular level: either the inopportune activation of an unaltered gene or the creation and transcription of a novel gene. The first process occurs predominantly in lymphoid malignancies. The translocation places a transcriptionally silent gene under the control of the promoter of a transcriptionally very active gene, e.g., immunoglobulin or T-cell receptor (TCR) genes in B- or T-lymphocytes, respectively [76]. This leads to the inappropriate transcription of a normal gene. Alternatively, balanced translocations and interstitial chromosome deletions or inversions can lead to the creation of novel, leukemogenic fusion genes. At each of the chromosomal breakpoints, a critical gene is disrupted; fragments of the two genes are brought together as a result of the translocation. Two hybrid fusion genes are created, one on each of the two chromosomes partnering in the translocation. Even if both chimeric genes are transcribed, only one is usually suspected as the transforming gene.

The following section is limited to those leukemia fusion genes, gene mutations, and instances of aberrant gene overexpression for which immunophenotypic data are available. While some antigen combinations can be viewed as specific for certain genetic lesions (e.g., $AML1/ETO^{POS}$ AML), others are indicative of a certain maturation stage of leukemic arrest (e.g., BAALC-overexpressing leukemias) or reflective of a specific cell of origin (e.g., NPM1-mutated AML).

Surrogate Antigen Profiles for Leukemia Fusion Genes

Specific associations have been established between the expression of single antigens or particular antigen expression patterns and cytogenetic-molecular abnormalities. While the first of such surrogate marker profiles were found rather serendipitously, i.e., that for t(15;17)/PML/RARα APL, antigen expression signatures of genetic lesions are increasingly sought in a planned fashion, in parallel to the genetic classification of the acute leukemias as well as due to developments in targeted therapy [16, 17]. Reliable surrogate marker profiles for genetic lesions are of clinical interest only when the associated genotype is prognostically significant and/or when targeted therapy for that genotype is available.

Outcome-based classification of the leukemias nowadays is based predominantly on cytogenetic aberrations and their molecular derivatives, whether recognizable by standard cytogenetics or requiring FISH analysis. Progressively, however, genetic and epigenetic profiling data provide a major source of information regarding perturbed pathogenetic pathways and potential therapeutic targets. The revolutionary discovery of BCR/ABL1-like or Ph-like B-lineage ALL is the best example for this development [18, 19, 30]. The advantage of having antigen profiles available, which can predict for the existence of, for example, gene mutation or gene silencing events, lies in the ease, speed, and low costs of flow cytometry. Appropriate situations of particular urgency arise when cytogenetics are unsuccessful or simply not performed, when chromosome structures are impaired, as in ALL, when only normal metaphases are seen, or when karyotyping, FISH analysis, and/or molecular analyses are not available at an institution. Surrogate marker profiles should not be used in lieu of molecular analyses, given that even the most reliable antigen combinations have shown some unexpected properties: (a) sensitivity to subtle antigenic alterations outside the core marker profile; for example, the antigen profile for t(8;21)-*AML1/ETO*^{POS} AML is invalid when the T-cell marker CD7 is also present on the surface of the myeloblasts; (b) precise alterations in response to variations in the global genetic lesion; for example, striking differences were found in the expression of CD25 and dual CD33/CD13 between the *e1a2* and *e13a2(b2a2)/e14a2(b3a2)* transcript forms in *BCR/ABL*^{POS} ALL, and absence of CD33/CD13 expression in the presence of a del(9p) in addition to the t(9;22); and (c) occasionally an overpowering effect of single antigens; for example, the expression of the T-cell marker CD2 by leukemic promyelocytes occasionally obviates the finding of the typical surrogate marker profile for *PML/RAR*α APL.

t(15;17)(q22;q12)-*PML/RAR*α^{POS} APL

Given the unmistakably hypergranular features of M3 leukemic promyelocytes, which rarely cause misreadings among morphologists, APL was the first leukemia for which characteristic immunophenotypic features were described. The history of the surrogate marker profile for APL is outlined in Table 15.1. The initial definition of an APL marker profile consisted of negativity for CD34 and HLA-DR. Subsequently, the profile was refined by adding the differential reactivity of CD15/CD15$_S$ antibodies, caused by the sialylation of the CD15 carbohydrate antigen in APL, weak expression of CD38 and CD45, expression of CD9, and lack of P-glycoprotein [17]. Two developments prompted the search for an improved profile: (1) the recognition of an ATRA-unresponsive AML subtype, termed natural killer cell AML, with morphologic similarities to M3v as well as CD34 and HLA-DR negativity, while expressing CD56, the neural cell adhesion molecule [77], and (2) the observation that CD56 expression by leukemic promyelocytes conferred inferior prognosis [78, 79]. The most recent surrogate marker profile for PML/RARα APL [29] is based predominantly on (a) lack of HLA-DR and CD133, two antigens expressed at differentiation levels more immature than that of promyelocytes during normal myelopoiesis; (b) absence of several adhesive molecules, such as CD11a (α_L subunit of the leukocyte integrin LFA-1), CD18 (β_2 subunit of LFA-1), and CD11b (α_M subunit of Mac-1 integrin); (c) expression of the carbohydrate structure, CD15, only in the sialylated form, CD15$_s$; and (d) faint expression of CD45, the common leukocyte antigen, and of CD38, a bifunctional ectoenzyme catalyzing involved in cell adhesion to endothelium. In summary, APL is characterized by absence or weak expression of adhesion molecules. CD117, a progenitor molecule associated predominantly with the myeloid lineage, is invariably expressed by leukemic promyelocytes, albeit occasionally at low levels [29, 59].

Table 15.1 History of the immunophenotype of *PML/RAR*α^{POS} APL

Earliest definition	Current definition	ECOG's new definition
Myeloid	Myeloid	Myeloid
HLA-DR NEG	HLA-DR NEG	HLA-DRNEG
CD34 HLA	CD34 NEG	CD11a NEG
	CD15 NEG	CD18NEG
	CH15s POS	CD133 NEG
	CD9 POS	CD45 WEAK
	CD38 LOW	CD38 WEAK
	Pgp WEAK/NEG	CD15 NEG

"Myeloid" defines the presence of a basic myeloid phenotype with expression of CD33 and CD13, occasional expression of CD65$_{(S)}$ and/or myeloperoxidase, and absence of lymphoid-specific antigens. *Pgp* P-glycoprotein, the multidrug resistance protein; *NEG* (negative) reflects absence of antigen-expressing cells; *POS* (positive) reflects expression of antigens by >10% of gated leukemic promyelocytes; *WEAK* reflects weak intensity of fluorescence of antibody staining

The (15;17) translocation involves the retinoic receptor α (RARA) gene on the long arm (q) of chromosome 17 and the promyelocytic leukemia (PML) gene on the q arm of chromosome 15. While the breakpoints in the RARA gene occur consistently in intron 2, differential breakpoints in the PML gene lead to the L- (Long, bcr1), S- (Short, bcr3), or the V- (Variable, bcr2) transcript isoform of PML/RARα. The HLA-DR^{LOW}, CD11a^{LOW}, CD18^{LOW} surrogate marker profile is applicable to all three molecular isoforms [29, 59]. However, the isoforms can be distinguished based on specific antigenic features outside this core antigen profile. While the antigen expression patterns in L- and V-form diseases are indistinguishable, they are clearly separable from S-isoform APL. Only leukemic promyelocytes that contain S-form transcripts variably express CD34, CD2, and CD56. The expression of CD2 together with the S-isoform correlates with poorer prognosis [80]. A potential explanation could be a higher incidence of extramedullary relapse in CD56^{POS} cases [81]. Furthermore, thrombotic events in APL were found to be associated with CD2^{POS} S-form disease with *FLT3-ITD* [82]. As discussed before, CD2^{POS} APL is hypothesized to be derived from a progenitor cell with myeloid/lymphoid potential [63, 83]. Note that while CD2 and/or CD56 on a patient's leukemic promyelocytes are highly suggestive of the S-isoform, because they are never seen in L- or V-isoform, there are S-isoform patients who lack these antigens. CD34 expression may be associated with the molecular isoform or the microgranular morphologic variant (see before). Even when expressed, the density of the CD34 antigen is significantly lower on the surface of leukemic promyelocytes than on non-APL myeloblasts [84]. CD2^{POS} APL occasionally may lack APL-typical antigenic features, something never seen in L- or V-form APL, thus possibly misleading laboratory investigators or pathologists when they interpret the data [16, 17]. It is recommended that any case of CD2^{POS} myeloid leukemia be immediately tested by PCR for *PML/RAR*α versus *CBF*β*/MYH11*, since APL [59] and inv(16)(p13q22)/t(16;16)(p13;q22) AML [62], respectively, are the two major AML subtypes found to express CD2, especially since these leukemia subdiagnoses require distinct therapies.

In addition to the *PML/RARα* fusion gene, which accounts for >98% of APL cases, a common segment 5′truncated *RARα* has been found to fuse with alternative genes [85]. Because such variant translocations are rare, clinical information regarding their responsiveness to ATRA is scarce; recurrent cases of *PLZF/RARα* (promyelocyte leukemia zinc finger), derived from t(11;17)(q23;q21), appear to lack ATRA responsiveness, while *NPM/RARα* (nucleophosmin) APL, derived from t(5;17)(q35;q21), is ATRA responsive. Despite their low frequency, the limited immunophenotypic observations available suggest that the main characteristic features of *PML/RARα* APL cells hold up for all currently known variant APL translocations that involve rearrangement of the *RARα* gene [59]. Novel variant *RARα* fusion genes keep appearing in the literature whereby ATRA sensitivity in individual cases appears to vary. Two pieces of evidence should prompt the search for the presence of an alternative *RARα* fusion gene in a patient: (a) the finding of APL-specific immunophenotypic features in a patient negative for *PML/RARα*, and (b) cytogenetic evidence of chromosome 17 abnormalities in such a patient. Occasionally, slight variations from the typical APL profile may be found. Gallagher et al. [86], for instance, found weak expression of CD133 in the only second case of *STATb/RARα*. If confirmed in further cases, this antigenic peculiarity may serve as a diagnostic tool for this particular APL variant.

t(8;21)(q22;q22)-*RUNX1/RUNX1T1* (formerly *AML1/ETO*)^{POS} AML

Leukemias with t(8;21) or inv(16)/t(16;16) belong to the core-binding factor (CBF) AMLs, which are a diagnostically and prognostically distinct subgroup [9]. Both of these chromosomal rearrangements result in the formation of fusion proteins, *RUNX1/RUNX1T1* and *CBFβ/MYH11*, respectively, that involve the disruption of one of the CBF transcription factor genes. The two genes involved in (8;21) translocation are the AML1 transcription factor, now called *RUNX1*, on chromosome 21q22.3, and the eight-twenty one oncoprotein (ETO) (now called *RUNX1T1*) on chromosome 8q22 [55]. The characteristic immunophenotype of t(8;21) AML allows for a correct prediction of this genetic aberration [87]. Distinctive features are expression of CD19, a B-lineage-associated antigen, and of CD56, the neural-cell adhesion molecule, by CD34^{POS} myeloblasts. Presence of CD56 may explain the increased incidence of granulocytic sarcomas observed in this disease [88, 89]. While CD19 is consistently present in the t(8;21) subtype and rarely found in other AMLs, expression of this antigen by myeloblasts is often very weak so that its detection can depend on the accurate choice of fluorochromes and an open mind on the part of the interpreting flow cytometrist. In fact, CD19 conjugated to fluorescein isothiocyanate (FITC) should be avoided at all costs. An example of CD19/CD56 double expression in a patient with *RUNX1/RUNX1T1*^{POS} AML is shown in Fig. 15.1. Although CD56 expression is promiscuous among myeloid leukemias and absent in a marked fraction of t(8;21) cases, the finding of both CD19 and CD56 against the background of a myeloid phenotype is highly suggestive of t(8;21) AML. As in the case of APL, an

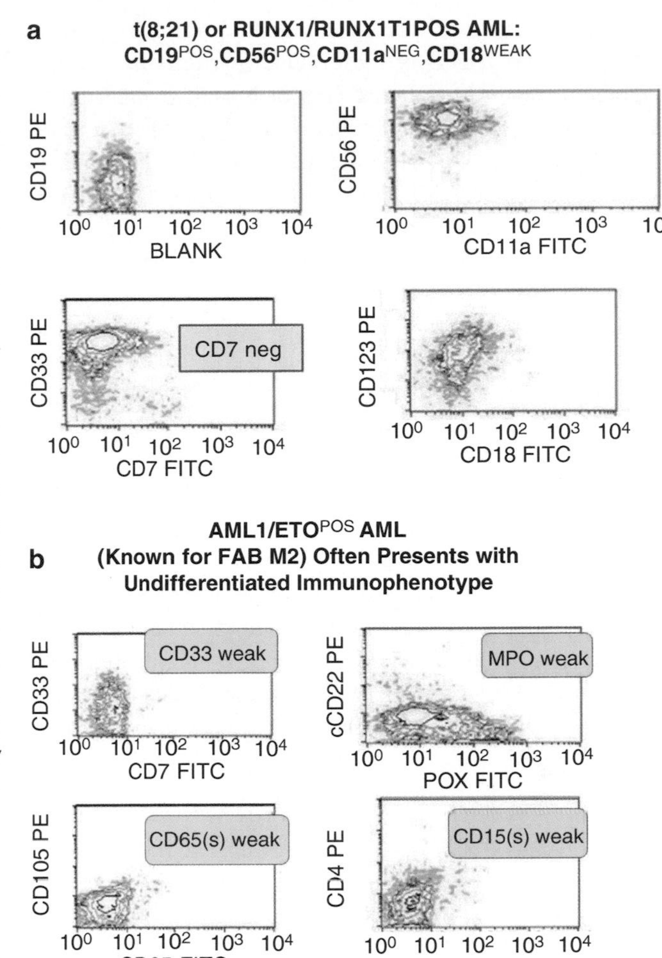

Fig. 15.1 (**a**) Dual-CD19 and -CD56 expression by t(8;21)-*RUNX1/RUNX1T1*^{POS} myeloblasts. Blasts were gated based on low side and forward scatter and all antigen expression shown reflects that of gated blasts. Antibody staining along the *X*-axis demonstrates fluorescence intensity of FITC-conjugated antibodies, whereas the *Y*-axis represents PE-conjugated antibody staining. (*A*) This contour plot demonstrates the weak though definite expression of CD19. (*B*) The same weakly CD19^{POS} blasts also strongly express CD56 but lack CD11a. (*C*) CD33 expression in this particular case of *RUNX1/RUNX1T1*^{POS} AML is strong, but notably there is no CD7 expression. (*D*) The blasts express the stem cell marker, CD123, but lack CD18. (**b**) This case of *RUNX1/RUNX1T1*^{POS} AML demonstrates the frequently found immature myeloid phenotype. Blasts were gated as described under 1.A. (*A*) Blasts only weakly express CD33 and lack CD7. (*B*) Myeloperoxidase expression is weak but there is no evidence of intracytoplasmic CD22. (*C*) Mature myeloid antigens CD65$_{(s)}$ and CD15 (*D*) are absent. The blasts also fail to stain for CD105, a marker of immature hematopoietic cells, and CD4, which is frequently expressed by monocytic cells. In the presence of CD19 staining (not shown for this case), this pattern of antigen expression may be confused with CD10^{NEG} B-lineage ALL. To exclude B-lineage ALL, myeloperoxidase and intracytoplasmic CD22 must be evaluated. Furthermore, CD10^{NEG} B-lineage ALL blasts preferentially express CD65/CD15 rather than CD33

increasingly accurate surrogate marker profile for t(8;21) AML has evolved over time. One particularly helpful diagnostic tool is the diminished or absent expression of CD11a/CD18 [59, 90], a member of the β2 integrin subfamily [69]. With the exception of t(8;21) or t(15;17) (and its variants), >90% of AML demonstrate expression of CD18. The absence of CD11a in t(8;21) AML is explained by the inhibition of Runx1-dependent CD11a transcription by the *RUNX1/RUNX1T1* fusion product [90].

Variable expression of CD11a is seen in AML with dual expression of CD19 and CD7, a T-lineage-affiliated antigen [58]. Previously, the incompatibility of t(8;21) with expression of CD7 had been reported [57]. More recently, CD19/CD7 double-positive AML has been associated with a predominantly normal karyotype and *FLT3-ITD* and *NPM1* mutations [58] (Fig. 15.2).

Aside from CD19, t(8;21) myeloblasts can also express two other B-lineage antigens, CD79a and PAX5 [56]. The *PAX5* gene encodes a paired box domain transcription factor, which is considered a crucial mediator of B-cell identity [91]. Tiacci et al. [56] hypothesized that the PAX5-dependent expression of CD19 and CD79a in t(8;21) AML results from the interaction and functional cooperation between the PAX5 and AML1/ETO proteins. Expression of CD56 is also not limited to the myeloid lineage [92] and in B-lineage ALL appears to be associated with BCR/ABL transcripts [93]. Taken together, these findings can lead to a misdiagnosis of B-lineage ALL, especially in view of the immaturity of the myeloid phenotype frequently encountered (as discussed before), as long as karyotypic and molecular data are unavailable. While in t(8;21) AML, the same blast population will co-express myeloperoxidase or surface myeloid antigens, e.g., CD13, weak CD33, and CD19, these blasts will not stain for cCD22. It is important to remember that dual absence of myeloperoxidase and cCD22 is consistent with AML.

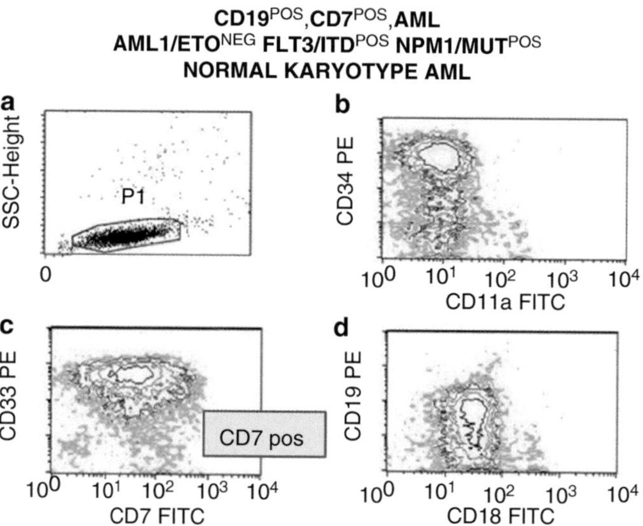

Fig. 15.2 Expression of CD7 by CD19^{POS} myeloblasts rules out t(8;21)-*RUNX1/RUNX1T1*^{POS} AML. (**a**) P1 is drawn around suspicious cells with low side (SSC) and forward scatter (FSC), reflecting lack of granularity and small-to-intermediate cell size. (**b**) In this biparametric contour plot, cells within gate P1 are found to contain a major population with high-intensity CD34 expression and a minor population with variable, weak CD34 expression; both populations lack CD11a. (**c**) Further characterization of gated cells reveals that both CD34^{HIGH} and CD34^{WEAK} cells belong to the leukemic population as they all express both CD33 and CD7. (**d**) These CD33^{POS}CD7^{POS} myeloblasts also express CD19 and lack CD18. In graphs b–d, a small population of residual normal T-lymphocytes is seen. In graph b to the right of the main CD34^{POS} cell population is a very small component of CD11a^{POS} cells; in graph c there is a small component of CD7^{POS} but CD33^{NEG} cells, and in graph d, there is a small population of CD18^{POS} but CD19^{NEG}, suggesting that they reflect a small number of normal T-lymphocytes, which had been inadvertently included in the P1 gate

t(9;22)(q34;q11)-*BCR/ABL*^{pos} ALL

The Philadelphia chromosome, t(9;22), which results in the *BCR/ABL* fusion gene, is the dominant negative prognostic factor in ALL [94]. Its incidence increases with age, accounting for 2–5% in children and up to 28% in adult patient cohorts [95]. The disappointing response of *BCR/ABL*^{POS} patients to standard therapy and the availability of specific inhibitors for the constitutively activated tyrosine kinase in BCR/ABL fusion proteins [96] have prompted separate trials for *BCR/ABL*^{POS} and *BCR/ABL*^{NEG} ALL, making it imperative that these patients are recognized accurately. It is important to differentiate between *BCR/ABL*^{POS} ALL and BCR/ABL1-like (or Ph-like) ALL (18,19), which will be discussed later.

Cytogenetic analyses in lymphoblasts are hampered by suboptimal chromosome structure [97], and, furthermore, approximately 10% of *BCR/ABL*^{POS} ALL lack evidence of the t(9;22) by chromosome banding [95]. Both karyotyping and molecular analyses by PCR require time, 1–2 weeks and, in most laboratories, at a minimum, 24 h, respectively. The first alleged antigenic signature for *BCR/ABL*^{POS} ALL relied solely on differences in staining intensity of antigens commonly found in B-lineage ALL, such as strong expression of CD10 and CD34 and weak expression of CD38 [98–100]. However, in 1997, a preliminary analysis of 144 patients enrolled in ECOG's phase III adult ALL trial, E2993, demonstrated an association between *BCR/ABL* positivity and expression of CD25, the α-chain of the interleukin-2 receptor [101]. This observation confirmed an earlier report of the incidental finding of CD25 in four patients with *BCR/ABL*^{POS} ALL [102]. The final analysis of E2993 [31] solidified the surrogate marker profile for *BCR/ABL*^{POS} lymphoblasts as CD25^{pos}CD34^{high} with frequent dual expression of myeloid antigens, CD33 and CD13. Despite the frequent expression of two myeloid antigens by *BCR/ABL*^{POS} lymphoblasts, this phenotype must not be considered biphenotypic, since *BCR/ABL*^{POS} lymphoblasts unequivocally belong to the B-cell lineage (cCD22^{POS}, myeloperoxidase^{NEG}). Approximately 60% of *BCR/ABL*^{POS} ALL cases (pediatric and adult) express additional cytogenetic aberrations [103, 104]. Rieder et al. [105] and Primo et al. [106] reported that patients with del(9)(p21), in addition to the t(9;22), lacked both CD33 and CD13. Among 11/156 *BCR/ABL^POS^* patients with del(9)(p11), del(9)(del(9)(p13), or del(9)(p21) on E2993, 8 lacked both CD33 and CD13, whereas the other 3 only showed decrease or loss of CD13 expression, thus supporting and expanding Primo's observation (Paietta E, personal observation). Wetzler et al. [104] could not confirm this association between myeloid marker expression and abnormalities of 9p. Of potential interest, a report from the pre-tyrosine kinase inhibitor (TKI) era indicated that *BCR/ABL^POS^* children with loss of the p-arm had a particularly poor outcome [103], confirming an early report from adult *BCR/ABL^POS^* patients [105].

The dual expression of myeloid antigens, CD33 and CD13 by *BCR/ABL^POS^* lymphoblasts, is not surprising, given that these blasts most commonly express immunophenotypic features of early pre-B-ALL (CD10^POS^). Ludwig et al. [107] have proposed that the expression of myeloid antigens in adult B-lineage ALL differs according to the level of B-lymphoblast maturation, analogous to what has been reported from pediatric ALL [108, 109]. Analysis of E2993 [110] confirmed but also expanded these associations. While pro/pre-pre-B-ALL, the immature CD10^NEG^ maturation stage, typically expressed $CD65_{(S)}$ and $CD15_{(S)}$, the CD10^POS^ early pre-B stage preferentially expressed the pan-myeloid antigens CD33 and CD13, which in normal myelopoiesis appear before $CD65_{(S)}/CD15_{(S)}$ on maturing myeloid cells. However, these relationships did not hold up in *BCR/ABL^POS^* cases; as given in Table 15.2, the paired expression of CD33/CD13 persisted irrespective of the maturation stage of BCR/ABL^POS^ lymphoblasts. CD33/CD13 positivity was seen whether *BCR/ABL^POS^* blasts lacked CD10 (pro/pre-pre-B stage) or expressed intracytoplasmic μ chains (pre-B stage). Importantly, *BCR/ABL^POS^* lymphoblasts never expressed $CD65_{(S)}/CD15_{(S)}$ even in those instances in which CD33 and/or CD13 were not expressed. It is important to realize that *BCR/ABL^POS^* cases with CD33/CD13 expression do not represent MPAL B/myeloid, as defined by the WHO classification [9], given that *BCR/ABL^POS^* ALL cells invariably contain intracytoplasmic CD22 (B-lineage-specific marker) and lack myeloperoxidase (myeloid-lineage-specific marker).

Table 15.2 *BCR/ABL^POS^* B-lineage ALL blasts frequently express both CD33 and CD13, irrespective of the maturation stage of the B-lymphoblasts (shown in **bold**)

BCR/ABL	B-ALL maturation	CD33	CD13	CD65	CD15
Negative	Pro-B /Pre-Pre-B	neg	neg	pos	pos
Positive	Pro-B/ Pre-Pre-B	**pos**	**pos**	neg	neg
Negative	Early Pre-B	*pos*	*pos*	neg	neg
Positive	Early Pre-B	**pos**	**pos**	neg	neg
Negative	Pre-B	neg	neg	neg	neg
Positive	Pre-B	**pos**	**pos**	neg	neg

While *BCR/ABL^NEG^* immature, CD10^*NEG*^ pro-B/pre-pre-B blasts commonly express CD65 and/or CD15, *BCR/ABL^POS^* pro-B/pre-pre-B blasts express CD33/CD13. The more mature pre-B blasts in *BCR/ABL^NEG^* ALL typically lack myeloid antigen expression

The (9;22)(q34;q11) translocation results in the actual Philadelphia chromosome, the derivative chromosome 22, in which the *BCR/ABL* fusion gene is located, and the derivative chromosome 9, where the reciprocal *ABL/BCR* fusion gene resides, which does not appear to contribute to the pathogenesis of this disease. Various isoforms of the *BCR/ABL* fusion gene are created dependent on the variable breakpoints in the *BCR* gene. All translated BCR/ABL proteins share a similar carboxy-terminal ABL tyrosine kinase domain (TKD), but differ in the portion of the BCR protein included in the fusion product, due to multiple breakpoint cluster regions in the *BCR* gene. In the majority of chronic myeloid leukemia (CML) cases and in one-third of *BCR/ABL^POS^* ALL, the break within the *BCR* gene occurs in the major breakpoint cluster region (M-bcr), resulting, when joined with a portion of *c-ABL* from chromosome 9, in a *e13a2 (b2a2)* or *e14a2 (b3a2)* fusion transcript encoding a protein of 210,000 Da molecular weight (p210^BCR-ABL^). A break in the minor breakpoint cluster region (m-bcr) forms the *e1a2* transcript encoding a 190,000 Da protein (p190^BCR-ABL^), found mostly in *BCR/ABL^POS^* ALL [111, 112]. Castor et al. [113] proposed a distict pattern of hematopoietic stem cell and committed B-cell progenitor involvement for major and minor *BCR/ABL* fusion ALLs, respectively.

The most striking observation with respect to CD25 and *BCR/ABL^POS^* ALL is that expression levels of CD25 are of prognostic significance predicting for a lower likelihood to achieve complete remission [31], and shorter overall (OS) [31] or event-free survival [114] among *BCR/ABL^POS^* patients. In other words, CD25 is unique in its dual function as a dependable marker of *BCR/ABL^POS^* ALL and an independent prognostic factor for outcome in this disease. Most recently, the mechanism of action of CD25 in *BCR/ABL^POS^* ALL was elucidated in detail [115]. The group of Markus Müschen [115] found that CD25 is a critical feedback regulator of the B-cell receptor (BCR) and a biomarker of tumor clones driven by oncogenic BCR mimics, including *BCR/ABL* and other *ABL1* fusion genes present in Ph-like ALL cases. This predicts that CD25-expressing B-cell malignancies may be sensitive to small-molecule inhibitors of the BCR signaling pathway (e.g., ibrutinib). In murine models for B-cell tumors, CD25 was crucial for the initiation of B-cell leukemia. Phosphorylation of the cytoplasmic tail of CD25 by protein kinase C δ (PKCδ) causes surface expression of CD25 which in turn coordinates a negative feedback by shuttling inhibitory phosphatases from the cytoplasm to the cell membrane (e.g., SHIP1). This recruitment of phosphatases stabilizes oncogenic tyrosine kinase signaling and mediates drug resistance. The mechanism of CD25 in BCR-driven lymphoid cells is illustrated in Fig. 15.3. Most importantly, CD25 inhibition sensitized CD25-expressing cells to conventional drug treatment. These preliminary data have

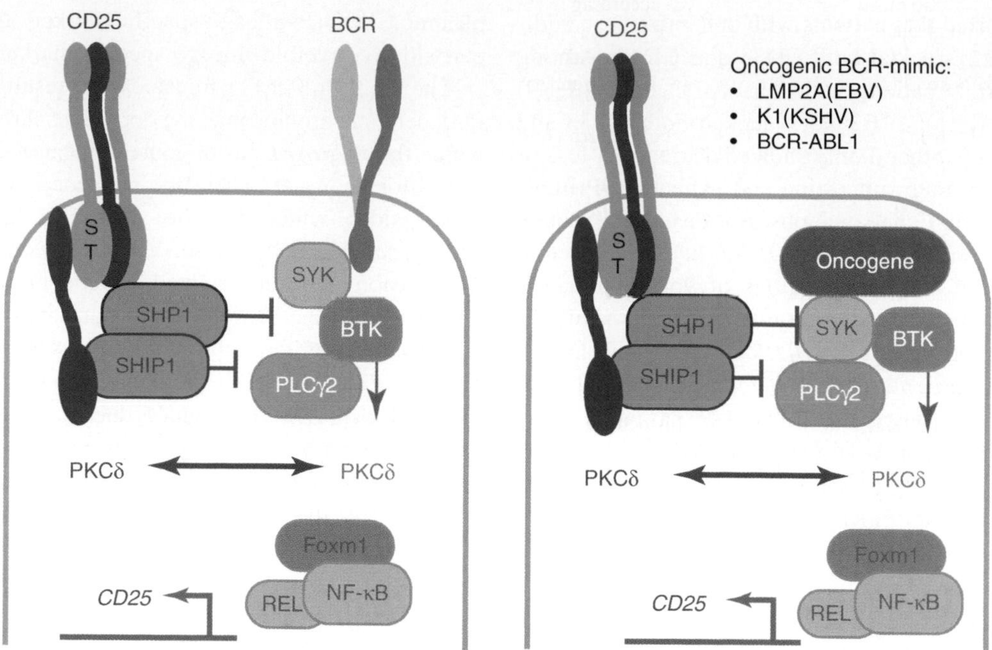

Fig. 15.3 *Left graph*: The left graph represents pre-B-cell receptor (BCR)-mediated signaling in normal B-cells. BCR signaling involves rapid activation of spleen tyrosine kinase (SYK), Bruton's tyrosine kinase (BTK), and phospholipase C γ-2 (PLCg2), which convert protein kinase C δ (PKCδ) from an inactive (*yellow*) to an activation state through phosphorylation (*blue*). Activated PCKδ (*blue*) is translocated from the cytoplasm to the plasma membrane. BCR also activates the proto-oncogene Foxm1, which encodes Forkhead box protein M1, and nuclear factor kappa B (NF-κB), a transcription factor which resides in the cytoplasm in an inactive complex. Müschen et al. have found that the genomic region of CD25 was occupied by several components of NF-κB, such as RELA and RELB, and able to interact with Foxm1. Once activated, NF-κB, and potentially also Foxm1, transcriptionally increases CD25 expression. Plasma membrane-located PKCδ (blue) recruits the newly synthesized CD25 to the cell surface via phosphorylation of the serine and threonine (ST) motif appended to the CD25 cytoplasmic tail. The now surface-located CD25 recruits phosphatases, such as Src homology region 2 domain-containing phosphatase-1 (SHP1) and phosphatidylinositol-3,4,5-triphosphate 5-phosphatase 1 (SHIP1), which counteract and stabilize BCR signaling. In normal pre-B- or B-cells, BCR signaling is transient and must be quelled by phosphatases such as SHP1 and SHIP1. *Right graph*: The right graph represents an ALL blast. ALL typically originates from pre-B-cells which critically depend on survival signals emanating from a functional pre-B-cell receptor (BCR). Oncogenes such as Epstein-Barr virus latent membrane protein 2A (LMP2A), the K1 protein of Kaposi's sarcoma-associated herpesvirus (K1), or BCR-ABL1 deregulate B-cell signal transduction by mimicking activated BCR. This "false" BCR signaling leads to constitutive activation of SYK, BTK, PLCg2, and NF-κB, which requires upregulation of surface CD25 expression via activation of PKCδ to stabilize signaling strength. With BCR mimics, BCR signaling is constitutive and excessive, a critical factor in the development of BCR-addicted leukemia and lymphoma (courtesy Dr. Markus Müschen)

led to a clinical trial using of ADCT-301, a human monoclonal antibody to CD25, linked to a pyrrolobenzodiazepine dimer toxin, in relapsed/refractory CD25^{POS} acute leukemias [NCT02588092]. As will be discussed later, CD25 also represents a most powerful prognostic factor in AML [32].

Though isolated case reports of *BCR/ABL^{POS}* ALL with T-lineage phenotype are still occasionally posted, all of the larger studies have reported that BCR/ABL rearrangements in pediatric and adult ALL are restricted to the B-cell lineage [31, 96, 116–118]. A substantial cohort of pediatric patients studied from various European groups found 3 T-ALLs among 61 *BCR/ABL^{POS}* patients [119]; unfortunately, no details were provided on the immunophenotypic diagnosis of those T-lineage cases, though it is apparent that cCD3 and cCD22 were not tested. The lack of demonstration of these lineage-specific antigens is the most likely reason for misdiagnosed *BCR/ABL^{POS}* T-cell phenotypes. A potential alternative cause is an apparent Philadelphia chromosome translocation by conventional karyotyping that does not yield the ABL-BCR juxtaposition on chromosome 9 [120]. While in the report by Fossa et al. [120] the leukemic phenotype was unequivocally T-lymphoid (cCD3^{POS}), an analogous case was seen in ECOG's E2993 trial, with a (9;22)(q34;q11.2) translocation that by FISH did not result in the *BCR/ABL* fusion but, as in Fossa's case, disrupted the *BCR* gene (ECOG Cytogenetics Committee, personal communication). The E2993 patient, however, expressed immunophenotypic features of pre-B-ALL. In summary, caution is definitely warranted when t(9;22)^{POS} or *BCR/ABL^{POS}* T-ALL cases are published.

t(4;11)(q22;q23)-*KMT2A (former MLL)/AF4^{POS}* B-Lineage ALL

The myeloid/lymphoid or mixed-lineage leukemia (*MLL*) gene has been renamed *KMT2A* gene, located at 11q23. *KMT2A* in humans encodes histone-lysine N-methyltransferase 2A. *KMT2A/AF4^{POS}* ALL is typically found in early infancy and also represents the most prevalent of the diverse *KMT2A* fusion genes in adult ALL [121–123]. Despite improved complete remission rates with modern treatments, overall survival in adults remains poor due to short remission duration [122–125]. There exists a striking difference in outcome by age group with the worst prognosis found in infants less than 6 months old as well as in adults [124]. *KMT2A/AF4^{POS}* ALL is associated with the immature pro/pre-pre-B-ALL maturation stage, defined by negativity for CD10. As a unique immunophenotypic feature among all ALL phenotypes, *KMT2A/AF4^{POS}* lymphoblasts show a tendency to express the more mature myeloid carbohydrate antigens, $CD65_{(S)}$ and $CD15_{(S)}$, while lacking CD33 and CD13, the pan-myeloid antigens expressed earlier in normal myelopoiesis [93, 123, 125, 126]. Overexpression of immature antigens, CD133 and CD135, further supports the immature state of this subtype [125]. On the other hand, CD33 and/or CD13 are found preferentially in CD10^{pos} early pre-B-ALL. Burmeister et al. [126] demonstrated that lymphoblasts from *KMT2*-rearranged adult ALL patients in general (55% with *KMT2A/AF4*) demonstrated significantly lower expression of CD10, CD33, and CD13 and more frequent expression of $CD65_{(S)}$ and $CD15_{(S)}$ irrespective of B-lineage differentiation stage. This report confirmed the observations from the E2993/UKALLXII trial [125]. Together with the myeloid antigen expression pattern in *BCR/ABL^{POS}*ALL, discussed before, these observations suggest that myeloid antigen expression in B-lineage ALL is determined by the underlying genetic defect rather than B-lymphoid developmental stage.

Cryptic t(12;21)(p13;q22)-*TEL(ETV6)/AML1(RUNX1)^{POS}* B-Lineage ALL

The cryptic (12;21)(p13;q22) translocation that results in the *TEL/AML1* fusion gene is the most common genetic aberration in pediatric ALL (>20%) and carries a favorable prognosis, especially with high-intensity therapy [127, 128]. In adults, this hybrid gene only accounts for <1–3% of ALL [95, 100, 129], thus precluding prognostic predictions. In children, the *TEL/AML1* fusion occurs exclusively in early pre-B-ALL with certain characteristic markers: high intensity of HLA-DR, CD40, and CD10 expression (early pre-B phenotype), commonly CD13^{POS} and/or CD33^{POS}, but CD9^{NEG}, CD20^{NEG}, and low expression of CD45, CD135, and CD86 [130–132]. A striking characteristic feature has recently been added, namely absence of CD11b, an integrin reported to confer poor response to therapy in B-lineage ALL [133]. Given the low incidence of *TEL/AML1^{POS}* ALL in adults, immunophenotypic information in this age group is scarce. The nine *TEL/AML1^{POS}* cases found among ECOG E2993 patients (1.4%) demonstrated the characteristic CD10^{POS} early pre-B phenotype, lacking CD20 and predominantly CD34, and frequently expressing CD33+CD13. However, in comparison to early pre-B-ALL with normal cytogenetics and molecularly negative for *TEL/AML1, BCR/ABL, MLL/AF4, and E2A/PBX1*, there was no difference in CD45, and the CD40 intensity was higher than the median value in normal karyotype controls in only half of the patients (Paietta E, unpublished observation). Although based on small numbers of patients, the most predictive immune profile applicable for both pediatric and adult *TEL/AML1^{POS}* B-lineage ALL, to date, is CD10^{POS}, CD20^{NEG}, CD34^{NEG}, cIgM^{NEG}, frequently CD33+CD13^{POS}, and possibly CD11b^{NEG}.

Inv(7)(p15q34) and t(7;7)(p15;q34)-*TRB@/HOXA*

As a result of two cryptic cytogenetic aberrations, inv(7)(p15q34) or t(7;7)(p15;q34), the TCRB locus (*TRB@*) at 7q34 is juxtaposed to the *HOXA@* at 7p15 (approximately <5% of pediatric and adult T-ALL), leading to transcriptional activation of several *HOXA* genes [134, 135]. The typical antigen expression patterns associated with the *TRB@/HOXA* rearrangement include negativity for CD2 and single expression of CD4, without CD8. It is important to emphasize that among surface antigens, CD7 is the only T-cell antigen universally expressed by T-cell lymphoblasts.

Antigens and Antigen Profiles Associated with Prognostic Gene Expression

FLT3 Mutations in AML

The *FLT3* gene encodes CD135, the FMS-like tyrosine kinase 3 (FLT-3) or receptor-type tyrosine-protein kinase FLT3, a cytokine receptor which belongs to the type 3 receptor tyrosine kinases and is expressed on the surface of normal hematopoietic progenitors and the leukemic blasts of most cases of AML. Upon binding of the FLT3 ligand, the receptor undergoes dimerization and subsequent autophosphorylation of the tyrosine kinase domains, leading to the induction of multiple intracellular signaling pathways involved in cell growth, differentiation, and survival [136]. There are two major clusters of mutations of the FMS-like tyrosine kinase-3 (*FLT3*) gene, those in the juxtamembrane domain that lead to internal tandem duplications (ITD) and point mutations in the tyrosine kinase domain (TKD. Both result in the activation of the transforming potential of *FLT3* [136, 137]. Activating mutations of the *FLT3* gene are the most common known genetic abnormalities in pediatric and adult AML, with *FLT3-ITD* found in approximately 20–35% of adults and 15% in children (ranging from 1.5% in infants to 20% at teenage age), while *FLT3-TKD* are present in about 7% of AML irrespective of age group. With respect to cytogenetic links, distinct differences are seen between *FLT3-ITDs* and *FLT3-TKDs*; *FLT3-ITDs* are particularly frequent in AML with normal cytogenetics, while *FLT3-TKDs* frequently occur in cases with inv(16)-*CBFβ/MYH11*. Both types of mutations are found in a large percentage of t(15;17)-*PML/RARα* APL with minimal impact on outcome, if treated according to modern strategies [138, 139]. In non-APL AML, the suggested negative clinical implications for *FLT3*-

ITD (e.g., increased relapse rate) vary with therapeutic intensities, allelic ratio (mutational burden), and size of ITD, and according to its genetic context [140, 141]. *FLT3-TKDs*, on the other hand, failed to confer unfavorable prognosis [142]; in fact, patients with high-level mutations (more than 25% mutant) experienced improved outcome [143]. The introduction of novel FLT3 inhibitors will certainly change the prognostic outlook of patients with FLT3 gene alterations [144].

The earliest description of a unique immunophenotype for *FLT3-ITD*^{POS} AML suggested a combination of increased CD123, decreased CD38, "mildly" decreased CD117, and loss of CD133 [145]. Subsequently, the same authors described the distinctive, cuplike nuclear morphology in *FLT3-ITD*^{POS} AML (which was discussed before) in association with loss of HLA-DR, CD34, and CD133 [73]. Falini et al. reported this paired absence of CD34/CD133 in *NPM1*-mutated AML in their groundbreaking publication in 2005 [146]. The frequent association of *FLT3-ITD* with *NPM1* mutations [114, 140, 141], therefore, suggests that the lack of CD34 and CD133 in *FLT3-ITD*^{POS} AML may be the result of the concomitant presence of mutated *NPM1*. Gönen et al. [32] reported that CD123 expression, but not CD34 or CD133, was significantly higher in CD25^{POS} AML which demonstrated a characteristic genotype of triple *FLT3-ITD/NPM1/DNMT3A* mutations. Co-association of *FLT3-ITD* with *DNMT3A* and *NPM1* mutations is well established [14, 147]. In mice, concurrent expression of *FLT3-ITD*, mutated *DNMT3A*, and mutated *NPM1* resulted in a fully penetrant leukemic phenotype, whereas any single or paired alleles led to incompletely penetrant disease [148]. Angelini et al. [149] also reported the combined expression of CD123 and CD25 as characteristic for *FLT3-ITD*^{POS} AML and, added CD99 (MIC-), a potential LSC marker, highly expressed in the LSC-enriched CD34^{POS}/CD38^{NEG} fraction compared to the bulk of blasts [150]. CD25^{POS} *FLT3-ITD*^{POS} AML patients on phase 3 trial E1900 [NCT00049517] had a significantly shorter overall survival than CD25^{NEG} FLT3-ITD^{POS} patients, whose survival did not differ from that of the *FLT3*-wild-type cohort [32].

FLT3-ITD^{POS} T-Lineage ALL

The rare subtype of CD117^{POS} T-lineage ALL with activating *FLT3* gene mutations [65, 151] belongs to the few known examples of gene mutations, which are predicted by the presence of a unique antigen expression pattern.

In pediatric ALL, *FLT3-TKDs* are common in cases with *KMT2A/MLL* rearrangements and those with hyperdiploid karyotype, while *FLT3* length mutations are extremely rare; still, high levels of FLT3 protein expression provide a target for therapeutic intervention [136, 140, 152, 153]. While in infant *KMT2A/MLL*-rearranged ALLs the presence of a *FLT3* mutation negatively affected outcome, there was no such effect seen in hyperdiploid cases [152]. *FLT3* mutations are even rarer in adult ALL. The analysis of ECOG study E2993 revealed an incidence of 1.9% *FLT3-ITD* among 511 patients [151]. Of the ten E2993 *FLT3-ITD*^{POS} patients, three belonged to the B- and the remaining seven to the T-cell lineage. No consistent immunophenotypic or cytogenetic features were shared by the three early pre-B patients. On the other hand, all *FLT3-ITD*^{POS} T-ALLs expressed a unique immunophenotype: CD5^{NEG}; surface CD3^{NEG}CD4^{NEG}CD8^{NEG} (triple-negative); positive for CD117, CD34, CD2, CD7, TdT, CD62L, CD13, CD135 (FLT3 protein); and positive for T-cell lineage-specific cCD3 [65]. CD117, the stem cell factor receptor, is much more frequently expressed by leukemic myeloblasts than lymphoblasts [154, 155]. In normal lymphopoiesis, a fraction of CD3/CD4/CD8-triple-negative CD34^{POS} thymocytes express high levels of CD117 [156, 157]. In these thymocytes, expression of CD117 coincides with that of CD135, the FLT3 receptor tyrosine kinase [136, 158]. Occasionally, up to 10% of cCD3^{POS}CD117^{POS}*FLT3-ITD*^{POS} blasts expressed myeloperoxidase, thus representing truly biphenotypic features [65]. This profile fits the most immature category of T-ALL [159–161], resembling earliest thymic precursors with both T- and myeloid lineage potential [162]. In further support of a T-lineage affiliation, FLT3-mutated T-lymphoblasts overexpressed *LYL1* and *LMO2* oncogenes [160]. In pediatric T-ALL, the LYL1-overexpressing, most immature cases demonstrate relative resistance to standard chemotherapy [160]. To the contrary, the *FLT3-ITD*^{POS}CD117^{POS}CD13^{POS} T-cell phenotype in adults does not carry inferior prognosis, though numbers were small [151]. This observation is remarkable given the negative prognostic impact of CD13 expression in CD117^{NEG} adult T-lineage ALL [151]. Neumann et al. [163] subsequently confirmed the CD2^{POS}/CD5^{NEG}/CD13^{POS}/CD33^{NEG} phenotype as a surrogate for mutated *FLT3* in T-cell ALL. They expanded the distinct gene expression pattern (aberrant expression of *IGFBP7*, *WT1*, *GATA3*) and mutational status (absence of *NOTCH1* mutations and a low frequency, 21%, of clonal TCR rearrangements). Despite the low frequency of *FLT3* gene mutations in adult ALL overall, the availability of a variety of FLT3-kinase inhibitors suggests a potential targeted approach in the treatment of this patient cohort. The potential of targeted therapy is the clinically important aspect in this ALL subtype and should supersede any discussions as to whether *FLT3*-mutated T-ALL represents a biphenotypic leukemia or an example for MPAL T/myeloid as defined by the WHO classification [9].

Van Vlierberghe et al. [164] reported that in pediatric T-ALL CD117 mRNA (not protein) expression was not invariably associated with *FLT3* gene mutations in that most pediatric cases expressed CD117 mRNA; this suggests that, similar to what has been reported for myeloperoxidase transcripts [165], CD117 mRNA might undergo posttranscriptional downregulation in ALL. Immunophenotypic profiles of the two pediatric *FLT3-ITD*^{POS} T-ALL patients identified by Van Vlierberghe et al. [164] were surface CD3^{NEG} but CD5^{POS}CD4^{POS} with partial CD13 expression. Furthermore, the authors stated that these blasts carried a "*HOX11L2* translocation," presumably leading to aberrant HOX11L2 expression. Taken together, these findings suggest arrest at an immature, though already single, CD4^{pos} differentiation level, distinct from the triple-negative stage seen in the adult cases [65]. Remarkably, another pediatric T-ALL case with *FLT3-ITD*, the only one among 59 children tested, identified by Ferrando et al. [160] belonged to the LYL^{POS} cluster, consistent with the findings in the adult cases.

Hoehn et al. concluded that the absence of CD117 expression in T-ALL precluded the presence of *FLT3* mutations, whereas the positive predictive value of CD117 for mutated *FLT3* was only 35% [166]. CD117^{pos} T-ALL lacking *FLT3* gene mutations were found in 2% of patients on E2993 [93]. Aside from CD117, their immunophenotype differed from that in *FLT3-ITD*^{POS} cases subtly but distinctly: the T-lymphoblasts expressed CD5, occasionally were single CD8^{POS}, frequently expressed CD33 instead of CD13, often were CD56^{POS}, and commonly lacked CD34 and CD62L, both markers of immaturity. A close association between CD117 and CD13 expression in surface CD3^{NEG} T-ALL has been previously reported [167]. Thus, while CD117 expression in adult T-lineage ALL might be considered a surrogate marker for *FLT3* gene mutations, this concept only applies for T-lymphoblasts arrested at the most immature stage of differentiation.

CD117^{POS}/*FLT3-ITD*^{POS} T-ALL represents a subtype of early T-cell precursor (ETP) leukemia, which, particularly in adults, has been demonstrated to be widely heterogeneous both in immunophenotype and genetic alterations [168–172].

Early T-cell Precursor (ETP) Leukemia

ETP ALL was initially characterized solely based on its immunophenotypic features, CD1a^{NEG}CD8^{NEG}CD5^{WEAK} with myeloid (e.g., CD33, CD13, CD11b, or CD65), and stem cell markers (e.g., CD34 and CD117), suggesting that this leukemia subtype may be part of a spectrum called stem-cell-like leukemias [173]. The name ETP was given to these leukemias because their immunophenotype appeared closely related to that of early T-cell precursors which retain their multilineage differentiation potential [162, 174, 175]. ETP-T-ALL accounts for approximately 10–15% of pediatric T-ALL [170] but has a much higher prevalence of 50% in adult T-ALL in some studies [168] but not others [176]. Though early data suggested that this subtype of T-ALL carried a very poor prognosis [173, 176–178], more recent results are encouraging [179–181].

Genetic alterations fueling ETP-ALL suggest that this leukemia has more in common with AML than with other types of ALL [168–170, 172, 182]. ETP-ALLs contain mutations in myeloid-specific oncogenes and tumor-suppressor genes, including *IDH1, IDH2, DNMT3A, FLT3, GATA3, ETV6*, and *NRAS*. On the other hand, ETP-ALLs showed a low incidence of alterations commonly seen in T-ALL, such as activating mutations in the *IL7R* gene and *NOTCH1*, while approximately 25% demonstrated co-occurrence of myeloid and T-typical mutations. In an analysis of ECOG trial E2993, Van Vlierberghe et al. [33] found that in these ETP-ALLs, mutations in *IDH1/IDH2* and *DNMT3A* were associated with poor prognosis. As much as ETP-ALL represents a grey zone with respect to its genetic affilations, it presents a challenge to us flow cytometrists. How many cases of ETP-ALL are indeed enrolled on AML treatment protocol because they were diagnosed as AML based on antigen profile? It has been suggested that ETP-ALL may benefit from myeloid therapy, though we will never get the answer to this if we do not establish a clear guideline for the immunophenotypic diagnosis of this subtype. I would like to suggest the following: any case with expression of surface CD7, CD2, and intracytoplasmic CD3; absence or weak surface expression of CD5; lack of surface CD3; expression of CD34, CD13, and/or CD33; and whether or not CD117 or myeloperoxidase are found should be considered ETP-ALL.

Whether or not an ETP ALL patient should be treated as ALL or AML is currently unclear. ALL COG study AALL0434 (NCT00408005) suggested that there was no difference in outcome between ETP, near-ETP, and not-ETP patients, whereby the distinction of near-ETP was based on elevated CD5 expression in otherwise ETP patients [179]. Induction failure, based on >25% blasts by morphology at the end of induction, was significantly higher in ETP and near-ETP patients. Day 29 bone marrow MRD levels of >0.01% were present in 81.4%, 64.8%, and 30.5% of ETP, near-ETP, and not-ETP patients. Day 29 MRD levels were used for risk stratification, whereby intermediate- (MRD <1%) and high-risk patients (MRD >1%) were randomized to receive or not receive nelarabine, delayed intensification, and maintenance. With this MRD-targeted approach, ETP patients had outcome identical to not-ETP patients.

However, there is the caveat when interpreting this study in that the immunophenotypic analysis for ETP-ALL status on AALL0434 was not completely assessed for all patients [183]. But can we solely rely on immunophenotypic features in defining ETP-ALL? Retrospective analyses of T-ALL samples with ETP-gene signature have not consistently been found to express the ETP-ALL immunophenotype [184, 185]. But what is the best way to identify ETP-ALL, or more importantly ETP-ALL with poor outcome? [186]. Bond et al. [187] reported that deregulation of homeobox (*HOX*) factor A was highly predictive of phenotypic immaturity, glucocorticoid resistance, and early treatment failure in T-ALL. However, while the entire *HOX*-activated group did not have an inferior outcome, poor prognosis was restricted to those patients who also had an ETP-like immunophenotype. Vice versa, ETP-ALL patients without *HOXA*-activation fared equally well as non-ETP patients. A subset analysis of AALL0434 [183], which included 10 patients who had failed induction therapy, corroborated the notion that *HOXA*-activated ETP-ALL, frequently acquired in *MLL (KMT2A)*-rearranged cases, is associated with induction failure, refractory disease, and relapse. Unfortunately, the detection of *HOX*-activated ETP-ALL carries its own pitfalls.

To date, alternative treatment options for ETP-ALL are limited. One could foresee, however, that a precision medicine approach be suggested in the near future, e.g., using a histone methyltransferase inhibitor to target *HOX* gene expression [188]. A phase 1 trial using EPZ-5676, an inhibitor of the DOT1-like histone H3 methyltransferase, in relapsed/refractory leukemia with *KMT2A* rearrangements has recently been completed (NCT02141828). So, when the time comes and a precise definition of ETP-ALL is important for targeted therapy, the burden will be in part on the flow cytometrist, the first one who could raise a suspicion of ETP-ALL in a new case of leukemia.

Association of T-ALL Differentiation Stages with Gene Expression

The changes brought about in the classification of T-cell ALL over the last 15 years have been dramatic, considering that where we started from was a mere distinction between CD2^{POS} and CD2^{NEG} T-ALL. In 2002, Ferrando et al. published gene expression signatures in pediatric T-ALLs which correlated with leukemic arrest at specific stages of normal thymocyte differentiation [160]. This elegant model was based on the unique, aberrant expression of oncogenic transcription factors in T-ALLs as a result of chromosomal translocations which typically juxtapose strong promoter and enhancer elements associated with *TCR* genes to a finite number of T-cell transcription factors. This T-ALL classification distinguished the early immature double-negative CD4^{NEG}CD8^{NEG}surface CD3^{NEG} stage with overexpression of transcription factor *LYL1* and *LMO2*, which corresponds to ETP-ALL with a transcriptional program related to hematopietic stem cells and specific genetic aberrations, as previously discussed. In contrast, the early cortical stage is characteristically CD1a^{POS} CD4^{POS}CD8^{POS}CD3^{WEAK}CD10^{POS} and frequently associated with cytogenetic translocations inducing activation of the *TLX1/HOX11* family of homeobox transcription factor oncogenes. Finally, the late cortical CD4^{POS}CD8^{POS}CD3^{HIGH} CD2^{POS}TCR^{POS} stage shows expression of the TAL1 transcription factor oncogenes. All of these stages precede that of mature single positive with either surface CD4 or CD8 expression. Constitutive expression of *TLX1/HOX11* has been associated with favorable prognosis in pediatric and adult T-lineage ALL [160, 189–191]. In the analysis of a large series of adult T-ALL enrolled on E2993 [151] all cases were tested for cCD3 and myeloperoxidase. Aside from cCD3, only surface CD7 was universally present. Attempts to stratify patients according to their maturation stage based on expression of CD3, CD2, or CD34, as suggested by the WHO classification system [9], failed to provide prognostic subsets. While the myeloid antigens CD13 and/or CD33 were found in approximately half of the patients, the carbohydrate antigens, CD65$_{(S)}$ and CD15$_{(S)}$, were detected in a minority of cases. The entire patient cohort could be divided into two prognostic subsets based on CD1a and CD13 expression: CD1a^{POS} T-ALL predominantly lacked CD34, CD13/CD33, and CD11b. These T-lymphoblasts, representative of intrathymic differentiation, frequently expressed the CD62L selectin and CD10, and were double positive for CD4 and CD8. CD1a^{POS} T-ALL did exceedingly well with an overall survival at 5 years of 64% (95% CI 48–80%). The other subtype with clinical significance was CD13^{POS} T-ALL. While the complete remission rate was similar to that of CD13^{NEG} patients, overall survival at 5 years was significantly shorter than for CD13^{NEG} patients ($p=0.0005$). CD13^{POS} or double-CD13/CD33^{POS} T-lymphoblasts preferentially expressed CD34 and CD11b and showed a tendency to be negative for CD4, CD8, surface CD3, or CD2. CD117^{POS} T-ALL was diagnosed in 18% of patients. Only 6/107 patients with unequivocal staining for cCD3 and negativity for cCD22 expressed CD19, occasionally in combination with CD10. Of potential interest, merely 17% of these patients survived for 5 years. In a follow-up analysis, Van Vlierberghe et al. [33] performed microarray gene expression profiling of these immunophenotypically characterized patients and described two clusters. The first corresponded to early immature leukemia (ETP) with a gene expression signature related to that of hematopoietic stem cells and myeloid progenitors. In contrast, the second cluster contained leukemias with gene expression signatures of cortical and mature thymocytes. Overall, the immature cohort was associated with poor prognosis and reduced overall survival compared with cortical/mature T-ALL ($p = 0.0112$). Notably, the poor prognostic effect of CD13 expression was restricted to the cortical/mature T-ALL, thus identifying a high-risk subgroup in an otherwise good prognosis subtype.

NPM1-Mutated AML

The *NPM1*-mutated AML subtype is characterized by high frequency of *FLT3-ITD*, association with normal karyotype, negativity for both CD34 and CD133, and good prognosis, especially in the absence of *FLT3ITD* [75]. Other reports have suggested additions and/or modifications to this phenotype. Nomdedeu et al. [192] concluded that the majority of cases showed high expression of CD33, CD13, HLA-DR, and CD123, and myelomonocytic traits in the morphologic appearance. On the other hand, Kern et al. [193] suggested high expression of myeloperoxidase and CD33 but lack of CD13, CD65, CD15, HLA-DR, and CD34, combined with minimal differentiation in 20 cases of *NPM1*-mutated AML. The rare immunophwnotypic subset of *NPM1*-mutated/*FLT3-ITD*^{POS} normal karyotype AML with dual-CD7/CD19 expression [58] presents with surprisingly high CD34 expression, higher than found in *NPM1*-mutated/*FLT3-ITD*^{POS}AML without this antigen profile or *NPM1*-mutated AML without *FLT3-ITD*. An informal analysis of the incidence of CD34^{POS} myeloblasts in 105 cases of *NPM1*-mutated AMLs suggested greater variability than previously appreciated with the percentage of CD34^{POS} blasts ranging from 0 to 99% (Paietta et al., unpublished observation). Taken together, these reports suggest that the immuneprofile of *NPM1*-mutated AML is not as homogenous as previously thought. Along the same line, LICs in *NPM1*-mutated AML have been located both in CD34^{POS} and CD34^{NEG} stem cell fractions [7]. Martelli et al. [194] reported that CD34^{POS} cells from *NPM1*-mutated cases harbored aberrant nucleophospmin expression in the cytoplasm. The *NPM1*-mutated gene and/or protein was also confirmed in the CD34^{POS} subfraction which expressed a stem cell-like phenotype, CD34^{POS}, CD38^{NEG}, CD123^{POS}, CD33^{POS}, and CD90^{NEG}. When transplanted into immunecompromised mice, these CD34^{POS} cells generated a leukemia indistinguishable from the original disease with *NPM1*-mutated CD34^{NEG} myeloblasts, suggesting that the CD34^{POS} cell fraction in *NPM1*-mutated leukemia contains cells with LIC properties.

BCR/ABL1-like or Ph-like B-lineage ALL

Just like T-lineage ALL, B-lineage ALL has undergone a major reclassification with strong prognostic and therapeutic implications. FAB classification of ALL has become obsolete [9, 47]. The standard subclassification of B-lineage ALL based on maturation stages lacks prognostic significance with modern chemotherapy [195]. The associations between level of maturation and major genetic subtype in B-lineage ALL have been discussed earlier for the historic genetic defects, *BCR/ABL, MLL/AF4,* and *TEL/AML1*. *E2A/PBX1* (now called *TCF3/PBX1*) transcripts, derived from the (1;19)(q23;p13) translocation, are more commonly associated with more mature pre-B ALL, characterized by the presence of intracytoplasmic IgM heavy chains. This subtype was previously considered as high risk, but is no longer included into the risk stratification as a result of modern treatment regimens [196]. It is difficult to distinguish mature B-ALL from the leukemic phase of Burkitt's lymphoma, as they share immunophenotypic features, clinical presentation, and cytogenetic abnormalities. In the prototype (8;14)(q24;q32) translocation, the c-myc proto-oncogene is translocated from chromosome 8 onto chromosome 14 and brought under the transcriptional control of the immunoglobulin heavy-chain locus. The variant translocations, t(2;8)(p12;q24) and t(8;22)(q24;q11), result in the positioning of portions of the κ and λ light chains, respectively, under the control of myc.

The revolution in B-lineage ALL classification started with the finding of alterations of the lymphoid transcription factor gene *IKZF1* (IKAROS) in B-ALL [170, 182]. *IKZF1* deletions and somatic mutations are the hallmark of *BCR/ABL*^{POS} ALL and confer poor prognosis in this disease [197–199]. Recently, Iacobucci et al. described surface expression of CD90 as a marker for *IKZF1* alterations in *BCR/ABL*^{POS} ALL [200]. CD90/Thy1 is a marker of hematopoietic stem cells [201]. In combination with surface CD25 expression [17, 31, 101], CD90 analysis affords the flow cytometrist to reliably predict the presence of *BCR/ABL* transcripts in B-ALL. As we discuss below, it is essential to exclude CRLF2-overexpressing *BCR/ABL1*-like ALL, which can present with both CD90 and CD25 expression [Paietta E, unpublished observation]. Noteworthy, however, neither CD25 nor CD90 will be expressed in a small percentage of *BCR/ABL*^{POS} patients, those with superior outcome [31]. The same is true for other immunophenotypic features published as associated with *BCR/ABL*^{POS} ALL, such as high CD34 and low CD38 expression and dual expression of CD13 and CD33 [98–100]. While in a case with B-lineage ALL, an immune profile with expression of both CD25 and CD90 and absence of CRLF2 expression, is highly predictive for the presence of *BCR/ABL* transcripts, I always advise to run the *BCR/ABL* PCR assay to confirm the immunophenotypic findings, if at all possible.

IKZF1 can also be deleted in *BCR/ABL*^{NEG} B-ALL, likewise associated with inferior outcome [199, 202]. Many of these *BCR/ABL*^{NEG}, *IKZF1*-mutated cases exhibit a gene expression profile similar to that of *BCR/ABL*^{POS} ALL with novel kinase-activating mutations (e.g., *JAK2, ABL1, PDGFRB, CSF1R*) or genetic alterations in signaling pathways (e.g., *EPOR, IL7R, SH2B3*), giving birth to the novel subtype of *BCR/ABL1*-like ALL (Ph-like ALL), which is incorporated into recent WHO revisions as a provisional category [13]. With continuously extended sequencing, the full repertoire of kinase-activating lesions and other rearrangements in Ph-like ALL awaits to be identified. Ph-like ALL has been characterized independently by two groups [199, 203]. Characteristically, these patients show high levels of MRD after induction and overall poor outcome. MRD-guided, risk-directed therapy, including allogeneic transplantation, may be able to abolish the adverse prognostic significance of Ph-like ALL, at least in children [204]. However, a recent report from German Multicenter ALL Working Group (GMALL) trials 06/99 and 07/03 suggested that adult Ph-like ALL patients, although they achieve complete hematologic remission (CR), relapse very rapidly after induction therapy, thus precluding stem cell transplantation in first CR, as had been stipulated in the protocols [205]. Fortunately, there are exciting genomic and preclinical findings which suggest that many patients with Ph-like ALL could be successfully treated with currently available lesion-specific kinase inhibitors [170, 182, 206, 207]. Tasian et al. [207] demonstrated the need for combinatorial treatment strategies which hit or ablate an entire multifaceted pathway affected in these patients using patient-derived xenograft models. About 15% of children present with Ph-like ALL and, just like with *BCR/ABL*^{POS} ALL, the incidence of Ph-like

ALL showed increase with age in a large study across various National Cancer Treatment Network groups in the USA [19]. In contrast, GMALL investigators reported the peak of Ph-like ALL among adolescents and young adults and a dramatic decrease in the incidence of Ph-like ALL with more advanced age [208].

Of utmost relevance to flow cytometrists, approximately 50% of Ph-like ALL patients harbor a rearrangement of *CRLF2* (cytokine receptor-like factor 2 or thymic stromal lymphopoietin receptor), either as an *IGH@-CRLF2* rearrangement or a focal deletion proximal to *CRLF2* that results in expression of the *P2RY8-CRLF2* fusion, both causing overexpression of *CRLF2* on the surface of the leukemic cells [209, 210]. Half of *CRLF2*-rearranged cases harbor concomitant activating *JAK1/2* mutations [209–211], and *CRLF2*-rearranged cases exhibit constitutively active JAK-STAT signaling and activation of the P13K/mTOR pathway making them sensitive to JAK mTOR inhibitors [170]. It is important to realize that CRLF2 overexpression occurs only in B-ALL cases which lack rearrangements of *TEL, MLL (KMT2A), TCF3*, and *BCR/ABL*. Rare cases of *CRLF2* overexpressing ALL patients without the molecular features of the Ph-like phenotype have been seen predominantly in children (Roberts K, personal communication). There are inconsistent data on the prognosis of *CRLF2*-rearranged Ph-like ALL cases [30, 212–214]. Whatever the prognostic power of CRLF2 overexpression, these patients may be treated with biologic treatment strategies and spared a stem cell transplant. Thus, the recognition of these cases is important and it is possible using a monoclonal antibody to CRLF2. This antibody must be included into any antibody panel used routinely by clinical laboratories in the evaluation of B-cell leukemias.

Antigens and Therapy

Acute leukemias provide a suitable testing environment for therapy with antibodies, which represent drugs with a clearly defined target, the specific antigen. There are several aspects to antigens and antibodies and their usefulness in therapy. Selected expression of antigens by leukemic cells is a first prerequisite. In the majority of cases, antibodies to antigens expressed by the leukemic cells are administered in in vivo treatment. Recently, adoptive immunotherapy with autologous chimeric antigen receptor-engineered T-cells (CAR-T-cells) has become a major focus of leukemia therapy, particularly in ALL. Antibodies are being incorporated into first-line therapies, to eliminate MRD, or during salvage attempts in relapsed/refractory patients [215–221]. Undoubtedly, with the documented benefits of antibody therapy, particularly in ALL, and ongoing optimization of CAR-T-cell therapy, antigen-specific immunotherapy strongly contributes to targeted or personalized therapy, thereby changing the paradigm of treatment of the acute leukemias.

Treatment with Monoclonal Antibodies

In vivo therapy with monoclonal antibodies aims at a specific antigen, which otherwise may be a part of a very diverse immunophenotype. Targeted delivery of these agents based on recognition of their relevant antigen on the surface of the leukemic cells improves efficacy and, optimally, minimizes off-target toxicity, provided that antigen distribution in normal tissues is well known (cytotoxic effects may be more widespread than intended). While there is a plethora of potential antibody targets on leukemic cells, only a select few have emerged as clinically successful. Reasons are multiple and include specificity of antigen expression on target tissue (i.e., the leukemic cell) and the question whether the target antigen is expressed by the LIC in individual patients. Monoclonal antibodies can be used naked, in unconjugated form (e.g., rituximab) and exert their effect via various mechanisms, including antibody-dependent or complement-dependent cytotoxicity or induction of apoptosis. Alternatively, conjugated antibodies are used, whereby they function as vehicles carrying immunotoxins or chemotherapeutic agents (e.g., calicheamicin-conjugated CD33 antibody), which requires knowledge that the target is internalized upon binding of the antibody [222]. Radioimmunotherapy, which adds radiobiological cytotoxicity to immunologic cytotoxicity by using monoclonal antibodies (e.g., CD45, CD33, CD22) conjugated to radioactive molecules, has been tested in AML or ALL, predominantly for its efficacy in intensifying the antileukemic effects of conditioning regimens prior to various types of stem cell transplantation [223]. T-cell engaging bi-specific antibodies use the host's cytotoxic T-cells to eliminate leukemic cells [215, 216, 219, 224].

CD20 Antibodies in B-ALL

In B-lineage ALL, CD20 expression depends on the maturation stage of malignant B-lymphoblasts with CD10^{NEG} pro-B/pre-pre-B lymphoblasts generally lacking CD2 [125], while CD20 expression by CD10^{POS} early pre-B-ALL blasts is variable [226]. But even when expressed, antigen density is usually quite low [110, 225]. Importantly, both the percentage of CD20^{POS} blasts and the intensity of staining are greatly affected by the choice of fluorochrome used in CD20 antibody binding in that CD20 antibody conjugated to fluorescein isothiocyanate (FITC) will yield much lower numbers than CD20 antibody conjugated to phycoerythrin (PE). This important information is not paid attention to in publications regarding the prognosis of CD20 expression in B-lineage ALL or the result of rituximab treatment [215, 216, 227]. Since the report of the trial, the Group for Research on Adult Acute Lymphoblastic Leukemia 2005 (GRAALL 2005), on rituximab in *BCR/ABL*^{NEG} CD20^{POS} B-lineage ALL at the plenary session of the American Society of Hematology meeting in 2015 and recently published in the New England Journal of Medicine [228], the addition of rituximab to the treatment of ALL has been accepted as standard of care. In this seminal trial, patients with <20% CD20^{POS} blasts were excluded and only those with at least 20% CD20^{POS} blasts were assigned to rituximab treatment or not. In this setting, and giving rituximab to all treatment phases, the rituximab group showed improved event-free survival and a reduction in the cumulative incidence of relapse when compared to the control group. Of note, CR rates were identical and MRD levels post-induction were comparable in the two groups suggesting that rituximab addition to induction therapy did not improve the quality of response. This is in contrast to the results of the GMALL Study 07/2003 [229] which also showed a comparable morphologic CR rate between patients treated with rituximab and those not receiving the antibody but in which the MRD load, measured by PCR, reduced significantly faster in the rituximab group. Interestingly, Thomas et al. [230] found that the benefit of rituximab addition to hyperCVAD therapy did not extent to patients ≥60 years old, suggesting that the high-risk features (e.g., unfavorable cytogenetics) more often encountered in the older patient population cannot be overcome with rituximab. Despite an upper age limit of 59 years, Maury et al. [228] also observed that older age remained significantly associated with shorter event-free survival in the rituximab group.

Unfortunately, in all of these studies, the definition of CD20 positivity was based on the arbitrary cutoff point of 20% CD20^{POS} blasts. There is no biologic basis for using a 20% cutoff level; this custom simply refers to a time when blast cells were not gated based on CD45 intensity and other means and the 20% threshold was used to account for contaminating normal cells [231]. Second, the choice of fluorochrome used in the CD20 conjugate is essential information. It is the common experience of flow cytometrists that CD20-FITC will yield fewer CD20^{POS} blasts than CD20-PE. This is particularly obvious in chronic lymphocytic leukemia (CLL) where the leukemic B-cells express CD20 at significantly lower density than normal B-lymphocytes. As a result CD20-FITC staining on B-CLL cells is frequently too weak for accurate quantification [232]. These comments do not advise against the use of CD20 in B-lineage ALL, they merely emphasize the importance of cautiously selecting fluorochromes and knowing the consequences of the particular selection. However, in clinical trials which use a certain threshold of antigen expression to leukemic cells to trigger the use of in vivo therapy with the relevant antibody, it is imperative to declare which fluorochrome was, is, or should be used to establish that threshold of antibody binding. Ideally, a trial should be designed to give rituxan to all patients with B-lineage ALL, irrespective of their CD20 expression which should be measured using various CD20 conjugates simultaneously; subsequently, a retrospective response-driven analysis would define the prognostically significant CD20 expression level with the various CD20 fluorochromes. UKALL14 (NCT01085617), conducted by the UK NCRI Adult ALL group, is a randomized trial which adds rituximab to the treatment of B-lineage ALL irrespective of the level of CD20 expression and the correlation of response with CD20 expression will be of great interest. There is evidence that the effectiveness of rituximab correlates with the level of CD20 expression by target tissues, at least in chronic B-cell leukemias [233]. In fact, Maury et al. [228] observed a more pronounced effect of rituximab in patients with higher CD20 expression. Dworzak et al. [225] found that a cutoff value for CD20 positivity at diagnosis of 20% was insufficient to predict rituximab-induced complement cytolysis of pediatric B-lymphoblasts in vitro. These investigators also reported upregulation of CD20 expression in a significant portion of patients by glucocorticoids as early as on day 8 of therapy. Stimulation of CD20 expression has also been reported with histone deacetylase inhibitors (e.g., valproic acid), demethylating agents (e.g., azacytidine), and farnesyltransferase inhibitors [234]. On the other hand, other therapies have been found to down-modulate CD20 expression (e.g., lenalidomide, bortezomib) [234]. Rituximab binding itself leads to the depletion of CD20-expressing B-cells which, just as up- and downregulation of the molecule, occurs through a variety of mechanisms [234]. In addition to surface CD20 expression, other factors may influence the clinical benefits of rituximab treatment and contribute to antibody resistance [235]. All of these considerations further question the use of arbitrary or any cutoff points of CD20^{POS} B-lymphoblasts for defining CD20 positivity, at least with respect to the decision to add rituximab to a treatment regimen. Biologic differences between patients may also account for the inconsistent data on the prognostic significance of CD20 expression in B-lineage ALL [236–240]. Similar to early findings in pediatric B-lineage ALL [241], our analysis of the adult E2993 trial found progressively higher intensity of CD20 staining, but not the percentage of CD20-expressing B-lymphoblasts, to be associated with increasingly reduced 5-year event-free survival [Paietta E, unpublished].

Second-generation CD20 antibodies, such as obinutuzumab [242], which act through mechanisms of action different from that of rituximab, have shown activity in rituximab-resistant patients [215, 216, 227]. Of potential importance with all anti-CD20 antibodies is the occurrence of soluble CD20 antigen, since high levels of circulating soluble antigens reduce the bioavailability and thus efficacy of administered antibody [243].

CD22 Antibodies in B-ALL

In contrast to CD20, CD22 is equally expressed across all maturation stages of B-lineage ALL [244, 245]. CD22 belongs to sialic-acid-binding immunoglobulin-like lectins (siglecs), which are endocytic receptors. As a result, cytotoxic agents conjugated to a CD22-antibody are immediately internalized without shedding into the extracellular environment [245]. Another advantage is that, when compared to CD20 antibodies, CD22 expression is maintained in patients treated with CD22-targeted therapy and levels of soluble CD22 are low [245]. Thus, CD22 is an ideal target for antibody-based therapy in B-cell malignancies.

Humanized CD22 antibody, epratuzumab, has been used both unconjugated and radiolabeled form. It has a unique mechanism of action in that it modulates B-cell activation and signaling rather than eliciting direct cytotoxicity [246, 247]. Re-induction chemoimmunotherapy with epratuzumab in relapsed ALL in COG trial ADVL04P2 (NCT00098839) did not improve the clinical response when compared to historical controls, but there was a trend towards improved MRD response when epratuzumab was administered more frequently [248]. Various trials in relapsed ALL are currently ongoing (www.clinicaltrials.gov).

Inotuzumab ozogamicin (INO) is a humanized CD22 antibody attached to a toxic natural calicheamicin, a potent DNA-binding cytotoxic antibiotic via an acid-labile linker. INO has shown encouraging results in relapsed/refractory B-lineage ALL [249, 250].

CD33 Monoclonal Antibodies

CD33 is a myeloid differentiation antigen which is expressed by the majority of blasts in AML, though with variable intensities [251, 252]. Unconjugated CD33 antibodies (e.g., lintuzumab) have shown disappointing activity (rev in [252]). However, though an antigen with endocytic properties, internalization is slow, making CD33 a challenging target. Several approaches to address this problem exist [252]. Nonetheless, I will focus on gemtuzumab ozogamicin (GO) as a humanized CD33 antibody, linked to a calicheamicin derivative, given its controversial history and biologic interests. In 2000, GO was granted accelerated approval by the US Food and Drug Administration for use in relapsed AML patients ≥60 years of age. GO was voluntarily withdrawn from the US marker in 2010 due to concerns of lack of efficacy in the presence of enhanced toxicity, which emerged during an interim analysis of S0106 [NCT00085709], a SWOG-led phase 3 trial in data untreated AML [253]. While there appears to be no beneficial effect of GO on the achievement of CR, there are compelling data suggesting that GO improves survival in cytogenetically favorable (CBF leukemias) and intermediate-risk leukemias [253–255], suggesting that reapproval of GO for risk-defined subsets of AML patients, as well as APL, may be warranted [256, 257]. Various additional biologic factors affect GO efficacy, such as the presence and activity of spleen tyrosine kinase (Syk) [258], CD33 expression levels [251, 259, 260], CD33 single-nucleotide polymorphisms [261], drug efflux, toxin release, and others (rev in [262]). Increasing Syk expression, e.g., with 5 azacytidine, can indirectly enhance CD33 antibody toxicity. Along the same line, the engagement of the SHP-1 tyrosine phosphatase in Syk regulation could be pharmacologically exploited by combining CD33 antibody with cytosine arabinoside and idarubicin [222]. There are case reports on the potential efficacy of GO in CD33^{POS} ALL, but no controlled studies have been conducted.

Of note, in a recent reanalysis of trial ALFA-0701 (NCT00927498), when the level of CD33 expression by myeloblasts was correlated with the outcome with GO, the cutoff of interest was found to be 70% CD33^{POS} blasts, in that a beneficial effect of GO was only observed in this response-defined high-CD33^{+} group [260]. Once again, this data strongly supports the view that cutoff points for defining the clinically relevant levels of antigen expression in immunotherapy can only be defined after the fact when response data are available. Whether or not such defined cutoff levels will hold true for other patient populations in future trials remains to be proven.

CD52 Antibody

CD52 is expressed on virtually all lymphocytes, monocytes, and natural killer cells. In ALL, the density of CD52 antigen expression varies by lymphoid lineage, with T-lymphoblasts demonstrating significantly lower amounts of CD52 on the cell surface [110]. Data with alemtuzumab in ALL are scarce, but suggestive of antileukemic activity [263, 264]. Gorin et al. [265] tested alemtuzumab together with G-CSF (to boost antibody-dependent cytotoxicity mediated by neutrophils) in refractory and heavily pretreated relapsed ALL (NCT00773149) and saw some responses though of short duration. ECOG performed a phase 2 trial of chemotherapy combined with alemtuzumab in relapsed/refractory ALL (NCT00262925); results have not yet been published.

CD25 Antibody

CD25, the α-chain of the interleukin 2 receptor, is a powerful negative prognostic indicator both in ALL [31] and AML [32]. Until recently, the mechanisms of action of CD25 in either of these diseases have been unknown, given that CD25 does not work as part of the interleukin-2 receptor on either lymphoblasts or myeloblasts [114]. CD25 is a transmembrane protein with a short, 13-amino acid-long cytoplasmic tail. Recent work by the Müschen group [114] has demonstrated that CD25 is a feedback regulator of the B-cell receptor (BCR) and a biomarker for disease driven by oncogenic BCR mimics. The tail of CD25 contains PKCδ substrate motifs. As a result, BCR signaling induces CD25 expression by PKCδ phosphorylation of the CD25 cytoplasmic tail which in turn leads to the membrane recruitment of phosphatases and robust oncogenic signaling (Fig. 15.2). Pharmacological activation of PKCδ, e.g., with the PKCδ agonist, diterpene ester ingenol-3-angelate (PEP005), induces rapid CD25 membrane translocation in patient-derived ALL cells. CD25 thereby mediates negative feedback signaling to stabilize oncogenic tyrosine kinase signaling and mediates drug resistance. Combinational treatment of CD25^{POS} leukemic B-lymphoblasts with PEP005- and CD25-directed immunotoxins may be a useful new approach to overcome drug resistance, for instance, in *BCR/ABL^{POS}* ALL. ADCT-301 is a human monoclonal antibody targeting CD25 linked with a pyrrolobenzodiazepine dimer toxin (CD25-ADC). CD25-ADC overcomes drug resistance in vivo when mice engrafted with CD25^{POS} human leukemic lymphoblasts are treated with this antibody conjugate. Based on this data, a clinical trial has been initiated using CD25-ADC in relapsed/refractory CD25-expressing ALL or AML (NCT02588092).

Bi-specific Antibodies

Bi-specific antibodies target leukemia-associated antigens while simultaneously activating antigens on cytotoxic effector cells or may otherwise potentiate the signaling events that will eventually lead to inhibition of leukemia cell growth. Bi-specific T-cell engagers (BiTE) form a new class of constructed antibodies, which direct the body's cytotoxic T-cells against tumor cells. One BiTE representative is blinatumomab (MT103), consisting of four immunoglobulin variable domains, of which two form the binding site for CD3 on the surface of T-cells, and the other two form the binding site for CD19 on the surface of the targeted B-cells [266]. Blinatumomab enables a patient's T-cells to recognize malignant B-lymphocytes and works by temporarily bridging these two cell types and activating the T-cells to exert cytotoxic activity against the malignant B-cells, causing redirected cell lysis, while nonspecific collateral killing effects have not been observed [267]. BiTE antibodies activate T-cells only in the presence of target cells, and nonspecific collateral killing effects have not been observed.

Blinatumomab [268] is currently indicated for *BCR/ABL^{NEG}* relapsed/refractory B-lineage ALL based on a single-arm study (NCT01209286) conducted by Topp et al. [269]. The US National Cancer Treatment Network leukemia groups are currently conducting a randomized phase 3 trial whereby patients with *BCR/ABL^{NEG}* B-ALL are randomized to blinatumomab or not at the time of complete hematologic remission based on MRD status (E1910/NCT02003222). The severe neurotoxicity seen in some blinatumomab-treated patients is not correlated with active CNS disease. Instead, variable expression of CD19 in neurons may make neurons susceptible to the inflammatory response from CD19-engaging T-cells [268]. Loss of the CD19 antigen, though rare, may contribute to resistance to blinatumomab as does extramedullary disease which probably reflects disease in sanctuary sites not penetrated by blinatumomab [268]. Duell et al. [270] recently reported that the frequency of CD4/CD25/FOXP3-expressing regulatory T-cells (Tregs), which inhibit T-cell proliferation, prior to blinatumomab administration, was able to predict blinatumomab responders. The authors also reported upregulation of CD69, CD25, and programmed death-1 (PD-1), an immune checkpoint receptor, by Tregs when incubated with blinatumomab and primary ALL blasts, suggesting a potential role of immune-inhibiting molecules, such as PD-1, in resistance to blinatumomab.

CD33/CD3-bi-specific T-cell-engaging antibody AMG 330 has shown promising ex vivo activity (rev in [271]) and has recently entered into a phase 1 trial in relapsed/refractory AML (NCT02520427). A dual-affinity-retargeting (DART) molecule generated from antibodies to CD3 and CD123 was designed to redirect T-cells against leukemic myeloblasts (also referred to as MGD006/S80880) [272]. CD123, the interleukin 3 receptor α, is highly expressed on the surface of AML blasts. Based on promising preclinical data, this antibody has entered into a phase 1 study in relapsed/refractory AML and high-risk MDS (NCT02152956).

Chimeric Antigen Receptor (CAR) T-Cells

CARs involve genetic engineering of a patient's own cells. In these molecules, an extracellular single-chain antigen recognition domain, usually derived from the variable fragment of a specific monoclonal antibody, such as CD19 (CART-19), is linked to the intracellular signaling domains of the T-cell receptor (TCR) [273]. Unlike the TCR, immunoglobulins can bind any antigen they encounter, independent of antigen processing and major histocompatibility complex. First-generation CARs, linked only to the intracellular CD3ζ signaling domain, were unable to adequately activate T-cells in vivo, and had limited clinical activity. Second-generation CARs contain costimulatory intracellular domains, such as CD28 or CD137 (4-1BB) in addition to CD3ζ [221, 274]. Third-generation CAR-T-cells which use two tandem costimulatory domains have also been reported [275]. Further improvement in efficacy and persistence of CAR-T-cells may derive from modifying these cells to express the proinflammatory cytokine, interleukin-12, or costimulatory ligands, 4-1BB and CD40L, thus "armoring" CAR-T-cells [276]. CART-19 cells have produced promising results in various B-cell malignancies, including B-ALL [221, 277–280].

Leukemia Escape After CD19-Targeted Therapies

Fascinating data are emerging concerning the potential adaptation of leukemia cells to CD19-directed immunotherapies, both with CD19/CD3 BiTE and CART-19. Relapses with CD19^{NEG} blasts have been seen both after blinatumomab and CART-19 treatment (rev in [281]). This experience demonstrates the potent selective pressure of these therapies that drives extreme and specific escape strategies by leukemic blasts. Alternatively, anti-CD19 treatment may result in the emergence of a CD19^{NEG} clone that had been present all along as a minor undetectable subclone among predominantly CD19^{POS} blasts, following the concept of oligoclonality [282, 283]. The loss of CD19 per se has a definite impact on MRD detection in these patients. Relying on side scatter characteristics, CD45 staining intensity and CD34 expression have been suggested as a way around third problem [284]. The National Cancer Institute initiated MRD Working Group has suggested gating strategies in these patients which do not rely on CD19 alone by combining CD20, CD22, CD10, and CD24, given that CD34 is frequently not expressed in B-ALL. Of course, it is essential to make sure that myeloid cells do not contribute to the gate, given that CD24 and CD10 are expressed by normal myeloid cells and CD22 by basophils.

The diversity of mechanisms which potentially contribute to the loss of the CD19 epitope on the cell surface is astounding. Sotillo et al. described *CD19* gene mutations and appearance of *CD19* splice variants which lacked the CAR-recognizing epitope after CART-19 treatment [285]. A complete loss of antigen, rather than epitope loss or splice variant, was suggested by Braig et al. [286] who did not detect CD19 by flow cytometry using CD19 antibodies with differential epitope recognition in one case of CD19^{NEG} relapse studied in detail. In that patient, the *CD19* gene had no mutations, and full-length CD19 messenger RNA was detected, excluding transcriptional regulation and splice variants for the loss of CD19. On flow cytometric analysis, ALL blasts lacked expression of CD81 and CD21, two molecules that form the B-cell co-receptor signal transduction complex with CD19 and CD225 on the cell surface of B-cells. CD81 regulates CD19 protein maturation and acts as a chaperone of CD19 during trafficking from the Golgi apparatus to the cell surface. Rather than caused by a genetic defect, as described in antibody deficiency syndrome [287], the lack of CD81 expression in the CD19^{NEG} relapse case was attributed to posttranscriptional regulation [286]. The finding of hypoglycosylated or deglycosylated CD19 indicated that in this case of CD19^{NEG} immune escape was the result of lack of CD81 expression, resulting in defective transport and/or maturation of CD19.

To date, the other escape variation described is myeloid lineage switch [281, 288]. While the exact mechanisms of lineage switch are still to be elucidated, it is important to note that the myeloid relapses appear to be clonally related to the pretreatment disease. Gardner et al. [289] described two distinct mechanisms leading to the myeloid relapse in two cases of *MLL (KMT2A)*-rearranged ALL treated with CART-19 therapy. Secondary therapy-related AML was excluded by the identification of cytogenetic abnormalities by conventional karyotyping or FISH which were shared between lymphoid blasts before and myeloid blasts after CAR-T-cell therapy. In one case, an identical rearranged *IGH* gene sequence that was identified in both lymphoid and myeloid blasts suggested a contribution from cell reprogramming or dedifferentiation of previously committed B lymphoid blasts. However, in the second case, absence of the original *IGH* rearrangement in the myeloblasts was consistent with myeloid differentiation of a non-committed stem cell clone or selection of a preexisting myeloid clone. These authors discussed as another alternative the outgrowth of a CD19^{NEG} myeloid clone in response to cytokines. Both patients with phenotypic switch had presented with severe cytokine release syndrome (CRS), including high serum levels of interleukin-6, a well-known complication of CAR-T-cell therapy [220, 221, 290, 291]. Other patients in the same treatment cohort, who did not experience phenotype switch, did not experience severe CRS [289]. In vitro IL-6 supplementation has been found to be a key factor in driving myeloid differentiation of a t(4;11) *MLL(KMT2A)*-rearranged B-ALL line [292], suggesting that high serum cytokine levels during CRS might contribute to the myeloid switch phenomenon encountered after CART-19 therapy. On the other hand, a clonal phenotypic switch was also described in a t(4;11) ALL patient following blinatumomab without any obvious sign of cytokine contribution [293].

How to deal with CD19 loss therapeutically or how to avoid it is a work in progress [221, 274, 281] and beyond the scope of this chapter.

Minimal Residual Disease Determination by Flow Cytometry

The topic of MRD in leukemia is comprised of several aspects, including (1) the most advantageous methodology for MRD assessment, (2) the selection of peripheral blood versus bone marrow and the issue of sample quality, (3) the timing of MRD assessments, (4) the clinically relevant level of MRD, and (5) the association of flow cytometry with other prognostic factors, in particular, genetic aberrations. This section of the chapter focuses on the flow cytometric detection of MRD and biologic parameters associated with or predictive of MRD.

MRD by definition refers to persistent disease after treatment that remains at levels too low to be detected by the human eye with light microscopy. MRD reflects the quality of response, serves as one of few post-therapy prognosticators, and has been found to prognostically significant at all time points though at different thresholds; furthermore, MRD thresholds will change with novel therapies and must be established with the introduction of new treatment strategies. The optimal way for detecting MRD has yet to be established, particularly in AML. Despite a lack of assay standardizations and the use of variable thresholds for defining MRD positivity, the prognostic effect of MRD has been confirmed universally indicating that this parameter is not easily swayed by technological aspects. There exist standard pre-therapeutic prognostic features, including cytogenetic aberrations, gene mutations, and immunophenotypic characteristics, which predict for the occurrence of MRD after therapy. However, within each conventional risk category, MRD status adds independent prognostic information. For example, patients with favorable cytogenetics will do much more poorly if they remain MRD^{POS} after therapy than favorable-risk patients who become MRD^{NEG}. On the other hand, intermediate-risk patients who become MRD^{NEG} with induction chemotherapy may do as well as MRD^{NEG} favorable-risk patients. In theory, early MRD assessment in the treatment course allows for refined risk stratification and tailored treatment. There are numerous reviews on MRD of which only a few recent ones are listed here, a list which by no means claims to be inclusive [34, 294–303].

New Definition of Complete Remission

It has almost become the standard of care to determine MRD in patients who after induction chemotherapy achieve a morphologic complete remission (CR). The implication that MRD might exist at the time of morphologic CR was raised by Bradstock et al. in 1981 [304] in patients with T-ALL, using the limited antibodies available at that time. It is quite unbelievable that despite 35 years of increasing evidence in favor of a prognostic significance of MRD in morphologic remitters, most clinical trials still define CR as the absence of blasts in the blood, normal trilineage hematopoiesis, ≤5% blasts in the marrow as recognized by the human eye with light microscopy, and absence of extramedullary disease [305]. We will discuss some of the reasons for this lag in reaction time, most of which appear to stem from lack of reliability in MRD measurements. Current CR subcategories, CR with incomplete blood count recovery (CRi), and its subset, CR with incomplete platelet recovery (CRp) [305], are associated with inferior long-term survival than patients in morphologic CR [306]. Chen et al. [307] found that MRD levels in marrows from CRi patients are significantly higher than in those from morphologic CR or CRp patients. Freeman et al. [308] had previously suggested a high incidence of MRD positivity in CRp patients and the loss of prognostic power for insufficient platelet count recovery in multivariate analysis after adjustment for MRD status. A major step in the direction of MRD has been taken by the European LeukemiaNet recommendations 2017 for the diagnosis and management of AML in adults [309] by introducing new response criteria, CR without MRD and the conventional morphologic CR with unknown or positive MRD. They also recommended that both multiparameter flow cytometry (MFC) and molecular techniques can be used to monitor MRD in AML. These recommendations will hopefully impact response criteria in clinical trials and individual patient treatment plans.

Of great importance are results from COG trial AAML03P1 [NCT0007017], which suggest that about 30% of children with AML who have a morphologically positive marrow after induction and are, therefore, considered induction failures are negative for MRD by MFC [310]. These children have an outcome superimposable to that of patients who were negative for MRD by both methods. Inaba et al. [311] similarly reported some AML patients who by morphologic examination of the bone marrow after induction had >5% blasts, while MFC-MRD did not detect residual leukemia. Percentage of myeloblasts by morphology did not affect the relation between MFC-MRD and treatment outcome marrows. These authors hypothesized that MFC-MRD negativity in morphologically positive marrows was due to therapy-induced differentiation of leukemic cells, resulting in the observed discordance between antigen expression and morphologic appearance. Since maturing blasts are doomed to undergo apoptosis, such patients would be expected to have a favorable outcome indistinguishable from that of MRD^{NEG} patients. In APL patients treated with all-*trans* retinoic acid, early MRD assessment by PCR for the *PML/RARα* transcript is not informative because the transcript persists in leukemic promyelocytes which undergo retinoic acid-induced maturation [312]. Such complication of MRD measurements does not occur in APL treated with arsenic trioxide [313]. However, a similar interference with MRD detection can be expected from other differentiation-inducing therapies, such as with inhibitors targeting *IDH2*-mutant AML [314]. Using real-time quantitative (RQ-PCR) for somatic receptor gene rearrangements, O'Connor et al. [315] analyzed end-of-induction MRD in pediatric ALL from

MRC trial, UKALL2003 [NCT00222612]. Of >3000 patients, only 1.9% were morphologic induction failures, and of those 59 patients, 6 had between 5 and 25% blasts by morphology (M2 marrow) but <0.01% MRD by PCR. These MRD$^{VERY\ LOW}$ patients had a 5-year event-free survival of 100%. These findings are surprising. What is surprising is the fact that despite the known limitations of morphology, these studies have not been done earlier and are still not being done in major trials. Going forward, every patient with AML and ALL, whether an induction failure by morphology or a morphologic remitter, must be evaluated for MRD by more sensitive methods to confirm or negate the morphologic result. Only then can we make sure that patients are treated according to their true depth of induction response.

The Choice Between Bone Marrow and Blood for MRD Detection

MRD determination by MFC invariably finds a lower percentage of blasts in bone marrow aspirates than in blood, provided that the aspirate is not diluted with blood. While this statement clearly applies to B-ALL, there may not exist such difference between marrow and blood in T-ALL [316]. This is in agreement with the fact that B-ALL (and AML, see below) are malignancies of the bone marrow, while T-ALL is of thymic origin. We have found in a large fraction of adult B-ALL patients that MRD by MFC was undetectable in the blood when up to 5% of blasts were measured in the marrow [317] and this experience continues in ongoing trial, E1910 [NCT02003222] (Paietta E unpublished observation). Along the same line, van der Velden et al. [318] found that RQ-PCR monitoring of immunoglobulin and T-cell receptor rearrangements yielded up to 1000 times higher levels of MRD in the bone marrow of children with B-ALL compared to levels in the blood. On the other hand, levels in the two tissues were comparable in T-ALL patients. Based on the available literature, MRD levels in the blood are 1–3 logs lower than in bone marrow in B-ALL and comparable or 1 log lower in T-ALL. Consequently, for both leukemia subtypes, bone marrow sampling was pronounced a prerequisite for accurate MRD monitoring (rev in [294, 297]).

Remarkably, a recent review stated that studies in ALL have already proven that assessment of bone marrow MRD could be replaced by peripheral blood MRD, without giving a reference or eluding further on the subject [296]. As stated above, this is not the case. However, there are some additional interesting data on this issue. Coustan-Smith et al. [316] reported from a small number of pediatric B-ALL that those patients with detectable MRD in both blood and marrow at the end of induction had a significantly higher incidence of relapse than patients with MRD in bone marrow only. It is important to mention here that their flow cytometric assay at the time only detected 1 leukemic cell in 10,000 normal cells, a sensitivity 10 times lower than what we are used to seeing now. Despite this limitation, their results suggested that peripheral blood MRD in B-ALL, though significantly lower than in the marrow, could provide prognostic information. An analysis of >2000 children with B-lineage ALL by Borowitz et al. [319] revealed that detection of bone marrow MRD at the end of induction helped to identify patients at high risk of relapse, but was not as useful for identifying patients at low risk. In multivariate analysis, MRD positivity (>0.01%) by MFC on day 29 (end of induction) was the most significant prognostic factor across all risk groups. While peripheral blood MRD was not equivalent to bone marrow MRD, the presence of MRD on day 8 in peripheral blood was associated with adverse outcome, with an increasingly bad outcome seen with progressively higher MRD levels. Strikingly, day 8 blood MRD^{NEG} patients had a better prognosis than patients who were bone marrow MRD^{NEG} on day 29. And the group of patients with the best outcome were MRD^{NEG} in blood on day 8 and had favorable cytogenetics. This prognostic significance of early blood MRD was also confirmed in a small study by Volejnikova et al. [320] using RQ-PCR for somatic receptor gene rearrangements. Once again, these authors confirmed a poor correlation between MRD levels in marrow and blood in B-ALL. However, they also found that a negative MRD result in the blood on day 15 identified a group of patients with excellent relapse-free survival. In summary, MRD levels in the blood are not equivalent to those in the marrow. Blood MRD status early on during induction chemotherapy in B-ALL, however, carries prognostic significance.

Measuring blood MRD on day 8 with MFC presents with a major challenge in that WBC counts will be markedly suppressed by chemotherapy. Rarely will it be possible to acquire the desired number of events (500,000–1 million), thus reducing sensitivity of MRD detection [319]. One clear advantage of blood when compared to bone marrow for MRD detection in B-ALL is the absence of normal B-cell precursor cells (hematogones) which occur in increased numbers in the marrow especially after consolidation therapy as part of marrow regeneration and which can be mistaken as persistent MRD [35, 297, 321]. In other words, the sensitivity of the blood MRD assay is lower compared to that of marrow MRD determination, while blood MRD has higher specificity due to the relative absence of normal progenitors in the blood. Next-generation sequencing (NGS) in paired bone marrow and blood samples from patients with B-lineage ALL also found that the leukemia burden in the blood was sixfold lower than in marrow [323]. However, due to the extremely high sensitivity of NGS, only 17% of paired samples had disease detectable in marrow but not peripheral blood and those were predominantly cases with marrow MRD ≤0.01% of total cells. These data suggest that with NGS, blood might be an alternative source tissue to marrow for MRD detection.

Regarding AML MRD, comparative data in blood and marrow are scarce. In 2007, Maurillo et al. [324] reported a strong concordance between MRD levels in blood and marrow by MFC and determined that a blood MRD level of 0.015% post-induction or post-consolidation correlated with outcome. Of the 50 patients studied, 43 had blood MRD levels higher than 0.015% after induction and 77% of those relapsed after a median of 10 months. Regarding biologic characteristics of this patient cohort, there was an overrepresentation of intermediate-risk karyotypes and cytogenetics had no effect on outcome. It is noteworthy that seven patients with detectable blood MRD after consolidation have remained in continuous remission, questioning whether the cutoff of 0.015% may be clinically relevant. There was no difference in overall survival between patients positive for blood MRD after induction and those with MRD >0.015%, though relapse-free survival was significantly shorter in the MRD^{POS} group. The same group of investigators use a threshold of 0.035% to define MRD positivity in the marrow [325]. Maurillo et al. [324] mentioned three patients in whom MRD levels in the blood were tenfold higher than in the marrow and these patients were monoblastic leukemias with extramedullary disease at the time of study. Zeijlmaker et al. [326] also reported one case with FAB M5 leukemia in whom MRD levels in the blood were 6.9 times higher than in the marrow, though extramedullary disease was not present. These investigators analyzed paired marrow and blood samples from 114 AML patients and found blood MRD levels to be 4–5 times lower in the blood based on MFC. Blood MRD was an independent predictor of response duration using a threshold of post-induction and post-consolidation MRD of 0.04% to distinguish between MRD^{NEG} and MRD^{POS} status, which was based on optimal specificity. This threshold agreed with the median of primitive marker-positive cells (CD34^{POS}, CD117^{POS}, or CD133^{POS}) in the blood of healthy individuals (0.038%) as compared to a median percentage of 0.88% in the marrow of these controls. Although the frequency of the primitive cell population itself was lower in the blood of AML patients, expression of aberrant markers by the primitive cells was not. With regard to the use of blood as an alternative source to marrow for MRD detection, they made the reasonable suggestion to monitor MRD in the blood and to assume that a patient is at high risk for relapse if the blood is MRD^{POS}. In cases in which the blood is MRD^{NEG}, an additional marrow aspiration should be performed to evaluate the true MRD status.

The Sample Quality Conundrum in MRD Determination

I cannot emphasize enough that it is the quality of the aspirate that determines the accuracy of MRD results. Several factors affect bone marrow quality and can be detrimental to accurate MRD determination. Many of those are out of the hands of the laboratory eventually performing MRD analysis. Those pre-analytical factors are sample storage after collection, delay in transport to the laboratory, or damaging conditions during transport (e.g., heat), resulting in degenerative changes with preferential loss of cell populations, possibly including the blasts in question. Hemodiluton of bone marrow samples, however, is probably the most significant and unfortunately too common problem. In an elegant, though mostly overlooked study, Helgestad et al. [327] demonstrated that the technique of bone marrow aspiration dramatically influenced MRD levels in ALL. Even the second pull from the same aspiration site reduced the leukemic fraction in the aspirate by almost 50% due to dilution with blood containing much fewer blasts. As a result, clinical trials in pediatric as well as adult B-ALL now emphasize the need of a first pull aspirate for MRD evaluation, or a separate pull from a distinct aspiration site after redirecting the needle, to avoid hemodilution at all costs as it leads to underestimation of leukemia involvement. Loken et al. [328] suggested a method to normalize aspirates for hemodilution flow cytometrically based on the proportion of dim-staining CD16^{POS} maturing myeloid cells, which, however, has not found widespread application. An intriguing suggestion as to how to resolve the problem of hemodilution in MRD detection was made by Terwijn et al. [329]. These investigators related the fraction of malignant primitive cells, those expressing aberrant markers (e.g., CD7) (aPC), to the total population of primitive cells, based on the dim expression of CD45, low side scatter characteristics, and expression of primitive markers, CD34, CD117, or CD133. In their experience, in contrast to MRD, the aPC fraction did not decrease upon dilution of the marrow with blood, because aPC fractions in peripheral blood and bone marrow were comparable.

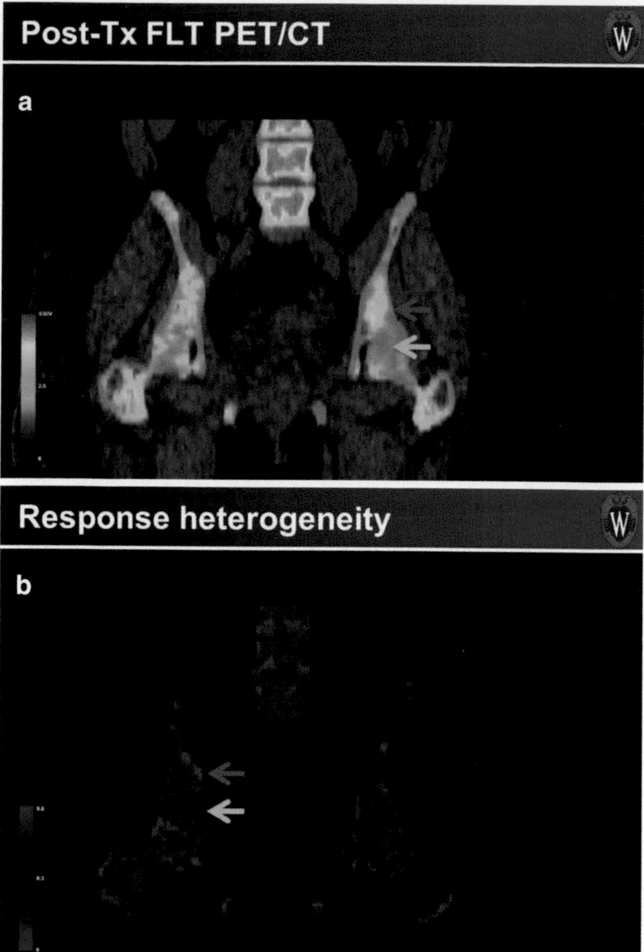

Fig. 15.4 FLT PET/CT images of posttreatment bone marrow in an AML patient. The patient was injected intravenously with 5 mCi FLT and scanned using a GE Discovery LS PET/CT scanner at the University of Wisconsin. PET/CT imaging began 45 min post-injection and extended inferiorly from the top of the skull to the distal femora. The pelvic region was chosen for display in this figure given that the iliac cristae are the most commonly used site for bone marrow aspiration and biopsy. PET activity concentrations were converted to standardized uptake values (SUV) by dividing the activity concentrations by the injected activity per patient mass. FLT PET images of bone marrow proliferative activity were extracted from full FLT PET/CT scans by first using the CT scans to extract the bone. These CT bone volumes were expanded to include the marrow resulting in bone and marrow CT masks. These masks were applied to the FLT PET images to isolate FLT PET voxels (volume elements of a scan) representing proliferative activity of bone marrow. An SUV threshold of 0.5 was applied to the masked FLT PET images to extract marrow FLT PET voxels, yielding FLT PET images of bone marrow proliferation. (**a**) Shows the FLT PET/CT of bone marrow in the pelvis and lower lumbar spine in an AML patient post-induction therapy. The SUV color bar reflects high proliferative activity in red (*red arrow* and red areas in the vertebrae) and low proliferative activity in blue (*blue arrow*). This scan demonstrates the heterogeneity of proliferative activity and thus distribution of residual disease in the pelvic regions. (**b**) Shows the spatial heterogeneity of bone marrow response to therapy in the same AML patient. The image represents a voxel-by-voxel ratio, whereby the values in the posttreatment FLT PET/CT were divided by the values in the pretreatment FLT PET/CT after co-registration of the pre- and posttreatment scans. Regions in red contained about 60% of the pretreatment activity, regions in black contained about 30%, and those in blue represent complete response. As can be seen from both images, there was substantial heterogeneity of residual bone marrow, as well as bone marrow response throughout the pelvic region, emphasizing the issues with a single-site bone marrow biopsy to assess treatment efficacy and response (courtesy Dr. Robert Jeraj)

Differential, heterogeneous distribution of the tumor load in different parts of the bone marrow, especially after treatment, could result in erroneously low MRD levels. In ALL, two independent bone marrow punctures at different locations showed comparable levels of MRD [330] strongly suggesting an equal distribution of ALL cells and indicating that it is sufficient to analyze MRD in a single bone marrow sample only. Substantial spatial heterogeneity in the bone marrow response after treatment for AML has been revealed by positron emission tomography (PET) with the proliferation marker, 3′-deoxy-3′-[^{18}F]fluoro-l-thymidine (FLT), in that response varied considerably throughout the pelvic region and in relation to other parts of the bone marrow [331]. Both during and after therapy, FLT uptake in the bone marrow of patients with residual disease, as assessed by bone marrow biopsy on day 14, was much higher and much more heterogeneous than in patients who achieved a morphologic CR. Figure 15.4 demonstrates the heterogeneous distribution of non-proliferating and actively proliferating bone marrow in the pelvis of an AML patient after induction chemotherapy (Fig. 15.4a). Figure 15.4b shows considerable spatial heterogeneity in the bone marrow response of an AML patient with refractory disease visualized by comparing pre- and posttreatment proliferative activity (disease) throughout the pelvis. Interestingly, there was a suggestion that elevated pretreatment FLT uptake may be predictive of poor response to induction, in agreement with data from Buck et al. who observed the highest FLT uptake in bone marrow of patients with refractory leukemia [332]. In other words, the accepted practice of performing single-point measurements for MRD in the bone marrow of treated AML patients could yield a false-negative result due to the heterogeneity in disease distribution. A similar study by Weindel Ibar Cribe et al. [333] also found a high degree of consistence between bone marrow response in AML patients to induction chemotherapy and the results of ^{18}F-fluorodeoxyglucose PET scans. These investigators speculated that a suboptimal PET response may be a predictor for an early relapse. The ECOG-ACRIN Cancer Research Group (Eastern Cooperative Oncology Group [ECOG], American College of Radiology Imaging Network [ACRIN]) is currently performing a trial to formally assess the value of FLT imaging in comparison to flow cytometric and morphologic MRD assessment in the marrow on day 28 of induction (EAI141, registered as NCT02392429).

A packed or concentrated marrow can be fully replaced by malignant cells at 100% cellularity leading to dry taps or the inability to obtain a suitable aspirate with spicules. Another etiology of dry taps can be reticulum fibrosis. Bone marrow fibrosis at diagnosis, as measured by reticulin fiber density, has been found to be more common in B- than T-ALL and has been associated with higher MRD levels on day 29 in B-ALL [334]. Packed marrows are much more common at diagnosis than after treatment and thus have less impact on MRD detection than hemodilution due to incorrect marrow aspiration.

MFC-MRD Versus Molecular MRD

The detection of MRD by MFC is based on the principle that leukemic cells express aberrant patterns of antigens which allow us to distinguish them from normal cells of same lineage and similar maturation stage [335–339]. The optimal method of MRD quantification and the best way to incorporate MRD information into risk-adapted strategies remain to be determined. The big advantage of MFC-based MRD assessment is its broad applicability. Leukemic blasts from approximately 90–95% of acute leukemia patients present with one or more antigen profiles which differ from the ordered pattern of antigen expression usually seen in normal hematopoiesis.

Flow cytometry looks at viable cells, which is an advantage over molecular techniques that may detect residual disease stemming from apoptotic or partially differentiated blast cells which have lost both aberrant phenotype and clonogenic potential. Inaba et al. [311] demonstrated this phenomenon when they compared MRD detection by MFC and qualitative PCR in CBF leukemias in which MRD by MFC after induction improved risk assessment, whereas the mere detection of the relevant transcripts by PCR did not. Low levels of molecular MRD may be compatible with long-term survival in CBF leukemias, again suggesting persistence of fusion transcripts in pre-leukemic cells or in differentiating leukemic cells without leukemogenic potential [340]. Complementary roles of MFC and RQ-PCR for the monitoring of MRD in CBF leukemias have been recently suggested [341].

With continuous improvements in the MFC methodology for MRD detection, differences in sensitivities between MFC and molecular techniques are diminishing. The standardized eight-color MFC-MRD procedure developed by the EuroFlow Consortium has proven a 98% concordance between MFC and RQ-PCR of immunoglobulin/TCR rearrangements in B-ALL [303], whereby the increased sensitivity of MFC was due to the availability of <4 million cells per antibody tube. Initially discordant cases were either due to overinterpretation of MFC-MRD (calling actually MRD^{NEG} cases MRD^{POS}) which were resolved by reanalysis or due to nonspecific amplification leading to false-positive RQ-PCR data. In those false-positive RQ-PCR cases, qualitative NGS analysis could not detect the involved leukemia-specific immunoglobulin/TCR rearrangements. The EuroFlow Consortium has reached extreme standardization of pre-analytical and MRD procedures (www.EuroFlow.org). Their EuroFlow quality assurance program helps to identify technical failures and inconsistencies [342]. Up until now, they have recommended using the Infinicyt software for analysis, which compares leukemic B-lymphoblasts with the nearest-normal B-cell precursors using automated population separator plots. Still, Theunissen et al. [303] concluded that interpretation of MFC-MRD, especially at very low levels, remains expert based. Being true to the term EuroFlow-based next-generation flow (NGF)-MRD strategy [294], EuroFlow now strives at developing new software tools to reduce subjectivity in MRD interpretation. The main limitation for MFC-based MRD evaluation, in fact, is the need for data interpretation which, in the hands of the untrained, is as subjective as the morphologic assessment of bone marrow smears. In other words, detailed knowledge of normal maturation for cells of the relevant lineage is an absolute prerequisite for the correct recognition of MRD by MFC [343, 344]. A recent first effort by the National Cancer Institute to standardize MFC-MRD for B-ALL in North America, using the COG-protocol for B-ALL as the gold standard, has demonstrated that a standardized methodology and continuous educational feedback helped improving the performance of participating laboratories [345]. While the COG protocol is based on the different-from-normal (DFN) approach, similar experience was reported by Feller et al. [346] who aimed at concordance of data in AML among five centers utilizing leukemia-associated immunophenotype (LAIP)-based MFC (DFN versus LAIP concepts of MFC-MRD determination will be discussed below). In both attempts, discordances were interpreter dependent, as previously observed in earlier European standardization efforts for B-ALL MRD assessments in multicenter settings [347, 348]. Since participants in all of these trainings were experienced in standard diagnostic flow cytometry of leukemias, these results suggest that immunophenotypic MRD assessment requires additional guided schooling.

Molecular studies are limited by the requirement of predefined targets, such as leukemia-specific, recurrent translocations leading to the creation of fusion transcripts (e.g., *BCR/ABL*), somatic gene mutations (e.g., *NPM1, FLT3, DNMT3A*), or, in ALL, creation of patient-specific primers for immunoglobulin and/or TCR gene rearrangements unique to the abnormal clone present at diagnosis. Good correlation has been found between RQ-PCR amplification of most frequent fusion transcripts in B-ALL and MFC-MRD [349]. Discordance between RQ-PCR MRD and MFC-MRD in *ETV6/RUNX1* (*TEL/AML1*) ALL affected only early time points of induction chemotherapy. It is possible that RQ-PCR detected *ETV6/RUNX1* carrying pre-leukemic clones (CD34^{POS}CD38^{NEG}CD19^{POS} pro-B-cells), which by MFC were not recognized as leukemic B-lymphoblasts [350]. Molecular signals may have derived from fusion transcripts present in nonviable or differentiating blast cells [340]. Huang et al. [349] speculated that the sensitivity of their six-color MFC-MRD assay could have been increased by adding additional antibodies to newly described markers to their panel [351]. Eight-color flow cytometry has yielded improved concordance with molecular MRD in BCR/ABL^{POS} ALL [352].

Ravandi et al. [353] reported that >50% of MRD specimens from their *BCR/ABL^{POS}* ALL patients were *BCR/ABL^{POS}* by PCR but negative by MFC. These findings are in agreement with those of others who found that MRD levels by MFC and/or PCR amplification of antigen receptor genes are largely equivalent but different from *BCR/ABL* transcript quantification [354]. It is conceivable that multi-lineage involvement with the presence of *BCR/ABL* in non-ALL cells is in part responsible for this finding [355]. More recently, the suppression of BCR/ABL protein translation in LSCs which carry *BCR/ABL* transcripts has been reported in imatinib-refractory chronic myeloid leukemia, resulting from the modulation of LSC metabolism by the environment in the stem cell niche [356]. The detection of MRD which is represented by residual LSCs is essential for long-term outcome in *BCR/ABL*^{POS} disease. A potential marker of *BCR/ABL*^{POS} LSC, dipeptidyl peptidase IV (CD26), has been proposed as a follow-up parameter at least in TKI-treated CML and lymphoid blast crisis of CML [357].

Correlations between MFC-MRD and molecular MRD in ALL have mainly focused on immunoglobulin/TCR gene rearrangements [340, 351, 358–360]. The two strategies were found to be complementary and (almost) comparable when properly standardized and the choice between these two methods is primarily dictated by costs, time, and expertise available. While fusion transcripts represent very stable targets for MRD determination, clonal evolution of immunoglobulin and TCR gene rearrangements is a frequent occurrence with therapy [361]. NGS, but not allele-specific oligonucleotide (ASO)-PCR, allows for the tracking of the evolution of all gene rearrangements during therapy [362–364]. Not surprisingly, deep sequencing by NGS measuring immunoglobulin heavy-chain variable, diversity, and joining DNA sequences proved superior to six-color MFC-MRD when tested prior to and early post-allogeneic stem cell transplantation [365]. With a sensitivity level 1000-fold lower than that of optimal MFC-MRD, pre-transplant NGS-MRD negativity, but not MFC-MRD negativity, was strongly correlated with relapse-free survival, raising the question whether the potential toxicities of allogeneic transplantation could be avoided in this patient cohort.

With respect to common gene mutations in AML, PCR- and sequencing-based MRD monitoring confirmed heterogeneity and clonal instability between diagnosis and relapse with selective outgrowth of mutated clones (oligoclonality), in particular, for *FLT3-ITD* [366], while *NPM1, DNMT3A*, and *IDH2* mutations were found to be more stable [282, 367–369]. Salipante et al. [369] reported *NPM1*-mutation-positive MRD by NGS in six out of six randomly selected AML patients after therapy though they were MFC-MRD negative, possibly reflecting persistence of mutated *NPM1* in a pre-leukemic clone, carrying also mutations in epigenetic landscaping genes (e.g., *DNMT3A, IDH1/IDH2*) [22]. Ivey et al. [370] found that in patients in molecular remission according to the *NPM1* mutation RQ-PCR assay, the coexisting *DNMT3A* mutations at arginine 882 (*DNMT3A*^{R882}) persisted, suggesting that they drive relapse [21]. The presence of *DNMT3A*^{R882} mutations predicted MRD measured by six-color MFC in AML patients in first remission, treated on phase 3 trial, E1900 [NCT00049517], underscoring their role in chemoresistance [148]. In that study, none of the other gene mutations analyzed, including mutated *NPM1* and *FLT3-ITD*, was associated with MFC-based MRD.

The relationship between *BCR/ABL1*-like genotype and MFC-MRD was studied by Roberts et al. in the St. Jude Total Therapy XV trial [204]. In that study, the majority of patients with *BCR/ABL1*-like ALL had an inferior initial response to treatment which triggered them being treated with intensified therapy. This MRD-guided risk assessment yielded comparable clinical results in *BCR/ABL1*-like and other B-ALL. Based on these findings, the authors proposed for centers that lack the capability to identify *BCR/ABL1*-like ALL that excellent overall treatment results can still be achieved, provided that reliable methods for monitoring MRD are available.

How to Define MRD Positivity and Negativity

In the study by Pulsipher et al. [365], ALL patients with even the lowest levels of residual disease by NGS (10^{-6} to 10^{-7}) benefitted from the allotransplant as patients with such low MRD levels who did not get a graft-versus-leukemia effect from the transplant relapsed. A strict correlation between the presence of quantifiable MRD pre-transplantation and outcome in ALL has also been reported by others [181, 371, 372], whereas this absolute need for MRD reduction may [373] or may not apply to AML [371, 374]. The power of pre-allotransplant MRD in AML has been demonstrated by a meta-analysis which demonstrated a strong relationship between pre-transplant MRD and post-transplant relapse and survival which was independent of the methodology used to determine MRD, the MRD threshold, as well as the conditioning regimen used [375].

MFC-MRD levels (threshold 0.01%) correlated with the outcome of myeloablative allogeneic stem cell transplantation in pediatric ALL with 3-year estimates of relapse being 17% and 38% and estimated 3-year overall survival being 68% and 40% for patients without and with MRD prior to transplant, respectively [376]. While these differences were highly statistically significant, they indicated that 17% of patients with <0.01% MFC-MRD relapsed within 3 years after transplant. This observation suggests that prognostic heterogeneity exists within the MRD^{NEG} group when defined by the 0.01% threshold. That the commonly used threshold of 0.01% to define MRD positivity in ALL, while usually achievable by MFC, may be set too high for clinical relevance in all ALL patients has also been suggested by PCR amplification of antigen-receptor genes at the end of remission induction [377]. On the other hand, in the first clinical trial in pediatric ALL that used MRD levels prospectively during and after remission induction therapy to guide risk-directed treatment, the St. Jude Total Therapy XV study (NCT00137111), the threshold for determining 10-year event-free survival was

≥1% of MFC-MRD on day 19 of induction [378]. However, at later time points of therapy, including prior to allotransplant, MRD^{NEG} status was defined with <0.01%. As pointed out by Campana and Coustan-Smith [340], the proportion of MRD^{POS} samples at any given time point during the course of treatment is highly dependent on the preceding therapy. Using a threshold of ≥0.01% to define MRD positivity, these authors stated that the prevalence of MRD positivity at the end of remission induction for ALL ranged from 19.4 to 83.5% in a variety of studies. This implicates that clinically meaningful MRD levels need to be determined with every new therapy. There is evidence that end-of-induction MFC-MRD is not as useful a determinant of outcome in T-lineage as in B-lineage ALL [379], consistent with PCR data which showed that T-ALL patients with MRD at the end of induction and even end of consolidation had a favorable outcome [380].

For MFC-based MRD in AML, the cut point used to define MRD positivity is, in general, ten times higher than in ALL (≥0.1%) [325, 381, 382]. To determine the cutoff of MRD positivity most relevant for relapse-free survival early during induction therapy, at the time of aplasia, Köhnke et al. [383] calculated hazard ratios for different cutoff values from 0.01 to 1% and arrived at 0.15% patients with ≥0.15% of mononuclear cells exhibiting the leukemia phenotypes(s) that were considered MRD^{POS}. Utilizing the same method, a cutoff of 0.3% was determined as to represent MRD positivity post-induction. Lowering the cutoff to 0.1% at that time point resulted in a nonsignificant correlation with survival.

In the pediatric AML02 trial (NCT00136084) [384], a rare example of MRD-guided therapy in AML, an MRD level of ≥1% after the first course of induction therapy was the determining factor for outcome in these high-risk patients, despite treatment intensification triggered by MRD results, suggesting that novel therapies might be indicated for this cohort. Patients with low MRD levels after induction 1 (0.1 to <1%) did as well as MRD^{NEG} patients, whereas any detectable MRD (>0.1%) after induction 2 was associated with poor outcome. Buccisano's group [385, 386] suggested that the clinically relevant threshold of MRD will differ with the intensity, in other words, the efficacy, of the therapies administered. In their experience, the MRD level that discriminated MRD^{NEG} from MRD^{POS} AML patients decreased from 0.1 to 0.035% in the bone marrow after intensification of the therapeutic schedule. On the other hand, high-dose versus low-dose cytarabine during induction did not affect post-induction MRD levels in pediatric AML, though this study demonstrated an MRD-lowering effect of gemtuzumab ozogamicin, the anti-CD33 antibody, when given after the first course of induction [384], and neither did doubling of the daunorubicin dose in adults [387], although the latter resulted in prolonged overall survival [388]. Similarly, there was a significantly better outcome in relapsed ALL children induced with mitoxantrone versus idarubicin without apparent difference in post-induction MRD levels [389]. Butturini et al. [390], however, warned about applying a definition of MRD status which was established in a given clinical situation in a random fashion to other settings. In other words, MRD thresholds that are prognostically significant in children with de novo ALL treated with standard therapy may not be applicable to children in relapse treated with experimental regimens. Yang et al. [391] identified germline variations which distinguished children at risk of relapse despite an excellent early response to therapy. Of the 134 single-nucleotide polymorphisms associated with relapse, 14 were associated with unfavorable pharmacokinetics of commonly used antileukemic drugs.

Intensification of induction chemotherapy may indeed lower the threshold to be used for defining MRD negativity to undetectable, given that patients who remain with detectable disease after highly cytotoxic therapy must be considered as having a low likelihood of benefitting from further cytotoxic therapy, most likely including transplantation [392]. Araki et al. [373] demonstrated that AML patients in MFC-MRD^{NEG} remission prior to myeloablative allogeneic transplantation had a cumulative risk of relapse of only 20–25% compared with a relapse risk of 65–70% for patients who underwent transplantation while in MRD^{POS} remission or patients with morphologically visible disease. Importantly, MRD negativity was defined as the absence of detectable MRD with ten-color MFC and the different-from-normal (DFN) MRD assay approach. Outcomes in patients with MFC-MRD^{POS} were unrelated to the level of MRD (<0.1% to >1%). The reason why about one-quarter of remitters relapsed posttransplant despite having been MRD^{NEG} prior to the procedure might at least in part be explained by the threshold of 0.1% to determine MRD negativity which falsely identified these patients as free of MRD.

Given the complex heterogeneity of AML, in addition to methodological disparities in MRD assays, it is probably reasonable to propose that the absence of detectable MRD, at any time point of treatment, should determine MRD negativity [393]. One of the main clinical uses of MRD determination is monitoring the kinetics of MRD reduction with treatment, rather than a single-time-point assessment. The usefulness of detecting recurring MRD in patients in continuous hematologic remission will depend on the availability of MRD-targeting preemptive therapeutic strategies [381].

Sample Preparation for MFC-MRD Determination

If MRD negativity is to be determined by the inability to detect MRD, then the lowest level of detection will dictate this definition. Consequently, unless everybody utilizes the same methodology for MFC-MRD assessment, it will continue to be impossible to compare studies. In addition to the caveat of threshold determination for MRD status and the choice of MRD assay, as discussed below, there are differences in sample preparation which can markedly affect results: for example, MRD determination in mononuclear cells versus whole bone marrow. While MFC-MRD data from mononuclear cells may be better comparable to those from molecular MRD analysis (nucleic acids are always prepared from mononuclear cells), there is the possibility that MRD cells are lost during density gradient centrifugation and/or antigen expression is altered during the procedure. Furthermore, Gaipa et al. [394] found that the impact of using either monucleated or total nucleated cells on the concordance of MFC with PCR results was minimal, and rather influenced by the time point at which MRD was measured. While direct antibody staining of MRD cells in whole, unseparated tissues is the preferred method nowadays, a no-wash procedure [395] is ill advised. It is imperative that excess antibodies be washed away after incubation and before red cell lysis and fixation prior to acquisition [297].

Optimally, a cluster of ten clearly aberrant cells can be sufficient for the recognition of MRD in a well-controlled assay. In that setting, for a limit of detection of 0.01%, the threshold currently utilized in B-lineage ALL to define MRD status, 1 million events must be acquired. Notably, in the presence of platelets, red cell fragments, tissue debris, or nonnucleated cells more events must be acquired, unless this noise can be excluded from the MRD enumeration. Other factors which can contribute to a suboptimal assay are nonspecific antibody binding or insufficiently cleaned flow cytometers. There is a lack of standardization of the denominator used for MRD enumeration. COG ALL-MRD assays maintain as denominator nucleated mononuclear cells [297], while others either relate MRD cells to total nucleated cells or total white cells, based on CD45 expression [396]. Dworzak et al. [347, 397] introduced the use of a live-cell-permeant nucleic acid-binding dye, such as Syto 16, a green fluorescent dye, to correct for nonnucleated cells and debris.

There are several other aspects of MRD determination, such as the choice of anticoagulant (EDTA or heparin is preferred) for the aspirate, use of cocktailed antibody combinations, and optimal ammonium chloride red cell lysis for white cell enrichment in the case of hypocellular marrow aspirates, a crucial step which is usually not paid attention to sufficiently. There are commercially available ACK (ammonium-chloride-potassium) lysing buffers and there are several home-brew recipes, which vary by temperature used during lysis (room temperature versus ice), speed during cell centrifugation after lysis, concentration of EDTA (ethylenediaminetetraacetic acid), and type of protein-containing buffer used to wash the white blood cells after lysis. I can only recommend that laboratories find the ACK buffer and lysing conditions which work best for their MRD assay, especially which avoid cell clumping.

The Two Philosophies of MFC-MRD Assays

MRD assays are widely applicable but require interpretive expertise. This notion is true whether MRD is based on leukemia-associated immunophenotypes (LAIP) [294, 303, 346, 382, 390, 396, 398, 399] established in the diagnostic specimen or the different-from-normal (DFN) approach [297, 301, 310, 343–345], which does not require knowledge of the presenting immunophenotype and relies on the recognition of cellular features that differ from those seen on normal cells of similar lineage and maturational stage. Cells that cluster in sites where normal cells are absent (the so-called empty spaces) are consequently defined as residual leukemic cells irrespective of the diagnostic phenotype of leukemia. Independent of the baseline phenotype, fixed antibody panels for leukemia population identification are used. Details regarding the methodology and antibody panels for all lineages have been published by B. Wood [399]. Which strategy to use is personal preference and a combination of the two might be the way to go. In fact, the contrast between these two philosophies appears to reflect more an individual conviction than actual scientific evidence. As Brent Wood [297] recently formulated, the use of LAIP is a simplified version of the DFN approach.

Preferentially, LAIPs consist of cell surface markers and combine antibodies which distinguish leukemic blasts from normal precursors; detect expression of lineage-foreign markers, e.g., lymphoid antigens on myeloblasts; detect altered density or lack of antigen expression; detect asynchronous expression of antigens (co-expression of antigens that are not concomitantly present during normal differentiation); or recognize antigens associated with particular genotypes (e.g., CD25 in BCR/ABL^{POS} ALL). Because of the dependence of LAIPs on the diagnosis immunophenotype, baseline and follow-up samples are ideally processed the same way and antibody combinations as well as fluorochrome choices for essential antibodies must be those used at diagnosis. LAIP-based MFC-MRD detection in the UK National Cancer Research Institute AML16 trial (NCT00454480) was performed in four reference laboratories with identical standard operating procedures, antibody panels, instrument type, and controls [400]. Still, these laboratories produced MRD values which were not identical. Especially in AML, multiple leukemic clones are frequently found requiring that equally multiple LAIPs be used in the MRD assay. However, it is recommended that only LAIPs expressed by a minimum of 10% of the leukemic blast population be monitored [401]. Though explained by the limits of sensitivity of MRD detection, this rule ignores the possibility that minor clones at presentation may dominate the remaining leukemia population at the time of MRD assessment or at relapse [282, 402]. Instability of even one of the LAIPs after treatment poses the risk of a false-negative MRD result.

The DFN-based analysis approach circumvents the problems of false negatives from phenotypic shifts and emerging subclones after treatment by using a fixed antibody panel. Most importantly, this approach avoids rigid gating predefined by the baseline specimen. Its independence from the diagnostic immunophenotype is very conveniently used in referral centers or commercial enterprises, when they receive samples for MRD determination without accompanying information on the baseline antigen profile. Both strategies are used in ALL and AML.

To reach satisfactory sensitivity against the background noise of antigen expression by normal bone marrow cells, leukemic immunophenotypes must be sufficiently aberrant to be present on less than 0.1 to 0.01% of normal lymphoid or myeloid marrow cells, so that in an adequate sample an MRD detection sensitivity threshold of 10^{-3} to 10^{-4} (1 in 1000 to 1 in 10,000 cells) can be achieved. However, for both LAIP and DFN methods, this signal-to-noise ratio is not a constant and varies with both treatment stage and leukemia subtype. The degree of abnormality in the population of interest is patient dependent. For leukemic phenotypes with a low degree of abnormality, the sensitivity of the MRD assay can be increased by acquiring more events (1,000,000 or even more) and the number of fluorochromes used per cell [303]. Furthermore, interference with the detection of MRD by normal cells will change with treatment stage. A simplified MRD assay in B-lineage ALL was based on the hypothesis that CD19^{POS}CD10^{POS}CD34$^{POS/NEG}$ cells detected early after initiation of treatment should be leukemic rather than normal, since normal bone marrow B-cell precursors (hematogones) with this phenotype are exquisitely sensitive to corticosteroids and thus eradicated during remission induction [403].

Hematogones and MFC-MRD Detection in B-lineage ALL

Hematogones are present in increased numbers during periods of hematopoietic regeneration, potentially causing interference with the detection of MRD [35, 36, 322]. In normal bone marrow, all differentiation stages of hematogones are present, whereby they exhibit a typical continuous differentiation spectrum that defines the normal evolution of B-cell precursors [35, 297, 322, 404]. This contrasts with discrete clusters of leukemic cells arrested at a certain stage of differentiation. In most studies, hematogones are differentiated from leukemic blasts by their expression pattern of CD45/CD19/CD10/CD20/CD38/CD22/CD34/CD58. As expected from normal B-lymphopoiesis, CD34 (and TdT) are present in the most immature stage of hematogones when CD10 is the highest and CD45 the lowest. With increasing maturation, hematogones lose CD10, and gain CD45, CD22, and some CD20. Zeidan et al. [405] demonstrated that the less mature hematogones express CD34 and lack CD123, whereas the more mature hematogones, with higher CD45 expression, lack CD34 but always express CD123. Given that the majority of B-ALL cases express both CD34 and CD123, this differential expression pattern was suggested to be helpful in distinguishing hematogones from leukemic blasts. As a side note, CD123 has been found to be overexpressed in B-lineage ALL patients with hyperdiploidy [351, 406]. It is also important to remember that leukemic lymphoblasts frequently express myeloid antigens, especially CD13 and/or CD33, which clearly allows the distinction from hematogones [407]. Based on differential gene expression between B-ALL and hematogones, Coustan-Smith et al. [351] found 22 markers which by flow cytometry were differentially expressed in the large majority of ALL cases tested, among them CD24, CD123, CD200, CD44, CD73, CD86, CD99, and BCL2. CD73 and CD86 have recently been confirmed as useful in differentiating B-lymphoblasts from hematogones [407]. While hematogones have been extensively studied in bone marrow, they are occasionally found in the blood (0.01–1.3%) according to Kroft et al. [408]. Chen et al. [409] identified a handful of proteins that were expressed in leukemic B-lymphoblasts at higher densities than in normal CD19^{POS}CD10^{POS}CD34^{POS} progenitors, including CD58 (LFA3), a ligand for CD2. Veltroni et al. [410] confirmed CD58 to be overexpressed by leukemic B-lymphoblasts when compared to regenerating and mature B-lymphocytes and no significant modulation of CD58 expression with treatment was noted.

While MRD detection in CD10^{POS} B-lineage ALL is plagued by the presence of hematogones, that in CD10^{NEG} B-ALL deals with the discrimination between leukemic cells and CD19^{POS}CD10^{NEG} plasma cells and plasmablasts. If one is lucky enough that the CD10^{NEG} leukemic blasts were CD34^{POS} at diagnosis, then CD34 negativity by suspicious cells together with high CD38 expression will definitely characterize those cells as plasma cells. CD38 expression by plasma cells exceeds by far that of leukemic B-lymphoblasts (or hematogones). CD138 (syndecan-1), a very useful marker of plasma cells, is usually not part of any MRD assay antibody panel. Plasmablasts, which may be found in marrow aspirates due to hemodilution, express CD38 at lower intensity than mature plasma cells, comparable to cases of CD10^{NEG} leukemic B-lymphoblasts, thus adding to a potential confusion. CD10^{NEG} pro-B or pre-pre-B-ALL blasts [44] vary in their expression of other B-cell differentiation antigens, such as CD22 and CD24, and CD20. Plasmablasts are CD20^{POS}, while plasma cells are CD20^{NEG}, CD24^{NEG}, but variably positive for CD22. Adding to a potential misinterpretation of CD10^{NEG} MRD is the infrequent finding of CD19 expression by natural killer cells [411]. Because MFC-based MRD identification is more difficult in CD10^{NEG} than CD10^{POS} ALL, standardized multicenter MRD testing demonstrated the highest discordant results between MFC- and PCR-MRD in CD10^{NEG} disease [348].

MFC-MRD Detection in T-lineage ALL

As mentioned before, the kinetic pattern of MRD response in T-lineage ALL is different from that in B-ALL with a slower rate of blast cell clearance in T-ALL, making end-of-induction MRD data less useful [379, 380]. Roshal et al. [412] reported that the main T-cell-associated antigens, surface CD3, CD2, CD4, CD5, CD7, and CD8, as well as CD45 remain relatively stable with treatment and thus can be reliably used in MRD detection. It is important to discriminate T-lymphoblasts from natural killer cells, which have variable expression of some T-cell antigens (especially CD7). Furthermore, the natural killer cell markers, CD16 and/or CD56, are occasionally expressed by T-ALL cells [413]. CD99 has been shown to be overexpressed in T-ALL when compared to hematopoietic stem cell and normal T-lymphocytes [412, 414, 415]. During T-lymphopoiesis, CD99 is downregulated with increasing expression of surface CD3 [416]. As a result, CD99 has been suggested as a very useful tool in MFC-MRD for T-ALL [414]. However, CD99 can be lost during therapy [412]. In fact, other markers of immaturity, such as TdT and CD34, dramatically decline during therapy of T-ALL as well [412].

MFC-MRD Detection in Myeloid Leukemias

Normal immunophenotypic patterns of maturation of hematopoietic lineages have been well described and they form the basis of MRD detection by the DFN approach [343]. While in lymphoid acute leukemias, the neoplastic population can be identified in most instances accurately even when present at very low levels, using either of the analysis approaches discussed, the situation is much more complicated in AML due to the heterogeneity of nonlymphoid acute leukemias and the multitude of differentiation stages to be encountered in follow-up samples [343]. A multitude of LAIPs have been proposed and utilized [346, 382, 417] and the DFN panel for MRD in AML has been published [399]. In APL, MFC-MRD determination is not very useful given the rather mature phenotype of leukemic promyelocytes and the ready availability of PCR-MRD monitoring for *PML/RARα* transcripts. Theoretically, one could utilize the expression (albeit often weak) of CD117 and the differential expression of CD15s and CD15 by leukemic and normal promyelocytes, respectively [29]. Monocytic leukemias present the biggest challenge because leukemic monocytes show considerable overlap in antigen expression with normal monocytes. Van Lochem et al. [418] have suggested various immunostainings for studying aberrant monocytic differentiation, which, however, also delineate their potential pitfalls. The European LeukemiaNet reported that the most common aberrations observed in AML are CD33^{POS}CD7^{POS} (±CD34^{POS}) and CD34^{POS}/CD11b^{POS} (±CD117^{POS}) [395]. Together with low CD45 expression and side scatter characteristics, it was suggested that a combination of four or five surface markers could reliably detect MRD in AML. The biggest handicap to this LAIP-based MRD approach is the multitude of LAIPs often present at diagnosis and the challenge to monitor all of them. While the DFN-based MRD approach has the definite advantage of not worrying about presenting LAIPs and being flexible enough to detect phenotypic changes, there is still a substantial incidence (about 25%) of false-negative MRD reports even with this methodology [310].

That tumor heterogeneity in AML makes this disease a moving target for the detection of MRD has been well described [402]. Despite its genetic and biologic heterogeneity, a common most primitive cell population with the Lin^{NEG}CD34^{POS}CD38^{NEG} phenotype was shown to be able to transfer AML to NOD-SCID mice [419]. Since these early studies, other markers have been detected on these LICs, including CD123, which is expressed by LICs at much higher levels than by normal hematopoietic stem cells [420]. Other differentiating markers of LICs are C-type lectin-like molecule-1 (CLL-1), CD96 (tactile), a member of the immunoglobulin gene family, CD47, the ligand for signal regulatory protein α, whose expression by LICs protects them from phagocytosis by macrophages and dendritic cells, and others [421]. However, there is marked variability in LIC antigen expression profiles among AML patients. LICs in *KMT2A(MLL)*-rearranged leukemias have variable surface antigen expression patterns dependent on gene fusion partners [8], also suggesting that the CD34^{POS}CD38^{NEG} cell pool may not uniquely contains LICs. Most importantly for MRD detection, the LIC compartment in AML is more heterogeneous than previously anticipated and includes cells with the surface phenotype of committed progenitors [421, 422]. This suggests that measuring CD34^{POS}CD38^{NEG} stem cells, as putative culprits of relapse, may not be entirely sufficient, although the frequency of these cells at diagnosis predicts for high MRD levels [423–426]. It is indeed surprising, though, that commonly used MFC-MRD assays, which solely measure residual cells from the original leukemic bulk, provide any clinically relevant information. The pre-leukemic stem cell clone, which has lost the major phenotype of bulk AML but contains the driver or founder mutations which led to the disease in the first place, survived standard treatment, thus persisted during remission, and eventually will lead to relapse (rev in [427]); this clone cannot (yet) be identified based on antigen expression. The mere evidence, however, that apparently mature myeloid cells in remission may be derived from leukemic progenitor cells [428, 429] makes MFC-based MRD measurements extremely difficult in AML.

Changes in Blast Cell Immunophenotypes with Treatment

Stability of LAIPs is a prerequisite for reliable LAIP-based MRD tracking. Despite the fact that differences in antigen expression levels between longitudinal studies during the treatment course of a patient may be due to technical aspects, like differences in analysis strategies or sample preparation, there is convincing evidence for true phenotypic changes. There is the reduction or disappearance of individual antigen expression and increments or gains in antigen expression; some phenotypes completely disappear while new abnormalities appear. The potential consequences of this phenomenon for MRD detection both in AML and ALL have been reviewed [402, 430]. Without question, changes in the immunophenotype of leukemic blasts with treatment and/or disease progression contribute to the approximately 25% of patients who relapse despite having been MRD$^{NEG/LOW}$ after induction or consolidation therapy.

Modern sequencing techniques have allowed us to prove beyond any doubt that the genetic landscape of leukemic subpopulations in a patient continues to evolve, either due to natural progression of the disease or in response to selective pressure from treatment [431, 432]. It is therefore not surprising if changes in surface phenotypes are observed between presentation and relapse but also early on during induction chemotherapy. Gaipa et al. [433] found the downregulation of CD10 and CD34, while CD19, CD11a, and CD20 were upregulated during the initial phase of induction treatment for pediatric B-lineage ALL, indicative of progressive maturation. These changes, which were found to be caused by glucocorticoid administration, were transitory. Remarkably, normal B-lymphocytes present in the specimens were equally affected. Rather than due to subclone selection or apoptosis-related artifacts, these changes (except for CD11a) were a direct result of drug-induced modulation [434]. Interestingly, the extent of phenotypic shift correlated positively with sensitivity to drug treatment [433]. Nonetheless, phenotypic shifts of highly relevant MRD antigens, like CD10 and CD34, returned to their initial aberrant expression levels after glucocorticoid-containing therapy was discontinued [434]. In addition, phenotypic modulation creates new combinations of aberrant expressions during follow-up, in particular based on upregulation of CD20. Genome-wide gene expression analysis revealed that glucocorticoid administration for 8 days resulted in decreased proliferative activity of the blast cells and a differentiation shift towards normal B-cells, both developments which may be the cause for the persistence of these blasts at day 8 of therapy as a result of drug resistance [435]. Rhein et al. [435] also reported increased expression of CD11b (MAC-1) integrin and CD119 (interferon gamma receptor-1) on day 8 B-lymphoblasts. The expression of CD11b in B-lineage ALL was found to confer a high risk of MRD when present on B-lymphoblasts at diagnosis [133]. Similar to B-lineage ALL, also leukemic T-lymphoblasts lose markers of immaturity during therapy, such as CD34, TdT, and CD99 [412].

Borowitz et al. [430] reviewed diagnostic and relapse immunophenotypes in children with ALL and found that although phenotypic shifts are common, they do not interfere with MRD detection, especially when the DFN approach is used. Of interest, these authors reported that the MRD-positive population at day 29 resembled the diagnostic specimen in 63% of cases, whereas in one-third of patients the day 29 MRD resembled the relapse phenotype, and in 2 out of 29 cases, day 29 MRD was unrelated to either phenotype. Surprisingly, time to relapse was identical in these groups. Contrary to what has been observed in ALL, phenotypic changes from diagnosis in AML point to a more immature state, through loss of CD11b and CD15 and frequent gain of CD34 and CD117 [298, 402]. A unique occurrence has been reported by Slamova et al. [436], a switch from CD2^{POS} B-ALL to acute leukemia of the monocytic lineage, associated with demethylation of the CEBPα gene and upregulation of this gene.

Epigenetic diversity within the LIC population and its progeny is an interesting alternative to permanent genetic modification as a cause of phenotypic changes, given that epigenetic modifications are dynamic and transient and allow the epigenetic status to return to its original status after selective pressure has been overcome. Although the actual mechanisms by which phenotype changes occur are unclear, the two most favored options are (1) spontaneous gains or loss of mutations in the primary tumor clone(s) present at the time of diagnosis and occurring during or after therapy and (2) selection of minor therapy-resistant subclones, already present but not routinely detected at diagnosis, which survived therapy and grew out to cause relapse [431].

With the increase in monoclonal antibody therapy, flow cytometrists face a novel situation, the potential of antigen loss or downregulation due to therapeutic antibody exposure. In patients treated with gemtuzumab ozogamicin, CD33 expression persisted at relapse in most cases [437]. In contrast, after rituximab therapy, more than one-third of cases lost CD20 expression [438]. With the bi-specific CD3/CD19-targeting antibody, blinatumomab, loss of CD19 expression occurred with treatment and at the time of relapse [439]. The mechanisms of CD19 loss after CD19-directed therapy have been discussed before.

As true for flow cytometry in general, MFC-based MRD determination cannot function in a vacuum, isolated from all other aspects of leukemia biology. Mooreman et al. [440] demonstrated that a subgroup of genetically good-risk ALL patients remained MRD^{POS} after induction, which was associated with more incidences of relapse but an overall survival of >90%. Rather than superseding other prognostic factors [441], MRD complements the power of genetic factors for risk stratification of patients with acute leukemia.

References

1. Lane SW, Scadden DT, Gilliland DG. The leukemic stem cell niche: current concepts and therapeutic opportunities. Blood. 2009;114:1150.
2. Wojiski S, Guibal FC, Kindler T, et al. PML-RARα initiates leukemia by conferring properties of self-renewal to committed promyelocytic progenitors. Leukemia. 2009;23:1462.
3. Lapidot T, Sirard C, Vormoor J, et al. A cell initiating acute myeloid leukaemia after transplantation into SCID mice. Nature. 1994;367:645.
4. van Rhenen A, van Dongen GA, Kelder A, et al. The novel AML stem cell associated antigen CLL-1 aids in discriminating between normal and leukaemic stem cells. Blood. 2007;110:2659.
5. Jin L, Lee EM, Ramshaw HS, et al. Monoclonal antibody-mediated targeting of CD123, IL-3 receptor alpha chain, eliminates human acute myeloid leukemic stem cells. Cell Stem Cell. 2009;5:31.
6. Majeti R, Chao MP, Alizadeh AA, et al. CD47 is an adverse prognostic factor and therapeutic antibody target on human acute myeloid leukemia stem cells. Cell. 2009;138:286.
7. Taussig DC, Vargaftig J, Miraki-Moud F, et al. Leukemia-initiating cells from some acute myeloid leukemia patients with mutated nucleophosmin reside in the CD34(−) fraction. Blood. 2010;115:1976.
8. Aoki Y, Watanabe T, Saito Y, et al. Identification of CD34^{+} and CD34^{-} leukemia-initiating cells in MLL-rearranged human acute lymphoblastic leukemia. Blood. 2014;125:967.
9. Swerdlow SH, Campo E, Harris NL, Jaffe ES, Pileri SA, Stein H, Thiele J, Vardiman JW, editors. WHO classification of tumours of haematopoietic and lymphoid tissues. 4th ed. Lyon: IARC; 2008.
10. Grimwade D, Ivey A, Huntly BJP. Molecular landscape of acute myeloid leukemia in younger adults and its clinical relevance. Blood. 2016;127:29.
11. Patel JP, Gönen M, Figueroa ME, et al. Prognostic relevance of integrated genetic profiling in acute myeloid leukemia. N Engl J Med. 2012;366:1079.
12. Klco JM, Spencer DH, Miller CA, et al. Functional heterogeneity of genetically defined subclones in acute myeloid leukemia. Cancer Cell. 2014;25:379.
13. Arber DA, Orazi A, Hasserjian R, et al. The 2016 revision to the World Health Organization classification of myeloid neoplasms and acute leukemia. Blood. 2016;127:2391.
14. Papaemmanuil E, Gerstung M, Bullinger L, et al. Genomic classification and prognosis in acute myeloid leukemia. N Engl J Med. 2016;374:2209.
15. Metzeler KH, Herold T, Rothenberg-Thurley M, et al. Spectrum and prognostic relevance of driver gene mutations in acute myeloid leukemia. Blood. 2016;128:686.
16. Paietta E. Phenotypic correlates of genetic abnormalities in acute and chronic leukemias. In: Detrick B, Hamilton RG, Folds JD, editors. Manual of molecular and clinical laboratory immunology, 7th ed. Washington, DC: ASM Press; 2006. p. 201.
17. Paietta E. Surrogate marker profiles for genetic lesions in acute leukemias. In: Paietta E, editor. Bailliere's best practice & research: clinical haematology, immunophenotyping in haematologic malignancies: state of the art, vol. 23. Amsterdam, Netherlands: Elsevier; 2010. p. 359–68.
18. Roberts K, Morin RD, Zhang J, et al. Genetic alterations activating kinase and cytokine receptor signaling in high-risk acute lymphoblastic leukemia. Cancer Cell. 2012;22:153.
19. Roberts KG, Gu Z, Payne-Turner D, McCastlain K, et al. High frequency and poor outcome of Ph-like acute lymphoblastic leukemia in adults. J Clin Oncol. 2017.; (In Press)
20. Jan M, Snyder TM, Corces-Zimmerman MR, et al. Clonal evolution of preleukemic hematopoietic stem cells precedes human acute myeloid leukemia. Sci Transl Med. 2012;4:149ra118.
21. Shlush LT, et al. Identification of pre-leukaemic haematopoietic stem cells in acute leukaemia. Nature. 2014;506:328.
22. Corces-Zimmerman MR, Hong W-J, Weissman IL, et al. Preleukemic mutations in human acute myeloid leukemia affect epigenetic regulators and persist in remission. Proc Natl Acad Sci. 2014;111:2548.
23. Xie M, Lu C, Wang J, et al. Age-related mutations associated with Clonal hematopoietic expansion and malignancies. Nat Med. 2014;20:1472.
24. Genovese G, Kähler AK, Handsaker RE, et al. Clonal hematopoiesis and blood-cancer risk inferred from blood DNA sequence. N Engl J Med. 2014;371:2477.
25. Jaiswal S, Fontanillas P, Flannick J, et al. Age-related Clonal hematopoiesis associated with adverse outcome. N Engl J Med. 2014;371:2488.
26. van der Akker EB, Pitts SJ, Deelen J, et al. Uncompromised 10-year survival of oldest old carrying somatic mutations in DNMT3A and TET2. Blood. 2016;127:1512.
27. Paietta E, Papenhausen P. Cytogenetic alterations and related molecular consequences in adult leukemia. In: Steele Jr GD, Phillips TL, Chabner BA, Gansler TS, editors. Adult leukemias, American Cancer Society: Atlas of clinical oncology series volume, Wiernik PH (series ed.). Hamilton, Canada: BC Decker; 2001. p. 161.
28. Falini B, Martelli MP, Tiacci E, et al. Immunohistochemical surrogates for genetic alterations of *CCDN1, PML, ALK*, and *NPM1* genes in lymphomas and acute myeloid leukemia. In: Paietta E, editor. Bailliere's best practice & research: clinical haematology, immunophenotyping in haematologic malignancies: state of the art, vol. 23. Amsterdam, Netherlands: Elsevier; 2010. p. 417–31.
29. Paietta E, Goloubeva O, Neuberg D, et al. A surrogate marker profile for PML/RARα expressing acute promyelocytic leukemia and the association of immunophenotypic markers with morphologic and molecular subtypes. Clin Cytometry. 2004;59B:1.
30. Harvey RC, Mullighan CG, Chen I-M, et al. Rearrangement of *CRLF2* is associated with mutation of *JAK* kinases, alteration if *IKZF1*, Hispanic/Latino ethnicity, and a poor outcome in pediatric B-progenitor acute lymphoblastic leukemia. Blood. 2010;115:5312.
31. Geng H, Brennan S, Milne TA, et al. Integrative epigenomic analysis of adult B-acute lymphoblastic leukemia identifies biomarkers and therapeutic targets. Cancer Discov. 2012;2:1004.
32. Gönen M, Sun Z, Figueroa ME, et al. CD25 expression status improves prognostic risk classification in AML independent of established biomarkers: ECOG phase III trial, E1900. Blood. 2012;120:2297.
33. Van Vlierberghe P, Ambesi-Impiombato A, De Keersmaeker K, et al. Prognostic relevance of integrated genetic profiling in adult T-cell acute lymphoblastic leukemia. Blood. 2013;122:74.
34. Paietta E, Litzow M. Minimal residual disease in acute leukemias: are we on the right path? In: Lazarus HM, Gale RP, Keating A, Bacigalupo A, Munker R, Atkinson K, editors. Hematopoietic cell transplants: concepts, controversies and future directions. Cambridge: Cambridge University Press; 2017. (in press).
35. Sevilla DW, Colovai AI, Emmons FN, et al. Hematogones: a review and update. Leuk Lymphoma. 2010;51:10.
36. Sedek L, Bulsa J, Sonsala A, et al. The immunophenotypes of blast cells in B-cell precursor acute lymphoblastic leukemia: how different are they from their normal counterparts? Cytometry B Clin Cytom. 2014;86:329.
37. Brown G, Sanchez-Garcia I. Is lineage-decision making restricted during tumoral reprogramming of haematopoietic stem cells. Oncotarget. 2015;6:43326.
38. He J, Abdel-Wahab O, Nahas MK, et al. Integrated genomic DNA/RNA profiling of hematologic malignancies in the clinical setting. Blood. 2016;127:3004.
39. McKerrell T, Moreno T, Ponstingl H, et al. Development and validation of a comprehensive genomic diagnostic tool for myeloid malignancies. Blood. 2016;128:e1.

40. www.lls.org/beat-aml: The Beat AML Master Trial
41. Kotrova M, Musilova A, Stuchly J, et al. Distinct bilineal leukemia immunophenotypes are not genetically determined. Blood. 2016;128:2263.
42. Dorantes-Acosta E, Pelayo R. Lineage switching in acute leukemias: a consequence of stem cell plasticity? Bone Marrow Res. 2012;2012:406796.
43. Regalo G, Leutz A. Hacking cell differentiation: transcriptional rerouting in reprogramming, lineage infidelity and metaplasia. EMBO Mol Med. 2013;5:1154.
44. Paietta E. Immunobiology of acute leukemia. In: Wiernik PH, Goldman JM, Dutcher JP, Kyle R, editors. Neoplastic diseases of the blood. 4th ed. Cambridge: Cambridge University Press; 2003. p. 194.
45. Paietta E: Immunobiology of acute leukemia. In: Wiernik PH, Dutcher J, Goldman J, Kyle R, editors. Neoplastic diseases of the blood. 5th ed. Springer: PA, 2012, pp 241-283.
46. Tuzuner NN, Bennett JM. Classification of the acute leukemias: Cytochemical and morphological considerations. In: Wiernik PH, Goldman JM, Dutcher JP, Kyle R, editors. Neoplastic diseases of the blood. 4th ed. Cambridge: Cambridge University Press; 2003. p. 176.
47. Harris NL, Jaffe ES, Diebold J, et al. World Health Organization classification of neoplastic diseases of the hematopoietic and lymphoid tissues: report of the clinical advisory committee meeting—Airlie House, Virginia, November 1997. J Clin Oncol. 1999;17:3835.
48. Schoch C, Schnittger S, Kern W, et al. Acute myeloid leukemia with recurring chromosome abnormalities as defined by the WHO-classification: incidence of subgroups, additional genetic abnormalities, FAB subtypes and age distribution in an unselected series of 1897 patients with acute myeloid leukemia. Haematologica. 2002;87:351.
49. Kornblau SM, Tibes R, Qiu YH, et al. Funcrional proteomic profiling of AML predicts response and survival. Blood. 2009;113:154.
50. Paietta E. Comments on the 2001 WHO proposal for the classification of haematopoietic neoplasms. Best Pract Res Clin Haematol. 2003;16:547.
51. Nucifora G, Dickstein JI, Torbenson V, et al. Correlation between cell morphology and expression of the AML1/ETO chimeric transcript in patients with acute myeloid leukemia without the t(8;21). Leukemia. 1994;8:1533.
52. Andrieu V, Radford-Weiss I, Troussard X, et al. Molecular detection of t(8;21)/AML1/ETO in AML M1/M2: correlation with cytogenetics, morphology and immunophenotype. Br J Haematol. 1996;92:855.
53. Fernandez HF, Sun Z, Yao X, et al. Anthracycline dose intensification improves overall survival in younger patients with acute myeloid leukemia: results of ECOG study E1900. N Engl J Med. 2009;351:1249.
54. Arber DA, Glackin C, Lowe G, et al. Presence of t(8;21)(q22;q22) in myeloperoxidase-positive, myeloid surface antigen-negative acute myeloid leukemia. Am J Clin Pathol. 1997;107:68.
55. Licht JD. AML1 and the AML1-ETO fusion protein in the pathogenesis of t(8;21) AML. Oncogene. 2001;20:5660.
56. Tiacci E, Pileri S, Orleth A, et al. PAX5 expression in acute leukemias: higher B-lineage specificity than CD79a and selective association with t(8;21)-acute myelogenous leukemia. Cancer Res. 2004;64:7399.
57. Paietta E, Wiernik PH, Andersen J. Immunophenotypic features of t(8;21)(q22;q22) acute myeloid leukemia in adults. Blood. 1993;81:1975.
58. Vevai XJ, O'Shea K, Keane S, et al. CD19/CD7 dual positive AML: a marker profile associated with FLT3-ITD positive, NPM1-mutated normal karyotype AML. Clin Cytometry. 2009;76B:406. #32
59. Paietta E. Expression of cell-surface antigens in acute promyelocytic leukemia. Best Pract Res Clin Haematol. 2003;16:369.
60. Grimwade D, Biondi A, Mozziconacci M-J, et al. Characterization of acute promyelocytic leukemia cases lacking the classic t(15;17): results of the European Working Party. Blood. 2000;96:1297.
61. Allford S, Grimwade D, Langabeer S, et al. Identification of the t(15;17) in AML FAB types other than M3: evaluation of the role of molecular screening for the PML/RARα rearrangement in newly diagnosed AML. Br J Haematol. 1999;105:198.
62. Adriaansen HJ, te Boekhorst PAW, Hagemeijer AM, et al. Acute myeloid leukemia M4 with bone marrow eosinophilia (M4Eo) and inv(16)(p13q22) exhibits a specific immunophenotype with CD2 expression. Blood. 1993;81:3043.
63. Schoch C, Kohlmann A, Schnittger S, et al. Acute myeloid leukemias with reciprocal rearrangements can be distinguished by specific gene expression profiles. Proc Natl Acad Sci U S A. 2002;99:10008.
64. Grimwade D, Outram SV, Flora R, et al. The T-lineage affiliated CD2 gene lies within the open chromatin environment in acute promyelocytic leukemia cells. Cancer Res. 2002;62:4730.
65. Paietta E, Ferrando AA, Neuberg D, et al. Activating FLT3 mutations in CD117/KIT(+) T-cell acute lymphoblastic leukemias. Blood. 2004;104:558.
66. Paietta E, Neuberg D, Bennett JM, et al. Low expression of the myeloid differentiation antigen CD65s, a feature of poorly differentiated AML in older adults: study of 711 patients enrolled in ECOG trials. Leukemia. 2003;17:1544.
67. Will B, Steidl U. Multiparameter fluorescence-activated cell sorting and analysis of stem and progenitor cells in myeloid malignancies. In: Paietta E, editor. Bailliere's best practice & research: clinical haematology, immunophenotyping in haematologic malignancies: state of the art, vol. 23(3); 2010. p. 391–401.
68. Muñoz L, Nomdedéu JF, López O, et al. Interleukin-3 receptor alpha chain (Cd123) is widely expressed in hematologic malignancies. Haematologica. 2001;86:1261.
69. Carlos TM, Harlan JM. Leukocyte-endothelial adhesion molecules. Blood. 1994;84:2068.
70. Terstappen LWMM, Loken MR. Myeloid cell differentiation in normal bone marrow and acute myeloid leukemia assessed by multidimensional flow cytometry. Anal Cell Pathol. 1990;2:229.
71. Elghetany MT. Surface marker abnormalities in the myelodysplastic syndromes. Haematologica. 1998;83:1104.
72. Paietta E, Andersen J, Yunis J, et al. Acute myeloid leukemia expressing the leucocyte integrin CD11b: a new leukemic syndrome with poor prognosis. Result of an ECOG database analysis. Br J Haematol. 1998;100:265.
73. Kussick SJ, Stirewalt DL, Yi HS, et al. A distinctive nuclear morphology in acute myeloid leukemia is strongly associated with loss of HLA-DR expression and FLT3 internal tandem duplication. Leukemia. 2004;18:1591.
74. Chen W, Rassidakis GZ, Li J, et al. High frequency of NPM1 gene mutations in acute myeloid leukemia with prominent nuclear invaginations "cuplike" nuclei. Blood. 2006;108:1783.
75. Falini B, Nicoletti I, Martelli MF, Mecucci C. Acute myeloid leukemia carrying cytoplasmic/mutated nucleophosmin (NPMc^{+}AML): biologic and clinical features. Blood. 2007;109:874.
76. Lieber MR. mechanisms of human lymphoid chromosomal translocations. Nature Reviews (Cancer). 2016;16:387.
77. Scott AA, Head DR, Kopecky KJ, et al. HLA-DR^{-}, CD33^{+}, CD56^{+}, CD16^{-} myeloid/natural killer cell acute leukemia: a previously unrecognized form of acute leukemia potentially misdiagnosed as French-American-British acute myeloid leukemia-M3. Blood. 1994;84:244.
78. Murray CK, Estey E, Paietta E, et al. CD56 expression in acute promyelocytic leukemia. A possible indicator of poor treatment outcome? J Clin Oncol. 1999;17:293.
79. Ferrara F, Morabito F, Martino B, et al. CD56 expression is an indicator of poor clinical outcome in patients with acute promyelocytic leukemia treated with simultaneous all-trans retinoic acid and chemotherapy. J Clin Oncol. 2000;18:1295.

80. Lin P, Hao S, Medeiros LJ, et al. Expression of CD2 in acute promyelocytic leukemia correlates with short form of PML/RARα transcripts and poorer prognosis. Am J Clin Pathol. 2004;121:402.
81. Ito S, Ishida Y, Oyake T, et al. Clinical and biological significance of CD56 antigen expression in acute promyelocytic leukemia. Leuk Lymphoma. 2004;45:1783.
82. Breccia M, Avvisati G, Latagliata R, et al. Occurrence of thrombotic events in acute promyelocytic leukemia correlates with consistent immunophenotypic and molecular features. Leukemia. 2007;21:79.
83. Chapiro E, Delabesse E, Asnafi V, et al. Expression of T-lineage-affiliated transcripts and TCR rearrangements in acute promyelocytic leukemia: implications for the cellular target of t(15;17). Blood. 2006;108:3484.
84. Paietta E, Andersen J, Racevskis J, et al. Significantly lower P-glycoprotein expression in acute promyelocytic leukemia than in other types of acute myeloid leukemia: immunological, molecular and functional analyses. Leukemia. 1994;8:968.
85. Redner RL. Variations on the theme: the alternate translocations in APL. Leukemia. 2002;16:1927.
86. Gallagher RE, Mak S, Paietta E, et al. Identification of a second acute promyelocytic leukemia (APL) patients with the STATb-RARalpha fusion gene among PML-RARalpha-negative Eastern Cooperative Oncology Group (ECOG) APL protocol registrants. Blood. 2004;104(11):821a. #3005
87. Ferrara F, Del Vecchio L. Acute myeloid leukemia with t(8;21)/AML1/ETO: a distinct biological and clinical entity. Haematologica. 2002;87:306.
88. Tallman MS, Hakimian D, Shaw JM, et al. Granulocytic sarcoma is associated with the 8;21 translocation in acute myeloid leukemia. J Clin Oncol. 1993;11:690.
89. Krishnan K, Ross CW, Adams PT, et al. Neural cell-adhesion molecule (CD 56)-positive, t(8;21) acute myeloid leukemia (AML, M-2) and granulocytic sarcoma. Ann Hematol. 1994;69:321.
90. Puig-Kröger A, Sánchez-Elsner T, Ruiz N, et al. RUNX/AML and C/EBP factors regulate CD11a integrin expression in myeloid cells through overlapping regulatory elements. Blood. 2003;102:3252.
91. Nutt SL, Heavey B, Rolink AG, et al. Commitment to the B-lymphoid lineage depends on the transcription factor Pax5. Nature. 1999;401:556.
92. Paietta E, Neuberg D, Richards S, et al. Rare adult acute lymphocytic leukemia with CD56 expression in the ECOG experience shows unexpected phenotypic and genotypic heterogeneity. Am J Hematol. 2001;66:189.
93. Paietta E. Unique subtypes in acute lymphoblastic leukemia. In: Advani A, Lazarus H, editors. Adult acute lymphocytic leukemia: biology and treatment. New York: Humana Press; 2011.
94. Fielding AK, Rowe JM, Richards SM, et al. Prospective outcome data on 267 unselected adult patients with Philadelphia chromosome-positive acute lymphoblastic leukemia confirms superiority of allogeneic transplantation over chemotherapy in the pre-imatinib era: results from the International ALL trial MRC UKALLXII/ECOG2993. Blood. 2009;113:4489.
95. Moorman AV, Harrison CJ, Buck GAN, et al. Karyotype is an independent prognostic factor in adult acute lymphoblastic leukemia (ALL): analysis of cytogenetic data from patients treated on the Medical Research Council (MRC) UKALLXII/Eastern Cooperative Oncology Group (ECOG) 2993 trial. Blood. 2007;109:3189.
96. Ottmann O, Dombret H, Martinelli G, et al. Dasatinib induces rapid hematologic and cytogenetic responses in adult patients with Philadelphia chromosome-positive acute lymphoblastic leukemia with resistance or intolerance to imatinib: interim results of a phase 2 study. Blood. 2007;110:2309. Yishai's protocol
97. Gersen SL, Keagle MB, editors. The principles of clinical cytogenetics. 2nd ed. Totowa, NJ: Humana Press; 2005.
98. Tabernero MD, Bortoluci AM, Alaejos I, et al. Adult precursor B-ALL with *BCR/ABL* gene rearrangements displays a unique immunophenotype based on the pattern of CD10, CD34, CD13 and CD38 expression. Leukemia. 2001;15:406.
99. Hrušák O, Porwit-MacDonald A. Antigen expression patterns reflecting genotype of acute leukemias. Leukemia. 2002;16:1233.
100. Mancini M, Scappaticci D, Cimino G, et al. A comprehensive genetic classification of adult acute lymphoblastic leukemia (ALL): analysis of the GIMEMA 0486 protocol. Blood. 2005;105:3434.
101. Paietta E, Racevskis J, Neuberg D, et al. Expression of CD25 (interleukin-2 receptor α chain) in adult acute lymphoblastic leukemia predicts for the presence of BCR/ABL fusion transcripts: results of a preliminary laboratory analysis of ECOG/MRC Intergroup Study E2993. Leukemia. 1997;11:1887.
102. Nakase K, Kita K, Otsuji A, et al. Diagnostic and clinical importance of interleukin-2 receptor alpha chain expression on non-T-cell acute leukemia cells. Br J Haematol. 1992;80:317.
103. Heerema NA, Harbott J, Galimberti S, et al. Secondary cytogenetic aberrations in childhood Philadelphia chromosome positive acute lymphoblastic leukemia are nonrandom and may be associated with outcome. Leukemia. 2004;18:693.
104. Wetzler M, Dodge RK, Mrózek K, et al. Additional cytogenetic abnormalities in adults with Philadelphia chromosome-positive acute lymphoblastic leukaemia: a study of the Cancer and Leukaemia Group B. Br J Haematol. 2004;124:275.
105. Rieder H, Ludwig WD, Gassmann W, et al. Prognostic significance of additional chromosome abnormalities in adult patients with Philadelphia chromosome positive acute lymphoblastic leukaemia. Br J Haematol. 1996;95:678.
106. Primo D, Tabernero MD, Perez JJ, et al. Genetic heterogeneity of *BCR/ABL*+ adult B-cell precursor acute lymphoblastic leukemia: impact on the clinical, biological and immunophenotypical disease characteristics. Leukemia. 2005;19:713.
107. Ludwig W-D, Rieder H, Bartram CR, et al. Immunophenotypic and genotypic features, clinical characteristics, and treatment outcome of adult pro-B acute lymphoblastic leukemia: results of the German multicenter trials GMALL 03/87 and 04/89. Blood. 1998;92:1898.
108. Putti MC, Rondelli R, Cocito MG, et al. Expression of myeloid markers lacks prognostic impact in children treated for acute lymphoblastic leukemia: Italian experience in AIEOP-ALL 88–91 studies. Blood. 1998;92:795.
109. Wilson GA, Vandenberghe EA, Pollitt RC, et al. Are aberrant BCR-ABL transcripts more common than previously thought? Br J Haematol. 2000;111:1109.
110. Paietta E, Li X, Richards S, et al. Implications for the use of monoclonal antibodies in future adult ALL trials: analysis of antigen expression in 505 B-lineage (B-lin) ALL patients (pts) on the MRC UKALLXII/ECOG2993 intergroup trial. Blood. 2008;112(11):666. #1907
111. Kurzrock R, Kantarjian HM, Druker BJ, Talpaz M. Philadelphia chromosome-positive leukemias: from basic mechanisms to molecular therapeutics. Ann Intern Med. 2003;138:819.
112. Quintas-Cardama A, Cortes A. Molecular biology of BCR-ABL1-positive chronic myeloid leukemia. Blood. 2009;113:1619.
113. Castor A, Nilsson L, Åstrand-Grundström I, et al. Distinct patterns of hematopoietic stem cell involvement in acute lymphoblastic leukemia. Nat Med. 2005;11:630.
114. Nakase K, Kita K, Miwa H, et al. Clinical and prognostic significance of cytokine receptor expression in adult acute lymphoblastic leukemia: interleukin-2 receptor α-chain predicts a poor prognosis. Leukemia. 2007;21:326.
115. Lee J-W, Geng H, Chen Z, et al. CD25 enables oncogenic BCR signaling and represents a therapeutic target in refractory B-cell malignancies. Blood. 2016;128:4088.

116. Aricó M, Valsecchi MG, Camitta B, et al. Outcome of treatment in children with Philadelphia chromosome-positive acute lymphoblastic leukemia. N Engl J Med. 2000;342:998.
117. Gleissner B, Gökbuget N, Bartram CR, et al. Leading prognostic relevance of the BCR-ABL translocation in adult acute B-lineage lymphoblastic leukemia: a prospective study of the German Multicenter Trial Group and confirmed polymerase chain reaction analysis. Blood. 2002;99:1536.
118. Dombret H, Gabert J, Boiron J-M, et al. Outcome of treatment in adults with Philadelphia chromosome-positive acute lymphoblastic leukemia-results of the prospective multicenter LALA-94 trial. Blood. 2002;100:2357.
119. Schrappe M, Aricó M, Harbott J, et al. Philadelphia chromosome-positive (Ph^+) childhood acute lymphoblastic leukemia: good initial steroid response allows early prediction of a favorable treatment outcome. Blood. 1998;92:2730.
120. Fossa A, Siebert R, Kasper C, et al. BCR rearrangement without juxtaposition of ABL in pre-T Acute lymphoblastic leukemia. Br J Haematol. 1996;93:403.
121. Kohlmann A, Schoch C, Dugas M, et al. New insights into MLL gene rearranged acute leukemias using gene expression profiling: shared pathways, lineage commitment, and partner genes. Leukemia. 2005;19:953.
122. Gleissner B, Goekbuget N, Rieder H, et al. $CD10^-$ pre-B acute lymphoblastic leukemia (ALL) is a distinct high-risk subgroup of adult ALL associated with a high frequency of MLL aberrations: results of the German Multicenter trials for adult ALL (GMALL). Blood. 2005;106:4054.
123. Harper DP, Aplan PD. Chromosomal rearrangements leading to MLL gene fusions: clinical and biological aspects. Cancer Res. 2008;68:10024.
124. Pui C-H, Campana D. Age-related differences in leukemia biology and prognosis: the paradigm of *MLL-AF4*-positive acute lymphoblastic leukemia. Leukemia. 2007;21:593.
125. Marks DI, Moorman AV, Chilton L, et al. The clinical characteristics, biology, therapy and outcome of 85 adults with acute lymphoblastic leukemia and t(4;11)(q21;q23)/*MLL-AFF1* uniformly treated on UKALLXII/ECOG2993. Haematologica. 2013;98:945.
126. Burmeister T, Meyer C, Schwartz S, et al. The *MLL* recombinome of adult CD10-negative B-cell precursor acute lymphoblastic leukemia: results from the GMALL study group. Blood. 2009;113:4011.
127. Pui C-H, Relling MV, Downing JR. Mechanisms of disease. Acute lymphoblastic leukemia. N Engl J Med. 2004;350:1535.
128. Rubnitz JE, Pui C-H, Downing JR. The role of TEL fusion genes in pediatric leukemias. Leukemia. 1999;13:6.
129. Aguiar RCT, Sohal J, van Rhee F, et al. TEL-AML1 fusion in acute lymphoblastic leukemia in adults. Br J Haematol. 1996;95:673.
130. Borowitz MJ, Rubnitz J, Nash M, et al. Surface antigen phenotype can predict TEL-AML1 rearrangement in childhood B-precursor ALL: a Pediatric Oncology Group study. Leukemia. 1998;12:1764.
131. De Zen L, Orfeo A, Cazzaniga G, et al. Quantitative multiparametric immunophenotyping in acute lymphoblastic leukemia: correlation with specific genotype. I. ETV6/AML1 ALLs identification. Leukemia. 2000;14:1225.
132. Alessandri AJ, Reid GS, Bader SA, et al. ETV6 (TEL)-AML1 pre-B acute lymphoblastic leukemia cells are associated with a distinct antigen-presenting phenotype. Br J Haematol. 2002;116:266.
133. Rhein P, Mitlohner R, Basso G, et al. CD11b is a therapy resistance- and minimal residual disease-specific marker in precursor B-cell acute lymphoblastic leukemia. Blood. 2010;115:3763.
134. Soulier J, Clappier E, Cayuela JM, et al. HOXA genes are included in genetic and biologic networks defining human acute T-cell leukemia (T-ALL). Blood. 2005;106:274.
135. Cauwelier B, Cave H, Gervais C, et al. Clinical, cytogenetic and molecular characteristics of 14 T-ALL patients carrying the TCRβ-HOXA rearrangement: a study of the Groupe Francophone de Cytogenetique Hematologique. Leukemia. 2007;21:121.
136. Gilliland DG, Griffin JD. The roles of FLT3 in hematopoiesis and leukemia. Blood. 2002;100:1532.
137. Kottaridis PD, Gale RE, Linch DC. FLT3 mutations and leukemia. Br J Haematol. 2003;122:523.
138. Barragan E, Montesinos P, Camos M, et al. Prognostic value of FLT3 mutations in patients with acute promyelocytic leukemia treated with all-trans retinoic acid and anthracycline monochemotherapy. Haematologica. 2011;96:1470.
139. Poiré X, Moser BK, Gallagher RE, et al. Arsenic trioxide in front-line therapy of acute promyelocytic leukemia (C9710): prognostic significance of FLT3 mutations and complex karyotype. Leuk Lymphoma. 2014;55:1523.
140. Levis M. FLT3 mutations in acute myeloid leukemia: what is the best approach in 2013? ASH Educ Book. 2013;2013:220.
141. Luskin MR, Lee J-W, Fernandez HF, et al. Benefit of high dose daunorubicin in AML induction extends across cytogenetic and molecular groups: updated analysis of E1900. Blood. 2016;127:1551.
142. Bacher U, Haferlach C, Kern W, et al. Prognostic relevance of FLT3-TKD mutations in AML: the combination matters-an analysis of 3082 patients. Blood. 2008;111:2527.
143. Mead AJ, Linch DC, Hills RK, et al. FLT3 tyrosine kinase domain mutations are biologically distinct from and have a significantly more favorable prognosis than FLT3 internal tandem duplications in patients with acute myeloid leukemia. Blood. 2007;110:1262.
144. Stein EM, Tallman MS. Emerging therapeutic drugs for AML. Blood. 2016;127:71.
145. Kussick SJ, Yi HS, Gerard AA, Brent BL. Acute myeloid leukemia bearing the Flt3 internal tandem duplication has a unique immunophenotype which enables its identification by flow cytometry. Blood. 2002;100:196a. #737
146. Falini B, Mecucci C, Tiacci E, et al. Cytoplasmic nucleophosmin in acute myelogenous leukemia with a normal karyotype. N Engl J Med. 2005;352:254.
147. Cancer Genome Atlas Research Network. Genomic and epigenomic landscapes of adult de novo acute myeloid leukemia. N Engl J Med. 2013;368:2059.
148. Guryanova OA, Shank K, Spitzer B, et al. DNMT3A mutations promote anthracycline resistance in acute myeloid leukemia via impaired nucleosome remodeling. Nat Med. 2016;22:1488.
149. Angelini DF, Ottone T, Guerrera G, et al. A leukemia-associated CD34/CD123/CD25/CD99+ immunophenotype identifies FLT3-mutated clones in acute myeloid leukemia. Clin Cancer Res. 2015;21:3977.
150. Chung SS, Tavakkoli M, Devlin SM, Park CY. CD99 is a therapeutic target on disease stem cells in acute myeloid leukemia and the myelodysplastic syndromes. Blood. 2013;122:2891.
151. Marks DI, Paietta E, Moorman AV, et al. T-cell acute lymphoblastic leukemia in adults: clinical features, immunophenotype, cytogenetics and outcome from the large randomized prospective trial (UKALL XII/ECOG 2993). Blood. 2009;114:5136.
152. Armstrong SA, Mabon ME, Silverman LB, et al. FLT3 mutation in childhood acute lymphoblastic leukemia. Blood. 2004;103:3544.
153. Brown P, Levis M, Shurtleff S, et al. FLT3 inhibition selectively kills childhood acute lymphoblastic leukemia cells with high levels of FLT3 expression. Blood. 2005;105:812.
154. Di Noto R, Lo Pardo C, Schiavone EM, et al. Stem cell factor receptor (c-kit, CD117) is expressed on blast cells from most immature types of acute myeloid malignancies but is also a characteristic of a subset of acute promyelocytic leukemia. Br J Haematol. 1996;92:562.
155. Nomdedéu JF, Mateu R, Altès A, et al. Enhanced myeloid specificity of CD117 compared with CD13 and CD33. Leuk Res. 1999;23:341.

156. Broudy VC. Stem cell factor and hematopoiesis. Blood. 1997;90:1345.
157. Sperling C, Schwartz S, Buchner T, et al. Expression of the stem cell factor receptor c-KIT (CD117) in acute leukemias. Haematologica. 1997;82:617.
158. Bertho J-M, Chapel A, Loilleux S, et al. CD135 (Flk2/Flt3) expression by human thymocytes delineates a possible role of FLT3-ligand in T-cell precursor proliferation and differentiation. Scand J Immunol. 2000;52:53.
159. Staal FJ, Weerkamp F, Langerak AW, et al. Transcriptional control of T lymphocyte differentiation. Stem Cells. 2001;19:165.
160. Ferrando AA, Neuberg DS, Staunton J, et al. Gene expression signatures define novel oncogenic pathways in T cell acute lymphoblastic leukemia. Cancer Cell. 2002;1:75.
161. Asnafi V, Beldjord K, Boulanger E, et al. Analysis of TCR, pTα, and RAG-1 in T-acute lymphoblastic leukemias improves understanding of early human T-lymphoid lineage commitment. Blood. 2003;101:2693.
162. Bell JJ, Bhandoola A. The earliest thymic progenitors for T cells possess myeloid lineage potential. Nature. 2008;452:764.
163. Neumann M, Coskun E, Fransecky L, et al. FLT3 mutations in early T-cell precursor ALL characterize a stem cell like leukemia and imply the clinical use of tyrosine kinase inhibitors. PLoS One. 2013;8:e53190.
164. Van Vlierberghe P, Meijerink JPP, Stam RW, et al. Activating *FLT3* mutations in CD4^{+}/CD8− pediatric T-cell acute lymphoblastic leukemias. Blood. 2005;106:4414.
165. Serrano J, Román J, Jiménez A, et al. Genetic, phenotypic and clinical features of acute lymphoblastic leukemias expressing myeloperoxidase mRNA detected by RT-PCR. Leukemia. 1999;13:175.
166. Hoehn D, Medeiros LJ, Chen SS, et al. CD117 expression is a sensitive but nonspecific predictor of *FLT3* mutation in T acute lymphoblastic leukemia and T/Myeloid acute leukemia. Am J Clin Pathol. 2012;137:213.
167. Nishii K, Kita K, Miwa H, et al. c-kit gene expression in CD7-positive acute lymphoblastic leukemia: close correlation with expression of myeloid-associated antigen CD13. Leukemia. 1992;6:662.
168. Van Vlierberghe P, Ambesi-Impiombato A, Perez-Garcia A, et al. *ETV6* mutations in early immature human T cell leukemias. J Exp Med. 2011;208:2571.
169. Zhang J, Ding L, Holmfeldt L, et al. The genetic basis of early T-cell precursor acute lymphoblastic leukaemia. Nature. 2012;481:157.
170. Mullighan CG. The molecular genetic makeup of acute lymphoblastic leukemia. Hematology. 2012;2012:389.
171. Haydu JE, Ferrando AA. Early T-cell precursor acute lymphoblastic leukemia (ETP T-ALL). Curr Opin Hematol. 2013;20:369.
172. Neumann M, Greif PA, Baldus CD. Mutational landscape of adult ETP-ALL. Oncotarget. 2013;4:954.
173. Coustan-Smith E, Mullighan CG, Onciu M, et al. Early T-cell precursor leukaemia: a subtype of very high-risk acute lymphoblastic leukaemia. Lancet Oncol. 2009;10:147.
174. Rothenberg EV, Moore JE, Yui MA. Launching the T-cell-lineage developmental programme. Nat Rev Immunol. 2008;8:9.
175. Wada H, Masuda K, Satoh R, et al. Adult T-cell progenitors retain myeloid potential. Nature. 2008;452:768.
176. Neumann M, Heesch S, Gökbuget N, et al. Clinical and molecular characterization of early T-cell precursor leukemia: a high-risk subgroup in adult T-ALL with a high frequency of FLT3 mutations. Blood Cancer J. 2012;2:e55.
177. Chopra A, Bakhshi S, Pramanik SK, et al. Immunophenotypic analysis of T-acute lymphoblastic leukemia. A CD5-based ETP-ALL perspective of non-ETP T-ALL. Eur J Haematol. 2014;92:211.
178. Jain N, Lamb AE, O'Brien S, et al. Early T-cell precursor acute lymphoblastic leukemia/lymphoma (ETP-ALL/LBL) in adolescents and adults: a high-risk subtype. Blood. 2016;127:1863.
179. Wood BL, Winter SS, Dunsmore KP, et al. T-lymphoblastic leukemia (T-ALL) shows excellent outcome, lack of significance of the early thymic precursor (ETP) immunophenotype, and validation of the prognostic value of end-induction minimal residual disease (MRD) in Children's Oncology Group (COG) Study AALL0434. Blood. 2014;124:1.
180. Patrick K, Wade R, Goulden N, et al. Outcome for children and young people with Early T-cell precursor acute lymphoblastic leukaemia treated on a contemporary protocol UKALL 2003. Br J Haematol. 2014;166:421.
181. Brammer JE, Saliba RM, Jorgensen JL, et al. Multi-center analysis of the effect of T-cell acute lymphoblastic leukemia subtype and minimal residual disease on allogeneic stem cell transplantation outcomes. Bone Marrow Transplant. 2017;52:20.
182. Chiaretti S, Gianfelici V, Ceglie G, Foá R. Genomic characterization of acute leukemias. Med Princ Pract. 2014;487
183. Matlawska-Wasowska K, Kang H, Devidas M, et al. MLL rearrangements impact outcome in HOXA-deregulated T-lineage acute lymphoblastic leukemia: A Children's Oncology Group study. Leukemia. 2016;30:1909.
184. Gutierrez A, Dahlberg SE, Neuberg DS, et al. Absence of biallelic TCRγ deletion predicts early treatment failure in pediatric T-cell acute lymphoblastic leukemia. J Clin Oncol. 2010;28:3816.
185. Zuurbier L, Gutierrez A, Mullighan CG, et al. Immature MEF2C-dysregulated T-ALL patients have an ETP-ALL gene signature and typically have non-rearranged T-cell receptors. Haematologica. 2014;99:94.
186. Meijerink JPP, Canté-Barrett K, Vroegindeweij E, Pieters R. HOXA-activated early T-cell progenitor acute lymphoblastic leukemia: predictor of poor outcome? Haematologica. 2016;101:654.
187. Bond J, Marchand T, Touzart A, et al. An early thymic precursor phenotype predicts outcome exclusively in HOXA-overexpressing adult T-cell acute lymphoblastic leukemia: A Group for Research in Adult Acute Lymphoblastic Leukemia study. Haematologica. 2016;101:732.
188. Chen CW, Armstrong SA. Targeting DOT1L and HOX gene expression in MLL-rearranged leukemia and beyond. Exp Hematol. 2015;43:673.
189. Asnafi V, Buzyn A, Thomas X, et al. Impact of TCR status and genotype on outcome in adult T-cell acute lymphoblastic leukemia: a LALA-94 study. Blood. 2005;105:3072.
190. Ferrando AA, Neuberg DS, Dodge RK, et al. Prognostic importance of TLX1 (HOX11) oncogene expression in adults with T-cell acute lymphoblastic leukemia. Lancet. 2004;363:535.
191. Meijerink JP. Genetic rearrangements in relation to immunophenotype and outcome in T-cell acute lymphoblastic leukaemia. Best Pract Res Clin Haematol. 2010;23:307.
192. Nomdedeu J, Bussaglia E, Villamore N, et al. Immunophenotype of acute myeloid leukemia with NPM mutations: Prognostic impact of the leukemic compartment size. Leuk Res. 2011;35:163.
193. Kern W, Haferlach C, Bacher U, et al. Flow cytometric identification of acute myeloid leukemia with limited differentiation and *NPM1* type A mutation: a new biologically defined entity. Leukemia. 2009;23:1361.
194. Martelli MP, Pettirossi V, Thiede C, et al. CD34+ cells from AML with mutated NPM1 harbor cytoplasmic mutated nucleophosmin and generate leukemia in immumocompromised mice. Blood. 2010;116:3907.
195. Litzow M, Buck G, Dewald G, et al. Outcome of 1,229 adult Philadelphia chromosome negative B acute lymphoblastic leukemia (B-ALL) patients (pts) from the international UKALLXII/E2993 trial: no difference in results between B cell immunophenotypic subgroups. Blood. 2010;116:524.

196. Schultz KR, Pullen J, Sather HN, et al. Risk- and response-based classification of childhood B-precursor acute lymphoblastic leukemia: a combined analysis of prognostic markers from the Pediatric Oncology Group (POG) and Children's Cancer Group (CCG). Blood. 2007;109:926.
197. Mullighan CG, Miller CB, Radtke I, et al. BCR-ABL1 lymphoblastic leukemia is characterized by the deletion of Ikaros. Nature. 2008;453:110.
198. Martinelli G, Iacobucci I, Storlazzi CT, et al. IKZF1 (Ikaros) deletions in BCR-ABL1-positive acute lymphoblastic leukemia are associated with short disease-free survival and high rate of cumulative incidence of relapse: a GIMEMA AL WP report. J Clin Oncol. 2009;27:5202.
199. Mullighan CG, Su X, Zhang J, et al. Children's Oncology Group: deletion of IKZF1 and prognosis in acute lymphoblastic leukemia. N Engl J Med. 2009;360:470.
200. Iacobucci I, Li Y, Roberts KG, et al. Truncated erythropoietin receptor rearrangements in acute lymphoblastic leukemia. Cancer Cell. 2016;29:186.
201. Tang DG. Understanding cancer stem cell heterogeneity and plasticity. Cell Res. 2012;22:457.
202. Kuiper RP, Waanders E, van der Velden VH, et al. IKZF1 deletions predict relapse in uniformly treated pediatric precursor B-ALL. Leukemia. 2010;24:1258.
203. Den Boer ML, van Slegtenhorst M, De Menezes RX, et al. A subtype of childhood acute lymphoblastic leukaemia with poor treatment outcome: a genome-wide classification study. Lancet Oncol. 209, 10:125.
204. Roberts KG, Pei D, Campana D, et al. Outcome of children with BCR-ABL1-like acute lymphoblastic leukemia treated with risk-directed therapy based on the levels of minimal residual disease. J Clin Oncol. 2014;32:3012.
205. Herold T, Schneider S, Metzeler KH, et al. Adults with Philadelphia chromosome-like acute lymphoblastic leukemia frequently have *IGH-CRLF2* and *JAK2* mutations, persistence of minimal residual disease and poor prognosis. Haematologica. 2017;102:130.
206. Roberts KG, Li Y, Payne-Turner D, et al. Targetable kinase activating lesions in Ph-like acute lymphoblastic leukemia. N Engl J Med. 2014;371:1005.
207. Tasian SK, Teachey DT, Li Y, et al. Potent efficacy of combined PI3K/mTOR and JAK or ABL inhibition in murine xenograft models of Ph-like acute lymphoblastic leukemia. Blood. 2017;129:177.
208. Herold T, Baldus CD, Gökbuget N. pH-like acute lymphoblastic leukemia in older adults. N Engl J Med (Correspondence). 2014:371, 23.
209. Mullighan CG, Collins-Underwood JR, Phillips LAA, et al. Rearrangement of *CRLF2* in B-progenitor and Down syndrome associated acute lymphoblastic leukemia. Nat Genet. 2009;41:1243.
210. Russell LJ, Capasso M, Vater I, et al. Deregulated expression of cytokine receptor gene, CRLF2, is involved in lymphoid transformation in B-cell precursor acute lymphoblastic leukemia. Blood. 2009;114:2688.
211. Hertzberg L, Vendramini E, Ganmore I, et al. Down syndrome acute lymphoblastic leukemia: a highly heterogenous disease in which aberrant expression of CRLF2 is associated with mutated JAK2: a report from the iBFM Study Group. Blood. 2010;115:1006.
212. Cario G, Zimmermann M, Romey R, et al. Presence of the *P2RY8-CRLF2* rearrangement is associated with a poor prognosis in non-high-risk precursor B-cell acute lymphoblastic leukemia in children treated according to the ALL-BFM 2000 protocol. Blood. 2010;115:5393.
213. Ensor HM, Schwab C, Russell LJ, et al. Demographic, clinical, and outcome features of children with acute lymphoblastic leukemia and *CRLF2* deregulation: results from the MRC ALL97 clinical trial. Blood. 2011;117:2129.
214. van der Veer A, Waanders E, Pieters R, et al. Independent prognostic value of BCR/ABL1-like signature and IKZF1 deletion, but not high CRLF2 expression, in children with B-cell precursor ALL. Blood. 2013;122:2622.
215. Farhadfar N, Litzow MR. New monoclonal antibodies for the treatment of acute lymphoblastic leukemia. Leuk Res. 2016;49:13.
216. Papadantonakis N, Advani AS. Recent advances and novel treatment paradigms in acute lymphocytic leukemia. Ther Adv Hematol. 2016;7:252.
217. Rashidi A, Walter RB. Antigen-specific immunotherapy for acute myeloid leukemia: where are we now, and where do we go from here? Expert Rev Hematol. 2016;9:335.
218. Garfin PM, Feldman EJ. Antibody-based treatment in acute myeloid leukemia. Curr Hematol Malig Rep. 2016;11:545.
219. Aldoss I, Bargou RC, Nagorsen D, et al. Redirecting T-cells to eradicate B-cell acute lymphoblastic leukemia: bispecific T-cell engagers and chimeric antigen receptors. Leukemia. 2016.; [Epub ahead of print]
220. Davila ML, Brentjens RJ. CD19-targeted CAR T cells as novel cancer immunotherapy for relapsed or refractory B-cell acute lymphoblastic leukemia. Clin Adv Hematol Oncol. 2016;14:802.
221. Frey NV, Porter DL. The promise of chimeric antigen receptor T-cell therapy. Oncology (Williston Park). 2016;30:880.
222. Wayne AS, FitzGerald DJ, Kreitman RJ, Pastan I. Immunotoxins for leukemia. Blood. 2014;123:2470.
223. Bodet-Milin C, Kraeber-Bodéré F, Eugéne T, et al. Radioimmunotherapy for treatment of acute leukemia. Semin Nucl Med. 2016;46:135.
224. Buckley SA, Walter RB. Update on antigen-specific immunotherapy of acute myeloid leukemia. Curr Hematol Malig Rep. 2015;10:65.
225. Dworzak M, Schumich A, Printz D, et al. CD20 up-regulation in pediatric B-cell precursor acute lymphoblastic leukemia during induction treatment: setting the stage for anti-CD20 directed immunotherapy. Blood. 2008;112:3982.
226. Gökbuget N, Hoelzer D. Treatment with monoclonal antibodies in acute lymphoblastic leukemia: current knowledge and future prospects. Ann Hematol. 2003;83:201.
227. Jabbour E, O'Brien S, Ravandi F, Kantarjian H. Monoclonal antibodies in acute lymphoblastic leukemia. Blood. 2015;125:4010.
228. Maury S, Chevret S, Thomas X, et al. Rituximab in B-lineage adult acute lymphoblastic leukemia. N Engl J Med. 2016;375:1044.
229. Hoelzer D, Huettmann A, Kaul F, et al. Immunochemotherapy with rituximab improves molecular CR rate and outcome in CD20+ B-lineage standard and high risk patients; results of 263 CD20+ patients studied prospectively in GMALL study 07/2003. Blood. 2010;116:170.
230. Thomas D, Faderl S, O'Brien S, et al. Chemoimmunotherapy with hyper-CVAD plus rituximab for the treatment of adult Burkitt and Burkitt-type lymphoma or acute lymphoblastic leukemia. Cancer. 2006;106:1569.
231. Paietta E, Andersen J, Wiernik PH. A new approach to analyzing the utility of immunophenotyping for predicting clinical outcome in acute leukemia. Leukemia. 1996;10:1.
232. Wang L, Abbasi F, Gaigalas AK, et al. Comparison of fluorescein and phycoerythrin conjugates for quantifying CD20 expression on normal and leukemic cells. Cytometry Part B: Clin Cytometry. 2006;70B:410.
233. Perz J, Topaly J, Fruehauf S, et al. Level of CD20-expression and efficacy of rituximab treatment in patients with resistant or relapsing B-cell prolymphocytic leukemia and B-cell chronic lymphocytic leukemia. Leuk Lymphoma. 2002;43:149.
234. Tomita A. Genetic and epigenetic modulation of CD20 expression in B-cell malignancies: molecular mechanisms and significance to rituximab resistance. J Clin Exp Hematop. 2016;56:89.

235. Henry C, Deschamps M, Rohrlich P-S, et al. Identification of an alternative CD20 transcript variant in B-cell malignancies coding for a novel protein associated to rituximab resistance. Blood. 2010;115:2420.
236. Jeha S, Behm F, Pei D, et al. Prognostic significance of CD20 expression in childhood B-cell precursor acute lymphoblastic leukemia. Blood. 2006;108:3302.
237. Thomas DA, O'Brien S, Jorgensen JL, et al. Prognostic significance of CD20 expression in adults with de novo precursor B-lineage acute lymphoblastic leukemia. Blood. 2009;113:6330.
238. Maury S, Huguet F, Leguay T, et al. Adverse prognostic significance of CD20 expression in adults with Philadelphia chromosome-negative B-cell precursor acute lymphoblastic leukemia. Haematologica. 2010;95:324.
239. Mannelli F, Gianfaldoni G, Intermesoli T, et al. CD20 expression has no prognostic role in Philadelphia-negative B-precursor acute lymphoblastic leukemia: new insights from the molecular study of minimal residual disease. Haematologica. 2012;97:568.
240. Ou DY, Luo JM, Ou DL. CD20 and outcome of childhood precursor B-cell acute lymphoblastic leukemia: a meta-analysis. J Pediatr Hematol Oncol. 2015;37:e138.
241. Borowitz MJ, Shuster J, Carroll AJ, et al. Prognostic significance of fluorescence intensity of surface marker expression in childhood B-precursor acute lymphoblastic leukemia. A Pediatric Oncology Group Study. Blood. 1997;89:3960.
242. Awasthi A, Ayello J, Van de Ven C, et al. Obinutuzumab (GA101) compared to rituximab significantly enhances cell death and antibody-dependent cytotoxicity and improves overall survival against CD20(+) rituximab-sensitive/-resistant Burkitt lymphoma (BL) and precursor B-acute lymphoblastic leukaemia (pre-B-ALL): potential targeted therapy in patients with poor risk CD20(+) BL and pre-B-ALL. Br J Haematol. 2015;171:763.
243. Manshouri T, Do K, Wang X, et al. Circulating CD20 is detectable in the plasma of patients with chronic lymphocytic leukemia and is of prognostic significance. Blood. 2003;101:2507.
244. Piccaluga P, Arpinati M, Candoni A, et al. Surface antigens analysis reveals significant expression of candidate targets for immunotherapy in adult acute lymphoid leukemia. Leuk Lymphoma. 2011;52:325.
245. Shah NN, Stetler-Stevenson M, Yuan CM, et al. Characterization of CD22 expression in acute lymphoblastic leukemia. Pediatr Blood Cancer. 2015;62:964.
246. Carnahan J, Wang P, Kendall R, et al. Epratuzumab, a humanized monoclonal antibody targeting CD22: characterization of in vitro properties. Clin Cancer Res. 2003;9:3982S.
247. Rossi EA, Goldenberg DM, Siegel AB, et al. Trogocytosis of multiple B-cell surface markers by CD22 targeting with epratuzumab. Blood. 2013;122:3020.
248. Raetz EA, Cairo MS, Borowitz MJ, et al. Re-induction chemoimmunotherapy with epratuzumab in relapsed acute lymphoblastic leukemia (ALL): Phase II results from Children's Oncology Group (COG) study ADVL04P2. Pediatr Blood Cancer. 2015;62:1171.
249. Yilmaz M, Richard S, Jabbour E. The clinical potential of inotuzumab ozogamicin in relapsed and refractory acute lymphocytic leukemia. Ther Adv Hematol. 2015;6:253.
250. Kantarjian HM, DeAngelo DJ, Stelljes M, et al. Inotuzumab ozogamicin versus standard therapy for acute lymphoblastic leukemia. N Engl J Med. 2016;375:740.
251. Pollard JA, Loken M, Gerbring RD, et al. CD33 expression and its association with gemtuzumab ozogamicin response: results from the randomized phase III Children's Oncology Group trial AAML0531. J Clin Oncol. 2016;34:747.
252. Walter RB. The role of CD33 as therapeutic target in acute myeloid leukemia. Expert Opinion Ther Targets. 2014;18:715.
253. Petersdorf SH, Kopecky KJ, Slovak M, et al. A phase 3 study of gemtuzumab ozogamicin during induction and postconsolidation therapy in younger patients with acute myeloid leukemia. Blood. 2013;121:4854.
254. Castaigne S, Pautas C, Terré C, et al. Effect of gemtuzumab ozogamicin on survival of adult patients with de-novo acute myeloid leukemia (ALFA-0701): a randomized, open-label, phse 3 study. Lancet. 2012;379:1508.
255. Burnett AK, Russell N, Hills RK, et al. The addition of gemtuzumab ozogamicin in induction chemotherapy improves survival in older patients with acute myeloid leukemia. J Clin Oncol. 2012;30:3924.
256. Ravandi F, Estey EH, Appelbaum FR, Lo-Coco F, Schiffer CA, Larson RA, Burnett AK, Kantarjian HM. Gemtuzumab ozogamicin: time to resurrect? J Clin Oncol. 2012;30:3921.
257. Hills RK, Castaigne S, Appelbaum FR, et al. Addition of gemtuzumab ozogamicin to induction chemotherapy of adult patient with acute myeloid leukemia: a meta-analysis of individual patient data from randomized controlled trials. Lancet Oncol. 2014;15:986.
258. Balaian L, Ball ED. Cytotoxic activity of gemtuzumab ozogamicin (Mylotarg) in acute myeloid leukemia correlates with the expression of protein kinase Syk. Leukemia. 2006;20:2093.
259. Olombel G, Guerin E, Guy J, et al. The level of blast CD33 expression positively impacts the effect of gemtuzumab ozogamicin in patients with acute myeloid leukemia. Blood. 2016;127:2157.
260. Khan N, Hills RK, Virgo P, et al. Expression of CD33 is a predictive factor for effect of gemtuzumab ozogamicin at different doses in adult acute myeloid leukemia. Leukemia. 2016; [Epub ahead of time].
261. Mortland L, Alonzo TA, Walter RB, et al. Clinical significance of CD33 non-synonymous single nucleotide polymorphisms (SNPs) in pediatric patients with acute myeloid leukemia treated with gemtuzumab-ozogamicin-containing chemotherapy. Clin Cancer Res. 2013;19:1620.
262. Walter RB, Appelbaum FR, Estey EH, Bernstein ID. Acute myeloid leukemia stem cells and CD33-targeted immunotherapy. Blood. 2012;119:6198.
263. Laporte JP, Isnard F, Garderet L, et al. Remission of adult acute lymphocytic leukemia with alemtuzumab. Leukemia. 2004;18:1557.
264. Piccaluga PP, Martinelli G, Malagola M, et al. Alemtuzumab in the treatment of relapsed acute lymphoid leukemia. Leukemia. 2005;19:135.
265. Gorin NC, Isnard F, Garderet L, et al. Administration of alemtuzumab and G-CSF to adults with relapsed or refractory acute lymphoblastic leukemia: results of a phase II study. Eur J Haematol. 2013;91:315.
266. Mølhøj M, Crommer S, Brischwein K, et al. CD19-/CD3-bispecific antibody of the BiTE class is far superior to tandem diabody with respect to redirected tumor cell lysis. Mol Immunol. 2007;44:1935.
267. Bargou R, Leo E, Zugmaier G, et al. Tumor regression in cancer patients by very low doses of a T cell-engaging antibody. Science. 2008;321(5891):974.
268. Benjamin JE, Stein AS. The role of blinatumomab in patients with relapsed/refractory acute lymphoblastic leukemia. Ther Adv Hematol. 2016;7:142.
269. Topp MS, Gökbuget N, Stein AS, et al. Safety and activity of blinatumomab for adult patients with relapsed or refractory B-precursor acute lymphoblastic leukaemia: a multicentre, single-arm, phase 2 study. Lancet Oncol. 2015;16:57.
270. Duell J, Dittrich M. Bedke T, et al. Leukemia: Frequency of regulatory T cells determines the outcome of the T-cell engaging antibody blinatumomab in patients with B precursor ALL; 2017. (Epub ahead of print)
271. Klinger M, Benjamin J, Kischel R, et al. Harnessing T cells to fight cancer with BiTE® antibody constructs—past developments and future directions. Immunol Rev. 2016;270:193.

272. Al-Hussaini M, Rettig MP, Ritchey JK, et al. Targeting CD123 in acute myeloid leukemia using a T-cell-directed dual-affinity retargeting platform. Blood. 2016;127:122.
273. Sadelain M, Brentjens R, Riviére I. The basic principles of chimeric antigen receptor design. Cancer Discov. 2013;3:388.
274. Khalil DN, Smith EL, Brentjens RJ, Wolchok JD. The future of cancer treatment: immunomodulation, CARs and combination immunotherapy. Nat Rev Clin Oncol. 2016;13:394.
275. Karlsson H, Svensson E, Gigg C, et al. Evaluation of intracellular signaling downstream chimeric antigen receptors. PLoS One. 2015;10:e0144787.
276. Yeku OO, Brentjens RJ. Armored CAR T-cells: utilizing cytokines and pro-inflammatory ligands to enhance CAR T-cell antitumour efficacy. Biochem Soc Trans. 2016;44:412.
277. Brentjens RJ, Davila ML, Riviére I, et al. CD19-targeted T cells rapidly induce molecular remissions in adults with chemotherapy-refractory acute lymphoblastic leukemia. Sci Transl Med. 2013;5:177ra38.
278. Grupp SA, Kalos M, Barrett D, et al. Chimeric antigen receptor-modified T cells for acute lymphoid leukemia. N Engl J Med. 2013;368:1509.
279. Maude SL, Frey N, Shaw PA, et al. Chimeric antigen receptor T cells for sustained remissions in leukemia. N Engl J Med. 2014;371:1507.
280. Hay KA, Turtle CJ. Chimeric antigen receptor (CAR) T cells: lessons learned from targeting of CD19 in B-cell malignancies. Drugs. 2017.; [Epub ahead of print]
281. Ruella M, Maus MV. Catch me if you can: leukemia escape after CD19-directed T cell immunotherapies. Comput Struct Biotechnol J. 2016;14:357.
282. Bachas C, Schuurhuis GJ, Assaraf YG, et al. The role of minor subpopulations within the leukemic blast compartment of AML patients at initial diagnosis in the development of relapse. Leukemia. 2012;26:1313.
283. Ruella M, Barrett DM, Kenderian SS, et al. Dual CD19 and CD123 targeting prevents antigen-loss relapses after CD19-directed immunotherapies. J Clin Invest. 2016;126:3814.
284. Yannakou CK, Came N, Bajel AR, Juneja S. CD19 negative relapse in B-ALL treated with Blinatumomab therapy: avoiding the Trap. Blood. 2015;126:4983.
285. Sotillo E, Barrett DM, Black KL, et al. Convergence of acquired mutations and alternative splicing of CD19 enables resistance to CART-19 immunotherapy. Cancer Discov. 2015;5:1282.
286. Braig F, Brandt A, Goebeler M, et al. Resistance to anti-CD19/CD3 BiTE in acute lymphoblastic leukemia may be mediated by disrupted CD19 membrane trafficking. Blood. 2017;129:129.
287. van Zelm MC, Smet J, Adams B, et al. CD81 gene defect in humans disrupts CD19 complex formation and leads to antibody deficiency. J Clin Invest. 2010;120:1265.
288. Jacoby E, Nguyen SM, Fountaine TJ, et al. CD19 CAR immune pressure induces B-precursor acute lymphoblastic leukemia lineage switch exposing inherent leukaemic plasticity. Nat Commun. 2016;7:12320.
289. Gardner R, Wu D, Cherian S, et al. Acquisition of a CD19 negative myeloid phenotype allows immune escape of MLL-rearranged B-ALL from CD19 CAR-T cell therapy. Blood. 2016;127:2406.
290. Brentjens RJ. Are chimeric antigen receptor T cells ready for prime time? Clin Adv Hematol Oncol. 2016;14:17.
291. Gill S, Maus MV, Porter DL. Chimeric antigen receptor T cell therapy. Blood Rev. 2016;30:157.
292. Cohen A, Petsche D, Grunberger T, Freedman MH. Interleukin 6 induces myeloid differentiation of a human biphenotypic leukemic cell line. Leuk Res. 1992;16(8):751–60.
293. Rayes A, McMasters RL, O'Brien MM. Lineage switch in MLL-rearranged infant leukemia following CD19-directed therapy. Pediatr Blood Cancer. 2016;63:1113.292.
294. van Dongen JJM, van der Velden VHJ, Brüggemann M, Orfao A. Minimal residual disease diagnostics in acute lymphoblastic leukemia: need for sensitive, fast, and standardized technologies. Blood. 2015;125:3996.
295. Health Quality Ontario. Minimal residual disease evaluation in childhood acute lymphoblastic leukemia: a clinical evidence review. Ont Health Technol Assess Ser. 2016;16:1.
296. Ossenkoppele G, Schuurhuis GJ. MRD In AML: does it already guide therapy decision-making? Hematol Am Soc Hematol Educ Program. 2016;2016:356.
297. Wood BL. Principles of minimal residual disease detection for hematopoietic neoplasms by flow cytometry. Cytometry Part B: Clin Cytometry. 2016;90:47.
298. Del Principe MI, Buccisano F, Maurillo L, et al. Minimal redidual disease in acute myeloid leukemia of adults: determination, prognostic impact and clinical applications. Mediterr J Hematol Infect Dis. 2016;8:e2016052.
299. Rocha JM, Zavier SG, de Lima Souza ME, et al. Current strategies for the detection of minimal residual disease in childhood acute lymphoblastic leukemia. Mediterr J Hematol Infect Dis. 2016;8:e2016024.
300. Athale UH, Gibson PJ, Bradley NM, et al. Minimal residual disease in childhood leukemia: standard of care recommendations from the Pediatric Oncology Group of Ontario MRD Working Group. Pediatr Blood Cancer. 2016;63:973.
301. Chen X, Wood BL. Monitoring minimal residual disease in acute leukemia: technical challenges and interpretive complexities. Blood Rev. 2016.; [Epub ahead of print]
302. Sung PJ, Luger SM. Minimal residual disease in acute myeloid leukemia. Curr Treat Options Oncol. 2017;18:1.
303. Theunissen P, Mejstrikova E, Sedek L, et al. Standardized flow cytometry for highly sensitive MRD measurements in B-cell acute lymphoblastic leukemia. Blood. 2017;129:347.
304. Bradstock KF, Janossy G, Tidman N, et al. Immunological monitoring of residual disease in treated thymic acute lymphoblastic leukemia. Leuk Res. 1981;5:301.
305. Cheson BD, Bennett JM, Kopecky KJ, et al. Revised recommendations of the International Working Group for Diagnosis, Standardization of Response Criteria, Treatment Outcomes, and Reporting Standards for Therapeutic Trials in Acute Myeloid Leukemia. J Clin Oncol. 2003;21:4642.
306. Walter RB, Kantarjian HM, Huang X, et al. Effect of complete remission and responses less than complete remission on survival in acute myeloid leukemia: a combined Eastern Cooperative Oncology Group, Southwest Oncology Group, and M.D. Anderson Cancer Center Study. J Clin Oncol. 2010;28:1766.
307. Chen X, Xie H, Wood BL, et al. The relation of clinical response and minimal residual disease and their prognostic impact on outcome in acute myeloid leukemia. J Clin Oncol. 2015;33:1258.
308. Freeman SD, Virgo P, Couzens S, et al. Prognostic relevance of treatment response measured by flow cytometric residual disease detection in older patients with acute myeloid leukemia. J Clin Oncol. 2013;31:4123.
309. Döhner H, Estey E, Grimwade D, et al. Diagnosis and management of AML in adults: 2017 ELN recommendations from an international expert panel. Blood. 2017;129:424.
310. Loken MR, Alonzo TA, Pardo L, et al. Residual disease detected by multidimensional flow cytometry signifies high relapse risk in patients with de novo acute myeloid leukemia: a report from Children's Oncology Group. Blood. 2012;120:1518.
311. Inaba H, Coustan-Smith E, Cao X, et al. Comparative analysis of different approaches measure treatment response in acute myeloid leukemia. J Clin Oncol. 2012;30:3625.
312. Grimwade D, Tallman M. Should minimal residual disease monitoring be the standard of care for all patients with acute promyelocytic leukemia? Leuk Res. 2011;35:3.

313. Matthews V, Chendamarai E, George B, et al. Treatment of acute promyelocytic leukemia with single-agent arsenic trioxide. Mediterr J Hematol Inf Dis. 2011;3:e2011056.
314. Wang F, Travis J, DeLaBarre B, et al. Targeted inhibition of mutant IDH2 in leukemia cells induces cellular differentiation. Science. 2013;340:622.
315. O'Connor D, Moorman AV, Wade R, et al. Use of minimal residual disease assessment to redefine induction failure in pediatric acute lymphoblastic leukemia. J Clin Oncol. 2017.; [Epub of print ahead]
316. Coustan-Smith E, Sancho J, Hancock ML, et al. Use of peripheral blood instead of bone marrow to monitor residual disease in children with acute lymphoblastic leukemia. Blood. 2002;100:2399.
317. Paietta E. Minimal residual disease in acute leukemia: a guide to precision medicine ready for prime time? In treatment strategies. Haematology. 2014;4:45.
318. van der Velden VH, Jacobs DC, Wijkhuijs AJ, et al. Minimal residual disease levels in bone marrow and peripheral blood are comparable in children with T cell acute lymphoblastic leukemia (ALL) but not in precursoe-B-ALL. Leukemia. 2002;16:1432.
319. Borowitz MJ, Devidas M, Hunger SP, et al. Clinical significance of minimal residual disease in childhood acute lymphoblastic leukemia and its relationship to other prognostic factors: a Children's Oncology Group study. Blood. 2008;111:5477.
320. Volejnikova J, Mejstrikova E, Valova T, et al. Minimal residual disease in peripheral blood at day 15 identifies a subgroup of childhood B-cell precursor acute lymphoblastic leukemia with superior prognosis. Haematologica. 2011;96:1815.
321. Chantepie SP, Cornet E, Salaün V, Reman O. Hematogones: an overview. Leuk Res. 2013;37:1404.
322. Sędek Ł, Bulsa J, Sonsala A, et al. The immunophenotypes of blast cells in B-cell precursor acute lymphoblastic leukemia: how different are they from normal counterparts? Cytometry Part B Clin Cytom. 2014;86:329.
323. Sala Torra O, Othus M, Williamson DW, et al. Next-generation sequencing in adult B cell acute lymphoblastic leukemia patients. Biol Blood Marrow Transplant. 2017.; [Epub ahead of print]
324. Maurillo L, Buccisano F, Spagnoli A, et al. Monitoring minimal residual disease in acute myeloid leukemia using peripheral blood as an alternative source to bone marrow. Haematologica. 2007;92:605.
325. Buccisano F, Maurillo L, Del Principe MI, et al. Prognostic and therapeutic implications of minimal residual disease detection in acute myeloid leukemia. Blood. 2012;119:332.
326. Zeijlemaker W, Kelder A, Oussoren-Brockhoff YJ, et al. Peripheral blood minimal residual disease may replace bone marrow minimal residual disease as an immunophenotypic biomarker for impending relapse in acute myeloid leukemia. Leukemia. 2016;30:7.
327. Helgestad J, Rosthoj S, Johansen P, et al. Bone marrow aspiration technique may have an impact on therapy stratification in children with acute lymphoblastic leukemia. Pediatr Blood Cancer. 2011;57:224.
328. Loken MR, Chu SC, Fritschle W, et al. Malization of bone marrow aspirates for hemodilution in flow cytometric analyses. Cytometry B Clin Cytom. 2009;76B:27.
329. Terwijn M, Kelder A, Snel AN, et al. Minimal residual disease detection defined as the malignant fraction of the total primitive stem cell compartment offers additional prognostic information in acuye myeloid leukemia. Int J Lab Hematol. 2012;34:432.
330. van der Velden VH, Hoogeveen PG, Pieters R, van Dongen JJ. Impact of two independent bone marrow samples on minimal residual disease monitoring in childhood acute lymphoblastic leukaemia. Br J Haematol. 2006;133:382.
331. Vanderhoek M, Juckett MB, Perlman SB, et al. Early assessment of treatment response in patients with AML using [^{18}F]FLT PET imaging. Leuk Res. 2011;35:310.
332. Buck AK, Bommer M, Juweid ME, et al. First demonstration of leukemia imaging with the proliferation marker 18F-fluorodeoxythymidine. J Nucl Med. 2008;49:1756.
333. Weindel Ibar Cribe A-S, Steenhof M, Werenberg Marcher C, et al. Extramedullary disease in patients with acute myeloid leukemia assessed by (18)F-FDG PET. Eur J Haematol. 2013;90:273.
334. Norén-Nyström U, Roos G, Bergh A, et al. Bone marrow fibrosis in childhood acute lymphoblastic leukemia correlates with biological factors, treatment response and outcome. Leukemia. 2008;22:504.
335. Orfao A, Ciudad J, Lopez-Berges MC, et al. Acute lymphoblastic leukemia (ALL): detection of minimal residual disease (MRD) at flow cytometry. Leuk Lymphoma. 1994;13(Suppl 1):87.
336. Weir EG, Cowan K, LeBeau P, Borowitz MJ. A limited antibody panel can distinguish B-precursor acute lymphoblastic leukemia from normal B precursors with four color flow cytometry: implications for residual disease detection. Leukemia. 1999;13:558.
337. Campana D, Neale GA, Coustan-Smith E, Pui CH. Detection of minimal residual disease in acute lymphoblastic leukemia: the St Jude experience. Leukemia. 2001;15:278.
338. Lucio P, Gaipa G, van Lochem EG, et al. BIOMED-I concerted action report: flow cytometric immunophenotyping of precursor B-ALL with standardized triple-stainings. BIOMED-1 concerted action investigation of minimal residual disease in acute leukemia: international standardization and clinical evaluation. Leukemia. 2001;15:1185.
339. zur Stadt U, Harms DO, Schluter S, et al. MRD at the end of induction therapy in childhood acute lymphoblastic leukemia: outcome prediction strongly depends on the therapeutic regimen. Leukemia. 2001;15:283.
340. Campana D, Coustan-Smith E. Measurements of treatment response in childhood acute leukemia. Korean J Hematol. 2012;47:245.
341. Ouyang J, Goswami M, Peng J, et al. Comparison of multiparameter flow cytometry immunophenotypic analysis and quantitative RT-PCR for the detection of minimal residual disease of core binding factor acute myeloid leukemia. Am J Clin Pathol. 2016;145:769.
342. Kalina T, Flores-Montero J, Lecrevisse Q, et al. Quality assessment program for EuroFlow protocols: summary results of four-year (2010–2013) quality assurance rounds. Cytometry A. 2015;87:145.
343. Wood B. Multicolor immunophenotyping: human immune system hematopoiesis. Methods Cell Biol. 2004;75:559.
344. Wood BL, Borowitz MJ. The flow cytometric evaluation of hematopoietic neoplasia. In: Clinical diagnosis and management by laboratory methods (Henry). Philadelphia, PA: WB Saunders; 2010.
345. Keeney M, Wood BL, Hedley BD, et al. Experience with a quality assurance program for MRD testing in pediatric B-ALL by flow cytometry: the challenge of interpretative discordance. Cytometry B Clin Cytom. 2017.; (in press)
346. Feller N, van der Velden VHJ, Brooimans RA, et al. Defining consensus leukemia-associated immunophenotypes for detection of minimal residual disease in acute myeloid leukemia in a multicenter setting. Blood Cancer. 2013;3:e129.
347. Dworzak MN, Gaipa G, Ratei R, et al. Standardization of flow cytometric minimal residual disease evaluation in acute lymphoblastic leukemia: multicentric assessment is feasible. Cytometry B Clin Cytom. 2008;74:331.
348. Irving J, Jesson J, Virgo P, et al. Establishment and validation of a standard protocol for the detection of minimal residual disease in

B lineage childhood acute lymphoblastic leukemia by flow cytometry in a multi-center setting. Haematologica. 2009;94:870.
349. Huang Y-J, Coustan-Smith E, Kao H-W, et al. Concordance of two approaches in monitoring of minimal residual disease in B-precursor acute lymphoblastic leukemia: fusion transcripts and leukemia-associated immunophenotypes. J Formos Med Assoc. 2017.; [Epub ahead of print]
350. Hong D, Gupta R, Ancliff P, et al. Initiating and cancer-propagating cells in *TEL-AML1*-associated childhood leukemia. Science. 2008;319:336.
351. Coustan-Smith E, Song G, Clark C, et al. New Markers for minimal residual disease detection in acute lymphoblastic leukemia. Blood. 2011;117:6267.
352. Weng XQ, Shen Y, Sheng Y, et al. Prognostic significance of monitoring leukemia-associated immunophenotypes by eight-color flow cytometry in adult B-acute lymphoblastic leukemia. Blood Cancer J. 2013;3:e133.
353. Ravandi F, Jorgensen JL, Thomas DA, et al. Detection of MRD may predict the outcome of patients with Philadelphia chromosome-positive ALL treated with tyrosine kinase inhibitors plus chemotherapy. Blood. 2013;122:1214.
354. Jeha S, Coustan-Smith E, Pei D, et al. Impact of tyrosine kinase inhibitors on minimal residual disease and outcome in childhood Philadelphia chromosome-positive acute lymphoblastic leukemia. Cancer. 2014;120:1514.
355. Schenk TM, Keyhani A, Böttcher S, et al. Multilineage involvement of Philadelphia chromosome positive acute lymphoblastic leukemia. Leukemia. 1998;12:666.
356. Rovida E, Peppicelli S, Bono S, et al. The metabolically-modulated stem cell niche: a dynamic scenario regulating cancer cell phenotype and resistance to therapy. Cell Cycle. 2014;13:3169.
357. Herrmann H, Sadovnik I, Cerny-Reiterer S, et al. Dipeptidylpeptidase IV (CD26) defines leukemic stem cells in chronic myeloid leukemia. Blood. 2014;123:3951.
358. Malec M, van der Velden VH, Bjorklund E, et al. Analysis of minimal residual disease in childhood acute lymphoblastic leukemia: comparison between RQ-PCR analysis of Ig/TcR gene rearrangements and multicolor flow cytometric immunophenotyping. Leukemia. 2004;18:1630.
359. Garand R, Beldjord K, Cave H, et al. Flow cytometry and IG/TCR quantitative PCR for minimal residual disease quantitation in acute lymphoblastic leukemia: a French multicenter prospective study on behalf of the FRALLE, EORTC and GRAALL. Leukemia. 2013;27:370.
360. Denys B, van der Sluijs-Gelling AJ, Homburg C, et al. Improved flow cytometric detection of minimal residual disease in childhood acute lymphoblastic leukemia. Leukemia. 2013;27:635.
361. Smirnova SY, Sidorova YV, Ryzhikova NY, et al. Evolution of tumor clones in adult acute lymphoblastic leukemia. Acta Nat. 2016;8:100.
362. Faham M, Zheng J, Moorhead M, et al. Deep-sequencing approach for minimal residual disease detection in acute lymphoblastic leukemia. Blood. 2012;120:5173.
363. Warren EH, Matsen FA IV, Chou J. High-throughput sequencing of B- and T-lymphocyte antigen receptors in hematology. Blood. 2013;122:19.
364. Wu D, Emerson RO, Sherwood A, et al. Detection of minimal residual disease in B lymphoblastic leukemia by high-throughput sequencing of IGH. Clin Cancer Res. 2014;20:4540.
365. Pulsipher MA, Carlson C, Langholz B, et al. IgH-V(D)J NGS-MRD measurement pre- and early post-allotransplant defines very low- and very high-risk ALL patients. Blood. 2015;125:3501.
366. Thol F, Kölking B, Damm F, et al. Next-generation sequencing for minimal residual disease monitoring in acute myeloid leukemia patients with FLT3-ITD or NPM1 mutations. Genes Chromosomes Cancer. 2012;51:689.
367. Hou H-A, Kuo Y-Y, Liu C-Y, et al. DNMT3A mutations in acute myeloid leukemia: stability during disease evolution and clinical implications. Blood. 2012;119:559.
368. Im AP, Sehgal AR, Carroll MP, et al. DNMT3A and IDH mutations in acute myeloid leukemia and other myeloid malignancies: associations with prognosis and potential treatment strategies. Leukemia. 2014;28:1774.
369. Salipante SJ, Fromm JR, Shendure J, et al. Detection of minimal residual disease in NPM1-mutated acute myeloid leukemia by next-generation sequencing. Mod Pathol. 2014;27:1438–46.
370. Ivey A, Hills RK, Simpson MA, et al. Assessment of minimal residual disease in standard-risk AML. N Engl J Med. 2016;374:422.
371. Leung W, Pui C-H, Coustan-Smith E, Yang J, Pei D, Gan K, et al. Detectable minimal residual disease before hematopoietic cell transplantation is prognostic but does not preclude cure for children with very-high-risk leukemia. Blood. 2012;120:468.
372. Gökbuget N, Kneba M, Raff T, et al. Adult patients with acute lymphoblastic leukemia and molecular failure display a poor prognosis and are candidates for stem cell transplantation and targeted therapies. Blood. 2012;120:1868.
373. Araki D, Wood BL, Othus M, et al. Allogeneic hematopoietic cell transplantation for acute myeloid leukemia: time to move toward a minimal residual disease-based definition of complete remission? J Clin Oncol. 2016;34:329.
374. Walter RB, Buckley SA, Pagel JM, Wood BL, Storer BE, Sandmaier BM, et al. Significance of minimal residual disease before myeloablative allogeneic hematopoietic cell transplantation for AML in first and second complete remission. Blood. 2013;122:1813–21.
375. Buckley SA, Wood BL, Othus M, et al. Minimal residual disease prior to allogeneic hematopoietic cell transplantation in acute myeloid leukemia: a meta-analysis. Haematologica. 2017;102. [Epub ahead of print]
376. Bar M, Wood BL, Radich JP, et al. Impact of minimal residual disease, detected by flow cytometry, on outcome of myeloablative hematopoietic cell transplantation for acute lymphoblastic leukemia. Leuk Res Treatment. 2014;2014:421723.
377. Stow P, Key L, Chen X, et al. Clinical significance of low levels of minimal residual disease at the end of remission induction therapy in childhood acute lymphoblastic leukemia. Blood. 2010;115:4657.
378. Pui C-H, Pei D, Coustan-Smith E, et al. Clinical utility of sequential minimal residual disease measurements in the context of risk-based therapy in childhood acute lymphoblastic leukemia: a prospective study. Lancet Oncol. 2015;16:465.
379. Parekh C, Gaynon PS, Abdel-Azim H. End of induction minimal residual disease alone is not a useful determinant for risk stratified therapy in pediatric T-cell acute lymphoblastic leukemia. Pediatr Blood Cancer. 2015;62:2040.
380. Schrappe M, Valsecchi MG, Bartram CR, et al. Late MRD response determines relapse risk overall and in subsets of childhood T-cell ALL: results of the AIEOP-BFM-ALL 2000 study. Blood. 2011;118:2077.
381. Paietta E. Minimal residual disease in AML: coming of age. Hematology. 2012;2012:35.
382. Al-Mawali A, Gillis D, Lewis I. The role of multiparameter flow cytometry for detection of minimal residual disease in acute myeloid leukemia. Am J Clin Pathol. 2015;131:16.
383. Köhnke T, Sauter D, Ringel K, et al. Early assessment of minimal residual disease in AML by flow cytometry during aplasia identifies patients at increased risk of relapse. Leukemia. 2015;29:377.

384. Rubnitz JE, Inaba H, Dahl G, et al. Minimal residual disease-directed therapy for childhood acute myeloid leukemia: results of the AML02 multicentre trial. Lancet. 2010;11:543–52.
385. Buccisano F, Maurillo L, Gattei V, et al. The kinetics of reduction of minimal residual disease impacts on duration of response and survival of patients with acute myeloid leukemia. Leukemia. 2006;20:1783.
386. Maurillo L, Buccisano F, Del Principe MI, et al. Toward optimization of postremission therapy for residual disease-positive patients with acute myeloid leukemia. J Clin Oncol. 2008;26:4944.
387. Ganzel C, Sun Z, Gönen M, et al. Minimal residual disease assessment by flow cytometry in AML is an independent prognostic factor even after adjusting for cytogenetic/molecular abnormalities. Blood. 2014;124:1016.
388. Fernandez HF, Sun Z, Yao X, et al. Anthracycline dose intensification in acute myeloid leukemia: results of ECOG Study E1900. N Engl J Med. 2009;361:1249.
389. Parker C, Waters R, Leighton C, et al. Effect of mitoxantrone on outcome of children with first relapse of acute lymphoblastic leukemia (ALL R3): an open-label randomized trial. Lancet. 2010;376:2009.
390. Butturini A, Klein J, Gale RP. Modeling minimal residual disease (MRD)-testing. Leuk Res. 2003;27:293.
391. Yang JJ, Cheng C, Devidas M, et al. Genome-wide association study identifies Germline polymorphisms associated with relapse of childhood acute lymphoblastic leukemia. Blood. 2012;120:4197–204.
392. Ravandi F, Jorgensen J, Borthakur G, et al. Persistence of minimal residual disease assessed by multiparameter flow cytometry is highly prognostic in younger patients with acute myeloid leukemia. Cancer. 2017;123:426.
393. Jaso JM, Wang SA, Jorgensen JL, Lin P. Multi-color flow cytometric immunophenotyping for detection of minimal residual disease in AML: past, present and future. Bone Marrow Transplant. 2014;49:1129.
394. Gaipa G, Cazzaniga G, Valsecchi MG, et al. Time point-dependent concordance of flow cytometry and RQ-PCR in minimal residual disease detection in childhood acute lymphoblastic leukemia. Haematologica. 2012;97:1582.
395. Bene MC, Kaeda JS. How and why minimal residual disease studies are necessary in leukemia: a review from WP10 and WP12 of the European LeukaemiaNet. Haematologica. 2009;94:1135.
396. Gaipa G, Basso G, Biondi A, Campana D. Detection of minimal residual disease in pediatric acute lymphoblastic leukemia. Cytometry B Clin Cytom. 2013;84B:359.
397. Dworzak MN, Fröschl G, Printz D, et al. Prognostic significance and modalities of flow cytometric minimal residual disease detection in childhood acute lymphoblastic leukemia. Blood. 2002;99:1952.
398. Karawajew L, Dworzak M, Ratei R, et al. Minimal residual disease analysis by eight-color flow cytometry in relapsed childhood acute lymphoblastic leukemia. Haematologica. 2015;100:935.
399. Wood BL. Flow cytometric monitoring of residual disease in acute leukemia. In: Czader M, editor. Hematological malignancies, methods in molecular biology, vol. 999; 2013. p. 123.
400. Grimwade D, Freeman SD. Defining minimal residual disease in acute myeloid leukemia: which platforms are ready for "prime time"? Blood. 2014;124:3345.
401. Reading CL, Estey EH, Huh YO, et al. Expression of unusual immunophenotype combinations in acute myelogenous leukemia. Blood. 1993;81:3083.
402. Zeijlmaker W, Gratama JW, Schuurhuis GJ. Tumor heterogeneity makes AML a "moving target" for detection of residual disease. Cytometry B Clin Cytom. 2014;86:3.
403. Coustan-Smith E, Ribeiro RC, Stow P, et al. A simplified flow cytometric assay identifies children with acute lymphoblastic leukemia who have a superior clinical outcome. Blood. 2006;108:97–102.
404. McKenna RW, Washington LT, Aquino BD, et al. Immunophenotypic analysis of hematogones (B-lymphocyte precursors) in 662 consecutive bone marrow specimens by 4-color flow cytometry. Blood. 2001;98:2498.
405. Zeidan MA, Kamal HM, EL Shabrawy DA, et al. Significance of CD34/CD123 expression in detection of minimal residual disease in B-acute lymphoblastic leukemia in children. Blood Cells Mol Dis. 2016;59:113.
406. Djokic M, Bjorklund E, Blennow E, et al. Overexpression of CD123 correlates with the hyperdiploid genotype in acute lymphoblastic leukemia. Haematologica. 2009;94:1016.
407. Tembhare PR, Ghogale S, Ghatwai N, et al. Evaluation of new markers for minimal residual disease monitoring in B-cell precursor acute lymphoblastic leukemia: CD73 and CD86 are the most relevant new markers to increase the efficacy of MRD. Cytometry B Clin Cytom. 2016.; [Epub ahead of print]
408. Kroft SH, Asplund SL, McKenna RW, Karandikar NJ. Haematogones in the peripheral blood of adults: a four-color flow cytometry study of 102 patients. Br J Haematol. 2004;126:209.
409. Chen J-S, Coustan-Smith E, Suzuki T, et al. Identification of novel markers for monitoring minimal residual disease in acute lymphoblastic leukemia. Blood. 2001;97:2115.
410. Veltroni M, De Zen L, Sanzari MC, et al. Expression of CD58 in normal, regenerating and leukemic bone marrow B cells: Implications for the detection of minimal residual disease in acute lymphocytic leukemia. Haematologica. 2003;88:1245.
411. Soma L, Wu D, Chen X, et al. Apparent CD19 expression by natural killer cells: a potential confounder for minimal residual disease detection by flow cytometry in B lymphoblastic leukemia. Cytometry B Clin Cytom. 2015;88:145.
412. Roshal M, Fromm JR, Winter S, et al. Immaturiry associated antigens are lost during induction for T cell lymphoblastic leukemia: implications for minimal residual disease detection. Cytometry B Clin Cytom. 2010;78:139.
413. Dalmazzo LF, Jacomo RH, Marinato AF, et al. The presence of CD56/CD16 in T-cell acute lymphoblastic leukaemia correlates with the expression of cytotoxic molecules and is associated with worse respobnse to treatment. Br J Haematol. 2009;144:223.
414. Dworzak MN, Fröschl G, Printz D, et al. CD99 expression in T-lineage ALL: implications for flow cytometric detection of minimal residual disease. Leukemia. 2004;18:703.
415. Cox CV, Diamanti P, Moppett JP, Blair A. Investigating CD99 expression in leukemia propagating cels in childhood T cell acute lymphoblastic leukemia. PLoS One. 2016;11:e0165210.
416. Dworzak MN, Fritsch G, Buchinger P, et al. Flow cytometric assessment of human MIC2 expression in bone marrow, thymus, and peripheral blood. Blood. 1994;83:415.
417. Zhou Y, Othus M, Araki D, et al. Pre- and post-transplant quantification of measurable ("minimal") residual disease via multiparameter flow cytometry in adult acute myeloid leukemia. Leukemia. 2016;30:1456.
418. van Lochem EG, van der Velden VHJ, Wind HK, et al. Immunophenotypic differentiation patterns of normal hematopoiesis in human bone marrow: reference patterns for age-related changes and disease-induced shifts. Cytometry B Clin Cytom. 2004;60B:1.
419. Bonnet D, Dick JE. Human acute myeloid leukemia is organized as a hierarchy that originates from a primitive hematopoietic cell. Nat Med. 1997;3:730.
420. Fajtova M, Babusikova O. Immunophenotype characterization of hematopoietic stem cells, progenitor cells restricted to myeloid lineage and their leukemia counterpart. Neoplasma. 2010;57:392.
421. Horton SJ, Huntly BJP. Recent advances in acute myeloid leukemia stem cell biology. Haematologica. 2012;97:966.
422. Goardon N, Marchi E, Atzberger A, et al. Coexistence of LMPP-like abd GMP-like leukemia stem cells in acute myeloid leukemia. Cancer Cell. 2011;19:138.

423. Witte K-E, Ahlers J, Schäfer I, et al. High proportion of leukemic stem cells at diagnosis is correlated with unfavorable prognosis in childhood acute myeloid leukemia. Pediatr Hematol Oncol. 2011;28:91.
424. Gerber JM, Smith BD, Ngwang B, et al. A clinically relevant population of leukemic CD34+CD38- cells in acute myeloid leukemia. Blood. 2012;119:3571.
425. Terwijn M, Zeijlemaker W, Kelder A, et al. Leukemic stem cell frequency: a strong biomarker for clinical outcome in acute myeloid leukemia. PLoS One. 2014;9:e107587.
426. Bradbury C, Houlton AE, Akiki S, et al. Prognostic value of monitoring a candidate immunophenotypic leukaemic stem/progenitor cell population in patients allografted for acute myeloid leukemia. Leukemia. 2015;29:988.
427. Koeffler HP, Leong G. Preleukemia: one name, many meanings. Leukemia. 2017.; [Epub ahead of print]
428. Corces-Zimmerman MR, Hong WJ, Weisman IL, et al. Preleukemic in buman acute myeloid leukemia affect epigenetic regulators and persist in remission. Proc Natl Acad Sci U S A. 2014;111:2548.
429. Bhatnagar B, Eisfeld AK, Nicolet D, et al. Persistence of DNMT3A R882 mutations during remission does not adversely affect outcomes of patients with acute myeloid leukaemia. Br J Haematol. 2016;175:226.
430. Borowitz MJ, Pullen DJ, Winick N, et al. Comparison of diagnostic and relapse flow cytometry phenotypes in childhood acute lymphoblastic leukemia: implications for residual disease detection: a report from the Children's Oncology Group. Cytometry B Clin Cytom. 2005;68B:18.
431. Ding L, Ley TJ, Larson DE, et al. Clonal evolution in relapsed acute myeloid leukemia revealed by whole-genome sequencing. Nature. 2012;481:506.
432. Shiba N, Yoshiba K, Shiraishi Y, et al. Whole-exome sequencing reveals the spectrum of gene mutations and the clonal evolution patterns in paediatric acute myeloid leukemia. Br J Haematol. 2016;175:476.
433. Gaipa G, Basso G, Aliprandi S, et al. Prednisone induces immunophenotypic modulation of cd10 and cd34 in nonapoptotic B-cell precursor acute lymphoblastic leukemia cells. Cytometry B Clin Cytom. 2008;74B:150.
434. Dworzak MN, Gaipa G, Schumich A, et al. Modulation of antigen expression in B-cell precursor acute lymphoblastic leukemia during induction therapy is partly transient: evidence for a drug-induced regulatory phenomenon. Results of the AIEOP-BFM-ALL-FLOW-MRD Study Group. Cytometry B Clin Cytom. 2010;78:147.
435. Rhein P, Scheid S, Ratei R, et al. Gene expression shift towards normal B cells, decreased proliferative capacity and distinct surface receptors characterize leukemic blasts persisting during induction therapy in childhood acute lymphoblastic leukemia. Leukemia. 2007;21:897.
436. Slamova L, Starkova J, Fronkova E, et al. CD2-positive B-cell precursor acute lymphoblastic leukemia with an early switch to the monocytic lineage. Leukemia. 2013;28:609.
437. Chevallier P, Robillard N, Ayari S, et al. Persistence of CD33 expression at relapse in CD33(+) acute myeloid leukaemia patients after receiving Gemtuzumab in the course of the disease. Br J Haematol. 2008;143:744.
438. Chu PG, Chen YY, Molina A, et al. Recurrent B-cell neoplasms after Rituximab therapy: an immunophenotypic and genotypic study. Leuk Lymphoma. 2002;43:2335.
439. Topp MS, Kufer P, Gökbuget N, et al. Targeted therapy with the T-cell-engaging antibody blinatumomab of chemotherapy-refractory minimal residual disease in B-lineage acute lymphoblastic leukemia patients results in high response rate and prolonged leukemia-free survival. J Clin Oncol. 2011;29:2493–8.
440. Moorman AV, Enshaei A, Schwab C, et al. A novel integrated cytogenetic and genetic classification refines risk stratification in pediatric acute lymphoblastic leukemia. Blood. 2014;124:1434.
441. Brüggemann M, Raff T, Kneba M. Has MRD monitoring superseded other prognostic factors in adult ALL? Blood. 2012;120:4470.

Cytogenetics of Acute Leukemia

16

Nyla A. Heerema and Susana Catalina Raimondi

Introduction

Cytogenetic abnormalities are an important factor in patient diagnosis, risk assessment, and treatment in acute leukemia. Characteristic genetic abnormalities are recognized as essential for disease classification and are a significant element of the 2008 World Health Organization (WHO) classification [1]. Some aberrations are involved in the initiation whereas others participate in the progression of different acute leukemias. Cytogenetic aberrations occur in most malignant cells, revealing acquired genomic changes that may have diagnostic and prognostic significance. This chapter reviews the most important cytogenetic and molecular genetic lesions in acute myeloid leukemia (AML) and acute lymphoblastic leukemia (ALL).

In acute leukemias, the bone marrow is the sample of choice to detect cytogenetic aberrations in malignant cells because cells of the bone marrow divide spontaneously; however, peripheral blood may also be studied if there is a significant number of circulating blasts. It should be noted that normal chromosomes in the periphery do not necessarily reflect a cytogenetically normal marrow because reactive rather than malignant cells may be dividing. Cytogenetic analysis involves either a direct procedure or culture of cells overnight to obtain dividing cells, which are necessary to observe chromosomes. Cells are exposed to colchicine to arrest the cells in division, when chromosomes are sufficiently contracted for visualization. The cells are fixed, banded, and analyzed. As only 20 completely analyzed metaphases are required for a cytogenetics evaluation, metaphase cytogenetics is limited in its sensitivity to detect abnormalities.

The sensitivity of cytogenetics has been greatly enhanced by the application of fluorescence in situ hybridization (FISH). FISH has notably advanced the field of cytogenetics by enabling the detection of numerical and structural aberrations in both hematologic malignancies and solid tumors. FISH is a molecular cytogenetic technique which uses a DNA probe to evaluate cells in either metaphase or interphase. Various types of probes are commercially available and are applied to detect gains, losses, and different types of cytogenetic rearrangements. The probes vary in size and can detect aberrations as small as 200 kb, although most clinically applied probes are much larger. This is in contrast to metaphase cytogenetics, in which most aberrations must be at least 2 Mb for detection. Technically, both the probe and the chromosomes are "denatured" (made single stranded), hybridization of the fluorescently labeled probe to its matching DNA on the chromosomes is allowed to occur, the excess probe is removed with several washings, and the preparations are analyzed using a fluorescence microscope. In addition to detecting much smaller aberrations, FISH is more sensitive than metaphase analysis because 200 interphase cells are generally analyzed. Furthermore, dividing cells are not required, so neither culturing nor live cells are necessary as for metaphase cytogenetics, making application to a wider range of tissues possible.

Different FISH probe "strategies" are used to detect different types of abnormalities. The ones commonly used in analysis of acute leukemias include probes for detection of rearrangements, gains, and losses. These include probes designed to detect specific loci, such as *TP53*, to detect centromeres, and to detect whole chromosomes (chromosome paints—metaphase analyses). The use of dual-color dual-fusion probes is another strategy to detect translocations. The breakpoints of each of the translocation partners are labeled in different colors, generally a red and a green, such that both probes are split when there is a translocation. Fusion of the two probes indicates the rearrangement, and since most

N.A. Heerema, Ph.D., F.A.C.M.G. (✉)
Department of Pathology, The Ohio State University, 1645 Neil Avenue, Columbus, OH 43210, USA
e-mail: nyla.heerema@osumc.edu

S.C. Raimondi, Ph.D., F.A.C.M.G.
Cytogenetics Laboratory, Department of Pathology, St. Jude Children's Research Hospital, 262 Danny Thomas Place, Memphis, TN 38105, USA
e-mail: susana.raimondi@stjude.org

P.H. Wiernik et al. (eds.), *Neoplastic Diseases of the Blood*, DOI 10.1007/978-3-319-64263-5_16

translocations are reciprocal, two fusions are typically present in addition to the two normal alleles. Thus, the pattern observed in abnormal cells with the translocation queried is two fusions, one red and one green signal. Break-apart probes have been designed to detect rearrangements of genes that frequently have different partners, such as *KMT2A* (formerly *MLL*). These probes are labeled with one color 5′ of the breakpoint, and a second color 3′ of the breakpoint, yielding two fusion signals in a normal cell. If the gene has been rearranged, one signal is split and one red, one green, and one fused signal will be detected in abnormal cells. In many cases, FISH should be performed on metaphase chromosome preparations, because there are many variations of each genetic abnormality at the DNA level and because analysis of only interphase nuclei can lead to misinterpretation of results. Furthermore, FISH analysis has shown that in several cases "balanced" translocations detected by conventional cytogenetics are not actually balanced, but rather associated with submicroscopic deletions. However, the clinical significance of these deletions remains unknown [2]. Use of FISH has become very common in the cytogenetic laboratory, as it is rapid and precise and gives a quick and accurate diagnosis. Because of its sensitivity, FISH is also useful to detect cytogenetically cryptic aberrations, such as the t(12;21)(p13;q22) found in ~25% of pediatric ALL. It also is frequently utilized to help define a complex karyotype or to confirm an abnormality suspected in a karyotype. However, FISH can only give results concerning the specific probes applied; the presence or absence of other aberrations is not detected.

Conventional cytogenetic methods, FISH and reverse transcriptase-polymerase chain reaction (RT-PCR), are complementary and can reliably identify clonal rearrangements of genes and aid in subclassification of disease subtypes in acute leukemias [3]. RT-PCR may be a useful adjunct to FISH when cytogenetic analysis is not possible because of a lack of dividing cells. For example, the cryptic t(12;21) generates an *ETV6–RUNX1* chimeric fusion that is easily identified by FISH or RT-PCR. Cytogenetic analyses of t(8;21), inv(16), or t(15;17) in patients with AML yield a low rate of false positives, but false negatives occur in rare cases when cryptic, complex rearrangements are not detected [4, 5]. Thus, it is clinically important to use FISH and RT-PCR separately or in combination to detect cryptic abnormalities, especially for disease subtypes such as acute promyelocytic leukemia (APL) wherein optimal therapy differs.

In some subgroups it may be difficult or not feasible to detect all translocations because of the diversity of partners (e.g., *KMT2A* with multiple partners) or because the genes involved are located near the telomeric regions of the chromosomes [e.g., *NUP98*(11p15.5), *RUNX1*(21q22), *ABL1*(9q34.1), *JAK2*(9p24), *ETV6*(12p13.2)]. For *KMT2A* cases, a long-distance inverse PCR method has been successfully used to identify any type of *KMT2A* rearrangement at the molecular level [6]. The rapid amplification of cDNA end PCR method can also be used to clone breakpoints of partner genes such as of *KMT2A*, or of *PDGFRB* in chronic myeloproliferative disorders or of *NUP98* in myeloid leukemias.

At present, newly developed methods such as array-comparative genomic hybridization (aCGH) and single-nucleotide polymorphism (SNP) arrays quantitatively analyze DNA copy number at high resolution and systematically detect changes on a genomic scale. The implementation of these technologies has improved the resolution with which genetic alterations, especially changes in copy number, can be localized to the human genome [7]. With novel emerging technologies aimed to genetic, immunophenotypic, epigenetic, and proteomic classification, as well as next-generation sequencing (NGS) approaches to aid the identification of new molecular subsets, the classification of acute leukemias will likely evolve to provide informative prognostic and biologic guidelines to clinicians and researchers.

Acute Myeloid Leukemia

AML, a malignant disorder of the bone marrow, develops because of the clonal transformation of a multipotent stem cell through the acquisition of chromosomal rearrangements and multiple mutations. Cure rates for AML have improved only moderately over the past few decades compared with those for ALL. Clonal, nonrandom chromosomal abnormalities have been observed by conventional cytogenetics in blast cells of 80% of children and adolescents and 60% of adults with AML.

Cytogenetic analysis is a primary component in the diagnosis and treatment of AML. According to the World Health Organization classification (WHO-2008) [1], results of diagnostic studies should correlate with clinical findings and be reported in a single, integrated report that includes the cytogenetic profile. In addition, a minimum of 20% blasts is typically required for the disease to be classified as AML. However, with t(8;21), inv(16)/t(16;16), and t(15;17), the disease is considered AML even if less than 20% blasts are present. WHO-2008 expanded the number of recognized chromosomal abnormalities associated with AML and for the first time included specific gene mutations (*CEBPA* and *NPM1*) as provisional categories [1] (Table 16.1). *FLT3* internal tandem duplication (*FLT3*-ITD) is included because of its recognized prognostic significance. In addition to cytogenetic abnormalities, with the advent of powerful high-throughput tools, these and other recurrent genetic mutations have been incorporated into clinical practice. A revision of the WHO classification

Table 16.1 World Health Organization 2008 classification of acute myeloid leukemias with recurrent genetic abnormalities

AML with t(8;21)(q22;q22)/*RUNX1-RUNX1T1 (AML1-ETO)*
AML with inv(16)(p13.1q22) or t(16;16)(p13.1q22)/*CBFB-MYH11*
APL with t(15;17)(q22;q21)/*PML-RARA*
AML with t(9;11)(p22;q23)/*MLLT3 -MLL* (specify other 11q23/*MLL* abnormality)
AML with t(6;9)(p23;q34)/*DEK-NUP214(CAN)*[a]
AML with inv(3)(q21q26.2) or t(3;3)(q21;q26.2)/*RPN1-MECOM*[a]
AML with t(1;22)(p13;q13)/*RBM15-MKL1(OTT-MAL)*[a]
Provisional entity: AML with mutated *NPM1*[a]
Provisional entity: AML with mutated *CEBPA*[a]

AML acute myeloid leukemia; *APL* acute promyelocytic leukemia
[a]Newly defined entities by WHO-2008 [1]

is under way to include the many lesions identified by genomic methods, which are either targetable for therapy or useful for prognostication. This update is expected to improve the risk classification for AML [8].

Favorable prognostic factors for patients with AML include low white blood cell (WBC) count; inv(16)/t(16;16); t(8;21); t(15;17); *NPM1* mutation (in the absence of *FLT3*-ITD or *DNMT3A* mutation); biallelic *CEBPA* mutation; Down syndrome (DS) in children up to 4 years old, mostly with acute megakaryoblastic leukemia (AMKL, AML-M7); and early response to treatment. Unfavorable prognostic factors include –7, –5/5q, t(6;9)(p23;q34), t(6;11)(q27;q23), and 3q abnormalities; complex karyotypes (≥3 unrelated cytogenetic abnormalities, excluding the categories described by WHO-2008); cryptic lesions mostly observed in children such as t(5;11)(q35;p15.5)/*NUP98–NSD1*, t(6;11)(q27;q23)/*KMT2A–MLLT4(MLL–AF6)*, inv(16)(p13.3q24.3)/*CBFA2T3–GLIS2*, t(11;12)(p15.5;p13.3)/*NUP98–KDM5A*, and t(7;12)(q36.3;p13.2)/*MNX1–ETV6*; as well as lesions found in all age groups, 17p/*TP53* deletion or mutation; *KMT2A(MLL)*-PTD and *FLT3*-ITD, particularly with a high allelic ratio; and *DNMT3A, ASXL1,* and *RUNX1* mutations. Intermediate-risk factors include normal and other karyotypes and genetic lesions excluding favorable and unfavorable abnormalities [1, 9–12].

AML represents 15–20% of all childhood leukemias and approximately 33% of adolescent and 50% of adult leukemias. The prognostic value of cytogenetics has been well established for all age groups [9, 10, 12, 13]. However, the distribution of recurrent chromosomal abnormalities observed in AML differs by age groups. In infants (<2 years old), chromosomal abnormalities most frequently include a breakpoint in 11q23 and involve *KMT2A(MLL)* in 60% of cases. The incidence decreases to 30% in children (2 to <13 years) and to 13% in adolescents (13 to <21 years), and is even lower in young adults (8%; 21 to <30 years) and adults (3%; ≥30 years) [13]. The t(1;22)(p13;q13) is specific for AMKL and is mostly seen in children younger than 2 years and rarely in adults. In older children (>10 years) and young adults (<60 years), the most frequent abnormalities are t(15;17), t(8;21), and inv(16). In older patients (>60 years) with AML, there is a low frequency of favorable core-binding factor chromosomal abnormalities but a higher incidence of complex aberrant karyotypes, which is attributed to both disease biology and host factors [14]. A previous study evaluating the effect of age on outcome of AML in children 21 years or younger suggested that age is an independent prognostic factor in childhood AML and that children younger than 10 years benefit more than older children from newer intensive therapies [15].

The following section describes the associations among specific recurring cytogenetic and molecular abnormalities in AML, distinct clinical subtypes of diseases, and treatment outcomes.

Specific Recurring Cytogenetic and Molecular Abnormalities

t(15;17)(q24;q21)/*PML–RARA*

The t(15;17)(q24;q21) is associated with APL, a distinct subtype of AML that is treated differently from other types of AML because of its marked sensitivity to the differentiating effects of all-*trans* retinoic acid (ATRA). The t(15;17) is found in 9% of children with AML; it is rarely observed in infants, and the incidence decreases with age in adults (rarely seen in adults 45 years or older) (Fig. 16.1). The t(15;17) generates the fusion gene *PML–RARA* to produce a chimeric protein. Patients with the t(15;17) and APL respond well to the combination therapy of ATRA and the chemotherapy agent arsenic trioxide (ATO) and have a favorable prognosis (cure rate 80%) [16–19].

A suspected diagnosis of APL should be treated as a medical emergency because immediate measures are needed to counteract coagulopathy and initiate ATRA therapy. Thus, a prompt genetic diagnosis by conventional cytogenetics, FISH with *PML–RARA* probes, RT-PCR, or anti-PML monoclonal antibodies, is essential for patients with suspected APL [18]. *Conventional G-banding* has helped to identify the t(15;17) in more than 90% of patients with APL, but it cannot detect the *PML–RARA* fusion resulting from cryptic rearrangements. However, cytogenetics facilitates the identification of rare variant translocations, including three-way translocations affecting *PML* and *RARA* or other aberrations affecting only *RARA*. FISH with commercially available probes is a rapid, highly sensitive, and specific method to confirm the presence of the *PML–RARA* fusion. However, in rare instances, fusion

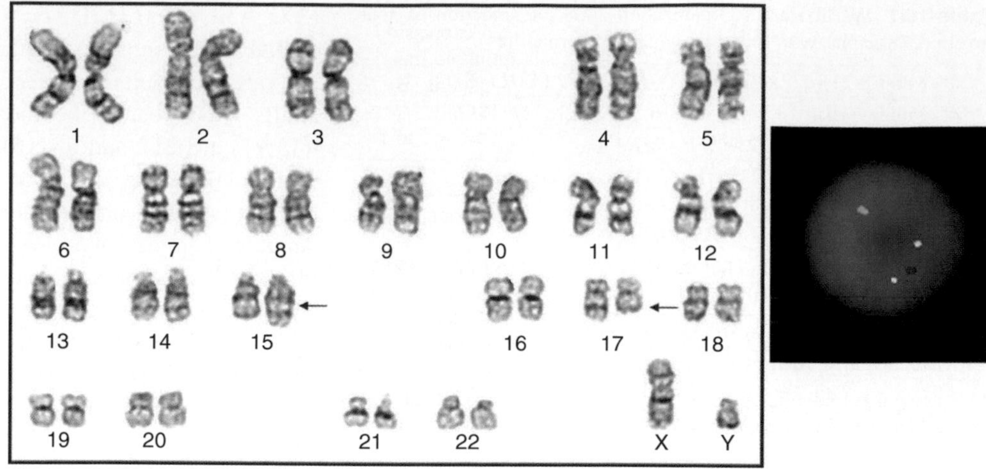

Fig. 16.1 *Left*: Karyogram of a cell from a patient with APL and the typical translocation between chromosomes 15 and 17 (*arrows*). The karyotype is 46,XY,t(15;17)(q24;q21). *Arrows* indicate abnormal chromosomes. *Right*: FISH with the dual-color dual-fusion *PML–RARA* probes (Abbott Molecular) showing 2 fusion (*yellow*), 1 *red*, and 1 *green* signals

signals might be different from those expected, because of deletion of sequences at translocation junctions or where *PML–RARA* is formed as a result of an insertion or a complex translocation [5]. FISH using *RARA* break-apart probes is useful to evaluate rearrangements in suspected cases that lack the *PML–RARA* fusion. *RT-PCR* is important to establish the type of *PML–RARA* isoform fusion transcript that will be the target to reliably monitor minimal residual disease. *Immunostaining* with anti-PML monoclonal antibodies on dry smears is also useful to establish a rapid diagnosis.

Small *PML–RARA* insertions can be missed by FISH when using very large probes; in such cases, it is more appropriate to use relatively small cosmid probes. Patients with APL in whom the *PML–RARA* fusion is generated due to variant three-way translocations or cryptic insertions respond to ATRA combination regimens in a similar manner as those with APL with the typical t(15;17) [5].

Other rare translocations involving *RARA* can also result in APL. Approximately 1% of patients with APL have variant translocations involving only *RARA*. The most common is t(11;17)(q23;q21)/*PLZF(ZBTB16)–RARA* (~20 patients) [20]. These patients and another patient with a rare inv(17)(q11.2q21)/*STAT5B-RARA* were partially resistant to ATRA [21]. Other variant translocations with *RARA* include *OBFC2A (NABP1)* (2q32), *TBL1XR1* (3q26), *FIPIL1* (4q12), *NPM1* (5q35), *NUMA1* (11q13), *ZBTB16* (11q23), *PRKAR1A* (17q24.2), and *BCOR* (Xp11.4) [20, 22, 23]. It is important to identify patients with such translocations, as the sensitivity for ATRA or ATO may vary.

Children with APL have a higher incidence of hyperleukocytosis (WBC count $\geq 10 \times 10^9$/L) than adults with APL, but the high WBC count is associated with poor outcome in both groups [18, 19]. *FLT3* mutations [either internal tandem duplications (ITDs) or kinase domain mutations] occur in up to 40% of patients with APL and are associated with high WBC counts; however, there is no clear correlation between the presence of *FLT3* mutations and outcome [19, 24, 25].

Core-Binding Factor Leukemias

In children and adults with AML, the highest complete response rates and longest survival times are associated with the two common aberrations, t(8;21) and either inv(16) or t(16;16). Both aberrations disrupt the core-binding protein complex, which plays a vital role in hematopoiesis, and are designated core-binding factor (CBF) leukemias. The t(8;21) targets *RUNX1*, and the inv(16)/t(16;16) targets *CBFB*. Several studies have shown an association between cooperating mutations and CBF leukemia; the most prevalent are *KIT* and *NRAS* mutations, but their prognostic significance remains debated [26].

t(8;21)(q22;q22)/*RUNX1(AML1, CBFA2)-RUNX1T1(ETO,MTG8)*

The t(8;21)(q22;q22) is among the most frequent recurrent abnormalities in AML (12% of children and 6% of adults). The t(8;21) juxtaposes *RUNX1* to *RUNX1T1* on the derivative chromosome 8, generating a chimeric gene *RUNX1–RUNX1T1* (*AML1–ETO*), which inhibits transcriptional activation by wild-type *RUNX1*. RT-PCR and *RUNX1–RUNX1T1* FISH probes are available to detect the t(8;21) and are useful especially when submicroscopic rearrangements are suspected or the sample does not yield metaphases for analysis. Additional cytogenetic aberrations are present in 68% of patients with t(8;21). The most frequent additional change in cases with t(8;21) is loss of a sex chromosome in approximately 40% of patients; the Y chromosome is lost in males more frequently (55%) than the X chromosome (33%) in females [27, 28]. A del(9q), rearrangement of 7q, +4, or +8, can also occur, but does not significantly affect the overall survival. However, a del(9q) was associated with lower complete remission and +4 with inferior outcome in a recent study [27]. The t(8;21) is associated with a favorable outcome, especially when the disease is treated with regimens containing high-dose cytarabine [27].

Presence of the *RUNX1–RUNX1T1* transcript in the bone marrow in adults and cord blood cells of children who do not have AML suggests that the t(8;21) is generated early in hematopoiesis. Some people may acquire secondary genetic alterations that lead to the development of AML [29], which is supported by the detection of *RUNX1–RUNX1T1* in neonatal blood spots of infants in whom AML subsequently developed (after >10 years) [30]. The most frequent genetic lesions identified are *KIT, ASXL2,* and Ras-pathway mutations [31].

inv(16)(p13.1q22) and t(16;16)(p13.1;q22)/*CBFB-MYH11(SMMHC)*

The inv(16) and t(16;16) result in fusion of *CBFB* at 16q22 to the smooth muscle myosin heavy-chain gene (*MYH11*) at 16p13.1. *CBFB* is the heterodimeric partner of *RUNX1*, which together form the transcriptional activating factor designated as CBF. The inv(16)/t(16;16) is strongly associated with the FAB M4Eo subtype and is observed in approximately 6% of children and adults with AML. FISH probes and RT-PCR are available to evaluate the status of fusion genes in patients with AML and can aid in the diagnosis of this subtle chromosomal abnormality. Additional abnormalities in leukemic cells with an inv(16) are found in up to 40% of patients, with +22, +8, and +21 being the most frequent. The inv(16)/t(16;16) confers a good prognosis in both children and adults with AML. The most frequent genetic lesions identified with inv(16)/t(16;16) are *KIT*, Ras-pathway mutations, and *FLT3*-ITD [32].

Other *RUNX1(AML1,CBFA2)* (21q22) Rearrangements

The *RUNX1* gene encodes a transcription factor that is important for hematopoiesis and is one of the most frequently mutated genes in acute leukemias. Chromosomal abnormalities include the t(12;21)(p13;q22)/*ETV6–RUNX1*(*TEL–AML1*) in ALL and many other *RUNX1* partner genes identified in AML, but several of them are reported for single cases (<1% of pediatric AML). One of the most frequently identified *RUNX1* partner genes is *MECOM(EVI1,MDS1)*, involved in the t(3;21)(q26.2;q22) associated with therapy-related MDS and CML in blast crisis [33]. The t(3;21) can generate fusion of *RUNX1* with several genes such as *EVI1, EAP*, and *MDS1*. In addition, other rearrangements of 3q26 (such as inv(3)(q21q26)) often lead to overexpression of *EVI1*, which is associated with poor prognosis, suggesting its role in the pathogenesis of AML [34]. Determination of *EVI1* expression is likely important, because it is overexpressed in cases with cryptic 3q26 rearrangements [35]. Another rare but recurrent translocation is the t(16;21)(q24;q22), mostly observed in patients with therapy-related acute leukemias and MDS but also in children and adults with de novo AML. The t(16;21) generates the fusion gene *RUNX1–CBFA2T(MTG16)*, which is similar to the *RUNX1–RUNX1T1* generated by the t(8;21). Of interest, a t(16;21)(p11;q22)/*FUS–ERG* is a rare recurrent abnormality associated with poor prognosis in AML. *RUNX1* mutations have been identified in AML with noncomplex karyotype and confer an unfavorable prognosis [36].

Other 3q26.2/*MECOM(EVI1, MDS1)* and 3q21.3/*GATA2/RPN1* Rearrangements

These aberrations are more frequently observed in adults with AML than in children with AML and are adverse prognostic factors [37, 38]. *EVI1*-rearranged AML is characterized by distinct molecular alterations [38, 39]. The molecular basis of inv(3)(q21q26.2) and t(3;3)(q21;q26.2) (observed frequently with −7) has been revised with the rearrangement of a *GATA2*(3q21.3) oncogenic enhancer element rather than of the *RPN1* gene with *MECOM(EVI1)* [8, 40]. Of interest, a recent study identified *GATA2* mutation as the most common germline defect predisposing to pediatric MDS, with a very high prevalence in adolescents with −7, but did not confer poor prognosis [41].

11q23/*KMT2A* (*MLL, MLL1, ALL1, TRX, HTRX1*)

Most myeloid blasts with an 11q23 abnormality have a *KMT2A* rearrangement and are associated with monocytic differentiation. Every *KMT2A* translocation results in gain of function by generating novel chimeric proteins coded by the N-terminus of *KMT2A* fused in-frame with one of many partner genes coding for diverse functions, and each oncogene is associated with a distinct form of leukemia. More than 120 translocations target *KMT2A* in acute leukemias, and approximately 80 partner genes for *KMT2A* have been cloned [42, 43]. Despite the diversity of chimeric proteins created, *KMT2A* fusions generate a characteristic gene expression profile, including upregulation of developmental homeobox genes such as *HOXA9* and *MEIS1*, suggesting that partner genes for *KMT2A* might be involved in regulating transcription elongation and chromatin structure remodeling.

Chromosomal rearrangements involving *KMT2A* in AML and in ALL include balanced and unbalanced translocations, inversions, insertions, amplifications, and partial tandem duplications (*KMT2A*(*MLL*)-PTD). These genetic mechanisms convert *KMT2A* into a chimeric transcription factor with leukemogenic properties. Some *KMT2A* gene rearrangements are not detected by conventional cytogenetic methods. In other *KMT2A* rearrangements, the precise breakpoint or gene partner is difficult to assign because different genes are mapped on chromosome regions with limited banding resolution, such as 10p and 19p [42]. FISH using commercially available dual-color *KMT2A* probes allows evaluation of derivatives of a translocation involving *KMT2A* in metaphase chromosomes and the splitting of signals in interphase nuclei (Fig. 16.2). In rare instances, FISH with this probe detects not only the reciprocal translocation but also a deletion of at least 190 kb from the 3′ region of *KMT2A*.

A *KMT2A* rearrangement is observed in up to 25% of children with AML, is prevalent in infants (~60%), and declines to less than 10% in older children with a median age of ~2 years. Pediatric patients with t(6;11)(q27;q23) and t(11;17)(q23;q21) are significantly older at presentation (12 years and 9 years, respectively). In contrast to the poor prognosis of infants with 11q23/*KMT2A*$^+$ ALL, the outcome of infants with 11q23/*KMT2A*$^+$ AML is not poorer than that of infants who do not have this rearrangement. The specific fusion partner of *KMT2A* may influence prognosis [44]. WHO-2008 has classified the t(9;11) as a separate category and recommends that partner genes be determined for patients with *KMT2A* rearrangements [1]. Several studies have reported a more favorable prognosis for children with t(9;11)(p22;q23)/*KMT2A-MLLT3* (50% of patients with *KMT2A* rearrangements) than children with other *KMT2A* rearrangements, but other studies have refuted these observations.

In a recent collaborative group study of 756 children with AML and an 11q23/*KMT2A* rearrangement, the overall 5-year event-free survival (EFS) was 44% [44]. The outcome of the subgroups varied greatly; for example, patients with a t(1;11)(q21;q23) (~3% of patients with *KMT2A* rearrangements) had an excellent outcome (5-year EFS, 92%), whereas those with a t(6;11)(q27;q23) (~9%) had the worst outcome (5-year EFS, 11%). Subgroups with a t(10;11)(p12;q23) (15%), t(4;11)(q21;q23) (<1%), and t(10;11)(p11.2;q23) (<1%) had 5-year EFS of 31%, 29%, and 17%, respectively [44]. A follow-up study by the international group reported that additional chromosomal abnormalities further influenced the outcome of children with *KMT2A* rearrangements, with complex karyotypes and trisomy 21 predicting poor outcome and trisomy 8 predicting a more favorable outcome [45].

A *KMT2A*-PTD is detected in approximately 10% of patients with AML, particularly those with trisomy 11 or a normal karyotype, and confers a poor prognosis [46]. In the 1990s, the use of epipodophyllotoxins was associated with the development of therapy-related AML (t-AML) with 11q23 abnormalities. The most frequently observed translocations were t(9;11)(p22;q23), t(11;19)(q23;p13.3), and t(11;16)(q23;p13.3). The t(11;16)(q23;p13.3), affecting *CREBBP*(*CBP*), was rarely seen in de novo AML. Subsequently, the dose and schedule of topoisomerase II inhibitors for treatment of acute leukemias were modified, which has reduced the occurrence of t-AML with a *KMT2A* rearrangement. Leukemias with *KMT2A* rearrangements are sensitive to BET, hDOTIL, and CDK6 inhibitors, which are currently being tested in an early clinical trial [12].

t(10;11)(p12;q14)/*PICALM*(*CALM*)–*MLLT10*(*AF10*)

The t(10;11)(p12;q14) is a rare recurrent abnormality seen in both adult and pediatric patients with AML or T-ALL and is often associated with a poor prognosis [47–49]. The t(10;11)(p12;q14) lacks a *KMT2A* rearrangement and can be difficult to differentiate microscopically from the t(10;11)(p12;q23)/*KMT2A–MLLT10*, and FISH or RT-PCR analysis is usually required to distinguish these two translocations with accuracy.

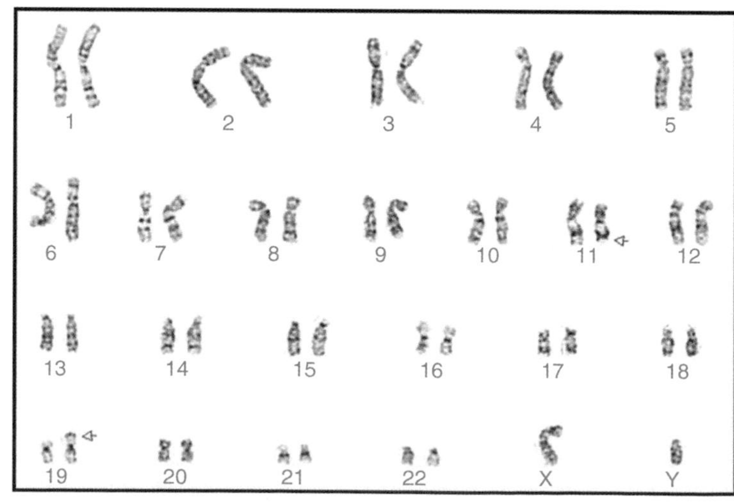

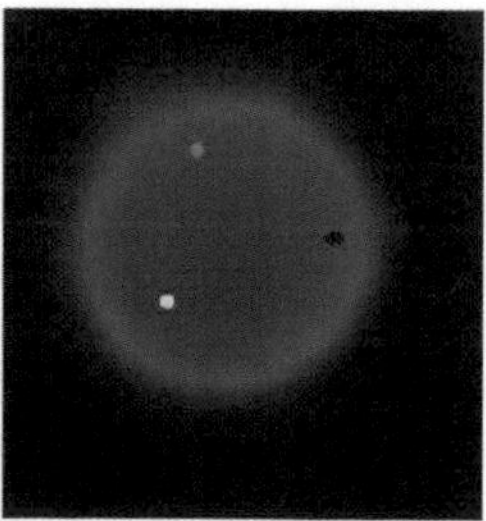

Fig. 16.2 *Left*: Karyogram of a cell with a t(11;19)(q23;p13.3), which occurs in both AML and ALL. *Arrows* indicate abnormal chromosomes. The karyotype is 46,XY,t(11;19)(q23;p13.3). *Right*: FISH with a *KMT2A* break-apart probe (Abbott Molecular) shows the separation of the 2 *KMT2A* signals (1 *red* and 1 *green*) and a normal fused (*yellow*) signal indicating a rearrangement of the *KMT2A* gene

t(1;22)(p13;q13)/*RBM15(OTT)–MKL1(MAL)*

The t(1;22)(p13;q13) is restricted to patients with AMKL and occurs in 33% of this subgroup, mostly in infants and young children. The t(1;22)(p13;q13) is rare in children with DS who develop AMKL. The t(1;22) juxtaposes the *RBM15(OTT)* on 1p13 to *MKL1(MAL)* on 22q13. Patients with this translocation present with hepatosplenomegaly and bone marrow fibrosis and can have high-hyperdiploid karyotypes. These patients were earlier classified as high risk, but the use of intensive therapy has significantly improved the prognosis [50–52].

t(3;5)(q25;q35)/*NPM1–MLF1*

The t(3;5)(q25;q35) is rare in young patients with AML and can present with trilineage dysplasia. However, patients with the t(3;5) have good outcomes [53, 54].

t(6;9)(p23;q34)/*DEK–NUP214(CAN)*

This translocation leads to formation of a leukemia-associated fusion protein DEK–NUP214(CAN), which occurs in up to 2% of children with AML. It is associated with relatively late onset (median age, 10.4 years) and male predominance. The t(6;9) presents with trilineage dysplasia and bone marrow basophilia and is the sole abnormality in 80% of the patients; the most common secondary changes are +8 or +13. The t(6;9) is strongly associated with *FLT3*-ITD mutations (up to 70% of patients), and has a poor prognosis [55]. Outcomes might improve with stem cell transplantation [56, 57].

t(X;6)(p11.2;q23.3)/*GATA1-MYB*

The t(X;6)(p11.2;q23.3) generates an *MYB–GATA1* fusion. The translocation is very rare, with few cases reported worldwide. It is predominantly seen in male infants presenting with basophilic leukemia, and most patients were in long-term complete remission at the time of reporting [58].

Recurrent Abnormalities of Chromosomes 5 and 7

Cytogenetic aberrations associated with unfavorable outcomes include monosomy 5 (−5) and del(5q)/5q−, monosomy 7 (−7), and complex abnormalities. These abnormalities occur more frequently in adults than in children. Patients with del(7q)/7q– are no longer considered to be at high risk of treatment failure [59]. Monosomy 7 is observed in approximately 2% of children with AML. The majority (72%) of adolescents with MDS and –7 carry an underlying *GATA2* deficiency, which does not confer poor prognosis [41]. In a large pediatric series, the prevalence of –5/del(5q) was 1.2%, the abnormality occurred in older children (median age, 12.5 years), it had a high incidence of undifferentiated blast morphology, and most patients had additional chromosomal abnormalities. The study confirmed the very poor prognosis of children with a –5/5q– [60].

t(8;16)(p11.2;p13.3)/*KAT6A(MOZ/MYST3)–CREBBP(CBP)*

Disruption of *KAT6A* at 8p11.2 is rare (~1%) and is seen in children (median age, 1.2 years), younger adults (median age, 45 years), and t-AML. It is associated with a poor prognosis [61]. The most frequent translocation is t(8;16)(p11.2;p13.3), which fuses *KAT6A* to *CREBBP*. Blast cell morphology is similar to that of acute myelomonocytic or monocytic leukemia, with the blast cells frequently (70%) displaying erythrophagocytosis. Patients with t(8;16)(p11.2;p13.3) can present with leukemia cutis (58%) and disseminated intravascular coagulation (39%); the coagulopathy may mimic that seen in APL [62, 63]. Importantly, spontaneous remissions occur in a subset of neonatal patients [28% of patients with a t(8;16) are diagnosed in the first month of life] and warrant a watch-and-wait strategy before initiating therapy [62]. The t(8;16) has a unique gene expression profile that clusters close to 11q23/*KMT2A* [62, 63]. Other *KAT6A* fusion partners are *NCOA2(TIF2)* in inv(8)(p11.2q13), *NCOA3* in t(8;20)(p11.2;q12), and *EP300* in t(8;22)(p11.2;q13.2). These partner genes encode proteins that have histone acetyltransferase activity and likely contribute to leukemogenesis by altering chromatin-mediated transcriptional control of unknown target genes. The *CREBBP(CBP)* (16p13.3) gene is also involved in other translocations in AML—t(10;16)(q22;p13.3)/*MYST4(MORF)–CREBBP* and t(11;16)(q23;p13.3)—which results in *KMT2A–CREBBP(CBP)* fusion and is strongly associated with treatment-related hematologic malignancies [64].

Complex Karyotype

The definition of a complex karyotype has not yet been standardized, but the current trend is to consider patients with three or more unrelated chromosomal abnormalities (excluding those recognized as categories by WHO-2008) in this category; adults with AML who have complex karyotypes have a significantly poorer prognosis than those without a complex karyotype [65]. The loss of 17p is among the most frequent abnormalities observed as part of a complex karyotype in hematologic disorders in adults, and it is strongly associated with abnormalities of chromosomes 5 or 7, or both [66]. The loss of 17p consistently creates a monoallelic loss of *TP53* and may be associated with *TP53* mutation or lack of expression, which is associated with a very poor prognosis; risk-adapted targeted therapies are being evaluated for patients in this category [67–69].

Cryptic Chromosomal Abnormalities and Submicroscopic Lesions

NUP98 (11p15.5)

Numerous partners have been identified for the *NUP98* (11p15.5) gene, and most partners are cryptic if the translocated genes are at the telomeric regions of the chromosomes involved. Chromosomal translocations involving *NUP98* occur in a wide range of hematopoietic malignancies. Patients harboring the cryptic t(5;11)(q35.2;p15.5)/*NUP98–NSD1* fusion usually present with a very high WBC count, have a high frequency of *FLT3*-ITD mutations, and have a dismal outcome. The overall prevalence of t(5;11)(q35.2;p15.5)/*NUP98–NSD1* is approximately 5% in children and 3% in adults with AML. Although most patients have normal cytogenetics, some can harbor +8 and del(5q) as secondary aberrations. In a large series of patients with *FLT3*-ITD, *NUP98–NSD1* was found in children (16%; median age, 10 years) and adults (8%; median age, 45 years). Among patients with normal karyotypes, *NUP98–NSD1* occurred in 8% of children and 4% of adults [70, 71]. The *NUP98–NSD1* has a distinct *HOXA/B* gene expression pattern and is associated with upregulation of other genes, including overexpression of *PRDM16(MEL1)* (mapped at 1p36.1) [72]. Of note, a cytogenetically cryptic t(11;12)(p15.5;p13.3)/*NUP98–KDM5A(JARID1A)* was recently identified in 11% of children with non-DS-AMKL (median age, 2 years). The cryptic translocation had a distinct *HOXA/B* gene overexpression signature and was associated with a poor outcome [50]. Of interest, a novel t(11;12)(p15.5;q13)/*NUP98–RARG* gene fusion was observed in a patient with AML, which resembled that seen in APL [73]. A frequent translocation in AML is the t(7;11)(p15.4;p15.5)/*NUP98–HOXA9*, with a preponderance in young adults (median age, 35 years) [74].

t(7;12)(q36.3;p13)/*MNX1–ETV6*

The t(7;12)(q36.3;p13) is seen in 20% of infants with AML, and patients harboring this translocation are younger than 2 years. The t(7;12) and *KMT2A(MLL)* rearrangements are mutually exclusive. The t(7;12) is a subtle chromosomal aberration and can be difficult to recognize; however, FISH with the *ETV6* probe can identify the rearrangement and detect the abnormality. Most patients with this translocation have an extra chromosome 19. The fusion predicts a poor clinical outcome in patients with AML [75, 76].

***ETV6* (12p13).** Other chromosomal abnormalities of 12p, such as deletion, balanced translocations, and unbalanced translocations, which may include the loss or rearrangement of *ETV6*, are rare in patients with AML (~3%) but have been associated with poor prognosis in children with AML [54, 77–79].

inv(16)(p13.3q24.3)/*CBFA2T3(MTG16/ETO2)–GLIS2*

The *CBFA2T3–GLIS2* fusion generated by the cryptic inv(16)(p13.3q24.3) was initially identified in 30% of children with non-DS-AMKL but not in adults. Subsequently, it was found in all morphological subtypes of AML, with an overall prevalence of 8% in pediatric AML, and in larger series, in 17% of patients with non-DS-AMKL [80, 81]. The *CBFA2T3–GLIS2* fusion occurs with normal karyotypes in 8% of children; it is rarely observed with other recurrent abnormalities such as 11q23, t(8;21)(q22;q22), or inv(16)/t(16;16)(p13.1;q22). There are very few common AML-associated mutations in these children, and the *CBFA2T3–GLIS2* fusion predicts an adverse outcome [80].

***CBFA2T3* (16q24.3)**. The *CBFA2T3* gene is also fused with *RUNX1(AML1)* in the t(16;21)(q24;q22), which is rarely identified in de novo and therapy-related AML [82]. The t(1;16)(p31;q24)/*NFIA–CBFA2T3* has been detected in young males with erythroleukemia [83].

14q32/*BCL11B*

The *BCL11B* gene is sometimes involved in mostly cryptic 14q32 translocations in AML; patients with *BCL11B* rearrangements concomitantly express myeloid and T-cell-specific biphenotypic markers and harbor *FLT3*-ITD. FISH with a break-apart *BCL11B* probe can reveal rearrangements of the 14q32 locus fused to different partner chromosomes (2q22, 6q25.3, and 8q24.21) [84, 85].

Acute Megakaryoblastic Leukemia

AMKL accounts for up to 15% of pediatric AML patients, but it is extremely rare in adults. AMKL can be divided into two subgroups: DS-AMKL and non-DS-AMKL. Non-DS-AMKL includes a heterogeneous group of patients who have poor outcomes despite receiving intensive chemotherapy

[51]. Many patients carry recurrent genetic lesions [86]. The t(1;22)(p13;q13)/*RBM15(OTT)–MKL1(MAL)* (13%) is the signature lesion for non-DS-AMKL. Other recurrent abnormalities include inv(16)(p13.3q24.3)/*CBFA2T3–GLIS2* (17 %), t(11;12)(p15.5;p13.3)/*NUP98–KDM5A(JARID1A)* (11%), and 11q23 *(KMT2A)(MLL)* (10%) [50, 80]. In general, DS-AMKL includes the majority of patients with DS who are younger than 4 years and develop AML. DS-AMKL is considered by WHO-2008 as a distinct subgroup [1]. The *GATA1* (Xp11.23) mutation is present in most patients with DS-AMKL, but it is rare in children with DS and other types of leukemias or in children with non-DS-AMKL. In patients with DS-AMKL, *GATA1* mutations confer increased sensitivity to regimens containing cytarabine. The therapy for these children is less intensive than that for AML, which results in superior outcomes (EFS > 80 %) [87, 88]. Children with DS-AMKL who are older than 4 years are usually treated on standard AML regimens and have a very poor prognosis [89].

Transient Abnormal Myelopoiesis

DS with transient myeloproliferative disorder (TMD) is observed in infants with DS and is characterized by a clonal expansion of myeloblasts that can be difficult to distinguish from that seen in AML. Most cases of TMD regress spontaneously within the first 3 months of life. TMD blasts are most commonly megakaryoblastic and have distinctive mutations involving *GATA1* (Xp11.23). TMD can occur in phenotypically normal infants with genetic mosaicism in the bone marrow for trisomy 21. Although patients with TMD rarely have other chromosomal abnormalities in addition to the +21, the presence of an aberration can predict an increased risk for developing AML [87, 90]. Approximately 20% of infants with DS and TMD eventually develop AML, most being diagnosed within the first 3 years of life [91]. This transformation likely occurs through the acquisition of additional mutations and clonal selection [86, 92].

Genetic Mutations and Cytogenetic Subgroups

Some recurrent mutations that are frequent in AML are mutually exclusive of the transcription-factor fusions generated by translocations or other structural aberrations, suggesting that a cooperating mutation such as *FLT3* might activate signal pathways important in triggering leukemogenesis. Mutations such as *NPM1, DNMT3A, IDH1,* and *TET2* are initiators of leukemogenesis. Clinically relevant mutations are usually not detected in the first years of life, but their prevalence increases with age.

FLT3 (13q12) Mutation

FLT3, a receptor tyrosine kinase expressed on hematopoietic progenitors, is frequently mutated in AML, mainly in patients with a normal karyotype and is associated with poor prognosis [93]. Mutations include internal tandem duplication (*FLT3*-ITD) and a less frequent mutation involving the region encoding the activation loop (tyrosine kinase domain, *FLT3*-TKD), leading to ligand-independent constitutive activation of FLT3 signaling. *FLT3*-ITD mutations occur in children (12%; rare in children younger than 10 years) and adults (30%) with AML. *FLT3*-TKD mutations have been identified in less than 10% of children and adults with AML, but their clinical significance is not clear [94, 95]. These mutations are particularly significant when both alleles are mutated or there is a high ratio of the mutant allele to the normal allele [96, 97]. Approximately 10% of *FLT3* mutations are either gained or lost at relapse, which suggests that they can be late subclonal events and are not always the driver mutation of prognosis and response [98]. *FLT3*-ITD mutations are particularly prevalent in APL (up to 40% of children and adults), but their prognostic impact is minimal [24]. There is also a strong association of *FLT3*-ITD mutations with t(6;9)(p23;q34)/*DEK–NUP214* (~70%) and t(5;11)(q35;p15.5)/*NUP98–NSD1* (~82%). Both abnormalities are associated with dismal outcome, but this is independent of the presence of *FLT3*-ITD [57, 71].

Isolated trisomy 13 is extremely rare in children, but has been reported in a low incidence in adults with AML or MDS. Such patients have a poor outcome; however, recent reports have shown that these patients may be sensitive to lenalidomide as are patients with low-risk MDS with the 5q- cytogenetic abnormality [99]. Trisomy 13 (chromosome 13 harbors *FLT3*) is strongly associated with *RUNX1*(*AML1*) mutations and increased *FLT3* expression in AML.

NPM1 (Nucleophosmin) (5q31) Mutation

The NPM1 protein has diverse functions in the cell, such as chromatin remodeling and ribosomal complex assembly. *NPM1* mutations are detected by immunohistochemical methods that show its cytoplasmic localization [100]. NPM1 mutations are found in up to 35% of adults and 8% of children with AML. These mutations are most frequent in cytogenetically normal AML (45–60% of patients), but can be associated with +4, +8, and del(9q) and additional gene mutations such as *FLT3*-ITD, *DNMT3*, *IDH1*, and *IDH2* [101]. *NPM1* mutations are a good marker to assess MRD [102]. *NPM1* mutations are associated with good prognosis if *FLT3*-ITD or *DNMT3* mutations are absent [103].

CEBPA (19q13.1) Mutation

CEBPA encoding a transcription factor involved in normal myelopoiesis is mutated in 10% of adults younger than 60 years and in 5% of children with AML [57]. *CEBPA* mutations are found in approximately 10% of patients with normal karyotypes and can occur in patients with abnormal karyotypes, but are mutually exclusive of recurrent chromosomal aberrations [104]. Reports suggest that only biallelic mutations of *CEBPA* associated with a normal karyotype predict a favorable outcome in the absence of *FLT3*-ITD mutations [105–107].

Summary

Conventional and molecular cytogenetics are among the most important features currently used to direct treatment randomization in AML. In the last 30 years, many recurrent genetic lesions have been identified, but no single mutation has been shown to be sufficient to cause leukemogenesis. Instead, cooperating mutations are believed to promote proliferation and survival of aberrant cells or block the differentiation necessary for leukemic transformation. Most of the recurrent chromosomal abnormalities identified in myeloid blast cells generate chimeric oncoproteins that inhibit differentiation. Recent molecular genetic studies have shown that the common molecular markers for subclasses of AML include genetic lesions that may or may not be associated with chromosome abnormalities as determined by conventional cytogenetics [108–110]. The advent of novel technologies available for the genomic sequencing of leukemic blasts will help enhance our understanding of the pathophysiology of acute leukemias and identify novel therapeutic targets. Collaborative trials are needed given the rarity of childhood AML, its biological heterogeneity, and the prospect of targeted therapeutics for small genetic subgroups [10, 111].

Acute Lymphoblastic Leukemia

ALL is the most common leukemia in children, where 80–85% of leukemias are ALL, and is much rarer in adults where only 20% of acute leukemia is ALL. The cytogenetics of ALL has long been known to be of prognostic relevance, and both the number of chromosomes (modal number) and some structural abnormalities are prognostic in both adult and pediatric ALL [112].

Both cytogenetic aberrations and outcome differ between children and adults with ALL. Children with ALL have a very good prognosis, with 5-year EFS rates approaching 90% [113]. On the other hand, adults with ALL have a much poorer outcome with an overall EFS of 40% [114]. This difference in outcome can in part be attributed to the different biology of ALL in the two age groups, some of which is demonstrated by cytogenetics. The frequencies of "good prognosis" cytogenetic aberrations are higher in children than in adults with ALL, and "poor prognosis" cytogenetic abnormalities are more frequent in adults than in children with ALL.

ALL also is differentiated by the cell type that becomes leukemic. Approximately 85% of children and 75–80% of adults with ALL have B-cell precursor (BCP) ALL, and the remaining have T-cell ALL (T-ALL) [115, 116]. The cytogenetics of BCP and T-ALL differ, although there are some overlaps, and will be discussed separately. (See Table 16.2 for summary of ALL cytogenetic aberrations.)

B-Cell Precursor ALL

Chromosome Numbers in ALL

Modal number (mn) is defined as the number of chromosomes in the most prevalent abnormal clone. However, in ALL, the mn for classification is considered the number of chromosomes in the simplest abnormal clone, regardless of the prevalence of the clone. The mn is prognostic in ALL. Modal number classification in ALL includes high hyperdiploidy (HH, 51–67 chromosomes), low hyperdiploidy (LH, 47–50 chromosomes), near-triploidy (68–79 chromosomes), near-tetraploidy (>79 chromosomes), pseudodiploidy (46 chromosomes with an abnormality, usually, although not always, structural), normal chromosomes, and hypodiploidy (HO, <46 chromosomes).

As per mn classification, patients with HH have the best outcome. About 35% of children with ALL have HH [unpublished Children's Oncology Group (COG) data], whereas <10% of adults have HH [117, 118]. Chromosomes X, 4, 6, 10, 14, 17, 18, and 21 are preferentially present in extra copy number in HH ALL [119, 120] (Fig. 16.3). Furthermore, the excellent prognosis of HH ALL can be attributed to the presence of specific extra chromosomes. The COG found that the simultaneous presence of extra copies of chromosomes 4, 10, and 17 was associated with an excellent prognosis [121], and the Medical Research Council (MRC) of the United Kingdom found that extra copies of chromosomes 10 and 18 were associated with an excellent prognosis [119]. The significance of specific extra chromosomes has not been studied in adults with ALL. Approximately 50% of children with HH ALL have a structural abnormality, most often a duplication of 1q, which does not have prognostic significance [122]. The only other recurring structural abnormality frequently found in pediatric HH ALL is a t(1;19)(q23;p13.3), which frequently does not have a *TCF3-PBX1* rearrangement. Adults with HH ALL, however, frequently have recurring structural abnormalities that are associated with an adverse outcome [118].

Table 16.2 Common recurring aberrations in ALL

B-cell precursor ALL						
	Frequency (%)					
Aberration	Adult	Pediatric	Genes	Prognosis	Cytogenetic variants	Comments
Numerical aberrations						
Hyperdiploidy, mn > 50	<10	25–30		Good		
Hyperdiploidy, mn > 46 < 51	15	15		Intermediate		Usually have structural abnormalities, ~50% recurrent
Pseudodiploidy				Intermediate		
Near-triploidy and mn 30–39	Rare			Poor		
Hypodiploidy, mn 44–45		7		Intermediate		Usually have structural abnormalities
Hypodiploidy, mn <44		1.7		Poor		Few structural abnormalities, frequent doubling in mn <40
Structural aberrations						
t(9;22)(q34.1;q11.2)	25	<4	*BCR-ABL1*	Intermediate with TKI therapy	5% complex	Frequency increases with age
t(12;21)(p13;q22)	Very rare	25	*ETV6-RUNX1*	Good		Cytogenetically cryptic. Many other *ETV6* rearrangements may differ in clinical characteristics and prognosis
t(4;11)(q21.3;q23)			*KMT2A-AFF1*	Poor	Insertions, three-way translocations	Frequent in infants. Outcome may differ with age
t(11;19)(q23;p13.3)			*KMT2A-MLLT1*	Poor		Also in T-ALL and AML
t(9;11)(p22;q23)			*KMT2A-MLLT3*	Adults better than other 11q23; children poor		
Other 11q23	5	5 >1 year 80 < 1 year	*KMT2A/other*	Poor		Frequent in infants. Outcome may differ with age and partner
t(1;19)(q23.3;p13.3)	3	6	*TCF3-PBX1*	Not prognostic	der(19)t(1;19)(q23.3;p13.3); t(17;19)(q22;p13.3)	*HLF-E2A* in t(17;19)—poor prognosis
der(21)/add(21)			*RUNX1*	Poor	der(21) appears in many guises	Amplification of *RUNX1* or near gene
del(9p)	30	6	*CDKN2A*	Unknown		
dic(9;12)(p13;p11.2)	Rare	Rare	50% *PAX5-ETV6*	Good		Not all have PAX5/ETV6 rearrangement
dic(9;20)(p12-p13;q11.2)	Rare	Rare	*Some PAX5-ASXL1*	Good		
dic(7;9)(p11.2;p13)	Rare	Rare				
t(8;14)(q24;q32.3)			*IGH-MYC*	Intermediate		Usually Burkitt leukemia/lymphoma
t(8;14)(q11.2;q32.3)			*IGH-CEBPD*	Good in Down syndrome		Prevalent in Down syndrome ALL
t(5;14)(q31;q32.3)	Rare	Rare	*IGH-IL3*	Poor		Associated with hypereosinophilia
Other 14q32.3			*IGH*			
del(6q)	7	1.5	*MYB* some cases	Not prognostic		Frequent in *ETV6-RUNX1* cases
del(5q)	Rare	Rare				
del(7p)	4	4		Poor		
del(12)(p11.2-p13)			*?ETV6*	Not prognostic		
Sole +8	3	3		Unknown		

(continued)

Table 16.2 (continued)

B-cell precursor ALL						
	Frequency (%)					
Aberration	Adult	Pediatric	Genes	Prognosis	Cytogenetic variants	Comments
Sole +X	Rare	Rare		Unknown		
Sole +21	Rare	Rare				
del(13q)monosomy 13	5	2		Unknown		
T-lineage ALL[a]						
14q11.2 rearrangement	35		*TRA/TRD*	Not prognostic	7p14, 7q34	*TRG,TRB*
t(1;14)(p32;q11.2)		10 translocations 30 deletions	*TRA/TRD-TAL1*	Favorable	del(1)(p32p32) cryptic	*TAL1-STIL*
t(11;14)(p13;q11.2)	5–10		*TRA/ TRD-LMO2*			
t(11;14)(p15;q11.2)	2		*TRA/ TRD-LMO1*			
t(10;14) (q24.32;q11.2)	5–10		*TRA/TRD-TLX1*	Favorable		
inv(7)(p15.2q34)	3–5		*TRB-HOXA*			
t(6;7)(q23;q34)	3		*TRA/TRD-MYB*			
t(6;11)(q27;q23)	Rare		*KMT2A-MLLT4*	Poor		Also in AML
t(11;19)(q23;p13.3)			*KMT2A-MLLT1*	Favorable		
ins(10;11) (p12;q23q13)			*KMT2A-MLLT10*	Poor		May be cryptic
t(10;11)(p12;q14)	2–3		*PICALM-MLLT10*	Poor		Also in AML
t(5;14)(q35.1;q32)	13	20	*TLX3-BCL11B*	Poor	*TLX3* rearranges with other partners	Cryptic
amp(*NUP421-ABL1*)	<6		*NUP214-ABL1*	Poor		Cryptic, FISH required, rearrangement on an episome
del(9)(p13-p22)	65		*CDKN2A-CDKN2B*			Frequently cryptic
del(6)	10–20		*?MYB*			

[a]When frequencies do not differ between children and adults, they are displayed in the adults column

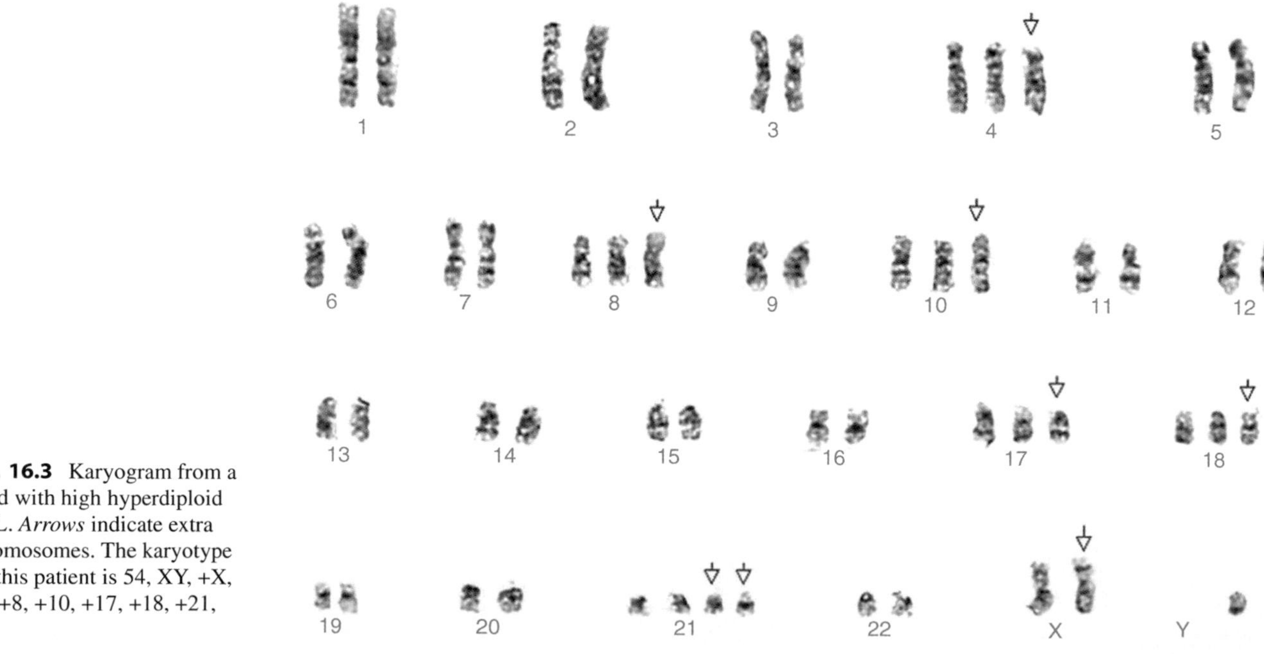

Fig. 16.3 Karyogram from a child with high hyperdiploid ALL. *Arrows* indicate extra chromosomes. The karyotype for this patient is 54, XY, +X, +4, +8, +10, +17, +18, +21, +21

Low hyperdiploidy is present in approximately 15% of both pediatric and adult ALL. These patients frequently have a recurring structural abnormality, and prognosis is associated with the recurring structural abnormality. The remaining patients with LH ALL have an intermediate prognosis [123, 124].

Near-tetraploidy is rare, occurring in <1% of pediatric and adult BCP ALL. It is more frequent in T-ALL. In pediatric BCP ALL, near-tetraploidy often also has an *ETV6-RUNX1(TEL-AML1)* rearrangement, which is associated with excellent prognosis (see in text to come). Because near-tetraploidy is rare, its prognostic significance in the absence of an *EVT6-RUNX1* rearrangement is unknown [117, 118].

Near-triploidy is also rare (<1% of pediatric ALL and 4% of adult ALL). These cases appear to be "true" near-triploids in pediatric ALL, with three copies of most chromosomes and only rarely structural abnormalities. Adult near-triploidy appears to be associated with hypodiploidy and represents a doubling of a hypodiploid clone. Cases with this karyotypic result are classified as hypodiploid cases in pediatric ALL. The prognosis of "true" near-triploidy is not known.

Pediatric ALL with hypodiploidy is further differentiated by mn. Seven percent of children with BCP ALL have 44 or 45 chromosomes. These cases usually have a structural abnormality, and prognostic significance is associated with the structural abnormality. Overall, these patients have an intermediate prognosis [125]. Patients with 43 and fewer chromosomes (1.7% of pediatric BCP ALL) have a dismal prognosis [125]. Cytogenetically, they can be classified as those with 40–43 chromosomes, with 30–39 chromosomes, or with 24–29 chromosomes [126, 127]. Patients with 40–43 chromosomes nearly always have a structural abnormality (>86%), and do not have doubling of the abnormal clone. Karyotypes of children with 30–39 chromosomes have doubling in 30–57% of cases and often (39–57% of cases) have structural abnormalities. Patients with 24–29 chromosomes (near-haploidy, 1% of pediatric BCP ALL) frequently also have doubling of the near-haploid clone (57–64% of cases), and structural abnormalities are found in only 14–25% of cases [126, 127]. Doubling of the hypodiploid clone can be masked, with only the doubled clone present. In such cases, additional studies, such as SNP microarray, are required to detect the abnormal clone and assure correct cytogenetic classification. Recent molecular studies of pediatric hypodiploid ALL have confirmed three categories of hypodiploidy differing in both modal number and types of mutations in the different groups [128]. Near-haploid cases (mn = 24–31) frequently have mutations in the signaling pathway, particularly in *NRAS*, *NF1*, and *IKZF3*. They also tend to be younger than hypodiploid patients with higher mn. Low hypodiploid cases (mn = 32–39) have mutations in *RB1* and *IKZF2* and significantly in *TP53*. Approximately half of the latter are germ line in origin, consistent with Li-Fraumeni syndrome. Adults with ALL with near-triploidy and hypodiploidy (30–39 chromosomes) are often classified together as the near-triploid clones usually represent doubling of the hypodiploid clone [117, 118]. Near-haploid adult ALL is extremely rare, and has not been reported in patients older than 40 years [117].

Recurring Structural Abnormalities in BCP ALL

Cytogenetic classification of BCP ALL is further classified on the basis of structural abnormalities. In cases with a recurring structural abnormality and a numerical abnormality, the case is generally classified by the structural abnormality.

Rearrangements Associated with Favorable Prognosis

The most common structural abnormality in pediatric BCP ALL is t(12;21)(p13;q22), which results in an *ETV6-RUNX1(TEL-AML1)* fusion gene. The abnormality is cryptic by standard cytogenetics, but can be detected by FISH using probes for *ETV6-RUNX1*. This rearrangement is present in 25% of children with BCP ALL and is associated with excellent prognosis [129]. It is rarely found in adult ALL, and then with rare exception, in patients younger than 30 years [130]. Although the t(12;21) is cryptic, 80% of these patients have cytogenetically visible aberrations [131]. The *ETV6-RUNX1* rearrangement is prenatal in origin [132]. It is not sufficient to cause leukemia, but appears to be an initiating event. A second event is required for expression of the disease [132]. The second event is often loss of the second *ETV6* allele, which is frequently detected by standard cytogenetics. This may explain early studies reporting either no prognostic significance or a good prognosis for patients with deletions of 12p.

Rearrangements Associated with Adverse Prognosis

Rearrangements of *KMT2A* (formerly *MLL*, 11q23) are associated with a poor prognosis in ALL. Although *KMT2A* rearrangements occur in both ALL and AML, some rearrangements are more common to each leukemia. *KMT2A* rearrangements are present in 2–7% of ALL patients older than 12 months. However, they are particularly common in infants, and up to 80% of infants younger than 12 months who are diagnosed with ALL have an *KMT2A* rearrangement. A t(4;11)(q21;q23)/*KMT2A-AFF1(AF4)* occurs in ALL, but the cells may have some myeloid markers [133]

(Fig. 16.4). It is the most common *KMT2A* rearrangement in infant ALL and is associated with a very poor prognosis [134]. The t(4;11) also occurs in pediatric and adult ALL, although at a much lower frequency (<2%), and also is associated with a poor prognosis. The etiology of the t(4;11) in infants and young children is prenatal [132]. Studies of monozygous twins with t(4;11) ALL show that they share identical molecular rearrangements, and studies of infant blood spots (Guthrie spots) from children with t(4;11) ALL show that these rearrangements can be detected in blood spots [132]. Also, cord blood investigations have shown that the rearrangement is much more prevalent than the development of leukemia [132]. These studies indicate that additional mutations are required for the development of ALL; even though a t(4;11) may occur prenatally, t(4;11) leukemia does not always develop, and when it does develop there is typically a time lag. The second most frequent *KMT2A* rearrangement in infant ALL is t(11;19)(q23;p13.3)/*KMT2A-MLLT1*(*ENL*), which also portends a poor prognosis, although it may not be as poor as t(4;11) infant ALL (Fig. 16.2). This rearrangement occurs in 3–7% of children and adults with ALL as well as in AML. A third common *KMT2A* rearrangement in ALL that occurs in all age groups is t(9;11)(p22;q23)/*KMT2A-MLLT3*(*AF9*), which is also very common in AML. Other *KMT2A* partners in ALL include Xq13.1/*FOXO4* (*AFX1*), 1p32/*EPS15*(*AF1P*), 5q31/*AFF4*(*AF5q31*), 6q27/*MLLT4*(*AF6*), 7p22.1/ *TNRC18*(*KIAA18856*), 10p12/*MLLT10*(*AF10*), 11q21 /*MAML2*, 11q23.3/*BCL9L*, 15q14/*CASC5*(*AF15Q14*), 16p13.3/*CREBBP*(*CBP*), 19p13.3/ *ASAH3*(*ACER1*), 19q13/ (*ACTN4*), 20q11/*MAPRE1*, and 22q11.21/*DEPT5*(*CDCREL*) [6].

Secondary ALL is a rare event, and most frequently has an *KMT2A* rearrangement. These secondary ALL generally occur after a patient has been treated with epipodophyllotoxins; they have a short lag time of 2–4 years and no preceding preleukemic phase. Patients with secondary ALL typically respond to therapy, but remissions are short and prognosis is poor. A t(4;11) is the most common *KMT2A* rearrangement in therapy-related ALL, but other *KMT2A* rearrangements, particularly t(9;11), also occur [6].

Philadelphia Chromosome (Ph+) and Philadelphia-like ALL

A Philadelphia chromosome (Ph), resulting from a t(9;22)(q34.1;q11.2) and a *BCR-ABL1* fusion, in ALL was associated with a very poor outcome in the past [114, 135] (Fig. 16.5). However, the poor outcome has been ameliorated by treatment with the tyrosine kinase inhibitor, imatinib mesylate [136, 137]. This translocation is present in less than 4% of children with ALL, but in 25% of adults with ALL. Its frequency increases with age, at least up to the fourth decade [117].

Philadelphia-like or *BCR-ABL1*-like ALL has an expression signature very much like that of Ph+ ALL, but without a t(9;22)(q34.1q11.2) [138, 139]. It is 3–4 times more common than Ph+ ALL in children, and its frequency increases with age. Outcome with traditional treatments is very poor. It is associated with *IKZF1* deletion, *CRLF2* rearrangements, and *JAK2* mutations. There are two different types of Ph-like ALL: those associated with *CRLF2* overexpression [140] and those with a variety of gene fusions targeting kinase

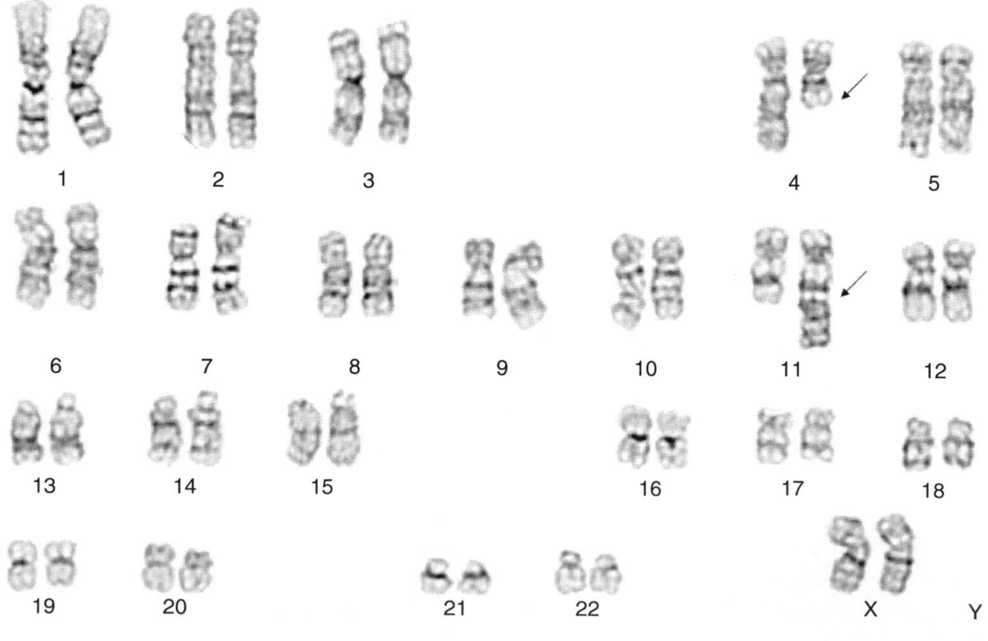

Fig. 16.4 Karyogram of patient with ALL and a t(4;11). *Arrows* indicate the abnormal chromosomes. The karyotype for this patient is 46,XX,t(4;11)(q21;q23)

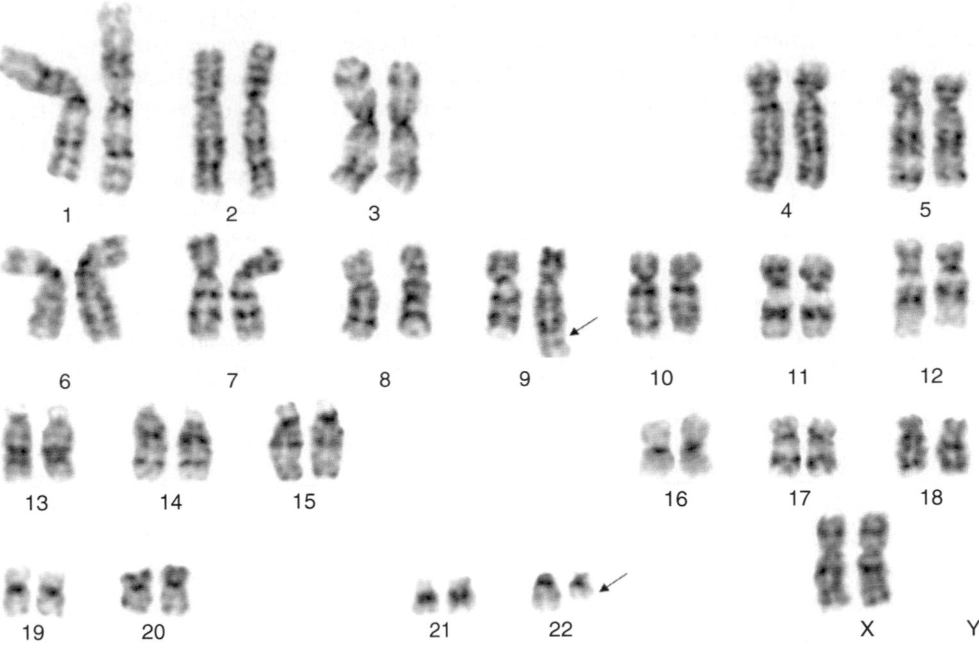

Fig. 16.5 Karyogram from a Philadelphia chromosome-positive ALL patient. *Arrows* indicate the abnormal chromosomes. The karyotype for this patient is 46,XX,t(9;22)(q34.1;q11.2)

genes, including *ABL1*, *ABL2*, *CSF1R*, *PDGFRB*, *EPOR*, and *JAK2* in a significant percentage of the remaining cases. Patients with these aberrations may be sensitive to tyrosine kinase inhibitors [141, 142]. Many of these gene fusions are cytogenetically cryptic, and molecular techniques are required to detect them. *CRLF2* is located in the pseudo-autosomal region of the X and Y chromosomes. CRLF2 overexpression results from a translocation with *IGH* or from a deletion of the sequences between *CRLF2* and *P2RY8*; both are cytogenically cryptic, and FISH or other molecular techniques are required for their detection. The *P2RY8-CRLF2* deletion is particularly common in children with DS [143]. Patients with a *CRLF2* rearrangement may be sensitive to ruxolitinib [142].

In addition to a t(12;21), the *ETV6-RUNX1* probes detect amplification of the *RUNX1* gene, resulting in an abnormality designated *iAMP21*. This may be detected with array studies, but is typically detected by FISH. By definition, amplification requires at least three extra copies of *RUNX1* on a single chromosome, usually an abnormal chromosome 21, resulting in a total of at least five *RUNX1* signals. It is not known whether the significant gene amplified in this region is *RUNX1*, as *RUNX1* is not overexpressed, although aCGH studies have shown that *RUNX1* is always included in the amplified region. The abnormality has been associated with a poor outcome [144, 145]. This aberration is more common in older children, but is rarely seen in adults with ALL [146].

Rearrangements Associated with Uncertain Prognostic Significance

A t(1;19)(q23.3;p13.3)/*TCF3*(*E2A*)-*PBX1* occurs both as a balanced t(1;19) and an unbalanced der(19)t(1;19) with two normal chromosomes 1. It is found in 6% of pediatric and 3% of adult ALL, typically with a pre-B-cell phenotype. It is only rarely prenatal in origin [132]. Early reports indicated an adverse prognosis for children with this aberration, but subsequent studies showed that it did not influence outcome, most likely due to more intense treatment in subsequent studies [130]. However, a t(1;19) may portend an adverse prognosis in adult ALL [147].

Deletions of 9p are frequent in ALL, occurring in up to 30% of adult ALL and up to 6% of pediatric ALL. Some are seen by traditional cytogenetics, but many are cryptic and cannot be detected by cytogenetics, so the frequency of this aberration may be much higher. The clinical significance of this abnormality has been controversial, with some studies showing an adverse prognosis [148] and others no impact on outcome [149]. The abnormality is thought to result in loss of the oncogene *CDKN2A*, which can be detected by FISH.

Interestingly, dicentric chromosomes are frequent in ALL, and they most often involve a chromosome 9. Although all dic(9;V) result in loss of 9p, the significance of dic(9;V) may be associated with a fusion gene rather than a deletion of 9p. A dic(9;12) is one of the more frequent dicentric chromosomes in ALL, although it is seen in less than 1% of children with ALL and very rarely in adults with ALL (usually in young adults) [150]. Approximately 50% of cases with dic(9;12) have a *PAX5-ETV6* rearrangement [151], and the remaining have an *ETV6-RUNX1* rearrangement instead [152]. The chromosome 12 involved in the dic(9;12) is not involved in the *ETV6-RUNX1* rearrangement, and the genes involved in the dic(9;12) in these cases have not yet been identified [152]. There is no consensus on the outcome of patients with dic(9;12); early reports of dic(9;12) indicated an excellent outcome [150], but studies by the Children's Cancer Group did not confirm this good prognosis [148].

A dic(9;20)(p12–p13;q11.2) is another frequent dicentric chromosome in ALL. This aberration is subtle and may be missed by traditional cytogenetics; cases with monosomy 20 need to be tested for the presence of this dicentric chromosome by FISH with probes for the centromeres of chromosomes 9 and 20 on either metaphases or interphases or using chromosome paints for chromosomes 9 and 20 on metaphases. The dic(9;20) has a peak incidence at age approximately 3 years and has a female predominance. It occurs in approximately 0.5% of adults and 2% of children with ALL and appears to have a favorable prognosis [153]. The molecular breakpoints of both partners of the dic(9;20) are heterogeneous—some 9p11–13 breakpoints occur in the repetitive region near the centromere and some involve *PAX5*. The 20q breakpoint frequently involves *ASXL1* [154].

Rearrangements of 14q32, usually involving the *IGH* gene, are recurrent in ALL. The t(8;14)(q22;q32.3)/*IGH-MYC* and its variants t(2;8)(p12;q22)/*IGK-MYC* and t(8;22)(q22;q11.2)/*IGL-MYC* generally indicate Burkitt leukemia. Although this aberration can occur in patients with BCP ALL, most are considered mature B-cell leukemias. Several rearrangements of 14q32.3, in addition to t(8;14)(q24;q32.3), are recurrent in ALL. They result in overexpression of the *IGH* partner gene. One such rearrangement is a t(8;14)(q11.2;q32.3)/*IGH-CEBPD*, which is more frequent in children with DS and ALL. In non-DS cases, trisomy 21 is often a secondary abnormality. Patients with DS and ALL who have this abnormality have an excellent prognosis [155]. Another *IGH* rearrangement in ALL is t(14;19)(q32.3;q13)/*IGH-CEBPA*. Additional *CEBP* genes also rearrange with *IGH*, indicating that overexpression of any of the several members of a gene family can contribute to ALL [156].

Recurrent Deletions and Single-Chromosome Aneusomies

Deletions of 12p are frequent in ALL. A del(12p) has been detected by cytogenetics in 9% of children and 4% of adults with ALL [118, 157]. It often includes deletion of *ETV6* and is sometimes associated with t(12;21) in pediatric ALL. When examined regardless of the presence of t(12;21), it has no prognostic significance [157]. Its clinical significance in the absence of t(12;21) remains to be investigated.

Deletion 6q is more frequent in adults (7%) than in children (1.5%) with ALL ([124] and COG unpublished data). It is often cryptic, and therefore its true incidence is not known. Whether the *MYB* oncogene is the significant gene deleted is controversial. When detected by traditional cytogenetics, del(6q) does not have prognostic significance in pediatric ALL [158], although it may have an adverse impact on prognosis in adult ALL [117, 159].

Deletions of 5q in ALL are rare (<2% of both children and adults). They do not appear to have prognostic significance in adults [160]. Children with ALL and a del(5q) have an adverse EFS, but not overall survival, indicating that they may respond to salvage therapy [161]. Whether the significant region of 5q lost in ALL is the same as that in AML remains to be investigated.

Monosomy 7 is rare but recurrent in ALL. It is frequently a secondary abnormality in Ph+ ALL. Deletions of chromosome 7 also occur, most frequently of 7p. When Ph+ cases are excluded, monosomy 7 or chromosome 7 deletions occur in approximately 5% of adults and children with ALL. Deletions of 7p appear to be an adverse prognostic factor in children but not adults with ALL [118, 162].

Trisomy 8 as a sole abnormality is also rare but recurrent in ALL, seen in approximately 3% of cases ([124] and COG unpublished data). There is no agreement on its prognostic significance: some studies have shown no prognostic significance [118], and others have shown an adverse outcome for patients with ALL and this abnormality [159].

Gain of an X chromosome in non-HH ALL is also recurrent, often in conjunction with another abnormality, such as the t(8;14)(q11.2;q32.3). As a sole cytogenetic abnormality, it is found in less than 1% of children with ALL (unpublished COG data), and its frequency in adults as a sole abnormality has not been reported. It does not appear to influence prognosis in adults when all cases with an extra X chromosome are considered [118].

Trisomy 21 in non-HH ALL is also recurrent. As with an extra X chromosome, it often occurs in conjunction with another abnormality, such as the t(12;21), wherein it is a frequent secondary abnormality. Sole trisomy 21 is rare in pediatric ALL, occurring in less than 1% of cases (unpublished COG data). Its frequency in adult ALL or its prognostic significance as a sole aberration in ALL has not been investigated.

Deletions of 13q and monosomy 13 occur in 5% of adults with ALL, and 2% of children with ALL have breakpoints in 13q12–14 [163]. In children, these aberrations contribute to a higher risk of treatment failure and are also associated with other adverse clinical features. Deletion 13/monosomy 13 does not appear to have prognostic significance in adults [118].

B-Cell Precursor ALL Summary

Frequencies of cytogenetic aberrations known to have the most significant impact on outcome differ in children and adults with ALL. The differences in frequencies of a Ph, an *ETV6-RUNX1* rearrangement, and HH contribute to the differences in outcome between pediatric and adult ALL. HH and an *ETV6-RUNX1* rearrangement, both rare in adults, have the best prognosis among all ALL cytogenetic aberrations. However, a Ph, which is much more common in adults than in children with ALL, predicts a poor prognosis, especially before the advent of treatment with tyrosine kinase inhibitors specific for this rearrangement. The frequencies of aberrations with less prognostic impact differ only slightly between adults and children with BCP ALL. Additional research is needed to elucidate the etiology of the differences in frequencies of ALL cytogenetic subsets between adults and children with ALL. Although the genes involved in many aberrations are known, many have not been identified. Identification of new aberrations, such as Ph-like ALL and development of treatments specific for genetic subsets of ALL will contribute to improved outcomes for these patients in the future.

T-Cell ALL

T-ALL is less common than BCP ALL, accounting for 10–15% of pediatric ALL and 25% of adult ALL, and is more frequent in males than in females [116]. It is cytogenetically distinct from BCP ALL, although both subtypes have some aberrations in common. It is typically subdivided according to the maturation status of the leukemic cells. Normal metaphase cytogenetics in T-ALL may in part be due to a high frequency of cryptic aberrations in T-ALL. Molecular approaches have shown that 90% of adults with T-ALL have aberrations [164]. Numeric changes are rare in pediatric T-ALL (<8%; unpublished COG data), but are more common in adult ALL (~30%) [118].

The most common cytogenetic aberrations in T-ALL involve the T-cell receptor (TCR) loci, *TRA/TRD* at 14q11.2, *TRB* at 7q34, and *TRG* at 7p14, and occur in 35% of cases of T-ALL [165]. Any of the TCRs can rearrange with each of the partner loci, and some partners appear to preferentially rearrange with different TCRs. As a result of these rearrangements, the translocation partner of the TCR is juxtaposed to the promoter or enhancer element of the TCR and is overexpressed. A t(1;14)(p32;q11.2)/*TRA/TRD-TAL1* results in overexpression of *TAL1*. This aberration is rare (3%) in T-ALL. However, a cryptic deletion of 1p, which results in loss of *SCL* and juxtaposition of *STIL* and *TAL1*, is much more common (17% of T-ALL) and also causes deregulation of *TAL1*. This rearrangement is associated with a good prognosis [166]. Other recurring translocations with the TCR loci are with 10q24/*TLX1*(*HOX11*), 9q34.3/*NOTCH1*, 11p13/*LMO2*, 11p15/*LMO1*, 7p15/*HOXA* cluster, 9q32/*TAL2*, 8q24/*MYC*, 19p13/*LYL1*, 1p34/*LCK*, 14q13/*NKX2.1*, and 12p13/*CCND2*. *TLX1* expression is generally associated with an improved outcome, and its expression also occurs in the absence of a *TLX1* rearrangement [167]. The prognostic significance of the other genes rearranged with TCR loci is not well established. The recurrent t(7;9)(q34;q34.3) led to the identification of Notch1 signaling in T-ALL pathogenesis, and *NOTCH1* activating mutations are now known to occur in 60% of T-ALL [168, 169]. Notch1 is important in regulating hematopoietic progenitor commitment to the T-cell lineage, consistent with *NOTCH1* mutations in 50–70% of T-ALL [170, 171].

Chimeric or fusion genes also recur in T-ALL, including *KMT2A* rearrangements, although these are rare (<5%; COG unpublished data and [116]). Interestingly, a t(11;19)(q23;p13.3) (*KMT2A-MLLT1*) rearrangement in T-ALL is associated with a relatively good prognosis [172] (Fig. 16.2). A t(10;11)(p12;q14)/*PICALM*(*CALM*)-*MLLT10* occurs in 2–3% of patients with T-ALL. It can be mistaken for a *KMT2A* rearrangement, as the breakpoints of different t(10;11) can be difficult to distinguish. These abnormalities can be detected by FISH. Patients with a *PICALM-MLLT10* fusion have a relatively good prognosis [116]. A t(5;14)(q35;q32)/*BCL11B-TLX3* is another cryptic rearrangement in T-ALL. *TLX3* also rearranges with other partners, including 14q11.2/*TRA/TRD*), 7q21/*CDK6*, and 5q34/*RANBP17*. As a result of these rearrangements, *TLX3* is overexpressed. The rearrangements are rare and previously appeared to predict a poor prognosis; however, with current therapies these patients may not have a poor prognosis [116, 173]. In most cases with *TLX3* expression, a chromosome 5 abnormality is present [173]. Amplification of a cryptic rearrangement of *NUP214-ABL1* is seen in 2–6% of patients with T-ALL. *NUP214* is slightly distal to *ABL1* on chromosome 9 band q34. This rearrangement is unique in that it is present as an episome (a small extrachromosomal circular body) with juxtaposition of these genes. The episomes are in the nucleoplasm. Although not detected by metaphase cytogenetics, this rearrangement can be detected by FISH with either a fusion probe for *NUP214-ABL1* or a probe for *ABL1* [174]. This aberration is also found in Ph-like B-precursor ALL [141]. There is some preliminary evidence that patients with this aberration may respond to imatinib therapy [175].

Deletions of 9p are very frequent in T-ALL; they are often cryptic and not detected by cytogenetics, and therefore FISH or PCR is needed for their detection. The genes deleted are *CDKN2A*, the primary target, and *CDKN2B*, also very frequently deleted. They are often homozygously deleted (65% of T-ALL) and less frequently hemizygously deleted (23%) [176]. In addition, they may be inactivated by methylation;

up to 93% of *CDKN2A* and 99% of *CDKN2B* may be inactivated at the protein level [177]. This aberration appears to have no prognostic significance [116]. Similarly, deletions of 6q are common, occurring in 30% of cases, but their prognostic significance is uncertain.

Although complexity has not been shown to be prognostic in BCP ALL, it may be prognostic in T-ALL, particularly in adults; 5–8% of adults with T-ALL have five or more abnormalities, and 15% have three or more abnormalities. In a large study, adults with T-ALL who had five or more abnormalities had a poor outcome [116].

T-ALL Summary

In normal development, T-cell progenitors originate in the bone marrow and migrate to the thymus, where they complete antigen-independent maturation. The thymus is encapsulated and has cortical and medullary areas. T-cell precursors enter the subcapsular cortical area where they proliferate and begin to differentiate. As the cells differentiate, they move from the cortex toward the medulla where differentiation continues, TCR rearrangement begins, and cells progress through differentiation stages; first expressing neither CD4 nor CD8, then expressing CD4 and CD8, and then either CD4 or CD8. The cells move to the cortico-medullary junction and maturation continues. When the cells are mature, they leave the thymus and enter the periphery.

Expression array studies of T-ALL have shown five different expression signatures, which correspond to differentiation stages and to cytogenetic aberrations [178]. The *TAL1/LMO* subgroup includes all rearrangements involving these genes (Table 16.2) and the T-cells are in an early stage of development, when neither CD4 nor CD8 is expressed. The *TLX1* subgroup includes cases with *TLX1* (10q24) rearrangements, typically affects cells at the early cortical thymocyte stage, and is associated with a good prognosis. The *TLX3* subgroup currently includes only *TLX3* (5q35) rearrangements. Although they do not have a unique differentiation profile, they do not have a mature immunophenotype. The fourth expression array subgroup is the *HOXA* subgroup and includes *PICALM-MLLT10*, *KMT2A*, inversion 7, and *SET-NUP214* rearrangements. *HOXA* genes are activated in this subgroup, and they generally have a mature immunophenotype. The *MYB* subgroup represents cases with expression of *MYB* through activation by a translocation with a TCR or by *MYB* amplification. The T-cell developmental stage of this subgroup has not been identified [178]. These expression array studies and their correlations with cytogenetic aberrations show a pattern of genetic lesions in T-ALL and a relationship to the differentiation status of the transformed T-cells. The different patterns of gene expression categorize many recurring T-ALL cytogenetic aberrations into groups, illustrating association of different abnormalities to each other, to T-cell differentiation, and to prognosis.

Summary

The use of conventional and molecular cytogenetics has led to many gene discoveries in cancer biology over the past several decades. The cloning of chromosome translocation breakpoints, like the t(8;21), inv(16), 11q23, t(12;21), t(9;22), and many others, has helped to identify the genes involved in these translocations and allowed the development of DNA probes for FISH and RT-PCR that are used to diagnose and monitor minimal residual disease. Many genetic lesions are currently used as tools for the diagnosis, classification, and management of patients with acute leukemia.

The advent of new DNA array and sequencing technologies has enabled the simultaneous detection of mutations, deletions, amplifications, and epigenetic changes; and RNA arrays have allowed the evaluation of associated biochemical pathways. Thus, the detection of additional tumor markers via innovative genetic technologies will help pinpoint the genes that act cooperatively in a particular malignant cell type, complementing the current WHO-2008 assignment of genetic lesions used in acute leukemias.

Currently known molecular genetic mutations as well as novel ones that remain to be identified are potential genetic markers that have clinical significance, underscoring the patient variability in and heterogeneity of acute leukemias. These genetic events alter cellular pathways and functions, which may in turn affect the clinical phenotype of the disease and treatment response, thereby facilitating individualized targeted therapy.

Acknowledgments We are unable to include the references for studies by several investigators because of limited space; only the latest references in various topics have been included in this chapter. Special thanks to Heather Breidenbach for assistance with the preparation of the chapter and to Vani Shanker for scientific editing of the chapter.

References

1. WHO. World health organization classification of tumours of haematopoietic and lymphoid tissues. Lyon: IARC Press; 2008.
2. Kolomietz E, Al-Maghrabi J, Brennan S, Karaskova J, Minkin S, Lipton J, Squire JA. Primary chromosomal rearrangements of leukemia are frequently accompanied by extensive submicroscopic deletions and may lead to altered prognosis. Blood. 2001;97(11):3581–8.
3. Gulley ML, Shea TC, Fedoriw Y. Genetic tests to evaluate prognosis and predict therapeutic response in acute myeloid leukemia. J Mol Diagn. 2010;12(1):3–16.
4. Mrozek K, Prior TW, Edwards C, Marcucci G, Carroll AJ, Snyder PJ, Koduru PR, Theil KS, Pettenati MJ, Archer KJ, Caligiuri MA,

Vardiman JW, Kolitz JE, Larson RA, Bloomfield CD. Comparison of cytogenetic and molecular genetic detection of t(8;21) and inv(16) in a prospective series of adults with de novo acute myeloid leukemia: a cancer and leukemia group b study. J Clin Oncol. 2001;19(9):2482–92.

5. Campbell LJ, Oei P, Brookwell R, Shortt J, Eaddy N, Ng A, Chew E, Browett P. Fish detection of pml-rara fusion in ins(15;17) acute promyelocytic leukaemia depends on probe size. Biomed Res Int. 2013;2013:164501.
6. Meyer C, Kowarz E, Hofmann J, Renneville A, Zuna J, Trka J, Ben Abdelali R, Macintyre E, De Braekeleer E, De Braekeleer M, Delabesse E, de Oliveira MP, Cave H, Clappier E, van Dongen JJ, Balgobind BV, van den Heuvel-Eibrink MM, Beverloo HB, Panzer-Grumayer R, Teigler-Schlegel A, Harbott J, Kjeldsen E, Schnittger S, Koehl U, Gruhn B, Heidenreich O, Chan LC, Yip SF, Krzywinski M, Eckert C, Moricke A, Schrappe M, Alonso CN, Schafer BW, Krauter J, Lee DA, Zur Stadt U, Te Kronnie G, Sutton R, Izraeli S, Trakhtenbrot L, Lo Nigro L, Tsaur G, Fechina L, Szczepanski T, Strehl S, Ilencikova D, Molkentin M, Burmeister T, Dingermann T, Klingebiel T, Marschalek R. New insights to the mll recombinome of acute leukemias. Leukemia. 2009;23(8):1490–9.
7. Eklund EA. Genomic analysis of acute myeloid leukemia: potential for new prognostic indicators. Curr Opin Hematol. 2010;17(2):75–8.
8. Dohner H, Weisdorf DJ, Bloomfield CD. Acute myeloid leukemia. N Engl J Med. 2015;373(12):1136–52.
9. Dohner H, Estey EH, Amadori S, Appelbaum FR, Buchner T, Burnett AK, Dombret H, Fenaux P, Grimwade D, Larson RA, Lo-Coco F, Naoe T, Niederwieser D, Ossenkoppele GJ, Sanz MA, Sierra J, Tallman MS, Lowenberg B, Bloomfield CD. Diagnosis and management of acute myeloid leukemia in adults: recommendations from an international expert panel, on behalf of the European leukemianet. Blood. 2010;115(3):453–74.
10. Creutzig U, van den Heuvel-Eibrink MM, Gibson B, Dworzak MN, Adachi S, de Bont E, Harbott J, Hasle H, Johnston D, Kinoshita A, Lehrnbecher T, Leverger G, Mejstrikova E, Meshinchi S, Pession A, Raimondi SC, Sung L, Stary J, Zwaan CM, Kaspers GJ, Reinhardt D, A. M. L. C. o. t. I. B. S. Group. Diagnosis and management of acute myeloid leukemia in children and adolescents: recommendations from an international expert panel. Blood. 2012;120(16):3187–205.
11. Schuback HL, Arceci RJ, Meshinchi S. Somatic characterization of pediatric acute myeloid leukemia using next-generation sequencing. Semin Hematol. 2013;50(4):325–32.
12. Grimwade D, Ivey A, Huntly BJ. Molecular landscape of acute myeloid leukemia in younger adults and its clinical relevance. Blood. 2016;127(1):29–41.
13. Creutzig U, Buchner T, Sauerland MC, Zimmermann M, Reinhardt D, Dohner H, Schlenk RF. Significance of age in acute myeloid leukemia patients younger than 30 years: a common analysis of the pediatric trials aml-bfm 93/98 and the adult trials amlcg 92/99 and amlsg hd93/98a. Cancer. 2008;112(3):562–71.
14. Chaudhury SS, Morison JK, Gibson BE, Keeshan K. Insights into cell ontogeny, age, and acute myeloid leukemia. Exp Hematol. 2015;43(9):745–55.
15. Razzouk BI, Estey E, Pounds S, Lensing S, Pierce S, Brandt M, Rubnitz JE, Ribeiro RC, Rytting M, Pui CH, Kantarjian H, Jeha S. Impact of age on outcome of pediatric acute myeloid leukemia: a report from 2 institutions. Cancer. 2006;106(11):2495–502.
16. Ortega JJ, Madero L, Martin G, Verdeguer A, Garcia P, Parody R, Fuster J, Molines A, Novo A, Deben G, Rodriguez A, Conde E, de la Serna J, Allegue MJ, Capote FJ, Gonzalez JD, Bolufer P, Gonzalez M, Sanz MA. Treatment with all-trans retinoic acid and anthracycline monochemotherapy for children with acute promyelocytic leukemia: a multicenter study by the pethema group. J Clin Oncol. 2005;23(30):7632–40.
17. Tallman MS, Altman JK. How i treat acute promyelocytic leukemia. Blood. 2009;114(25):5126–35.
18. Sanz MA, Grimwade D, Tallman MS, Lowenberg B, Fenaux P, Estey EH, Naoe T, Lengfelder E, Buchner T, Dohner H, Burnett AK, Lo-Coco F. Management of acute promyelocytic leukemia: recommendations from an expert panel on behalf of the European leukemianet. Blood. 2009;113(9):1875–91.
19. Iland HJ, Bradstock K, Supple SG, Catalano A, Collins M, Hertzberg M, Browett P, Grigg A, Firkin F, Hugman A, Reynolds J, Di Iulio J, Tiley C, Taylor K, Filshie R, Seldon M, Taper J, Szer J, Moore J, Bashford J, Seymour JF, Australasian L, Lymphoma G. All-trans-retinoic acid, idarubicin, and iv arsenic trioxide as initial therapy in acute promyelocytic leukemia (apml4). Blood. 2012;120(8):1570–80. quiz 1752
20. Adams J, Nassiri M. Acute promyelocytic leukemia: a review and discussion of variant translocations. Arch Pathol Lab Med. 2015;139(10):1308–13.
21. Grimwade D, Mrozek K. Diagnostic and prognostic value of cytogenetics in acute myeloid leukemia. Hematol/Oncol Clin N Am. 2011;25(6):1135–61, vii
22. Won D, Shin SY, Park CJ, Jang S, Chi HS, Lee KH, Lee JO, Seo EJ. Obfc2a/rara: a novel fusion gene in variant acute promyelocytic leukemia. Blood. 2013;121(8):1432–5.
23. Chen Y, Li S, Zhou C, Li C, Ru K, Rao Q, Xing H, Tian Z, Tang K, Mi Y, Wang B, Wang M, Wang J. Tblr1 fuses to retinoid acid receptor alpha in a variant t(3;17)(q26;q21) translocation of acute promyelocytic leukemia. Blood. 2014;124(6):936–45.
24. Souza Melo CP, Campos CB, Dutra AP, Neto JC, Fenelon AJ, Neto AH, Carbone EK, Pianovski MA, Ferreira AC, Assumpcao JG. Correlation between flt3-itd status and clinical, cellular and molecular profiles in promyelocytic acute leukemias. Leuk Res. 2015;39(2):131–7.
25. Renneville A, Roumier C, Biggio V, Nibourel O, Boissel N, Fenaux P, Preudhomme C. Cooperating gene mutations in acute myeloid leukemia: a review of the literature. Leukemia. 2008;22(5):915–31.
26. Manara E, Bisio V, Masetti R, Beqiri V, Rondelli R, Menna G, Micalizzi C, Santoro N, Locatelli F, Basso G, Pigazzi M. Core-binding factor acute myeloid leukemia in pediatric patients enrolled in the aieop aml 2002/01 trial: screening and prognostic impact of c-kit mutations. Leukemia. 2014;28(5):1132–4.
27. Klein K, Kaspers G, Harrison CJ, Beverloo HB, Reedijk A, Bongers M, Cloos J, Pession A, Reinhardt D, Zimmerman M, Creutzig U, Dworzak M, Alonzo T, Johnston D, Hirsch B, Zapotocky M, De Moerloose B, Fynn A, Lee V, Taga T, Tawa A, Auvrignon A, Zeller B, Forestier E, Salgado C, Balwierz W, Popa A, Rubnitz J, Raimondi S, Gibson B. Clinical impact of additional cytogenetic aberrations, ckit and ras mutations, and treatment elements in pediatric t(8;21)-aml: results from an international retrospective study by the international berlin-frankfurt-munster study group. J Clin Oncol. 2015;33(36):4247–58.
28. Mrozek K, Marcucci G, Paschka P, Bloomfield CD. Advances in molecular genetics and treatment of core-binding factor acute myeloid leukemia. Curr Opin Oncol. 2008;20(6):711–8.
29. Basecke J, Cepek L, Mannhalter C, Krauter J, Hildenhagen S, Brittinger G, Trumper L, Griesinger F. Transcription of aml1/eto in bone marrow and cord blood of individuals without acute myelogenous leukemia. Blood. 2002;100(6):2267–8.
30. Wiemels JL, Xiao Z, Buffler PA, Maia AT, Ma X, Dicks BM, Smith MT, Zhang L, Feusner J, Wiencke J, Pritchard-Jones K, Kempski H, Greaves M. In utero origin of t(8;21) aml1-eto translocations in childhood acute myeloid leukemia. Blood. 2002;99(10):3801–5.
31. Micol JB, Duployez N, Boissel N, Petit A, Geffroy S, Nibourel O, Lacombe C, Lapillonne H, Etancelin P, Figeac M, Renneville A, Castaigne S, Leverger G, Ifrah N, Dombret H, Preudhomme C, Abdel-Wahab O, Jourdan E. Frequent asxl2 mutations in acute myeloid leukemia patients with t(8;21)/runx1-runx1t1 chromosomal translocations. Blood. 2014;124(9):1445–9.
32. Paschka P, Du J, Schlenk RF, Gaidzik VI, Bullinger L, Corbacioglu A, Spath D, Kayser S, Schlegelberger B, Krauter J, Ganser A,

Kohne CH, Held G, von Lilienfeld-Toal M, Kirchen H, Rummel M, Gotze K, Horst HA, Ringhoffer M, Lubbert M, Wattad M, Salih HR, Kundgen A, Dohner H, Dohner K. Secondary genetic lesions in acute myeloid leukemia with inv(16) or t(16;16): a study of the german-austrian aml study group (amlsg). Blood. 2013;121(1):170–7.

33. Nucifora G, Begy CR, Kobayashi H, Roulston D, Claxton D, Pedersen-Bjergaard J, Parganas E, Ihle JN, Rowley JD. Consistent intergenic splicing and production of multiple transcripts between aml1 at 21q22 and unrelated genes at 3q26 in (3;21)(q26;q22) translocations. Proc Natl Acad Sci U S A. 1994;91(9):4004–8.
34. Levy ER, Parganas E, Morishita K, Fichelson S, James L, Oscier D, Gisselbrecht S, Ihle JN, Buckle VJ. Dna rearrangements proximal to the evi1 locus associated with the 3q21q26 syndrome. Blood. 1994;83(5):1348–54.
35. Lugthart S, van Drunen E, van Norden Y, van Hoven A, Erpelinck CA, Valk PJ, Beverloo HB, Lowenberg B, Delwel R. High evi1 levels predict adverse outcome in acute myeloid leukemia: prevalence of evi1 overexpression and chromosome 3q26 abnormalities underestimated. Blood. 2008;111(8):4329–37.
36. Schnittger S, Dicker F, Kern W, Wendland N, Sundermann J, Alpermann T, Haferlach C, Haferlach T. Runx1 mutations are frequent in de novo aml with noncomplex karyotype and confer an unfavorable prognosis. Blood. 2011;117(8):2348–57.
37. Luesink M, Hollink IH, van der Velden VH, Knops RH, Boezeman JB, de Haas V, Trka J, Baruchel A, Reinhardt D, van der Reijden BA, van den Heuvel-Eibrink MM, Zwaan CM, Jansen JH. High gata2 expression is a poor prognostic marker in pediatric acute myeloid leukemia. Blood. 2012;120(10):2064–75.
38. Groschel S, Sanders MA, Hoogenboezem R, Zeilemaker A, Havermans M, Erpelinck C, Bindels EM, Beverloo HB, Dohner H, Lowenberg B, Dohner K, Delwel R, Valk PJ. Mutational spectrum of myeloid malignancies with inv(3)/t(3;3) reveals a predominant involvement of ras/rtk signaling pathways. Blood. 2015;125(1):133–9.
39. Lavallee VP, Gendron P, Lemieux S, D'Angelo G, Hebert J, Sauvageau G. Evi1-rearranged acute myeloid leukemias are characterized by distinct molecular alterations. Blood. 2015;125(1):140–3.
40. Groschel S, Sanders MA, Hoogenboezem R, de Wit E, Bouwman BA, Erpelinck C, van der Velden VH, Havermans M, Avellino R, van Lom K, Rombouts EJ, van Duin M, Dohner K, Beverloo HB, Bradner JE, Dohner H, Lowenberg B, Valk PJ, Bindels EM, de Laat W, Delwel R. A single oncogenic enhancer rearrangement causes concomitant evi1 and gata2 deregulation in leukemia. Cell. 2014;157(2):369–81.
41. Wlodarski MW, Hirabayashi S, Pastor V, Stary J, Hasle H, Masetti R, Dworzak M, Schmugge M, van den Heuvel-Eibrink M, Ussowicz M, De Moerloose B, Catala A, Smith OP, Sedlacek P, Lankester AC, Zecca M, Bordon V, Matthes-Martin S, Abrahamsson J, Kuhl JS, Sykora KW, Albert MH, Przychodzien B, Maciejewski JP, Schwarz S, Gohring G, Schlegelberger B, Cseh A, Noellke P, Yoshimi A, Locatelli F, Baumann I, Strahm B, Niemeyer CM, Ewog MDS. Prevalence, clinical characteristics, and prognosis of gata2-related myelodysplastic syndromes in children and adolescents. Blood. 2016;127(11):1387–97.
42. Meyer C, Hofmann J, Burmeister T, Groger D, Park TS, Emerenciano M, Pombo de Oliveira M, Renneville A, Villarese P, Macintyre E, Cave H, Clappier E, Mass-Malo K, Zuna J, Trka J, De Braekeleer E, De Braekeleer M, Oh SH, Tsaur G, Fechina L, van der Velden VH, van Dongen JJ, Delabesse E, Binato R, Silva ML, Kustanovich A, Aleinikova O, Harris MH, Lund-Aho T, Juvonen V, Heidenreich O, Vormoor J, Choi WW, Jarosova M, Kolenova A, Bueno C, Menendez P, Wehner S, Eckert C, Talmant P, Tondeur S, Lippert E, Launay E, Henry C, Ballerini P, Lapillone H, Callanan MB, Cayuela JM, Herbaux C, Cazzaniga G, Kakadiya PM, Bohlander S, Ahlmann M, Choi JR, Gameiro P, Lee DS, Krauter J, Cornillet-Lefebvre P, Te Kronnie G, Schafer BW, Kubetzko S, Alonso CN, zur Stadt U, Sutton R, Venn NC, Izraeli S, Trakhtenbrot L, Madsen HO, Archer P, Hancock J, Cerveira N, Teixeira MR, Lo Nigro L, Moricke A, Stanulla M, Schrappe M, Sedek L, Szczepanski T, Zwaan CM, Coenen EA, van den Heuvel-Eibrink MM, Strehl S, Dworzak M, Panzer-Grumayer R, Dingermann T, Klingebiel T, Marschalek R. The mll recombinome of acute leukemias in 2013. Leukemia. 2013;27(11):2165–76.
43. Lavallee VP, Baccelli I, Krosl J, Wilhelm B, Barabe F, Gendron P, Boucher G, Lemieux S, Marinier A, Meloche S, Hebert J, Sauvageau G. The transcriptomic landscape and directed chemical interrogation of mll-rearranged acute myeloid leukemias. Nat Genet. 2015;47(9):1030–7.
44. Balgobind BV, Raimondi SC, Harbott J, Zimmermann M, Alonzo TA, Auvrignon A, Beverloo HB, Chang M, Creutzig U, Dworzak MN, Forestier E, Gibson B, Hasle H, Harrison CJ, Heerema NA, Kaspers GJ, Leszl A, Litvinko N, Nigro LL, Morimoto A, Perot C, Pieters R, Reinhardt D, Rubnitz JE, Smith FO, Stary J, Stasevich I, Strehl S, Taga T, Tomizawa D, Webb D, Zemanova Z, Zwaan CM, V. d. H.-E. MM. Novel prognostic subgroups in childhood 11q23/mll-rearranged acute myeloid leukemia: results of an international retrospective study. Blood. 2009;114(12):2489–96.
45. Coenen EA, Raimondi SC, Harbott J, Zimmermann M, Alonzo TA, Auvrignon A, Beverloo HB, Chang M, Creutzig U, Dworzak MN, Forestier E, Gibson B, Hasle H, Harrison CJ, Heerema NA, Kaspers GJ, Leszl A, Litvinko N, Lo NL, Morimoto A, Perot C, Reinhardt D, Rubnitz JE, Smith FO, Stary J, Stasevich I, Strehl S, Taga T, Tomizawa D, Webb D, Zemanova Z, Pieters R, Zwaan CM, V. d. H.-E. MM. Prognostic significance of additional cytogenetic aberrations in 733 de novo pediatric 11q23/mll-rearranged aml patients: results of an international study. Blood. 2011;117(26):7102–11.
46. Shimada A, Taki T, Tabuchi K, Taketani T, Hanada R, Tawa A, Tsuchida M, Horibe K, Tsukimoto I, Hayashi Y. Tandem duplications of mll and flt3 are correlated with poor prognoses in pediatric acute myeloid leukemia: a study of the Japanese childhood aml cooperative study group. Pediatr Blood Cancer. 2008;50(2):264–9.
47. Savage NM, Kota V, Manaloor EJ, Kulharya AS, Pierini V, Mecucci C, Ustun C. Acute leukemia with picalm-mllt10 fusion gene: diagnostic and treatment struggle. Cancer Genet Cytogenet. 2010;202(2):129–32.
48. van Grotel M, Meijerink JP, van Wering ER, Langerak AW, Beverloo HB, Buijs-Gladdines JG, Burger NB, Passier M, van Lieshout EM, Kamps WA, Veerman AJ, van Noesel MM, Pieters R. Prognostic significance of molecular-cytogenetic abnormalities in pediatric t-all is not explained by immunophenotypic differences. Leukemia. 2008;22(1):124–31.
49. Caudell D, Aplan PD. The role of calm-af10 gene fusion in acute leukemia. Leukemia. 2008;22(4):678–85.
50. de Rooij JD, Hollink IH, Arentsen-Peters ST, van Galen JF, Berna Beverloo H, Baruchel A, Trka J, Reinhardt D, Sonneveld E, Zimmermann M, Alonzo TA, Pieters R, Meshinchi S, van den Heuvel-Eibrink MM, Zwaan CM. Nup98/jarid1a is a novel recurrent abnormality in pediatric acute megakaryoblastic leukemia with a distinct hox gene expression pattern. Leukemia. 2013;27(12):2280–8.
51. Inaba H, Zhou Y, Abla O, Adachi S, Auvrignon A, Beverloo HB, de Bont E, Chang TT, Creutzig U, Dworzak M, Elitzur S, Fynn A, Forestier E, Hasle H, Liang DC, Lee V, Locatelli F, Masetti R, De Moerloose B, Reinhardt D, Rodriguez L, Van Roy N, Shen S, Taga T, Tomizawa D, Yeoh AE, Zimmermann M, Raimondi SC. Heterogeneous cytogenetic subgroups and outcomes in childhood acute megakaryoblastic leukemia: a retrospective international study. Blood. 2015;126(13):1575–84.
52. Rubnitz JE, Crews KR, Pounds S, Yang S, Campana D, Gandhi VV, Raimondi SC, Downing JR, Razzouk BI, Pui CH, Ribeiro RC. Combination of cladribine and cytarabine is effective for child-

hood acute myeloid leukemia: results of the st jude aml97 trial. Leukemia. 2009;23(8):1410–6.

53. Lim G, Choi JR, Kim MJ, Kim SY, Lee HJ, Suh JT, Yoon HJ, Lee J, Lee S, Lee WI, Park TS. Detection of t(3;5) and npm1/mlf1 rearrangement in an elderly patient with acute myeloid leukemia: clinical and laboratory study with review of the literature. Cancer Genet Cytogenet. 2010;199(2):101–9.
54. Harrison CJ, Hills RK, Moorman AV, Grimwade DJ, Hann I, Webb DK, Wheatley K, De Graaf SS, van den BE, Burnett AK, Gibson BE. Cytogenetics of childhood acute myeloid leukemia: United Kingdom medical research council treatment trials aml 10 and 12. J Clin Oncol. 2010;28(16):2674–81.
55. Slovak ML, Gundacker H, Bloomfield CD, Dewald G, Appelbaum FR, Larson RA, Tallman MS, Bennett JM, Stirewalt DL, Meshinchi S, Willman CL, Ravindranath Y, Alonzo TA, Carroll AJ, Raimondi SC, Heerema NA. A retrospective study of 69 patients with t(6;9)(p23;q34) aml emphasizes the need for a prospective, multicenter initiative for rare 'poor prognosis' myeloid malignancies. Leukemia. 2006;20(7):1295–7.
56. Sandahl JD, Coenen EA, Forestier E, Harbott J, Johansson B, Kerndrup G, Adachi S, Auvrignon A, Beverloo HB, Cayuela JM, Chilton L, Fornerod M, de Haas V, Harrison CJ, Inaba H, Kaspers GJ, Liang DC, Locatelli F, Masetti R, Perot C, Raimondi SC, Reinhardt K, Tomizawa D, von Neuhoff N, Zecca M, Zwaan CM, van den Heuvel-Eibrink MM, Hasle H. T(6;9)(p22;q34)/dek-nup214-rearranged pediatric myeloid leukemia: an international study of 62 patients. Haematologica. 2014;99(5):865–72.
57. Tarlock K, Alonzo TA, Moraleda PP, Gerbing RB, Raimondi SC, Hirsch BA, Ravindranath Y, Lange B, Woods WG, Gamis AS, Meshinchi S. Acute myeloid leukaemia (aml) with t(6;9)(p23;q34) is associated with poor outcome in childhood aml regardless of flt3-itd status: a report from the Children's Oncology Group. Br J Haematol. 2014;166(2):254–9.
58. Quelen C, Lippert E, Struski S, Demur C, Soler G, Prade N, Delabesse E, Broccardo C, Dastugue N, Mahon FX, Brousset P. Identification of a transforming myb-gata1 fusion gene in acute basophilic leukemia: a new entity in male infants. Blood. 2011;117(21):5719–22.
59. Hasle H, Alonzo TA, Auvrignon A, Behar C, Chang M, Creutzig U, Fischer A, Forestier E, Fynn A, Haas OA, Harbott J, Harrison CJ, Heerema NA, van den Heuvel-Eibrink MM, Kaspers GJ, Locatelli F, Noellke P, Polychronopoulou S, Ravindranath Y, Razzouk B, Reinhardt D, Savva NN, Stark B, Suciu S, Tsukimoto I, Webb DK, Wojcik D, Woods WG, Zimmermann M, Niemeyer CM, Raimondi SC. Monosomy 7 and deletion 7q in children and adolescents with acute myeloid leukemia: an international retrospective study. Blood. 2007;109(11):4641–7.
60. Johnston DL, Alonzo TA, Gerbing RB, Hirsch B, Heerema NA, Ravindranath Y, Woods WG, Lange BJ, Gamis AS, Raimondi SC. Outcome of pediatric patients with acute myeloid leukemia (aml) and -5/5q- abnormalities from five pediatric aml treatment protocols: a report from the Children's Oncology Group. Pediatr Blood Cancer. 2013;60(12):2073–8.
61. Gervais C, Murati A, Helias C, Struski S, Eischen A, Lippert E, Tigaud I, Penther D, Bastard C, Mugneret F, Poppe B, Speleman F, Talmant P, VanDen Akker J, Baranger L, Barin C, Luquet I, Nadal N, Nguyen-Khac F, Maarek O, Herens C, Sainty D, Flandrin G, Birnbaum D, Mozziconacci MJ, Lessard M. Acute myeloid leukaemia with 8p11 (myst3) rearrangement: an integrated cytologic, cytogenetic and molecular study by the groupe francophone de cytogenetique hematologique. Leukemia. 2008;22(8):1567–75.
62. Coenen EA, Zwaan CM, Reinhardt D, Harrison CJ, Haas OA, de Hass V, Mihal V, De MB, Jeison M, Rubnitz JE, Tomizawa D, Johnston D, Alonzo TA, Hasle H, Auvrignon A, Dworzak M, Pession A, van der Velden VH, Swansbury J, Wong KF, Terui K, Savasan S, Winstanley M, Vaitkeviciene G, Zimmermann M, Pieters R, van den Heuvel-Eibrink MM. Pediatric acute myeloid leukemia with t(8;16)(p11;p13), a distinct clinical and biological entity: a collaborative study by the international-berlin-frankfurt-munster aml-study group. Blood. 2013;122(15):2704–13.
63. Diab A, Zickl L, Abdel-Wahab O, Jhanwar S, Gulam MA, Panageas KS, Patel JP, Jurcic J, Maslak P, Paietta E, Mangan JK, Carroll M, Fernandez HF, Teruya-Feldstein J, Luger SM, Douer D, Litzow MR, Lazarus HM, Rowe JM, Levine RL, Tallman MS. Acute myeloid leukemia with translocation t(8;16) presents with features which mimic acute promyelocytic leukemia and is associated with poor prognosis. Leuk Res. 2013;37(1):32–6.
64. Glassman AB, Hayes KJ. Translocation (11;16)(q23;p13) acute myelogenous leukemia and myelodysplastic syndrome. Ann Clin Lab Sci. 2003;33(3):285–8.
65. Appelbaum FR, Gundacker H, Head DR, Slovak ML, Willman CL, Godwin JE, Anderson JE, Petersdorf SH. Age and acute myeloid leukemia. Blood. 2006;107(9):3481–5.
66. Haferlach C, Dicker F, Herholz H, Schnittger S, Kern W, Haferlach T. Mutations of the tp53 gene in acute myeloid leukemia are strongly associated with a complex aberrant karyotype. Leukemia. 2008;22(8):1539–41.
67. Rucker FG, Schlenk RF, Bullinger L, Kayser S, Teleanu V, Kett H, Habdank M, Kugler CM, Holzmann K, Gaidzik VI, Paschka P, Held G, von Lilienfeld-Toal M, Lubbert M, Frohling S, Zenz T, Krauter J, Schlegelberger B, Ganser A, Lichter P, Dohner K, Dohner H. Tp53 alterations in acute myeloid leukemia with complex karyotype correlate with specific copy number alterations, monosomal karyotype, and dismal outcome. Blood. 2012;119(9):2114–21.
68. Volkert S, Kohlmann A, Schnittger S, Kern W, Haferlach T, Haferlach C. Association of the type of 5q loss with complex karyotype, clonal evolution, tp53 mutation status, and prognosis in acute myeloid leukemia and myelodysplastic syndrome. Genes Chromosomes Cancer. 2014;53(5):402–10.
69. Nahi H, Selivanova G, Lehmann S, Mollgard L, Bengtzen S, Concha H, Svensson A, Wiman KG, Merup M, Paul C. Mutated and non-mutated tp53 as targets in the treatment of leukaemia. Br J Haematol. 2008;141(4):445–53.
70. Hollink IH, van den Heuvel-Eibrink MM, Arentsen-Peters ST, Pratcorona M, Abbas S, Kuipers JE, van Galen JF, Beverloo HB, Sonneveld E, Kaspers GJ, Trka J, Baruchel A, Zimmermann M, Creutzig U, Reinhardt D, Pieters R, Valk PJ, Zwaan CM. Nup98/nsd1 characterizes a novel poor prognostic group in acute myeloid leukemia with a distinct Hox gene expression pattern. Blood. 2011;118(13):3645–56.
71. Ostronoff F, Othus M, Gerbing RB, Loken MR, Raimondi SC, Hirsch BA, Lange BJ, Petersdorf S, Radich J, Appelbaum FR, Gamis AS, Alonzo TA, Meshinchi S. Nup98/nsd1 and flt3/itd coexpression is more prevalent in younger aml patients and leads to induction failure: a cog and swog report. Blood. 2014;124(15):2400–7.
72. Shiba N, Ohki K, Kobayashi T, Hara Y, Yamato G, Tanoshima R, Ichikawa H, Tomizawa D, Park MJ, Shimada A, Sotomatsu M, Arakawa H, Horibe K, Adachi S, Taga T, Tawa A, Hayashi Y. High prdm16 expression identifies a prognostic subgroup of pediatric acute myeloid leukaemia correlated to flt3-itd, kmt2a-ptd, and nup98-nsd1: the results of the japanese paediatric leukaemia/lymphoma study group aml-05 trial. Br J Haematol. 2016;172(4):581–91.
73. Gough SM, Slape CI, Aplan PD. Nup98 gene fusions and hematopoietic malignancies: common themes and new biologic insights. Blood. 2011;118(24):6247–57.
74. Wei S, Wang S, Qiu S, Qi J, Mi Y, Lin D, Zhou C, Liu B, Li W, Wang Y, Wang M, Wang J. Clinical and laboratory studies of 17 patients with acute myeloid leukemia harboring t(7;11)(p15;p15) translocation. Leuk Res. 2013;37(9):1010–5.
75. Beverloo HB, Panagopoulos I, Isaksson M, van Wering E, van Drunen E, de Klein A, Johansson B, Slater R. Fusion of the homeo-

box gene hlxb9 and the etv6 gene in infant acute myeloid leukemias with the t(7;12)(q36;p13). Cancer Res. 2001;61(14):5374–7.

76. Von Bergh AR, van Drunen E, Van Wering ER, van Zutven LJ, Hainmann I, Lonnerholm G, Meijerink JP, Pieters R, Beverloo HB. High incidence of t(7;12)(q36;p13) in infant aml but not in infant all, with a dismal outcome and ectopic expression of hlxb9. Genes Chromosomes Cancer. 2006;45(8):731–9.
77. von Neuhoff C, Reinhardt D, Sander A, Zimmermann M, Bradtke J, Betts DR, Zemanova Z, Stary J, Bourquin JP, Haas OA, Dworzak MN, Creutzig U. Prognostic impact of specific chromosomal aberrations in a large group of pediatric patients with acute myeloid leukemia treated uniformly according to trial aml-bfm 98. J Clin Oncol. 2010;28(16):2682–9.
78. Haferlach C, Bacher U, Schnittger S, Alpermann T, Zenger M, Kern W, Haferlach T. Etv6 rearrangements are recurrent in myeloid malignancies and are frequently associated with other genetic events. Genes Chromosomes Cancer. 2012;51(4):328–37.
79. De Braekeleer E, Douet-Guilbert N, Morel F, Le Bris MJ, Basinko A, De Braekeleer M. Etv6 fusion genes in hematological malignancies: a review. Leuk Res. 2012;36(8):945–61.
80. Gruber TA, Larson Gedman A, Zhang J, Koss CS, Marada S, Ta HQ, Chen SC, Su X, Ogden SK, Dang J, Wu G, Gupta V, Andersson AK, Pounds S, Shi L, Easton J, Barbato MI, Mulder HL, Manne J, Wang J, Rusch M, Ranade S, Ganti R, Parker M, Ma J, Radtke I, Ding L, Cazzaniga G, Biondi A, Kornblau SM, Ravandi F, Kantarjian H, Nimer SD, Dohner K, Dohner H, Ley TJ, Ballerini P, Shurtleff S, Tomizawa D, Adachi S, Hayashi Y, Tawa A, Shih LY, Liang DC, Rubnitz JE, Pui CH, Mardis ER, Wilson RK, Downing JR. An inv(16)(p13.3q24.3)-encoded cbfa2t3-glis2 fusion protein defines an aggressive subtype of pediatric acute megakaryoblastic leukemia. Cancer Cell. 2012;22(5):683–97.
81. Masetti R, Pigazzi M, Togni M, Astolfi A, Indio V, Manara E, Casadio R, Pession A, Basso G, Locatelli F. Cbfa2t3-glis2 fusion transcript is a novel common feature in pediatric, cytogenetically normal aml, not restricted to fab m7 subtype. Blood. 2013;121(17):3469–72.
82. Lavallee VP, Lemieux S, Boucher G, Gendron P, Boivin I, Armstrong RN, Sauvageau G, Hebert J. RNA-sequencing analysis of core binding factor aml identifies recurrent zbtb7a mutations and defines runx1-cbfa2t3 fusion signature. Blood. 2016;127(20):2498–501.
83. Micci F, Thorsen J, Panagopoulos I, Nyquist KB, Zeller B, Tierens A, Heim S. High-throughput sequencing identifies an nfia/cbfa2t3 fusion gene in acute erythroid leukemia with t(1;16)(p31;q24). Leukemia. 2013;27(4):980–2.
84. Abbas S, Sanders MA, Zeilemaker A, Geertsma-Kleinekoort WM, Koenders JE, Kavelaars FG, Abbas ZG, Mahamoud S, Chu IW, Hoogenboezem R, Peeters JK, van Drunen E, van Galen J, Beverloo HB, Lowenberg B, Valk PJ. Integrated genome-wide genotyping and gene expression profiling reveals bcl11b as a putative oncogene in acute myeloid leukemia with 14q32 aberrations. Haematologica. 2014;99(5):848–57.
85. Torkildsen S, Gorunova L, Beiske K, Tjonnfjord GE, Heim S, Panagopoulos I. Novel zeb2-bcl11b fusion gene identified by rna-sequencing in acute myeloid leukemia with t(2;14)(q22;q32). PLoS One. 2015;10(7):e0132736.
86. Gruber TA, Downing JR. The biology of pediatric acute megakaryoblastic leukemia. Blood. 2015;126(8):943–9.
87. Massey GV, Zipursky A, Chang MN, Doyle JJ, Nasim S, Taub JW, Ravindranath Y, Dahl G, Weinstein HJ. A prospective study of the natural history of transient leukemia (tl) in neonates with down syndrome (ds): Children's Oncology Group (cog) study pog-9481. Blood. 2006;107(12):4606–13.
88. Malinge S, Izraeli S, Crispino JD. Insights into the manifestations, outcomes, and mechanisms of leukemogenesis in down syndrome. Blood. 2009;113(12):2619–28.
89. Gamis AS, Woods WG, Alonzo TA, Buxton A, Lange B, Barnard DR, Gold S, Smith FO. Increased age at diagnosis has a significantly negative effect on outcome in children with down syndrome and acute myeloid leukemia: a report from the Children's Cancer Group Study 2891. J Clin Oncol. 2003;21(18):3415–22.
90. Forestier E, Izraeli S, Beverloo B, Haas O, Pession A, Michalova K, Stark B, Harrison CJ, Teigler-Schlegel A, Johansson B. Cytogenetic features of acute lymphoblastic and myeloid leukemias in pediatric patients with down syndrome: an ibfm-sg study. Blood. 2008;111(3):1575–83.
91. Klusmann JH, Creutzig U, Zimmermann M, Dworzak M, Jorch N, Langebrake C, Pekrun A, Macakova-Reinhardt K, Reinhardt D. Treatment and prognostic impact of transient leukemia in neonates with Down syndrome. Blood. 2008;111(6):2991–8.
92. Yoshida K, Toki T, Okuno Y, Kanezaki R, Shiraishi Y, Sato-Otsubo A, Sanada M, Park MJ, Terui K, Suzuki H, Kon A, Nagata Y, Sato Y, Wang R, Shiba N, Chiba K, Tanaka H, Hama A, Muramatsu H, Hasegawa D, Nakamura K, Kanegane H, Tsukamoto K, Adachi S, Kawakami K, Kato K, Nishimura R, Izraeli S, Hayashi Y, Miyano S, Kojima S, Ito E, Ogawa S. The landscape of somatic mutations in down syndrome-related myeloid disorders. Nat Genet. 2013;45(11):1293–9.
93. Scholl C, Gilliland DG, Frohling S. Deregulation of signaling pathways in acute myeloid leukemia. Semin Oncol. 2008;35(4):336–45.
94. Meshinchi S, Alonzo TA, Stirewalt DL, Zwaan M, Zimmerman M, Reinhardt D, Kaspers GJ, Heerema NA, Gerbing R, Lange BJ, Radich JP. Clinical implications of flt3 mutations in pediatric aml. Blood. 2006;108(12):3654–61.
95. Mrozek K, Marcucci G, Paschka P, Whitman SP, Bloomfield CD. Clinical relevance of mutations and gene-expression changes in adult acute myeloid leukemia with normal cytogenetics: are we ready for a prognostically prioritized molecular classification? Blood. 2007;109(2):431–48.
96. Fitzgibbon J, Smith LL, Raghavan M, Smith ML, Debernardi S, Skoulakis S, Lillington D, Lister TA, Young BD. Association between acquired uniparental disomy and homozygous gene mutation in acute myeloid leukemias. Cancer Res. 2005;65(20):9152–4.
97. Gale RE, Green C, Allen C, Mead AJ, Burnett AK, Hills RK, Linch DC. The impact of flt3 internal tandem duplication mutant level, number, size, and interaction with npm1 mutations in a large cohort of young adult patients with acute myeloid leukemia. Blood. 2008;111(5):2776–84.
98. Bachas C, Schuurhuis GJ, Hollink IH, Kwidama ZJ, Goemans BF, Zwaan CM, van den Heuvel-Eibrink MM, de Bont ES, Reinhardt D, Creutzig U, de Haas V, Assaraf YG, Kaspers GJ, Cloos J. High-frequency type i/ii mutational shifts between diagnosis and relapse are associated with outcome in pediatric AML: implications for personalized medicine. Blood. 2010;116(15):2752–8.
99. Fehniger TA, Byrd JC, Marcucci G, Abboud CN, Kefauver C, Payton JE, Vij R, Blum W. Single-agent lenalidomide induces complete remission of acute myeloid leukemia in patients with isolated trisomy 13. Blood. 2009;113(5):1002–5.
100. Falini B, Mecucci C, Tiacci E, Alcalay M, Rosati R, Pasqualucci L, La Starza R, Diverio D, Colombo E, Santucci A, Bigerna B, Pacini R, Pucciarini A, Liso A, Vignetti M, Fazi P, Meani N, Pettirossi V, Saglio G, Mandelli F, Lo-Coco F, Pelicci PG, Martelli MF. Cytoplasmic nucleophosmin in acute myelogenous leukemia with a normal karyotype. N Engl J Med. 2005;352(3):254–66.
101. Haferlach C, Mecucci C, Schnittger S, Kohlmann A, Mancini M, Cuneo A, Testoni N, Rege-Cambrin G, Santucci A, Vignetti M, Fazi P, Martelli MP, Haferlach T, Falini B. Aml with mutated npm1 carrying a normal or aberrant karyotype show overlapping biologic, pathologic, immunophenotypic, and prognostic features. Blood. 2009;114(14):3024–32.

102. Grimwade D, Freeman SD. Defining minimal residual disease in acute myeloid leukemia: which platforms are ready for "Prime time"? Blood. 2014;124(23):3345–55.
103. Gale RE, Lamb K, Allen C, El-Sharkawi D, Stowe C, Jenkinson S, Tinsley S, Dickson G, Burnett AK, Hills RK, Linch DC. Simpson's paradox and the impact of different dnmt3a mutations on outcome in younger adults with acute myeloid leukemia. J Clin Oncol. 2015;33(18):2072–83.
104. Ho PA, Alonzo TA, Gerbing RB, Pollard J, Stirewalt DL, Hurwitz C, Heerema NA, Hirsch B, Raimondi SC, Lange B, Franklin JL, Radich JP, Meshinchi S. Prevalence and prognostic implications of cebpa mutations in pediatric acute myeloid leukemia (aml): a report from the Children's Oncology Group. Blood. 2009;113(26):6558–66.
105. Wouters BJ, Lowenberg B, Erpelinck-Verschueren CA, van Putten WL, Valk PJ, Delwel R. Double cebpa mutations, but not single cebpa mutations, define a subgroup of acute myeloid leukemia with a distinctive gene expression profile that is uniquely associated with a favorable outcome. Blood. 2009;113(13):3088–91.
106. Dufour A, Schneider F, Metzeler KH, Hoster E, Schneider S, Zellmeier E, Benthaus T, Sauerland MC, Berdel WE, Buchner T, Wormann B, Braess J, Hiddemann W, Bohlander SK, Spiekermann K. Acute myeloid leukemia with biallelic cebpa gene mutations and normal karyotype represents a distinct genetic entity associated with a favorable clinical outcome. J Clin Oncol. 2010;28(4):570–7.
107. Schlenk RF, Dohner K, Krauter J, Frohling S, Corbacioglu A, Bullinger L, Habdank M, Spath D, Morgan M, Benner A, Schlegelberger B, Heil G, Ganser A, Dohner H. Mutations and treatment outcome in cytogenetically normal acute myeloid leukemia. N Engl J Med. 2008;358(18):1909–18.
108. Dohner K, Dohner H. Molecular characterization of acute myeloid leukemia. Haematologica. 2008;93(7):976–82.
109. Frankfurt O, Licht JD, Tallman MS. Molecular characterization of acute myeloid leukemia and its impact on treatment. Curr Opin Oncol. 2007;19(6):635–49.
110. Mrozek K, Bloomfield CD. Chromosome aberrations, gene mutations and expression changes, and prognosis in adult acute myeloid leukemia. Hematology Am Soc Hematol Educ Program. 2006:169–77.
111. Zwaan CM, Kolb EA, Reinhardt D, Abrahamsson J, Adachi S, Aplenc R, De Bont ES, De Moerloose B, Dworzak M, Gibson BE, Hasle H, Leverger G, Locatelli F, Ragu C, Ribeiro RC, Rizzari C, Rubnitz JE, Smith OP, Sung L, Tomizawa D, van den Heuvel-Eibrink MM, Creutzig U, Kaspers GJ. Collaborative efforts driving progress in pediatric acute myeloid leukemia. J Clin Oncol. 2015;33(27):2949–62.
112. Third international workshop on chromosomes in leukemia 1980 (1981). Clinical significance of chromosomal abnormalities in acute lymphoblasic leukemia. Cancer Genet Cytogenet. 1981;4:111–37.
113. Pui CH, Yang JJ, Hunger SP, Pieters R, Schrappe M, Biondi A, Vora A, Baruchel A, Silverman LB, Schmiegelow K, Escherich G, Horibe K, Benoit YC, Izraeli S, Yeoh AE, Liang DC, Downing JR, Evans WE, Relling MV, Mullighan CG. Childhood acute lymphoblastic leukemia: progress through collaboration. J Clin Oncol. 2015;33(27):2938–48.
114. Pullarkat V, Slovak ML, Kopecky KJ, Forman SJ, Appelbaum FR. Impact of cytogenetics on the outcome of adult acute lymphoblastic leukemia: results of southwest oncology group 9400 study. Blood. 2008;111(5):2563–72.
115. Heerema NA, Sather HN, Sensel MG, Kraft P, Nachman JB, Steinherz PG, Lange BJ, Hutchinson RS, Reaman GH, Trigg ME, Arthur DC, Gaynon PS, Uckun FM. Frequency and clinical significance of cytogenetic abnormalities in pediatric t-lineage acute lymphoblastic leukemia: a report from the Children's Cancer Group. J Clin Oncol. 1998;16(4):1270–8.
116. Marks DI, Paietta EM, Moorman AV, Richards SM, Buck G, DeWald G, Ferrando A, Fielding AK, Goldstone AH, Ketterling RP, Litzow MR, Luger SM, McMillan AK, Mansour MR, Rowe JM, Tallman MS, Lazarus HM. T-cell acute lymphoblastic leukemia in adults: clinical features, immunophenotype, cytogenetics, and outcome from the large randomized prospective trial (ukall xii/ecog 2993). Blood. 2009;114(25):5136–45.
117. Moorman AV, Chilton L, Wilkinson J, Ensor HM, Bown N, Proctor SJ. A population-based cytogenetic study of adults with acute lymphoblastic leukemia. Blood. 2010;115(2):206–14.
118. Moorman AV, Harrison CJ, Buck GA, Richards SM, Secker-Walker LM, Martineau M, Vance GH, Cherry AM, Higgins RR, Fielding AK, Foroni L, Paietta E, Tallman MS, Litzow MR, Wiernik PH, Rowe JM, Goldstone AH, Dewald GW. Karyotype is an independent prognostic factor in adult acute lymphoblastic leukemia (all): analysis of cytogenetic data from patients treated on the medical research council (mrc) ukallxii/eastern cooperative oncology group (ecog) 2993 trial. Blood. 2007;109(8):3189–97.
119. Moorman AV, Richards SM, Martineau M, Cheung KL, Robinson HM, Jalali GR, Broadfield ZJ, Harris RL, Taylor KE, Gibson BE, Hann IM, Hill FG, Kinsey SE, Eden TO, Mitchell CD, Harrison CJ. Outcome heterogeneity in childhood high-hyperdiploid acute lymphoblastic leukemia. Blood. 2003;102(8):2756–62.
120. Heerema NA, Raimondi SC, Anderson JR, Biegel J, Camitta BM, Cooley LD, Gaynon PS, Hirsch B, Magenis RE, McGavran L, Patil S, Pettenati MJ, Pullen J, Rao K, Roulston D, Schneider NR, Shuster JJ, Sanger W, Sutcliffe MJ, van Tuinen P, Watson MS, Carroll AJ. Specific extra chromosomes occur in a modal number dependent pattern in pediatric acute lymphoblastic leukemia. Genes Chromosomes Cancer. 2007;46(7):684–93.
121. Sutcliffe MJ, Shuster JJ, Sather HN, Camitta BM, Pullen J, Schultz KR, Borowitz MJ, Gaynon PS, Carroll AJ, Heerema NA. High concordance from independent studies by the Children's Cancer Group (ccg) and pediatric oncology group (pog) associating favorable prognosis with combined trisomies 4, 10, and 17 in children with nci standard-risk b-precursor acute lymphoblastic leukemia: a Children's Oncology Group (cog) initiative. Leukemia. 2005;19(5):734–40.
122. Heerema N, Sensel M, Sather H, Lee M, Hutchinson R, Nachman J, Lange B, Steinherz P, Bostrom B, Gaynon P, Uckun F. Chromosome1 abnormalities in childhood acute lymphoblastic leukemia (all). J Clin Oncol. 2000;19:582a.
123. Heerema N, Sather H, Reaman G, Hutchinson R, Lange B, Nachman J, Stinherz P, Uckun F, Gaynon P, Trigg M, Arthur D. Cytogenetic studies of acute lymphoblastic leukemia: clinical correlations results from the Children's Cancer Group. J Assoc Genet Technol. 1998;24:206–12.
124. Secker-Walker LM, Prentice HG, Durrant J, Richards S, Hall E, Harrison G. Cytogenetics adds independent prognostic information in adults with acute lymphoblastic leukaemia on mrc trial ukall xa. Mrc adult leukaemia working party. Br J Haematol. 1997;96(3):601–10.
125. Nachman JB, Heerema NA, Sather H, Camitta B, Forestier E, Harrison CJ, Dastugue N, Schrappe M, Pui CH, Basso G, Silverman LB, Janka-Schaub GE. Outcome of treatment in children with hypodiploid acute lymphoblastic leukemia. Blood. 2007;110(4):1112–5.
126. Heerema NA, Nachman JB, Sather HN, Sensel MG, Lee MK, Hutchinson R, Lange BJ, Steinherz PG, Bostrom B, Gaynon PS, Uckun F. Hypodiploidy with less than 45 chromosomes confers adverse risk in childhood acute lymphoblastic leukemia: a report from the Children's Cancer Group. Blood. 1999;94(12):4036–45.
127. Harrison CJ, Moorman AV, Broadfield ZJ, Cheung KL, Harris RL, Reza Jalali G, Robinson HM, Barber KE, Richards SM, Mitchell CD, Eden TO, Hann IM, Hill FG, Kinsey SE, Gibson BE, Lilleyman J, Vora A, Goldstone AH, Franklin IM, Durrant J,

Martineau M. Three distinct subgroups of hypodiploidy in acute lymphoblastic leukaemia. Br J Haematol. 2004;125(5):552–9.
128. Holmfeldt L, Wei L, Diaz-Flores E, Walsh M, Zhang J, Ding L, Payne-Turner D, Churchman M, Andersson A, Chen SC, McCastlain K, Becksfort J, Ma J, Wu G, Patel SN, Heatley SL, Phillips LA, Song G, Easton J, Parker M, Chen X, Rusch M, Boggs K, Vadodaria B, Hedlund E, Drenberg C, Baker S, Pei D, Cheng C, Huether R, Lu C, Fulton RS, Fulton LL, Tabib Y, Dooling DJ, Ochoa K, Minden M, Lewis ID, To LB, Marlton P, Roberts AW, Raca G, Stock W, Neale G, Drexler HG, Dickins RA, Ellison DW, Shurtleff SA, Pui CH, Ribeiro RC, Devidas M, Carroll AJ, Heerema NA, Wood B, Borowitz MJ, Gastier-Foster JM, Raimondi SC, Mardis ER, Wilson RK, Downing JR, Hunger SP, Loh ML, Mullighan CG. The genomic landscape of hypodiploid acute lymphoblastic leukemia. Nat Genet. 2013;45(3):242–52.
129. Uckun FM, Pallisgaard N, Hokland P, Navara C, Narla R, Gaynon PS, Sather H, Heerema N. Expression of tel-aml1 fusion transcripts and response to induction therapy in standard risk acute lymphoblastic leukemia. Leuk Lymphoma. 2001;42(1-2):41–56.
130. Burmeister T, Gokbuget N, Schwartz S, Fischer L, Hubert D, Sindram A, Hoelzer D, Thiel E. Clinical features and prognostic implications of tcf3-pbx1 and etv6-runx1 in adult acute lymphoblastic leukemia. Haematologica. 2010;95(2):241–6.
131. Raynaud SD, Dastugue N, Zoccola D, Shurtleff SA, Mathew S, Raimondi SC. Cytogenetic abnormalities associated with the t(12;21): a collaborative study of 169 children with t(12;21)-positive acute lymphoblastic leukemia. Leukemia. 1999;13(9):1325–30.
132. Greaves MF, Wiemels J. Origins of chromosome translocations in childhood leukaemia. Nat Rev Cancer. 2003;3(9):639–49.
133. Raimondi SC, Peiper SC, Kitchingman GR, Behm FG, Williams DL, Hancock ML, Mirro J Jr. Childhood acute lymphoblastic leukemia with chromosomal breakpoints at 11q23. Blood. 1989;73(6):1627–34.
134. Dreyer ZE, Dinndorf PA, Camitta B, Sather H, La MK, Devidas M, Hilden JM, Heerema NA, Sanders JE, McGlennen R, Willman CL, Carroll AJ, Behm F, Smith FO, Woods WG, Godder K, Reaman GH. Analysis of the role of hematopoietic stem-cell transplantation in infants with acute lymphoblastic leukemia in first remission and mll gene rearrangements: a report from the Children's Oncology Group. J Clin Oncol. 2011;29(2):214–22.
135. Arico M, Camitta B, Scrappe M, Chessells J, Baruchel A, Gaynon P, Silverman L, Janka-Schaub G, Kamps W, Pui C-H, Masera G, Conter V, Riehm H, Heerema N, Sallan S, Auclerc M-F, Pullen J, Shuster J, Carroll A, Raimondi S, Richards S. Outcome of treatment in children with Philadelphia chromosome-positive acute lymphoblastic leukemia. N Engl J Med. 2000;342:998–1006.
136. Schultz KR, Bowman WP, Aledo A, Slayton WB, Sather H, Devidas M, Wang C, Davies SM, Gaynon PS, Trigg M, Rutledge R, Burden L, Jorstad D, Carroll A, Heerema NA, Winick N, Borowitz MJ, Hunger SP, Carroll WL, Camitta B. Improved early event-free survival with imatinib in Philadelphia chromosome-positive acute lymphoblastic leukemia: a Children's Oncology Group study. J Clin Oncol. 2009;27(31):5175–81.
137. Schultz KR, Carroll A, Heerema NA, Bowman WP, Aledo A, Slayton WB, Sather H, Devidas M, Zheng HW, Davies SM, Gaynon PS, Trigg M, Rutledge R, Jorstad D, Winick N, Borowitz MJ, Hunger SP, Carroll WL, Camitta B, C. S. O. Group. Long-term follow-up of imatinib in pediatric philadelphia chromosome-positive acute lymphoblastic leukemia: Children's Oncology Group Study aall0031. Leukemia. 2014;28(7):1467–71.
138. Den Boer ML, van Slegtenhorst M, De Menezes RX, Cheok MH, Buijs-Gladdines JG, Peters ST, Van Zutven LJ, Beverloo HB, Van der Spek PJ, Escherich G, Horstmann MA, Janka-Schaub GE, Kamps WA, Evans WE, Pieters R. A subtype of childhood acute lymphoblastic leukaemia with poor treatment outcome: a genome-wide classification study. Lancet Oncol. 2009;10(2):125–34.
139. Harvey RC, Mullighan CG, Wang X, Dobbin KK, Davidson GS, Bedrick EJ, Chen IM, Atlas SR, Kang H, Ar K, Wilson CS, Wharton W, Murphy M, Devidas M, Carroll AJ, Borowitz MJ, Bowman WP, Downing JR, Relling M, Yang J, Bhojwani D, Carroll WL, Camitta B, Reaman GH, Smith M, Hunger SP, Willman CL. Identification of novel cluster groups in pediatric high-risk b-precursor acute lymphoblastic leukemia with gene expression profiling: correlation with genome-wide DNA copy number alterations, clinical characteristics, and outcome. Blood. 2010;116(23):4874–84.
140. Russell LJ, Capasso M, Vater I, Akasaka T, Bernard OA, Calasanz MJ, Chandrasekaran T, Chapiro E, Gesk S, Griffiths M, Guttery DS, Haferlach C, Harder L, Heidenreich O, Irving J, Kearney L, Nguyen-Khac F, Machado L, Minto L, Majid A, Moorman AV, Morrison H, Rand V, Strefford JC, Schwab C, Tonnies H, Dyer MJ, Siebert R, Harrison CJ. Deregulated expression of cytokine receptor gene, crlf2, is involved in lymphoid transformation in b-cell precursor acute lymphoblastic leukemia. Blood. 2009;114(13):2688–98.
141. Roberts KG, Morin RD, Zhang J, Hirst M, Zhao Y, Su X, Chen SC, Payne-Turner D, Churchman ML, Harvey RC, Chen X, Kasap C, Yan C, Becksfort J, Finney RP, Teachey DT, Maude SL, Tse K, Moore R, Jones S, Mungall K, Birol I, Edmonson MN, Hu Y, Buetow KE, Chen IM, Carroll WL, Wei L, Ma J, Kleppe M, Levine RL, Garcia-Manero G, Larsen E, Shah NP, Devidas M, Reaman G, Smith M, Paugh SW, Evans WE, Grupp SA, Jeha S, Pui CH, Gerhard DS, Downing JR, Willman CL, Loh M, Hunger SP, Marra MA, Mullighan CG. Genetic alterations activating kinase and cytokine receptor signaling in high-risk acute lymphoblastic leukemia. Cancer Cell. 2012;22(2):153–66.
142. Roberts KG, Li Y, Payne-Turner D, Harvey RC, Yang YL, Pei D, McCastlain K, Ding L, Lu C, Song G, Ma J, Becksfort J, Rusch M, Chen SC, Easton J, Cheng J, Boggs K, Santiago-Morales N, Iacobucci I, Fulton RS, Wen J, Valentine M, Cheng C, Paugh SW, Devidas M, Chen IM, Reshmi S, Smith A, Hedlund E, Gupta P, Nagahawatte P, Wu G, Chen X, Yergeau D, Vadodaria B, Mulder H, Winick NJ, Larsen EC, Carroll WL, Heerema NA, Carroll AJ, Grayson G, Tasian SK, Moore AS, Keller F, Frei-Jones M, Whitlock JA, Raetz EA, White DL, Hughes TP, Guidry Auvil JM, Smith MA, Marcucci G, Bloomfield CD, Mrózek K, Kohlschmidt J, Stock W, Kornblau SM, Konopleva M, Paietta E, Pui CH, Jeha S, Relling MV, Evans WE, Gerhard DS, Gastier-Foster JM, Mardis E, Wilson RK, Loh ML, Downing JR, Hunger SP, Willman CL, Zhang J, Mullighan CG. Targetable kinase-activating lesions in pH-like acute lymphoblastic leukemia. N Engl J Med. 2014;371(11):1005–15.
143. Mullighan CG, Collins-Underwood JR, Phillips LA, Loudin MG, Liu W, Zhang J, Ma J, Coustan-Smith E, Harvey RC, Willman CL, Mikhail FM, Meyer J, Carroll AJ, Williams RT, Cheng J, Heerema NA, Basso G, Pession A, Pui CH, Raimondi SC, Hunger SP, Downing JR, Carroll WL, Rabin KR. Rearrangement of crlf2 in b-progenitor- and down syndrome-associated acute lymphoblastic leukemia. Nat Genet. 2009;41(11):1243–6.
144. Heerema NA, Carroll AJ, Devidas M, Loh ML, Borowitz MJ, Gastier-Foster JM, Larsen EC, Mattano LA, Maloney KW, Willman CL, Wood BL, Winick NJ, Carroll WL, Hunger SP, Raetz EA. Intrachromosomal amplification of chromosome 21 is associated with inferior outcomes in children with acute lymphoblastic leukemia treated in contemporary standard-risk Children's Oncology Group studies: a report from the Children's Oncology Group. J Clin Oncol. 2013;31(27):3397–402.
145. Moorman AV, Robinson H, Schwab C, Richards SM, Hancock J, Mitchell CD, Goulden N, Vora A, Harrison CJ. Risk-directed treatment intensification significantly reduces the risk of relapse among children and adolescents with acute lymphoblastic leukemia and intrachromosomal amplification of chromosome 21: a

comparison of the mrc all97/99 and ukall2003 trials. J Clin Oncol. 2013;31(27):3389–96.
146. Penther D, Preudhomme C, Talmant P, Roumier C, Godon A, Mechinaud F, Milpied N, Bataille R, Avet-Loiseau H. Amplification of aml1 gene is present in childhood acute lymphoblastic leukemia but not in adult, and is not associated with aml1 gene mutation. Leukemia. 2002;16(6):1131–4.
147. Landau H, Lamanna N. Clinical manifestations and treatment of newly diagnosed acute lymphoblastic leukemia in adults. Curr Hematol Malig Rep. 2006;1(3):171–9.
148. Heerema NA, Sather HN, Sensel MG, Liu-Mares W, Lange BJ, Bostrom BC, Nachman JB, Steinherz PG, Hutchinson R, Gaynon PS, Arthur DC, Uckun FM. Association of chromosome arm 9p abnormalities with adverse risk in childhood acute lymphoblastic leukemia: a report from the Children's Cancer Group. Blood. 1999;94(5):1537–44.
149. van Zutven LJ, van Drunen E, de Bont JM, Wattel MM, Den Boer ML, Pieters R, Hagemeijer A, Slater RM, Beverloo HB. Cdkn2 deletions have no prognostic value in childhood precursor-b acute lymphoblastic leukaemia. Leukemia. 2005;19(7):1281–4.
150. Behrendt H, Charrin C, Gibbons B, Harrison CJ, Hawkins JM, Heerema NA, Horschler-Botel B, Huret JL, Lai JL, Lampert F, et al. Dicentric (9;12) in acute lymphocytic leukemia and other hematological malignancies: report from a dic(9;12) study group. Leukemia. 1995;9(1):102–6.
151. Strehl S, Konig M, Dworzak MN, Kalwak K, Haas OA. Pax5/etv6 fusion defines cytogenetic entity dic(9;12)(p13;p13). Leukemia. 2003;17(6):1121–3.
152. Gastier-Foster JM, Carroll AJ, Ell D, Harvey R, Chen I-M, Ketterling R, Meloni-Ehrig A, Opheim KE, Patil S, Pettenati M, Rao K, Wu S, Heerema NA. Two distinct subsets of dic(9;12) (p12;p11.2) among children with b-cell precursor acute lymphoblastic leukemia (all): Pax5-etv6 and etv6-runx1 rearrangements: a report from the Children's Oncology Group. ASH Ann Meeting Abstr. 2007;110(11):1439.
153. Pichler H, Moricke A, Mann G, Teigler-Schlegel A, Niggli F, Nebral K, Konig M, Inthal A, Krehan D, Dworzak MN, Janousek D, Harbott J, Schrappe M, Gadner H, Strehl S, Haas OA, Panzer-Grumayer R, Attarbaschi A. Prognostic relevance of dic(9;20) (p11;q13) in childhood b-cell precursor acute lymphoblastic leukaemia treated with berlin-frankfurt-munster (bfm) protocols containing an intensive induction and post-induction consolidation therapy. Br J Haematol. 2010;
154. An Q, Wright SL, Moorman AV, Parker H, Griffiths M, Ross FM, Davies T, Harrison CJ, Strefford JC. Heterogeneous breakpoints in patients with acute lymphoblastic leukemia and the dic(9;20) (p11-13;q11) show recurrent involvement of genes at 20q11.21. Haematologica. 2009;94(8):1164–9.
155. Messinger YH, Higgins R, Devidas M, Hunger SP, Carroll AJ, Heerema NA. Acute lymphoblastic leukemia (all) with t(8;14) (q11.2;q32): B-lineage disease with high proportion of down syndrome. A Children's Oncology Group (cog) study. ASH Ann Meeting Abstr. 2008;112(11):1477.
156. Harrison CJ. Cytogenetics of paediatric and adolescent acute lymphoblastic leukaemia. Br J Haematol. 2009;144(2):147–56.
157. Heerema NA, Sather HN, Sensel MG, Lee MK, Hutchinson R, Nachman JB, Lange BJ, Steinherz PG, Bostrom B, Gaynon PS, Uckun FM. Prognostic significance of cytogenetic abnormalities of chromosome arm 12p in childhood acute lymphoblastic leukemia: a report from the Children's Cancer Group. Cancer. 2000;88(8):1945–54.
158. Heerema NA, Sather HN, Sensel MG, Lee MK, Hutchinson R, Lange BJ, Bostrom BC, Nachman JB, Steinherz PG, Gaynon PS, Uckun FM. Clinical significance of deletions of chromosome arm 6q in childhood acute lymphoblastic leukemia: a report from the Children's Cancer Group. Leuk Lymphoma. 2000;36(5–6):467–78.
159. Wetzler M, Dodge RK, Mrozek K, Carroll AJ, Tantravahi R, Block AW, Pettenati MJ, Le Beau MM, Frankel SR, Stewart CC, Szatrowski TP, Schiffer CA, Larson RA, Bloomfield CD. Prospective karyotype analysis in adult acute lymphoblastic leukemia: the cancer and leukemia group b experience. Blood. 1999;93(11):3983–93.
160. Dabaja BS, Faderl S, Thomas D, Cortes J, O'Brien S, Nasr F, Pierce S, Hayes K, Glassman A, Keating M, Kantarjian HM. Deletions and losses in chromosomes 5 or 7 in adult acute lymphocytic leukemia: incidence, associations and implications. Leukemia. 1999;13(6):869–72.
161. Rao K, Heerema N, Sather H, Sensel M, Lee M, Hutchinson R, Nachman J, Lange B, Steinherz P, Bostrom B, Gaynon P, Uckun F. Deletions of chromosome arm 5q in childhood acute lymphoblastic leukemia (all). Proc Am Soc Clin Oncol. 2000;19:589a.
162. Heerema NA, Nachman JB, Sather HN, La MK, Hutchinson R, Lange BJ, Bostrom B, Steinherz PG, Gaynon PS, Uckun FM. Deletion of 7p or monosomy 7 in pediatric acute lymphoblastic leukemia is an adverse prognostic factor: a report from the Children's Cancer Group. Leukemia. 2004;18(5):939–47.
163. Heerema NA, Sather HN, Sensel MG, Lee MK, Hutchinson RJ, Nachman JB, Reaman GH, Lange BJ, Steinherz PG, Bostrom BC, Gaynon PS, Uckun FM. Abnormalities of chromosome bands 13q12 to 13q14 in childhood acute lymphoblastic leukemia. J Clin Oncol. 2000;18(22):3837–44.
164. Gorello P, La Starza R, Varasano E, Chiaretti S, Elia L, Pierini V, Barba G, Brandimarte L, Crescenzi B, Vitale A, Messina M, Grammatico S, Mancini M, Matteucci C, Bardi A, Guarini A, Martelli MF, Foa R, Mecucci C. Combined interphase fluorescence in situ hybridization elucidates the genetic heterogeneity of t-cell acute lymphoblastic leukemia in adults. Haematologica. 2010;95(1):79–86.
165. Cauwelier B, Dastugue N, Cools J, Poppe B, Herens C, De Paepe A, Hagemeijer A, Speleman F. Molecular cytogenetic study of 126 unselected t-all cases reveals high incidence of tcrbeta locus rearrangements and putative new t-cell oncogenes. Leukemia. 2006;20(7):1238–44.
166. Janssen JW, Ludwig WD, Sterry W, Bartram CR. Sil-tal1 deletion in t-cell acute lymphoblastic leukemia. Leukemia. 1993;7(8):1204–10.
167. Kees UR, Heerema NA, Kumar R, Watt PM, Baker DL, La MK, Uckun FM, Sather HN. Expression of hox11 in childhood t-lineage acute lymphoblastic leukaemia can occur in the absence of cytogenetic aberration at 10q24: a study from the Children's Cancer Group (ccg). Leukemia. 2003;17(5):887–93.
168. Weng AP, Ferrando AA, Lee W, Morris JP, Silverman LB, Sanchez-Irizarry C, Blacklow SC, Look AT, Aster JC. Activating mutations of notch1 in human t cell acute lymphoblastic leukemia. Science. 2004;306(5694):269–71.
169. Ellisen LW, Bird J, West DC, Soreng AL, Reynolds TC, Smith SD, Sklar J. Tan-1, the human homolog of the drosophila notch gene, is broken by chromosomal translocations in t lymphoblastic neoplasms. Cell. 1991;66(4):649–61.
170. Maillard I, Pear WS. Immunology. Keeping a tight leash on notch. Science. 2007;316(5826):840–2.
171. Mansour MR, Linch DC, Foroni L, Goldstone AH, Gale RE. High incidence of notch-1 mutations in adult patients with t-cell acute lymphoblastic leukemia. Leukemia. 2006;20(3):537–9.
172. Pui CH, Evans WE. Treatment of acute lymphoblastic leukemia. N Engl J Med. 2006;354(2):166–78.
173. Ballerini P, Blaise A, Busson-Le Coniat M, Su XY, Zucman-Rossi J, Adam M, van den Akker J, Perot C, Pellegrino B, Landman-Parker J, Douay L, Berger R, Bernard OA. Hox11l2 expression defines a clinical subtype of pediatric t-all associated with poor prognosis. Blood. 2002;100(3):991–7.
174. Graux C, Cools J, Melotte C, Quentmeier H, Ferrando A, Levine R, Vermeesch JR, Stul M, Dutta B, Boeckx N, Bosly A, Heimann

P, Uyttebroeck A, Mentens N, Somers R, MacLeod RA, Drexler HG, Look AT, Gilliland DG, Michaux L, Vandenberghe P, Wlodarska I, Marynen P, Hagemeijer A. Fusion of nup214 to abl1 on amplified episomes in t-cell acute lymphoblastic leukemia. Nat Genet. 2004;36(10):1084–9.
175. Quintas-Cardama A, Tong W, Manshouri T, Vega F, Lennon PA, Cools J, Gilliland DG, Lee F, Cortes J, Kantarjian H, Garcia-Manero G. Activity of tyrosine kinase inhibitors against human nup214-abl1-positive t cell malignancies. Leukemia. 2008;22(6):1117–24.
176. Bertin R, Acquaviva C, Mirebeau D, Guidal-Giroux C, Vilmer E, Cave H. Cdkn2a, cdkn2b, and mtap gene dosage permits precise characterization of mono- and bi-allelic 9p21 deletions in childhood acute lymphoblastic leukemia. Genes Chromosomes Cancer. 2003;37(1):44–57.
177. Omura-Minamisawa M, Diccianni MB, Batova A, Chang RC, Bridgeman LJ, Yu J, Pullen J, Bowman WP, Yu AL. Universal inactivation of both p16 and p15 but not downstream components is an essential event in the pathogenesis of t-cell acute lymphoblastic leukemia. Clin Cancer Res. 2000;6(4):1219–28.
178. Van Vlierberghe P, Pieters R, Beverloo HB, Meijerink JP. Molecular-genetic insights in paediatric t-cell acute lymphoblastic leukaemia. Br J Haematol. 2008;143(2):153–68.

Diagnosis and Treatment of Childhood Acute Lymphoblastic Leukemia

17

Melinda Pauly and Lewis B. Silverman

Introduction

Acute lymphoblastic leukemia (ALL) is the most common malignancy of childhood, accounting for 25–30% of all pediatric cancer cases [1]. Leukemias arise from genetic changes that occur in a single lymphoid progenitor cell at various stages of maturation, resulting in a clonal expansion. The single-cell origin of ALL is demonstrated by the finding of clonal rearrangements of immunoglobulin (Ig) or T-cell receptor (TCR) genes in most lymphoblasts [2]. Malignant lymphoblasts possess the immunophenotypic and genetic characteristics of either B- or T-lymphoid precursors [3, 4]. The inability of these lymphoid progenitors to differentiate as well as their resistance to cell death leads to their accumulation in the marrow compartment and spread throughout the body. By the time of diagnosis, lymphoblasts have usually occupied much of the bone marrow microenvironment at the expense of normal hematopoietic cells, resulting in anemia, thrombocytopenia, and/or neutropenia. Effective treatment for the majority of patients consists of multiagent chemotherapy administered for 2–3 years, resulting in clonal eradication; the intensity of therapy is stratified based on presenting features, leukemia genetics, and early response to therapy.

M. Pauly, M.D. (✉)
Division of Hematology/Oncology, Department of Pediatrics, Emory University, Aflac Cancer and Blood Disorder's Center, Atlanta, GA 30338, USA
e-mail: melinda.pauly@choa.org

L.B. Silverman, M.D.
Division of Pediatric Hematology-Oncology, Department of Pediatric Oncology, Dana-Farber Cancer Institute, Boston Children's Hospital, Boston, MA 02215, USA
e-mail: lewis_silverman@dfci.harvard.edu

Incidence

Of the approximately 6600 new cases of ALL diagnosed in the USA per year, 57% of cases are under the age of 20 years and 15.6% of death from ALL occur in this age group [5]. ALL is the most common malignancy diagnosed in patients younger than 15 years, representing 23% of all cancers and 76% of leukemias in this age group [6]. Over the last 30 years, the incidence of ALL in the USA and Europe has steadily increased [1, 7]. The incidence of ALL is highest between ages 2 and 5 years, and is higher in boys than in girls (especially for T-ALL), although girls have a slightly higher (1.5 times) incidence in the first year of life [8].

Predisposing Factors

Risk factors for developing leukemia include family history, underlying genetic conditions, and (rarely) certain environmental exposures. For the vast majority of cases of childhood ALL, predisposing factors cannot be identified.

Fraternal twins and siblings of children with leukemia have a two- to fourfold greater risk of developing leukemia during the first decade of life [9, 10]. The concordance rate of ALL in monozygotic twins ranges from 5 to 25%, depending on subtype and age that the first twin develops leukemia. When one twin develops infant ALL (typically with a *KMT2A* gene rearrangement), ALL almost invariably develops in the other twin with a short latency (generally within a few months), likely reflecting transfer of ALL cells via the placental circulation [11–14]. The concordance rate in twins with ALL with the *ETV6-RUNX1* fusion is much lower at 10% and the postnatal latency period is longer, suggesting that cooperating genetic events are required postnatally for leukemic transformation in this subtype of ALL [15, 16].

Only a small proportion (<5%) of cases of ALL are associated with hereditary genetic abnormalities. The most common condition associated with the development of ALL is Down syndrome (trisomy 21). Children with Down syndrome

P.H. Wiernik et al. (eds.), *Neoplastic Diseases of the Blood*, DOI 10.1007/978-3-319-64263-5_17

have a 20-fold greater risk of ALL compared with non-Down syndrome children [17, 18]. The ALL observed in children with Down syndrome appears biologically distinctive, with a higher frequency of *CRLF2* overexpression and *JAK2* mutations, and a lower frequency of other recurrent genetic abnormalities, such as *ETV6-RUNX1*, high hyperdiploidy, *KMT2A*-rearrangement, and *BCR-ABL1* [19–23].

Other genetic disorders associated with an increased risk of ALL include ataxia telangiectasia and Bloom's syndrome [18, 24, 25]. Patients with ataxia telangiectasia have a 70-fold greater risk of leukemia, particularly T-ALL [26]. Nearly 90% of pediatric cases of low hypodiploid ALL (32–39 chromosomes), a rare subtype, have a TP53 mutation (compared with <5% of non-low-hypodiploid ALL); almost half of the TP53 mutations observed in low hypodiploid ALL are germline [27].

Genome-wide association studies (GWAS) have identified a number of germline polymorphisms associated with increased risk for developing childhood ALL. The first SNPs which GWAS technology identified as significantly associated with ALL were *ARIDB5, IKZF1,* and *CEBPE* [28, 29]. Additional variants in *CDKN2A, BMI1-PIP4K2A,* and *GATA3* have been identified and verified as increasing the host's risk for childhood ALL [30–32]. In addition, it is now known that specific susceptibility variants are associated with either molecular subtypes of ALL and/or ancestry. For instance, the risk alleles of *ARID5B*, a gene that encodes a transcriptional factor important in embryonic development, are associated with the development of the high hyperdiploid B-ALL subtype, and the susceptibility associated with *CEBPE* and *CDKN2A* polymorphisms is only seen in Europeans [33]. While a number of polymorphisms have been identified, the effect size of these genetic variants is relatively small, and very few childhood ALL cases are associated with them.

In utero exposure to diagnostic X-rays is associated with a slightly increased risk of ALL, proportional to the number of exposures [34]. The association between leukemia and maternal exposure to potential mutagens, parental use of medications and drugs, proximity to electromagnetic fields, parental smoking, exposure to petrochemical air pollution, and administration of vitamin K in the neonatal period have been studied, but findings have been contradictory and/or inconclusive [10, 35–40]. For instance, one study found that in utero exposure to DNA-damaging drugs, herbal medicines, or pesticides was significantly associated with infant leukemia with *KMT2A* rearrangements [41], but a Children's Oncology Group study found no association with pesticides and infant ALL [42].

Clinical and Laboratory Features at Diagnosis

Rarely ALL is detected during routine examination in the absence of signs or symptoms, but in most cases some symptoms are present for a few days to a few weeks prior to diagnosis. Patients typically present with the clinical signs of pancytopenia due to replacement of normal hematopoiesis by leukemic cells. Symptoms may include pallor, fatigue, or dizziness from anemia, and bruising and/or petechiae from thrombocytopenia. Fever is common and can be caused by infection or by pyrogenic cytokines released by the leukemic cells. In addition, leukemic infiltration of the marrow is often a painful process and patients may present with bone pain and arthralgias, frequently with a limp and complaints of back pain. Abnormalities of the bone, such as metaphyseal banding, periosteal reactions, osteolysis, osteosclerosis, or osteopenia, can be revealed by radiography in many patients. As these changes do not affect treatment and outcome, routine diagnostic imaging studies (except for chest radiograph to rule out mediastinal mass) are not necessary.

The complete blood count generally reveals abnormalities in more than one lineage; anemia, neutropenia, and thrombocytopenia are all usually present to various degrees. Hemoglobin is commonly <8 g/dL. Profound neutropenia (<500/mm^3) occurs in 40% of patients, putting them at a high risk of infection. Initial leukocyte counts may range from very low to extremely high; presenting leukocyte counts are >10,000/mm^3 in slightly over 50% of patients and >50,000/mm^3 in approximately 20% of patients. Patients with T-ALL are more likely to present with elevated leukocyte counts than those with B-ALL [43, 44]. Leukemic blast cells are frequently, but always, observed on peripheral blood smears, and their absence does not rule out a diagnosis of acute leukemia in a patient with pancytopenia. Hypereosinophilia, generally reactive, may be present at diagnosis; hypereosinophilia in B-ALL can also be associated with the t(5;14)(q31;q32) translocation involving the IL-3 gene on chromosome 5 and the Ig heavy-chain (IgH) gene on chromosome 14 [45].

Extramedullary sites of leukemic involvement include the liver, spleen, thymus, lymph nodes, and kidney. Hepatosplenomegaly is a common physical exam finding at diagnosis, as is lymphadenopathy. Painless enlargement of the scrotum can be a sign of testicular leukemia or hydrocele resulting from lymphatic obstruction; these two causes can usually be distinguished by ultrasound.

Leukemic infiltration of the thymus can lead to the development of an anterior mediastinal mass, observed on diagnostic chest X-ray in approximately 10% of newly diagnosed patients, almost always associated with T-cell immunophenotype. Anterior mediastinal masses can lead to life-threatening airway compression as well as superior vena cava (SVC) syndrome (facial and upper limb swelling, venous distension in neck, upper chest, and arms). Pleural and pericardial effusions can also be associated with mediastinal masses, which can exacerbate respiratory distress and cardiovascular compromise.

CNS involvement at diagnosis is usually asymptomatic and is diagnosed by cerebrospinal fluid (CSF) examination.

Lymphoblasts are identified morphologically at diagnosis in the CSF in over 20% of patients, most of whom have no neurologic symptoms [46]. Rarely, patients present with signs of increased intracranial pressure (vomiting, headache, papilledema, and lethargy) related to CSF pleocytosis or cranial nerve palsy related to leukemic infiltration. Ophthalmologic examination may reveal leukemic infiltration of the anterior ocular chamber, retinal hemorrhage and/or detachment, and optic nerve infiltration, especially in patients presenting with hyperleukocytosis.

Rapid turnover of leukemia cells at the time of diagnosis, especially in patients with high leukemic cell burden, can lead to elevations in serum uric acid, potassium, phosphorus, and lactate dehydrogenase (LDH). Patients with high levels of uric acid are at risk for the development of acute renal failure secondary to uric acid deposition in the kidney. Hypercalcemia at diagnosis has been observed but is uncommon; it appears to be related to elevated levels of parathyroid hormone-related peptide and has been associated with the rare t(17;19) translocation (*E2A-HLF*) [47]. Disseminated intravascular coagulation (DIC) may also occur at diagnosis, more commonly in T-ALL than B-ALL, and is only rarely associated with severe hemorrhage [48]. Coagulopathy has also been associated with the t(17;19) translocation [49].

Differential Diagnosis

Many of the presenting features of ALL are common to other childhood illnesses. Infection due to Epstein–Barr virus, cytomegalovirus, and other viruses can present with fever, lymphadenopathy, hepatomegaly, or splenomegaly, along with atypical lymphocytes that can be confused as lymphoblasts on peripheral blood smear. Patients with pertussis or parapertussis may have marked lymphocytosis, although composed by mature lymphocytes rather than lymphoblasts.

Patients with idiopathic thrombocytopenic purpura (ITP) can present with petechiae and bruising. In contrast to ALL, ITP typically presents with isolated thrombocytopenia, often with large platelets seen on blood smear, as opposed to abnormalities in other cell lines and smear findings suggestive of marrow infiltration observed with ALL.

Aplastic anemia may present with pancytopenia, but usually without the extramedullary findings frequently noted in ALL, such as hepatosplenomegaly and lymphadenopathy. Bone pain, arthralgia, and occasionally arthritis may mimic juvenile rheumatoid arthritis, rheumatic fever, other rheumatologic diseases, or osteomyelitis; because of the difficulty in distinguishing some rheumatologic conditions from ALL, bone marrow examination should be considered before initiating corticosteroid therapy. Solid tumors with extensive marrow metastatic involvement, including neuroblastoma and rhabdomyosarcoma, may also present similarly to ALL.

The definitive diagnosis of ALL requires morphologic examination of the bone marrow along with immunophenotyping. Cytogenetics and molecular analyses should be sent from diagnostic specimens for further classification of the leukemia. While the diagnosis of ALL can usually be made from a bone marrow aspirate, it is sometimes difficult to obtain an adequate aspirate sample (due to marrow fibrosis), in which case the diagnosis can be made by morphologic examination and immunohistochemical staining of a bone marrow biopsy specimen. For patients presenting with high peripheral blast count, peripheral blood flow cytometry may also be useful.

Diagnostic Classification

Morphology and Cytochemistry

ALL is diagnosed when more than 25% of the cells in the bone marrow are lymphoblasts. Morphologic analysis distinguishes three subtypes of ALL (L1, L2, and L3) as classified by the French–American–British (FAB) schema [50]. L1 lymphoblasts are small with scant cytoplasm. The cells are characterized by a large nucleus often with clefts along the membrane and prominent nucleoli. Approximately 90% of childhood ALL cases exhibit this morphology. In contrast, L2 lymphoblasts are much larger with more abundant cytoplasm and may resemble M1 myeloblasts. The L2 morphology is present in 5–10% of pediatric ALL. The distinction between L1 and L2 lymphoblasts, however, has no prognostic relevance with contemporary therapy [51]. L3 lymphoblasts occur in 1–2% of all cases; these cells exhibit vacuoles throughout deep blue cytoplasm. L3 lymphoblasts are nearly always associated with surface immunoglobulin expression and translocations involving the *MYC* gene, and are more effectively treated with regimens for advanced-stage Burkitt lymphoma.

Immunophenotype

The immunophenotype of ALL cells refers to the compilation of specific surface antigens which reveals both the lineage and maturation stage of the lymphoid progenitor cell from which the leukemia originated (Table 17.1). Lymphoblasts can be divided into two main immunophenotypic groups: B-ALL and T-ALL. Patients with B-ALL may be further subdivided into pro-B, early pre-B, pre-B, and mature B subtypes, as discussed below.

B-ALL

Approximately 80–85% of children with ALL present with B-ALL immunophenotype, characterized by the expression of the B-cell markers CD19, CD22, and CD79a [52]. The cells lack expression of cytoplasmic (or surface) CD3 and of myeloperoxidase (by cytochemistry and antibody staining). While

Table 17.1 Immunophenotypic subgroups of childhood ALL

Antigen expression (% of cases positive)										
Subtype	CD19	CD22	CD79a	CD10	CD7	CD5	CD3	cIgM	sIgM	sIg κ or λ	Prevalence (%)
Early pre-B	100	>95[a]	>95	95	5	0	0	0	0	0	60–65
Pre-B	100	100[a]	100	>95	0	<2	0	100[b]	0	0	20–25
Mature B	100	100[a]	100	50	0	0	0	>95	>95	>95	2–3
T	<5	0	30	45	100	95	100[a]	0	0	0	10-15

Source: Campana and Behm [52]

cIgM cytoplasmic immunoglobulin μ heavy chain; *sIgM* surface IgM; *sIg* κ *or* λ surface immunoglobulin κ or λ light chains

[a]Detectable only in the cytoplasm in some cases

[b]IgM heavy chains only

aberrant expression of myeloid antigens is not uncommon in B-ALL, co-expression of T-lineage antigens is rare [53].

Pro-B ALL is thought to be derived from a very immature B-cell precursor. It is most frequently observed in infants with ALL, especially those with *KMT2A* (*MLL*) rearrangements, and is characterized by absence of both CD10 surface expression and cytoplasmic immunoglobulin. In cases with *KMT2A* rearrangements, myeloid antigen co-expression is common [54, 55].

Early pre-B-ALL is the most common subtype of B-ALL seen in pediatric patients. Expression of CD10 and terminal deoxynucleotidyl transferase (TdT) is found in at least 90% of cases, and CD34 is expressed in more than 75% of cases [52]. CD20 (a marker of a more mature B-cell) can be detected at diagnosis in approximately 50% of cases [56], although its expression may increase during induction treatment [57]. Cytoplasmic and surface immunoglobulin are typically absent.

Pre-B-ALL, defined by the presence of cytoplasmic IgM heavy chains without detectable surface immunoglobulins, represents approximately 20–25% of cases of B-ALL [52]. In rare cases, IgM heavy chains without κ or λ light chains are also detectable on the cell surface [58], but can be distinguished from Burkitt-type leukemia by the absence of c-*MYC* translocations. Like early pre-B-ALL, pre-B-ALL cells usually express CD10 and TdT [52]. The *TCF3-PBX1* gene fusion is associated with pre-B immunophenotype; this cytogenetic abnormality is found in 20–25% of pre-B-ALL cases but in only 1% of cases with early pre-B-ALL [52, 53].

Mature B-cell ALL, which occurs in 1–2% of childhood ALL cases, is characterized by the expression of surface immunoglobulin. Cells are generally recognizable by FAB L3 morphology, as described above. CD20 is frequently expressed and CD34 is typically negative [52]. Mature B-cell ALL is characterized by the presence of c-*MYC* rearrangements caused by the translocation of this gene on chromosome 8 with one of the chromosomes containing an immunoglobulin gene, such as t(8;14)(q24;q32), t(2;8)(p12;q24), and t(8;22)(q24;q11) [59]. Mature B-cell ALL should be treated as advanced-stage Burkitt lymphoma rather than on regimens intended for childhood B-ALL [60].

T-ALL

Approximately 10–15% of children with ALL present with T-cell immunophenotype. Compared with B-ALL, T-ALL is more frequently associated with older age at diagnosis higher presenting leukocyte counts, and male predominance [44]. Mediastinal masses, when present in children with ALL, are almost exclusively observed in patients with T-cell immunophenotype.

The cell surface markers most consistently expressed in T-ALL are CD7 and CD3. Expression of the latter is confined to the cytoplasm in approximately two-thirds of cases [61]; approximately half of these cases also express cytoplasmic TCR proteins (TCRβ, TCRα, or both). In the remaining third of T-ALL cases, CD3 is expressed on the cell surface together with TCR proteins, TCRαβ, or, less commonly, TCRγδ [62]. Other markers usually expressed in T-ALL include CD2, CD5, and TdT; CD1a is detected in approximately half of the cases and two-thirds expressing CD4 and/or CD8 [52, 63]. Aberrant myeloid antigen expression may be seen in up to 15% of T-ALL [63].

Early T-cell precursor (ETP) ALL is a distinct subset of T-ALL that was first identified by gene expression profiling studies [64]. This subtype is characterized by a gene expression profile similar to that of normal thymic ETP cells, a population of recent immigrants from the bone marrow to the thymus which retains multi-lineage differentiation potential [65, 66]. ETP ALL expresses a specific immunophenotype that lacks CD1a and CD8 expression, has weak or absent CD5 expression, and expresses at least one stem cell or myeloid-associated antigen (e.g., CD34, CD117, CD13, CD33, and CD11b) [64]. ETP-ALL represents approximately 10–15% of childhood T-ALL cases and was initially thought to have an extremely poor prognosis [64, 67], although subsequent reports suggest that its outcome may not be significantly different than other cases of T-ALL [68].

Myeloid Antigen Co-expression

Up to 20–30% of lymphoblasts in childhood ALL co-express myeloid antigens. Myeloid antigen co-expression is associated with certain chromosomal abnormalities (both favorable and unfavorable), such as *KMT2A* rearrangements, *BCR-ABL1*, and *ETV6-RUNX1*. Older studies suggested that myeloid co-expression was associated with an inferior outcome [69], but more recent reports have indicated that myeloid antigen co-expression lacks independent prognostic significance [70–72]. Distinction is made between ALL with myeloid co-expression and leukemia of ambiguous lineage or MPAL (mixed-phenotype acute leukemia), another leukemia subtype in which a predominant lineage cannot be determined. To be classified as MPAL, the 2008 WHO classification system requires that cells co-express at least two of the following three groups of lineage-defining antigens: [1] myeloid: myeloperoxidase or evidence of monocytic differentiation; [2] T-cell: cytoplasmic CD3; and [3] B-cell surface markers CD19, CD79a, CD22, and/or CD10 [73].

Table 17.3 Classification of ALL according to the 2008 revision of the World Health Organization classification of myeloid neoplasms and acute leukemia

B lymphoblastic leukemia
B lymphoblastic leukemia, not otherwise specified
B lymphoblastic leukemia with recurrent genetic abnormalities
B lymphoblastic leukemia with t(9;22)(q34;q11.2); *BCR-ABL1*
B lymphoblastic leukemia with t(v;11q23); *MLL (KMT2A)* rearranged
B lymphoblastic leukemia with t(12;21)(p13;q22); *TEL-AML1 (ETV6-RUNX1)*
B lymphoblastic leukemia with hyperdiploidy
B lymphoblastic leukemia with hypodiploidy
B lymphoblastic leukemia with t(5;14)(q31;q32); *IL3-IGH*
B lymphoblastic leukemia with t(1;19)(q23;p13.3); *TCF3-PBX1*
T lymphoblastic leukemia

Source: Modified from Vardiman et al., 2009 [73]

Cytogenetics and Molecular Genetics

There are several recurrent cytogenetic abnormalities that have been identified in childhood ALL, many with important prognostic implications, as summarized in Table 17.2. The 2008 World Health Organization (WHO) classification of ALL is based on immunophenotype and cytogenetics, as shown in Table 17.3 [73].

Cytogenetic abnormalities in childhood ALL can be subdivided into those involving [1] abnormalities in chromosome number (ploidy) and [2] chromosomal translocations and gains/deletions of chromosomal segments.

Table 17.2 Recurrent cytogenetic abnormalities in childhood B-ALL and their relation to prognosis with contemporary therapy[a]

Abnormality	Frequency[a]	Prognostic impact
Hyperdiploidy 51–65 chromosomes	33%	Favorable
t(12;21)(p13;q22) [*ETV6-RUNX1*]	25%	Favorable
t(1;19)(q23;p13) [*TCF3-PBX1*]	4%	Neutral
t(9;22)(q34;q11)	3%	Unfavorable
iAMP21	2%	Unfavorable
KMT2A (11q23) rearrangements	2% [~80% of infants]	Unfavorable
Hypodiploidy (including near haplopidy, low hypodiploidy)	1–2%	Unfavorable
t(17;19)(q22;p13) [*TCF3-HLF*]	<1%	Unfavorable
IKZF1 deletions	15%[b]	Unfavorable

[a]Frequency from Moorman et al., 2010 [77], except frequencies of *IKZF1* deletions

[b]Frequency from Clappier et al. 2015 [110]

Abnormalities of Chromosomal Number

Hyperdiploid ALL

The most common recurrent chromosomal abnormality in childhood ALL is high hyperdiploidy (defined as 51–65 chromosomes, or DNA index $\geq$ 1.16), occurring in 25–30% of cases [74]. High hyperdiploidy is characterized by nonrandom gains of chromosomes, with trisomies and tetrasomies occurring most often (listed in order of frequency) in chromosomes 21, X, 14, 18, 4, 17, 10, and 8 [75]. High hyperdiploidy frequently occurs as the sole cytogenetic abnormality, without other karytotypic aberrations, but can also be observed along with chromosomal translocations, including *BCR-ABL1* and *TCF3-PBX1*. Whole-genome and whole-exome sequencing of high-hyperdiploid ALL revealed aberrations of receptor tyrosine kinase (RTK)/Ras pathway signaling (*KRAS, NRAS, FLT3, PTPN11*) and histone modifiers (including *CREBBP* and *WHSC1*) in the majority of cases [76]. High-hyperdiploid ALL occurs more frequently in children with "low-risk" presenting features (age 1–10 years, presenting leukocyte count <50,000/mm^3), and when it occurs in the absence of other prognostically significant abnormalities (such as *BCR-ABL1* fusion), it has been identified as an independent predictor of favorable outcome [75, 77]. High hyperdiploid patients with trisomies of chromosomes 4, 10, and 17 have been reported to have particularly favorable outcomes [75, 78].

Near triploidy (68–80 chromosomes) and near tetraploidy (>80 chromosomes) occur in approximately 1–2% of cases of childhood ALL, and are biologically distinctive from high hyperdiploidy [79, 80]. Compared with high hyperdiploidy, near trisomy/tetraploidy is more often associated with the *ETV6-RUNX1* fusion and more frequently occurs in T-ALL patients [79–81].

Hypodiploidy

Hypodiploidy (<45 chromosomes) is much less common than hyperdiploidy in childhood ALL, and has been associated with an unfavorable outcome [82, 83]. The chromosome loss is not random; disomies of chromosomes X/Y, 8, 10, 14, 18, and 21 are preserved in the majority of cases [84]. Rather than representing a single subtype of ALL, hypodiploid ALL consists of two distinct biologic subsets, near haploidy (24–31 chromosomes) and low hypodiploidy (32–39 chromosomes), which differ strikingly on a molecular basis from each other [27]. In near haploidy, genetic alterations in RTK/Ras pathway signaling (including *NRAS*, *KRAS*, *NF1*, *MAPK*, *FLT3*, and *PTPN11*) and the lymphoid transcription factor *IKZF3* are common, while low hypodiploidy is characterized by alterations in *TP53* (observed in 90% of cases), *IKZF2*, and *RB1*. Of note, almost half of the *TP53* mutations in pediatric low-hypodiploid ALL appear to be germline [27].

Doubling of the chromosome content in hypodiploid lymphoblasts can occur, resulting in a pseudo-hyperdiploid clone. These "masked hypodiploid" cases are biologically and prognostically indistinguishable from other cases of low hypodiploidy [27]. At diagnosis, both the hypodiploid and pseudo-hyperdiploid clone may be evident; however, the doubled hypodiploid clone may be the only one detectable at diagnosis, and can be confused with true hyperdiploidy. Given the very different expected outcomes of near-haploid/low-hypodiploid (poor prognosis) and high-hyperdiploid ALL (favorable prognosis), cases of masked hypodiploidy need to be distinguished from true high hyperdiploidy for risk stratification and treatment allocation. By karyotype, the "extra" chromosomes in masked hypodiploidy mostly occur as tetrasomies from the doubling of retained disomies, while in true high hyperdiploidy, trisomies are more common then tetrasomies [84].

Chromosomal Translocations and Gains/ Deletions of Chromosomal Segments

ETV6-RUNX1

The *ETV6-RUNX1* fusion is the most frequent chromosomal rearrangement in childhood ALL. It is found in approximately 20–25% of childhood ALL, occurring nearly exclusively in B-ALL [85]. It is caused by the t(12;21)(p13;q22) which juxtaposes the 5′ portion of the *ETV6* (*TEL*) gene and the nearly complete *RUNX1* (*AML1*) gene [86]. This translocation is usually cryptic by conventional karyotyping; the abnormality is typically detected only by fluorescence in situ hybridization (FISH) or reverse transcriptase-polymerase chain reaction (RT-PCR) [86–88]. The non-translocated *ETV6* allele is frequently deleted [81, 89]. Like high hyperdiploidy, *ETV6-RUNX1* is more frequent in children aged 1–10 years [87, 90, 91] and has been shown to be an independent predictor of favorable outcome [77, 90].

The widely expressed *ETV6* gene belongs to the *Ets* family of transcription factors and *RUNX1* encodes a transcription factor that binds DNA as a heterodimer with core-binding factor (CBF) β; both *ETV6* and *RUNX1* are essential for normal hematopoietic development [92, 93]. There is evidence that the gene fusion occurs prenatally, giving rise to a preleukemic clone that requires additional postnatal genetic events for the development of ALL. For instance, analyses of neonatal blood spots of healthy babies indicated that *ETV6-RUNX1* was detectable at a 100 times the frequency of this ALL subtype in the general population [94]. Additionally, studies of five monozygotic twin pairs with concordant *ETV6-RUNX1* ALL revealed that there was discordance within each twin pair for genome-wide copy number alterations considered "driver" mutations [95].

BCR-ABL1

BCR-ABL1-positive ALL (also known as Philadelphia chromosome-positive or Ph+ ALL) occurs in 3–5% of cases of childhood ALL. The *BCR-ABL1* fusion gene results from the t(9;22)(q34;q11), which juxtaposes the 5′ portion of *BCR* and the 3′ portion of *ABL1*, encoding a constitutively activated tyrosine kinase [96]. The fusion protein varies in size, depending on the breakpoint in the *BCR* gene. In ALL, the translocation occurs most often in the minor breakpoint cluster regions, resulting in a *BCR-ABL1* fusion protein of 190 kD (p190), while in chronic myelogenous leukemia (CML), the major breakpoint cluster region is typically involved, resulting in a larger fusion protein of 210 kD (p210) [97]. Deletions of *IKZF1*, a gene that encodes Ikaros, a lymphoid transcription factor, have been observed in approximately 70% of cases *BCR-ABL1*-positive ALL [98].

BCR-ABL1 positivity in childhood ALL is associated with older age at diagnosis and higher presenting leukocyte counts [99]. Historically, patients with this subtype had a significantly worse outcome than other children with ALL, and were typically allocated to hematopoietic stem cell transplant (HSCT) after achieving complete remission [77, 100]. More recent clinical trials have indicated that the addition of imatinib, a selective inhibitor of the *BCR-ABL1* tyrosine kinase, to an intensive chemotherapy backbone may improve the prognosis for pediatric *BCR-ABL1*-positive patients and obviate the need for HSCT in first complete remission for the majority of patients [101, 102].

BCR-ABL1-Like Subtype, IKZF1 Deletions, and CRLF2 Overexpression

Lymphoblasts from approximately 15% of pediatric ALL patients have been found to have a gene expression profile similar to *BCR-ABL1*-positive ALL, but lacking the *BCR-ABL1* fusion [103–107]. This subtype, termed *BCR-ABL1*-like (or Ph-like) ALL, is more common in older children and adolescents, and has been associated with an adverse outcome [106, 107]. *BCR-ABL1*-like ALL is characterized by a high frequency of *IKZF1* deletions, as well as overexpression of cytokine receptor-like factor 2 (*CRLF2*). Detailed genomic analyses have identified kinase-activating alterations in over 90% of patients with *BCR-ABL1*-like ALL [106], suggesting the potential for targeted interventions with tyrosine kinase inhibitors. Kinase-activating alterations appear to primarily impact the ABL-class signaling pathway (with fusions involving *ABL1*, *ABL2*, *CSF1R*, or *PDGFRB*) and JAK-STAT signaling pathway (including rearrangements of *JAK2*, *EPOR*, and/or *CRLF2*) [106, 108, 109].

IKZF1 deletions, including deletions of the entire gene and deletions of specific exons, are present in approximately 15% of pediatric B-ALL, with increased frequency in older children and adolescents, those with higher presenting leukocyte counts, and patients with Down syndrome [104, 110, 111]. *IKZF1* deletions are detectable in the majority of patients with *BCR-ABL1*-positive ALL [98, 112], and in 40–60% of cases with the *BCR-ABL1*-like subtype [103, 106, 107]; however, many patients with *IKZF1* deletions have neither of these abnormalities [107]. Several studies have indicated that *IKZF1* deletions independently predict the outcome in B-ALL, even when controlling for other adverse features, including *BCR-ABL1* status and high levels of minimal residual disease (MRD) [107, 110, 113, 114]. *IKZF1* deletions have also been shown to predict inferior outcome in biologically favorable subtypes, such as high hyperdiploidy [110]. Some reports indicate that the presence of an *ERG* gene deletion, observed in 3–5% of cases of B-ALL, may abrogate the adverse prognostic significance of *IKZF1* deletions when the two co-occur [115, 116].

Genomic alterations in *CRLF2*, located on the pseudoautosomal regions of the sex chromosomes, have been identified in 5–10% of cases of B-ALL and in approximately 50% of cases of the *BCR-ABL1*-like subtype [117, 118]. They are strongly associated with *IKZF1* deletions and *JAK* mutations [118–121], and are more common in children with Down syndrome, occurring in 50–60% of cases [121, 122]. They have also been reported to be more common in Hispanic patients [119]. Two alterations have been described, both of which lead to *CRLF2* overexpression: (i) a cryptic chromosomal translocation involving the *CRLF2* gene and IgH locus on chromosome 14, and (ii) interstitial deletions juxtaposing *CRLF2* with the *P2RY8* promoter in pseudoautosomal regions of the sex chromosomes, resulting in a *P2RY8-CRLF2* fusion [117–120]. Although univariate analyses have suggested that *CRLF2* abnormalities may have adverse prognostic significance, these alterations have not been shown to be independent predictors of outcome in most studies when controlling for other factors, such as *IKZF1* deletion and *BCR-ABL1*-like status [107, 119].

KMT2A (MLL) Gene Rearrangements

Rearrangements involving the *KMT2A* (*MLL*) gene occur in approximately 5% of childhood ALL cases, but in up to 80% of infants with ALL. The most common rearrangement is the t(4;11)(q21;q23) which fuses the *KMT2A* (chromosome 11) and *AFF1* (chromosome 4) genes, but multiple other fusion partners have been identified. *KMT2A* translocations are also found in AML, but particular translocations show lineage predominance; for instance the t(4;11) is found most often in ALL while the t(9;11) is more common in AML.

In ALL cases, *KMT2A* rearrangements are associated with high presenting leukocyte counts, CD10-negative B-cell immunophenotype (pro-B), and myeloid antigen coexpression [123]. Even with intensified chemotherapy regimens, infants with *KMT2A* rearrangements have an adverse prognosis, particularly those who present at a very young age (<6 months) and with extremely high leukocyte counts [124]. The prognosis of older (non-infant) pediatric patients with *KMT2A* rearrangements is not as well established, but it appears that such patients fare better than infant *KMT2A*-rearranged patients but not as well as other non-infant B-ALL patients lacking these aberrations [77, 125]. There is also controversy regarding the prognostic significance of various fusion partners. For infants with *KMT2A* rearrangements, outcome appears similarly unfavorable regardless of fusion partner [124, 125], but for older children, some (but not all) studies have found that the t(4;11) confers a worse prognosis than other translocations [125]. In one report, the t(11;19), involving *KMT2A* and *MLLT1* (*ENL*) was associated with a poor outcome in infants (all with B-ALL) but appeared to be associated with a relatively favorable progress in non-infant patients with T-ALL [126].

Gene expression profile studies indicate that *KMT2A*-rearranged ALL is characterized by overexpression of a number of genes, including *FLT3*, *LMO2*, HOX genes (e.g., *HOXA9*, *HOXA5*, *HOXA4*, and *HOXC6*), *NRAS*, and *KRAS* [127, 128]. The unique biology of *KMT2A*-rearranged ALL appears to be driven primarily by epigenetic dysregulation rather than somatic mutations. Whole-genome sequencing has revealed that *KMT2A*-rearranged infant ALL has one of the lowest frequencies of somatic mutations of any cancer [127]; in non-infant *KMT2A*-rearranged ALL, frequent mutations in epigenetic regulators (but not other somatic mutations) have been identified [127]. Wild-type *KMT2A* possesses a methyltransferase domain which regulates expression of multiple genes, including HOX genes; *KMT2A* rearrangements lead to disruptions in *KMT2A*'s normal epigenetic function, resulting in overexpression of multiple genes through transcriptional dysregulation [129, 130].

TCF3 Rearrangements

Approximately 5% of pediatric B-ALL cases have the balanced t(1;19)(q23;p13) or the unbalanced der [19]t(1;19) (q23;p13), both of which juxtapose the *TCF3* (*E2A*) gene on chromosome 19 and the *PBX1* gene on chromosome 1 [131–133]. The resulting *TCF3-PBX1* fusion protein contains the transcriptional activation domains of *TCF3* linked to the DNA-binding domain of *PBX1*, thereby inappropriately activating the transcription of genes normally regulated by *PBX1*, as well as reducing wild-type *TCF3* activity [134, 135].

The *TCF3-PBX1* fusion had previously been considered a predictor of inferior outcome [136], but with contemporary therapy, it lacks prognostic significance and in general is no longer considered a high-risk feature [131, 137]. Some investigators have reported a higher rate of CNS relapse in patients with the t(1;19) [138], but this has not been confirmed by others [131].

Another fusion observed in childhood ALL involving *TCF3* is the t(17;19)(q22;p13), resulting in the fusion of *TCF3* with *HLF*, a gene that encodes another transcription factor [139, 140]. The *TCF3-HLF* fusion is rare, occurring in fewer than 1% of pediatric ALL cases, and is associated with a very poor prognosis [47, 77, 141]. ALL with the *TCF3-HLF* fusion presents with disseminated intravascular coagulation and hypercalcemia [47, 141]. Genomic profiling has revealed that *TCF3-HLF*-positive ALL is characterized by deletions in genes involved in B-cell development (*PAX5*, *BTG1*, and *VPREB1*) and by mutations in RAS pathway genes (*NRAS*, *KRAS*, and *PTPN11*) [142].

Intrachromosomal Amplification of Chromosome 21 (iAMP21)

Intrachromosomal amplification of the RUNX1 gene on chromosome 21 (iAMP21) occurs in approximately 2% of childhood ALL (almost exclusively B-ALL), and has been associated with older age at diagnosis (median age approximately 10 years) and with lower presenting leukocyte count (less than 50,000 cells/mm^3) [77, 87, 143]. It is diagnosed primarily by FISH, and is defined as three or more extra copies of RUNX1 on a single chromosome 21 (a total of five or more RUNX1 signals per cell). Initial retrospective analyses suggested that children with iAMP21 had a markedly inferior event-free survival compared with other patients [144, 145]. Subsequent reports have indicated that, with more intensive treatment, patients with iAMP21 may not have as high a risk of relapse as suggested in these initial studies [143, 146, 147].

Genetic Subtypes of T-cell ALL

T-ALL can be subdivided into multiple genetically distinct subsets, but most do not appear to be prognostically significant and are not used for treatment stratification.

Translocations involving one of the T-cell receptor loci [chromosome 14q11 (TCRα and TCRδ), 7q34 (TCRβ), or 7p14 (TCRγ)] have been observed in approximately 35% of cases of T-ALL [148]. The translocations include rearrangements of transcriptional factors to the TCR loci that are often not visible by karyotype but can be identified by FISH. Some of the more common translocations involve rearrangements of *LMO1* (11p15), *LMO2* (11p13), *TAL1*(1p32), and *HOX11L2/TLX3* (5q35) to TCRδ, *TLX1* (10q24) to TCRδ or TCRβ, and *HOXA* (7p15) to TCRβ [149]. In addition, aberrant expression of these transcription factors can occur in the absence of T-cell receptor loci rearrangements; for instance, the *TLX3/HOX11L2* locus is recurrently translocated to T-cell regulatory sequences in the proximity of the *BCL11B* locus, small intrachromosomal deletions in chromosome 1p32 result in *TAL1* overexpression, and cryptic deletions in chromosome 11p13 can lead to activation of the *LMO2* oncogene [149].

Activating mutations in the *NOTCH1* gene are present in over 50% of T-ALL cases [150]. Additionally, *FBXW7* mutations, observed in about 15% of T-ALL, lead to constitutive activation of *NOTCH1* signaling by impairing degradation of activated *NOTCH1* [151]. The prognostic significance of *NOTCH1*-activating mutations is not clear. While some investigators have reported that these lesions are associated with a favorable early response (e.g., increased sensitivity to corticosteroid prophase) and/or a decreased risk of relapse, most studies have not demonstrated that these lesions have any prognostic significance [152–155].

Other common genetic lesions observed in T-ALL include deletions in the *CDKN2A* locus at chromosome 9p21, observed in 70% of cases, and deletions of *PTEN* (5–10% of cases), which is a negative regulator of the PI3K-AKT signaling pathway [156, 157]. Additional activating mutations of *PI3K* and *AKT* genes have also been reported, suggesting that up to 40–50% of T-ALL patients may have genetic alterations impacting this signaling pathway [156]. *ABL1* rearrangements occur in about 8% of T-ALL, including the *NUP214-ABL1* fusion (the most frequent *ABL1* abnormality), a cytogenetically cryptic, complex rearrangement seen on FISH on amplified episomes [158, 159].

The early T-cell precursor (ETP) subtype appears to be molecularly heterogeneous, but distinct from other cases of T-ALL. Compared with other T-ALL cases, ETP ALL has a lower rate of *NOTCH1* mutations and significantly higher frequencies of alterations in genes regulating cytokine receptors and RAS signaling, hematopoietic development, and histone modification [160].

Prognostic Factors

Several factors have been identified as significant predictors of outcome in childhood ALL, including age, presenting leukocyte count, immunophenotype, chromosomal abnormalities, presence of morphologically detectable lymphoblasts in the spinal fluid at diagnosis, and early response to initial therapy [161]. These factors are used to stratify the intensity of therapy, with stronger, potentially more toxic treatments reserved for those presenting with adverse prognostic features. Ultimately, the prognostic significance of any factor is treatment dependent, and the importance of a particular presenting feature in predicting the outcome may vary, depending on the therapy delivered to that patient.

Age

Age at diagnosis is a long-established prognostic factor in B-ALL, but not T-ALL [162–165]. Its prognostic significance likely reflects age-related differences in the frequencies of various underlying biologic subsets. For instance, the two cytogenetic abnormalities associated with the most favorable outcome in childhood ALL, *ETV6-RUNX1* and high hyperdiploidy, occur most frequently in children aged 1–10 years, the age group with the best prognosis: approximately 80% of children with B-ALL diagnosed between the ages of 2 and 7 years have one of these two abnormalities [91].

Infants are the age group with the worst prognosis in pediatric ALL. Nearly 80% of infants present with rearrangements of the *KMT2A* gene, compared with <5% of older children [54, 55, 124, 162]. Even when treated with intensified regimens, infants with *KMT2A* rearrangements have an unfavorable prognosis, with long-term event-free survival rates less than 50% [124, 125, 166]. Infants whose leukemia lacks a *KMT2A* rearrangement fare better, with event-free survival rates that are closer to those observed in older children [124].

Older children and adolescents (10–21 years of age) with ALL also have a less favorable outcome than children aged 1–10 years at diagnosis, although not as poor as infants. Compared with younger children, adolescents with ALL more frequently present with higher risk biologic subtypes, including T-cell immunophenotype, *BCR-ABL1* fusion, *IKZF1* deletions, and *BCR-ABL*-like subtype, and less often with more favorable cytogenetic aberrations, such as high hyperdiploidy and the *ETV6/RUNX1* fusion [106, 107, 110, 162, 167]. Multiple retrospective studies have shown that adolescents fare better with pediatric ALL regimens than on treatments designed for adults with ALL [167–170].

Leukocyte Count

The initial peripheral blood leukocyte count is a significant predictor of treatment outcome, with outcomes worsening as the leukocyte count increases [161]. The relationship between leukocyte count and risk of subsequent relapse is more firmly established for B-ALL than T-ALL [43, 44, 171]. Based on a cutoff established by Cancer Therapy Evaluation Program (CTEP) of the National Cancer Institute (NCI), many clinical trials utilize a leukocyte count of 50,000 cells/mm^3 as the cutoff to differentiate between high versus low presenting leukocyte count [161].

Immunophenotype

Historically, immunophenotype was considered an important prognostic factor, with inferior outcomes observed in patients with T-ALL. However, if treated with more intensive regimens, children with T-ALL fare as well as those with B-ALL [44]. Myeloid antigen coexpression was previously thought to be associated with an inferior outcome, but more recent reports have indicated that it is not an independent prognostic factor [72, 172].

Central Nervous System (CNS) Disease at Diagnosis

Approximately 15–20% of children with ALL present with detectable lymphoblasts in their cerebrospinal fluid [173, 174]. Some children, such as those diagnosed in infancy and those with T-cell ALL, have a higher incidence of morphologically evident CNS leukemia at diagnosis [162].

CNS status at presentation is usually classified as CNS-1 (no blast cells in spinal fluid), CNS-2 (fewer than five leukocytes per microliter with blast cells), and CNS-3 (five or more leukocytes per microliter with blast cells or cranial nerve palsy) [161]. With more frequent dosing of intrathecal chemotherapy, the prognosis of patients with CNS-2 status appears similar to those who are CNS-1 [174, 175]. CNS-3 status at diagnosis (observed in approximately 5% of patients) is associated with a higher risk of relapse (both CNS-involved and marrow-only), and is typically treated with more intensive systemic and CNS-directed therapies [174].

Traumatic lumbar punctures with lymphoblasts on cytospin have also been associated with an adverse prognosis [174, 176]. Like those with CNS-2 status, patients with traumatic lumbar punctures with lymphoblasts at diagnosis may also benefit from additional doses of intrathecal chemotherapy early in treatment [174].

Chromosomal Abnormalities and Other Genetic Lesions

Recurrent chromosomal abnormalities in childhood ALL are detailed above. Several of these have been shown to be significant predictors of outcome. Two abnormalities, the cryptic t(12;21) (*ETV6/RUNX1* fusion) and high hyperdiploidy (51–65 chromosomes or a DNA index ≥1.16), have each been associated with a favorable prognosis [77].

The most favorable outcomes in high-hyperdiploid ALL patients have been associated with the presence of trisomies of chromosomes 4, 10, and 17 [177–179]. Both *ETV6-RUNX1* and high hyperdiploidy occur more most commonly in younger, non-infant patients with B-ALL, with decreased frequency in adolescents, and are usually mutually exclusive [81, 91].

Chromosomal abnormalities associated with an unfavorable prognosis include low hypodiploidy [82, 83, 180], rearrangements of the *KMT2A* (*MLL*) gene [125, 180, 181], and *BCR-ABL1* fusion (Philadelphia chromosome) [77, 100]. The use of imatinib and other tyrosine kinase inhibitors, given in conjunction with intensified chemotherapy, appears to have favorably impacted the outcome of *BCR-ABL1*-positive ALL [101, 102]. Intrachromosomal amplification of chromosome 21 (iAMP21) has also been associated with a higher risk of relapse [144, 145], although the adverse prognostic significance of this abnormality appears to be abrogated when patients are treated on more intensive, "high-risk" therapy [143, 146, 147].

Patients with *BCR-ABL1*-like ALL (defined by gene expression profile) and/or *IKZF1* gene deletions (each representing approximately 15% of B-ALL, with a large overlap between the two groups) have an inferior outcome; each has been shown to be an independent adverse prognostic factor [106, 107, 110, 113, 114].

Early Response to Therapy

The rapidity with which a patient responds to initial chemotherapy is a significant predictor of long-term outcome. Early response to therapy has been evaluated using morphologic measures (residual microscopically detectable disease in blood or marrow) and more sensitive minimal residual disease (MRD) techniques to quantitate submicroscopic levels of disease, such as flow cytometry, PCR, and next-generation sequencing (NGS).

Morphologic Response to Therapy

On trials run by the Berlin-Frankfurt-Munster (BFM) group and several other clinical trial consortia, patients begin treatment with 1 week of corticosteroid monotherapy (and one dose of intrathecal methotrexate) prior to beginning multiagent induction chemotherapy; poor peripheral blood response at the end of that week (defined as an absolute blast count of 1000/mm^3) is an independent predictor of adverse outcome [182]. Similarly, the persistence of leukemia in bone marrow specimens obtained 7 or 14 days after beginning multiagent chemotherapy strongly correlates with increased relapse risk [183], although intensification of therapy can abrogate the adverse prognostic significance of slow early morphologic marrow response [184].

Patients who require two or more cycles of induction chemotherapy to achieve complete remission (CR) have a much worse prognosis than those who achieve CR after the first induction attempt [185–187].

Minimal Residual Disease

Minimal residual disease (MRD) evaluation involves the measurement of very low levels of leukemia using sensitive assays, such as specialized multiparameter flow cytometry, PCR, or NGS techniques. Leukemic cells are identified using targets identified at diagnosis, including leukemia-specific immunophenotypes (for flow cytometry-based assays), chromosomal translocations, or lymphoblast-specific immunoglobulin or T-cell antigen receptor gene rearrangements (for PCR- and NGS-based assays). Using these techniques, leukemia cells have been identified at levels as low as 1 in 1000 to 1 in 100,000 cells [188–192].

Many studies have demonstrated that MRD status at early time points in treatment is a significant and independent predictor of long-term outcome for patients with both B-ALL and T-ALL [188, 193–197]. For patients achieving a morphologic remission at the end of the first month of treatment, those with higher levels of marrow MRD at that time point have a higher risk of relapse than those with lower or undetectable MRD [188, 193–195, 197–201]. MRD levels measured in the peripheral blood as early as 8 days after starting multiagent chemotherapy have also been shown to be prognostically significant, especially in patients with B-ALL presenting with standard-risk features (age between 1 and 10 years, leukocyte count <50,000/mm^3) [199].

MRD levels obtained 10–12 weeks after the start of therapy (at the end of the second phase of treatment) have also been shown to be prognostically important; patients with high levels of MRD at this time point have a significantly inferior EFS compared with other patients [200–202]. The AIEOP-BFM group has defined three prognostically distinct groups of patients based on MRD measurements: (1) patients with low end-induction MRD (best outcome); (2) patients with high end-induction MRD but low MRD after the second phase of treatment (intermediate outcome); and (3) patients with persistently high MRD after the second phase of treatment (worst outcome) [200, 201].

Intensifying therapy for patients with high MRD has been shown to improve the outcome [203, 204]. MRD measurements, in conjunction with other presenting features, have also been used to identify subsets of patients with an extremely low risk of relapse. The Children's Oncology Group reported a very favorable outcome (5-year EFS of 97%) for B-ALL patients with non-high-risk presenting features (age between 1 and 10 years, leukocyte count <50,000/mm^3, CNS-1 status, and either high hyperdiploidy with favorable trisomies or *ETV6-RUNX1* fusion) and MRD levels of less than 0.01% at both day 8 (from peripheral blood) and end induction (from bone marrow) [199].

Other Prognostic Factors

Gender

In some studies, boys appear to fare slightly worse than girls. This observation cannot be entirely explained by the rates of isolated testicular relapse, which are relatively low with contemporary treatment regimens [205, 206].

Race and Ethnicity

Lower event-free survival (EFS) rates have been reported for African-American, Hispanic, and Native American patients, even after adjustment for differences in prognostically significant presenting features [207–209]. This finding may be in part related to differences in the frequency of prognostically relevant biologic subtypes amongst racial and ethnic groups. For example, compared with Caucasians, African-American children have a higher incidence of T-ALL and lower rates of high hyperdiploidy [210]. Hispanic children also have a lower frequency of *ETV6-RUNX1*-rearranged ALL [211], and, in one study, were noted to have a higher incidence of ALL with *CRLF2* rearrangements, a finding that is associated with the *BCR-ABL1*-like subtype [119]. Lower rates of adherence to oral 6-mercaptopurine, a critical component of ALL treatment, have also been observed in African-American, Hispanic, and Asian-American patients [212, 213].

Down Syndrome

Results from several studies have indicated that children with Down syndrome have inferior outcomes compared with other pediatric ALL patients. Down syndrome patients have been reported to have both higher rates of treatment-related mortality (with significantly increased risk of infections and other treatment complications) and relapse [23, 214–216]. The increased risk of relapse may be due in part to the lower frequency of favorable biologic features (such as *ETV6-RUNX1* and high hyperdiploidy) observed in Down syndrome patients [23, 214, 216]. ALL arising in Down syndrome patients is characterized by a higher incidence of *IKZF1* deletions, *CRLF2* aberrations, and *JAK* mutations [19, 111, 122]; the presence of *IKZF1* deletions (but not *CRLF2* aberrations and *JAK* mutations) has been associated with an inferior outcome in Down syndrome patients [111, 217].

Treatment Adherence

Poor adherence to oral 6-mercaptopurine (6-MP), a key component of maintenance therapy in childhood ALL, is an important predictor of relapse [212, 213, 218]. Using an electronic cap to record the date and time of 6-MP bottle openings, investigators from the Children's Oncology Group (COG) demonstrated that there was a progressive increase in relapse rate with decreasing adherence that remained statistically significant after adjusting for NCI risk classification, chromosomal abnormalities, and other prognostically relevant variables. When 6MP adherence was lower than 90%, the risk of relapse was nearly fourfold increased [212]. Factors associated with higher risk of nonadherence included older age (≥12 years), non-white race/ethnicity, low annual household income, low parental education, single-parent households, and absence of a routine surrounding pill taking [212, 213].

Treatment

Historical Background

Over the last several decades, there has been a dramatic improvement in the prognosis of children with ALL. Improvement in cure rates can be attributed to many factors, including [1] identification of active agents and development of complex chemotherapeutic regimens designed to achieve clonal eradication and prevent emergence of drug-resistant clones; [2] improvements in supportive care; [3] recognition of the central nervous system (CNS) as a sanctuary site; and [4] identification of prognostic factors and application of risk-adapted therapy.

Prior to 1947, when the first complete remission in childhood ALL was attained by Farber and colleagues using the folate antagonist aminopterin [219], the disease was uniformly fatal with a median duration of survival of 2 months from the time of diagnosis [220]. During the 1950s, drugs such as 6-mercaptopurine, methotrexate, and corticosteroids were found to be active and induced complete remissions in the majority of patients, but cure rates remained very low due to extremely high rates of relapse [221–224]. Additional active drugs were introduced in the 1960s and 1970s, including the anthracyclines (doxorubicin and daunorubicin), L-asparaginase, and epipodophyllotoxins (etoposide and teniposide) [225–227].

In the 1960s, as effective systemic chemotherapy combinations were identified, the incidence of the CNS as an initial site of relapse became increasingly more common [228, 229]. It was hypothesized that leukemia cells, even if not morphologically evident, were present in the CNS in all patients, and that these cells were protected by the blood-brain barrier from many of the systemically administered chemotherapy agents used at the time. Thus, the concept of the CNS as a sanctuary site emerged, prompting the inclusion of CNS-directed therapy to prevent relapse. With the introduction of cranial radiation to treat subclinical CNS leukemia in the 1970s, long-term disease-free survival rates in childhood ALL dramatically increased to 50% [230]. Although nearly all pediatric patients are now treated without prophylactic cranial radiation, the inclusion of CNS-directed therapies (such as intrathecal chemotherapy and high-dose methotrexate) remains a universal component of all successful treatment regimens.

Risk-Adapted Therapy

After the addition of CNS-directed therapy improved cure rates in the 1970s, investigators compared presenting features in patients who relapsed and those who had not to establish clinically relevant prognostic factors. Subsequent clinical trials used these prognostic factors to stratify therapy. More intensive therapy was administered to those patients considered to be at the highest risk of relapse. In contrast, some of the more morbid components of therapy were modified or eliminated for those children considered to have the best prognosis. The goal of risk-adapted therapy is to treat away adverse presenting features, so that higher and lower risk patients have similar cure rates.

For many years, pediatric clinical trials consortia applied prognostic factors differently when defining risk categories. A more uniform approach to risk classification was proposed and agreed upon at an NCI-sponsored workshop held in 1993 [161]. For patients with B-ALL, the NCI standard-risk category was defined as age between 1 and 10 years and initial leukocyte count lower than 50,000/mm^3. The remaining patients were considered to have NCI high-risk ALL. Other characteristics used by cooperative groups to classify patients as high risk include T-cell phenotype, CNS-3 status at diagnosis, and high peripheral blast count after a week of steroid monotherapy (and a single dose of intrathecal methotrexate), cytogenetics, and MRD levels obtained after the first one or two treatment phases into risk group stratification. In some cases, only cytogenetics and early response (as assessed by MRD), and not other factors, such as age and leukocyte count, are considered when assigning risk groups [200].

Treatment Phases

In general, treatment regimens for children with ALL consist of 2–3 years of multiagent chemotherapy. Treatment consists of the three main parts: (1) remission induction, (2) post-induction consolidation, and (3) continuation (or maintenance). CNS-directed therapies are included throughout all phases. With contemporary regimens, event-free survival rates exceed 80%, and overall survival rates are approximately 90% [200, 204, 231, 232] (Table 17.4).

Table 17.4 Results of selected clinical trials in childhood ALL

Study	Time period	No. of patients	5-year EFS (%)	5-year OS (%)	References
AIEOP-BFM 2000[a]	2000–2006	4016	80[b]	92[b]	[200]
COG	2000–2005	7153	–	90	[232]
DCOG ALL-10	2004–2012	778	87	92	[204]
DFCI 05-001	2005–2010	551	85	91	[231]
NOPHO ALL-2000	2002–2007	1023	79	89	[372]
SJCRH Total XV	2000–2007	498	86	93	[138]
MRC UK-ALL 2003	2003–2011	3126	87	92	[203]

EFS Event-free survival, *OS* Overall survival, *AIEOP-BFM*, Associazione Italiana di Ematologia Pediatrica-Berlin Frankfurt-Munster; *COG* Children's Oncology Group, *DCOG* Dutch Childhood Oncology Group, *DFCI* Dana–Farber Cancer Institute ALL Consortium, *NOPHO* Nordic Society of Pediatric Hematology and Oncology, *SJCRH* St. Jude Children's Research Hospital, *MRC UK* Medical Research Council United Kingdom

[a]B-ALL only

[b]7-year estimates

[c]5-year overall survival

Remission Induction

The goal of the first phase of treatment, remission induction, is to induce complete morphologic remission. Complete remission is defined as attainment of a bone marrow with normal cellular elements but fewer than 5% lymphoblasts, return of normal peripheral blood counts, and resolution of other bulk sites of disease. The remission induction phase typically lasts for 4–5 weeks, and consists of glucocorticoid (prednisone, prednisolone, or dexamethasone), vincristine, and L-asparaginase; some regimens include an anthracycline (daunorubicin or doxorubicin) for all patients while others reserve its use for higher risk patients. About 1–2% of patients die of disease- or treatment-related complications during the first month of treatment, and about 1–2% fail to fully respond and have morphologically detectable disease at the completion of the remission induction phase [231, 233, 234]. Induction failure rates tend to be higher in patients with high presenting leukocyte counts and/or T-cell phenotype [185, 186]. Overall, more than 95% of pediatric patients with newly diagnosed ALL achieve complete remission at the end of the first month of treatment, with slightly lower rates in T-ALL compared with B-ALL [138, 164, 165, 231, 235–244].

Several randomized trials have compared two glucocorticoids, prednisone and dexamethasone, during remission induction and subsequent treatment phases. Potential advantages of dexamethasone include more potent in vitro antileukemic activity, higher free plasma levels, and better CNS penetration [245–247]. In nearly all of the randomized trials, dexamethasone was associated with superior event-free survival [234, 248, 249], although in one trial (which closed early due to toxicity concerns with dexamethasone), no advantage was demonstrated for adolescents [250]. Dexamethasone during the remission induction phase has also associated with higher rates of infection, myopathy, hyperglycemia, and behavioral issues [234, 248–250].

Most patients with initial induction failure will eventually achieve complete remission; however the chance for subsequent relapse is quite high, leading to low rates of long-term survival [185–187]. Allogeneic hematopoietic stem cell transplantation (HSCT) after complete remission is achieved (as opposed to continued chemotherapy) may improve the outcome of patients with initial induction failure [251]. In a large retrospective series, a trend for superior overall survival with allogeneic HSCT compared with chemotherapy alone was observed in patients with initial induction failure and either T-ALL (any age) or B-ALL and age greater than 6 years [187].

Post-induction Consolidation

After achieving complete remission, patients typically receive several phases of treatment designed to further decrease levels of residual disease. The intensity of post-induction consolidation is stratified by risk group, with higher risk patients receiving stronger therapy.

A commonly used post-induction consolidation regimen was first introduced by the German Berlin-Frankfurt-Munster (BFM) study group [182], and this scheme has subsequently been adopted by several other large cooperative groups, with variations in some of the doses and agents used. The BFM-type consolidation regimen generally includes (1) a "consolidation" course consisting of cyclophosphamide, low-dose cytarabine, and a thiopurine (mercaptopurine or thioguanine), followed by (2) multiple doses of either high-dose or escalating doses of methotrexate with or without leucovorin rescue, and then (3) a reinduction (or delayed intensification) course, which typically include the same agents used during the initial induction/consolidation cycles [182]. This backbone has been modified on some protocols to eliminate or truncate some of the chemotherapy courses for lower risk patients, and intensified for high-risk patients by more doses of some agents (such as vincristine, pegaspargase, and methotrexate) and/or a second delayed intensification phase [184, 242, 252–256]. Alternative post-induction regimens have been adopted by some groups, with similarly favorable outcome results as those achieved using the BFM-type backbone. For instance, the consolidation phase on trials conducted by the DFCI ALL Consortium includes 20–30 weeks of consecutively dosed L-asparaginase along with frequent pulses of vincristine and corticosteroid, and doxorubicin for higher risk patients [231, 257, 258].

Continuation (Maintenance)

A standard feature of all treatment regimens for childhood ALL is a prolonged continuation or maintenance phase, consisting of daily mercaptopurine and weekly low-dose methotrexate. The importance of this phase is highlighted by results of studies indicating that patients who are compliant with less than 95% of their prescribed mercaptopurine doses have a significantly higher risk of subsequent relapse [212, 213, 218]. Pulses of vincristine and corticosteroid are frequently added to this maintenance backbone, although their benefit remains controversial [259–262]. When vincristine/corticosteroid pulses are used, it appears that dexamethasone is superior to prednisone [248, 249, 258], but also associated with increased risk of behavioral problems and skeletal toxicities [249, 258].

6-Thioguanine has been investigated as an alternative to 6-mercaptopurine during the continuation phase, with conflicting results regarding its impact on event-free survival [263–265]. The use of 6-thioguanine during maintenance has been associated with significant hepatotoxicity, including veno-occlusive disease and cirrhosis, as well as higher remission death rates, primarily caused by infection [263, 264], and so it is not typically used in this phase.

Approximately 0.5–1% of patients have an inherited homozygous deficiency of thiopurine *S*-methyltransferase (TPMT), which catalyzes the inactivation of mercaptopurine [266]. These patients are at increased risk for acute hematologic and hepatic toxicities when given standard doses of mercaptopurine, and can only tolerate much lower dosages [267, 268]. Patients who are heterozygous for this mutation (approximately 10% of the population) have intermediate levels of enzyme activity, generally tolerate mercaptopurine better than those with homozygous deficiencies, but still require dose reductions more frequently than patients who do not carry any mutant allele [267, 268]. Polymorphisms of the *NUTD15* gene, observed most frequently in Hispanic and East Asian patients, have also been associated with extreme sensitivity to mercaptopurine, necessitating significant dose reductions to avoid severe hematologic and hepatic toxicity [269].

On most treatment protocols, maintenance chemotherapy is administered until patients have received a total of 2–2.5 years of treatment from the time of diagnosis. Previous studies suggested that boys might benefit from a more prolonged continuation phase [270], so on some regimens, boys are treated for an additional year; however, the benefit of this approach with more contemporary regimens is not clear. Attempts to shorten therapy duration from 2 years have not been successful. In a randomized comparison of 18 versus 24 months of treatment, patients receiving the shorter duration had a higher rate of relapse [271]. Similarly, very high relapse rates were observed in a nonrandomized trial on which patients received intensified therapy for only

12 months, suggesting that truncated therapy, even if intensive, is inadequate for most children with ALL [272].

CNS-Directed Therapy

Because the central nervous system (CNS) is a sanctuary site into which many of the systemically administered agents used to treat childhood ALL do not effectively penetrate, treatment that is specifically directed at treating CNS leukemia is an essential component of all treatment regimens. Options for CNS-directed therapies include cranial radiation, intrathecal chemotherapy, and CNS penetrant systemic chemotherapy, such as high-dose methotrexate with leucovorin rescue, escalating-dose methotrexate, and dexamethasone. The type of CNS-directed therapy that is used is based on a patient's risk of CNS relapse, with higher risk patients receiving more intensive treatments.

Radiation therapy was the first treatment approach successfully used to prevent CNS relapses. In the 1960s and 1970s, studies performed at St. Jude Children's Research Hospital (SJCRH) documented the effectiveness of CNS radiation (cranial or craniospinal) in children with ALL [273, 274]. Subsequent studies demonstrated that 2400 cGy cranial radiation with intrathecal methotrexate was as effective in preventing CNS relapse as craniospinal radiation without intrathecal chemotherapy [275, 276]. Because craniospinal radiation was associated with increased toxicity, including excessive myelosuppression and spinal growth retardation, cranial radiation administered with intrathecal chemotherapy became the standard form of CNS treatment in the 1970s. Increased recognition of late effects associated with 2400 cGy cranial radiation led to the use of a lower dose (1200–1800 cGy) in trials conducted in the 1980s and 1990s [258, 277, 278].

The proportion of patients receiving cranial radiation has decreased significantly over the last few decades. With contemporary regimens, nearly all pediatric patients are treated without cranial radiation, relying on other CNS-directed therapies, including multiple doses of intrathecal chemotherapy, for CNS prophylaxis. When it is used, radiation is administered only to those patients considered to be at highest risk of subsequent CNS relapse, such as those with CNS-3 status at diagnosis and T-ALL patients with high presenting leukocyte counts and/or slow early response to initial therapy.

Several nonrandomized studies have been conducted in which cranial radiation was omitted for all patients, regardless of risk group status [138, 279, 280]. These trials intensified other CNS-directed therapies for higher risk patients, including additional doses of high-dose methotrexate and/or high-dose cytarabine and increased frequency of intrathecal chemotherapy. Predictors of subsequent CNS relapse on these trials included T-cell phenotype and the presence of blasts in spinal fluid at diagnosis [138]. In a meta-analysis of aggregated data from more than 16,000 patients treated between 1996 and 2007 by ten cooperative groups, only patients with CNS-3 status at diagnosis appeared to benefit from cranial radiation therapy [281]. In this analysis, CNS-3 patients who received cranial radiation had a significantly lower rate of relapses involving the CNS compared with nonirradiated CNS-3 patients; however, the overall 5-year mortality rate for CNS-3 patients was similar whether or not they received radiation.

Treatment Sequelae

As cure rates for childhood ALL have improved over the last several decades, late effects related to the disease and its treatment have become increasingly evident. A number of late effects have been documented in long-term survivors, including neurocognitive sequelae, short stature, obesity, cardiac dysfunction, cataracts, osteonecrosis, and second malignant neoplasms.

Neurocognitive Late Effects

Long-term neurocognitive sequelae have been well documented in survivors of childhood ALL. The frequency and severity of impairments vary by treatment and patient characteristics. Children treated at a younger age, and, in some studies, female patients, are at higher risk for developing neurocognitive late effects [282–288]. The most severely impaired long-term survivors are those who received relatively high cranial radiation doses (24–28 Gy) in the 1970s. Low and low average intelligence quotients (IQs) have been frequent findings in these patients [282, 283, 289], and they also exhibit a high frequency of neuropsychological deficits, including a slow speed of processing information, distractibility, and difficulty in dealing with complex or conceptually demanding material [285, 290]. Long-term survivors treated with lower dose (18 Gy) radiation, especially those who were 3 years or older at diagnosis, appear to fare better, with less severe neurocognitive late effects. In some studies, this group of survivors does not demonstrate any significant cognitive deficits, although subtle effects can be observed in some of these patients with detailed neuropsychological testing [284, 291].

Intrathecal chemotherapy and CNS-penetrant systemic treatments (such as high-dose methotrexate) also appear to contribute to neurocognitive late effects. There is evidence that cognitive deficits are present in long-term survivors treated without cranial radiation [291–294], but these deficits do not tend to be severe and their neurocognitive function is generally within the normal range [288, 295]. In most studies of long-term survivors, nonirradiated patients have fewer and less severe impairments than those who received cranial radiation [283, 296], although with current chemotherapy regimens and lower doses of radiation, differences between the two groups may be subtle [291]. For nonirradiated patients, greater treatment intensity of systemic and intrathecal chemotherapy has been associated with a higher frequency of neuropsychologic deficits and difficulties at school [297].

Skeletal Toxicities

Osteonecrosis, which is observed in 5–10% of children treated for ALL, is a disabling bone toxicity resulting from treatment with glucocorticoids. It is typically diagnosed during the maintenance phase or soon after the completion of therapy, frequently involves multiple joints, and can lead to chronic pain and loss of function, sometimes requiring joint replacement and other surgeries [298–300]. Rates of osteonecrosis are significantly higher in adolescents than in younger children [258, 298, 300]. Adults with ALL do not seem to have as high an incidence of symptomatic osteonecrosis as teenagers, suggesting that the hormonal and physiologic changes of puberty may render adolescents more susceptible to this complication [301]. In addition to age, other risk factors for the development of osteonecrosis include higher total doses of glucocorticoids, female sex, and high body mass index [298, 300]. In some studies, dexamethasone (when used instead of prednisone) has been associated with a higher risk of osteonecrosis, particularly in adolescents [299].

Several studies have shown that children with ALL develop osteopenia during therapy [302, 303], most likely secondary to glucocorticoid exposure, resulting in an increased risk for fractures during and immediately after treatment [304, 305]. It appears that bone mineral density improves once therapy is completed, although some degree of residual osteopenia may persist [306–309].

Cardiac Late Effects

Anthracyclines, such as doxorubicin and daunorubicin, have been associated with cardiotoxicity in long-term survivors, including left ventricular wall thinning and depressed contractility [310]. Patients treated at a young age, females, and those with Down syndrome appear to be more vulnerable to developing anthracycline-associated cardiac toxicity [311, 312]. The severity of cardiac dysfunction is correlated with higher cumulative doses of anthracycline and higher dose rates [311–314]. Over the last few decades, therapeutic regimens have been modified so that patients receive lower cumulative dosages of anthracyclines; as a consequence, symptomatic congestive heart failure has become increasingly uncommon and now only rarely occurs in long-term survivors of childhood ALL [312, 314]. However, asymptomatic echocardiographic abnormalities can still occur, sometimes developing many years after completion of therapy, and may be progressive over time [315]. Randomized clinical trials have demonstrated that use of the cardioprotectant agent dexrazoxane can reduce the frequency of long-term cardiotoxicity in patients receiving relatively high doses of anthracycline without adversely impacting event-free survival rates [316–318].

Second Malignant Neoplasms

Long-term survivors of childhood ALL are at risk for developing second malignant neoplasms (SMNs), including brain tumors, acute myelogenous leukemia (AML), non-Hodgkin's lymphomas, and carcinomas of the parotid and thyroid glands [319–321]. The overall cumulative incidence of SMNs reported in the literature ranges from 1 to 6%, depending on the treatment regimen and length of follow-up [319, 320]. In a retrospective study of 2169 patients treated between 1962 and 1998 (median follow-up 18.7 years), the overall cumulative incidence of SMN was approximately 4% at 15 years and 11% at 30 years [320]. When benign neoplasms, such as basal cell carcinoma and meningioma, were excluded from that analysis, the cumulative incidence of SMNs at 30 years was approximately 6%.

Malignant gliomas and nonmalignant meningiomas occur almost exclusively in patients who received cranial or craniospinal radiation [319, 320]. The cumulative incidence of malignant glioma in irradiated survivors appears to plateau approximately 15–20 years after diagnosis; conversely, even with 30 years of follow-up, a plateau in the incidence of meningiomas has not been observed [320]. Cranial radiation has also been associated with the development of vascular malformations, which can lead to neurological symptoms and intracranial hemorrhage [322]. Rates of secondary AML are increased in patients who receive higher total (and/or more frequent) doses of epipodophyllotoxins and alkylating agents [323–325]. Some studies have suggested that secondary leukemia risk may also be increased in patients with homozygous or heterozygous deficiencies in thiopurine methyltransferase (an enzyme involved in the metabolism of mercaptopurine) [326].

Relapse

Approximately 15% of children with ALL who achieve complete remission will subsequently relapse. Relapses tend to occur during the first 5 years after initial diagnosis, but can occur as late as 10 years [327]. The most common site of relapse is the bone marrow, with or without overt extramedullary involvement; more uncommonly, relapse can sometimes only be detectable only in an extramedullary site, such as the CNS or testes.

Duration of initial remission is one of the most important prognostic factors at the time of relapse, with significantly worse outcomes observed in patients with shorter initial remissions [328–330]. Site of relapse also has prognostic importance, with superior outcomes observed for patients experiencing isolated extramedullary relapses compared with marrow relapses [329, 330]. Some studies have suggested that patients with combined marrow and extramedullary relapses have a better prognosis than those with isolated marrow relapses [328, 330], although this has not been consistently demonstrated [329]. T-cell phenotype and age older than 10 years at initial diagnosis have also been associated with an adverse prognosis after relapse [328–330], as has response to initial reinduction chemotherapy assessed by sensitive minimal residual disease (MRD) tests [331, 332].

Marrow Relapse

Approximately 80–90% of children experiencing a marrow relapse will achieve a second complete remission, often with agents similar to those used at the time of initial diagnosis [333, 334]; second complete remission rates are lower in those relapsing early and/or with T-ALL [328, 333, 335, 336]. Patients with persistent morphologic disease at the end of the first month of reinduction have a very poor prognosis, even if they subsequently achieve a second remission [337].

For B-ALL patients with early marrow relapses (defined as those occurring earlier than 30–36 months from initial diagnosis), allogeneic hematopoietic stem cell transplant (HSCT) has consistently been shown to be superior to chemotherapy-only approaches, although even with HSCT, long-term survival rates are less than 50% [338–340]. Patients with T-ALL, regardless of timing of relapse, are also generally treated with allogeneic HSCT because of poor survival rates with chemotherapy-only salvage therapy [341].

For B-ALL patients with a late marrow relapse, a chemotherapy-only approach leads to survival rates of approximately 50%, and it not clear that allogeneic HSCT is associated with superior outcome [328, 329, 338, 342]. End-reinduction minimal residual disease (MRD) levels strongly predict the prognosis of late-relapsing patients treated with chemotherapy only [331, 332]. Those with low MRD at this time point fare relatively well (event-free survival rates exceeding 70%), while those with higher MRD levels have a significantly greater risk of subsequent relapse [331, 332]. In one study, allogeneic stem cell transplant was associated with an improved outcome (compared to historic controls treated with chemotherapy only) in late-relapsing patients with high MRD levels at the end of reinduction [343].

For relapsed ALL patients who proceed to allogeneic HSCT, the components of the preparative regimen appear to impact the outcome; several studies have shown that regimens that include total body irradiation (TBI) are associated with better outcomes than those that do not [338, 344]. MRD levels at the time of transplant are also highly prognostic; patients with MRD-detectable disease just prior to HSCT fare worse than those with non-detectable levels [345–348].

Isolated Extramedullary Relapses

Isolated extramedullary relapses occur in fewer than 5% of patients. Using sensitive molecular techniques, submicroscopic marrow disease can be demonstrated in most children at the time of an isolated extramedullary relapse [349]. Thus, successful treatment strategies must address both the local site of relapse and submicroscopic systemic disease.

For patients with isolated CNS relapses, therapy typically involves intensive systemic chemotherapy with cranial radiation [350–352]. As with marrow relapses, patients experiencing late isolated CNS relapses have a better prognosis than those whose relapses occur earlier [329, 351–353], although a different cutoff is used to distinguish early versus late because of the overall more favorable outcome associated with extramedullary relapses. On two consecutive clinical trials conducted by the Pediatric Oncology Group, children with B-ALL and a late isolated CNS relapse (defined as initial remission duration of at least 18 months) had EFS rates exceeding 75% when treated with intensive chemotherapy and delayed cranial radiation, while patients with earlier relapses fared less well [351, 352]. It is not clear that allogeneic HSCT is associated with a survival advantage for patients with an isolated CNS relapse, even those with early relapses [354, 355]. Patients whose initial therapy included cranial radiation may have a worse prognosis after an isolated CNS relapse than previously unirradiated patients [350].

Isolated testicular relapses are uncommon, occurring in less than 1% of boys with ALL [239, 240]. For boys with isolated testicular relapses, systemic chemotherapy and testicular radiation and/or orchiectomy have resulted in prolonged second remissions in more than 80% of patients with late-occurring relapses [356, 357], with worse outcomes reported for those with earlier relapses [356, 358].

Future Directions

The improvement in cure rates for childhood ALL over the last several decades is due to the development of effective multiagent chemotherapy regimens, enhanced supportive care, successful implementation of risk-adapted therapy, and advances in the understanding of disease biology. Despite this remarkable progress, some leukemia subtypes still respond poorly, and for patients who are successfully treated, therapy remains, to the large part, nonspecific and associated with multiple acute and long-term toxicities. Thus, there remains a need to further refine risk stratification and to develop more effective and potentially less toxic therapies.

Investigations of the genomic landscape of ALL have identified biologically distinctive subsets that may supplement or replace the currently applied clinical risk factors in order to identify those patients at highest risk of treatment failure [27, 64, 103, 104, 160, 359]. Druggable molecular lesions identified in various ALL subsets may lead to incorporation of targeted therapies, such as ABL-kinase and/or JAK-STAT inhibitors for *BCR-ABL1*-like ALL and epigenetic-modifying agents for *KMT2A*-rearranged ALL [109, 360]. In addition, research focused on germline genetic variation and pharmacogenomics may identify patient-related factors that affect the outcome and vulnerability to treatment-related toxicities, leading to more individualized therapy [361, 362]. The use of more sensitive molecular measures to assess minimal residual disease levels may enhance evaluation of early response [192, 348].

Novel therapies with the potential to improve outcomes include immunotherapeutic approaches. Although varying in their mechanisms of action, all of these approaches target cell surface antigens expressed on lymphoblasts, including CD19 and CD22 (nearly universally expressed in B-ALL), and thus represent a more targeted treatment strategy than current, nonspecific cytotoxic chemotherapy agents. Rituximab (anti-CD20 monoclonal antibody) has demonstrated benefit in adults with newly diagnosed CD20-positive ALL when given in combination with chemotherapy [363], and administration of single-agent inotuzumab ozogamycin, a recombinant immunotoxin consisting of humanized anti-CD22 antibody linked to calicheamicin, led to high complete remission rates in relapsed, refractory adult B-ALL patients [364]. Blinatumomab, a bi-specific (anti-CD3-anti-CD19 antibody) T-cell engager, has demonstrated single-agent activity in adult and pediatric relapsed B-ALL patients, and also has been shown to reduce minimal residual disease in those who had already achieved complete remission [365–367].

Cellular therapy using genetically engineered autologous chimeric antigen receptor (CAR) T-cells is an emerging and very promising immunotherapeutic approach. CAR T-cell therapy involves collection of autologous T-cells from patients, ex vivo genetic engineering to induce expression of ALL-specific chimeric antigen receptors along with additional co-stimulatory domains, and then reinfusion into the patient, typically after a chemotherapy preparative regimen [368, 369]. Phase 1 and 2 trials of CD19-directed CAR T-cells in relapsed/refractory pediatric and adult B-ALL patients have demonstrated high response rates, with some patients achieving sustained remissions without further treatment [369–371]. While there are many unanswered questions regarding CAR T-cells (duration of response, mechanisms of resistance, prevention of acute toxicities, potential long-term sequelae), the promising early outcome results highlight the potential of this treatment approach to transform therapy for relapsed and high-risk newly diagnosed ALL patients.

References

1. Smith MA, Seibel NL, Altekruse SF, Ries LA, Melbert DL, O'Leary M, et al. Outcomes for children and adolescents with cancer: challenges for the twenty-first century. J Clin Oncol. 2010;28(15):2625–34.
2. van Dongen JJ, Wolvers-Tettero IL. Analysis of immunoglobulin and T cell receptor genes. Part II: Possibilities and limitations in the diagnosis and management of lymphoproliferative diseases and related disorders. Clin Chim Acta. 1991;198(1–2):81.
3. Bernt KM, Armstrong SA. Leukemia stem cells and human acute lymphoblastic leukemia. Semin Hematol. 2009;46(1):33–8.
4. Bernt KM, Hunger SP, Neff T. The functional role of PRC2 in early T-cell precursor acute lymphoblastic leukemia (ETP-ALL)—mechanisms and opportunities. Front Pediatr. 2016;4:49.
5. SEER Cancer Statistics Review, 1975–2013 [Internet]. 2015 [cited August 2016].
6. Siegel RL, Miller KD, Jemal A. Cancer statistics, 2016. CA Cancer J Clin. 2016;66(1):7–30.
7. Kaatsch P, Steliarova-Foucher E, Crocetti E, Magnani C, Spix C, Zambon P. Time trends of cancer incidence in European children (1978–1997): report from the Automated Childhood Cancer Information System project. Eur J Cancer. 2006;42(13):1961–71.
8. Spector LG, Ross JA. Infant leukemia: finding the needle in the haystack. Cancer Epidemiol Biomark Prev. 2006;15(12):2331.
9. Couto E, Chen B, Hemminki K. Association of childhood acute lymphoblastic leukaemia with cancers in family members. Br J Cancer. 2005;93(11):1307–9.
10. Spector LG, Ross JA, Robison LL, Bhatia S. Epidemiology and etiology. In: Pui CH, editor. Childhood leukemias. 2nd ed. Cambridge: Cambridge University Press; 2006. p. 48–66.
11. Greaves M. In utero origins of childhood leukaemia. Early Hum Dev. 2005;81(1):123–9.
12. Greaves MF, Maia AT, Wiemels JL, Ford AM. Leukemia in twins: lessons in natural history. Blood. 2003;102(7):2321–33.
13. Maia AT, Ford AM, Jalali GR, Harrison CJ, Taylor GM, Eden OB, et al. Molecular tracking of leukemogenesis in a triplet pregnancy. Blood. 2001;98(2):478–82.
14. Wiemels JL, Cazzaniga G, Daniotti M, Eden OB, Addison GM, Masera G, et al. Prenatal origin of acute lymphoblastic leukaemia in children. Lancet. 1999;354(9189):1499–503.
15. Greaves M. Infection, immune responses and the aetiology of childhood leukaemia. Nat Rev Cancer. 2006;6(3):193–203.
16. Hong D, Gupta R, Ancliff P, Atzberger A, Brown J, Soneji S, et al. Initiating and cancer-propagating cells in TEL-AML1-associated childhood leukemia. Science. 2008;319(5861):336–9.
17. Ross JA, Spector LG, Robison LL, Olshan AF. Epidemiology of leukemia in children with Down syndrome. Pediatr Blood Cancer. 2005;44(1):8–12.
18. Sandler DP, Ross JA. Epidemiology of acute leukemia in children and adults. Semin Oncol. 1997;24(1):3–16.

19. Bercovich D, Ganmore I, Scott LM, Wainreb G, Birger Y, Elimelech A, et al. Mutations of JAK2 in acute lymphoblastic leukaemias associated with Down's syndrome. Lancet. 2008;372(9648):1484–92.
20. Gaikwad A, Rye CL, Devidas M, Heerema NA, Carroll AJ, Izraeli S, et al. Prevalence and clinical correlates of JAK2 mutations in Down syndrome acute lymphoblastic leukaemia. Br J Haematol. 2009;144(6):930–2.
21. Kearney L, Gonzalez De Castro D, Yeung J, Procter J, Horsley SW, Eguchi-Ishimae M, et al. Specific JAK2 mutation (JAK2R683) and multiple gene deletions in Down syndrome acute lymphoblastic leukemia. Blood. 2009;113(3):646–8.
22. Mullighan CG, Zhang J, Harvey RC, Collins-Underwood JR, Schulman BA, Phillips LA, et al. JAK mutations in high-risk childhood acute lymphoblastic leukemia. Proc Natl Acad Sci U S A. 2009;106(23):9414–8.
23. Maloney KW, Carroll WL, Carroll AJ, Devidas M, Borowitz MJ, Martin PL, et al. Down syndrome childhood acute lymphoblastic leukemia has a unique spectrum of sentinel cytogenetic lesions that influences treatment outcome: a report from the Children's Oncology Group. Blood. 2010;116(7):1045–50.
24. Bhatia S, Neglia JP. Epidemiology of childhood acute myelogenous leukemia. J Pediatr Hematol Oncol. 1995;17(2):94–100.
25. Louie S, Schwartz RS. Immunodeficiency and the pathogenesis of lymphoma and leukemia. Semin Hematol. 1978;15(2):117–38.
26. Liberzon E, Avigad S, Stark B, Zilberstein J, Freedman L, Gorfine M, et al. Germ-line ATM gene alterations are associated with susceptibility to sporadic T-cell acute lymphoblastic leukemia in children. Genes Chromosomes Cancer. 2004;39(2):161–6.
27. Holmfeldt L, Wei L, Diaz-Flores E, Walsh M, Zhang J, Ding L, et al. The genomic landscape of hypodiploid acute lymphoblastic leukemia. Nat Genet. 2013;45(3):242–52.
28. Papaemmanuil E, Hosking FJ, Vijayakrishnan J, Price A, Olver B, Sheridan E, et al. Loci on 7p12.2, 10q21.2 and 14q11.2 are associated with risk of childhood acute lymphoblastic leukemia. Nat Genet. 2009;41(9):1006–10.
29. Trevino LR, Yang W, French D, Hunger SP, Carroll WL, Devidas M, et al. Germline genomic variants associated with childhood acute lymphoblastic leukemia. Nat Genet. 2009;41(9):1001–5.
30. Migliorini G, Fiege B, Hosking FJ, Ma Y, Kumar R, Sherborne AL, et al. Variation at 10p12.2 and 10p14 influences risk of childhood B-cell acute lymphoblastic leukemia and phenotype. Blood. 2013;122(19):3298–307.
31. Sherborne AL, Hosking FJ, Prasad RB, Kumar R, Koehler R, Vijayakrishnan J, et al. Variation in CDKN2A at 9p21.3 influences childhood acute lymphoblastic leukemia risk. Nat Genet. 2010;42(6):492–4.
32. Xu H, Yang W, Perez-Andreu V, Devidas M, Fan Y, Cheng C, et al. Novel susceptibility variants at 10p12.31-12.2 for childhood acute lymphoblastic leukemia in ethnically diverse populations. J Natl Cancer Inst. 2013;105(10):733–42.
33. Moriyama T, Relling MV, Yang JJ. Inherited genetic variation in childhood acute lymphoblastic leukemia. Blood. 2015;125(26):3988–95.
34. Doll R, Wakeford R. Risk of childhood cancer from fetal irradiation. Br J Radiol. 1997;70:130–9.
35. Ahlbom A, Day N, Feychting M, Roman E, Skinner J, Dockerty J, et al. A pooled analysis of magnetic fields and childhood leukaemia. Br J Cancer. 2000;83(5):692–8.
36. Buffler PA, Kwan ML, Reynolds P, Urayama KY. Environmental and genetic risk factors for childhood leukemia: appraising the evidence. Cancer Investig. 2005;23(1):60–75.
37. Chang JS. Parental smoking and childhood leukemia. Methods Mol Biol. 2009;472:103–37.
38. Orsi L, Rudant J, Ajrouche R, Leverger G, Baruchel A, Nelken B, et al. Parental smoking, maternal alcohol, coffee and tea consumption during pregnancy, and childhood acute leukemia: the ESTELLE study. Cancer Causes Control. 2015;26(7):1003–17.
39. Slater ME, Linabery AM, Blair CK, Spector LG, Heerema NA, Robison LL, et al. Maternal prenatal cigarette, alcohol and illicit drug use and risk of infant leukaemia: a report from the Children's Oncology Group. Paediatr Perinat Epidemiol. 2011;25(6):559–65.
40. Weng HH, Tsai SS, Chiu HF, Wu TN, Yang CY. Association of childhood leukemia with residential exposure to petrochemical air pollution in Taiwan. Inhal Toxicol. 2008;20(1):31–6.
41. Alexander FE, Patheal SL, Biondi A, Brandalise S, Cabrera ME, Chan LC, et al. Transplacental chemical exposure and risk of infant leukemia with MLL gene fusion. Cancer Res. 2001;61(6):2542–6.
42. Slater ME, Linabery AM, Spector LG, Johnson KJ, Hilden JM, Heerema NA, et al. Maternal exposure to household chemicals and risk of infant leukemia: a report from the Children's Oncology Group. Cancer Causes Control. 2011;22(8):1197–204.
43. Pullen J, Shuster JJ, Link M, Borowitz M, Amylon M, Carroll AJ, et al. Significance of commonly used prognostic factors differs for children with T cell acute lymphocytic leukemia (ALL), as compared to those with B-precursor ALL. A Pediatric Oncology Group (POG) study. Leukemia. 1999;13(11):1696–707.
44. Goldberg JM, Silverman LB, Levy DE, Dalton VK, Gelber RD, Lehmann L, et al. Childhood T-cell acute lymphoblastic leukemia: the Dana-Farber Cancer Institute acute lymphoblastic leukemia consortium experience. J Clin Oncol. 2003;21(19):3616–22.
45. Hogan TF, Koss W, Murgo AJ, Amato RS, Fontana JA, VanScoy FL. Acute lymphoblastic leukemia with chromosomal 5;14 translocation and hypereosinophilia: case report and literature review. J Clin Oncol. 1987;5(3):382–90.
46. Levinsen M, Marquart HV, Groth-Pedersen L, Abrahamsson J, Albertsen BK, Andersen MK, et al. Leukemic blasts are present at low levels in spinal fluid in one-third of childhood acute lymphoblastic leukemia cases. Pediatr Blood Cancer. 2016;63(11):1935–42.
47. Inukai T, Hirose K, Inaba T, Kurosawa H, Hama A, Inada H, et al. Hypercalcemia in childhood acute lymphoblastic leukemia: frequent implication of parathyroid hormone-related peptide and E2A-HLF from translocation 17;19. Leukemia. 2007;21(2):288–96.
48. Ribeiro RC, Pui CH. The clinical and biological correlates of coagulopathy in children with acute leukemia. J Clin Oncol. 1986;4(8):1212–8.
49. Raimondi SC, Privitera E, Williams DL, Look AT, Behm F, Rivera GK, et al. New recurring chromosomal translocations in childhood acute lymphoblastic leukemia. Blood. 1991;77(9):2016–22.
50. Bennett JM, Catovsky D, Daniel MT, Flandrin G, Galton DA, Gralnick HR, et al. Proposals for the classification of the acute leukaemias. French-American-British (FAB) co-operative group. Br J Haematol. 1976;33(4):451–8.
51. van Eys J, Pullen J, Head D, Boyett J, Crist W, Falletta J, et al. The French-American-British (FAB) classification of leukemia. The Pediatric Oncology Group experience with lymphocytic leukemia. Cancer. 1986;57(5):1046–51.
52. Campana D, Behm FG. Immunophenotyping of leukemia. J Immunol Methods. 2000;243(1–2):59–75.
53. Seegmiller AC, Kroft SH, Karandikar NJ, McKenna RW. Characterization of immunophenotypic aberrancies in 200 cases of B acute lymphoblastic leukemia. Am J Clin Pathol. 2009;132(6):940–9.
54. Chen CS, Sorensen PH, Domer PH, Reaman GH, Korsmeyer SJ, Heerema NA, et al. Molecular rearrangements on chromosome 11q23 predominate in infant acute lymphoblastic leukemia and are associated with specific biologic variables and poor outcome. Blood. 1993;81(9):2386–93.
55. Pui CH, Behm FG, Downing JR, Hancock ML, Shurtleff SA, Ribeiro RC, et al. 11q23/MLL rearrangement confers a poor prognosis in infants with acute lymphoblastic leukemia. J Clin Oncol. 1994;12(5):909–15.
56. Jeha S, Behm F, Pei D, Sandlund JT, Ribeiro RC, Razzouk BI, et al. Prognostic significance of CD20 expression in childhood B-cell precursor acute lymphoblastic leukemia. Blood. 2006;108(10):3302–4.

57. Dworzak MN, Schumich A, Printz D, Potschger U, Husak Z, Attarbaschi A, et al. CD20 up-regulation in pediatric B-cell precursor acute lymphoblastic leukemia during induction treatment: setting the stage for anti-CD20 directed immunotherapy. Blood. 2008;112(10):3982–8.
58. Koehler M, Behm FG, Shuster J, Crist W, Borowitz M, Look AT, et al. Transitional pre-B-cell acute lymphoblastic leukemia of childhood is associated with favorable prognostic clinical features and an excellent outcome: a Pediatric Oncology Group study. Leukemia. 1993;7(12):2064–8.
59. Dalla-Favera R, Bregni M, Erikson J, Patterson D, Gallo RC, Croce CM. Human c-myc onc gene is located on the region of chromosome 8 that is translocated in Burkitt lymphoma cells. Proc Natl Acad Sci U S A. 1982;79(24):7824–7.
60. Patte C, Auperin A, Michon J, Behrendt H, Leverger G, Frappaz D, et al. The Societe Francaise d'Oncologie Pediatrique LMB89 protocol: highly effective multiagent chemotherapy tailored to the tumor burden and initial response in 561 unselected children with B-cell lymphomas and L3 leukemia. Blood. 2001;97(11):3370–9.
61. Campana D, Thompson JS, Amlot P, Brown S, Janossy G. The cytoplasmic expression of CD3 antigens in normal and malignant cells of the T lymphoid lineage. J Immunol. 1987;138(2):648–55.
62. Campana D, van Dongen JJ, Mehta A, Coustan-Smith E, Wolvers-Tettero IL, Ganeshaguru K, et al. Stages of T-cell receptor protein expression in T-cell acute lymphoblastic leukemia. Blood. 1991;77(7):1546–54.
63. Han YS, Xue YQ, Zhang J. Clinical and molecular cytogenetic studies of a case of B-lineage acute lymphoblastic leukemia with t(14;14)(q11;q32). Zhonghua Yi Xue Yi Chuan Xue Za Zhi. 2012;29(2):137–40.
64. Coustan-Smith E, Mullighan CG, Onciu M, Behm FG, Raimondi SC, Pei D, et al. Early T-cell precursor leukaemia: a subtype of very high-risk acute lymphoblastic leukaemia. Lancet Oncol. 2009;10(2):147–56.
65. Bell JJ, Bhandoola A. The earliest thymic progenitors for T cells possess myeloid lineage potential. Nature. 2008;452(7188):764–7.
66. Rothenberg EV, Moore JE, Yui MA. Launching the T-cell-lineage developmental programme. Nat Rev Immunol. 2008;8(1):9–21.
67. Inukai T, Kiyokawa N, Campana D, Coustan-Smith E, Kikuchi A, Kobayashi M, et al. Clinical significance of early T-cell precursor acute lymphoblastic leukaemia: results of the Tokyo Children's Cancer Study Group Study L99-15. Br J Haematol. 2012;156(3):358–65.
68. Patrick K, Wade R, Goulden N, Mitchell C, Moorman AV, Rowntree C, et al. Outcome for children and young people with Early T-cell precursor acute lymphoblastic leukaemia treated on a contemporary protocol, UKALL 2003. Br J Haematol. 2014;166(3):421–4.
69. Wiersma SR, Ortega J, Sobel E, Weinberg KI. Clinical importance of myeloid-antigen expression in acute lymphoblastic leukemia of childhood. N Engl J Med. 1991;324(12):800–8.
70. Pui CH, Behm FG, Singh B, Rivera GK, Schell MJ, Roberts WM, et al. Myeloid-associated antigen expression lacks prognostic value in childhood acute lymphoblastic leukemia treated with intensive multiagent chemotherapy. Blood. 1990;75(1):198–202.
71. Uckun FM, Sather HN, Gaynon PS, Arthur DC, Trigg ME, Tubergen DG, et al. Clinical features and treatment outcome of children with myeloid antigen positive acute lymphoblastic leukemia: a report from the Children's Cancer Group. Blood. 1997;90(1):28–35.
72. Pui CH, Rubnitz JE, Hancock ML, Downing JR, Raimondi SC, Rivera GK, et al. Reappraisal of the clinical and biologic significance of myeloid-associated antigen expression in childhood acute lymphoblastic leukemia. J Clin Oncol. 1998;16(12):3768–73.
73. Vardiman JW, Thiele J, Arber DA, Brunning RD, Borowitz MJ, Porwit A, et al. The 2008 revision of the World Health Organization (WHO) classification of myeloid neoplasms and acute leukemia: rationale and important changes. Blood. 2009;114(5):937–51.
74. Paulsson K, Johansson B. High hyperdiploid childhood acute lymphoblastic leukemia. Genes Chromosomes Cancer. 2009;48(8):637–60.
75. Paulsson K, Forestier E, Andersen MK, Autio K, Barbany G, Borgstrom G, et al. High modal number and triple trisomies are highly correlated favorable factors in childhood B-cell precursor high hyperdiploid acute lymphoblastic leukemia treated according to the NOPHO ALL 1992/2000 protocols. Haematologica. 2013;98(9):1424–32.
76. Paulsson K, Forestier E, Lilljebjorn H, Heldrup J, Behrendtz M, Young BD, et al. Genetic landscape of high hyperdiploid childhood acute lymphoblastic leukemia. Proc Natl Acad Sci U S A. 2010;107(50):21719–24.
77. Moorman AV, Ensor HM, Richards SM, Chilton L, Schwab C, Kinsey SE, et al. Prognostic effect of chromosomal abnormalities in childhood B-cell precursor acute lymphoblastic leukaemia: results from the UK Medical Research Council ALL97/99 randomised trial. Lancet Oncol. 2010;11(5):429–38.
78. Schultz KR, Pullen DJ, Sather HN, Shuster JJ, Devidas M, Borowitz MJ, et al. Risk- and response-based classification of childhood B-precursor acute lymphoblastic leukemia: a combined analysis of prognostic markers from the Pediatric Oncology Group (POG) and Children's Cancer Group (CCG). Blood. 2007;109(3):926–35.
79. Raimondi SC, Zhou Y, Shurtleff SA, Rubnitz JE, Pui CH, Behm FG. Near-triploidy and near-tetraploidy in childhood acute lymphoblastic leukemia: association with B-lineage blast cells carrying the ETV6-RUNX1 fusion, T-lineage immunophenotype, and favorable outcome. Cancer Genet Cytogenet. 2006;169(1):50–7.
80. Lemez P, Attarbaschi A, Bene MC, Bertrand Y, Castoldi G, Forestier E, et al. Childhood near-tetraploid acute lymphoblastic leukemia: an EGIL study on 36 cases. Eur J Haematol. 2010;85(4):300–8.
81. Attarbaschi A, Mann G, Konig M, Dworzak MN, Trebo MM, Muhlegger N, et al. Incidence and relevance of secondary chromosome abnormalities in childhood TEL/AML1+ acute lymphoblastic leukemia: an interphase FISH analysis. Leukemia. 2004;18(10):1611–6.
82. Heerema NA, Nachman JB, Sather HN, Sensel MG, Lee MK, Hutchinson R, et al. Hypodiploidy with less than 45 chromosomes confers adverse risk in childhood acute lymphoblastic leukemia: a report from the Children's Cancer Group. Blood. 1999;94(12):4036–45.
83. Nachman JB, Heerema NA, Sather H, Camitta B, Forestier E, Harrison CJ, et al. Outcome of treatment in children with hypodiploid acute lymphoblastic leukemia. Blood. 2007;110(4):1112–5.
84. Safavi S, Paulsson K. Near-haploid and low-hypodiploid acute lymphoblastic leukemia: two distinct subtypes with consistently poor prognosis. Blood. 2017;129(4):420–3.
85. Shurtleff SA, Buijs A, Behm FG, Rubnitz JE, Raimondi SC, Hancock ML, et al. TEL/AML1 fusion resulting from a cryptic t(12;21) is the most common genetic lesion in pediatric ALL and defines a subgroup of patients with an excellent prognosis. Leukemia. 1995;9(12):1985–9.
86. Romana SP, Mauchauffe M, Le Coniat M, Chumakov I, Le Paslier D, Berger R, et al. The t(12;21) of acute lymphoblastic leukemia results in a tel-AML1 gene fusion. Blood. 1995;85(12):3662–70.
87. Loh ML, Goldwasser MA, Silverman LB, Poon WM, Vattikuti S, Cardoso A, et al. Prospective analysis of TEL/AML1-positive patients treated on Dana-Farber Cancer Institute Consortium Protocol 95-01. Blood. 2006;107(11):4508–13.
88. Harrison CJ, Moorman AV, Barber KE, Broadfield ZJ, Cheung KL, Harris RL, et al. Interphase molecular cytogenetic screening for chromosomal abnormalities of prognostic significance in childhood acute lymphoblastic leukaemia: a UK Cancer Cytogenetics Group Study. Br J Haematol. 2005;129(4):520–30.
89. Forestier E, Andersen MK, Autio K, Blennow E, Borgstrom G, Golovleva I, et al. Cytogenetic patterns in ETV6/RUNX1-positive pediatric B-cell precursor acute lymphoblastic leukemia: a Nordic series of 245 cases and review of the literature. Genes Chromosomes Cancer. 2007;46(5):440–50.

90. Rubnitz JE, Wichlan D, Devidas M, Shuster J, Linda SB, Kurtzberg J, et al. Prospective analysis of TEL gene rearrangements in childhood acute lymphoblastic leukemia: a Children's Oncology Group study. J Clin Oncol. 2008;26(13):2186–91.
91. Forestier E, Schmiegelow K. The incidence peaks of the childhood acute leukemias reflect specific cytogenetic aberrations. J Pediatr Hematol Oncol. 2006;28(8):486–95.
92. Hock H, Meade E, Medeiros S, Schindler JW, Valk PJ, Fujiwara Y, et al. Tel/Etv6 is an essential and selective regulator of adult hematopoietic stem cell survival. Genes Dev. 2004;18(19):2336–41.
93. Zelent A, Greaves M, Enver T. Role of the TEL-AML1 fusion gene in the molecular pathogenesis of childhood acute lymphoblastic leukaemia. Oncogene. 2004;23(24):4275–83.
94. Mori H, Colman SM, Xiao Z, Ford AM, Healy LE, Donaldson C, et al. Chromosome translocations and covert leukemic clones are generated during normal fetal development. Proc Natl Acad Sci U S A. 2002;99(12):8242–7.
95. Bateman CM, Colman SM, Chaplin T, Young BD, Eden TO, Bhakta M, et al. Acquisition of genome-wide copy number alterations in monozygotic twins with acute lymphoblastic leukemia. Blood. 2010;115(17):3553–8.
96. Hermans A, Gow J, Selleri L, von Lindern M, Hagemeijer A, Wiedemann LM, et al. bcr-abl oncogene activation in Philadelphia chromosome-positive acute lymphoblastic leukemia. Leukemia. 1988;2(10):628–33.
97. Hermans A, Heisterkamp N, von Linden M, van Baal S, Meijer D, van der Plas D, et al. Unique fusion of bcr and c-abl genes in Philadelphia chromosome positive acute lymphoblastic leukemia. Cell. 1987;51(1):33–40.
98. van der Veer A, Zaliova M, Mottadelli F, De Lorenzo P, Te Kronnie G, Harrison CJ, et al. IKZF1 status as a prognostic feature in BCR-ABL1-positive childhood ALL. Blood. 2014;123(11):1691–8.
99. Uckun FM, Nachman JB, Sather HN, Sensel MG, Kraft P, Steinherz PG, et al. Clinical significance of Philadelphia chromosome positive pediatric acute lymphoblastic leukemia in the context of contemporary intensive therapies: a report from the Children's Cancer Group. Cancer. 1998;83(9):2030–9.
100. Arico M, Schrappe M, Hunger SP, Carroll WL, Conter V, Galimberti S, et al. Clinical outcome of children with newly diagnosed Philadelphia chromosome-positive acute lymphoblastic leukemia treated between 1995 and 2005. J Clin Oncol. 2010;28(31):4755–61.
101. Biondi A, Schrappe M, De Lorenzo P, Castor A, Lucchini G, Gandemer V, et al. Imatinib after induction for treatment of children and adolescents with Philadelphia-chromosome-positive acute lymphoblastic leukaemia (EsPhALL): a randomised, open-label, intergroup study. Lancet Oncol. 2012;13(9):936–45.
102. Schultz KR, Carroll A, Heerema NA, Bowman WP, Aledo A, Slayton WB, et al. Long-term follow-up of imatinib in pediatric Philadelphia chromosome-positive acute lymphoblastic leukemia: Children's Oncology Group study AALL0031. Leukemia. 2014;28(7):1467–71.
103. Den Boer ML, van Slegtenhorst M, De Menezes RX, Cheok MH, Buijs-Gladdines JG, Peters ST, et al. A subtype of childhood acute lymphoblastic leukaemia with poor treatment outcome: a genome-wide classification study. Lancet Oncol. 2009;10(2):125–34.
104. Mullighan CG, Su X, Zhang J, Radtke I, Phillips LA, Miller CB, et al. Deletion of IKZF1 and prognosis in acute lymphoblastic leukemia. N Engl J Med. 2009;360(5):470–80.
105. Palmi C, Savino AM, Silvestri D, Bronzini I, Cario G, Paganin M, et al. CRLF2 over-expression is a poor prognostic marker in children with high risk T-cell acute lymphoblastic leukemia. Oncotarget. 2016;7(37):59260–72.
106. Roberts KG, Li Y, Payne-Turner D, Harvey RC, Yang YL, Pei D, et al. Targetable kinase-activating lesions in Ph-like acute lymphoblastic leukemia. N Engl J Med. 2014;371(11):1005–15.
107. van der Veer A, Waanders E, Pieters R, Willemse ME, Van Reijmersdal SV, Russell LJ, et al. Independent prognostic value of BCR-ABL1-like signature and IKZF1 deletion, but not high CRLF2 expression, in children with B-cell precursor ALL. Blood. 2013;122(15):2622–9.
108. Maude SL, Tasian SK, Vincent T, Hall JW, Sheen C, Roberts KG, et al. Targeting JAK1/2 and mTOR in murine xenograft models of Ph-like acute lymphoblastic leukemia. Blood. 2012;120(17):3510–8.
109. Roberts KG, Morin RD, Zhang J, Hirst M, Zhao Y, Su X, et al. Genetic alterations activating kinase and cytokine receptor signaling in high-risk acute lymphoblastic leukemia. Cancer Cell. 2012;22(2):153–66.
110. Clappier E, Grardel N, Bakkus M, Rapion J, De Moerloose B, Kastner P, et al. IKZF1 deletion is an independent prognostic marker in childhood B-cell precursor acute lymphoblastic leukemia, and distinguishes patients benefiting from pulses during maintenance therapy: results of the EORTC Children's Leukemia Group study 58951. Leukemia. 2015;29(11):2154–61.
111. Buitenkamp TD, Pieters R, Gallimore NE, van der Veer A, Meijerink JP, Beverloo HB, et al. Outcome in children with Down's syndrome and acute lymphoblastic leukemia: role of IKZF1 deletions and CRLF2 aberrations. Leukemia. 2012;26(10):2204–11.
112. Mullighan CG, Miller CB, Radtke I, Phillips LA, Dalton J, Ma J, et al. BCR-ABL1 lymphoblastic leukaemia is characterized by the deletion of Ikaros. Nature. 2008;453(7191):110–4.
113. Dorge P, Meissner B, Zimmermann M, Moricke A, Schrauder A, Bouquin JP, et al. IKZF1 deletion is an independent predictor of outcome in pediatric acute lymphoblastic leukemia treated according to the ALL-BFM 2000 protocol. Haematologica. 2013;98(3):428–32.
114. Olsson L, Ivanov Ofverholm I, Noren-Nystrom U, Zachariadis V, Nordlund J, Sjogren H, et al. The clinical impact of IKZF1 deletions in paediatric B-cell precursor acute lymphoblastic leukaemia is independent of minimal residual disease stratification in Nordic Society for Paediatric Haematology and Oncology treatment protocols used between 1992 and 2013. Br J Haematol. 2015;170(6):847–58.
115. Clappier E, Auclerc MF, Rapion J, Bakkus M, Caye A, Khemiri A, et al. An intragenic ERG deletion is a marker of an oncogenic subtype of B-cell precursor acute lymphoblastic leukemia with a favorable outcome despite frequent IKZF1 deletions. Leukemia. 2014;28(1):70–7.
116. Zaliova M, Zimmermannova O, Dorge P, Eckert C, Moricke A, Zimmermann M, et al. ERG deletion is associated with CD2 and attenuates the negative impact of IKZF1 deletion in childhood acute lymphoblastic leukemia. Leukemia. 2014;28(1):182–5.
117. Cario G, Zimmermann M, Romey R, Gesk S, Vater I, Harbott J, et al. Presence of the P2RY8-CRLF2 rearrangement is associated with a poor prognosis in non-high-risk precursor B-cell acute lymphoblastic leukemia in children treated according to the ALL-BFM 2000 protocol. Blood. 2010;115(26):5393–7.
118. Ensor HM, Schwab C, Russell LJ, Richards SM, Morrison H, Masic D, et al. Demographic, clinical, and outcome features of children with acute lymphoblastic leukemia and CRLF2 deregulation: results from the MRC ALL97 clinical trial. Blood. 2010;117(7):2129–36.
119. Harvey RC, Mullighan CG, Chen IM, Wharton W, Mikhail FM, Carroll AJ, et al. Rearrangement of CRLF2 is associated with mutation of JAK kinases, alteration of IKZF1, Hispanic/Latino ethnicity, and a poor outcome in pediatric B-progenitor acute lymphoblastic leukemia. Blood. 2010;115(26):5312–21.
120. Loh ML, Zhang J, Harvey RC, Roberts K, Payne-Turner D, Kang H, et al. Tyrosine kinome sequencing of pediatric acute lymphoblastic leukemia: a report from the Children's Oncology Group TARGET Project. Blood. 2013;121(3):485–8.

121. Mullighan CG, Collins-Underwood JR, Phillips LA, Loudin MG, Liu W, Zhang J, et al. Rearrangement of CRLF2 in B-progenitor- and Down syndrome-associated acute lymphoblastic leukemia. Nat Genet. 2009;41(11):1243–6.
122. Hertzberg L, Vendramini E, Ganmore I, Cazzaniga G, Schmitz M, Chalker J, et al. Down syndrome acute lymphoblastic leukemia, a highly heterogeneous disease in which aberrant expression of CRLF2 is associated with mutated JAK2: a report from the International BFM Study Group. Blood. 2010;115(5):1006–17.
123. Pui CH, Frankel LS, Carroll AJ, Raimondi SC, Shuster JJ, Head DR, et al. Clinical characteristics and treatment outcome of childhood acute lymphoblastic leukemia with the t(4;11)(q21;q23): a collaborative study of 40 cases. Blood. 1991;77(3):440–7.
124. Pieters R, Schrappe M, De Lorenzo P, Hann I, De Rossi G, Felice M, et al. A treatment protocol for infants younger than 1 year with acute lymphoblastic leukaemia (Interfant-99): an observational study and a multicentre randomised trial. Lancet. 2007;370(9583):240–50.
125. Pui CH, Gaynon PS, Boyett JM, Chessells JM, Baruchel A, Kamps W, et al. Outcome of treatment in childhood acute lymphoblastic leukaemia with rearrangements of the 11q23 chromosomal region. Lancet. 2002;359(9321):1909–15.
126. Rubnitz JE, Camitta BM, Mahmoud H, Raimondi SC, Carroll AJ, Borowitz MJ, et al. Childhood acute lymphoblastic leukemia with the MLL-ENL fusion and t(11;19)(q23;p13.3) translocation. J Clin Oncol. 1999;17(1):191–6.
127. Andersson AK, Ma J, Wang J, Chen X, Gedman AL, Dang J, et al. The landscape of somatic mutations in infant MLL-rearranged acute lymphoblastic leukemias. Nat Genet. 2015;47(4):330–7.
128. Armstrong SA, Staunton JE, Silverman LB, Pieters R, den Boer ML, Minden MD, et al. MLL translocations specify a distinct gene expression profile that distinguishes a unique leukemia. Nat Genet. 2002;30(1):41–7.
129. Krivtsov AV, Armstrong SA. MLL translocations, histone modifications and leukaemia stem-cell development. Nat Rev Cancer. 2007;7(11):823–33.
130. Krivtsov AV, Feng Z, Lemieux ME, Faber J, Vempati S, Sinha AU, et al. H3K79 methylation profiles define murine and human MLL-AF4 leukemias. Cancer Cell. 2008;14(5):355–68.
131. Andersen MK, Autio K, Barbany G, Borgstrom G, Cavelier L, Golovleva I, et al. Paediatric B-cell precursor acute lymphoblastic leukaemia with t(1;19)(q23;p13): clinical and cytogenetic characteristics of 47 cases from the Nordic countries treated according to NOPHO protocols. Br J Haematol. 2011;155(2):235–43.
132. Felice MS, Gallego MS, Alonso CN, Alfaro EM, Guitter MR, Bernasconi AR, et al. Prognostic impact of t(1;19)/ TCF3-PBX1 in childhood acute lymphoblastic leukemia in the context of Berlin-Frankfurt-Munster-based protocols. Leuk Lymphoma. 2011;52(7):1215–21.
133. Kamps MP, Look AT, Baltimore D. The human t(1;19) translocation in pre-B ALL produces multiple nuclear E2A-Pbx1 fusion proteins with differing transforming potentials. Genes Dev. 1991;5(3):358–68.
134. Aspland SE, Bendall HH, Murre C. The role of E2A-PBX1 in leukemogenesis. Oncogene. 2001;20(40):5708–17.
135. DiMartino JF, Selleri L, Traver D, Firpo MT, Rhee J, Warnke R, et al. The Hox cofactor and proto-oncogene Pbx1 is required for maintenance of definitive hematopoiesis in the fetal liver. Blood. 2001;98(3):618–26.
136. Crist WM, Carroll AJ, Shuster JJ, Behm FG, Whitehead M, Vietti TJ, et al. Poor prognosis of children with pre-B acute lymphoblastic leukemia is associated with the t(1;19)(q23;p13): a Pediatric Oncology Group study. Blood. 1990;76(1):117–22.
137. Uckun FM, Sensel MG, Sather HN, Gaynon PS, Arthur DC, Lange BJ, et al. Clinical significance of translocation t(1;19) in childhood acute lymphoblastic leukemia in the context of contemporary therapies: a report from the Children's Cancer Group. J Clin Oncol. 1998;16(2):527–35.
138. Pui CH, Campana D, Pei D, Bowman WP, Sandlund JT, Kaste SC, et al. Treating childhood acute lymphoblastic leukemia without cranial irradiation. N Engl J Med. 2009;360(26):2730–41.
139. Hunger SP, Ohyashiki K, Toyama K, Cleary ML. Hlf, a novel hepatic bZIP protein, shows altered DNA-binding properties following fusion to E2A in t(17;19) acute lymphoblastic leukemia. Genes Dev. 1992;6(9):1608–20.
140. Inaba T, Roberts WM, Shapiro LH, Jolly KW, Raimondi SC, Smith SD, et al. Fusion of the leucine zipper gene HLF to the E2A gene in human acute B-lineage leukemia. Science. 1992;257(5069):531–4.
141. Minson KA, Prasad P, Vear S, Borinstein S, Ho R, Domm J, et al. t(17;19) in Children with acute lymphocytic leukemia: a report of 3 cases and a review of the literature. Case Rep Hematol. 2013;2013:563291.
142. Fischer U, Forster M, Rinaldi A, Risch T, Sungalee S, Warnatz HJ, et al. Genomics and drug profiling of fatal TCF3-HLF-positive acute lymphoblastic leukemia identifies recurrent mutation patterns and therapeutic options. Nat Genet. 2015;47(9):1020–9.
143. Harrison CJ, Moorman AV, Schwab C, Carroll AJ, Raetz EA, Devidas M, et al. An international study of intrachromosomal amplification of chromosome 21 (iAMP21): cytogenetic characterization and outcome. Leukemia. 2014;28(5):1015–21.
144. Moorman AV, Richards SM, Robinson HM, Strefford JC, Gibson BE, Kinsey SE, et al. Prognosis of children with acute lymphoblastic leukemia (ALL) and intrachromosomal amplification of chromosome 21 (iAMP21). Blood. 2007;109(6):2327–30.
145. Attarbaschi A, Mann G, Panzer-Grumayer R, Rottgers S, Steiner M, Konig M, et al. Minimal residual disease values discriminate between low and high relapse risk in children with B-cell precursor acute lymphoblastic leukemia and an intrachromosomal amplification of chromosome 21: the Austrian and German acute lymphoblastic leukemia Berlin-Frankfurt-Munster (ALL-BFM) trials. J Clin Oncol. 2008;26(18):3046–50.
146. Moorman AV, Robinson H, Schwab C, Richards SM, Hancock J, Mitchell CD, et al. Risk-directed treatment intensification significantly reduces the risk of relapse among children and adolescents with acute lymphoblastic leukemia and intrachromosomal amplification of chromosome 21: a comparison of the MRC ALL97/99 and UKALL2003 trials. J Clin Oncol. 2013;31(27):3389–96.
147. Heerema NA, Carroll AJ, Devidas M, Loh ML, Borowitz MJ, Gastier-Foster JM, et al. Intrachromosomal amplification of chromosome 21 is associated with inferior outcomes in children with acute lymphoblastic leukemia treated in contemporary standard-risk Children's Oncology Group studies: a report from the children's oncology group. J Clin Oncol. 2013;31(27):3397–402.
148. Cauwelier B, Dastugue N, Cools J, Poppe B, Herens C, De Paepe A, et al. Molecular cytogenetic study of 126 unselected T-ALL cases reveals high incidence of TCRbeta locus rearrangements and putative new T-cell oncogenes. Leukemia. 2006;20(7):1238–44.
149. Van Vlierberghe P, Ferrando A. The molecular basis of T cell acute lymphoblastic leukemia. J Clin Invest. 2012;122(10):3398–406.
150. Weng AP, Ferrando AA, Lee W, Morris JP, Silverman LB, Sanchez-Irizarry C, et al. Activating mutations of NOTCH1 in human T cell acute lymphoblastic leukemia. Science. 2004;306(5694):269–71.
151. O'Neil J, Grim J, Strack P, Rao S, Tibbitts D, Winter C, et al. FBW7 mutations in leukemic cells mediate NOTCH pathway activation and resistance to gamma-secretase inhibitors. J Exp Med. 2007;204(8):1813–24.
152. Breit S, Stanulla M, Flohr T, Schrappe M, Ludwig WD, Tolle G, et al. Activating NOTCH1 mutations predict favorable early treatment response and long-term outcome in childhood precursor T-cell lymphoblastic leukemia. Blood. 2006;108(4):1151–7.

153. Larson Gedman A, Chen Q, Kugel Desmoulin S, Ge Y, LaFiura K, Haska CL, et al. The impact of NOTCH1, FBW7 and PTEN mutations on prognosis and downstream signaling in pediatric T-cell acute lymphoblastic leukemia: a report from the Children's Oncology Group. Leukemia. 2009;23(8):1417–25.
154. Zuurbier L, Homminga I, Calvert V, te Winkel ML, Buijs-Gladdines JG, Kooi C, et al. NOTCH1 and/or FBXW7 mutations predict for initial good prednisone response but not for improved outcome in pediatric T-cell acute lymphoblastic leukemia patients treated on DCOG or COALL protocols. Leukemia. 2010;24(12):2014–22.
155. Clappier E, Collette S, Grardel N, Girard S, Suarez L, Brunie G, et al. NOTCH1 and FBXW7 mutations have a favorable impact on early response to treatment, but not on outcome, in children with T-cell acute lymphoblastic leukemia (T-ALL) treated on EORTC trials 58881 and 58951. Leukemia. 2010;24(12):2023–31.
156. Gutierrez A, Sanda T, Grebliunaite R, Carracedo A, Salmena L, Ahn Y, et al. High frequency of PTEN, PI3K, and AKT abnormalities in T-cell acute lymphoblastic leukemia. Blood. 2009;114(3):647–50.
157. Palomero T, Sulis ML, Cortina M, Real PJ, Barnes K, Ciofani M, et al. Mutational loss of PTEN induces resistance to NOTCH1 inhibition in T-cell leukemia. Nat Med. 2007;13(10):1203–10.
158. Graux C, Cools J, Melotte C, Quentmeier H, Ferrando A, Levine R, et al. Fusion of NUP214 to ABL1 on amplified episomes in T-cell acute lymphoblastic leukemia. Nat Genet. 2004;36(10):1084–9.
159. Hagemeijer A, Graux C. ABL1 rearrangements in T-cell acute lymphoblastic leukemia. Genes Chromosomes Cancer. 2010;49(4):299–308.
160. Zhang J, Ding L, Holmfeldt L, Wu G, Heatley SL, Payne-Turner D, et al. The genetic basis of early T-cell precursor acute lymphoblastic leukaemia. Nature. 2012;481(7380):157–63.
161. Smith M, Arthur D, Camitta B, Carroll AJ, Crist W, Gaynon P, et al. Uniform approach to risk classification and treatment assignment for children with acute lymphoblastic leukemia. J Clin Oncol. 1996;14(1):18–24.
162. Moricke A, Zimmermann M, Reiter A, Gadner H, Odenwald E, Harbott J, et al. Prognostic impact of age in children and adolescents with acute lymphoblastic leukemia: data from the trials ALL-BFM 86, 90, and 95. Klin Padiatr. 2005;217(6):310–20.
163. Eden OB, Harrison G, Richards S, Lilleyman JS, Bailey CC, Chessells JM, et al. Long-term follow-up of the United Kingdom Medical Research Council protocols for childhood acute lymphoblastic leukaemia, 1980–1997. Medical Research Council Childhood Leukaemia Working Party. Leukemia. 2000;14(12):2307–20.
164. Maloney KW, Shuster JJ, Murphy S, Pullen J, Camitta BA. Long-term results of treatment studies for childhood acute lymphoblastic leukemia: Pediatric Oncology Group studies from 1986 to 1994. Leukemia. 2000;14(12):2276–85.
165. Pui CH, Sandlund JT, Pei D, Campana D, Rivera GK, Ribeiro RC, et al. Improved outcome for children with acute lymphoblastic leukemia: results of Total Therapy Study XIIIB at St Jude Children's Research Hospital. Blood. 2004;104(9):2690–6.
166. Hilden JM, Dinndorf PA, Meerbaum SO, Sather H, Villaluna D, Heerema NA, et al. Analysis of prognostic factors of acute lymphoblastic leukemia in infants: report on CCG 1953 from the Children's Oncology Group. Blood. 2006;108(2):441–51.
167. Barry E, DeAngelo DJ, Neuberg D, Stevenson K, Loh ML, Asselin BL, et al. Favorable outcome for adolescents with acute lymphoblastic leukemia treated on Dana-Farber Cancer Institute Acute Lymphoblastic Leukemia Consortium Protocols. J Clin Oncol. 2007;25(7):813–9.
168. Boissel N, Auclerc MF, Lheritier V, Perel Y, Thomas X, Leblanc T, et al. Should adolescents with acute lymphoblastic leukemia be treated as old children or young adults? Comparison of the French FRALLE-93 and LALA-94 trials. J Clin Oncol. 2003;21(5):774–80.
169. de Bont JM, Holt B, Dekker AW, van der Does-van den Berg A, Sonneveld P, Pieters R. Significant difference in outcome for adolescents with acute lymphoblastic leukemia treated on pediatric vs adult protocols in the Netherlands. Leukemia. 2004;18(12):2032–5.
170. Stock W, La M, Sanford B, Bloomfield CD, Vardiman JW, Gaynon P, et al. What determines the outcomes for adolescents and young adults with acute lymphoblastic leukemia treated on cooperative group protocols? A comparison of Children's Cancer Group and Cancer and Leukemia Group B studies. Blood. 2008;112(5):1646–54.
171. Vaitkeviciene G, Forestier E, Hellebostad M, Heyman M, Jonsson OG, Lahteenmaki PM, et al. High white blood cell count at diagnosis of childhood acute lymphoblastic leukaemia: biological background and prognostic impact. Results from the NOPHO ALL-92 and ALL-2000 studies. Eur J Haematol. 2011;86(1):38–46.
172. Putti MC, Rondelli R, Cocito MG, Arico M, Sainati L, Conter V, et al. Expression of myeloid markers lacks prognostic impact in children treated for acute lymphoblastic leukemia: Italian experience in AIEOP-ALL 88-91 studies. Blood. 1998;92(3):795–801.
173. Mahmoud HH, Rivera GK, Hancock ML, Krance RA, Kun LE, Behm FG, et al. Low leukocyte counts with blast cells in cerebrospinal fluid of children with newly diagnosed acute lymphoblastic leukemia. N Engl J Med. 1993;329(5):314–9.
174. Burger B, Zimmermann M, Mann G, Kuhl J, Loning L, Riehm H, et al. Diagnostic cerebrospinal fluid examination in children with acute lymphoblastic leukemia: significance of low leukocyte counts with blasts or traumatic lumbar puncture. J Clin Oncol. 2003;21(2):184–8.
175. Pui CH, Mahmoud HH, Rivera GK, Hancock ML, Sandlund JT, Behm FG, et al. Early intensification of intrathecal chemotherapy virtually eliminates central nervous system relapse in children with acute lymphoblastic leukemia. Blood. 1998;92(2):411–5.
176. Gajjar A, Harrison PL, Sandlund JT, Rivera GK, Ribeiro RC, Rubnitz JE, et al. Traumatic lumbar puncture at diagnosis adversely affects outcome in childhood acute lymphoblastic leukemia. Blood. 2000;96(10):3381–4.
177. Harris MB, Shuster JJ, Carroll A, Look AT, Borowitz MJ, Crist WM, et al. Trisomy of leukemic cell chromosomes 4 and 10 identifies children with B-progenitor cell acute lymphoblastic leukemia with a very low risk of treatment failure: a Pediatric Oncology Group study. Blood. 1992;79(12):3316–24.
178. Heerema NA, Sather HN, Sensel MG, Zhang T, Hutchinson RJ, Nachman JB, et al. Prognostic impact of trisomies of chromosomes 10, 17, and 5 among children with acute lymphoblastic leukemia and high hyperdiploidy (> 50 chromosomes). J Clin Oncol. 2000;18(9):1876–87.
179. Sutcliffe MJ, Shuster JJ, Sather HN, Camitta BM, Pullen J, Schultz KR, et al. High concordance from independent studies by the Children's Cancer Group (CCG) and Pediatric Oncology Group (POG) associating favorable prognosis with combined trisomies 4, 10, and 17 in children with NCI Standard-Risk B-precursor Acute Lymphoblastic Leukemia: a Children's Oncology Group (COG) initiative. Leukemia. 2005;19(5):734–40.
180. Chessells JM, Swansbury GJ, Reeves B, Bailey CC, Richards SM. Cytogenetics and prognosis in childhood lymphoblastic leukaemia: results of MRC UKALL X. Medical Research Council Working Party in Childhood Leukaemia. Br J Haematol. 1997;99(1):93–100.
181. Behm FG, Raimondi SC, Frestedt JL, Liu Q, Crist WM, Downing JR, et al. Rearrangement of the MLL gene confers a poor prognosis in childhood acute lymphoblastic leukemia, regardless of presenting age. Blood. 1996;87(7):2870–7.
182. Moricke A, Zimmermann M, Reiter A, Henze G, Schrauder A, Gadner H, et al. Long-term results of five consecutive trials in childhood

acute lymphoblastic leukemia performed by the ALL-BFM study group from 1981 to 2000. Leukemia. 2010;24(2):265–84.

183. Gaynon PS, Desai AA, Bostrom BC, Hutchinson RJ, Lange BJ, Nachman JB, et al. Early response to therapy and outcome in childhood acute lymphoblastic leukemia: a review. Cancer. 1997;80(9):1717–26.
184. Nachman JB, Sather HN, Sensel MG, Trigg ME, Cherlow JM, Lukens JN, et al. Augmented post-induction therapy for children with high-risk acute lymphoblastic leukemia and a slow response to initial therapy. N Engl J Med. 1998;338(23):1663–71.
185. Silverman LB, Gelber RD, Young ML, Dalton VK, Barr RD, Sallan SE. Induction failure in acute lymphoblastic leukemia of childhood. Cancer. 1999;85(6):1395–404.
186. Oudot C, Auclerc MF, Levy V, Porcher R, Piguet C, Perel Y, et al. Prognostic factors for leukemic induction failure in children with acute lymphoblastic leukemia and outcome after salvage therapy: the FRALLE 93 study. J Clin Oncol. 2008;26(9):1496–503.
187. Schrappe M, Hunger SP, Pui CH, Saha V, Gaynon PS, Baruchel A, et al. Outcomes after induction failure in childhood acute lymphoblastic leukemia. N Engl J Med. 2012;366(15):1371–81.
188. van Dongen JJ, Seriu T, Panzer-Grumayer ER, Biondi A, Pongers-Willemse MJ, Corral L, et al. Prognostic value of minimal residual disease in acute lymphoblastic leukaemia in childhood. Lancet. 1998;352(9142):1731–8.
189. Coustan-Smith E, Behm FG, Sanchez J, Boyett JM, Hancock ML, Raimondi SC, et al. Immunological detection of minimal residual disease in children with acute lymphoblastic leukaemia. Lancet. 1998;351(9102):550–4.
190. Weir EG, Cowan K, LeBeau P, Borowitz MJ. A limited antibody panel can distinguish B-precursor acute lymphoblastic leukemia from normal B precursors with four color flow cytometry: implications for residual disease detection. Leukemia. 1999;13(4):558–67.
191. Li A, Zhou J, Zuckerman D, Rue M, Dalton V, Lyons C, et al. Sequence analysis of clonal immunoglobulin and T-cell receptor gene rearrangements in children with acute lymphoblastic leukemia at diagnosis and at relapse: implications for pathogenesis and for the clinical utility of PCR-based methods of minimal residual disease detection. Blood. 2003;102(13):4520–6.
192. Ladetto M, Bruggemann M, Monitillo L, Ferrero S, Pepin F, Drandi D, et al. Next-generation sequencing and real-time quantitative PCR for minimal residual disease detection in B-cell disorders. Leukemia. 2014;28(6):1299–307.
193. Cave H, van der Werff ten Bosch J, Suciu S, Guidal C, Waterkeyn C, Otten J, et al. Clinical significance of minimal residual disease in childhood acute lymphoblastic leukemia. European Organization for Research and Treatment of Cancer--Childhood Leukemia Cooperative Group. N Engl J Med. 1998;339(9):591–8.
194. Coustan-Smith E, Sancho J, Hancock ML, Boyett JM, Behm FG, Raimondi SC, et al. Clinical importance of minimal residual disease in childhood acute lymphoblastic leukemia. Blood. 2000;96(8):2691–6.
195. Nyvold C, Madsen HO, Ryder LP, Seyfarth J, Svejgaard A, Clausen N, et al. Precise quantification of minimal residual disease at day 29 allows identification of children with acute lymphoblastic leukemia and an excellent outcome. Blood. 2002;99(4):1253–8.
196. Panzer-Grumayer ER, Schneider M, Panzer S, Fasching K, Gadner H. Rapid molecular response during early induction chemotherapy predicts a good outcome in childhood acute lymphoblastic leukemia. Blood. 2000;95(3):790–4.
197. Zhou J, Goldwasser MA, Li A, Dahlberg SE, Neuberg D, Wang H, et al. Quantitative analysis of minimal residual disease predicts relapse in children with B-lineage acute lymphoblastic leukemia in DFCI ALL Consortium Protocol 95-01. Blood. 2007;110(5):1607–11.
198. Brisco MJ, Condon J, Hughes E, Neoh SH, Sykes PJ, Seshadri R, et al. Outcome prediction in childhood acute lymphoblastic leukaemia by molecular quantification of residual disease at the end of induction. Lancet. 1994;343(8891):196–200.
199. Borowitz MJ, Devidas M, Hunger SP, Bowman WP, Carroll AJ, Carroll WL, et al. Clinical significance of minimal residual disease in childhood acute lymphoblastic leukemia and its relationship to other prognostic factors: a Children's Oncology Group study. Blood. 2008;111(12):5477–85.
200. Conter V, Bartram CR, Valsecchi MG, Schrauder A, Panzer-Grumayer R, Moricke A, et al. Molecular response to treatment redefines all prognostic factors in children and adolescents with B-cell precursor acute lymphoblastic leukemia: results in 3184 patients of the AIEOP-BFM ALL 2000 study. Blood. 2010;115(16):3206–14.
201. Schrappe M, Valsecchi MG, Bartram CR, Schrauder A, Panzer-Grumayer R, Moricke A, et al. Late MRD response determines relapse risk overall and in subsets of childhood T-cell ALL: results of the AIEOP-BFM-ALL 2000 study. Blood. 2011;118(8):2077–84.
202. Borowitz MJ, Wood BL, Devidas M, Loh ML, Raetz EA, Salzer WL, et al. Prognostic significance of minimal residual disease in high risk B-ALL: a report from Children's Oncology Group study AALL0232. Blood. 2015;126(8):964–71.
203. Vora A, Goulden N, Mitchell C, Hancock J, Hough R, Rowntree C, et al. Augmented post-remission therapy for a minimal residual disease-defined high-risk subgroup of children and young people with clinical standard-risk and intermediate-risk acute lymphoblastic leukaemia (UKALL 2003): a randomised controlled trial. Lancet Oncol. 2014;15(8):809–18.
204. Pieters R, de Groot-Kruseman H, Van der Velden V, Fiocco M, van den Berg H, de Bont E, et al. Successful therapy reduction and intensification for childhood acute lymphoblastic leukemia based on minimal residual disease monitoring: Study ALL10 From the Dutch Childhood Oncology Group. J Clin Oncol. 2016;34(22):2591–601.
205. Chessells JM, Richards SM, Bailey CC, Lilleyman JS, Eden OB. Gender and treatment outcome in childhood lymphoblastic leukaemia: report from the MRC UKALL trials. Br J Haematol. 1995;89(2):364–72.
206. Shuster JJ, Wacker P, Pullen J, Humbert J, Land VJ, Mahoney DH Jr, et al. Prognostic significance of sex in childhood B-precursor acute lymphoblastic leukemia: a Pediatric Oncology Group Study. J Clin Oncol. 1998;16(8):2854–63.
207. Bhatia S, Sather HN, Heerema NA, Trigg ME, Gaynon PS, Robison LL. Racial and ethnic differences in survival of children with acute lymphoblastic leukemia. Blood. 2002;100(6):1957–64.
208. Kadan-Lottick NS, Ness KK, Bhatia S, Gurney JG. Survival variability by race and ethnicity in childhood acute lymphoblastic leukemia. JAMA. 2003;290(15):2008–14.
209. Pui CH, Pei D, Pappo AS, Howard SC, Cheng C, Sandlund JT, et al. Treatment outcomes in black and white children with cancer: results from the SEER database and St Jude Children's Research Hospital, 1992 through 2007. J Clin Oncol. 2012;30(16):2005–12.
210. Pollock BH, DeBaun MR, Camitta BM, Shuster JJ, Ravindranath Y, Pullen DJ, et al. Racial differences in the survival of childhood B-precursor acute lymphoblastic leukemia: a Pediatric Oncology Group Study. J Clin Oncol. 2000;18(4):813–23.
211. Aldrich MC, Zhang L, Wiemels JL, Ma X, Loh ML, Metayer C, et al. Cytogenetics of Hispanic and White children with acute lymphoblastic leukemia in California. Cancer Epidemiol Biomark Prev. 2006;15(3):578–81.
212. Bhatia S, Landier W, Hageman L, Kim H, Chen Y, Crews KR, et al. 6MP adherence in a multiracial cohort of children with acute lymphoblastic leukemia: a Children's Oncology Group study. Blood. 2014;124(15):2345–53.
213. Bhatia S, Landier W, Shangguan M, Hageman L, Schaible AN, Carter AR, et al. Nonadherence to oral mercaptopurine and risk

of relapse in Hispanic and non-Hispanic white children with acute lymphoblastic leukemia: a report from the children's oncology group. J Clin Oncol. 2012;30(17):2094–101.

214. Buitenkamp TD, Izraeli S, Zimmermann M, Forestier E, Heerema NA, van den Heuvel-Eibrink MM, et al. Acute lymphoblastic leukemia in children with Down syndrome: a retrospective analysis from the Ponte di Legno study group. Blood. 2014;123(1):70–7.
215. Whitlock JA, Sather HN, Gaynon P, Robison LL, Wells RJ, Trigg M, et al. Clinical characteristics and outcome of children with Down syndrome and acute lymphoblastic leukemia: a Children's Cancer Group study. Blood. 2005;106(13):4043–9.
216. Arico M, Ziino O, Valsecchi MG, Cazzaniga G, Baronci C, Messina C, et al. Acute lymphoblastic leukemia and Down syndrome: presenting features and treatment outcome in the experience of the Italian Association of Pediatric Hematology and Oncology (AIEOP). Cancer. 2008;113(3):515–21.
217. Hanada I, Terui K, Ikeda F, Toki T, Kanezaki R, Sato T, et al. Gene alterations involving the CRLF2-JAK pathway and recurrent gene deletions in Down syndrome-associated acute lymphoblastic leukemia in Japan. Genes Chromosomes Cancer. 2014;53(11):902–10.
218. Bhatia S, Landier W, Hageman L, Chen Y, Kim H, Sun CL, et al. Systemic exposure to thiopurines and risk of relapse in children with acute lymphoblastic leukemia: a Children's Oncology Group Study. JAMA Oncol. 2015;1(3):287–95.
219. Farber S, Diamond LK, Mercer RD, Sylvester RF, Wolff JA. Temporary remissions in acute leukemia in children produced by folic acid antagonist, 4-aminopteroyl-glutamic acid (aminopterin). N Engl J Med. 1948;238:787–93.
220. Frei E 3rd. Acute leukemia in children. Model for the development of scientific methodology for clinical therapeutic research in cancer. Cancer. 1984;53(10):2013–25.
221. Elion GB, Hitchings GH. Metabolic basis for the actions of analogs of purines and pyrimidines. Adv Chemother. 1965;2:91–177.
222. Burchenal JH, Murphy ML, Ellison RR, Sykes MP, Tan TC, Leone LA, et al. Clinical evaluation of a new antimetabolite, 6-mercaptopurine, in the treatment of leukemia and allied diseases. Blood. 1953;8(11):965–99.
223. Frei E 3rd, Holland JF, Schneiderman MA, Pinkel D, Selkirk G, Freireich EJ, et al. A comparative study of two regimens of combination chemotherapy in acute leukemia. Blood. 1958;13(12):1126–48.
224. Freireich EJ, Frei E 2nd. Recent advances in acute leukemia. Prog Hematol. 1964;4:187–202.
225. Blum RH, Carter SK. Adriamycin. A new anticancer drug with significant clinical activity. Ann Intern Med. 1974;80(2):249–59.
226. Tallal L, Tan C, Oettgen H, Wollner N, McCarthy M, Helson L, et al. E. coli L-asparaginase in the treatment of leukemia and solid tumors in 131 children. Cancer. 1970;25(2):306–20.
227. Jaffe N, Traggis D, Das L, Kim BS, Won H, Hann L, et al. Comparison of daily and twice-weekly schedule of L-asparaginase in childhood leukemia. Pediatrics. 1972;49(4):590–5.
228. Pinkel D, Hernandez K, Borella L, Holton C, Aur R, Samoy G, et al. Drug dosage and remission duration in childhood lymphocytic leukemia. Cancer. 1971;27(2):247–56.
229. Evans AE, Gilbert ES, Zandstra R. The increasing incidence of central nervous system leukemia in children. (Children's Cancer Study Group A). Cancer. 1970;26(2):404–9.
230. Rivera GK, Pinkel D, Simone JV, Hancock ML, Crist WM. Treatment of acute lymphoblastic leukemia. 30 years' experience at St. Jude Children's Research Hospital. N Engl J Med. 1993;329(18):1289–95.
231. Place AE, Stevenson KE, Vrooman LM, Harris MH, Hunt SK, O'Brien JE, et al. Intravenous pegylated asparaginase versus intramuscular native Escherichia colil-asparaginase in newly diagnosed childhood acute lymphoblastic leukaemia (DFCI 05-001): a randomised, open-label phase 3 trial. Lancet Oncol. 2015;16(16):1677–90.
232. Hunger SP, Lu X, Devidas M, Camitta BM, Gaynon PS, Winick NJ, et al. Improved survival for children and adolescents with acute lymphoblastic leukemia between 1990 and 2005: a report from the children's oncology group. J Clin Oncol. 2012;30(14):1663–9.
233. Prucker C, Attarbaschi A, Peters C, Dworzak MN, Potschger U, Urban C, et al. Induction death and treatment-related mortality in first remission of children with acute lymphoblastic leukemia: a population-based analysis of the Austrian Berlin-Frankfurt-Munster study group. Leukemia. 2009;23(7):1264–9.
234. Moricke A, Zimmermann M, Valsecchi MG, Stanulla M, Biondi A, Mann G, et al. Dexamethasone vs. prednisone in induction treatment of pediatric ALL: results of the randomized trial AIEOP-BFM ALL 2000. Blood. 2016;127(17):2101–12.
235. Chessells JM, Harrison G, Richards SM, Gibson BE, Bailey CC, Hill FG, et al. Failure of a new protocol to improve treatment results in paediatric lymphoblastic leukaemia: lessons from the UK Medical Research Council trials UKALL X and UKALL XI. Br J Haematol. 2002;118(2):445–55.
236. Conter V, Arico M, Valsecchi MG, Basso G, Biondi A, Madon E, et al. Long-term results of the Italian Association of Pediatric Hematology and Oncology (AIEOP) acute lymphoblastic leukemia studies, 1982-1995. Leukemia. 2000;14(12):2196–204.
237. Duval M, Suciu S, Ferster A, Rialland X, Nelken B, Lutz P, et al. Comparison of Escherichia coli-asparaginase with Erwinia-asparaginase in the treatment of childhood lymphoid malignancies: results of a randomized European Organisation for Research and Treatment of Cancer-Children's Leukemia Group phase 3 trial. Blood. 2002;99(8):2734–9.
238. Kamps WA, Bokkerink JP, Hakvoort-Cammel FG, Veerman AJ, Weening RS, van Wering ER, et al. BFM-oriented treatment for children with acute lymphoblastic leukemia without cranial irradiation and treatment reduction for standard risk patients: results of DCLSG protocol ALL-8 (1991–1996). Leukemia. 2002;16(6):1099–111.
239. Moghrabi A, Levy DE, Asselin B, Barr R, Clavell L, Hurwitz C, et al. Results of the Dana-Farber Cancer Institute ALL Consortium Protocol 95-01 for children with acute lymphoblastic leukemia. Blood. 2007;109(3):896–904.
240. Moricke A, Reiter A, Zimmermann M, Gadner H, Stanulla M, Dordelmann M, et al. Risk-adjusted therapy of acute lymphoblastic leukemia can decrease treatment burden and improve survival: treatment results of 2169 unselected pediatric and adolescent patients enrolled in the trial ALL-BFM 95. Blood. 2008;111(9):4477–89.
241. Pui CH, Boyett JM, Rivera GK, Hancock ML, Sandlund JT, Ribeiro RC, et al. Long-term results of Total Therapy studies 11, 12 and 13A for childhood acute lymphoblastic leukemia at St Jude Children's Research Hospital. Leukemia. 2000;14(12):2286–94.
242. Seibel NL, Steinherz PG, Sather HN, Nachman JB, Delaat C, Ettinger LJ, et al. Early postinduction intensification therapy improves survival for children and adolescents with high-risk acute lymphoblastic leukemia: a report from the Children's Oncology Group. Blood. 2008;111(5):2548–55.
243. Tsuchida M, Ohara A, Manabe A, Kumagai M, Shimada H, Kikuchi A, et al. Long-term results of Tokyo Children's Cancer Study Group trials for childhood acute lymphoblastic leukemia, 1984–1999. Leukemia. 2010;24(2):383–96.
244. Vilmer E, Suciu S, Ferster A, Bertrand Y, Cave H, Thyss A, et al. Long-term results of three randomized trials (58831, 58832, 58881) in childhood acute lymphoblastic leukemia: a CLCG-EORTC report. Children Leukemia Cooperative Group. Leukemia. 2000;14(12):2257–66.
245. Balis FM, Lester CM, Chrousos GP, Heideman RL, Poplack DG. Differences in cerebrospinal fluid penetration of corticosteroids:

possible relationship to the prevention of meningeal leukemia. J Clin Oncol. 1987;5(2):202–7.

246. Ito C, Evans WE, McNinch L, Coustan-Smith E, Mahmoud H, Pui CH, et al. Comparative cytotoxicity of dexamethasone and prednisolone in childhood acute lymphoblastic leukemia. J Clin Oncol. 1996;14(8):2370–6.
247. Jones B, Freeman AI, Shuster JJ, Jacquillat C, Weil M, Pochedly C, et al. Lower incidence of meningeal leukemia when prednisone is replaced by dexamethasone in the treatment of acute lymphocytic leukemia. Med Pediatr Oncol. 1991;19(4):269–75.
248. Bostrom BC, Sensel MR, Sather HN, Gaynon PS, La MK, Johnston K, et al. Dexamethasone versus prednisone and daily oral versus weekly intravenous mercaptopurine for patients with standard-risk acute lymphoblastic leukemia: a report from the Children's Cancer Group. Blood. 2003;101(10):3809–17.
249. Mitchell CD, Richards SM, Kinsey SE, Lilleyman J, Vora A, Eden TO. Benefit of dexamethasone compared with prednisolone for childhood acute lymphoblastic leukaemia: results of the UK Medical Research Council ALL97 randomized trial. Br J Haematol. 2005;129(6):734–45.
250. Larsen EC, Devidas M, Chen S, Salzer WL, Raetz EA, Loh ML, et al. Dexamethasone and high-dose methotrexate improve outcome for children and young adults with high-risk B-acute lymphoblastic leukemia: A Report From Children's Oncology Group Study AALL0232. J Clin Oncol. 2016;34(20):2380–8.
251. Balduzzi A, Valsecchi MG, Uderzo C, De Lorenzo P, Klingebiel T, Peters C, et al. Chemotherapy versus allogeneic transplantation for very-high-risk childhood acute lymphoblastic leukaemia in first complete remission: comparison by genetic randomisation in an international prospective study. Lancet. 2005;366(9486):635–42.
252. Arico M, Valsecchi MG, Conter V, Rizzari C, Pession A, Messina C, et al. Improved outcome in high-risk childhood acute lymphoblastic leukemia defined by prednisone-poor response treated with double Berlin- Frankfurt-Muenster protocol II. Blood. 2002;100(2):420–6.
253. Lange BJ, Bostrom BC, Cherlow JM, Sensel MG, La MK, Rackoff W, et al. Double-delayed intensification improves event-free survival for children with intermediate-risk acute lymphoblastic leukemia: a report from the Children's Cancer Group. Blood. 2002;99(3):825–33.
254. Vora A, Goulden N, Wade R, Mitchell C, Hancock J, Hough R, et al. Treatment reduction for children and young adults with low-risk acute lymphoblastic leukaemia defined by minimal residual disease (UKALL 2003): a randomised controlled trial. Lancet Oncol. 2013;14(3):199–209.
255. Gaynon PS, Angiolillo AL, Carroll WL, Nachman JB, Trigg ME, Sather HN, et al. Long-term results of the children's cancer group studies for childhood acute lymphoblastic leukemia 1983-2002: a Children's Oncology Group Report. Leukemia. 2010;24(2):285–97.
256. Matloub Y, Bostrom BC, Hunger SP, Stork LC, Angiolillo A, Sather H, et al. Escalating intravenous methotrexate improves event-free survival in children with standard-risk acute lymphoblastic leukemia: a report from the Children's Oncology Group. Blood. 2011;118(2):243–51.
257. Silverman LB, Stevenson KE, O'Brien JE, Asselin BL, Barr RD, Clavell L, et al. Long-term results of Dana-Farber Cancer Institute ALL Consortium protocols for children with newly diagnosed acute lymphoblastic leukemia (1985–2000). Leukemia. 2010;24(2):320–34.
258. Vrooman LM, Neuberg DS, Stevenson KE, Supko JG, Sallan SE, Silverman LB. Dexamethasone and individualized asparaginase dosing are each associated with superior event-free survival in childhood acute lymphoblastic leukemia: Results from the DFCI-ALL Consortium. Blood. 2009;114(22):136. (abstract 321)
259. Bleyer WA, Sather HN, Nickerson HJ, Coccia PF, Finklestein JZ, Miller DR, et al. Monthly pulses of vincristine and prednisone prevent bone marrow and testicular relapse in low-risk childhood acute lymphoblastic leukemia: a report of the CCG-161 study by the Childrens Cancer Study Group. J Clin Oncol. 1991;9(6):1012–21.
260. Conter V, Valsecchi MG, Silvestri D, Campbell M, Dibar E, Magyarosy E, et al. Pulses of vincristine and dexamethasone in addition to intensive chemotherapy for children with intermediate-risk acute lymphoblastic leukaemia: a multicentre randomised trial. Lancet. 2007;369(9556):123–31.
261. De Moerloose B, Suciu S, Bertrand Y, Mazingue F, Robert A, Uyttebroeck A, et al. Improved outcome with pulses of vincristine and corticosteroids in continuation therapy of children with average risk acute lymphoblastic leukemia (ALL) and lymphoblastic non-Hodgkin lymphoma (NHL): report of the EORTC randomized phase 3 trial 58951. Blood. 2010;116(1):36–44.
262. Eden T, Pieters R, Richards S. Systematic review of the addition of vincristine plus steroid pulses in maintenance treatment for childhood acute lymphoblastic leukaemia—an individual patient data meta-analysis involving 5659 children. Br J Haematol. 2010;149(5):722–33.
263. Stork LC, Matloub Y, Broxson E, La M, Yanofsky R, Sather H, et al. Oral 6-mercaptopurine versus oral 6-thioguanine and veno-occlusive disease in children with standard-risk acute lymphoblastic leukemia: report of the Children's Oncology Group CCG-1952 clinical trial. Blood. 2010;115(14):2740–8.
264. Vora A, Mitchell CD, Lennard L, Eden TO, Kinsey SE, Lilleyman J, et al. Toxicity and efficacy of 6-thioguanine versus 6-mercaptopurine in childhood lymphoblastic leukaemia: a randomised trial. Lancet. 2006;368(9544):1339–48.
265. Escherich G, Richards S, Stork LC, Vora AJ. Meta-analysis of randomised trials comparing thiopurines in childhood acute lymphoblastic leukaemia. Leukemia. 2011;25(6):953–9.
266. Relling MV, Pui CH, Cheng C, Evans WE. Thiopurine methyltransferase in acute lymphoblastic leukemia. Blood. 2006;107(2):843–4.
267. Relling MV, Hancock ML, Rivera GK, Sandlund JT, Ribeiro RC, Krynetski EY, et al. Mercaptopurine therapy intolerance and heterozygosity at the thiopurine S-methyltransferase gene locus. J Natl Cancer Inst. 1999;91(23):2001–8.
268. Andersen JB, Szumlanski C, Weinshilboum RM, Schmiegelow K. Pharmacokinetics, dose adjustments, and 6-mercaptopurine/methotrexate drug interactions in two patients with thiopurine methyltransferase deficiency. Acta Paediatr. 1998;87(1):108–11.
269. Yang JJ, Landier W, Yang W, Liu C, Hageman L, Cheng C, et al. Inherited NUDT15 variant is a genetic determinant of mercaptopurine intolerance in children with acute lymphoblastic leukemia. J Clin Oncol. 2015;33(11):1235–42.
270. Ravindranath Y, Soorya DT, Schultz GE, Lusher JM. Long-term survivors of acute lymphoblastic leukemia--risk of relapse after cessation of therapy. Med Pediatr Oncol. 1981;9(3):209–18.
271. Schrappe M, Reiter A, Zimmermann M, Harbott J, Ludwig WD, Henze G, et al. Long-term results of four consecutive trials in childhood ALL performed by the ALL-BFM study group from 1981 to 1995. Berlin-Frankfurt-Munster Leukemia. 2000;14(12):2205–22.
272. Toyoda Y, Manabe A, Tsuchida M, Hanada R, Ikuta K, Okimoto Y, et al. Six months of maintenance chemotherapy after intensified treatment for acute lymphoblastic leukemia of childhood. J Clin Oncol. 2000;18(7):1508–16.
273. Hustu HO, Aur RJ, Verzosa MS, Simone JV, Pinkel D. Prevention of central nervous system leukemia by irradiation. Cancer. 1973;32(3):585–97.
274. Simone J, Aur RJ, Hustu HO, Pinkel D. "Total therapy" studies of acute lymphocytic leukemia in children. Current results and prospects for cure. Cancer. 1972;30(6):1488–94.
275. Aur RJ, Simone JV, Hustu HO, Verzosa MS. A comparative study of central nervous system irradiation and intensive chemotherapy

early in remission of childhood acute lymphocytic leukemia. Cancer. 1972;29(2):381–91.

276. Nesbit ME, Sather H, Robison LL, Donaldson M, Littman P, Ortega JA, et al. Sanctuary therapy: a randomized trial of 724 children with previously untreated acute lymphoblastic leukemia: A Report from Children's Cancer Study Group. Cancer Res. 1982;42(2):674–80.
277. Nesbit ME Jr, Sather HN, Robison LL, Ortega J, Littman PS, D'Angio GJ, et al. Presymptomatic central nervous system therapy in previously untreated childhood acute lymphoblastic leukaemia: comparison of 1800 rad and 2400 rad. A report for Children's Cancer Study Group. Lancet. 1981;1(8218):461–6.
278. Schrappe M, Reiter A, Henze G, Niemeyer C, Bode U, Kuhl J, et al. Prevention of CNS recurrence in childhood ALL: results with reduced radiotherapy combined with CNS-directed chemotherapy in four consecutive ALL-BFM trials. Klin Padiatr. 1998;210(4):192–9.
279. Veerman AJ, Kamps WA, van den Berg H, van den Berg E, Bokkerink JP, Bruin MC, et al. Dexamethasone-based therapy for childhood acute lymphoblastic leukaemia: results of the prospective Dutch Childhood Oncology Group (DCOG) protocol ALL-9 (1997-2004). Lancet Oncol. 2009;10(10):957–66.
280. Sirvent N, Suciu S, Rialland X, Millot F, Benoit Y, Plantaz D, et al. Prognostic significance of the initial cerebro-spinal fluid (CSF) involvement of children with acute lymphoblastic leukaemia (ALL) treated without cranial irradiation: results of European Organization for Research and Treatment of Cancer (EORTC) Children Leukemia Group study 58881. Eur J Cancer. 2011;47(2):239–47.
281. Vora A, Andreano A, Pui CH, Hunger SP, Schrappe M, Moericke A, et al. Influence of cranial radiotherapy on outcome in children with acute lymphoblastic leukemia treated with contemporary therapy. J Clin Oncol. 2016;34(9):919–26.
282. Meadows AT, Gordon J, Massari DJ, Littman P, Fergusson J, Moss K. Declines in IQ scores and cognitive dysfunctions in children with acute lymphocytic leukaemia treated with cranial irradiation. Lancet. 1981;2(8254):1015–8.
283. Jankovic M, Brouwers P, Valsecchi MG, Van Veldhuizen A, Huisman J, Kamphuis R, et al. Association of 1800 cGy cranial irradiation with intellectual function in children with acute lymphoblastic leukaemia. ISPACC. International Study Group on Psychosocial Aspects of Childhood Cancer. Lancet. 1994;344(8917):224–7.
284. Waber DP, Shapiro BL, Carpentieri SC, Gelber RD, Zou G, Dufresne A, et al. Excellent therapeutic efficacy and minimal late neurotoxicity in children treated with 18 grays of cranial radiation therapy for high-risk acute lymphoblastic leukemia: a 7-year follow-up study of the Dana-Farber Cancer Institute Consortium Protocol 87-01. Cancer. 2001;92(1):15–22.
285. Waber DP, Gioia G, Paccia J, Sherman B, Dinklage D, Sollee N, et al. Sex differences in cognitive processing in children treated with CNS prophylaxis for acute lymphoblastic leukemia. J Pediatr Psychol. 1990;15(1):105–22.
286. Waber DP, Tarbell NJ, Kahn CM, Gelber RD, Sallan SE. The relationship of sex and treatment modality to neuropsychologic outcome in childhood acute lymphoblastic leukemia. J Clin Oncol. 1992;10(5):810–7.
287. Mulhern RK, Fairclough D, Ochs J. A prospective comparison of neuropsychologic performance of children surviving leukemia who received 18-Gy, 24-Gy, or no cranial irradiation. J Clin Oncol. 1991;9(8):1348–56.
288. Harila-Saari AH, Lahteenmaki PM, Pukkala E, Kyyronen P, Lanning M, Sankila R. Scholastic achievements of childhood leukemia patients: a nationwide, register-based study. J Clin Oncol. 2007;25(23):3518–24.
289. Rowland JH, Glidewell OJ, Sibley RF, Holland JC, Tull R, Berman A, et al. Effects of different forms of central nervous system prophylaxis on neuropsychologic function in childhood leukemia. J Clin Oncol. 1984;2(12):1327–35.
290. Butler RW, Hill JM, Steinherz PG, Meyers PA, Finlay JL. Neuropsychologic effects of cranial irradiation, intrathecal methotrexate, and systemic methotrexate in childhood cancer. J Clin Oncol. 1994;12(12):2621–9.
291. Waber DP, Turek J, Catania L, Stevenson K, Robaey P, Romero I, et al. Neuropsychological outcomes from a randomized trial of triple intrathecal chemotherapy compared with 18 Gy cranial radiation as CNS treatment in acute lymphoblastic leukemia: findings from Dana-Farber Cancer Institute ALL Consortium Protocol 95-01. J Clin Oncol. 2007;25(31):4914–21.
292. Copeland DR, Moore BD 3rd, Francis DJ, Jaffe N, Culbert SJ. Neuropsychologic effects of chemotherapy on children with cancer: a longitudinal study. J Clin Oncol. 1996;14(10):2826–35.
293. Buizer AI, de Sonneville LM, van den Heuvel-Eibrink MM, Veerman AJ. Behavioral and educational limitations after chemotherapy for childhood acute lymphoblastic leukemia or Wilms tumor. Cancer. 2006;106(9):2067–75.
294. Krull KR, Brinkman TM, Li C, Armstrong GT, Ness KK, Srivastava DK, et al. Neurocognitive outcomes decades after treatment for childhood acute lymphoblastic leukemia: a report from the st jude lifetime cohort study. J Clin Oncol. 2013;31(35):4407–15.
295. Kingma A, van Dommelen RI, Mooyaart EL, Wilmink JT, Deelman BG, Kamps WA. Slight cognitive impairment and magnetic resonance imaging abnormalities but normal school levels in children treated for acute lymphoblastic leukemia with chemotherapy only. J Pediatr. 2001;139(3):413–20.
296. Spiegler BJ, Kennedy K, Maze R, Greenberg ML, Weitzman S, Hitzler JK, et al. Comparison of long-term neurocognitive outcomes in young children with acute lymphoblastic leukemia treated with cranial radiation or high-dose or very high-dose intravenous methotrexate. J Clin Oncol. 2006;24(24):3858–64.
297. Conklin HM, Krull KR, Reddick WE, Pei D, Cheng C, Pui CH. Cognitive outcomes following contemporary treatment without cranial irradiation for childhood acute lymphoblastic leukemia. J Natl Cancer Inst. 2012;104(18):1386–95.
298. te Winkel ML, Pieters R, Hop WC, de Groot-Kruseman HA, Lequin MH, van der Sluis IM, et al. Prospective study on incidence, risk factors, and long-term outcome of osteonecrosis in pediatric acute lymphoblastic leukemia. J Clin Oncol. 2011;29(31):4143–50.
299. Vrooman LM, Stevenson KE, Supko JG, O'Brien J, Dahlberg SE, Asselin BL, et al. Postinduction dexamethasone and individualized dosing of Escherichia Coli L-asparaginase each improve outcome of children and adolescents with newly diagnosed acute lymphoblastic leukemia: results from a randomized study--Dana-Farber Cancer Institute ALL Consortium Protocol 00-01. J Clin Oncol. 2013;31(9):1202–10.
300. Mattano LA Jr, Devidas M, Nachman JB, Sather HN, Hunger SP, Steinherz PG, et al. Effect of alternate-week versus continuous dexamethasone scheduling on the risk of osteonecrosis in paediatric patients with acute lymphoblastic leukaemia: results from the CCG-1961 randomised cohort trial. Lancet Oncol. 2012;13(9):906–15.
301. Patel B, Richards SM, Rowe JM, Goldstone AH, Fielding AK. High incidence of avascular necrosis in adolescents with acute lymphoblastic leukaemia: a UKALL XII analysis. Leukemia. 2008;22(2):308–12.
302. Halton JM, Atkinson SA, Fraher L, Webber C, Gill GJ, Dawson S, et al. Altered mineral metabolism and bone mass in children during treatment for acute lymphoblastic leukemia. J Bone Miner Res. 1996;11(11):1774–83.
303. Arikoski P, Komulainen J, Riikonen P, Jurvelin JS, Voutilainen R, Kroger H. Reduced bone density at completion of chemotherapy for a malignancy. Arch Dis Child. 1999;80(2):143–8.

304. Hogler W, Wehl G, van Staa T, Meister B, Klein-Franke A, Kropshofer G. Incidence of skeletal complications during treatment of childhood acute lymphoblastic leukemia: comparison of fracture risk with the General Practice Research Database. Pediatr Blood Cancer. 2007;48(1):21–7.
305. van der Sluis IM, van den Heuvel-Eibrink MM, Hahlen K, Krenning EP, de Muinck Keizer-Schrama SM. Altered bone mineral density and body composition, and increased fracture risk in childhood acute lymphoblastic leukemia. J Pediatr. 2002;141(2):204–10.
306. Arikoski P, Komulainen J, Voutilainen R, Riikonen P, Parviainen M, Tapanainen P, et al. Reduced bone mineral density in long-term survivors of childhood acute lymphoblastic leukemia. J Pediatr Hematol Oncol. 1998;20(3):234–40.
307. Kadan-Lottick N, Marshall JA, Baron AE, Krebs NF, Hambidge KM, Albano E. Normal bone mineral density after treatment for childhood acute lymphoblastic leukemia diagnosed between 1991 and 1998. J Pediatr. 2001;138(6):898–904.
308. Mandel K, Atkinson S, Barr RD, Pencharz P. Skeletal morbidity in childhood acute lymphoblastic leukemia. J Clin Oncol. 2004;22(7):1215–21.
309. Kaste SC, Rai SN, Fleming K, McCammon EA, Tylavsky FA, Danish RK, et al. Changes in bone mineral density in survivors of childhood acute lymphoblastic leukemia. Pediatr Blood Cancer. 2006;46(1):77–87.
310. Harake D, Franco VI, Henkel JM, Miller TL, Lipshultz SE. Cardiotoxicity in childhood cancer survivors: strategies for prevention and management. Futur Cardiol. 2012;8(4):647–70.
311. Lipshultz SE, Lipsitz SR, Mone SM, Goorin AM, Sallan SE, Sanders SP, et al. Female sex and drug dose as risk factors for late cardiotoxic effects of doxorubicin therapy for childhood cancer. N Engl J Med. 1995;332(26):1738–43.
312. Krischer JP, Epstein S, Cuthbertson DD, Goorin AM, Epstein ML, Lipshultz SE. Clinical cardiotoxicity following anthracycline treatment for childhood cancer: the Pediatric Oncology Group experience. J Clin Oncol. 1997;15(4):1544–52.
313. Lipshultz SE, Colan SD, Gelber RD, Perez-Atayde AR, Sallan SE, Sanders SP. Late cardiac effects of doxorubicin therapy for acute lymphoblastic leukemia in childhood. N Engl J Med. 1991;324(12):808–15.
314. Sorensen K, Levitt G, Bull C, Chessells J, Sullivan I. Anthracycline dose in childhood acute lymphoblastic leukemia: issues of early survival versus late cardiotoxicity. J Clin Oncol. 1997;15(1):61–8.
315. Lipshultz SE, Lipsitz SR, Sallan SE, Dalton VM, Mone SM, Gelber RD, et al. Chronic progressive cardiac dysfunction years after doxorubicin therapy for childhood acute lymphoblastic leukemia. J Clin Oncol. 2005;23(12):2629–36.
316. Asselin BL, Devidas M, Chen L, Franco VI, Pullen J, Borowitz MJ, et al. Cardioprotection and safety of dexrazoxane in patients treated for newly diagnosed T-cell acute lymphoblastic leukemia or advanced-stage lymphoblastic non-hodgkin lymphoma: A Report of the Children's Oncology Group Randomized Trial Pediatric Oncology Group 9404. J Clin Oncol. 2016;34(8):854–62.
317. Lipshultz SE, Rifai N, Dalton VM, Levy DE, Silverman LB, Lipsitz SR, et al. The effect of dexrazoxane on myocardial injury in doxorubicin-treated children with acute lymphoblastic leukemia. N Engl J Med. 2004;351(2):145–53.
318. Lipshultz SE, Scully RE, Lipsitz SR, Sallan SE, Silverman LB, Miller TL, et al. Assessment of dexrazoxane as a cardioprotectant in doxorubicin-treated children with high-risk acute lymphoblastic leukaemia: long-term follow-up of a prospective, randomised, multicentre trial. Lancet Oncol. 2010;11(10):950–61.
319. Bhatia S, Sather HN, Pabustan OB, Trigg ME, Gaynon PS, Robison LL. Low incidence of second neoplasms among children diagnosed with acute lymphoblastic leukemia after 1983. Blood. 2002;99(12):4257–64.
320. Hijiya N, Hudson MM, Lensing S, Zacher M, Onciu M, Behm FG, et al. Cumulative incidence of secondary neoplasms as a first event after childhood acute lymphoblastic leukemia. JAMA. 2007;297(11):1207–15.
321. Schmiegelow K, Levinsen MF, Attarbaschi A, Baruchel A, Devidas M, Escherich G, et al. Second malignant neoplasms after treatment of childhood acute lymphoblastic leukemia. J Clin Oncol. 2013;31(19):2469–76.
322. Morris B, Partap S, Yeom K, Gibbs IC, Fisher PG, King AA. Cerebrovascular disease in childhood cancer survivors: A Children's Oncology Group Report. Neurology. 2009;73(22):1906–13.
323. Pui CH, Behm FG, Raimondi SC, Dodge RK, George SL, Rivera GK, et al. Secondary acute myeloid leukemia in children treated for acute lymphoid leukemia. N Engl J Med. 1989;321(3):136–42.
324. Winick NJ, McKenna RW, Shuster JJ, Schneider NR, Borowitz MJ, Bowman WP, et al. Secondary acute myeloid leukemia in children with acute lymphoblastic leukemia treated with etoposide. J Clin Oncol. 1993;11(2):209–17.
325. Tucker MA, Meadows AT, Boice JD Jr, Stovall M, Oberlin O, Stone BJ, et al. Leukemia after therapy with alkylating agents for childhood cancer. J Natl Cancer Inst. 1987;78(3):459–64.
326. Schmiegelow K, Al-Modhwahi I, Andersen MK, Behrendtz M, Forestier E, Hasle H, et al. Methotrexate/6-mercaptopurine maintenance therapy influences the risk of a second malignant neoplasm after childhood acute lymphoblastic leukemia: results from the NOPHO ALL-92 study. Blood. 2009;113(24):6077–84.
327. Rivera GK, Hudson MM, Liu Q, Benaim E, Ribeiro RC, Crist WM, et al. Effectiveness of intensified rotational combination chemotherapy for late hematologic relapse of childhood acute lymphoblastic leukemia. Blood. 1996;88(3):831–7.
328. Einsiedel HG, von Stackelberg A, Hartmann R, Fengler R, Schrappe M, Janka-Schaub G, et al. Long-term outcome in children with relapsed ALL by risk-stratified salvage therapy: results of trial acute lymphoblastic leukemia-relapse study of the Berlin-Frankfurt-Munster Group 87. J Clin Oncol. 2005;23(31):7942–50.
329. Gaynon PS, Qu RP, Chappell RJ, Willoughby ML, Tubergen DG, Steinherz PG, et al. Survival after relapse in childhood acute lymphoblastic leukemia: impact of site and time to first relapse--the Children's Cancer Group Experience. Cancer. 1998;82(7):1387–95.
330. Nguyen K, Devidas M, Cheng SC, La M, Raetz EA, Carroll WL, et al. Factors influencing survival after relapse from acute lymphoblastic leukemia: a Children's Oncology Group study. Leukemia. 2008;22(12):2142–50.
331. Eckert C, von Stackelberg A, Seeger K, Groeneveld TW, Peters C, Klingebiel T, et al. Minimal residual disease after induction is the strongest predictor of prognosis in intermediate risk relapsed acute lymphoblastic leukaemia— long-term results of trial ALL-REZ BFM P95/96. Eur J Cancer. 2013;49(6):1346–55.
332. Coustan-Smith E, Gajjar A, Hijiya N, Razzouk BI, Ribeiro RC, Rivera GK, et al. Clinical significance of minimal residual disease in childhood acute lymphoblastic leukemia after first relapse. Leukemia. 2004;18(3):499–504.
333. Raetz EA, Borowitz MJ, Devidas M, Linda SB, Hunger SP, Winick NJ, et al. Reinduction platform for children with first marrow relapse of acute lymphoblastic leukemia: A Children's Oncology Group Study. J Clin Oncol. 2008;26(24):3971–8.
334. Parker C, Waters R, Leighton C, Hancock J, Sutton R, Moorman AV, et al. Effect of mitoxantrone on outcome of children with first relapse of acute lymphoblastic leukaemia (ALL R3): an open-label randomised trial. Lancet. 2010;376(9757):2009–17.
335. von Stackelberg A, Hartmann R, Buhrer C, Fengler R, Janka-Schaub G, Reiter A, et al. High-dose compared with intermediate-dose methotrexate in children with a first relapse of acute lymphoblastic leukemia. Blood. 2008;111(5):2573–80.

336. Hijiya N, Gajjar A, Zhang Z, Sandlund JT, Ribeiro RC, Rubnitz JE, et al. Low-dose oral etoposide-based induction regimen for children with acute lymphoblastic leukemia in first bone marrow relapse. Leukemia. 2004;18(10):1581–6.
337. von Stackelberg A, Volzke E, Kuhl JS, Seeger K, Schrauder A, Escherich G, et al. Outcome of children and adolescents with relapsed acute lymphoblastic leukaemia and non-response to salvage protocol therapy: a retrospective analysis of the ALL-REZ BFM Study Group. Eur J Cancer. 2011;47(1):90–7.
338. Eapen M, Raetz E, Zhang MJ, Muehlenbein C, Devidas M, Abshire T, et al. Outcomes after HLA-matched sibling transplantation or chemotherapy in children with B-precursor acute lymphoblastic leukemia in a second remission: a collaborative study of the Children's Oncology Group and the Center for International Blood and Marrow Transplant Research. Blood. 2006;107(12):4961–7.
339. Borgmann A, von Stackelberg A, Hartmann R, Ebell W, Klingebiel T, Peters C, et al. Unrelated donor stem cell transplantation compared with chemotherapy for children with acute lymphoblastic leukemia in a second remission: a matched-pair analysis. Blood. 2003;101(10):3835–9.
340. Uderzo C, Valsecchi MG, Bacigalupo A, Meloni G, Messina C, Polchi P, et al. Treatment of childhood acute lymphoblastic leukemia in second remission with allogeneic bone marrow transplantation and chemotherapy: ten-year experience of the Italian Bone Marrow Transplantation Group and the Italian Pediatric Hematology Oncology Association. J Clin Oncol. 1995;13(2):352–8.
341. Burke MJ, Verneris MR, Le Rademacher J, He W, Abdel-Azim H, Abraham AA, et al. Transplant outcomes for children with T Cell acute lymphoblastic leukemia in second remission: A Report from the Center for International Blood and Marrow Transplant Research. Biol Blood Marrow Transplant. 2015;21(12):2154–9.
342. Rivera GK, Zhou Y, Hancock ML, Gajjar A, Rubnitz J, Ribeiro RC, et al. Bone marrow recurrence after initial intensive treatment for childhood acute lymphoblastic leukemia. Cancer. 2005;103(2):368–76.
343. Eckert C, Henze G, Seeger K, Hagedorn N, Mann G, Panzer-Grumayer R, et al. Use of allogeneic hematopoietic stem-cell transplantation based on minimal residual disease response improves outcomes for children with relapsed acute lymphoblastic leukemia in the intermediate-risk group. J Clin Oncol. 2013;31(21):2736–42.
344. Davies SM, Ramsay NK, Klein JP, Weisdorf DJ, Bolwell B, Cahn JY, et al. Comparison of preparative regimens in transplants for children with acute lymphoblastic leukemia. J Clin Oncol. 2000;18(2):340–7.
345. Knechtli CJ, Goulden NJ, Hancock JP, Grandage VL, Harris EL, Garland RJ, et al. Minimal residual disease status before allogeneic bone marrow transplantation is an important determinant of successful outcome for children and adolescents with acute lymphoblastic leukemia. Blood. 1998;92(11):4072–9.
346. Bader P, Kreyenberg H, Henze GH, Eckert C, Reising M, Willasch A, et al. Prognostic value of minimal residual disease quantification before allogeneic stem-cell transplantation in relapsed childhood acute lymphoblastic leukemia: the ALL-REZ BFM Study Group. J Clin Oncol. 2009;27(3):377–84.
347. Sramkova L, Muzikova K, Fronkova E, Krejci O, Sedlacek P, Formankova R, et al. Detectable minimal residual disease before allogeneic hematopoietic stem cell transplantation predicts extremely poor prognosis in children with acute lymphoblastic leukemia. Pediatr Blood Cancer. 2007;48(1):93–100.
348. Pulsipher MA, Carlson C, Langholz B, Wall DA, Schultz KR, Bunin N, et al. IgH-V(D)J NGS-MRD measurement pre- and early post-allotransplant defines very low- and very high-risk ALL patients. Blood. 2015;125(22):3501–8.
349. Hagedorn N, Acquaviva C, Fronkova E, von Stackelberg A, Barth A, zur Stadt U, et al. Submicroscopic bone marrow involvement in isolated extramedullary relapses in childhood acute lymphoblastic leukemia: a more precise definition of "isolated" and its possible clinical implications, a collaborative study of the Resistant Disease Committee of the International BFM study group. Blood. 2007;110(12):4022–9.
350. Ribeiro RC, Rivera GK, Hudson M, Mulhern RK, Hancock ML, Kun L, et al. An intensive re-treatment protocol for children with an isolated CNS relapse of acute lymphoblastic leukemia. J Clin Oncol. 1995;13(2):333–8.
351. Ritchey AK, Pollock BH, Lauer SJ, Andejeski Y, Barredo J, Buchanan GR. Improved survival of children with isolated CNS relapse of acute lymphoblastic leukemia: a pediatric oncology group study. J Clin Oncol. 1999;17(12):3745–52.
352. Barredo JC, Devidas M, Lauer SJ, Billett A, Marymont M, Pullen J, et al. Isolated CNS relapse of acute lymphoblastic leukemia treated with intensive systemic chemotherapy and delayed CNS radiation: a pediatric oncology group study. J Clin Oncol. 2006;24(19):3142–9.
353. Roy A, Cargill A, Love S, Moorman AV, Stoneham S, Lim A, et al. Outcome after first relapse in childhood acute lymphoblastic leukaemia—lessons from the United Kingdom R2 trial. Br J Haematol. 2005;130(1):67–75.
354. Borgmann A, Hartmann R, Schmid H, Klingebiel T, Ebell W, Gobel U, et al. Isolated extramedullary relapse in children with acute lymphoblastic leukemia: a comparison between treatment results of chemotherapy and bone marrow transplantation. BFM Relapse Study Group. Bone Marrow Transplant. 1995;15(4):515–21.
355. Eapen M, Zhang MJ, Devidas M, Raetz E, Barredo JC, Ritchey AK, et al. Outcomes after HLA-matched sibling transplantation or chemotherapy in children with acute lymphoblastic leukemia in a second remission after an isolated central nervous system relapse: a collaborative study of the Children's Oncology Group and the Center for International Blood and Marrow Transplant Research. Leukemia. 2008;22(2):281–6.
356. Uderzo C, Grazia Zurlo M, Adamoli L, Zanesco L, Arico M, Calculli G, et al. Treatment of isolated testicular relapse in childhood acute lymphoblastic leukemia: an Italian multicenter study. Associazione Italiana Ematologia ed Oncologia Pediatrica. J Clin Oncol. 1990;8(4):672–7.
357. Wofford MM, Smith SD, Shuster JJ, Johnson W, Buchanan GR, Wharam MD, et al. Treatment of occult or late overt testicular relapse in children with acute lymphoblastic leukemia: a Pediatric Oncology Group study. J Clin Oncol. 1992;10(4):624–30.
358. Finklestein JZ, Miller DR, Feusner J, Stram DO, Baum E, Shina DC, et al. Treatment of overt isolated testicular relapse in children on therapy for acute lymphoblastic leukemia. A report from the Childrens Cancer Group. Cancer. 1994;73(1):219–23.
359. Mullighan CG, Goorha S, Radtke I, Miller CB, Coustan-Smith E, Dalton JD, et al. Genome-wide analysis of genetic alterations in acute lymphoblastic leukaemia. Nature. 2007;446(7137):758–64.
360. Bernt KM, Zhu N, Sinha AU, Vempati S, Faber J, Krivtsov AV, et al. MLL-rearranged leukemia is dependent on aberrant H3K79 methylation by DOT1L. Cancer Cell. 2011;20(1):66–78.
361. Kager L, Evans WE. Pharmacogenomics of acute lymphoblastic leukemia. Curr Opin Hematol. 2006;13(4):260–5.
362. Yang JJ, Cheng C, Yang W, Pei D, Cao X, Fan Y, et al. Genome-wide interrogation of germline genetic variation associated with treatment response in childhood acute lymphoblastic leukemia. JAMA. 2009;301(4):393–403.
363. Maury S, Chevret S, Thomas X, Heim D, Leguay T, Huguet F, et al. Rituximab in B-Lineage Adult Acute Lymphoblastic Leukemia. N Engl J Med. 2016;375(11):1044–53.
364. Kantarjian HM, DeAngelo DJ, Stelljes M, Martinelli G, Liedtke M, Stock W, et al. Inotuzumab ozogamicin versus standard therapy for acute lymphoblastic leukemia. N Engl J Med. 2016;375(8):740–53.

365. Kantarjian H, Stein A, Gokbuget N, Fielding AK, Schuh AC, Ribera JM, et al. Blinatumomab versus chemotherapy for advanced acute lymphoblastic leukemia. N Engl J Med. 2017;376(9):836–47.
366. von Stackelberg A, Locatelli F, Zugmaier G, Handgretinger R, Trippett TM, Rizzari C, et al. Phase I/Phase II Study of Blinatumomab in pediatric patients with relapsed/refractory acute lymphoblastic leukemia. J Clin Oncol. 2016;34(36):4381–9.
367. Topp MS, Kufer P, Gokbuget N, Goebeler M, Klinger M, Neumann S, et al. Targeted therapy with the T-cell-engaging antibody blinatumomab of chemotherapy-refractory minimal residual disease in B-lineage acute lymphoblastic leukemia patients results in high response rate and prolonged leukemia-free survival. J Clin Oncol. 2011;29(18):2493–8.
368. Grupp SA, Kalos M, Barrett D, Aplenc R, Porter DL, Rheingold SR, et al. Chimeric antigen receptor-modified T cells for acute lymphoid leukemia. N Engl J Med. 2013;368(16):1509–18.
369. Maude SL, Frey N, Shaw PA, Aplenc R, Barrett DM, Bunin NJ, et al. Chimeric antigen receptor T cells for sustained remissions in leukemia. N Engl J Med. 2014;371(16):1507–17.
370. Lee DW, Kochenderfer JN, Stetler-Stevenson M, Cui YK, Delbrook C, Feldman SA, et al. T cells expressing CD19 chimeric antigen receptors for acute lymphoblastic leukaemia in children and young adults: a phase 1 dose-escalation trial. Lancet. 2015;385(9967):517–28.
371. Gardner RA, Finney O, Annesley C, Brakke H, Summers C, Leger K, et al. Intent to treat leukemia remission by CD19CAR T cells of defined formulation and dose in children and young adults. Blood. 2017;129(25):3322–31.
372. Schmiegelow K, Forestier E, Hellebostad M, Heyman M, Kristinsson J, Soderhall S, et al. Long-term results of NOPHO ALL-92 and ALL-2000 studies of childhood acute lymphoblastic leukemia. Leukemia. 2010;24(2):345–54.

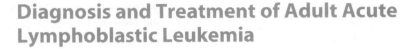

18 Diagnosis and Treatment of Adult Acute Lymphoblastic Leukemia

Nicola Gökbuget and Dieter Hoelzer

Introduction

Acute lymphoblastic leukemia (ALL) is the most frequent neoplastic disease in childhood and accounts for about 20% of the acute leukemias in adults. An early peak of ALL incidence occurs at the age of 4–5 years and the overall incidence is 1.4 with a male predominance. It is relatively infrequent in younger adults but the incidence seems to increase in adults aged over 50 (Chap. 13). The median age of patients in most adult ALL studies ranges from 25 to 39 years.

In the past decades substantial progress has been made in the treatment of ALL mainly based on intensified chemotherapy regimens adopted from pediatric protocols, stem cell transplantation, risk- and subgroup-adjusted therapy, and improved supportive care. With contemporary regimens complete remission (CR) rates of 90% and cure rates of 40–70% depending on age can be achieved [1]. More recently individualized treatment according to minimal residual disease (MRD) has been implemented into treatment protocols. Targeted therapy particularly with tyrosine kinase inhibitors in Ph/BCR–ABL-positive ALL but also antibody therapy has contributed to further improved outcome in subgroups of ALL.

Clinical Features

The clinical presentation of adult ALL is almost always acute and the patient usually has symptoms of only a few weeks' duration. Patients show a rapid decline in general condition and feel generally ill. In rare cases, ALL may also develop from a transient preceding pancytopenia.

Most of the symptoms of adult patients with ALL are nonspecific and are not usually severe. The patients may complain of progressive malaise with lethargy, fatigue, and occasionally weight loss. They may also complain of fever and night sweats in the absence of clinical infection. In older patients complications of anemia such as dyspnea, angina, and dizziness may dominate the clinical picture. Adult ALL patients may have minor arthralgias and bone pain but much less frequently than in children. One-third of the patients have infections or fever. As infections, hemorrhages are also less frequent than in acute myeloid leukemia (AML). There may be a history of some easy bruising and mucosal hemorrhage. In a series of 1273 consecutive ALL patients (15–65 years) treated in the German Multicenter Trials for Adult ALL (GMALL) one-third had some signs of minor bleeding tendency such as petechiae. Fever or infections had the same frequency. A few patients may present with neurological symptoms such as headache, alteration of mental function, or cranial nerve palsies due to leukemic infiltration.

An outline of the clinical approach to a patient with adult ALL is given in Table 18.1. Physical examination will show some degree of organomegaly in most adult patients with ALL: lymphadenopathy, usually cervical, is present in about half of the patients (57%) and palpable splenomegaly (56%) or hepatomegaly (47%) also in about half. A thymic mass can be found from chest roentgenograms or computer tomograms in 15% of all adult ALL patients. The majority of these patients have a T-cell ALL, but patients with other subtypes may occasionally also present with a mediastinal mass. Massive thymic enlargement can cause dyspnea, especially when associated with large pleural effusions. Some patients with mediastinal enlargement have pericardial effusions as well.

Presentation with clinically detectable signs related to leukemic infiltration of the central nervous system (CNS) occurs in about 5–10% of adult ALL patients [2]. Risk factors for CNS involvement include a high initial white blood cell (WBC) count, T-cell phenotype, and L3 or Burkitt's morphology. CNS involvement may manifest as raised intracranial pressure with headache and papilledema without

N. Gökbuget, M.D. (✉) • D. Hoelzer, M.D., Ph.D.
Department of Medicine II, Goethe University Hospital, Theodor Stern Kai 7, Frankfurt 60590, Germany
e-mail: goekbuget@em.uni-frankfurt.de; hoelzer@em.uni-frankfurt.de

P.H. Wiernik et al. (eds.), *Neoplastic Diseases of the Blood*, DOI 10.1007/978-3-319-64263-5_18

Table 18.1 Adult ALL: clinical approach and laboratory investigation

Complete medical history, including
• Past medical history, especially heart, lung, liver, or renal disease, and diabetes mellitus (comorbidity score)
• Family history
• Occupational history
Complete physical examination, with special attention to lymphadenopathy and hepatosplenomegaly
• Temperature
• Potential sites of infection including lungs, oropharynx, and perineum
• Signs of abnormal hemorrhage
• Optic fundi
• Full neurological examination including the cranial and peripheral nerves
Diagnostic hematological studies
• Full blood examination including hemoglobin, platelet count, and white blood cell count (total and differential)
• Bone marrow aspirate and trephine biopsy
• Bone marrow cytology
• Immunological markers: T-cell, B-cell, immunological subtypes
• Cytogenetic analysis
• Molecular analysis, for prognostic markers, therapy targets, and MRD markers
Biochemical studies
• Including renal and hepatic function, serum uric acid, serum electrolytes including calcium and phosphate, blood glucose, and serum LDH
Coagulation studies
• Including prothrombin ratio, partial thromboplastin time, fibrinogen, and ATIII
Cardiac assessment
• Including electrocardiograph, echocardiogram, and other noninvasive tests of myocardial function if indicated
Chest roentgenogram: posterior–anterior and lateral
Computer tomograph, if mediastinal lymph nodes, tumor or abdominal masses are suspected
Serological studies
• ABO and Rh blood group
• HLA typing
Microbiological studies
• Culture from any infected site or lesion
• Surveillance cultures
• Serum for antibody titers, CMV, EBV, HIV, candida, aspergillosis
CSF examination
• Examination for cell count and cytocentrifuge preparation for morphology and, if necessary, immunophenotyping
Pregnancy test
Information about fertility preservation

HLA human leukocyte antigen; *PA* posterior–anterior; *CMV* cytomegalovirus; *EBV* Epstein–Barr virus; *HIV* human immunodeficiency virus

focal neurological signs or, rarely, as cranial nerve palsies, the sixth and seventh cranial nerves being most frequently involved. Careful examination of the ocular fundus must be made for leukemic infiltration as well as for hemorrhages due to thrombocytopenia.

Virtually any organ can be involved by infiltration of leukemic cells. The presence of bone lesions could be found in the earlier mentioned ALL series in only 1.2%. Also the initial involvement of the testis was very rare (0.3%). Other leukemic infiltrations were observed in the retina (0.9%), skin (0.9%), tonsils (0.5%), lung (0.5%), and kidney (0.5%). These organ manifestations present a typical clinical pattern of non-Hodgkin's lymphoma (NHL). They occur more frequently in mature B-cell ALL (32%) and T-ALL.

Diagnostic Procedures

The diagnosis of ALL is made by examination of the peripheral blood and bone marrow. Other investigations also need to be performed to further categorize and subclassify the disease and in preparation for therapy. These include cytochemical stains, immunological markers, cytogenetic analysis, and molecular genetic methods.

Peripheral Blood

Peripheral blood examination characteristically shows anemia, thrombocytopenia, and neutropenia (Table 18.2) although the total white blood cell count (WBC) is variable. The reduction in the level of hemoglobin is mild to moderate, but nearly one-third of the patients have a hemoglobin level below 8 g/dL. Although clinical bleeding due to thrombocytopenia is not very common, about half of the patients have a platelet count below 50×10^9/L. The proportion (30%) of adult ALL patients having had some history of hemorrhage corresponds well with the 30% of patients with a platelet count below 25×10^9/L. The proportion of patients with a granulocyte count below 0.5×10^9/L, usually associated with high risk of infection, was only one-fifth in this series. Only a small minority of patients had clotting defects and of these 5% had an initially decreased fibrinogen level, which might be of relevance if an immediate l-asparaginase treatment is anticipated. The WBC was reduced in 27%, and normal or modestly elevated in 60%, and 16% had a marked leukocytosis (WBC count > 100×10^9/L) at presentation. However, even in the cases where the WBC was reduced or normal, characteristic lymphoblasts could be identified on a well-stained blood smear in more than 90% (Table 18.2).

Table 18.2 Laboratory findings at diagnosis of adult ALL

	1273 patients (%)
Total leukocytes (×10⁹/L)	
<5	27
5–10	14
10–50	31
50–100	12
>100	16
Granulocytes (×10⁹/L)	
<0.5	22
0.5–1.0	14
1.0–1.5	9
>1.5	55
Hemoglobin (g/dL)	
<6	8
6–8	20
8–10	26
10–12	24
>12	22
Thrombocytes (×10⁹/L)	
<25	30
25–50	22
50–150	33
>150	16
Fibrinogen (mg/dL)	
<100	5
>100	95
Leukemic blast cells in PB	
Present	92
Absent	8
Leukemic blast cells in BM	
<50%	4
51–90%	25
>90%	71

Data from unpublished GMALL studies

Bone Marrow

Bone marrow examination provides further material for diagnostic assessment including morphology, cytochemical stains, immunological markers, and cytogenetic and molecular analysis. Smears of the bone marrow aspirate show markedly hypercellular particles. The majority of cells are leukemic lymphoblasts. A total of 97% of the adult ALL patients had a bone marrow infiltration with leukemic lymphoblasts above 50% (Table 18.2). The normal hematopoietic elements are greatly reduced or absent but, in contrast to AML, they have essentially normal morphology. The trephine biopsy of the bone marrow will further demonstrate marked hypercellularity with replacement of fat spaces and normal marrow elements by infiltration with leukemic cells. A slight increase in marrow reticulin is seen in a small proportion of patients with ALL but much less commonly than with AML. If an adequate bone marrow aspiration is available, it remains open whether an additional biopsy should be done. In our hands a biopsy was necessary when aspiration was not possible due to heavily packed leukemic cells or increased reticulin fibers.

Laboratory Investigations

The laboratory investigations that should be performed at the time of diagnosis (Table 18.1) will serve as a baseline for subsequent studies during the induction period, and may also document metabolic abnormalities that require correction before the start of treatment or modification of drug dosage. Renal impairment, hyperuricemia, and electrolyte imbalance should be corrected if possible before treatment is begun. Serum lactic dehydrogenase (LDH) levels are markedly elevated in most patients with ALL. A full hemostatic profile should be performed to detect the very occasional adult ALL patients with disseminated intravascular coagulation or with an incidental clotting abnormality related to preexisting liver disease or liver infiltration. Besides cultures from any clinically infected site, surveillance cultures from the nose, throat, axillae, groin, vagina, perianal area, and sputum and urine are taken to detect clinically occult infection and to provide useful information about microbiological etiology if septicemia or severe infection subsequently develops. In patients with a past medical history of heart disease and in older patients where treatment with an anthracycline is anticipated, an echocardiogram with myocardial function, including the ejection fraction, should be carried out.

Cerebrospinal Fluid

The examination of the cerebrospinal fluid (CSF) is an essential diagnostic procedure in ALL to exclude or confirm initial CNS disease. There are different opinions as to when the first lumbar puncture should be done. Early recognition of CNS disease is clinically important because more aggressive CNS therapy is required for such patients. Therefore a diagnostic puncture should be done if possible before initiation of systemic chemotherapy. This procedure is restricted to patients with an adequate platelet count which can be achieved by platelet transfusion (>20 × 10^9/L), an absence of manifest clinical hemorrhages, and without a high WBC. For safety reasons patients should receive intrathecal methotrexate at the first lumbar puncture. Clearly this procedure necessitates an atraumatic lumbar puncture and should only be performed by experienced physicians since in childhood ALL blood contamination of the CSF was associated with a higher relapse risk. In pediatric studies nowadays CNS disease at diagnosis is classified into four groups: CNS1 (no blasts in CSF), CNS2 (<5 WBC/μL with blasts), CNS3 (≥5 WBC/μL with blasts), and TLP+ (traumatic lumbar puncture with ≥10 RBC/μL with blasts) [2]. CNS involvement in adult ALL is generally defined as CNS3 or the presence of signs of CNS involvement in CT or MRT or neurological symptoms not otherwise explainable, e.g., cranial nerve palsies.

Differential Diagnosis

Difficulty is rarely experienced in establishing the diagnosis of ALL. Viral infection may cause lymphadenopathy and hepatosplenomegaly with lymphocytosis in the blood and bone marrow and, although the distinction can usually be made on clinical and morphological grounds, the results of viral antibody titers, lymphocyte surface markers, and cytogenetic analyses may be required. The leukemic phase of non-Hodgkin's lymphoma can mostly be recognized by clinical and morphological features, by the type and pattern of immunological cell surface markers, and by the degree and distribution of bone marrow infiltration. In the rare cases with a low bone marrow infiltration an arbitrary distinction between ALL and lymphoblastic lymphoma is usually chosen according to the degree of infiltration, above or below 25%. With more advanced immunological marker application, mixed leukemias having myeloid as well as lymphoid surface markers are diagnosed, which might be allocated to a treatment strategy for either ALL or AML; recent data show more favorable outcomes with ALL regimens for biphenotypic leukemias [3]. They have to be distinguished from cases with ALL and coexpression of myeloid markers, which is rather frequent in immature subtypes such as pro-B-ALL or early T-ALL. These patients are treated with ALL strategies.

Occasionally, difficulties can occur in distinguishing Ph/BCR–ABL-positive ALL from primary lymphoid blast crisis of CML. Sometimes final diagnosis can be done only after treatment initiation. In ALL patients achieving complete clinical remission (CR), the peripheral blood count shows normal values, whereas CML cases may revert to a chronic phase with pathological left shift.

Classification

There is a wide heterogeneity within ALL. Therefore accurate morphological classification, determination of the immunological phenotype, and cytogenetic and molecular genetic analysis, which are of prognostic and therapeutic relevance, should be performed in every case of ALL, including older ALL patients. In addition, in all patients, material from the time point of diagnosis should be sent to a reference laboratory in order to identify individual markers for detection of minimal residual disease.

Morphology and Cytochemistry

Bone marrow aspirates and blood smears are stained with Wright's or Wright's-Giemsa stain and the blast cells may be classified according to the French–American–British (FAB) classification. Clinical relevance of FAB subtypes is limited to the detection of the L3 FAB subtype which is characteristic for mature B-ALL. This subtype is important to identify since different treatment approaches are used. In the new WHO classification ALL is classified together with lymphoblastic lymphoma into B-precursor lymphoblastic leukemia/lymphoma, T-precursor lymphoblastic leukemia/lymphoma, and Burkitt's leukemia/lymphoma [4]. The further subclassification is of less relevance for management of adult ALL.

The cytochemical stains to discriminate between AML and ALL are Sudan black, myeloperoxidase, and chloracetate or nonspecific esterase. These reactions are negative in ALL, negativity being usually defined as less than 3% of leukemic blast cells positive. Cytochemical stains to confirm ALL are periodic acid-Schiff (PAS) and acid phosphatase. The PAS stain will show coarse granules or block positivity in at least some cells of most patients with adult ALL of the L1 or L2 type, the incidence of positivity being approximately 60–70% in both groups. The acid phosphatase reaction is positive in 20–30% of all ALL being more specific for T-ALL. About 70% of patients with T-ALL will show strong and localized paranuclear staining with acid phosphatase. PAS or acid phosphatase reactivity is, however, not restricted to ALL and since it can be positive in some cases (M5) of AML the additional reactions for peroxidase and acetate esterase must be negative.

Immunophenotyping

The main aim of immunophenotyping of leukemic blast cells is to distinguish between AML and within the ALL between B- or T-lineage ALL by using monoclonal antibodies to pan-B (CD19), pan-T (CD7), and pan-myeloid surface antigens (CD13, CD33, CDw65). To detect early lymphoid or myeloid differentiation, lineage-specific markers which are first exhibited in the cytoplasm (cy) of B-cell (cyCD22), T-cell (cyCD3), and myeloid precursor cells (myeloperoxidase) are used. To define further maturational stages within the B- and T-cell lineages, markers more specific for

Table 18.3 Immunological, morphological, cytogenetic, and molecular characterization of ALL[a]

Subtypes	Marker	Incidence[a] (%)	FAB subtype	Frequent cytogenetic aberrations	Fusion transcripts and mutations
B-lineage ALL	**HLA-DR$^+$, TdT$^+$, CD19$^+$and/or CD79a$^+$and/or CD22$^+$**	**76**			
Pro B-ALL	No additional differentiation markers	12	L1, L2	t(4;11)(q21;q23)	70% ALL1-AF4 (20% Flt3 in MLL+)
Common ALL	**CD10+**	49	L1, L2	t(9;22)(q34;q11) del(6q)	33% BCR–ABL (30–50% in c/preB) 4% t(1;19)/PBX-E2A 10–20% BCR-ABL-like[c]
Pre-B-ALL	CD10±, **cyIg+**	11	L1, L2	t(9;22)(q34;q11) t(1;19)(q23;p13)	
Mature B-ALL	CD10 ±, sIg+	4	L3	t(8;14)(q24;q32) t(2;8)(p12;q24) t(8;22)(q24;q11)	
T-lineage ALL	**cyCD3 orsCD3**	**23**			
Early T-ALL Cortical T-ALL Mature T-ALL	No additional differentiation markers, mostly CD2– **CD1a+**, sCD3 ± sCD3+, **CD1a–**	6 12 5	L1, L2	t/del(9p) t(10;14)(q24;q11) t(11;14)(p13;q11)	5% NUP214-ABL1[b] 30% TLX1[b] >60% Notch1[b]

[a]N = 946 adult ALL patients [7]
[b][8]
[c][9]

particular maturational stages are used: for B-lineage CD20, cy immunoglobulin μ heavy chain (cyIgM), and surface immunoglobulin (sIg), and for T-lineage CD1, CD2, CD4, CD8, and surface sCD3. The maturation stages are not identified by the presence or absence of a single antigen but by a pattern of antigen expression. One widely used classification system for immunologic subtypes in ALL has been proposed by the EGIL group [5]. More recently early T-precursor ALL has been described as a specific subtype of T-ALL, characterized by a unique gene expression and surface marker profile [6]. For further details on immunobiology of ALL refer to Chap. 15.

With the availability of more specific monoclonal antibodies 98–99% of the acute leukemias can now be reliably classified by immunological marker analysis. In addition, ALL can be subdivided according to various maturational stages of B- or T-lineage, whereby it is assumed that they are in differentiation arrest corresponding to normal maturational stages. Immunological classification of ALL subtypes is summarized in Table 18.3.

B-Lineage ALL

With the analysis of CD10 (the common ALL antigen), cyIgM, and sIg, the B-lineage ALL can be subdivided into three subgroups of B-cell-precursor ALL and mature B-ALL. Virtually all B-precursor ALLs are positive for HLA-DR and TdT. Pro-B-ALL (also termed pre-pre-B-ALL, null-ALL, CD10-negative ALL) is the most immature subtype of the B-ALL lineage. This subtype is characterized by the expression of CD19, cyCD22, and mostly CD24, while CD10, cyIgM, and SIg are negative. Common ALL, the major immunological subtype in childhood as well as in adult ALL, is characterized by the expression of CD10 in combination with CD19, cy or sCD22, and CD24. Common ALL blast cells do not carry markers of relatively mature B-cells such as cyIgM or sIg. Pre-B-ALL is characterized by the expression of cyIgM, being negative in common ALL but otherwise identical with all other markers, such as CD19, cy or sCD22, CD24, and only very rarely CD10 may be absent in this subtype. In most adult clinical studies pre-B-ALL is included in the common ALL category. In most studies common ALL is defined by surface antigen expression of CD10 on 20% or more of leukemic cells and the diagnosis of pre-B-ALL by cyIgM in 10% or more of blast cells.

Leukemic blast cells in mature B-ALL, also termed Burkitt's leukemia, express sIg and B-cell antigens including CD19, CD20, CD22, CD24, and usually CD10. In contrast to the B-precursor ALLs, leukemic cells in B-ALL are mostly negative for TdT. Most B-ALLs can be identified morphologically as L3 FAB subtype.

T-Lineage ALL

Early T-ALL is characterized by the expression of cyCD3 with no additional differentiation markers. CD2 is generally negative. In cases positive for CD2 but negative for CD4, CD8, sCD3, and CD1a, an early T-ALL is present as well. Cortical T-ALL, also referred to as thymic T-ALL, is characterized by the expression of CD1 in combination with CD7, CD5, and CD2, and sometimes also sCD3, CD4, and CD8. Mature T-ALL is characterized by positivity for sCD3, CD7,

CD5, and CD2 while CD1 is negative. CD4 and CD8 are present in most cases. In the newly described entity of early T-precursor ALL (ETP) by definition, blasts in ETP ALL express CD7 but lack CD1a and CD8, and are positive for one or more of the myeloid/stem cell markers [4].

Myeloid Antigen-Positive ALL (My + ALL)

Immunophenotyping has shown the existence of acute leukemia cases in which the blast cells express markers supposedly specific for or associated with another cell lineage. The myeloid-antigen-associated monoclonal antibodies that are used for the detection of My + ALL are CD13, CD14, CD15, CD33, and CDw65. The reported frequencies of My + ALL differ widely, ranging from 5 to 46% depending on the definition, and an approximate figure for adult My + ALL may be 18%. Commonly a case is considered as My + ALL if 20% or more of the blast cells are reactive with the myeloid-lineage-associated monoclonal antibodies. The expression of myeloid antigens is associated with certain subtypes of ALL such as pro B-ALL or early T-ALL. Myeloid coexpression should be differentiated from biphenotypic leukemia. The EGIL group has proposed a score for identification of biphenotypic acute leukemia [5].

Table 18.4 Characteristics of immunological subtypes of adult ALL[a]

Subgroup	Clinical/laboratory characteristics	Relapse kinetics and localization
B-lineage		
Pro-B-ALL	– t(4;11)/ALL1-AF4 (70%) – High WBC (>100/mL) (26%) – Frequent myeloid coexpression (>50%)	– Mainly BM (>90%)
c-ALL/ pre-B-ALL	– Higher age (24% > 50 year) – Ph/BCR–ABL (40–50%) – m-BCR (70%), M-BCR (30%)	– Mainly BM (>90%) – Prolonged relapse kinetics (up to 5–7 year)
B-ALL	– Higher age (27% > 50 year) – Frequent organ involvement (32%) – Frequent CNS involvement (13%)	– Frequent CNS (10%) – Short relapse kinetics (up to 1–1½ years)
T-lineage		
	– Younger age (90% < 50 year) – Frequent mediastinal tumors (60%) – Frequent CNS involvement (8%) – High WBC (>50/mL) (46%)	– Frequent CNS (10%)/ extramedullary (6%) – Intermediate relapse kinetics (up to 3–4 years)

[a]Data based on German multicenter trials of adult ALL

Frequency and Clinical Features of Immunological Subtypes

The frequency of immunological subtypes in adult ALL shows distinct differences from that in childhood ALL. Approximately 84% of the children have a B-precursor ALL and common ALL is, with 63%, the most frequent subtype, whereas this subtype is only observed in one-half of adult ALL patients. There is a significantly higher proportion of the pro-B-ALL, with 12% in adults compared to only 5% in children. Mature B-ALL is rare in both childhood and adult ALL. Adult T-ALL, with 23%, has a twofold higher incidence in adults than the 13% observed in children. As in the B-lineage the most immature form, pre-T-ALL, has a higher incidence in adults compared to children.

The clinical features of the immunological subtypes of ALL are quite distinct. The immature pro-B-ALL has a peak in infants less than 1 year old and is associated with high WBC, massive hepatosplenomegaly, CNS disease, and myeloid coexpression, and approximately 70% of the patients show t(4;11). Nearly one-half of the patients with c-ALL or pre-B-ALL show the translocation t(9;22) and the incidence increases with age. Mature B-ALL is characterized by frequent abdominal tumor masses, often organ involvement, an increased incidence of CNS leukemia, and a male preponderance. T-ALL is associated with mediastinal masses in nearly half of the patients, occasionally associated with pleural and pericardial effusions, an increased incidence of organomegaly, a higher incidence of CNS disease, a high WBC count, and male prevalence. The major clinical differences between immunological subtypes of adult ALL are summarized in Table 18.4.

Cytogenetics and Molecular Genetics

Cytogenetic and molecular genetics abnormalities are independent prognostic variables for predicting the outcome of adult ALL (Chap. 16). In several multicenter studies, clonal chromosomal aberrations could be detected in approximately 62–85% of adult ALL patients. The most frequent numerical chromosomal aberrations are hypodiploid karyotype with less than 46 chromosomes (4–8%), hyperdiploid karyotype with 47–50 chromosomes (7–15%), or greater than 50 chromosomes (7–8%). The most frequent structural aberration is the translocation t(9;22)/Philadelphia chromosome (P+ ALL). Other translocations occur less frequently and are mostly associated with distinct immunological subtypes such as t(4;11) (3–4%) in pro-B-ALL, t(8;14) (5%) in mature B-ALL, t(1;19) (2–3%) in pre-B-ALL, and t(10;14) (3%), 9p– (5–15%), 6q– (4–6%), and 12p aberrations (4–5%) mainly in T-ALL.

The Ph chromosome t(9;22)(q34;q11) results from a translocation involving the breakpoint cluster region of the BCR gene on chromosome 22 and the ABL gene on chromosome 9. One-third of adult ALL patients with a Ph chromosome show M-BCR rearrangements (resulting in a 210 kDa protein), similar to patients with CML, whereas two-thirds have m-BCR rearrangements (resulting in a 190 kDa protein).

Currently a new subgroup with prognostic and therapeutic relevance is discussed. The "Ph-like" or "BCR-ABL-like" ALL is characterized by a gene expression profile similar to Ph-positive ALL. A part of the patients also show translocations or mutations of ABL or JAK genes, which can potentially be targeted by tyrosine kinase inhibitors [9, 10]. Patients with this subtype of ALL show an inferior prognosis in childhood and adults with lower rates of molecular responses [9–11]. A prospective and validated diagnostic identification of Ph-like ALL is currently not possible but identification of targetable lesions may be helpful in individual patients with refractory disease.

The most frequent form of 11q23 abnormalities in ALL is t(4;11)(q21;q23). The translocation is frequently detected in infant leukemia and in patients with the pro-B-ALL subtype (CD10 negative). The overall incidence in adults is approximately 5%. Typical molecular aberrations in ALL with associated cytogenetic translocations and immunological subtypes are summarized in Table 18.3.

Blasts cells with a low hypodiploid karyotype represent another high-risk entity which is frequently associated with TP53 mutations [12].

Overall the observed incidence of the majority of cytogenetic aberrations is very low and therefore the options of correlation to clinical outcome and even more therapeutic consequences are limited. The most relevant markers can be identified by molecular analysis as well. Nevertheless, cytogenetic analysis is still recommended as a routine diagnostic method in ALL. It is highly recommended to store biomaterials from each ALL patient for potential future analyses, e.g., focused on targetable lesions.

Detection of Minimal Residual Disease

Conventional microscopic evaluation of bone marrow smears has a detection limit of 5%. With methods for detection of MRD, residual blast cells can be detected and measured quantitatively below this level with a sensitivity of 10^{-4}–10^{-6}. With these methods individual follow-up analyses can be performed in patients with clinical and morphological CR. ALL is an "ideal" disease for detection of MRD since more than 90% of the patients show individual clonal markers. Most experience has been accumulated with MRD detection by flow cytometry and PCR (overview in [13]).

MRD detection by flow cytometry targets individual leukemia-specific combinations of surface antigens and reaches a sensitivity of 10^{-4}. PCR detection may target the expression of leukemia-specific fusion genes such as BCR–ABL, which may be detected in 30–40 of adult ALL cases. A more widespread applicability is reached with detection of clonal rearrangements of immunoglobulin heavy-chain (IgH) or T-cell receptor (TCR- β, −δ, −γ) gene rearrangements. This method reaches a sensitivity of 10^{-4}–10^{-6} and combinations of two or more target structures can be identified in more than 80% of ALL patients. For this method the best level of standardization has been reached regarding methodology and reporting and interpretation of results for clinical trials [14]. MRD detection with any method should be restricted to experienced laboratories, which participate in quality control rounds taking place on an international level.

Markers for MRD detection have to be established at the time of first diagnosis. Therefore diagnostic material has to be provided to a specialized laboratory.

Supportive Care

The management of adult patients undergoing induction therapy for ALL requires intensive treatment of initial complications and supportive care to prevent and manage the infectious, hemorrhagic, metabolic, and psychological problems that may arise.

Metabolic Abnormalities

A few general measures can be started at once. Sufficient fluid intake to guarantee urine production of at least 100 mL/h throughout induction therapy reduces the risk of uric acid formation. This may require parenteral fluid administration when the patient's oral intake is inadequate because of nausea or difficulty in swallowing. If the venous system does not offer an easy approach, access by catheter or port is advantageous when anticipating a longer period of induction therapy or when part of the therapy will be carried out on an outpatient basis.

Hyperuricemia is frequently present at diagnosis; it may worsen following the initiation of chemotherapy and, if not treated, can lead to renal failure. Adequate doses of allopurinol (300–600 mg/day) should be given and the urine alkalinized before chemotherapy. Allopurinol has to be reduced when 6-mercaptopurine is given. In patients with high risk of tumor lysis, uratoxidase may be used for prevention of hyperurikemia.

In patients presenting with renal impairment, an attempt must be made to reestablish renal function before chemotherapy is started. Renal failure is often observed in patients with Burkitt's lymphoma or B-ALL with abdominal tumor masses and can be resolved by a gentle pretreatment with cyclophosphamide (C) combined with dexamethasone (P) or dexamethasone (DX) or steroids alone.

The acute tumor lysis syndrome is most frequently seen in patients with B-ALL or T-ALL but may also occur in other subtypes with high WBC or large tumor mass. Massive and rapid tumor cell lysis leads to hyperkalemia, hyperphosphatemia, hyperuricemia, and hypocalcemia, which can largely be prevented by the C + P/DX treatment.

Infections

Approximately one-third of adult ALL patients present with infections at diagnosis. Fever or infection at the time of admission is mainly associated with severe granulocytopenia, especially if the granulocyte count is less than 5×10^9/L but may also be due to immunological deficiency (e.g., CD4 lymphopenia) or mucosal lesions. Combination chemotherapy causes additional hematological toxicity and at least 50% of adults undergoing induction treatment will experience severe or life-threatening infections. The incidence of infections with gram-positive bacteria has increased—especially those due to more frequent use of indwelling catheters. Fungal infections also occur more frequently.

Much attention has been paid to prophylactic measures against infection. They include oral hygiene using antiseptic soaps and mouthwashes and disinfection of the anogenital region. Other precautions include reverse protective isolation and air filtration, if available, which can reduce especially the risk of Aspergillus infections. Simple precautions that can always be carried out are no live plants in the room, no humidifiers, no i.m./s.c. injections if avoidable, no uncooked vegetables, no unpeeled fruits, and no visitors having any kind of infection. Prevention and management of infections are discussed in detail in Chaps. 49 and 51.

Hematopoietic Growth Factors

The use of hematopoietic growth factors (HPGFs) such as colony-stimulating factor–granulocyte (G-CSF) is a valuable component of supportive therapy during the treatment of ALL. There is no indication that these CSFs stimulate leukemic cell growth in a clinically significant manner. The majority of clinical trials demonstrate that the prophylactic administration of G-CSF significantly accelerates neutrophil recovery and several prospective randomized studies also showed that this is associated with a substantially reduced incidence and duration of febrile neutropenia and of severe infections [15, 16]. The enhanced marrow recovery allows closer adherence to the dose and schedule of chemotherapeutic regimens.

The advantage of G-CSF administration is particularly evident in patients at high risk for prolonged granulocytopenia. Furthermore, scheduling appears to be important. When CSFs are first given at the end of a 4-week chemotherapy regimen, potential benefits are limited. Therefore it is noteworthy that G-CSF may be given in parallel with chemotherapy without aggravating the myelotoxicity of these specific regimens [15, 16] and that this scheduling is an important determinant of the clinical efficacy.

Hemorrhage

The thrombocytopenia present in one-third of the patients at diagnosis will worsen following chemotherapy, requiring transfusion of platelet concentrates. Platelet transfusions should be given for bleeding and to prevent bleeding when platelet counts are below 20×10^9/L especially during febrile periods, which interfere with platelet function. When a long induction period is anticipated and there is a likelihood that a patient will need frequent platelet transfusions it might be preferable to start with HLA-matched platelets immediately, if this is logistically possible (technical facilities, costs), to avoid refractoriness to random platelets. The issue of platelet transfusions is discussed in detail in Chap. 54.

L-Asparaginase treatment leads to a decrease in fibrinogen and ATIII and may thereby enhance the risk of thrombosis and bleeding. So far no standards have been defined for substitution of both factors although it is done in many trials.

Chemotherapy

The approach to therapy of adult ALL has evolved along similar lines to that successfully employed in childhood ALL. An induction therapy is followed by a postremission or consolidation therapy. Whereas the induction phase of therapy is usually well defined, the postremission therapy may consist of different consolidation cycles, including reinduction or stem cell transplantation. In addition there is a CNS prophylaxis throughout the whole therapy and maintenance treatment.

Traditionally successful treatment protocols for adult ALL are based on pediatric approaches. The overall outcome is evident from the published studies in younger ALL patients listed in Table 18.5. Complete remission (CR) rates in modern protocols reach 90% with approximately 5% early

Table 18.5 Results of recent trials with pediatric based regimens in adult ALL

Study	Year	*N*	Median age (range)	CR rate (%)	Survival (%)
Ribera et al.[a] [17]	2008	81	29 (15–30)[a]	98	69 (6 years)
Huguet et al. [18]	2009	225	31 (15–60)	93	60 (3 years)
Rijneveld et al. [19]	2011	54	26 (17–40)	91	72 (2 years)
Stock et al. [20]	2014	296	24 (17–39)	nr	78 (2 years)
Rytting et al. [21]	2014	84	21 (13–39)	94	74 (4 years)
De Angelo et al. [22]	2015	92	28 (18–50)	85	67 (4 years)

[a]Standard risk only

death during induction and 5% failure to achieve a remission. Overall survival and leukemia-free survival range between 40 and 70% with a large variability according to subgroups of ALL with around 30–50% survival for high risk, 40–70% for standard risk, 50–70% for Ph+ ALL, and 70–80% for mature B-ALL.

Initial Treatment

In patients with a large leukemic cell burden, that is, a high WBC and/or massive organomegaly, cell reduction with a cautious preinduction therapy is recommended. In patients with high WBC count (>100 × 10^9/L), where hyperviscosity due to leukostasis with cerebral impairment may occur, leukopheresis may be considered. However, such technical facilities may not be available and these patients can also be managed with a gentle prephase chemotherapy consisting of vincristine or cyclophosphamide and prednisone or dexamethasone in nearly all cases without complications. Prephase treatment is suitable anyway in order to stabilize the patients and complete all diagnostic procedures before the start of induction treatment.

Remission Induction

Standard induction therapy for ALL includes prednisone, vincristine, anthracyclines, mostly daunorubicin, and also L-asparaginase. Further drugs, such as cyclophosphamide, cytarabine (either conventional or high dose), mercaptopurine, and others, are added in many protocols, sometimes named as early intensification.

Steroids such as prednisone and prednisolone have been most frequently administered. Dexamethasone shows a higher antileukemic activity in vitro and a better penetration of the cerebrospinal fluid. Extensive use of DX without interruptions may, however, be associated with an increased risk of septicemias and fungal infections, which may be circumvented if treatment time is reduced.

The most frequently used anthracycline is *daunorubicin* (DNR). Several study groups have replaced the usual weekly applications, as in the BFM-based protocols, by higher doses of DNR (45–80 mg/m^2) on subsequent days. In one recent trial the intensified use of daunorubicin failed to improve response rates [23]. Thus it remains open whether intensified anthracyclines are beneficial for adult ALL at all, for all subgroups and age groups. Intensive anthracycline therapy may be associated with an increased induction mortality. Therefore, intensive supportive care and probably the use of growth factors are recommended with these types of protocols.

Asparaginase (A) does not affect the CR rate but improves LFS. If not used during induction therapy, it is often included as part of the consolidation treatment. Three different A preparations with significantly different half-lives are available: native *E. coli* A (1.2 days), Erwinia A (0.65 days), and pegylated *E. coli* A (PEG-L-A) (5.7 days). The availability may vary between different countries. In order to reach equal efficacy, the application schedule has to be adapted and is generally daily for Erwinia, every second day for *E. coli*, and 1–2 weeks for PEG-L-A. The latter asparaginase preparation has the advantage of less frequent administrations and more even activity distribution. In a considerable proportion of adult ALL patients A induces laboratory changes, e.g., coagulation disorders and liver transaminases with unclear clinical impact [24] and in fewer patients severe complications such as hepatopathies or pancreatitis. A-induced toxicities are not always predictable and may lead to treatment delays in individual patients. Consistent management of toxicities is essential [25]. On the other hand, ASP is recognized as an extremely important drug for the treatment of ALL due to its unique mechanism of action and resistance. Optimization of A therapy is therefore a major aim for management of adult ALL.

Definition of Complete Remission

Complete remission is defined as a state in which there is no clinical or laboratory manifestation of leukemia. The peripheral blood count and bone marrow appearances are within normal limits except for abnormalities attributable to chemotherapy; the marrow blast cell count is less than 5%; also examination of the CSF shows no blast cells. CR includes also the disappearance of organomegalies, but it should be noted that the persistence of splenomegaly is not always due to leukemic infiltration.

Table 18.6 Definition of response in ALL

Conventional definition		Evaluation of MRD	
Complete remission	• <5% blasts in bone marrow smear and • Regeneration of peripheral blood count and • Disappearance of all extramedullary manifestations	Molecular remission	Negative MRD status detected with a standardized method and a minimum sensitivity of 0.01%
		Molecular failure	Positive MRD-status above 0.01%
Relapse	• Detection of more than 5% blasts in bone marrow after prior achievement of CR[a] or • Reappearance of extramedullary manifestations	Molecular relapse	Increase of MRD above 0.01% after prior achievement of molecular CR

[a]In case of 5–10% blasts in regenerating marrow a repeated bone marrow assessment is recommended in order to distinguish blasts form hematogones

Definition of complete remission was recently extended by the definition of MRD response or molecular response. An international consensus workshop has defined technical prerequisites for MRD-based response evaluation mainly for PCR-based measurement of individual gene rearrangements. In patients with a marker with sensitivity of at least 10^{-4}, complete MRD response is defined as a negative status of MRD. MRD failure is defined as MRD level above 10^{-4} [14]. MRD response is strongly associated with prognosis. Therefore MRD-based response evaluation is a new endpoint for clinical trials (Table 18.6).

Failure of Induction Therapy

With current protocols failure rates after induction are generally around 10%. The rate of early death depends on age and ranges from <3% in adolescents to 20% in patients >60 years of age. The main cause of death in approximately two-thirds of the patients is infection, in part fungal infection. Beyond mortality also morbidity, e.g., due to extended cytopenias and subsequent infections such as fungal pneumonias, has to be considered which may compromise further treatment and dose intensity. The remaining nonresponders may achieve a partial remission or may be refractory to standard treatment. These patients have an extremely poor prognosis. They are therefore candidates for experimental treatment approaches or consideration for an SCT, even if not in CR but in good partial remission.

Consolidation Therapy

When in ALL CR is achieved, treatment has to be continued in order to eliminate residual leukemia after induction chemotherapy and thereby prevent relapse as well as emergence of drug-resistant cells because a high percentage of patients show MRD after induction therapy. Continuation or postremission therapy consists of intensification or consolidation and maintenance. Consolidation/intensification refers either to high-dose therapy, the use of multiple new agents, or readministration of the induction regimen (reinduction). SCT is also included in postremission therapy in many trials. In most studies that involve repeated consolidation cycles over the entire treatment period, it is difficult to analyze critically the effect of the different treatment phases on outcome.

Intensive consolidation is standard in the treatment of ALL although consolidation cycles in large studies are very variable and it is impossible to evaluate their individual efficacy. In general it seems that intensive application of high-dose methotrexate (HDMTX) is beneficial. Depending on age, in adults dosages are probably limited at 1.5–3 g/m^2 if given as 24-h infusion. Otherwise toxicities, particularly mucositis, may lead to subsequent treatment delays and decreased compliance. From pediatric ALL trials there is increasing evidence that intensified application of asparaginase leads to improved overall results. In adult ALL this approach appears to be useful particularly in consolidation, where less toxicity can be expected compared to induction. Several studies have also demonstrated that a reinduction improves outcome.

The most important feature of consolidation is probably to administer rotating cycles with short intervals. However after several consolidation cycles some adult patients tend to develop prolonged cytopenias, which lead to delays of subsequent chemotherapies. Therefore a balance between bone marrow toxic and less toxic cycles may be important. For future studies in adult ALL stricter adherence to protocols with fewer delays, dose reductions, and omissions would be an important contribution to therapeutic progress.

Maintenance

Maintenance up to a total treatment duration of 2½ years even after intensive induction and consolidation is still standard for adult ALL; all attempts to omit maintenance led to inferior outcome. MTX preferably given intravenously (i.v.) or orally and mercaptopurine (MP) given orally are the backbone of maintenance. It may be important to aim for leukocyte counts below 3000/μL during maintenance [26]. Intensification cycles with vincristine and steroids did not provide additional benefit at least in pediatric trials using intensive reinduction [27]. Furthermore in adults prolonged steroid therapy may lead to an increase of late effects such as osteonecrosis. Randomized trials also failed to demonstrate an advantage of intensified maintenance with HD cycles although the compliance in these trials is unclear.

Adults often show poor compliance to intensive maintenance due to toxicities and moreover social reasons. Even for conventional maintenance compliance may be a problem. In Ph+ ALL maintenance with kinase inhibitors appears to be of utmost importance after chemotherapy as well as after stem cell transplantation. Overall, for further improvement of outcome the physicians' and patients' compliance to maintenance therapy seems to be essential.

Central Nervous System Therapy

Prophylactic CNS Therapy

Without some form of prophylactic CNS therapy, around 30% of adults with ALL will develop overt CNS leukemia [2]. Prophylactic CNS therapy in ALL is essential due to several reasons: CNS leukemia is more easily prevented than treated; once CNS leukemia has developed, it is generally followed by systemic relapse shortly after; and effective CNS prophylaxis also prevents systemic relapse.

Several treatment options are available for prevention of CNS relapse: intrathecal (i.th.) therapy, cranial irradiation (CRT), and systemic high-dose chemotherapy (overviews in Ref [2]). I.th. therapy is usually based on MTX as single drug but combinations with AC and/or steroids are used in some studies. The route of application is generally lumbar puncture. CRT (18–24 Gy in 12 fractions over 16 days) may be administered with or without parallel i.th. therapy. Systemic HD chemotherapy may comprise HdAC or HdMTX since both drugs reach cytotoxic drug levels in the CSF and showed effectivity in overt CNS leukemia.

Various combinations of these approaches have been used in adult ALL trials but the issue of CNS prophylaxis has not been addressed prospectively. For analysis of published trials, it has to be considered that most authors only report the frequency of isolated CNS relapses. However, in a significant proportion of adult ALL patients combined CNS and bone marrow relapses occur. Overall there is evidence that CNS relapse rates decrease with increasing intensity of prophylaxis and with the number of applied modalities.

The role of CNS irradiation in different subtypes of adult ALL remains to be determined. In pediatric patients considerable late effects of CNS irradiation are observed and effective CNS prophylaxis is achieved by high doses of systemic methotrexate treatment. In adults similar doses cannot be administered due to toxicities. Therefore the role of CNS irradiation may be different; in addition there are no reports on similar late effects compared to those observed in children.

In current trials with effective CNS prophylaxis the incidence of CNS relapse is below 5–10%. It is influenced by several risk factors such as immunophenotype (T-ALL, B-ALL), extreme leukocytosis, high leukemia cell proliferation rate, high serum LDH levels, and extramedullary organ involvement. Risk-adapted CNS prophylaxis may be based on these features.

Recently a liposomal preparation of cytarabine has been used for treatment of CNS relapse of lymphoma and ALL and was evaluated in several protocols for prophylaxis of CNS relapse. Due to the preparation a prolonged cytotoxic activity and a more even distribution in the CSF are observed [28]. Therefore fewer applications, i.e., every 2 weeks are required. However combination regimens of liposomal cytarabine with systemic high-dose therapy have to be defined carefully since neurological toxicities may occur [29].

Therapy of Established CNS Disease

About 5–10% of adult ALL patients present with manifestations of CNS leukemia. The incidence is correlated to the immunological subtype and is higher in T-ALL and mature B-ALL. Treatment of overt CNS leukemia is usually undertaken with either i.th. MTX alone, in combination with AC or hydrocortisone, or CRT. I.th. MTX is administered 2–3 times per week and until two consecutive CSF examinations show no evidence of leukemic infiltration. Following the establishment of a remission there is some evidence that continued maintenance i.th. chemotherapy at less frequent intervals is beneficial in prolonging the duration of CNS remission. When adult ALL patients with CNS leukemia at diagnosis are treated adequately, they have no inferior outcome with regard to LFS or CNS relapse rate. However there might be an increased risk of prolonged cytopenias during induction due to the systemic effects of intensified intrathecal therapy.

Stem Cell Transplantation

SCT is an integral part of treatment strategy for adult ALL. Bone marrow and to an increasing extent peripheral blood are used as stem cell source. Despite a great number of trials the indications for SCT in first CR, scheduling, and procedures are still not defined satisfactorily. The potential advantages of SCT (short treatment duration, favorable outcome in some trials) must be balanced to the disadvantages (mortality of 20–30%, morbidity, late complications, reduced quality of life) and assessed in relation to the improving outcome of conventional and targeted chemotherapy regimens.

The role of SCT in postremission therapy is one major question in the management of adult ALL. The recommended indications for SCT varied over the time [30–32]. With the broader application of pediatric based regimens the indication is defined more restrictively. More recently, the guidelines and many prospective trials are in favor of transplantation in patients with high-risk features. This applies particularly for younger patients treated with intensive pediatric based chemotherapy. In older patients, due to increasing transplant-related mortality, only dose-reduced conditioning regimens can be considered. Future clinical trials will show whether this approach would be superior to chemotherapy regimens.

Overall according to guidelines overall survival for high-risk patients (with varying definitions) was superior for SCT compared to chemotherapy, whereas the role of SCT in standard risk remained open. The need for SCT in specific genetically defined groups of ALL, such as BCR-ABL1-positive or MLL-positive cases, remains to be defined. Allogeneic SCT is currently carried out for MLL-rearranged ALL in most trials and, in the largest study conducted to date, better results have been observed compared with chemotherapy [33]. In younger standard-risk patients, treated with pediatric based regimens, SCT is not recommended by most groups in order to avoid acute mortality and long-term effects.

MRD is considered as the most important factor to guide the decision of chemotherapy or SCT after consolidation. Data from recent studies have shown that SCT offers better results than chemotherapy in patients with high MRD levels after consolidation, regardless of the conventional risk factors at baseline [34]. The question remains open whether SCT is justified in patients with conventional high-risk features but low or negative MRD after consolidation, for whom OS rates >50% are expected with chemotherapy. An analysis of the French group demonstrated an advantage of SCT in patients with MRD-positive ALL only [35]. Since historical trials mostly did not consider MRD as a decision tool for SCT, future prospective studies are required to answer this question.

Finally there is a general agreement that SCT is clearly the best therapeutic option for patients in second or later CR [30, 31, 36]. A summary of current indication is given in Table 18.7. Since the outcome of ALL with and without SCT is influenced by numerous factors such as type of SCT, donor match, posttransplant regimens, age, MRD status, and availability of targeted therapies, the indication may change over time.

Table 18.7 Recommendations for SCT in adult ALL (modified from [32, 36])

Treatment phase	Transplant option	Recommendations
CR1	Allogeneic SCT	• Recommended in all patients with persistent MRD • Not recommended in standard-risk patients with sustained molecular remission • Unclear indication in high-risk patients with sustained molecular remission
CR1	Autologous SCT	• Inferior compared to allogeneic SCT and chemotherapy in randomized trials • Maintenance therapy after transplant and negative MRD status may improve outcomes
CR ≥ 2	Allogeneic SCT	• Allogeneic SCT recommended in all patients

Donor Type for Allogeneic SCT

There is sufficient evidence that sibling and very-well-matched, unrelated donors (MUD) SCT can be considered equivalent options in terms of results, and therefore MUD SCT can be offered to patients lacking a sibling donor [32, 36]. Umbilical cord blood can be an alternative source when an HSCT is needed urgently or when the search for a very-well-matched, unrelated donor is unsuccessful [30, 37]. Haploidentical SCT could be an option in patients without a matched sibling or MUD, but prospective comparative studies are lacking. Particularly new approaches for haploidentical SCT with post-transplantation cyclophosphamide provide promising results [38]. Autologous SCT is considered inferior to chemotherapy and to allogeneic SCT [39]. The intensity of pretreatment has an important impact on the outcome of autologous SCT, since it leads to reduction of tumor load. It may still be an option in MRD-negative patients unfit for allogeneic SCT and was successful in Ph-positive ALL [40]. Maintenance therapy after autologous SCT, e.g., with MP and MTX, or imatinib in Ph+ ALL—particularly in MRD-positive patients—is also a useful approach.

Conditioning Regimens

There is no standard MAC regimen, but total body irradiation-based regimens seem to have better antileukemic activity than busulfan-based preparative regimens [30, 41]. Regimens with reduced intensity (RIC) are increasingly considered as an option for older patients with high-risk ALL or patients with contraindications for myeloablative conditioning [42], but no prospective comparative studies between these two types of preparative regimens have been conducted in young, fit patients.

Factors for Outcome of SCT

Relapse rate and transplant-related mortality both range between 25 and 30%. Although TRM is strongly correlated with age, the upper age limit for SIB–SCT has increased continuously up to 50–55 years. There is evidence that a graft-versus-leukemia (GvL) effect is also present in ALL, as indicated by several observations, such as lower relapse risk in patients with acute and/or chronic GvHD, lower relapse risk after matched unrelated donor SCT, and induction of remission by withdrawal of prophylaxis against GvHD or donor lymphocyte infusions (DLI) in single patients with relapsed ALL.

Furthermore posttransplant monitoring of MRD is of increasing importance to improve the outcome of SCT.

Prognostic Factors in ALL

ALL is not a uniform disease but characterized by subgroups with different biological and clinical features and cure rates. For various parameters prognostic value for either the achievement of remission or for remission duration has been established in adult ALL [1]. At the present time the following are the most important prognostic features: age, initial WBC, immunophenotype, abnormal cytogenetics, or molecular genetics, and to an increasing extent response criteria such as time to achieve CR and MRD (refer to Table 18.10 discussed later in this chapter).

Age

Age is probably the most important prognostic factor. There is a continuous decrease in outcome with increasing age from childhood to elderly ALL patients. In adults, OS ranges up to 70% below 30 years to 20–30% above 50–60 years. In contrast to other prognostic factors age cannot be used to identify patients who could benefit from SCT as done by some groups because outcome of SCT also decreases with increasing age. Actually improved treatment strategies have to be claimed for older patients as well as for young adults with ALL.

Older Patients with ALL

The median survival time in older ALL patients is 3–14 months. There are several reasons that may account for this. Increased hematological and nonhematological toxicity (e.g., hepato- and cardiotoxicity) results in a higher morbidity and mortality during induction therapy. The death rate during induction therapy for older patients above 65 years reaches 20–30%. Incomplete drug administration and extended intervals between cycles of therapy may lead to inferior long-term results. There is a higher frequency of adverse biological features in adults; thus the incidence of Ph+ ALL patients increases from 3% in children to 20–30% in patients above 50 years. The incidence of unfavorable immunophenotypes such as early T-ALL and pro-B-ALL is also higher in older patients. There is, however, no good evidence that within an identical biological subtype of ALL the leukemic blast cells in elderly ALL patients are more resistant than in younger patients.

The optimal treatment for older ALL patients remains to be defined. Registries give an impression on the overall outcome of unselected older ALL patients [43–46]. Survival rates in patients older than 60 years were 10–25% [44, 45] (Table 18.8) with only marginal improvement over the past decades.

30–70% of the older patients are allocated to palliative therapy mainly due to poor performance status at diagnosis. Most studies have shown an advantage of more intensive therapy (Table 18.8). There is no evidence that palliative approaches are associated with lower rates of early mortality or better quality of life.

If older patients are treated according to protocols designed for younger patients, one major problem is the toxicity and early mortality [47]. Patients may acquire severe infections, non-predefined treatment modifications occur frequently, and treatments may be interrupted or even stopped due to severe complications.

More recently several study groups have developed protocols specifically for older ALL patients (Table 18.9) that have the theoretical aim to provide a chance of cure on the one hand and to limit toxicity, early mortality, and hospitalization duration on the other and thereby maintain as much quality of life as possible. Specifically asparaginase seems to be less well tolerated in older patients during induction [48, 49]. Therefore it would be advisable to start asparaginase in older patients later during consolidation.

Table 18.8 Outcome of different strategies to treatment of older ALL patients (adapted from [51])

Approach	Age	*N* studies	*N* patients	CR (%)	Early death (%)	Survival
Population based	≥65	*4*	*n.r.*	40	n.r.	6–30%
Palliative	60–91	4	94	43	24	7 months
Intensive	60–92	12	519	56	23	14%
Age specific	55–85	11	653	72	18	42%

Table 18.9 Prospective specific studies for older ALL patients (adapted from [51])

Author	Year	Age	Patients (N)	CR rate (%)	Early death (%)	OS[a] (%)
Bassan et al. [52]	1996	60–73 (64)	22	59	18	20 (2 years)
Delannoy et al. [53]	1997	55–86 (67)	40	85	n.r.	16 (2 years)
Delannoy et al. [54]	2002	65 (55–81)	58	43	10	n.r.
Offidani et al. [55]	2004	69 (61–79)	17	76	17	38 (2 years)
Sancho et al. [48]	2007	65 (56–77)	33	58	36	39 (1 year)
Kao et al. [56]	2008	66 (60–78)	17	71	29	71 (1 year)
Gökbuget et al. [57]	2008	66 (56–73)	54	85	0	61 (1 year)
Hunault-Berger et al. [58]	2010					
	Arm 1	68 (55–77)	31	90	7	35 (2 years)
	Arm 2	66 (60–80)	29	72	10	24 (2 years)
Gökbuget et al. [50]	2012	57 (55–85)	268	76	14	23 (5 years)
Fathi et al. [49]	2016	58 (51–72)	30	67	3	52 (2 years)
Ribera et al. [59]	2016	66 (56–79)	54	74	14	12; 30 (2 years)[b]

Abbreviations: Ph + Ph/BCR-ABL1-positive ALL included yes or no, Arm 1 continuous infusion doxorubicin, Arm 2 pegylated doxorubicin, *CCR* continuous complete remission, *DFS* disease-free survival, *OS* overall survival

[a]Probability

[b]Estimated from Kaplan–Meier curve

The majority of complications in older ALL patients are observed during induction; thus there is still space for intensification of consolidation therapy. Based on this assumption a consensus treatment protocol for older patients with ALL was defined by the European Working Group for Adult ALL (EWALL) based on a pediatric based protocol developed by the German Multicenter Study Group for Adult ALL (GMALL). The median age of this cohort was 65 years [55–85]. In 268 patients the CR rate was 76%, early death rate 14%, mortality in CR 6%, continuous remission 32%, and survival 23% at 5 years [50]. Patients younger than 75 years with an ECOG performance status below 2 had 86% CR rate, 10% early death, and 36% survival at 3 years.

Overall, pediatric based regimens in ALL are undoubtedly successful and should be scheduled with prospectively defined adaptations with respect to tolerability in older patients. The most important modification of induction therapy in older patients is probably omission of asparaginase, and flexible, reduced dose of anthracyclines. In consolidation, intensified treatment should be attempted and during this treatment phase even asparaginase may be surprisingly well tolerated at moderate doses.

Adolescents and Young Adults with ALL

Several groups have published data comparing the outcome of young adults with "pediatric" protocols to those with so-called adult protocols (most recently in [60]). The reason to select specifically these protocols for comparison is not evident because compared treatment regimens were rather different. The "adult" protocols used for comparison often yielded results below the average; one reason may be that several of these protocols were focused on SCT. In contrast to the studies selected for comparison, several other study groups for adult ALL already apply modified pediatric protocols (Table 18.5) with survival rates of 60% and more in young adults up to 30 years.

These regimens are associated with considerable side effects in adults, particularly liver toxicities and pancreatitis due to asparaginase, polyneuropathies due to vincristine, and avascular bone necrosis. Results are promising at short follow-up but it remains open whether this approach will be feasible, up to which age, at less experienced centers, how selection of patients is handled, and whether it will lead to an improvement of overall results.

On the other hand the attempt of adult ALL study groups to define uniform protocols for ALL ranging from 18 to 75 years is not successful. Currently study groups for adult ALL develop into two directions and [1] either use unmodified pediatric protocols for young adults up to the age of 25–30 years or [2] use modified pediatric protocols, e.g., the BFM-based GMALL protocol for the whole group or adult ALL with additional intensification in young adults. One important aim is dose intensification with a better adherence to time schedules with as few as possible. Another aim is to integrate more successful treatment elements from pediatric trials such as vincristine, dexamethasone, asparaginase, reinduction therapy, and maintenance. The opportunity to use targeted therapies developed in adult ALL studies is useful also for young adults.

White Blood Cell Count

Elevated WBC at diagnosis (>30–50,000/μL) as poor prognostic feature has been confirmed in various trials. The biological reason for the highly resistant behavior of B-precursor ALL with high WBC is unclear. Probably in the future additional molecular markers can help to clarify the underlying mechanisms. Due to the high relapse rate evaluation of MRD, use of experimental drugs and SCT modalities seems particularly important.

Immunophenotype

Immunologic subtypes are associated with different presentation and prognosis and distinct cytogenetic and/or molecular aberrations.

Pro-B-ALL/t(4;11)

Pro-B-ALL and/or t(4;11)-positive ALL is considered as high-risk subgroup in nearly all trials [33]. It appears to be particularly susceptible to high-dose cytarabine-based regimens and SCT as reported from the GMALL studies [61].

Common/Pre-B-ALL

Common(c)/pre-B-ALL bears a large proportion of Ph+ ALL. Based on prognostic factors it can be subdivided into an SR and an HR group with significantly different outcome of 50–60% and 30–40% OS, respectively; 40–50% of patients with common/pre-B-ALL show expression of CD20 on the cell surface. It has been demonstrated that CD20 expression is associated with poorer outcome [62]. Recently promising results have been reported for the addition of rituximab to chemotherapy with a benefit regarding LFS and OS particularly in younger patients [63]. Recently a randomized study confirmed the benefit of rituximab in combination with chemotherapy, which did not impact the CR rates but contributed to higher molecular response rates and improved long-term outcome [64].

T-ALL

Outcome of T-lineage ALL is generally considered superior compared to B-lineage [65]. It comprises the subtypes early T-ALL, thymic (cortical T-ALL), and mature T-ALL with inferior outcome for early T-ALL and favorable outcome for thymic T-ALL. Some groups consider very high WBC (>100.000) also a poor prognostic feature in T-ALL [66].

The biological relevance of immunophenotype is underlined by the fact that overexpression of HOX11, HOX11L2, SIL-TAL1, and CALM-AF10 is associated with subtypes, i.e., maturation states of thymocytes (reviewed in [8]). Some groups observed inferior outcomes for early T-ALL [67, 68] and high expression of the transcription factors ERG and/or BAALC [69]. Low expression of ERG and BAALC was associated with favorable outcome [69] as well as overexpression of HOX11, which is associated with thymic T-ALL [70]. Notch1-activating mutations were identified in up to 50% of T-ALL cases [71, 72]. Notch mutations are correlated with thymic T-ALL and a favorable prognosis. An alternative risk model for T-ALL defines cases with mutations of Notch1 or FBXW7 lacking RAS or PTEN mutations as a favorable subgroup whereas patients with RAS or PTEN mutations lacking Notch1 or FBWW7 mutations are considered as high-risk ALL [73]. The prognostic impact of early T-precursor ALL within early T-ALL remains to be defined [68]. Overall the question of which risk model is most suitable depends on treatment strategies and their historical development in study groups.

Five percent of T-ALL shows the NUP214-ABL1 aberration, which may identify a target population for imatinib therapy [74]. The variety of new prognostic markers can impossibly be integrated in current risk models but may moreover serve to identify pathogenetic mechanisms and therapeutic targets.

With current treatment regimens CR rates of more than 90% and an LFS 50–70% can be achieved in T-ALL. The role of stem cell transplantation within T-ALL remains to be defined [35].

Mature B-ALL

Mature B-ALL is grouped according to the WHO classification together with Burkitt's lymphoma and treated according to a specific concept. Treatment is based on childhood B-cell ALL studies that significantly improved outcome. The drugs responsible for the improvement were high doses of fractionated cyclophosphamide, ifosfamide, HDMTX (0.5–8 g/m^2), and HDAC in conjunction with the conventional drugs for remission induction in ALL, given in short cycles at frequent intervals over a period of 6 months.

The application of these childhood B-cell ALL protocols in original or modified form also brought a substantial improvement for adult patients with B-cell ALL. More than 80% of the cases of mature B-ALL or Burkitt's lymphoma express CD20 on their surface. Further significant improvement of survival rates to 80–90% was achieved by the application of rituximab in combination with chemotherapy [75].

B-cell ALL has a higher incidence of CNS involvement at diagnosis, and of CNS relapse. Therefore, effective measures against CNS disease, such as HDMTX and HDAC as well as intrathecal therapy, are important components of treatment regimens. On the other hand, maintenance treatment has been omitted. Because relapses occur almost exclusively within the first year in childhood as well as in adult B-cell ALL studies, patients thereafter can be considered as cured.

Ph/BCR–ABL-Positive ALL

The translocation t(9;22) and the respective fusion gene BCR–ABL until recently marked the most unfavorable subgroup of adult ALL. Ph/BCR–ABL (Ph+) ALL nearly exclusively occurs in conjunction with B-precursor ALL (c-ALL, pre-B-ALL). The incidence increases with age. In Ph+ leukemia the BCR–ABL fusion gene is causally involved in leukemogenesis and is considered to be essential for leukemic transformation. With a selective inhibitor of the ABL tyrosine kinase (imatinib) cellular proliferation of BCR–ABL-positive CML and ALL cells can be inhibited selectively. Phase II trial demonstrated a CR rate of 29% in relapsed/refractory Ph+ ALL with imatinib as single drug [76].

The use of imatinib in combination with chemotherapy contributed to a significant improvement in the outcome of newly diagnosed Ph+ ALL. As compared with the pre-imatinib era, CR rates improved from 60–70% to 80–90% or even higher and outcome was much better, with survival reaching approximately 50%, compared with ≤20% in the pre-imatinib era [77–82]. Imatinib in combination with chemotherapy is now considered the standard treatment of Ph-positive ALL.

Historically a subsequent stem cell transplantation was considered as the only chance of cure in patients with Ph+ ALL. It remains a matter of debate whether this is still true in the imatinib era. A recent report confirmed that allogeneic SCT is still associated with a better relapse-free survival in younger Ph+ ALL patients [83]. Younger patients may receive standard myeloablative conditioning, but the role of reduced-intensity conditioning (RIC)-SCT in older patients remains to be prospectively evaluated. After SCT prophylactic imatinib maintenance is probably the best option to prevent post-SCT relapse [84]. The optimal TKI for first-line treatment, and the question whether in patients with favorable response to treatment SCT may be avoided remains matter of discussion.

The incidence of Ph+ ALL increases with age and older patients are usually not candidates for allogeneic SCT. Nowadays, older patients with Ph+ ALL may have a better chance to achieve a CR than patients with Ph-negative ALL. The GMALL study group conducted a first randomized study to evaluate the efficacy of imatinib single-drug induction compared to chemotherapy. The remission rates were 96% and 50%, respectively [85]. The Italian study group focused on first-line therapy with TKI and steroids only. With imatinib (800 mg) and prednisone for induction followed by imatinib single-drug treatment the CR rate, survival, and disease-free survival were 100, 74, and 48% after 1 year [86]. A subsequent trial with dasatinib (140 mg) and prednisone followed by dasatinib single-drug treatment was not specifically designed for older patients (range 24–76 years). The CR rate was 92% and survival was 69%. Post-remission therapy was at the discretion of the treating physician and 14 of 19 patients with TKI monotherapy relapsed with a high frequency of T315I mutations [87].

The largest prospective study so far in older patients with Ph+ ALL used an EWALL chemotherapy backbone with vincristine, dexamethasone, and dasatinib (140 mg) for induction. Consolidation and maintenance according to the EWALL backbone were combined with intermittent dasatinib applications. In 71 patients the CR rate was 96%. The regimen was feasible and the survival after 5 years of follow-up was 36%, which is promising. Persistent MRD above 0.1% after induction and consolidation was associated with a poorer remission duration of only 5 months [88]. A subsequent EWALL trial with a similar backbone but nilotinib (400 mg BID) instead of dasatinib was started subsequently. Again a high CR rate of 97% was reported. Thirty percent of patients achieved a complete molecular remission after induction [89]. Overall, there is increasing evidence that second-generation TKIs in combination with dose-reduced chemotherapy can induce very high CR rates with low mortality in older patients. The rate of molecular remissions appears to be higher compared to imatinib-based regimens. Moderate intensive consolidation therapies in combination with TKIs are tolerated well. Long-term results have to be assessed after 5 or more years and show a still high rate of relapses. New approaches may include reduced intensity SCT, MRD-based change of TKI, or use of new immunotherapies.

Also in younger patients there is a trend towards dose-reduced chemotherapy in induction. A randomized trial showed lower early mortality and higher CR rate in patients receiving imatinib, combined with less intensive chemotherapy compared with those receiving HyperCVAD/imatinib [83]. Once CR has been reached, autologous SCT might also be a good option, at least in patients who have reached a good MRD response, or in those who cannot tolerate allogeneic SCT [83, 90].

In patients with persistent MRD or progressive disease, the recommendation is to switch to another TKI while screening for TKI resistance mutations, and then to adapt TKI choice according to the resistance profile. The third-generation TKI ponatinib is currently the only option in patients progressing with the T315I mutation. First results with ponatinib in newly diagnosed Ph+ ALL are promising but toxicity risks have to be considered, particularly in older, comorbid patients [91].

Treatment Response and Minimal Residual Disease

Longitudinal minimal residual disease (MRD) evaluation during treatment with the aim to assess individual response identifies one of the most important available prognostic factors. The role of MRD as independent prognostic factor has been confirmed in large cohorts of pediatric and adult ALL (reviewed in [13]). MRD evaluation has two major applications in the management of adult ALL, (1) redefinition of clinical response, failure, and relapse and (2) utilization as prognostic factor, and both are finally used for treatment decisions.

Redefinition of Response

In contemporary trials for adult ALL, CR rates of 85–90% can be reached. The cytological response rate is often favorable, but MRD evaluation reveals differences in subgroups [34]. The molecular CR may be defined as a negative MRD status below 10^{-4} (0.01%) after induction and ranges in adult ALL from 50% for Ph+ ALL treated with imatinib to 80% for SR ALL. Thus molecular CR rate defined according to international standards [14] is an important new endpoint for efficacy evaluation after induction but also after consolidation or salvage cycles (Table 18.6).

During treatment and follow-up molecular relapse, defined as MRD above 10^{-4} after prior achievement of molecular CR, is highly predictive of cytological relapse [34]. Molecular bone marrow relapse is also often present in patients with apparently isolated extramedullary relapse. In clinical trials it should be treated similarly to cytological relapse.

If MRD-based endpoints are used in clinical trials, standardization of methods and definitions is extremely important. It is so far achieved for PCR analysis of individual gene rearrangements [14] and BCR–ABL whereas for flow cytometry or newer methods based on next-generation sequencing international standards for MRD evaluation were not defined so far.

MRD as Prognostic Factor

MRD is a significant prognostic marker at any time point. Early achievement of molecular CR identifies a subgroup of patients with very favorable prognosis. However in the GMALL studies these were only 12% of SR patients [92]. Adult ALL patients reach molecular CR later than children and later time points are more predictive of relapse risk. In the GMALL studies 25–30% of the patients did not achieve molecular CR after induction and first consolidation and nearly all of them relapsed [34]. Similar results were reported by others (reviewed in [13]). SCT can contribute to an improved outcome of patients with high persistent MRD [34, 93]. However patients with high MRD before SCT or persisting MRD after SCT have a poorer outcome [94].

The application of MRD as prognostic factor is complicated by the fact that it has to be combined with "conventional" factors. MRD identifies additional HR patients in those with conventional SR but also good-risk patients in those with conventional HR features, who are usually scheduled for SCT. Thus MRD as prognostic factor depends on time point, treatment protocol, general risk stratification, and planned therapeutic consequences.

Integrated Risk Classification

All risk factors are to a certain extent specific for a defined treatment protocol and used with variations by different study groups. Beyond established factors and factors suggested by individual study groups (Table 18.10), a variety of molecular markers newly detected by microarray analysis have been proposed as prognostic factors [32]. All of these factors can

Table 18.10 Prognostic factors for risk stratification of adult ALL[a]

	Good	Adverse	
		B-lineage	T-lineage
At diagnosis			
Clinical parameters	**WBC < 30,000/μL**	**WBC > 30,000/μL**	WBC > 100,000/μL
Immunophenotype	Thymic T	**Pro B** (CD10−) Pre B (CD10−)	Early T (CD1a−, sCD3−) Mature T (CD1a−, sCD3+)
Cytogenetics/molecular genetics/gene expression profiles	TEL-AML1 HOX11[a] NOTCH-1 9p del Hyperdiploid	**t(9;22)/BCR–ABL** **t(4;11)/ALL1-AF4** t(1;19)/E2A-PBX Complex aberrations Low hypodiploid/near tetraploid	HOX11L2 CALM-AF4 Complex aberrations Low hypodiploid/near tetraploid
Individual response during treatment			
Prednisone response	Good	Poor	
Time to CR	**Early**	**Late (>8–12 weeks)**	
MRD after induction	**Negative/< 10^{-4}**	**Positive > 10^{-4}**	
Age			
	<25 years, <35 years	**>35 years, >55 years, >70 years**	

[a]Generally accepted factors are printed in *bold*

impossibly be integrated in a conventional risk model, which mainly aims to identify patients for SCT in CR1. They may rather stimulate analysis of underlying mechanisms, drug targets, or invention of treatment adaptations. The major aim of future risk stratification in ALL is therefore to identify at diagnosis patients with an increased risk of relapse who are candidates for a stem cell transplantation. The second aim is to identify treatment targets for the use of targeted therapy approaches. During the course of disease the individual response of the patients can be considered by MRD evaluation. This may lead to reconsideration of the indication for SCT, e.g., not to offer a patient with high-risk factors the transplant if he or she is MRD negative or to transfer patients to SCT despite the lack of high-risk factors if he or she remains MRD positive. In the future additional factors such as pharmacogenomic markers or resistance patterns may be considered for treatment stratification.

Treatment of Relapsed or Refractory ALL

Published data show response rates to first salvage of around 40% and overall survival rates below 20% [95, 96]. Patients with late relapse respond to repeated induction therapy in more than 70% of the cases. However, in adult ALL the majority of relapses occur early and the CR rate is clearly below 40%. This was confirmed in a recent international reference analysis [97]. In early relapse the apparent chemotherapy resistance may be overcome by new immunotherapies.

In more than 90% of the cases of B-precursor ALL CD19 is expressed on the surface of blast cells. The bi-specific antibody blinatumomab is directed to CD19 and on the other hand attracts with a CD3 domain cytotoxic T-cells. These cells come in close proximity to the CD19-positive target cells and induce serial killing. A phase II trial in unfavorable cases of relapsed/refractory ALL showed in 189 patients a CR rate of 43% with 82% molecular remissions [98]. The median survival was 6.1 months. In a randomized trial in a similar patient population with early or refractory relapses the CR rate was 44% for blinatumomab compared to 25% for standard chemotherapy. Survival rates were 7.7 months for blinatumomab compared to 4.0 months with standard chemotherapy [99]. More favorable response rates and superior survival were achieved in patients with molecular failure or molecular relapse. The molecular response rate was 78% and the median survival 36 months [100] indicating that the MRD setting is optimal for response and long-term outcome.

Also CD22 is expressed in more than 90% of the cases of B-precursor ALL. The CD22 antibody inotuzumab is conjugated to the cytotoxin calicheamicin. In a randomized trial in relapsed/refractory ALL CR rates of 81% compared to 29% with high-dose cytarabine-based chemotherapy were described. The median survival for patients treated with inotuzumab was 7.7. months [101].

Another promising option is immunotherapy with genetically modified T-cells. These so called chimeric antigen receptor (CAR) T-cells are produced ex vivo from patient-derived T-cells and carry an antigen receptor directed to lymphatic blasts such as CD19 together with several signal transduction elements. The cells are infused after a cytoreductive and immunosuppressive chemotherapy. First results in smaller trials mostly in pediatric ALL cohorts are promising but also demonstrated considerable toxicity [102].

Future treatment of relapsed B-precursor ALL will strongly depend on immunotherapy. However, despite improved response rates, the long-term survival is only around 6 months and the chance of cure strongly depends on subsequent stem cell transplantation. The optimal use of potent new antibody and cell therapies still has to be defined. For individual patients the relapse treatment should be selected based on availability of targeted therapies, age, general condition, type of involvement, and availability of donors. Any longer treatment-free intervals should be avoided. By consequent measurement of MRD and early therapeutic intervention, relapses may be at least partly avoided.

Long-Term Follow-Up and Late Effects

As a result of improved survival rates, more patients with adult ALL are long-term survivors. In pediatric ALL and to a lesser extent adult ALL patients long-term effects of treatment can occur and they should be considered during aftercare of the patients [103]. This includes cataract, infertility, bone necrosis, fatigue, secondary malignancy, hormonal disorder, or psychiatric diseases.

References

1. Bassan R, Hoelzer D. Modern therapy of acute lymphoblastic leukemia. J Clin Oncol. 2011;29(5):532–43.
2. Pui CH, Thiel E. Central nervous system disease in hematologic malignancies: historical perspective and practical applications. Semin Oncol. 2009;36(4 Suppl 2):S2–S16.
3. Wolach O, Stone RM. Mixed-phenotype acute leukemia: current challenges in diagnosis and therapy. Curr Opin Hematol. 2017;24(2):139–45.
4. Arber DA, Orazi A, Hasserjian R, et al. The 2016 revision to the World Health Organization classification of myeloid neoplasms and acute leukemia. Blood. 2016;127(20):2391–405.
5. Bene MC, Castoldi G, Knapp W, et al. Proposal for the immunological classification of acute leukemias. Leukemia. 1995;9:1783–6.
6. Coustan-Smith E, Mullighan CG, Onciu M, et al. Early T-cell precursor leukaemia: a subtype of very high-risk acute lymphoblastic leukaemia. Lancet Oncol. 2009;10(2):147–56.
7. Ludwig WD, Raghavachar A, Thiel E. Immunophenotypic classification of acute lymphoblastic leukemia. Baillieres Clin Haematol. 1994;7(2):235.
8. Belver L, Ferrando A. The genetics and mechanisms of T cell acute lymphoblastic leukaemia. Nat Rev Cancer. 2016;16(8):494–507.
9. Roberts KG, Gu Z, Payne-Turner D, et al. High frequency and poor outcome of Philadelphia chromosome-like acute lymphoblastic leukemia in adults. J Clin Oncol. 2017;35(4):394–401.

10. Roberts KG, Li Y, Payne-Turner D, et al. Targetable kinase-activating lesions in Ph-like acute lymphoblastic leukemia. N Engl J Med. 2014;371(11):1005–15.
11. Herold T, Schneider S, Metzeler KH, et al. Adults with Philadelphia chromosome-like acute lymphoblastic leukemia frequently have IGH-CRLF2 and JAK2 mutations, persistence of minimal residual disease and poor prognosis. Haematologica. 2017;102(1):130–8.
12. Stengel A, Schnittger S, Weissmann S, et al. TP53 mutations occur in 15.7% of ALL and are associated with MYC-rearrangement, low hypodiploidy, and a poor prognosis. Blood. 2014;124(2):251–8.
13. van Dongen JJ, van der Velden VH, Bruggemann M, Orfao A. Minimal residual disease diagnostics in acute lymphoblastic leukemia: need for sensitive, fast, and standardized technologies. Blood. 2015;125(26):3996–4009.
14. Bruggemann M, Schrauder A, Raff T, et al. Standardized MRD quantification in European ALL trials: proceedings of the Second International Symposium on MRD assessment in Kiel, Germany, 18-20 September 2008. Leukemia. 2010;24(3):521–35.
15. Larson RA, Dodge RK, Linker CA, et al. A randomized controlled trial of filgrastim during remission induction and consolidation chemotherapy for adults with acute lymphoblastic leukemia: CALGB study 9111. Blood. 1998;92(5):1556–64.
16. Ottmann OG, Hoelzer D, Gracien E, et al. Concomitant granulocyte colony-stimulating factor and induction chemoradiotherapy in adult acute lymphoblastic leukemia: a randomized phase III trial. Blood. 1995;86(2):444–50.
17. Ribera JM, Oriol A, Sanz MA, et al. Comparison of the results of the treatment of adolescents and young adults with standard-risk acute lymphoblastic leukemia with the Programa Espanol de Tratamiento en Hematologia pediatric-based protocol ALL-96. J Clin Oncol. 2008;26(11):1843–9.
18. Huguet F, Leguay T, Raffoux E, et al. Pediatric-inspired therapy in adults with philadelphia chromosome-negative acute lymphoblastic leukemia: The GRAALL-2003 Study. J Clin Oncol. 2009;27(6):911–8.
19. Rijneveld AW, van der Holt B, Daenen SM, et al. Intensified chemotherapy inspired by a pediatric regimen combined with allogeneic transplantation in adult patients with acute lymphoblastic leukemia up to the age of 40. Leukemia. 2011;25(11):1697–703.
20. Stock W, Luger S, Advani A, et al. Favorable outcomes for older adolescents and young adults (AYA) with acute lymphoblastic leukemia (ALL): early results of U.S. Intergroup Trial C10403. Blood. 2014;124(21):796a.
21. Rytting ME, Thomas DA, O'Brien SM, et al. Augmented Berlin-Frankfurt-Munster therapy in adolescents and young adults (AYAs) with acute lymphoblastic leukemia (ALL). Cancer. 2014;120(23):3660–8.
22. DeAngelo DJ, Stevenson KE, Dahlberg SE, et al. Long-term outcome of a pediatric-inspired regimen used for adults aged 18–50 years with newly diagnosed acute lymphoblastic leukemia. Leukemia. 2015;29(3):526–34.
23. Stock W, Johnson JL, Stone RM, et al. Dose intensification of daunorubicin and cytarabine during treatment of adult acute lymphoblastic leukemia: results of Cancer and Leukemia Group B Study 19802. Cancer. 2013;119(1):90–8.
24. Douer D, Aldoss I, Lunning MA, et al. Pharmacokinetics-based integration of multiple doses of intravenous pegaspargase in a pediatric regimen for adults with newly diagnosed acute lymphoblastic leukemia. J Clin Oncol. 2014;32(9):905–11.
25. Stock W, Douer D, DeAngelo DJ, et al. Prevention and management of asparaginase/pegasparaginase-associated toxicities in adults and older adolescents: recommendations of an expert panel. Leuk Llymphoma. 2011;52(12):2237–53.
26. Schmiegelow K, Nielsen SN, Frandsen TL, Nersting J. Mercaptopurine/methotrexate maintenance therapy of childhood acute lymphoblastic leukemia: clinical facts and fiction. J Pediatr Hematol Oncol. 2014;36(7):503–17.
27. Conter V, Valsecchi MG, Silvestri D, et al. Pulses of vincristine and dexamethasone in addition to intensive chemotherapy for children with intermediate-risk acute lymphoblastic leukaemia: a multicentre randomised trial. Lancet. 2007;369(9556):123–31.
28. Howell SB. Liposomal cytarabine for the treatment of lymphomatous meningitis. Biol Therapy Lymphoma. 2003;6:10–4.
29. Jabbour E, O'Brien S, Kantarjian H, et al. Neurologic complications associated with intrathecal liposomal cytarabine given prophylactically in combination with high-dose methotrexate and cytarabine to patients with acute lymphocytic leukemia. Blood. 2007;109(8):3214–8.
30. Dhawan R, Marks DI. Who should receive a transplant for acute lymphoblastic leukaemia? Curr Hematol Malig Rep. 2017;12(2):143–52.
31. NCCN Clinical Practice Guidelines in Oncology (NCCN Guidelines®). Acute Lymphoblastic Leukemia. Version 2.2016 (NCCN.org). 2016.
32. Hoelzer D, Bassan R, Dombret H, et al. Acute lymphoblastic leukaemia in adult patients: ESMO Clinical Practice Guidelines for diagnosis, treatment and follow-up. Ann Oncol. 2016;27(Suppl 5):v69–82.
33. Marks DI, Moorman AV, Chilton L, et al. The clinical characteristics, therapy and outcome of 85 adults with acute lymphoblastic leukemia and t(4;11)(q21;q23)/MLL-AFF1 prospectively treated in the UKALLXII/ECOG2993 trial. Haematologica. 2013;98(6):945–52.
34. Gokbuget N, Kneba M, Raff T, et al. Adult patients with acute lymphoblastic leukemia and molecular failure display a poor prognosis and are candidates for stem cell transplantation and targeted therapies. Blood. 2012;120(9):1868–76.
35. Dhedin N, Huynh A, Maury S, et al. Role of allogeneic stem cell transplantation in adult patients with Ph-negative acute lymphoblastic leukemia. Blood. 2015;125(16):2486–96. quiz 2586
36. Oliansky DM, Camitta B, Gaynon P, et al. The role of cytotoxic therapy with hematopoietic stem cell transplantation in the treatment of pediatric acute lymphoblastic leukemia: update of the 2005 evidence-based review. ASBMT Position Statement. Biol Blood Marrow Transplant. 2012;18(7):979–81.
37. Marks DI, Woo KA, Zhong X, et al. Unrelated umbilical cord blood transplant for adult acute lymphoblastic leukemia in first and second complete remission: a comparison with allografts from adult unrelated donors. Haematologica. 2014;99(2):322–8.
38. Robinson TM, O'Donnell PV, Fuchs EJ, Luznik L. Haploidentical bone marrow and stem cell transplantation: experience with post-transplantation cyclophosphamide. Semin Hematol. 2016;53(2):90–7.
39. Goldstone AH, Richards SM, Lazarus HM, et al. In adults with standard-risk acute lymphoblastic leukemia (ALL) the greatest benefit is achieved from a matched sibling allogeneic transplant in first complete remission (CR) and an autologous transplant is less effective than conventional consolidation/maintenance chemotherapy in All patients : final results of the international ALL trial (MRC UKALL XII/ ECOG E2993). Blood. 2008;111(4):1827–33.
40. Wetzler M, Watson D, Stock W, et al. Autologous transplantation for Philadelphia chromosome-positive acute lymphoblastic leukemia achieves outcomes similar to allogeneic transplantation: results of CALGB Study 10001 (Alliance). Haematologica. 2014;99(1):111–5.
41. Yanada M, Naoe T, Iida H, et al. Myeloablative allogeneic hematopoietic stem cell transplantation for Philadelphia chromosome-positive acute lymphoblastic leukemia in adults: significant roles of total body irradiation and chronic graft-versus-host disease. Bone Marrow Transplant. 2005;36(10):867–72.
42. Mohty M, Labopin M, Volin L, et al. Reduced-intensity versus conventional myeloablative conditioning allogeneic stem cell

transplantation for patients with acute lymphoblastic leukemia: a retrospective study from the European Group for Blood and Marrow Transplantation. Blood. 2010;116(22):4439–43.

43. Altekruse SF, Kosary CL, Krapcho M, et al. Seer Cancer Statistics Review 1975–2007. Bethesda, MD: National Cancer Institute; 2007; https://seer.cancer.gov/archive/csr/1975_2007/.
44. Moorman AV, Chilton L, Wilkinson J, Ensor HM, Bown N, Proctor SJ. A population-based cytogenetic study of adults with acute lymphoblastic leukemia. Blood. 2010;115(2):206–14.
45. Juliusson G, Karlsson K, Hallbook H. Population-based analyses in adult acute lymphoblastic leukemia. Blood. 2010;116(6):1011. author reply 1012
46. Toft N, Schmiegelow K, Klausen TW, Birgens H. Adult acute lymphoblastic leukaemia in Denmark. A national population-based retrospective study on acute lymphoblastic leukaemia in Denmark 1998–2008. Br J Haematol. 2012;157(1):97–104.
47. Sive JI, Buck G, Fielding A, et al. Outcomes in older adults with acute lymphoblastic leukaemia (ALL): results from the international MRC UKALL XII/ECOG2993 trial. Br J Haematol. 2012;157(4):463–71.
48. Sancho JM, Ribera JM, Xicoy B, et al. Results of the PETHEMA ALL-96 trial in elderly patients with Philadelphia chromosome-negative acute lymphoblastic leukemia. Eur J Haematol. 2007;78(2):102–10.
49. Fathi AT, DeAngelo DJ, Stevenson KE, et al. Phase 2 study of intensified chemotherapy and allogeneic hematopoietic stem cell transplantation for older patients with acute lymphoblastic leukemia. Cancer. 2016;122(15):2379–88.
50. Gökbuget N, Beck J, Brüggemann M, et al. Moderate intensive chemotherapy including CNS-prophylaxis with liposomal cytarabine is feasible and effective in older patients with ph-negative acute lymphoblastic leukemia (ALL): Results of a Prospective Trial From the German Multicenter Study Group for Adult ALL (GMALL). Blood. 2012;120:1493.
51. Gokbuget N. Treatment of older patients with acute lymphoblastic leukemia. Hematology Am Soc Hematol Educ Program. 2016;2016(1):573–9.
52. Bassan R, Di BE, Lerede T, et al. Age-adapted moderate-dose induction and flexible outpatient postremission therapy for elderly patients with acute lymphoblastic leukemia. LeukLymphoma. 1996;22(3–4):295–301.
53. Delannoy A, Sebban C, Cony-Makhoul P, et al. Age-adapted induction treatment of acute lymphoblastic leukemia in the elderly and assessment of maintenance with interferon combined with chemotherapy. A multicentric prospective study in forty patients. Leukemia. 1997;11:1429–34.
54. Delannoy A, Cazin B, Thomas X, et al. Treatment of acute lymphoblastic leukemia in the elderly: an evaluation of interferon alpha given as a single agent after complete remission. Leuk Lymphoma. 2002;43(1):75–81.
55. Offidani M, Corvatta L, Malerba L, et al. Comparison of two regimens for the treatment of elderly patients with acute lymphoblastic leukaemia (ALL). Blood. 2004;104(11):4490.
56. Kao S, Xu W, Gupta V, et al. Outcome of patients aged 60 and over with acute lymphoblastic leukemia (ALL) treated with a modified pediatric protocol. Blood. 2008;112:3962a.
57. Gökbuget N, Leguay T, Hunault M, et al. First European chemotherapy schedule for elderly patients with acute lymphoblastic leukemia: promising remission rate and feasible moderate dose intensity consolidation. ASH Annual Meeting Abstracts. 2008;112(11):304.
58. Hunault-Berger M, Leguay T, Thomas X, et al. A randomized study of pegylated liposomal doxorubicin versus continuous-infusion doxorubicin in elderly patients with acute lymphoblastic leukemia: the GRAALL-SA1 study. Haematologica. 2011;96(2):245–52.
59. Ribera JM, Garcia O, Oriol A, et al. Feasibility and results of subtype-oriented protocols in older adults and fit elderly patients with acute lymphoblastic leukemia: Results of three prospective parallel trials from the PETHEMA group. Leuk Res. 2016;41:12–20.
60. Dombret H, Cluzeau T, Huguet F, Boissel N. Pediatric-like therapy for adults with ALL. Curr Hematol Malig Rep. 2014;9(2):158–64.
61. Gleissner B, Gökbuget N, Rieder H, et al. CD10-negative pre-B acute lymphoblastic leukemia (ALL): a distinct high-risk subgroup of adult ALL associated with a high frequency of MLL aberrations. Results of the German Multicenter Trials for Adult ALL (GMALL). Blood. 2005;106(13):4054–6.
62. Maury S, Huguet F, Leguay T, et al. Adverse prognostic significance of CD20 expression in adults with Philadelphia chromosome-negative B-cell precursor acute lymphoblastic leukemia. Haematologica. 2010;95(2):324–8.
63. Thomas DA, O'Brien S, Faderl S, et al. Chemoimmunotherapy with a modified hyper-CVAD and rituximab regimen improves outcome in de novo philadelphia chromosome-negative precursor B-lineage acute lymphoblastic leukemia. J Clin Oncol. 2010;28(24):3880–9.
64. Maury S, Chevret S, Thomas X, et al. Rituximab in B-lineage adult acute lymphoblastic leukemia. N Engl J Med. 2016;375(11):1044–53.
65. Marks DI, Rowntree C. Management of adults with T-cell lymphoblastic leukemia. Blood. 2017;129(9):1134–42.
66. Marks DI, Paietta EM, Moorman AV, et al. T-cell acute lymphoblastic leukemia in adults: clinical features, immunophenotype, cytogenetics, and outcome from the large randomized prospective trial (UKALL XII/ECOG 2993). Blood. 2009;114(25):5136–45.
67. Vitale A, Guarini A, Ariola C, et al. Adult T-cell acute lymphoblastic leukemia: biologic profile at presentation and correlation with response to induction treatment in patients enrolled in the GIMEMA LAL 0496 protocol. Blood. 2006;107(2):473–9.
68. Jain N, Lamb AV, O'Brien S, et al. Early T-cell precursor acute lymphoblastic leukemia/lymphoma (ETP-ALL/LBL) in adolescents and adults: a high-risk subtype. Blood. 2016;127(15):1863–9.
69. Baldus CD, Martus P, Burmeister T, et al. Low ERG and BAALC expression identifies a new subgroup of adult acute T-lymphoblastic leukemia with a highly favorable outcome. JClinOncol. 2007;25(24):3739–45.
70. Baak U, Gökbuget N, Orawa H, et al. Thymic adult T-cell acute lymphoblastic leukemia stratified in standard- and high-risk group by aberrant HOX11L2 expression: experience of the German multicenter ALL study group. Leukemia. 2008;22(6):1154–60.
71. Baldus CD, Thibaut J, Gökbuget N, et al. Prognostic implications of NOTCH1 and FBXW7 mutations in adult acute T-lymphoblastic leukemia. Haematologica. 2009;94(10):1383–90.
72. Ben Abdelali R, Asnafi V, Leguay T, et al. Pediatric-inspired intensified therapy of adult T-ALL reveals the favorable outcome of NOTCH1/FBXW7 mutations, but not of low ERG/BAALC expression: a GRAALL study. Blood. 2011;118(19):5099–107.
73. Trinquand A, Tanguy-Schmidt A, Ben Abdelali R, et al. Toward a NOTCH1/FBXW7/RAS/PTEN-based oncogenetic risk classification of adult T-cell acute lymphoblastic leukemia: a Group for Research in Adult Acute Lymphoblastic Leukemia study. J Clin Oncol. 2013;31(34):4333–42.
74. Burmeister T, Gökbuget N, Reinhardt R, Rieder H, Hoelzer D, Schwartz S. NUP214-ABL1 in adult T-ALL: the GMALL study group experience. Blood. 2006;108(10):3556–9.
75. Hoelzer D, Walewski J, Dohner H, et al. Improved outcome of adult Burkitt lymphoma/leukemia with rituximab and chemotherapy: report of a large prospective multicenter trial. Blood. 2014;124(26):3870–9.
76. Ottmann OG, Druker BJ, Sawyers CL, et al. A phase II study of Imatinib Mesylate (Glivec) in patients with relapsed or refractory Philadelphia chromosome-positive acute lymphoid leukemias. Blood. 2002;100(6):1965–71.

77. Fielding AK, Rowe JM, Richards SM, et al. Prospective outcome data on 267 unselected adult patients with Philadelphia chromosome-positive acute lymphoblastic leukemia confirms superiority of allogeneic transplantation over chemotherapy in the pre-imatinib era: results from the International ALL Trial MRC UKALLXII/ECOG2993. Blood. 2009;113(19):4489–96.
78. Thomas DA, Faderl S, Cortes J, et al. Treatment of Philadelphia chromosome-positive acute lymphocytic leukemia with hyper-CVAD and imatinib mesylate. Blood. 2004;103(12):4396–407.
79. de Labarthe R. P, Huguet-Rigal F, et al. Imatinib combined with induction or consolidation chemotherapy in patients with de novo Philadelphia chromosome-positive acute lymphoblastic leukemia: results of the GRAAPH-2003 study. Blood. 2007;109(4):1408–13.
80. Ribera JM, Oriol A, Gonzalez M, et al. Concurrent intensive chemotherapy and imatinib before and after stem cell transplantation in newly diagnosed Philadelphia chromosome-positive acute lymphoblastic leukemia. Final results of the CSTIBES02 trial. Haematologica. 2010;95(1):87–95.
81. Fielding AK, Rowe JM, Buck G, et al. UKALLXII/ECOG2993: addition of imatinib to a standard treatment regimen enhances long-term outcomes in Philadelphia positive acute lymphoblastic leukemia. Blood. 2014;123(6):843–50.
82. Bassan R, Rossi G, Pogliani EM, et al. Chemotherapy-phased imatinib pulses improve long-term outcome of adult patients with Philadelphia chromosome-positive acute lymphoblastic leukemia: Northern Italy Leukemia Group protocol 09/00. J Clin Oncol. 2010;28(22):3644–52.
83. Chalandon Y, Thomas X, Hayette S, et al. Randomized study of reduced-intensity chemotherapy combined with imatinib in adults with Ph-positive acute lymphoblastic leukemia. Blood. 2015;125(24):3711–9.
84. Pfeifer H, Wassmann B, Bethge W, et al. Randomized comparison of prophylactic and minimal residual disease-triggered imatinib after allogeneic stem cell transplantation for BCR-ABL1-positive acute lymphoblastic leukemia. Leukemia. 2013;27(6):1254–62.
85. Ottmann OG, Wassmann B, Pfeifer H, et al. Imatinib compared with chemotherapy as front-line treatment of elderly patients with Philadelphia chromosome-positive acute lymphoblastic leukemia (Ph+ALL). Cancer. 2007;109(10):2068–76.
86. Vignetti M, Fazi P, Cimino G, et al. Imatinib plus steroids induces complete remissions and prolonged survival in elderly Philadelphia chromosome-positive acute lymphoblastic leukemia patients without additional chemotherapy: results of the GIMEMA LAL0201-B protocol. Blood. 2007;109(9):3676–8.
87. Foa R, Vitale A, Vignetti M, et al. Dasatinib as first-line treatment for adult patients with Philadelphia chromosome-positive acute lymphoblastic leukemia. Blood. 2011;118(25):6521–8.
88. Rousselot P, Coude MM, Gokbuget N, et al. Dasatinib and low-intensity chemotherapy in elderly patients with Philadelphia chromosome-positive ALL. Blood. 2016;128(6):774–82.
89. Ottmann OG, Pfeifer H, Cayuela J-M, et al. Nilotinib (Tasigna®) and chemotherapy for first-line treatment in elderly patients with de novo Philadelphia Chromosome/BCR-ABL1 Positive Acute Lymphoblastic Leukemia (ALL): A Trial of the European Working Group for Adult ALL (EWALL-PH-02). Blood. 2014;124(21):798.
90. Giebel S, Labopin M, Gorin NC, et al. Improving results of autologous stem cell transplantation for Philadelphia-positive acute lymphoblastic leukaemia in the era of tyrosine kinase inhibitors: a report from the Acute Leukaemia Working Party of the European Group for Blood and Marrow Transplantation. Eur J Cancer. 2014;50(2):411–7.
91. Jabbour E, Kantarjian H, Ravandi F, et al. Combination of hyper-CVAD with ponatinib as first-line therapy for patients with Philadelphia chromosome-positive acute lymphoblastic leukaemia: a single-centre, phase 2 study. Lancet Oncol. 2015;16(15):1547–55.
92. Bruggemann M, Raff T, Flohr T, et al. Clinical significance of minimal residual disease quantification in adult patients with standard-risk acute lymphoblastic leukemia. Blood. 2006;107(3):1116–23.
93. Beldjord K, Chevret S, Asnafi V, et al. Oncogenetics and minimal residual disease are independent outcome predictors in adult patients with acute lymphoblastic leukemia. Blood. 2014;123:3739–49.
94. Spinelli O, Peruta B, Tosi M, et al. Clearance of minimal residual disease after allogeneic stem cell transplantation and the prediction of the clinical outcome of adult patients with high-risk acute lymphoblastic leukemia. Haematologica. 2007;92(5):612–8.
95. Gokbuget N, Stanze D, Beck J, et al. Outcome of relapsed adult lymphoblastic leukemia depends on response to salvage chemotherapy, prognostic factors, and performance of stem cell transplantation. Blood. 2012;120(10):2032–41.
96. Fielding AK, Richards SM, Chopra R, et al. Outcome of 609 adults after relapse of acute lymphoblastic leukemia (ALL); an MRC UKALL12/ECOG 2993 study. Blood. 2007;109(3):944–50.
97. Gokbuget N, Dombret H, Ribera JM, et al. International reference analysis of outcomes in adults with B-precursor Ph-negative relapsed/refractory acute lymphoblastic leukemia. Haematologica. 2016;101(12):1524–33.
98. Topp MS, Gokbuget N, Stein AS, et al. Safety and activity of blinatumomab for adult patients with relapsed or refractory B-precursor acute lymphoblastic leukaemia: a multicentre, single-arm, phase 2 study. Lancet Oncol. 2015;16(1):57–66.
99. Kantarjian H, Stein A, Gokbuget N, et al. Blinatumomab versus chemotherapy for advanced acute lymphoblastic leukemia. N Engl J Med. 2017;376(9):836–47.
100. Gökbuget N, Dombret H, Bonifacio M, et al. Long-Term outcomes after blinatumomab treatment: Follow-up of a Phase 2 Study in Patients (Pts) with minimal residual disease (MRD) Positive B-cell precursor acute lymphoblastic leukemia (ALL). Blood. 2015;126:23.
101. Kantarjian HM, DeAngelo DJ, Stelljes M, et al. Inotuzumab ozogamicin versus standard therapy for acute lymphoblastic leukemia. N Engl J Med. 2016;375(8):740–53.
102. Sadelain M. CAR therapy: the CD19 paradigm. J Clin Invest. 2015;125(9):3392–400.
103. Silverman LB. Balancing cure and long-term risks in acute lymphoblastic leukemia. Hematology Am Soc Hematol Educ Program. 2014;2014(1):190–7.

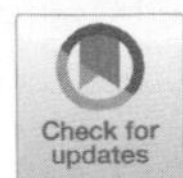

19 Diagnosis and Treatment of Acute Myeloid Leukemia in Children

Brenton G. Mar and Barbara A. Degar

Introduction

Acute myeloid leukemia (AML) accounts for 15–20% of acute leukemias diagnosed in children and about 5% of childhood cancer diagnoses. Less than 1000 new cases of AML are diagnosed in children each year in the United States [1]. In the past 30 years, survival rates for children with AML have progressively improved, although not as dramatically as for children with acute lymphoblastic leukemia (ALL) [2]. During this period, the components of AML therapy have remained essentially unchanged. Incremental improvements in outcome are attributable to a number of factors including increased treatment intensity, optimized supportive care, and application of stem cell transplantation. With recent advances in molecular diagnostics and the emergence of targeted approaches, AML therapy is poised to enter a new age of accelerated progress. This chapter focuses on factors specifically relevant to AML in children.

Epidemiology and Pathogenesis

AML is primarily a disease of adults, with the median age at diagnosis in the seventh decade of life. In children, the incidence of ALL far exceeds the incidence of AML [1]. Within the pediatric population, the incidence of AML varies by age with a small peak in the first 2 years of life and then gradual rise after the second decade of life, as depicted in Fig. 19.1.

Although the vast majority of pediatric AML is thought to be sporadic in nature, the contribution of inherited leukemia predisposition has become significantly more appreciated over the past decade as more familial myelodysplastic syndrome (MDS), acute leukemia, and marrow failure syndromes have been described. A large genomic study of germline material from 1120 pediatric cancer patients found that 8.5% of all patients and 4% of leukemia patients had a pathogenic or probably pathogenic mutation in a cancer predisposition gene [3]. Importantly, a positive family history of cancer was only present in 40%, demonstrating that germline predisposition remains an underappreciated and under-evaluated concern, which can impact future risk of relapse, second malignancy and other sequelae, transplant conditioning, and transplant donor selection. Although germline screening for predisposition is not (yet) universally recommended for pediatric AML patients, clinicians should have a high index of suspicion for considering a germline workup in the right clinical context. A comprehensive review of these disorders and their diagnostic workup is beyond the scope of this chapter, but we highlight several important syndromes and concepts.

First, there exist cancer predisposition syndromes in which hematological neoplasms are merely one class of several cancers which are at significantly increased risk. These include Bloom syndrome, ataxia telangiectasia, neurofibromatosis type I, and others. In addition, familial MDS and AML syndromes associated with germline mutations have also been described, which can be organized into three groups. In the first group are those with thrombocytopenia, platelet dysfunction, and an increased risk of myeloid and other hematopoietic neoplasms, including constitutional mutations in RUNX1 [4], ANKRD26 [5], and ETV6 [6]. A second group has increased risk of MDS/AML with associated organ manifestations, which include GATA2, TP53, TERT, and TERC. A final group, which includes mutations in CEBPA, SRP72, and DDX41, has increased risk of MDS/AML and no thrombocytopenia and organ dysfunction. Lastly there are bone marrow failure syndromes, including Fanconi anemia, Shwachman-Diamond syndrome ,and dyskeratosis congenita, which also have an elevated risk for transformation to MDS or AML.

Although not familial, Down syndrome deserves special attention as a germline syndrome associated with increased risk of leukemia. Babies with Down syndrome (DS) exhibit

B.G. Mar (✉) • B.A. Degar, M.D.,
Dana Farber/Boston Children's Cancer and Blood Disorders Center, 450 Brookline Ave, Boston, MA 02215-5450, USA
e-mail: brenton_mar@dfci.harvard.edu

P.H. Wiernik et al. (eds.), *Neoplastic Diseases of the Blood*, DOI 10.1007/978-3-319-64263-5_19

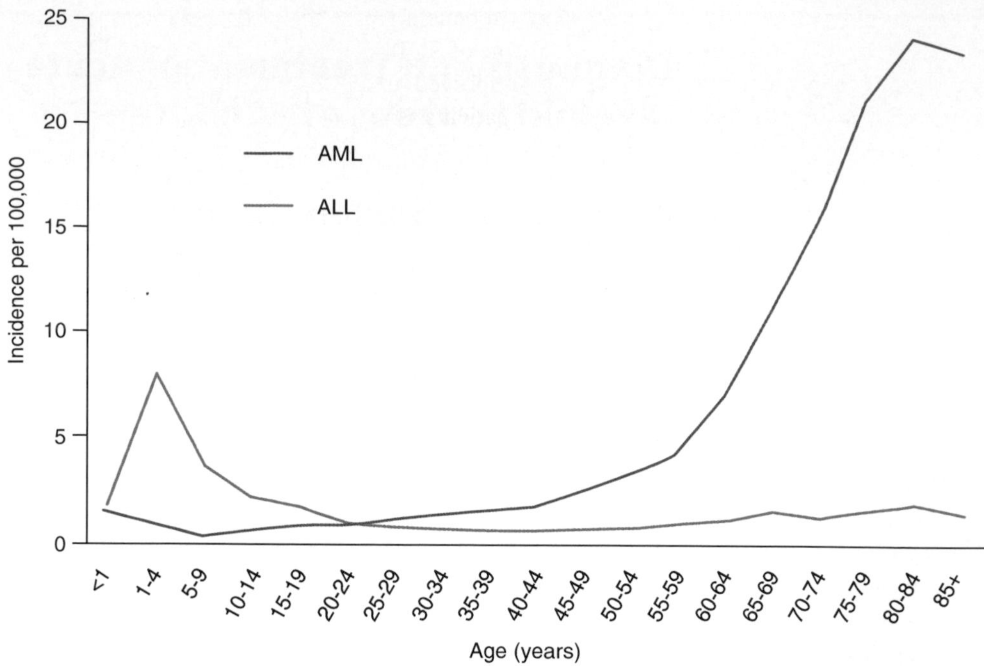

Fig. 19.1 Incidence per 100,000 of acute lymphoblastic leukemia (ALL) and acute myeloid leukemia (AML) by age. Data from Surveillance, Epidemiology, and End Results Program (SEER) 1975–2011

a unique pattern of abnormal myelopoiesis in the neonatal period which is usually transient and self-resolving. Myelodysplastic syndrome (MDS) and/or AML (also known as myeloid leukemia of Down Syndrome, or ML-DS) develops later in some of these babies. After the first few years of life, the incidence of AML declines to non-DS baseline levels concomitant with a rise in the incidence of ALL in children with DS (see ML-DS below).

Increased AML risk is also associated with exposure to DNA-damaging agents in the form of chemotherapy or therapeutic, diagnostic, or environmental radiation. As the number of survivors of childhood and adult cancer grows, the population at risk for this complication increases. The risk period for the development of myelodysplasia and overt AML is influenced by the therapeutic class of the genotoxic therapy previously administered. Also, both cumulative dose and administration schedule appear to matter [7]. Secondary leukemias that arise after exposure to topoisomerase II inhibitors, such as epipodophyllotoxins and anthracyclines, characteristically present as overt AML, without a preceding phase of myelodysplasia. These leukemias occur relatively early, peaking at 2–3 years after drug exposure. Balanced translocations, especially rearrangements involving the MLL (KMT2A) gene at chromosome 11q23, are characteristic of AMLs that occur in association with these agents [8]. Frequent, intermittent schedule of administration of etoposide is associated with a higher risk of treatment-related leukemia [9]. In contrast, exposure to alkylating agents is characteristically associated with leukemias that evolve in the setting of MDS occurring more than 5 years after drug exposure. Deletions involving chromosomes 5 and 7 are often observed [8].

Other environmental and lifestyle factors do not appear to contribute strongly to the incidence of AML in children. Studies linking childhood AML to exposure to environmental toxins, pesticides, fetal exposure to cigarettes, drugs or alcohol, parental age, and birth weight have been suggestive but so far inconclusive [10].

Clinical Presentation

Children with acute leukemia, whether AML or ALL, typically present with symptoms related to bone marrow infiltration, including pallor, fatigue, fever, petechiae, and bruising. Hepatosplenomegaly is common. Less often, AML cells can also form solid masses, referred to as myeloid sarcoma or chloroma, or infiltrate tissues such as the gingiva and skin. This may occur with or without concomitant peripheral blood or bone marrow involvement. Extramedullary involvement is associated in particular with young age, monoblastic differentiation, and certain cytogenetic abnormalities [11].

In children with AML, the white blood cell count at presentation may be low, normal, or high and circulating blasts may be present or absent. 15–20% of children present with a white blood cell count of 100,000 cells/μL or more [12–14]. Rarely, circulating blasts are detected on screening blood work performed in the absence of symptoms. When the white blood cell count is extremely elevated, patients may experience signs and symptoms related to impaired tissue perfusion that results from hyperviscosity and microvascular obstruction. Leukostasis is a significant risk in AML patients with white blood cell counts over 100,000. Respiratory compromise and central nervous system (CNS) manifestations are of primary concern. Concomitant renal dysfunction and metabolic derangement due to spontaneous tumor lysis syndrome and hemorrhagic diathesis due to thrombocytopenia and disseminated intravascular coagulopathy (DIC) exacerbate the problem. As in adults, DIC with or without hyperleukocytosis is a particularly prominent feature of acute promyelocytic leukemia (APL). The role of leukapheresis remains controversial in children with hyperleukocytosis. In conjunction with prompt initiation of cytoreductive chemotherapy and aggressive management of tumor lysis syndrome, the procedure might reduce the risk of early death in selected patients with very high WBC (>200,000) and monoblastic leukemia [15]. Due to risk of bleeding, leukapheresis is discouraged in patients with APL [16].

The diagnosis of AML may be established when leukemic blasts are circulating in the peripheral blood. However, bone marrow aspiration/biopsy is usually recommended to fully characterize the leukemia. In every new case of AML, the possibility of APL must be considered, since this entity demands urgent initiation of specific therapy (see below). Leukemia cytogenetics, FISH, and molecular tests for subchromosomal genetic alterations, such as FLT3-ITD, should be obtained. Although institutional protocols may differ on which exact studies are sent, molecular studies are increasingly important in determining treatment and predicting prognosis. The option to bank leukemia samples for future studies should always be offered when possible.

Examination of CSF is an important part of the diagnostic evaluation in new-onset leukemia, although it may be delayed or deferred in the setting of coagulopathy. CSF sampling is usually performed in conjunction with administration of intrathecal chemotherapy when the diagnosis of acute leukemia has been established. A summary of commonly recommended studies for the diagnostic evaluation of pediatric AML is shown in Table 19.1.

Table 19.1 Diagnostic evaluation of suspected pediatric AML

Initial workup and staging
• History and physical exam, including family history for malignancies and hematological disorders
• Complete blood count with differential
• Electrolytes, including calcium, phosphorous, uric acid, and lactate dehydrogenase
• Liver function tests, including AST, ALT, bilirubin
• Prothrombin time (PT), partial thromboplastin time (PTT), international normalized ratio (INR), fibrinogen, d-dimer
• Peripheral blood flow cytometry, if circulating blasts are present
• HLA typing for potential transplant
• Chest radiograph
• Ophthalmology exam
• Echocardiogram, electrocardiogram
• Consider central access options
• Consider fertility-preservation options
• Consider research specimen banking, if available
• Bone marrow aspirate
– Morphology, flow cytometry, karyotype, FISH for prognostic AML cytogenetics including t(8;21), inv. [16], MLL, t(15;17), −7, +8
– FLT3 internal tandem duplication
– PML/RAR if suspected or confirmed APL (consider also from blood)
• Bone marrow biopsy
• If no coagulopathy, diagnostic/therapeutic lumbar puncture

Classification

AML is a morphologically, cytogenetically, and molecularly heterogeneous set of diseases and its classification strongly influences prognosis and therapy. Many classification schema have been developed over time, for example, the French-American-British (FAB) classification system, which used morphologic criteria to divide AML into eight groups (M0: acute myeloblastic leukemia with minimal differentiation, M1: acute myeloblastic leukemia without maturation, M2: acute myeloblastic leukemia with maturation, M3: acute promyelocytic leukemia, M4: acute myelomonocytic leukemia, M5: acute monocytic leukemia, M6: acute erythroid leukemia, and M7; acute megakaryocytic leukemia) [17, 18]. However, with increasing understanding of AML biology, particularly in adults, recurrent genetic and cytogenetic alterations have become integrated with classification. This is reflected in the introduction of World Health Organization (WHO) classification of myeloid neoplasms and acute leukemia in 2001, which was revised in 2008 and again in 2016 (Table 19.2).

Because AML is primarily a disease of adults, it is not surprising that the WHO classification schema has limited applicability to pediatric AML. This is illustrated by the fact that in a study of 639 children with AML, AML-NOS (not otherwise specified) is the largest group [19].

Cytogenetic and Molecular Features of Childhood AML and Their Role in Risk Stratification

In large part, the limited applicability in pediatric AML of the genetic and cytogenetic approach driving the WHO classification is driven by age-related differences in the molecular features of adult and childhood AML. Many of the common cytogenetic abnormalities vary considerably by age (Fig. 19.2), and common pediatric alterations that are uncommon in adult AML are not well represented in the WHO classification. For example, although *KMT2A (MLL)* has over 120 described fusion partners [6, 7] and is translocated in

Table 19.2 World Health Organization 2016 classification of myeloid neoplasms and acute leukemia

Acute myeloid leukemia (AML) and related neoplasms
AML with recurrent genetic abnormalities
AML with t(8;21)(q22;q22.1);RUNX1-RUNX1T1
AML with inv. [16](p13.1q22) or t(16;16)(p13.1;q22);CBFB-MYH11
APL with PML-RARA
AML with t(9;11)(p21.3;q23.3);MLLT3-KMT2A
AML with t(6;9)(p23;q34.1);DEK-NUP214
AML with inv. [3](q21.3q26.2) or t(3;3)(q21.3;q26.2); GATA2, MECOM
AML (megakaryoblastic) with t(1;22)(p13.3;q13.3);RBM15-MKL1
Provisional entity: AML with BCR-ABL1
AML with mutated NPM1
AML with biallelic mutations of CEBPA
Provisional entity: AML with mutated RUNX1
AML with myelodysplasia-related changes
Therapy-related myeloid neoplasms
AML, NOS
AML with minimal differentiation
AML without maturation
AML with maturation
Acute myelomonocytic leukemia
Acute monoblastic/monocytic leukemia
Pure erythroid leukemia
Acute megakaryoblastic leukemia
Acute basophilic leukemia
Acute panmyelosis with myelofibrosis
Myeloid sarcoma
Myeloid proliferations related to Down syndrome
Transient abnormal myelopoiesis (TAM)
Myeloid leukemia associated with Down syndrome
Acute leukemias of ambiguous lineage
Acute undifferentiated leukemia
Mixed-phenotype acute leukemia (MPAL) with t(9;22)(q34.1;q11.2); BCR-ABL1
MPAL with t(v;11q23.3); KMT2A rearranged
MPAL, B/myeloid, NOS
MPAL, T/myeloid, NOS

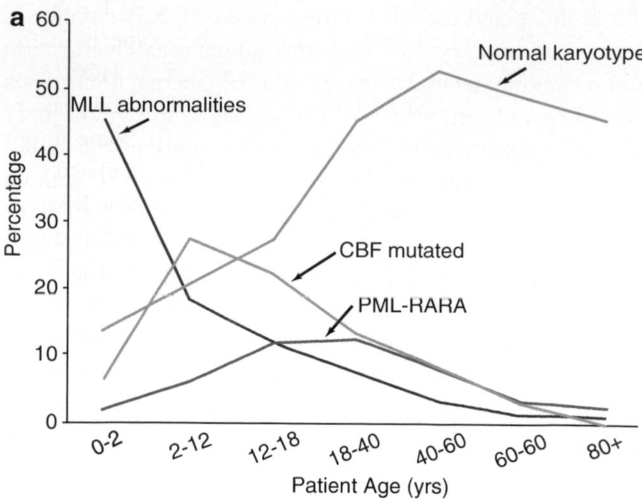

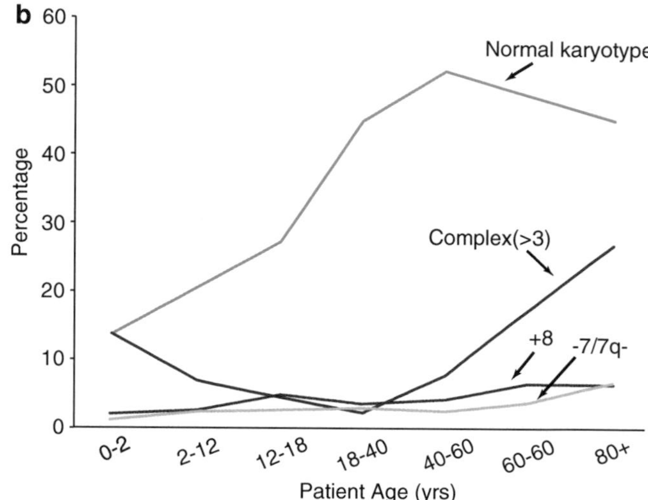

Fig. 19.2 Frequency of molecular abnormalities in AML by age. (**a**) Abnormalities more common in pediatric AML, with normal karyotype AML as a reference. (**b**) Abnormalities more common in adult AML. Data summarized from Cruetzig et al. Cancer 2016

50% of infants and 25% of children with AML, it is uncommon in older adults. As a consequence, the WHO criteria in 2008 and 2016 recognize only the most common fusion protein, t(9;11)(p21.3;q23.3); MLLT3-KMT2A (previously known as MLL-AF9) [8], leading AMLs with other KMT2A translocations to be classified as AML-NOS, despite their differential impact on prognosis.

Other pediatric centric molecular features are recognized however, for example, the favorable risk core-binding factor (CBF) group, with t(8;21) or inv.(16) and t(16;16), is very common (>25%) in childhood AML, while uncommon in older adults with AML. PML-RAR is common (>10%) in adolescents and young adults with AML, while uncommon in young children and older adults over 60. In contrast, cytogenetically normal, complex karyotype and losses of 5q and 7 are more common in older adults.

Although the frequencies of specific cytogenetic abnormalities vary, most abnormalities retain a similar clinical meaning in pediatric compared to adult AML (Table 19.3). However there are a few notable exceptions. Both monosomy 7 and 7q- are poor risk markers in adults, while children with 7q- do relatively well compared to those with monosomy 7 [19–21]. Since 11q23 rearrangement is more common in children, more data is available regarding the prognostic impact of specific KMT2A translocations in pediatric AML, which is variable. The t(6;11)(q27;q23), t(10;11)(p12;q23), and t(10;11)(p11.2;q23) translocations have been specifically associated with unfavorable outcomes, while

Table 19.3 Prognostic cytogenetic alterations in pediatric acute myeloid leukemia

Favorable	
t(8;21)(q22;q22)/RUNX1-RUNX1T1	[21, 24]
Inv(16)(p13.1;q22)/CBFb-MYH11	[21, 24]
Mutated NPM1 without FLT3-ITD	[25, 26]
Biallelic mutations of CEBPA	[27, 28]
t(1;11)(q21;q23)/MLLT11-KMT2A	[22]
t(15;17)/PML-RARA	[24]
Intermediate or unclear	
t(9;11)(p12;q23)/MLLT3-KMT2A	[22]
Other KMT2A fusions	[22]
Unfavorable	
t(6;11)(q27;q23)/MLLT4-KMT2A	22
t(10;11)(p12;q23)/MLLT10-KMT2A	[22]
t(10;11)(p11.2;q23)/ABI1-KMT2A	[22]
t(6;9)(p23;q34)/DEK-NUP214	[29, 30]
t(5;11)(q35;p15.5)/NUP98-NSD1 with FLT3-ITD	[31, 32]
Inv(16)(p13.3q24.3)/CBFA2T3-GLIS2	[33, 34]
FLT3-ITD	[26, 35]
Monosomy 7	[19, 20, 21]
t(9;22)/BCR-ABL	[21]
5q abnormalities	[21]

t(1;11)(q21;q23) is favorable, and others appear to have little impact on prognosis [22]. The prognostic significance of other cytogenetic lesions is emerging in pediatric AML, but is not yet validated [23].

In addition to cytogenetic alterations, nearly all cases of adult AML have multiple pathogenic somatic single-nucleotide variants (mutations) and some copy number variants that can be identified by next-generation sequencing techniques, with the most frequently altered including *FLT3, NPM1, DNMT3A, IDH1, IDH2, TET2, RUNX1, TP53, CEBPA, WT1, KIT*, the Ras pathway (*NRAS, KRAS, PTPN11*), splicing (*U2AF1, SF3B1, ZRSF2*), and the cohesion complex (*STAG2, SMC3, RAD21*) [36]. Although studies have been limited to small cohorts, often assaying only a few genes, variants in most of these genes have been far less common. For example, *FLT3-ITD* (25% vs. 12%) and mutations in *CEBPA* (35% vs. 8%), *IDH1* or *IDH2* (17% vs. 2%), and *DNMTA* (22% vs. 0%) [37] are all significantly more frequent in adult versus childhood AML patients.

The cell of origin, order, number, and which combinations of mutations are required for AML development remain an active field of investigation, beyond the scope of this chapter. Gilliland and colleagues previously proposed a model in which AML develops from a combination of "class II" mutations, which primarily cause a differentiation arrest and increased self-renewal, with "class I" mutations that cause increased proliferation and survival [38]. Such class I mutations include activating mutations in the Ras pathway as well as constitutive activation of receptor or cytoplasmic tyrosine kinases such as *FLT3* and *KIT*. The contribution of many recently described mutations, such as those in epigenetic regulators, splicing, and cohesin complex, are incompletely understood and their effects on differentiation, self-renewal, and proliferation are under investigation.

Increasing evidence is accumulating that some of these somatic variants, particularly in *DNMT3A, TET2, ASXL1, JAK2*, and *SF3B1*, may be an initial event in the pathogenesis of adult AML. Several studies [39–41] have now documented the existence of detectable, pathogenic, persistent, and typically subclonal variants in these genes in the blood of healthy volunteers, which likely represent the expansion of mutated hematopoietic stem cells and is now termed clonal hematopoiesis of indeterminate potential (CHIP) [42, 43]. These mutations are associated with an increased risk of transformation to a hematopoietic malignancy; they are more frequent in patients with unexplained cytopenias [44] and have been documented in non-leukemic hematopoietic stem cells of leukemic patients [45] and the blood samples of patients prior to the development of AML [46]. The prevalence of CHIP increases dramatically with age, with over 10% affected of those over 70 years or older, but is rare in healthy adults under 40 [39], which is thought to be related to age-related accumulation of DNA damage. The near absence of these variants in healthy young people and low prevalence in childhood AML suggest that most childhood AML may have a very different etiology than most adult AML.

Immunophenotype Analysis at Diagnosis in Pediatric AML

The diagnosis of AML, to be distinguished from ALL and MPAL, has been greatly assisted by the advent of flow cytometry and immunophenotyping. An aberrant immunophenotype can be detected on myeloid blasts in 95% of cases [47] at diagnosis, commonly with expression of myeloid and stem cell markers CD13, CD15, CD33, CD34, CD56, and CD117 as well as lymphoid markers such as CD7, CD10, and CD19. Some specific immunophenotypes are correlated to cytogenetics or outcomes and should be noted.

Minimally differentiated M0 FAB subtype of AML is rare and a poor prognostic marker [48]. The good prognostic t(8;21)(q22;q22) translocation is more frequently found in pediatric patients, in the FAB M2 subtype, and often associated with extramedullary tumors, chloromas, and splenomegaly. They also have a specific immunophenotype, with positivity for the B-cell cell-associated marker CD19, as well as CD13, CD34, CD56, and HLA-DR, while CD2 and CD7 are rarely expressed and CD33 is weak [49].

In FAB M3, acute promyelocytic leukemia (APL) blasts co-express CD13, CD33, and CD9 but are negative for HLA-DR, CD15, CD10, or CD11b. In addition to distinct morphologic features, this immunophenotype will be one of the earliest hints that a newly presenting patient has APL and could benefit from the early initiation of tretinoin (see below).

M6 erythroleukemia is rare in childhood AML but associated with a poor outcome, particularly induction failure and death [50]. The megakaryocytic M7 FAB subtype may be suspected based on morphology or histochemistry, and is confirmed by immunophenotypic analysis (identification of platelet or megakaryocytic antigens CD41 and CD61) [18]. It is frequently associated with Down syndrome, and is in fact the most common type of AML in young children with Down syndrome, where it has a favorable prognosis. In contrast, M7 AML in non-Down syndrome patients is rare and carries a poor prognosis [50].

Loken and colleagues [51] recently described a pediatric restricted high-risk immunophenotype with bright CD56, dim to negative CD45 and CD38, and a lack of HLA-DR, named the RAM phenotype (after a particular patient's initials). These patients were significantly younger (1.26 years old vs. 10.1) and lacked FLT3-ITD, CEBPA, or NPM1 mutations and were all considered standard-risk cytogenetics; however, they were more frequently MRD positive (84% vs. 33%), had lower EFS (16% vs. 51%), and OS (26% vs. 66%) compared to the non-RAM cohort.

Treatment

Treatment of AML in children is similar to adults, but outcomes in children are superior in all risk groups [12, 52]. Overall survival for pediatric AML exceeds 60% with current treatment protocols [23]. Treatment is separated into two phases: remission induction and post-remission consolidation. Approximately 90% of children achieve remission after one or two cycles of intensive induction chemotherapy [53]. The choice of post-remission consolidation is determined by risk group which is, in turn, based on the combination of disease characteristics and treatment response. Broadly speaking, lower risk patients in first complete remission are allocated to receive additional cycles of combination chemotherapy while higher risk patients are typically referred for allogeneic hematopoietic cell transplantation (HCT). Allocation to HCT is not based solely on the existence of a matched family donor, as it was in the past. For AML patients who relapse, HCT in second remission is generally considered the best option for the possibility of cure.

Remission Induction

For decades, the combination of cytarabine plus an anthracycline has remained the mainstay of induction therapy for newly diagnosed AML. Multiple clinical trials in childhood AML have examined different cytarabine doses and schedules, different anthracyclines, and addition of a third agent. Despite these efforts, no clear optimal combination and schedule have been defined. Currently in the United States, induction therapy typically consists of cytarabine, daunorubicin, and etoposide (ADE 10 + 3 + 5) based on the series of trials conducted by the United Kingdom Medical Research Council (MRC) [54, 55]. Bone marrow examination is performed to assess response to chemotherapy around days 21–28 of induction I. If residual leukemia is present, a second cycle of chemotherapy may be immediately initiated. Otherwise, induction II begins when peripheral blood counts recover. Morphologic assessment of early treatment response is notoriously challenging. Application of multiparameter flow cytometry and molecular studies significantly improves the accuracy of the hematopathologists' interpretation [56]. Depending on genetic and clinical factors, response to induction I, and provider preference, a second cycle of ADE or a more intensive combination, such as high-dose cytarabine with mitoxantrone [13], is administered in induction II. After two cycles of induction chemotherapy, about 90% of children with de novo AML will achieve remission, defined as <5% marrow blasts by morphology and/or flow cytometry. Among the subset of patients who do not achieve this milestone, refractory disease is the cause in the majority, in most studies. However, early death due to toxicity is also a significant problem [14, 57, 58].

Monitoring Treatment Response

In addition to the initial immunophenotypic, cytogenetic, and genetic features, response to therapy is a strong predictor for relapse and long-term outcome. Morphologic induction failure, unquestionably, portends a dismal prognosis, but occurs in only a small minority of cases and unfortunately nearly half of patients that achieve complete remission (CR) will eventually relapse. Modern assessment of treatment response involves the measurement of minimal residual disease (MRD), which is typically performed by sensitive multidimensional flow cytometry after induction chemotherapy; however RT-PCR analysis of leukemia-specific transcripts [59] and genomic DNA assessment of mutation clearance have been studied as well.

Flow cytometry for aberrant immunophenotypes post-induction is the most generalizable method and has been shown to be prognostic in childhood AML and predicts relapse risk in multiple studies. For example, in the St. Jude AML02 trial [58], the presence of high MRD by flow after one course of induction was associated with a 3-year cumulative incidence of relapse of 39% compared with only 17% for patients with no detectable MRD. The relapse rate was particularly high for patients with MRD >1% after one course of therapy and for those with any detectable MRD (>0.1%) after two courses of induction chemotherapy.

At relapse, 88% of pediatric AML cases demonstrated an antigenic shift in at least one marker [60]. Because immunophenotype can vary greatly and aberrancy can be subtle, it is important to perform multiparameter flow cytometry, especially in cases of minimal disease detection, which should not be restricted to the immunophenotype detected at presentation. In contrast to adult AML trials, flow-based MRD is well accepted and used by most pediatric cooperative group to determine which patients receive high-risk therapy (in combination with clinical, cytogenetic, and genetic features).

Consolidation Chemotherapy

Consolidation therapy for pediatric AML in first complete remission is determined by risk group. It is generally agreed that the core-binding factor (CBF) leukemias have a reasonably good chance of cure with chemotherapy alone. For these patients with so-called low-risk cytogenetics, the up-front toxicity of HCT in first complete remission is not warranted [61, 62]. On the opposite end of the spectrum, high-risk AML is variably defined among cooperative groups and the definition continues to evolve. General consensus has emerged for many of the more frequent subtypes and scenarios, taking into account both disease features and response to therapy. High-risk characteristics include poor response to initial therapy, AML arising in the setting of MDS or prior treatment, presence of FLT3-ITD with high allelic ratio, and presence of adverse cytogenetics such as monosomy 7, monosomy 5, del5q, and other specific rare translocations [14, 55, 63–65]. HCT from the best available donor is typically, although not universally, considered the treatment of choice for children with high-risk AML in first complete remission, even though a clear benefit from HCT has been difficult to demonstrate in prospective [66] and retrospective trials [67]. A loosely defined intermediate-risk group is comprised of patients with neither low-risk nor high-risk features. For this population, the risk-benefit analysis related to consolidation chemotherapy versus HCT is closer to neutral. Individual factors, such as the availability of a matched family donor, may be taken into consideration in selecting the best consolidation strategy.

For patients who do not proceed to HCT in first remission, post-remission treatment usually consists of additional cycles of intensive consolidation chemotherapy, including some exposure to cytarabine at high dose (≥1 g/m^2/dose) [65, 68]. Although the optimal number of cycles is not determined, a total of four cycles of multiagent chemotherapy is relatively standard in the United States at this time. This is primarily based on results from the MRC AML12 trial which demonstrated that three cycles of consolidation chemotherapy did not improve event-free or overall survival in comparison to two cycles [55]. With current intensive chemotherapy, children with CBF leukemia can expect event-free survival in the range of 80% and overall survival in the range of 90% at 3 years [13, 58]. The influence of risk group on outcome is depicted in Fig. 19.3 [58]. Maintenance chemotherapy has no proven benefit in childhood AML [69, 70], with the exception of APL [71].

Extramedullary Disease

The incidence of central nervous system (CNS) involvement is higher in children with AML compared to ALL. However, the impact that it has on prognosis, and therefore on treatment, is less important. CNS involvement in AML is associated with higher presenting WBC count, younger age, and certain karyotypic abnormalities. CNS-directed therapy in the form of intrathecal chemotherapy, in addition to CNS-penetrant systemic chemotherapy is incorporated into all contemporary treatment protocols for pediatric AML. Prophylactic cranial radiation is not routinely used. CNS3 status, which is defined as ≥5 WBC/μL and blasts present on cytospin, occurs in about 10% of children with AML [72]. For these children, intensification of intrathecal chemotherapy is recommended. The management of CNS2 status (<5 WBC with blasts seen) is variable. Although CNS involvement does not appear to confer a significant impact on overall prognosis, it is associated with a higher risk of CNS relapse [72, 73].

Soft-tissue masses, referred to as myeloid sarcoma or chloroma, are identified occasionally in children with newly diagnosed AML. The pattern and prognostic impact of this are linked to associated karyotypic changes. As mentioned above, cutaneous involvement ("leukemia cutis") is characteristically seen in babies with *KMT2A (MLL)*-rearranged AML (Fig. 19.4). Orbital, parameningeal, and CNS masses

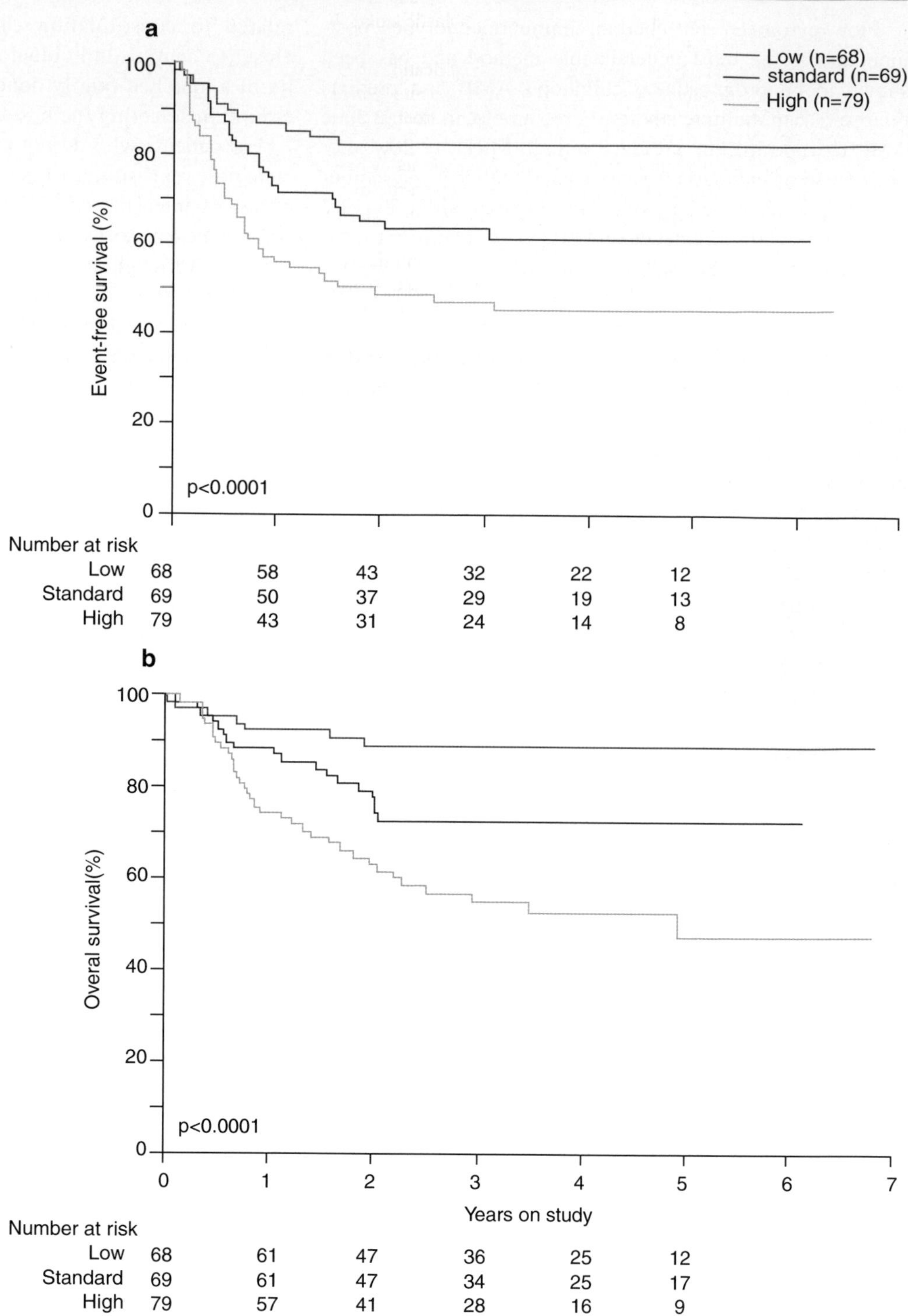

Fig. 19.3 Treatment outcome according to risk group on St. Jude AML02. Reproduced with permission from Rubnitz, et al. Lancet Oncology 2010

are characteristic of AML in older children in association with favorable cytogenetics [74]. Although focal radiation may have a role in selected cases for the acute management of myeloid tumors that threaten permanent consequences due to their location or in the palliative setting, there is no established benefit to addition of focal radiation to myeloid tumors that respond well to chemotherapy [75]. Apparently "isolated" extramedullary disease is viewed as a harbinger of systemic illness both at initial diagnosis and at relapse and should be treated as such [76].

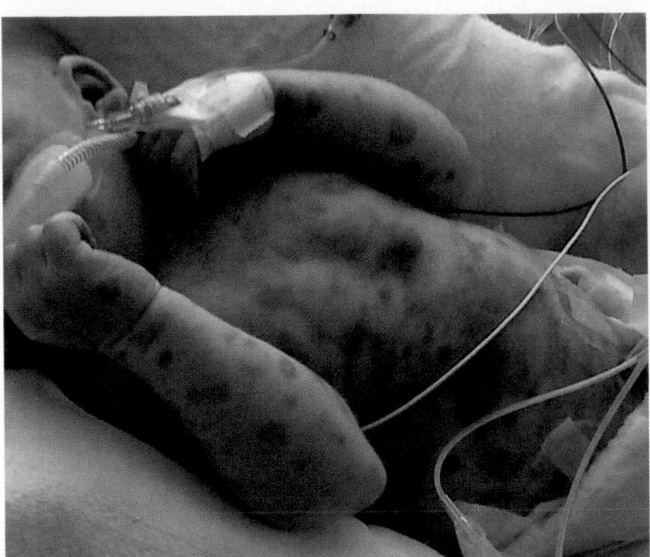

Fig. 19.4 Leukemia cutis in a newborn infant with KMT2A (MLL)-rearranged AML

Newer and Targeted Agents

Due to the suboptimal outcomes in pediatric AML, novel therapies targeting a broad variety of mechanisms are in development. These include second-generation nucleoside analogs, such as clofarabine, which is more resistant to deamination than classical agents such as cytarabine [77], new formulations of traditional chemotherapy, such as CPX-351, a liposomal formulation of daunorubicin and cytarabine, and targeted agents such as kinase inhibitors, monoclonal antibodies, epigenetic modulators, and others. Since AML is much more common in adults, novel therapies are generally studied and often shown to have activity in adults before being used in pediatric studies.

As noted above, the presence of the FLT3 internal tandem duplication is an adverse prognostic feature in children [35, 78] as it is in adults. Several FLT3 inhibitors that range in specificity and potency already exist that have been, or are being, tested in adult AML. These drugs include midostaurin, sorafenib, quizartinib, gilteritinib, and crenolanib [79]. The multikinase inhibitor midostaurin was approved for adults with AML with certain FLT3 mutations in 2017, however data in children is limited at this time. The multikinase inhibitor sorafinab, which is FDA approved for certain solid tumors, also has activity against some FLT3 mutations, with reported clinical activity in relapsed pediatric AML [80] and some use in the post transplant setting [81].

Gemtuzumab ozogamicin is a humanized monoclonal antibody directed against CD33, a protein that is expressed on the surface of a high proportion of AML blasts but not on hematopoietic stem cells. The antibody is covalently linked to an antitumor antibiotic, calicheamicin. The drug was approved in 2017 for AML in patients aged 2 and older [82]. Children's Oncology Group (COG) AAML 0531 [14] demonstrated that addition of gemtuzumab was associated with a statistically significant positive effect on event-free survival through reduction of relapse. High expression of the target antigen, CD33, is associated with response to the drug [83]. Additional immunoconjugates, including vadastuximab talirine (SGN-CD33A) [84], are in development for AML.

Many other classes of agents show promise in AML and are currently under investigation. Epigenetic modifiers are a broad class including drugs that inhibit histone deacetylase (vorinostat) and DNA methyltransferase (azacitidine and decitabine) which are being studied in relapsed pediatric and adult AML. DOT1L inhibition is being studied in children and adults for KMT2A (MLL)-rearranged AML. Other strategies being investigated with new clinical agents include IDH1 and IDH2 inhibition, proteasomal inhibition, exportin inhibition, ubiquitination modulation, and chimeric antigen receptor T-cell therapy [53, 85].

Acute Promyelocytic Leukemia

Acute promyelocytic leukemia (APL) is a unique AML subtype characterized by the presence of reciprocal translocation involving chromosomes 15 and 17 leading to the production of a promyelocytic leukemia (*PML*)-retinoic acid receptor alpha (*RARA*) fusion protein. APL is a disease of older children and young adults. APL accounts for about 10% of pediatric AML and it is distinctly uncommon in children under 10 years. The molecular features of APL are described above and elsewhere in this text. In children as in adults, the treatment of APL differs significantly from other AML subtypes and the overall prognosis is markedly better. But APL is associated with a high risk of early death, due primarily to hemorrhage. Therefore, clinicians must be on alert for this entity because prompt and accurate diagnosis is critical to successful management.

APL is characterized morphologically by the appearance of large hypergranular myeloid blasts with prominent Auer rods. The hypogranular variant (M3v), which is more common in children [86], may be more difficult to distinguish from other AML subtypes. Typically, the blasts co-express CD13, CD33, and CD9 but do not express HLA-DR, CD15, CD10, or CD11b. Blasts of the hypogranular variant typically express CD2 [87]. Demonstration of the molecular fusion of PML gene on chromosome 17 and the RARA gene on chromosome 15 by RT-PCR, FISH, or karyotype is the key to diagnosis. RT-PCR is the preferred modality since it is rapid, specific, and quantitative.

Disseminated intravascular coagulopathy (DIC) is a significant and potentially life-threatening feature of new-onset APL. Transfusions should be provided to maintain the platelet count ≥30–50 K and fibrinogen level ≥100–150 mg/dL. To address the underlying cause of the bleeding diathesis, emergent initiation of leukemia-directed therapy in the form of tretinoin is recommended at the first suspicion of the disease [16]. Delay in starting tretinoin is associated with a higher risk of early hemorrhagic death [88]. In children, there is an estimated 7.4% risk of death within the first 7 days of APL diagnosis [89].

The introduction of tretinoin into the treatment of APL in the late 1980s transformed the management and the prognosis of this disease. Tretinoin is now a standard component of APL therapy in children. Tretinoin causes differentiation of malignant promyelocytes, sometimes leading to marked increase in the peripheral leukocyte count. Differentiation syndrome occurs in 10–20% of children being treated with tretinoin for APL [90–92]. Higher presenting WBC is a risk factor for the development of this complication of therapy which is characterized by fever, hypotension, pulmonary infiltrates, and renal insufficiency. Aggressive supportive care, administration of dexamethasone, and early introduction of cytotoxic chemotherapy are recommended. Temporary interruption of tretinoin is indicated in severe cases. Pseudotumor cerebri is an important side effect of tretinoin that occurs more commonly in children than in adults [90–92] warranting the use of a lower starting dose of tretinoin in children.

While it is true that APL is associated with an unacceptably high risk of early morbidity and mortality, the overall prognosis for children with APL is significantly better than most other AML subtypes. Treatment with combination of chemotherapy and tretinoin results in event-free and overall survival in the range of 75 and 90%, respectively [90, 91]. As in adults, the intensity of treatment is risk stratified based on presenting white blood cell (WBC) count, with high risk defined as presenting WBC >10,000 cells/dL. Although highly effective, these chemotherapy regimens are lengthy (almost 3 years in duration due to inclusion of a maintenance phase) and associated with potential for significant late effects (especially cardiotoxicity related to high cumulative anthracycline exposure). Exciting recent studies in adults have demonstrated that APL can be cured in many cases with combination of tretinoin and arsenic trioxide with little or no cytotoxic chemotherapy [93]. Arsenic has been shown to be effective and tolerable in children with relapsed APL [94] and in small series of children with newly diagnosed APL [95, 96]. Ongoing clinical trials are examining the use of arsenic and tretinoin as up-front therapy for pediatric APL with concomitant reduction or omission of cytotoxic agents and shortening of treatment duration.

Myeloid Leukemia of Down Syndrome

Children with Down syndrome (DS) are at a 10–20-fold increased risk for developing leukemia. The pattern of disease is unique, comprising neonatal transient abnormal myelopoiesis (TAM), MDS/AML, and ALL. In the first 5 years of life, the risk of myeloid leukemia is about 150 times higher in DS children compared with non-DS children [97].

Myeloid blasts are identified in the peripheral blood smears of approximately 10–15% of newborns with DS. The blasts typically, but not always, express immunophenotypic markers of megakaryoblasts, including CD41, CD42b, and CD61 [98]. Despite the fact that the abnormal cells are morphologically and immunophenotypically indistinguishable from acute megakaryoblastic leukemia (AML M7), they almost always disappear with little or no specific treatment. This process, known as transient abnormal myelopoiesis (also called transient leukemia or transient myeloproliferative disorder) is unique to babies with constitutional and mosaic trisomy 21. In the context of trisomy 21, acquisition of a truncating mutation in the GATA-1 transcription factor in a fetal liver-derived hematopoietic stem or progenitor cell results in expansion of the myeloid blast population. GATA-1 mutation is invariably present in DS babies with clinical TAM. Surprisingly, GATA-1 mutation was also detected in about 20% of DS infants without clinical evidence of TAM. These babies have so-called silent TAM [99].

The main clinical feature of TAM is leukocytosis with circulating blasts. There is currently no defined absolute blast threshold for the diagnosis of TAM. In a systematic review of 48 patients with TAM, the median age at diagnosis was 1 week, median WBC was about 30x10e9/L, and median peripheral blast percentage was 25%. Hepatosplenomegaly was present in more than half and liver dysfunction occurred in about one-third. Even though circulating blasts resolved in nearly all of the patients within a mean of 2 months, almost 20% of the patients died. Mortality in babies with TAM is most often attributed to hepatic fibrosis and liver failure [98]. Survival is associated with the absence of both hepatomegaly and life-threatening symptoms [100]. Treatment with very-low-dose cytarabine appears to decrease the risk of death in babies with severe TAM. However, chemotherapy treatment has never been shown to influence the risk of ML-DS later in childhood [101].

About 20% of TAM patients go on to develop myeloid leukemia before the age of 4 years. As in TAM, immunophenotypic markers of megakaryoblastic differentiation are observed in most cases and GATA-1 mutation is present in all cases. In association with evolution to ML-DS, additional "cooperating" mutations involving genes that encode cohesin complex components, epigenetic regulators, and/or signaling molecules are acquired [102]. In some children with ML-DS, a history of clinical TAM is absent. Presumably, these patients previously experienced undiagnosed "silent" TAM. Taking the incidence of silent TAM into account, it is estimated that progression to ML-DS occurs in about 5–10% of TAM cases [103] (Fig. 19.5).

ML-DS is a subtype of childhood AML that is clinically distinct and warrants distinct treatment. The median age at presentation is in the second year of life and the onset of the disease is often indolent, with gradual progression of cytopenias. ML-DS patients who do not meet the AML threshold of 20% blasts in blood or marrow often fulfill WHO criteria for MDS. In contrast to TAM, successful treatment of ML-DS requires chemotherapy. However, the intensity of chemotherapy necessary to cure ML-DS is less than de novo AML in children without DS. In fact, in an analysis performed by the Children's Cancer Group, higher intensity chemotherapy led to significant treatment-related toxicity in children with ML-DS, substantially offsetting the potential benefit in terms of leukemia control [57]. Since the late 1990s, treatment protocols designed specifically for children with ML-DS have progressively reduced treatment intensity while preserving good results with overall and event-free survival at around 80% [104–106]. Older age, higher presenting white blood cell count, and "normal" karyotype are associated with a significantly worse prognosis [107, 106].

Relapsed and Refractory AML

AML that is refractory to initial treatment or recurs after initial treatment represents a significant therapeutic challenge. Refractory disease occurs in about 5% and relapse affects about 30% [108]. Approximately half of relapses occur within 1 year, and almost all occur within 4 years of initial diagnosis [109, 110]. Long-term disease control can be accomplished in a minority of these patients but, in general, requires attainment of remission followed by HCT. For patients with relapsed AML, favorable cytogenetics [111], longer duration of first complete remission (i.e., ≥1 year from initial diagnosis), and receipt of HCT after relapse are associated with better outcomes [112].

There is currently no standard re-induction protocol for children with relapsed AML. Like up-front therapy, relapsed therapy mainly relies on the use of cytarabine with or without an anthracycline. Newer agents, including the purine analogues fludarabine, clofarabine, and cladribine, are incorporated into some regimens. Several combinations have been tested in children including fludarabine, cytarabine, idarubicin (Ida-FLAG) [113], mitoxantrone, cytarabine [114], fludarabine, cytarabine +/− liposomal daunorubicin [115], clofarabine, and cytarabine [116]. With any combination,

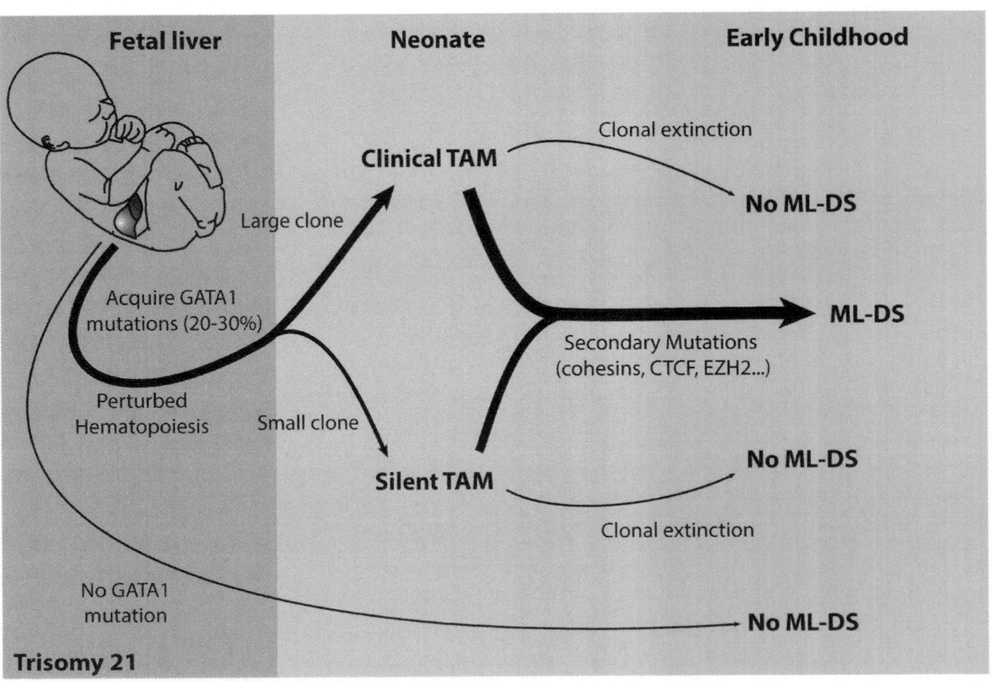

Fig. 19.5 Progression of transient abnormal myelopoiesis to Down syndrome-myeloid leukemia

complete remission is achieved in about 60–70% and many of these patients are able to proceed to HCT. MRD before HCT is a strong predictor of survival [117]. Both subsequent relapse and high treatment-related toxicity are major obstacles to overall survival. Treatment with novel and/or targeted agents, preferably in the context of clinical trials, may be an option for some patients.

The prognosis for patients with relapsed APL is much more favorable than for other relapsed AML subtypes. A role for autologous HCT has been demonstrated for those patients who achieve a second molecular remission [118]. In contrast, relapsed/refractory ML-DS is associated with a dismal prognosis [119].

Treatment Toxicity and Supportive Care

Improved survival in childhood AML is the product of maximizing treatment intensity in coordination with optimizing supportive care. Current treatment protocols appear to be reaching the inevitable limit of dose intensification. The severity and importance of treatment-related risks differ in children compared to adults. In general, children have fewer comorbidities and they tolerate myelosuppression better than adults. However, effects on growth and development matter much more. For children under 1 year of age and those who have a body surface area of less than 0.6 m^2, cytotoxic chemotherapy doses are adjusted, either as percent reduction or by basing calculations on weight instead of body surface area.

All children undergoing treatment for AML experience repeated episodes of prolonged and profound myelosuppression. Infections are the main cause of treatment-related morbidity and mortality. Unsurprisingly, the incidence of infection correlates with treatment intensity [120]. The use of bacterial and fungal prophylaxis is now recommended [121] as this does appear to reduce the rate of severe bacterial and invasive fungal infections [122]. In addition, prophylaxis against pneumocystis pneumonia is advised. The benefit of granulocyte colony-stimulating factor (filgrastim) remains controversial. When addition of prophylactic filgrastim was studied in a randomized fashion in the context of intensive chemotherapy in the Berlin-Frankfurt-Muenster (BFM)-98 study, the duration of neutropenia was shortened but the rate of severe infections was not reduced. However, in an analysis of the COG AAML0531 study, in which infections were collected and monitored prospectively, filgrastim prophylaxis was associated with a statistically significantly lower rate of bacterial infections [123]. However, its use is not without risk. A higher incidence of relapse was observed in children treated with filgrastim whose AML expressed a specific G-CSF receptor isoform [124]. At this time, routine use of filgrastim is not recommended.

Most children treated for AML receive substantial cumulative exposure to anthracyclines, often greater than 360 mg/m^2. As a consequence, survivors are at high risk of long-term cardiac sequelae [125, 126]. Dexrazoxane has not been extensively studied in pediatric AML, but it might reduce cardiotoxicity [127]. Cardiotoxicity is a particular concern for children with DS [128]. After completion of treatment, patients should be monitored for cardiac late effects according to established guidelines [129].

Conclusions

Among pediatricians, it is often said that children are not just small adults. Although pediatric and adult AML share many features, there are important differences in terms of epidemiology, etiology, cytogenetics, and molecular genetics which influence therapy and outcome. Today, childhood AML is a curable disease in more than half of the cases. From the "glass is half-full" perspective, this fact unquestionably represents a major accomplishment. But, much more progress needs to be made to improve outcomes for all children and to reduce the burden of treatment. Progress is needed in many areas including molecular diagnostics, refinement of risk stratification, optimization of chemotherapy, development of targeted agents, and application of conventional and novel transplant strategies. Better outcomes also depend on advances in supportive care and implementation of best clinical practices. The way forward requires cooperation among pediatric oncology providers, scientists, and the pharmaceutical industry and on our patient's ability to access and participate in well-designed clinical trials.

References

1. Cancer Stat Facts: Acute Myeloid Leukemia (AML). http://seer.cancer.gov/statfacts/html/amyl.html.
2. Pui CH, Carroll WL, Meshinchi S, Arceci RJ. Biology, risk stratification, and therapy of pediatric acute leukemias: an update. J Clin Oncol. 2011;29(5):551–65.
3. Zhang J, Walsh MF, Wu G, et al. Germline mutations in predisposition genes in pediatric cancer. N Engl J Med. 2015;373(24):2336–46.
4. Song WJ, Sullivan MG, Legare RD, et al. Haploinsufficiency of CBFA2 causes familial thrombocytopenia with propensity to develop acute myelogenous leukaemia. Nat Genet. 1999;23(2):166–75.
5. Noris P, Perrotta S, Seri M, et al. Mutations in ANKRD26 are responsible for a frequent form of inherited thrombocytopenia: analysis of 78 patients from 21 families. Blood. 2011;117(24):6673–80.
6. Zhang MY, Churpek JE, Keel SBB, et al. Germline ETV6 mutations in familial thrombocytopenia and hematologic malignancy. Nat Genet. 2015;47(2):180–5.

7. Hijiya N, Ness KK, Ribeiro RC, Hudson MM. Acute leukemia as a secondary malignancy in children and adolescents: current findings and issues. Cancer. 2009;115(1):23–35.
8. Andersen MK, Johansson B, Larsen SO, Pedersen-Bjergaard J. Chromosomal abnormalities in secondary MDS and AML. Relationship to drugs and radiation with specific emphasis on the balanced rearrangements. Haematologica. 1998;83(6):483–8.
9. Smith MA, Rubinstein L, Anderson JR, et al. Secondary leukemia or myelodysplastic syndrome after treatment with epipodophyllotoxins. J Clin Oncol. 1999;17(2):569–77.
10. Puumala SE, Ross JA, Aplenc R, Spector LG. Epidemiology of childhood acute myeloid leukemia. Pediatr Blood Cancer. 2013;60(5):728–33.
11. Kobayashi R, Tawa A, Hanada R, et al. Extramedullary infiltration at diagnosis and prognosis in children with acute myelogenous leukemia. Pediatr Blood Cancer. 2007;48(4):393–8.
12. Gibson BE, Wheatley K, Hann IM, et al. Treatment strategy and long-term results in paediatric patients treated in consecutive UK AML trials. Leukemia. 2005;19(12):2130–8.
13. Creutzig U, Zimmermann M, Bourquin JP, et al. Second induction with high-dose cytarabine and mitoxantrone: different impact on pediatric AML patients with t(8;21) and with inv(16). Blood. 2011;118(20):5409–15.
14. Gamis AS, Alonzo TA, Meshinchi S, et al. Gemtuzumab ozogamicin in children and adolescents with de novo acute myeloid leukemia improves event-free survival by reducing relapse risk: results from the randomized phase III Children's Oncology Group trial AAML0531. J Clin Oncol. 2014;32(27):3021–32.
15. Creutzig U, Rossig C, Dworzak M, et al. Exchange transfusion and leukapheresis in pediatric patients with AML with high risk of early death by bleeding and leukostasis. Pediatr Blood Cancer. 2016;63(4):640–5.
16. Sanz MA, Grimwade D, Tallman MS, et al. Management of acute promyelocytic leukemia: recommendations from an expert panel on behalf of the European LeukemiaNet. Blood. 2009;113(9):1875–91.
17. Behm FG. Diagnosis of childhood acute myeloid leukemia. Clin Lab Med. 1999;19(1):187.
18. Bennett JM, Catovsky D, Daniel MT, et al. Proposed revised criteria for the classification of acute myeloid leukemia. A report of the French-American-British Cooperative Group. Ann Intern Med. 1985;103(4):620–5.
19. Sandahl JD, Kjeldsen E, Abrahamsson J, et al. The applicability of the WHO classification in paediatric AML. A NOPHO-AML study. Br J Haematol. 2015;169(6):859–67.
20. Hasle H, Alonzo TA, Auvrignon A, et al. Monosomy 7 and deletion 7q in children and adolescents with acute myeloid leukemia: an international retrospective study. Blood. 2007;109(11):4641–7.
21. Harrison CJ, Hills RK, Moorman AV, et al. Cytogenetics of childhood acute myeloid leukemia: United Kingdom Medical Research Council Treatment trials AML 10 and 12. J Clin Oncol. 2010;28(16):2674–81.
22. Balgobind BV, Raimondi SC, Harbott J, et al. Novel prognostic subgroups in childhood 11q23/MLL-rearranged acute myeloid leukemia: results of an international retrospective study. Blood. 2009;114(12):2489–96.
23. Zwaan CM, Kolb EA, Reinhardt D, et al. Collaborative efforts driving progress in pediatric acute myeloid leukemia. J Clin Oncol. 2015;33(27):2949–62.
24. von Neuhoff C, Reinhardt D, Sander A, et al. Prognostic impact of specific chromosomal aberrations in a large group of pediatric patients with acute myeloid leukemia treated uniformly according to trial AML-BFM 98. J Clin Oncol. 2010;28(16):2682–9.
25. Brown P, McIntyre E, Rau R, et al. The incidence and clinical significance of nucleophosmin mutations in childhood AML. Blood. 2007;110(3):979–85.
26. Staffas A, Kanduri M, Hovland R, et al. Presence of FLT3-ITD and high BAALC expression are independent prognostic markers in childhood acute myeloid leukemia. Blood. 2011;118(22):5905–13.
27. Ho PA, Alonzo TA, Gerbing RB, et al. Prevalence and prognostic implications of CEBPA mutations in pediatric acute myeloid leukemia (AML): a report from the Children's Oncology Group. Blood. 2009;113(26):6558–66.
28. Matsuo H, Kajihara M, Tomizawa D, et al. Prognostic implications of CEBPA mutations in pediatric acute myeloid leukemia: a report from the Japanese Pediatric Leukemia/Lymphoma Study Group. Blood Cancer J. 2014;4(7):e226.
29. Sandahl JD, Coenen EA, Forestier E, et al. T(6;9)(p22;q34)/DEK-NUP214-rearranged pediatric myeloid leukemia: an international study of 62 patients. Haematologica. 2014;99(5):865–72.
30. Tarlock K, Alonzo TA, Moraleda PP, et al. Acute myeloid leukaemia (AML) with t(6;9)(p23;q34) is associated with poor outcome in childhood AML regardless of FLT3-ITD status: a report from the Children's Oncology Group. Br J Haematol. 2014;166(2):254–9.
31. Hollink I, van den Heuvel-Eibrink MM, Arentsen-Peters S, et al. NUP98/NSD1 characterizes a novel poor prognostic group in acute myeloid leukemia with a distinct HOX gene expression pattern. Blood. 2011;118(13):3645–56.
32. Ostronoff F, Othus M, Gerbing RB, et al. NUP98/NSD1 and FLT3/ITD coexpression is more prevalent in younger AML patients and leads to induction failure: a COG and SWOG report. Blood. 2014;124(15):2400–7.
33. Gruber TA, Larson Gedman A, Zhang J, et al. An Inv(16)(p13.3q24.3)-encoded CBFA2T3-GLIS2 fusion protein defines an aggressive subtype of pediatric acute megakaryoblastic leukemia. Cancer Cell. 2012;22(5):683–97.
34. Masetti R, Pigazzi M, Togni M, et al. CBFA2T3-GLIS2 fusion transcript is a novel common feature in pediatric, cytogenetically normal AML, not restricted to FAB M7 subtype. Blood. 2013;121(17):3469–72.
35. Meshinchi S, Alonzo TA, Stirewalt DL, et al. Clinical implications of FLT3 mutations in pediatric AML. Blood. 2006;108(12):3654–61.
36. Cancer Genome Atlas Research N. Genomic and epigenomic landscapes of adult de novo acute myeloid leukemia. N Engl J Med. 2013;368(22):2059–74.
37. Ho PA, Kutny MA, Alonzo TA, et al. Leukemic mutations in the methylation-associated genes DNMT3A and IDH2 are rare events in pediatric AML: a report from the Children's Oncology Group. Pediatr Blood Cancer. 2011;57(2):204–9.
38. Kelly LM, Gilliland DG. Genetics of myeloid leukemias. Annu Rev Genomics Hum Genet. 2002;3:179–98.
39. Jaiswal S, Fontanillas P, Flannick J, et al. Age-related clonal hematopoiesis associated with adverse outcomes. N Engl J Med. 2014;371(26):2488–98.
40. Xie M, Lu C, Wang J, et al. Age-related mutations associated with clonal hematopoietic expansion and malignancies. Nat Med. 2014;20(12):1472–8.
41. Genovese G, Kähler AK, Handsaker RE, et al. Clonal hematopoiesis and blood-cancer risk inferred from blood DNA sequence. N Engl J Med. 2014;371(26):2477–87.
42. Jan M, Ebert BL, Jaiswal S. Clonal hematopoiesis. Semin Hematol. 2017;54(1):43–50.
43. Steensma DP, Bejar R, Jaiswal S, et al. Clonal hematopoiesis of indeterminate potential and its distinction from myelodysplastic syndromes. Blood. 2015;126(1):9–16.

44. Kwok B, Hall JM, Witte JS, et al. MDS-associated somatic mutations and clonal hematopoiesis are common in idiopathic cytopenias of undetermined significance. Blood. 2015;126(21):2355–61.
45. Shlush LI, Zandi S, Mitchell A, et al. Identification of pre-leukaemic haematopoietic stem cells in acute leukaemia. Nature. 2014;506(7488):328–33.
46. Wong TN, Ramsingh G, Young AL, et al. Role of TP53 mutations in the origin and evolution of therapy-related acute myeloid leukaemia. Nature. 2015;518(7540):552–5.
47. van der Velden VH, van der Sluijs-Geling A, Gibson BE, et al. Clinical significance of flowcytometric minimal residual disease detection in pediatric acute myeloid leukemia patients treated according to the DCOG ANLL97/MRC AML12 protocol. Leukemia. 2010;24(9):1599–606.
48. Amadori S, Venditti A, Del Poeta G, et al. Minimally differentiated acute myeloid leukemia (AML-M0): a distinct clinico-biologic entity with poor prognosis. Ann Hematol. 1996;72(4):208–15.
49. Kita K, Nakase K, Miwa H, et al. Phenotypical characteristics of acute myelocytic leukemia associated with the t(8;21)(q22;q22) chromosomal abnormality: frequent expression of immature B-cell antigen CD19 together with stem cell antigen CD34. Blood. 1992;80(2):470–7.
50. Barnard DR, Alonzo TA, Gerbing RB, Lange B, Woods WG. Group Cs. Comparison of childhood myelodysplastic syndrome, AML FAB M6 or M7, CCG 2891: report from the Children's Oncology Group. Pediatr Blood Cancer. 2007;49(1):17–22.
51. Eidenschink Brodersen L, Alonzo TA, Menssen AJ, et al. A recurrent immunophenotype at diagnosis independently identifies high-risk pediatric acute myeloid leukemia: a report from Children's Oncology Group. Leukemia. 2016;30(10):2077–80.
52. Wheatley K, Burnett AK, Goldstone AH, et al. A simple, robust, validated and highly predictive index for the determination of risk-directed therapy in acute myeloid leukaemia derived from the MRC AML 10 trial. United Kingdom Medical Research Council's Adult and Childhood Leukaemia Working Parties. Br J Haematol. 1999;107(1):69–79.
53. Rubnitz JE. Current management of childhood acute myeloid leukemia. Paediatr Drugs. 2017;19(1):1–10.
54. Hann IM, Stevens RF, Goldstone AH, et al. Randomized comparison of DAT versus ADE as induction chemotherapy in children and younger adults with acute myeloid leukemia. Results of the Medical Research Council's 10th AML trial (MRC AML10). Adult and childhood Leukaemia Working Parties of the Medical Research Council. Blood. 1997;89(7):2311–8.
55. Gibson BE, Webb DK, Howman AJ, et al. Results of a randomized trial in children with acute myeloid Leukaemia: medical research council AML12 trial. Br J Haematol. 2011;155(3):366–76.
56. Inaba H, Coustan-Smith E, Cao X, et al. Comparative analysis of different approaches to measure treatment response in acute myeloid leukemia. J Clin Oncol. 2012;30(29):3625–32.
57. Lange BJ, Kobrinsky N, Barnard DR, et al. Distinctive demography, biology, and outcome of acute myeloid leukemia and myelodysplastic syndrome in children with Down syndrome: Children's Cancer Group Studies 2861 and 2891. Blood. 1998;91(2):608–15.
58. Rubnitz JE, Inaba H, Dahl G, et al. Minimal residual disease-directed therapy for childhood acute myeloid leukaemia: results of the AML02 multicentre trial. Lancet Oncol. 2010;11(6):543–52.
59. Ivey A, Hills RK, Simpson MA, et al. Assessment of minimal residual disease in standard-risk AML. N Engl J Med. 2016;374(5):422–33.
60. Langebrake C, Brinkmann I, Teigler-Schlegel A, et al. Immunophenotypic differences between diagnosis and relapse in childhood AML: implications for MRD monitoring. Cytometry Part B: Clin Cytometry. 2005;63(1):1–9.
61. Horan JT, Alonzo TA, Lyman GH, et al. Impact of disease risk on efficacy of matched related bone marrow transplantation for pediatric acute myeloid leukemia: the Children's Oncology Group. J Clin Oncol. 2008;26(35):5797–801.
62. Niewerth D, Creutzig U, Bierings MB, Kaspers GJ. A review on allogeneic stem cell transplantation for newly diagnosed pediatric acute myeloid leukemia. Blood. 2010;116(13):2205–14.
63. Creutzig U, Zimmermann M, Bourquin JP, et al. Randomized trial comparing liposomal daunorubicin with idarubicin as induction for pediatric acute myeloid leukemia: results from Study AML-BFM 2004. Blood. 2013;122(1):37–43.
64. Abrahamsson J, Forestier E, Heldrup J, et al. Response-guided induction therapy in pediatric acute myeloid leukemia with excellent remission rate. J Clin Oncol. 2011;29(3):310–5.
65. Tsukimoto I, Tawa A, Horibe K, et al. Risk-stratified therapy and the intensive use of cytarabine improves the outcome in childhood acute myeloid leukemia: the AML99 trial from the Japanese childhood AML Cooperative Study Group. J Clin Oncol. 2009;27(24):4007–13.
66. Klusmann JH, Reinhardt D, Zimmermann M, et al. The role of matched sibling donor allogeneic stem cell transplantation in pediatric high-risk acute myeloid leukemia: results from the AML-BFM 98 study. Haematologica. 2012;97(1):21–9.
67. Kelly MJ, Horan JT, Alonzo TA, et al. Comparable survival for pediatric acute myeloid leukemia with poor-risk cytogenetics following chemotherapy, matched related donor, or unrelated donor transplantation. Pediatr Blood Cancer. 2014;61(2):269–75.
68. Stevens RF, Hann IM, Wheatley K, Gray RG. Marked improvements in outcome with chemotherapy alone in paediatric acute myeloid leukemia: results of the United Kingdom Medical Research Council's 10th AML trial. MRC Childhood Leukaemia Working Party. Br J Haematol. 1998;101(1):130–40.
69. Wells RJ, Woods WG, Buckley JD, et al. Treatment of newly diagnosed children and adolescents with acute myeloid leukemia: a Childrens Cancer Group study. J Clin Oncol. 1994;12(11):2367–77.
70. Perel Y, Auvrignon A, Leblanc T, et al. Treatment of childhood acute myeloblastic leukemia: dose intensification improves outcome and maintenance therapy is of no benefit--multicenter studies of the French LAME (Leucemie Aigue Myeloblastique Enfant) Cooperative Group. Leukemia. 2005;19(12):2082–9.
71. Fenaux P, Chastang C, Chevret S, et al. A randomized comparison of all transretinoic acid (ATRA) followed by chemotherapy and ATRA plus chemotherapy and the role of maintenance therapy in newly diagnosed acute promyelocytic leukemia. The European APL Group. Blood. 1999;94(4):1192–200.
72. Johnston DL, Alonzo TA, Gerbing RB, Lange BJ, Woods WG. The presence of central nervous system disease at diagnosis in pediatric acute myeloid leukemia does not affect survival: a Children's Oncology Group Study. Pediatr Blood Cancer. 2010;55(3):414–20.
73. Abbott BL, Rubnitz JE, Tong X, et al. Clinical significance of central nervous system involvement at diagnosis of pediatric acute myeloid leukemia: a single institution's experience. Leukemia. 2003;17(11):2090–6.
74. Johnston DL, Alonzo TA, Gerbing RB, Lange BJ, Woods WG. Superior outcome of pediatric acute myeloid leukemia patients with orbital and CNS myeloid sarcoma: a report from the Children's Oncology Group. Pediatr Blood Cancer. 2012;58(4):519–24.
75. Felice MS, Zubizarreta PA, Alfaro EM, et al. Good outcome of children with acute myeloid leukemia and t(8;21)(q22;q22), even when associated with granulocytic sarcoma: a report from a single institution in Argentina. Cancer. 2000;88(8):1939–44.
76. Reinhardt D, Creutzig U. Isolated myelosarcoma in children--update and review. Leuk Lymphoma. 2002;43(3):565–74.
77. Ghanem H, Kantarjian H, Ohanian M, Jabbour E. The role of clofarabine in acute myeloid leukemia. Leuk Lymphoma. 2013;54(4):688–98.

78. Meshinchi S, Woods WG, Stirewalt DL, et al. Prevalence and prognostic significance of Flt3 internal tandem duplication in pediatric acute myeloid leukemia. Blood. 2001;97(1):89–94.
79. Pratz KW, Levis M. How I treat FLT3-mutated AML. Blood. 2016;129(5):565–71.
80. Watt TC, Cooper T. Sorafenib as treatment for relapsed or refractory pediatric acute myelogenous leukemia. Pediatr Blood Cancer. 2012;59(4):756–7.
81. Tarlock K, Chang B, Cooper T, et al. Sorafenib treatment following hematopoietic stem cell transplant in pediatric FLT3/ITD acute myeloid leukemia. Pediatr Blood Cancer. 2015;62(6):1048–54.
82. Petersdorf SH, Kopecky KJ, Slovak M, et al. A phase 3 study of gemtuzumab ozogamicin during induction and postconsolidation therapy in younger patients with acute myeloid leukemia. Blood. 2013;121(24):4854–60.
83. Pollard JA, Loken M, Gerbing RB, et al. CD33 expression and its association with gemtuzumab ozogamicin response: results from the randomized phase III Children's Oncology Group Trial AAML0531. J Clin Oncol. 2016;34(7):747–55.
84. Fathi AT, Erba HP, Lancet JE, et al. Vadastuximab Talirine plus hypomethylating agents: a well-tolerated regimen with high remission rate in frontline older patients with acute myeloid leukemia (AML). Blood. 2016;128:591. Oral Abstract 591
85. Faulk K, Gore L, Cooper T. Overview of therapy and strategies for optimizing outcomes in de novo pediatric acute myeloid leukemia. Paediatr Drugs. 2014;16(3):213–27.
86. Rovelli A, Biondi A, Cantu Rajnoldi A, et al. Microgranular variant of acute promyelocytic leukemia in children. J Clin Oncol. 1992;10(9):1413–8.
87. Guglielmi C, Martelli MP, Diverio D, et al. Immunophenotype of adult and childhood acute promyelocytic leukaemia: correlation with morphology, type of PML gene breakpoint and clinical outcome. A cooperative Italian study on 196 cases. Br J Haematol. 1998;102(4):1035–41.
88. Visani G, Gugliotta L, Tosi P, et al. All-trans retinoic acid significantly reduces the incidence of early hemorrhagic death during induction therapy of acute promyelocytic leukemia. Eur J Haematol. 2000;64(3):139–44.
89. Fisher BT, Singh S, Huang YS, et al. Induction mortality, ATRA administration, and resource utilization in a nationally representative cohort of children with acute promyelocytic leukemia in the United States from 1999 to 2009. Pediatr Blood Cancer. 2014;61(1):68–73.
90. de Botton S, Coiteux V, Chevret S, et al. Outcome of childhood acute promyelocytic leukemia with all-trans-retinoic acid and chemotherapy. J Clin Oncol. 2004;22(8):1404–12.
91. Testi AM, Biondi A, Lo Coco F, et al. GIMEMA-AIEOPAIDA protocol for the treatment of newly diagnosed acute promyelocytic leukemia (APL) in children. Blood. 2005;106(2):447–53.
92. Ortega JJ, Madero L, Martin G, et al. Treatment with all-trans retinoic acid and anthracycline monochemotherapy for children with acute promyelocytic leukemia: a multicenter study by the PETHEMA Group. J Clin Oncol. 2005;23(30):7632–40.
93. Lo-Coco F, Avvisati G, Vignetti M, et al. Retinoic acid and arsenic trioxide for acute promyelocytic leukemia. N Engl J Med. 2013;369(2):111–21.
94. Fox E, Razzouk BI, Widemann BC, et al. Phase 1 trial and pharmacokinetic study of arsenic trioxide in children and adolescents with refractory or relapsed acute leukemia, including acute promyelocytic leukemia or lymphoma. Blood. 2008;111(2):566–73.
95. George B, Mathews V, Poonkuzhali B, Shaji RV, Srivastava A, Chandy M. Treatment of children with newly diagnosed acute promyelocytic leukemia with arsenic trioxide: a single center experience. Leukemia. 2004;18(10):1587–90.
96. Zhou J, Zhang Y, Li J, et al. Single-agent arsenic trioxide in the treatment of children with newly diagnosed acute promyelocytic leukemia. Blood. 2010;115(9):1697–702.
97. Fong CT, Brodeur GM. Down's syndrome and leukemia: epidemiology, genetics, cytogenetics and mechanisms of leukemogenesis. Cancer Genet Cytogenet. 1987;28(1):55–76.
98. Massey GV, Zipursky A, Chang MN, et al. A prospective study of the natural history of transient leukemia (TL) in neonates with Down syndrome (DS): Children's Oncology Group (COG) Study POG-9481. Blood. 2006;107(12):4606–13.
99. Roberts I, Alford K, Hall G, et al. GATA1-mutant clones are frequent and often unsuspected in babies with Down syndrome: identification of a population at risk of leukemia. Blood. 2013;122(24):3908–17.
100. Gamis AS, Alonzo TA, Gerbing RB, et al. Natural history of transient myeloproliferative disorder clinically diagnosed in Down syndrome neonates: a report from the Children's Oncology Group Study A2971. Blood. 2011;118(26):6752–9. quiz 6996
101. Klusmann JH, Creutzig U, Zimmermann M, et al. Treatment and prognostic impact of transient leukemia in neonates with Down syndrome. Blood. 2008;111(6):2991–8.
102. Gruber TA, Downing JR. The biology of pediatric acute megakaryoblastic leukemia. Blood. 2015;126(8):943–9.
103. Bhatnagar N, Nizery L, Tunstall O, Vyas P, Roberts I. Transient abnormal myelopoiesis and AML in Down syndrome: an update. Curr Hematol Malig Rep. 2016;11(5):333–41.
104. Creutzig U, Reinhardt D, Diekamp S, Dworzak M, Stary J, Zimmermann M. AML patients with Down syndrome have a high cure rate with AML-BFM therapy with reduced dose intensity. Leukemia. 2005;19(8):1355–60.
105. Sorrell AD, Alonzo TA, Hilden JM, et al. Favorable survival maintained in children who have myeloid leukemia associated with Down syndrome using reduced-dose chemotherapy on Children's Oncology Group Trial A2971: a report from the Children's Oncology Group. Cancer. 2012;118(19):4806–14.
106. Blink M, Zimmermann M, von Neuhoff C, et al. Normal karyotype is a poor prognostic factor in myeloid leukemia of Down syndrome: a retrospective, international study. Haematologica. 2014;99(2):299–307.
107. Gamis AS, Woods WG, Alonzo TA, et al. Increased age at diagnosis has a significantly negative effect on outcome in children with Down syndrome and acute myeloid leukemia: a report from the Children's Cancer Group Study 2891. J Clin Oncol. 2003;21(18):3415–22.
108. Kaspers GJ, Creutzig U. Pediatric acute myeloid leukemia: international progress and future directions. Leukemia. 2005;19(12):2025–9.
109. Webb DK. Management of relapsed acute myeloid leukaemia. Br J Haematol. 1999;106(4):851–9.
110. Rubnitz JE, Inaba H, Leung WH, et al. Definition of cure in childhood acute myeloid leukemia. Cancer. 2014;120(16):2490–6.
111. Sander A, Zimmermann M, Dworzak M, et al. Consequent and intensified relapse therapy improved survival in pediatric AML: results of relapse treatment in 379 patients of three consecutive AML-BFM trials. Leukemia. 2010;24(8):1422–8.
112. Rubnitz JE, Razzouk BI, Lensing S, Pounds S, Pui CH, Ribeiro RC. Prognostic factors and outcome of recurrence in childhood acute myeloid leukemia. Cancer. 2007;109(1):157–63.
113. Fleischhack G, Hasan C, Graf N, Mann G, Bode U. IDA-FLAG (idarubicin, fludarabine, cytarabine, G-CSF), an effective remission-induction therapy for poor-prognosis AML of childhood prior to allogeneic or autologous bone marrow transplantation: experiences of a phase II trial. Br J Haematol. 1998;102(3):647–55.
114. Wells RJ, Adams MT, Alonzo TA, et al. Mitoxantrone and cytarabine induction, high-dose cytarabine, and etoposide intensification for pediatric patients with relapsed or refractory acute myeloid leukemia: Children's Cancer Group Study 2951. J Clin Oncol. 2003;21(15):2940–7.
115. Kaspers GJ, Zimmermann M, Reinhardt D, et al. Improved outcome in pediatric relapsed acute myeloid leukemia: results of a

randomized trial on liposomal daunorubicin by the International BFM Study Group. J Clin Oncol. 2013;31(5):599–607.
116. Cooper TM, Alonzo TA, Gerbing RB, et al. AAML0523: a report from the Children's Oncology Group on the efficacy of clofarabine in combination with cytarabine in pediatric patients with recurrent acute myeloid leukemia. Cancer. 2014;120(16):2482–9.
117. Leung W, Pui CH, Coustan-Smith E, et al. Detectable minimal residual disease before hematopoietic cell transplantation is prognostic but does not preclude cure for children with very-high-risk leukemia. Blood. 2012;120(2):468–72.
118. Yanada M, Tsuzuki M, Fujita H, et al. Phase 2 study of arsenic trioxide followed by autologous hematopoietic cell transplantation for relapsed acute promyelocytic leukemia. Blood. 2013;121(16):3095–102.
119. Hitzler JK, He W, Doyle J, et al. Outcome of transplantation for acute myelogenous leukemia in children with Down syndrome. Biol Blood Marrow Transplant. 2013;19(6):893–7.
120. Sung L, Gamis A, Alonzo TA, et al. Infections and association with different intensity of chemotherapy in children with acute myeloid leukemia. Cancer. 2009;115(5):1100–8.
121. Freifeld AG, Bow EJ, Sepkowitz KA, et al. Clinical practice guideline for the use of antimicrobial agents in neutropenic patients with cancer: 2010 update by the Infectious Diseases Society of America. Clin Infect Dis. 2011;52(4):427–31.
122. Yeh TC, Liu HC, Hou JY, et al. Severe infections in children with acute leukemia undergoing intensive chemotherapy can successfully be prevented by ciprofloxacin, voriconazole, or micafungin prophylaxis. Cancer. 2014;120(8):1255–62.
123. Sung L, Aplenc R, Alonzo TA, Gerbing RB, Lehrnbecher T, Gamis AS. Effectiveness of supportive care measures to reduce infections in pediatric AML: a report from the Children's Oncology Group. Blood. 2013;121(18):3573–7.
124. Ehlers S, Herbst C, Zimmermann M, et al. Granulocyte colony-stimulating factor (G-CSF) treatment of childhood acute myeloid leukemias that overexpress the differentiation-defective G-CSF receptor isoform IV is associated with a higher incidence of relapse. J Clin Oncol. 2010;28(15):2591–7.
125. Temming P, Qureshi A, Hardt J, et al. Prevalence and predictors of anthracycline cardiotoxicity in children treated for acute myeloid leukaemia: retrospective cohort study in a single centre in the United Kingdom. Pediatr Blood Cancer. 2011;56(4):625–30.
126. Tukenova M, Guibout C, Oberlin O, et al. Role of cancer treatment in long-term overall and cardiovascular mortality after childhood cancer. J Clin Oncol. 2010;28(8):1308–15.
127. Sanchez-Medina J, Gonzalez-Ramella O, Gallegos-Castorena S. The effect of dexrazoxane for clinical and subclinical cardiotoxicity in children with acute myeloid leukemia. J Pediatr Hematol Oncol. 2010;32(4):294–7.
128. O'Brien MM, Taub JW, Chang MN, et al. Cardiomyopathy in children with Down syndrome treated for acute myeloid leukemia: a report from the Children's Oncology Group Study POG 9421. J Clin Oncol. 2008;26(3):414–20.
129. Group CsO. Long-term follow-up guidelines for survivors of childhood, adolescent, and young adult cancers. http://www.survivorshipguidelines.org/.

Diagnosis and Treatment of Adult Acute Myeloid Leukemia Other than Acute Promyelocytic Leukemia

20

Peter H. Wiernik

Introduction

Acute myeloid leukemia (AML) includes all acute leukemias characterized by cells of other than lymphoid origin. AML subgroups with special clinical features have been defined by morphologic, immunologic, cytogenetic, and molecular techniques as discussed in Chaps. 14, 15, and 16. All subtypes other than acute progranulocytic leukemia (APL) are discussed in this chapter and APL is discussed in Chap. 21.

From a patient management point of view, the most serious pathologic consequence of AML is usually pancytopenia, rather than the production of leukemic cells. Therefore, management of AML requires prophylaxis and treatment of life-threatening complications of the absence of normal blood elements as well as eradication of the neoplastic clone from which the leukemic cells are derived. Prevention and treatment of the challenges to health posed by pancytopenia are discussed in the section "Supportive Care." It will be evident from those chapters that the management of a patient with AML is complicated and must be provided by a coordinated team of healthcare professionals thoroughly versed in the clinical nuances and complications of the disease, treatment of the disease, and impact of this catastrophic illness on patient, family, and society if optimal results are to be achieved. Such care is usually available only at major institutions and it is strongly recommended that, in general, the patient with AML be referred to such an institution immediately after the diagnosis is made. Some patients may not wish to be treated with curative intent and therefore need not be referred.

P.H. Wiernik, M.D., D.hc., FASCO
Cancer Research Foundation, Chappaqua, New York, NY 10514, USA
e-mail: pwiernik@aol.com

Clinical Features of AML at Presentation

AML is diagnosed primarily in adults, although it can occur at any age. The median age at diagnosis in most large series is in the fifth or sixth decade, and the sexes have an approximately equal incidence. There is usually only a vague history of lethargy or lassitude prior to diagnosis, but approximately one-fourth of patients present with a serious infection of soft tissue or the lower respiratory tract associated on occasion with septicemia. Most patients have petechiae as evidence of intracutaneous capillary bleeding, but rarely more serious bleeding may be present initially. Bleeding gums after teeth brushing lead to the diagnosis in some cases. Lymphadenopathy is unusual in AML and splenomegaly is found in less than 25% of patients. If hepatomegaly is present it is almost always due to a cause other than AML in a de novo patient. Gingival hypertrophy (Fig. 20.1) is found in approximately half of patients with acute monocytic (FAB M5) or myelomonocytic (FAB M4) subtypes of AML. M4 and M5 patients have the highest incidence of all forms of extramedullary infiltration including leukemia cutis, and central nervous system (CNS) disease [1]. In some series granulocytic sarcoma is more common in patients with the M2 subtype of AML who demonstrate the t(8;21) cytogenetic abnormality. Perirectal lesions such as fissures or abscesses [2] may be present initially or during severe granulocytopenia at any time, especially in patients with M4 and M5 subtypes. The FAB subtypes defined by morphology and histochemistry, and the distribution of the subtypes among patients with AML, are identified in Table 20.1. More recent classifications based on cytogenetics and molecular characteristics are shown in Tables 20.2 and 20.3.

An elevated white blood cell (WBC) count is found in approximately one-third of patients with AML at diagnosis, and an equal number of patients have a normal WBC count or leukopenia. Hyperleukocytosis (WBC count >100,000 cells/μL) is uncommon, but may require special therapeutic interventions when present (see text to come). Blast forms

P.H. Wiernik et al. (eds.), *Neoplastic Diseases of the Blood*, DOI 10.1007/978-3-319-64263-5_20

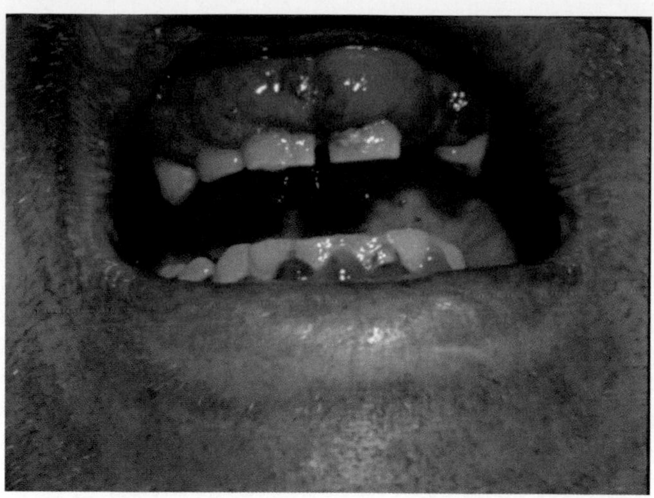

Fig. 20.1 Gingival hypertrophy in a patient with FAB M5 subtype of AML. Leukemic infiltration is the cause

Table 20.1 The French–American–British (FAB) Classification for AML

FAB type	Definition	% of adult AML patients
M0	Undifferentiated AML	5
M1	AML with minimal maturation	15
M2	AML with maturation	25
M3	Acute promyelocytic leukemia	10
M4	Acute myelomonocytic leukemia	20
M4E	Acute myelomonocytic leukemia with eosinophilia	5
M5	Acute monocytic leukemia	10
	(a) Monoblastic (b) Monocytic	
M6	Acute erythroid leukemia	5
M7	Acute megakaryocytic leukemia	5

Table 20.2 WHO Classification of AML with recurrent genetic abnormalities [3]

Karyotype abnormalities	Gene abnormalities
AML with t(8;21)(q22;q22)	RUNX1-RUNX1T1
AML with inv(16)(p13.1q(22) or t(16;16)(p13.1q22)	CBEB-MYH11
APL with t(15;17)(q22;q12)	PML-RARα
AML with t(9;11)(p22;q23)	MLLT3-KMT2A
AML with t(6;9)(p23;q34)	DEK-NUP214
AML with inv(3)(q21.3q26.2) or t(3;3)(q21.3;q26.2)	GATA2, MECOM
Acute megakaryoblastic leukemia with t(1;22)(p13.3;q13.3)	RBM15-MKL1
AML with	Mutated NPM1
AML with biallelic mutations of	CEBPA
Provisional: AML with	BCR-ABL1

Table 20.3 European LeukemiaNet Risk Stratification of AML [4, 5]

Risk groups	Included
Favorable	t(8;21); RUNX1-RUNX1T1
	Inv(16) or t(16;16); CBFB-MYH11
	Mutated NPM1 without FLT3-ITD and normal karyotype
	Biallelic mutated CEBPA and normal karyotype
Intermediate I	All cases with a normal karyotype except those in the favorable-risk group
	Wild-type NPM1 with or without FLT3-ITD
	Mutated NPM1 without FLT3-ITD
Intermediate II	t(9;11); KMT2A
	Cytogenetic abnormalities not favorable or adverse
Adverse	GATA2-MECOM (EVI1)
	T(6;9); DEK-NUP214
	T(v;11)(v;q23); KMT2A rearranged
	−5, or del 5(q); −7; abnl (17p)
	Complex karyotype without t(8;21), inv(16) or t(16;16), t(9;11) or other favorable abnormalities

are present in the peripheral blood of 85% of patients with AML before treatment. Therefore, about 15% of patients will not have a firm diagnosis made by examination of peripheral blood alone. The absolute granulocyte count is reduced in virtually all patients with AML and is less than 500 cells/ μL in approximately half of patients on the first examination. Thrombocytopenia is virtually universal and as many as one-third of patients will present with a platelet count <20,000/μL and they are candidates for immediate prophylactic platelet transfusion. Moderate anemia is the rule, but severe anemia may be found in patients with active bleeding other than petechial, or in patients in whom the diagnosis was delayed.

All patients with AML require bone marrow aspiration and biopsy. A biopsy is necessary to determine marrow cellularity. While the marrow is usually markedly hypercellular in de novo patients it may be hypocellular, especially in older patients, patients with secondary AML after treatment of another neoplasm with chemotherapy or radiotherapy, or patients who have developed AML after certain nonmalignant hematologic entities such as paroxysmal nocturnal hemoglobinuria [6]. Obviously, the marrow specimen must be obtained from a previously unirradiated site. It is important to assess marrow cellularity before and after treatment so that meaningful comparisons can be made. The pretreatment and subsequent marrow aspirates should be examined for morphology, histochemical reactions, immunophenotype, karyotype, and certain genetic mutations as discussed in this and other chapters in this section. Marrow aspirates submitted for immunological, cytogenetic, and molecular studies must be collected in heparin or acid citrate dextrose (ACD).

Leukemic blast cells account for at least one-half of marrow-nucleated elements in approximately 75% of AML patients at presentation. In elderly patients the leukemic cells may be less numerous. Usually, a diagnosis of AML is not made unless blasts account for at least 30% of the marrow white cells. Serial examinations in some patients will be necessary to determine the correct diagnosis and the rate of progression of the marrow infiltration. Rarely, the number of marrow blasts may increase slowly in some patients over several months or longer. It may be possible to withhold chemotherapy temporarily in some patients under those circumstances, especially elderly patients, as long as they are clinically well and the blood platelet and granulocyte counts are not dangerously low (<20,000/μL and <1000/μL, respectively).

The marrow aspirate may reveal other abnormalities in addition to leukemic cell infiltration. In patients with the M4 subtype relative erythroid hyperplasia is often present, despite anemia. There may be increased numbers of eosinophil precursors, especially in the M4E variant. Megakaryocytes are usually reduced in number except in secondary leukemia developing in a patient with polycythemia vera or primary thrombocytosis. Patients with the M7 subtype may have morphologically recognizable megakaryocytosis, but more often cell surface immunological or electron microscopic studies will be necessary to establish the lineage of the leukemic cells. Bone marrow necrosis may be evident prior to therapy [7], or discovered after therapy [8], especially in septic patients, and myelofibrosis may be detected in secondary leukemia or the FAB M7 subtype. Both marrow necrosis and myelofibrosis impair prognosis.

A minimal or moderate elevation in serum uric acid concentration is found in at least 50% of patients with AML. Serum lactate dehydrogenase levels may be elevated, especially in M4 or M5 subtypes, but usually to a lesser degree than in patients with acute lymphocytic leukemia (ALL). Lysozyme (muramidase) is elevated in the serum [9, 10] and urine of patients with M4 and M5 subtypes. As is the case with serum uric acid, levels of lysozyme directly reflect the body burden of tumor. Serial determinations of lysozyme may aid in evaluating response to therapy in patients with initial elevations [10].

AML is not simply a disease of the bone marrow and blood. Dysfunction of a number of organs may result directly from leukemic infiltration or indirectly from other consequences of the disease, and may dominate the clinical picture. Petechiae resulting from capillary hemorrhage secondary to thrombocytopenia are the most common skin and mucous membrane lesions. They tend to occur on dependent or traumatized areas of the body surface and may become confluent over some areas, especially in obese patients. Petechiae also occur on the surface and in the parenchyma of internal organs, but such lesions are usually clinically silent. Painless, nontender, small, raised nodules of leukemic cells may be palpable on the skin (leukemia cutis) of a small minority of patients with AML, especially those with M4 or M5 subtypes [11, 12], and approximately half of patients with leukemia cutis have an NPM1 mutation in their leukemia cells [13]. Such lesions are usually pink in color and not pruritic (Fig. 20.2). On rare occasion, leukemia cutis may be evident before bone marrow or other evidence of the disease is discovered [11], or it may be the first sign of relapse. Leukemia cutis has rarely been noted solely around central venous catheter exit sites or other injection sites [14, 15]. Leukemia cutis does not alter prognosis, but can be disturbing to the patient or even grossly disfiguring [16]. The lesions usually involve the entire corium, and the cells comprising them may have a different phenotype than the leukemic marrow cells [11]. The discordance may be due to partial differentiation of the skin lesion cells into macrophages [11].

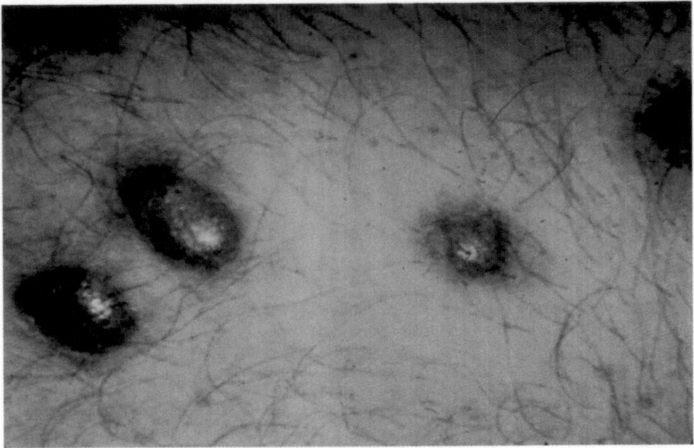

Fig. 20.2 Leukemia cutis in a patient with FAB M4 subtype of AML. The raised papules are due to leukemic infiltration of all layers of the corium

The lesions almost always respond to systemic chemotherapy rapidly, even if a complete remission is not ultimately obtained.

Rarely, a patient, especially a young patient, with AML will present with or develop a large subcutaneous or other mass of leukemic cells termed a granulocytic or myeloid sarcoma. On occasion, there is no other evidence of acute leukemia [17, 18]. Such lesions may also arise from subperiosteal areas of bone, particularly ribs, sternum, and orbit [19]. Granulocytic sarcoma of bone is rare, and other bone lesions such as radiographically seen metaphyseal lines that occur frequently in children with ALL are even rarer in adults.

Granulocytic sarcomas may occur in ovary [20], uterus [21], breast [22], cranial or spinal dura [23] (Fig. 20.3), and gastrointestinal tract [24] including liver [25], lung [26], mediastinum [27], prostate [28], and other organs and may present diagnostic difficulties in the absence of the usual manifestations of AML [17, 29]. Such lesions may present as primary tumors of the organs involved, or suggest the diagnosis of lymphoma, plasmacytoma, or eosinophilic granuloma [30]. Typical AML may be discovered simultaneously, later, or never. A Wright-stained touch preparation of the lesion may help immeasurably in establishing the correct diagnosis. Immunohistochemical studies of fixed tissue may also be helpful in addition to routine histological studies [31, 32]. When isolated granulocytic sarcomas occur without other evidence of AML, radiotherapy [33] or surgery may be indicated. Although there is some evidence that treatment of an isolated granulocytic sarcoma with systemic chemotherapy will prevent the later occurrence of typical AML [34], this is not always the case and it is best to withhold systemic therapy until frank leukemia develops unless the granulocytic sarcoma cannot be treated locally.

Granulocytic sarcomas may occur more frequently in patients with M2 AML and t(8;21) [23, 35, 36], but it is clear that they also occur in patients with other cytogenetic abnormalities [37]. Their increased frequency as paraspinal tumors with t(8;21) may be related to the co-expression of a neural cell adhesion molecule (CD56) expressed by leukemic cells with that karyotype [38].

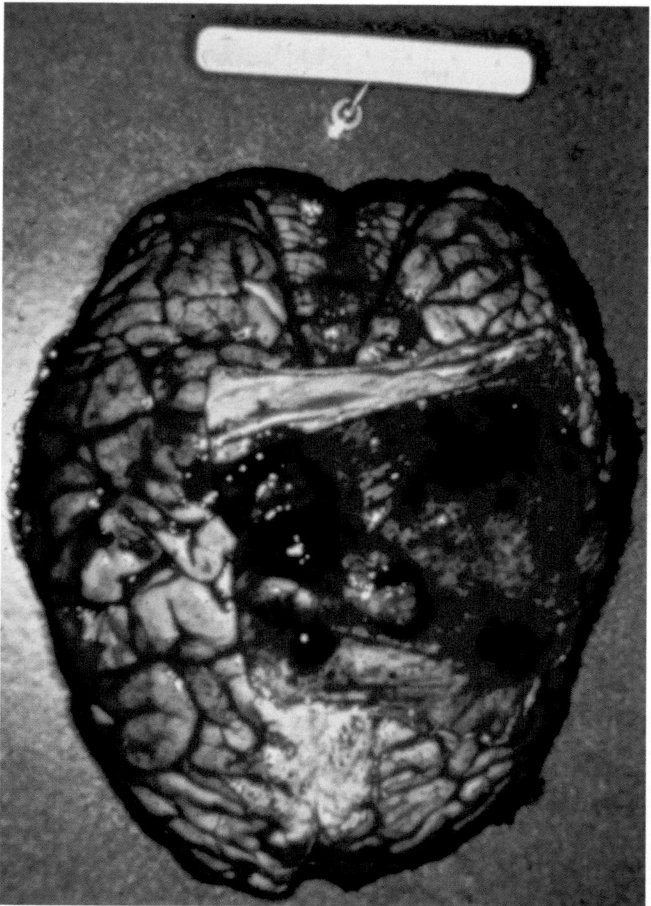

Fig. 20.3 A granulocytic sarcoma arising from the dura of the brain in a patient with FAB M2 subtype of AML with t(8;21) karyotype. The dura has been retracted to expose several dark nodules of tumor, which were *dark green*, due to myeloperoxidase contained in the cytoplasmic granules of the myeloid blast cells. The color fades when exposed to light

Acute febrile neutrophilic dermatosis (Sweet's syndrome) is a rare skin disorder that occurs in 1% of patients with AML for unknown reasons. It is more common in AML patients with FLT3 mutations [39]. The syndrome is characterized by fever, multiple painful papular and erythematous cutaneous eruptions, and a dense dermal infiltrate of mature granulocytes [40, 41]. A rapid response to glucocorticoids is usually obtained [42].

Fundic hemorrhage (Fig. 20.4) due to thrombocytopenia or leukemic infiltration of the retina may be found in patients of all ages with acute leukemia [43], including adults with AML [44].

Retinal leukemic infiltration is uncommon, is essentially confined to those patients with extreme hyperleukocytosis (blood blast count >200,000/μL), and is seen as one or more Roth-like spots with surrounding hemorrhage upon fundoscopic examination. Such lesions should be immediately irradiated if sight in the affected eye is to be preserved, but hemorrhage alone responds to successful platelet transfusion [44]. Other fundoscopic findings, such as cotton-wool spots; central vein obstruction; and vitreous, choroidal, or macular hemorrhage, are occasionally found [43, 44]. Certain treatments, such as high-dose cytarabine, may cause conjunctival and corneal pathology that results in impaired visual acuity [45]. The lesions resolve and normal visual acuity returns after discontinuation of the drug, and the problem can be prevented or attenuated with glucocorticoid ophthalmic drops administered during cytarabine treatment in most patients [46].

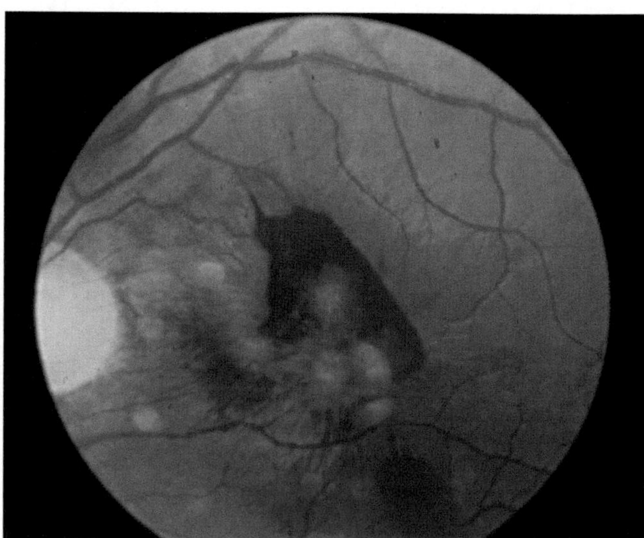

Fig. 20.4 Fundic hemorrhage in an AML patient with thrombocytopenia

Pulmonary dysfunction in patients with AML usually results from infection, which is discussed in Chaps. 53 and 54. A rare patient may develop dyspnea with or without an asthma-like syndrome due to pulmonary capillary leukostasis [47]. Such patients often have high blood blast counts [48, 49] and usually have the M3, M4, or M5 subtype of AML, but the frequency of this syndrome in patients with moderate degrees of leukocytosis may be underestimated [47]. The chest radiograph may be normal, show a ground-glass appearance suggestive of hemorrhage, or reveal diffuse alveolar consolidations [50]. This complication is frequently not recognized premortem, especially in patients with unrevealing chest radiographs [51]. Therefore, a therapeutic trial of bilateral low-dose whole-lung irradiation should be considered in an AML patient who has inexplicably developed progressively deteriorating pulmonary function [52–54]. A special form of this problem may occur after all-*trans* retinoic acid (ATRA) or arsenic trioxide therapy for acute promyelocytic leukemia and is fully discussed in Chap. 23. Severe and often fatal bilateral pulmonary hemorrhage may occur in end-stage patients who are thrombocytopenic and refractory to platelet transfusion, or in patients with a coagulopathy. This problem rarely arises during initial treatment. Although such hemorrhage has usually been ascribed to severe thrombocytopenia it may occur after successful platelet transfusion and other evidence suggests that its cause may be multifactorial. Diffuse alveolar cell damage may precede the hemorrhage, and cytoplasmic swelling and bleb formation have been noted in both capillary endothelial and alveolar lining cells in such patients [55]. While it is possible that these histologic changes represent toxic effects of extravascular blood, similar changes have resulted from cytarabine administration [56] or sepsis [57].

Heart conduction defects, murmurs, pericarditis, and congestive heart failure secondary to leukemic infiltration have been reported in AML [58–60]. Rarely, leukemic cardiac infiltration may occur in the absence of other evidence of AML [61]. These lesions are quite responsive to radiotherapy, which should be considered when leukemic infiltration of the heart cannot be ruled out [33].

It is important to have a dentist examine a patient with AML prior to therapy. Periodontal infections are common when AML is diagnosed and they may result in septicemia in a granulocytopenic patient. Dental extractions may be required [62] before initiation of chemotherapy, but often dental infections can be managed medically without interruption of leukemia treatment [63]. Other problems experienced by patients with AML in the region of the head and neck include leukemic infiltration of or hemorrhage into oropharyngeal structures that result in dysphagia or obstruction [64–66]. Leukemic infiltration of the inner, middle, and external ear has also been reported [67, 68].

As noted earlier, perirectal abscess and rectal fissure may develop in AML patients especially with the M4 or M5 FAB types. A small mucosal tear exquisitely painful on defecation or examination associated with fever may be the only indication of this potentially serious problem in a granulocytopenic patient, since infiltration and inflammation are often minimal [69]. Such lesions are usually the result of infection with gram-negative organisms, and bacteremia is frequent if proper treatment is delayed.

Necrotizing enterocolitis, or typhlitis, previously thought to occur primarily in children with acute leukemia, is described with increasing frequency in adults with AML who have been treated intensively [70]. Common symptoms include abdominal pain and distention with or without lower gastrointestinal bleeding. Abdominal radiographs may show only a nonspecific bowel gas pattern or lesions as serious as pneumatosis intestinalis, usually in the right colon. The lesions consist of mucosal ulcerations with inflammatory or leukemic infiltrates and usually involve the cecum but may also involve the ileum or the ascending colon. Bacteremia or fungemia frequently accompanies these lesions. Medical management may suffice [71], but surgery, which is usually successful when appropriate supportive care is available, may be required in some cases [72].

Renal dysfunction secondary to leukemic infiltration of the kidney or urate nephropathy is uncommon in adults with AML. Leukemic infiltration of the prostate [73] may obstruct the flow of urine and may rarely require irradiation. In most instances, however, induction chemotherapy will completely resolve the problem. Rarely, prostatic infiltration may be the first and only evidence of AML. Under no circumstances should a urinary catheter remain in place in a granulocytopenic AML patient.

Testicular relapse is common in ALL, especially in children, and has also been reported in adults with AML [74]. Postrelapse survival is frequently compromised in such patients.

Potassium wasting and other evidence of renal tubular dysfunction may occur in patients with the M4 and M5 subtypes who excrete lysozyme (muramidase), which is toxic to the proximal renal tubular epithelium [10]. The problem resolves with reduction of the tumor cell mass with chemotherapy. Lactic acidosis is a rare but difficult problem in AML [75]. Patients usually have large, vacuolated leukemic cells that may be difficult to accurately classify histologically. The etiology of the acidosis is obscure. Most patients have poorly controlled disease, and many have significant hepatic leukemic infiltration. The acidosis may require phenomenal quantities of alkali for control even after a partial remission of the leukemia is obtained.

Patients with AML may develop hypercalcemia [76], but hypocalcemia is more common. The latter may be a result of increased endogenous phosphorus production secondary to destruction of leukemic cells by either ineffective leukopoiesis, chemotherapy, or both, but septicemia and nephrotoxic antibiotics are frequently contributing factors [77]. On rare occasion, hypocalcemia and hypophosphatemia may result from accelerated bone formation stimulated by leukemic cells [78].

Patients with AML subtypes M4 and M5 often present with hypocholesterolemia, which is thought to be due to increased low-density lipoprotein catabolism by mature monocytic phagocytes. Cholesterol levels return to normal with remission, and fall again with relapse of the leukemia [79].

Rarely, an AML patient presents with a markedly elevated peripheral blood blast cell count (>200,000 blasts/μL). This is a medical emergency since such a patient has approximately a 25% chance of a fatal intracerebral hemorrhage within a day or two [80–82]. This potential catastrophe is the result of intracerebral leukostasis secondary to increased blood viscosity. The hyperviscous blood causes sludging of blast cells at the low-pressure venous end of the capillary bed, which leads to plugging and eventual rupture of the vessel. The bleeding that then occurs would go unnoticed in most organs, but not in the brain. Those patients who undergo induction therapy with hyperleukocytosis are at risk for tumor lysis syndrome, which can be fatal even if recognized early [83]. Therefore, prophylactic emergency treatment directed at rapidly lowering the blood blast count and destroying established intracerebral foci of leukemic cells must be initiated at once (see discussion to come). A more common manifestation of CNS leukemia is meningeal infiltration with leukemia cells, which may arise from petechial hemorrhage in the meninges. Less than 2% of AML patients will have CNS leukemia at diagnosis. They are usually <45 years old, have a high WBC count of at least 50,000/μL, and have M4 or M5 FAB type (1). With proper treatment CNS leukemia at presentation does not impair prognosis. However, an isolated CNS relapse carries a poorer prognosis [1].

Many patients with AML are anergic to a battery of intradermal skin tests. This finding is of little clinical significance today since modern therapy has eliminated cutaneous anergy as a poor prognostic factor in AML. Some AML patients have decreased serum concentration of IgG and increased IgM concentration of unknown significance at presentation. Immunoglobulin levels usually normalize during induction therapy. On rare occasions, a serum paraprotein is present initially, which disappears after chemotherapy [84, 85]. Most patients with AML have a normal ability to raise a secondary antibody response [86, 87].

Diagnosis of AML

A thorough evaluation of a patient suspected of having AML must be conducted in a systematic fashion. A complete history should be taken with emphasis on exposure to medications, chemicals, and radiation, and the presence or absence of other diseases associated with an increased incidence of AML, including other neoplasms. A thorough family history should be taken, since a surprising number of patients with AML have a history of hematologic disorders in the family.

A complete physical examination is essential. If the patient is febrile, a thorough search for a focus of infection (periodontal disease, hemorrhoids, sinusitis, otitis, pharyngitis, pneumonia, abscess) must be made. The presence or absence of lymphadenopathy, splenomegaly, optic fundus pathology, CNS leukemia including cranial nerve palsy, and bleeding must be established. Granulocytopenic patients should not routinely undergo digital rectal examination.

Required peripheral blood studies include hematocrit, WBC count, platelet count, and differential WBC count. The peripheral blood smear should be examined by an oncologist or hematologist with experience in hematologic malignancies. A bone marrow biopsy and aspiration should be obtained from the posterior iliac crest with a Jamshidi needle or similar instrument. If it is impossible to obtain a posterior iliac crest aspirate, an attempt to obtain one from the sternum just under the ridge of the sternal angle with an Illinois or similar needle should be made. It is important to learn to perform these procedures properly from someone with experience. The biopsy is necessary to determine marrow cellularity and to assess the extent of the leukemic infiltrate. The aspirate should be examined after thin air-dried preparations are made, preferably on cover slips. No anticoagulant should be added to the aspirate obtained for routine staining and histochemistry, since some anticoagulants cause morphologic abnormalities in the leukemic cells, such as vacuolization, which may lead to diagnostic confusion. Aspirate smears should be stained with Wright's stain and a battery of histochemical reactions as detailed in Chap. 16. Such stains facilitate differentiation among the various AML subgroups, and between AML and ALL, and are required for proper French–American–British (FAB) classification. An iron stain should also be obtained on the biopsy to assess iron stores, and on the aspirate to identify sideroblasts often found in secondary AML, especially after treatment for Hodgkin's disease or multiple myeloma, and ringed sideroblasts that may be found in erythroleukemia (FAB M6).

An aspirate anticoagulated with heparin or ACD should be sent for immunophenotypic, cytogenetic, and molecular studies. The importance of these studies in the diagnosis of AML is detailed in Chaps. 17 and 18, and may give important prognostic information as discussed below.

Certain blood chemistry studies are required for proper assessment of the patient. Serum electrolytes, uric acid, lactate dehydrogenase, creatinine, lysozyme, and blood urea nitrogen should be determined. Routine coagulation studies and a plasma fibrinogen concentration are especially important in a patient suspected of having the M3 subtype of AML. Since hypogranular variants of that subtype exist, it is important to study all patients initially. It should be remembered that some antibiotics commonly used in leukemia patients may cause abnormalities of coagulation unless vitamin K is administered prophylactically.

It is only necessary to examine the cerebrospinal fluid (CSF) routinely in asymptomatic AML patients with the M4 subtype. A lumbar puncture should only be performed in thrombocytopenic patients after a successful platelet transfusion has elevated the platelet count to 75,000/μL or more and in patients with a coagulopathy only after the plasma fibrinogen level has risen above 100 mg percent. Only 25-gauge needles should be used. The CSF obtained should be studied for routine parameters and, in addition, a cytocentrifuged specimen should be studied after staining with Wright's stain. Some training is required to accurately assess such specimens. Occasionally ependymal and other cells will be seen that may be mistaken for leukemic cells by the untrained observer. An elevated β_2-microglobulin CSF concentration may suggest occult CNS leukemia [88].

A posteroanterior and lateral chest radiograph should be obtained primarily as a baseline in an asymptomatic patient. Rarely, a mediastinal mass will be observed. This finding may confuse the observer unless one is aware of this rare manifestation of granulocytic sarcoma in AML [27].

Finally, the patient's blood should be typed and at least two packed red cell units cross matched with the patient's blood should be available at all times. If the patient has circulating lymphocytes the HLA type should be determined so that this information is available if bone marrow transplantation is contemplated in the future or if HLA-compatible platelet transfusions become necessary. At the same time, family members who agree to donate platelets, granulocytes, or bone marrow to the patient should also be HLA typed.

Preparation for Induction Therapy

It may not be necessary to begin induction chemotherapy immediately upon the diagnosis of AML. It is best to spend a day or two diagnosing the leukemic disorder precisely and resolving whatever medical emergencies are evident or developing.

Thrombocytopenic hemorrhage is more easily prevented than treated. Therefore, an AML patient with a platelet count less than 15,000–20,000/μL is a candidate for prophylactic platelet transfusion, which is discussed fully in Chap. 57. Prophylactic platelet transfusion has virtually eliminated hemorrhage as a cause of death during induction therapy. Platelet transfusion should not be given to a patient with a coagulopathy until low-dose heparin therapy is begun, or the coagulopathy may be aggravated.

An AML patient with a serious, uncontrolled infection at the time induction therapy is begun has a greatly reduced chance of remission. Therefore, documented or suspected infection should be under treatment and showing clear evidence of resolution before the institution of chemotherapy whenever possible. It is especially important not to begin chemotherapy until infection is controlled if the patient has circulating granulocytes. If absolute granulocytopenia exists in an infected patient, chemotherapy and antibacterial antibiotic therapy should be started simultaneously. Empiric broad-spectrum antibiotic therapy should be instituted immediately in a febrile granulocytopenic AML patient [89]. It should be remembered that fever may be the only clue to a serious infection in such a patient since the usual signs and symptoms of infection, which are largely due to granulocytic infiltration of infected tissues, may be absent [90]. Infection prevention and treatment for patients with AML are fully discussed in Chaps. 52 and 53, respectively.

The prophylaxis of intracerebral hemorrhage secondary to hyperleukocytosis [91] usually consists of emergency irradiation to the entire cranium with 600 cGy in a single dose and the administration of oral hydroxyurea (3 g/m^2 given daily for 2 days). The former will resolve already established intracerebral foci of leukemia, and the latter will rapidly reduce the blood blast count and thereby reduce blood viscosity, which is necessary to prevent reformation of intracapillary collections of blasts. Emergency leukapheresis has also been reported to be effective in this setting [92]. The procedure requires the availability of a blood cell separator and has not been demonstrated to be more effective than simple hydroxyurea administration. Management of hyperleukocytosis solely with hydration, urinary alkalinization, and allopurinol has been reported to be effective in infants [93] but is not recommended for adults.

Urate nephropathy is unusual in AML, except in patients with hyperleukocytosis or organomegaly due to leukemic infiltration. However, it is prudent to begin allopurinol (300 mg orally, daily for 1 or 2 days) before induction therapy and equally prudent to discontinue the drug after the marrow has become hypocellular following chemotherapy. Unnecessary prolongation of allopurinol administration may result in cutaneous eruption, which occurs with about 20% of prolonged courses of the agent or, on rare occasion, permanent marrow aplasia [94]. Patients who present with elevated serum uric acid concentration and an unusually large tumor load due to hyperleukocytosis or granulocytic sarcoma will require double or triple the usual allopurinol course initially, or treatment with recombinant urate oxidase (rasburicase) [95, 96].

Infection prevention methods should be instituted before induction therapy. The patient should be placed in strict reverse isolation in a meticulously cleaned room with air supplied only through high-efficiency particulate (HEPA) air filtration systems.

A triple-lumen Hickman catheter or similar device should be installed prior to treatment to facilitate blood drawing and intravenous therapy. If at all possible, the catheter should be placed at a time when the patient has circulating granulocytes, and use of the catheter should be restricted to personnel who have been specifically trained in the proper use and care of such devices.

Special consideration needs to be given to the pregnant patient with AML. Commonly administered induction agents other than idarubicin [97] can be given with relative safety to mother and fetus during the third and probably the second trimester [98–100] and should be given at doses based on actual body weight [101]. Children born to mothers undergoing induction therapy for AML during those trimesters have experienced only minor problems at birth and after long-term follow-up [98–102]. However, the use of lipophilic idarubicin during pregnancy may result in neutropenia and/or cardiac dysfunction in the neonate [97]. Induction therapy during the first trimester is very likely to result in abortion [99], and the diagnosis of AML itself in the first trimester may cause spontaneous pregnancy loss [101]. It may therefore be prudent to induce abortion under controlled circumstances in the first trimester. Rarely, spontaneous temporary remission of untreated AML may occur after cesarean section [22], or other event, usually a pyogenic infection [103].

Chemotherapy for AML

Chemotherapy for AML is administered in two stages: induction therapy followed by consolidation therapy. Allogeneic or autologous bone marrow transplantation may follow consolidation therapy in some circumstances, or consolidation therapy may be followed by or replaced by long-term maintenance therapy in other circumstances. The latter approach is not commonly used, although there is a rationale for it [104–106]. The purpose of induction therapy is to achieve complete clinical and hematological remission, which is defined as the absence of all clinical evidence of leukemia as well as a normocellular marrow devoid of leukemic cells and with normal trilineage hematopoiesis. Peripheral blood counts and differential WBC count are usually within the normal range in patients in complete remission, although in a minority of cases the platelet count may not recover to normal levels [107, 108]. Patients without complete platelet recovery may have impaired long-term survival compared with others [108, 109]. In patients whose AML is characterized by a specific gene mutation, quantitation of that mutation in marrow or peripheral blood cells [110] after complete hematologic remission is obtained may yield significant prognostic information with regard to the likelihood of relapse and even drive postremission therapy decisions. Such minimal residual disease testing is likely to become standard in the near future, once technical details are worked out [111–113]. The purpose of postremission therapy is to reduce the body burden of subclinical leukemia to, theoretically, zero. There is overwhelming evidence to support the concept of postremission therapy in that in virtually all studies in which outcome with and without postremission therapy has been prospectively compared, disease-free and overall survivals are greater in patients who continue treatment while in complete remission. Furthermore, most available data demonstrate a dose–response relationship for postremission therapy so that, in general, cure rates are higher with postremission dose-intense regimens than with regimens of lesser dose intensity. While there is no question that intensive postremission therapy is currently necessary in order to achieve optimal results, some studies have suggested that intensification of induction therapy may improve disease-free and overall survival despite no improvement in remission rate [114].

Although there is little evidence that the major FAB subtypes respond differently to standard induction therapy for AML, the development of ATRA therapy for the M3 subtype suggests that more subtype-specific therapy for AML may be developed in the future and that remission induction by mechanisms other than leukemia cell kill may be possible. There is already evidence that some dose-intense postremission regimens may be more beneficial in AML patients with favorable cytogenetics than in others [115].

There is no need for CNS prophylaxis in adult AML. The frequency of overt CNS leukemia is less than 1–2%, and cytarabine is virtually always used during induction therapy in intravenous doses that result in therapeutic CSF levels.

Results of induction therapy vary depending on a variety of prognostic factors. Patient age is the oldest recognized such factor. Patients over the age of 60–65 years have significantly lower complete response rates to induction therapy in most studies. Cytogenetic abnormalities are divided into favorable, intermediate, and unfavorable groups with respect to prognosis for complete response to therapy, and overall survival. The favorable group includes inv(16), t(8;21) without kit mutations, and t(15;17). A normal karyotype has an intermediate prognosis as does t(8;21) with kit mutation, and monosmy 5 or 7 (usually seen in secondary AML) as well as a complex karyotype have an unfavorable effect on prognosis [115]. See Tables 20.2 and 20.3.

More recently a number of genetic aberrations that affect prognosis in AML patients treated with currently available therapy have been identified [116]. In some instances, new treatments have been devised that partially offset the poor prognosis associated with some of these mutations. FLT3 mutation is one of the most common mutations seen in AML. The fems-like receptor tyrosine kinase (FLT3) expressed by immature hematopoietic cells is important for the normal development of hematopoietic stem cells. Activating mutations caused by either an internal tandem duplication (ITD) or multiple amino acids in the juxtamembrane region or point mutation in the activation loop of the tyrosine kinase domain (TKD) are present in approximately 30% of patients with de novo AML. FLT3-ITD mutation is the most common molecular abnormality associated with adult AML. FLT3-ITD mutation occurs in patients with all FAB and cytogenetic designations, but is most common in patients with FAB M3. Such mutations have a negative impact on disease-free and overall survival in patients with a normal karyotype but have little influence on prognosis of patients with favorable or unfavorable cytogenetics. Recently developed inhibitors of these mutations given with standard induction therapy partially neutralize the activity of FLT3 mutations in the laboratory [117, 118] and partially negate the impaired prognosis conferred by these mutations in the clinic [119–121].

A number of other molecular prognostically significant factors have recently been identified, such as NPM1, CEBPA, IDH1, IDH2, and WT1 mutations, and they have the potential for becoming therapeutic targets in the future. NMP1 is frequently mutated in AML and preclinical studies suggest that cells with the mutation may undergo apoptosis with retinoic acid or arsenic trioxide treatment [122]. In a study of 148 AML patients 60 years old or older with normal cytogenetics, Becker et al. [123] reported that 56% of the patients had NPM1 mutations and those patients had a higher complete response rate [84% vs. 48% for patients without the mutation ($p < 0.001$)] as well as significantly longer disease-free and overall survival. The prognostic impact of the mutation was observed predominantly in patients at least 70 years old. Others have reported similar results [124]. See Table 20.4.

Damm et al. [125] found that patients with normal cytogenetics and a single-nucleotide polymorphism located in the mutational hot spot of the WT1 gene had improved relapse-free and overall survival compared with others, and Dufour et al. [126] reported that patients with normal karyotype biallelic CEBPA gene mutations, compared with those with monoallelic mutations or wild-type CEBPA, had significantly better overall survival after standard therapy. Conversely, Kornblau et al. [127] reported that highly phosphorylated Foxhead transcription factor (FOXO) in leukemic cells is a significant negative prognostic factor for survival in AML, independent of karyotype. Phosphorylated FOXO levels were higher in patients with FLT3 mutations, and were associated with higher WBC counts and a higher percent of blood and marrow blast cells.

In general, approximately 65–70% of unselected patients with de novo AML will achieve complete remission after one course of induction therapy. At least 30%, and perhaps as many as 40%, of complete responders will be cured after appropriate postremission therapy. In some studies long-term results are significantly better in women [128] and in virtually all studies they are better in patients <60 years old. Results of induction therapy are likely to improve as inhibitors of diver mutations are developed.

An excellent review of the molecular biology of AML has recently appeared [129].

Table 20.4 Examples of gene alterations affecting prognosis in AML [111, 129–135]

Gene	Prognostic effect	FAB type
FLT3-ITD	Poor with intermediate karyotype	
RUNX1	Poor	43% in M0
TP53	Poor-almost always with complex karyotype	36% in M6
FOXO phosphorylated	Poor	
EVI1	Poor	
IDH1, IDH2	Conflicting data	
DNMT3A	Poor if normal karyotype	26% in M2
KIT	Poor in CBF AML	
MLL-PTD	Poor	
TET2	Poor with intermediate karyotype	
TET2 hypomethylation	Very favorable	
NPM1	Favorable in FLT3-ITD mutation negative	42% in M1 57% in M4 49% in M5a 70% in M5b
CEBPA biallelic	Favorable	
WT1	Favorable if other than normal karyotype Unfavorable with normal karyotype	

PTD partial tandem duplication, *CBF* core-binding factor

Induction Therapy

The standard induction regimen for adults with AML for decades has been the two-drug combination of daunorubicin and cytarabine, and complete response rates on the order of 65% in unselected patients have regularly been reported with that combination [136–140] in unselected patients. Patients over the age of 60 years usually have a lower response rate. In a prospective, randomized ECOG study elderly patients treated with a standard induction regimen plus GM-CSF had a higher response rate, lower rate of infection, and lower death rate [141]. However, a similar study utilizing an investigational GM-CSF derived from *Escherichia coli* showed no advantage for the growth factor [142]. The ECOG study demonstrated that GM-CSF does not stimulate leukemia when used after marrow hypoplasia occurs, since patients receiving the growth factor did not have shorter disease-free or overall survival [141].

A commonly used induction regimen is a continuous intravenous 7-day infusion of cytarabine given at the rate of 100 mg/m^2 per day, plus daunorubicin given as 3 daily bolus injections of 45 mg/m^2 each, beginning on the first day of treatment. However, recent data suggest that much larger doses of daunorubicin may be more efficacious than standard doses. Fernandez et al. [143] randomly allocated 657 patients with previously untreated AML aged 17–60 years to cytarabine, 100 mg/m^2/day as a continuous 7-day I.V. infusion plus daunorubicin 45 mg/m^2 daily for 3 days or daunorubicin 90 mg/m^2 on the same schedule. The results were recently reported after more than 80-month median follow-up [144]. The higher daunorubicin dose resulted in a higher complete response rate (71% vs. 59%) and improved overall survival (median 25.4 months vs. 16.6 months, respectively). Only patients aged <50 years benefited from the high-dose therapy. The median overall survival with high-dose daunorubicin was 44.7 months compared with 20.7 months for the standard-dose patients younger than age 50. Patients with favorable cytogenetics benefited the most from the high-dose regimen but those with intermediate and unfavorable cytogenetics may have done so as well, but his could not be confirmed on univariate analysis. Patients with FLT3-ITD, NPM1, IDH, or DNMT3A mutations benefited as well from high-dose daunorubicin, and the high-dose induction regimen was required for the favorable impact of the NPM1 mutation on the disease to be evident. The rates of serious adverse events were similar in the two groups, but longer follow-up of survivors will be needed before that fact can be verified. Löwenberg et al. [145] conducted a similar study in older patients. They randomized 813 newly diagnosed AML or high-risk refractory anemia patients aged 60–83 years to receive daunorubicin at one of the two doses used in the Fernandez study [143] and cytarabine, 200 mg/m^2/day in a continuous 7-day infusion. The CR rate was 64% with the 90 mg/m^2 daunorubicin dose and 54% with the 45 mg/m^2 dose. Overall survival was similar in the two groups, but patients aged 60–65 years had greater event-free (29% vs. 14%) and overall (38% vs. 23%) survival with the 90 mg/m^2 dose of daunorubicin. A Korean study using the same regimens reported a higher complete response rate, and longer event-free and overall survival with similar toxicity in 383 patients ≤60 years old [146]. These three studies are interesting, but they need to be viewed critically. In many published studies the response rates with standard-dose daunorubicin are better than those reported in at least one of these studies [143] and similar to the results obtained with the daunorubicin 90 mg/m^2 dose. Patients who receive a total of 270 mg/m^2 daunorubicin with one course of the high-dose daunorubicin will probably not be able to receive retreatment in the future with an anthracycline should the need arise. Furthermore, the long-term toxicity of the high-dose daunorubicin regimen is unknown.

Burnett et al. [147] randomized 1206 patients, mostly younger than 60 years, with previously untreated AML or high-risk myelodysplastic syndrome to receive daunorubicin, 90 or 60 mg/m^2 on days 1, 3, and 5, combined with cytarabine, 100 mg/m^2/day as a 10-day continuous infusion. All patients received a second induction course with daunorubicin, 50 mg/m^2 on days 1, 3, and 5. There was no difference in complete response rate overall or 2-year overall survival in any subgroup. However, 60-day mortality was significantly increased in the patients who received daunorubicin, 90 mg/m^2. Although there are differences in the design of this study and the Fernandez study described above [143, 144] the results of the two studies are completely at odds with each other, especially with respect to toxicity of daunorubicin, 90 mg/m^2. Other smaller studies have addressed the question of daunorubicin dosage intensification. Prebet et al. [148] concluded from a retrospective study of AML newly diagnosed patients with core-binding factor that relapse-free survival was significantly better with daunorubicin 90 mg/m^2 than with daunorubicin 60 mg/m^2 and that there was a trend ($p = 0.07$) for a superior 2-year overall survival with the former. Another small retrospective study concluded that daunorubicin 90 mg/m^2 improved overall survival compared with daunorubicin 60 mg/m^2 [149]. Pautas et al. [150] compared daunorubicin 80 mg/m^2 daily for 3 days with idarubicin 12 mg/m^2 daily for 3 days or, in another group, daily for 4 days in 468 patients with ages ranging from 50 to 70 years. All patients received cytarabine as well. Both idarubicin schedules resulted in a significantly higher complete response rate than did daunorubicin, but there was no difference in relapse rate, event-free survival, or overall survival among the treatments.

From a meta-analysis of six randomized controlled trials Gong et al. [151] found significant improvement in complete response rate, event-free survival, and overall survival with daunorubicin 90 mg/m^2 compared with lower daunorubicin doses, but no differences in disease-free survival, relapse rate, or toxicity. Another meta-analysis found that both high-dose daunorubicin (90 mg/m^2 × 3 and 50 mg/m^2 × 5 studies lumped together) and idarubicin, 12 mg/m^2 × 3, achieve 5-year survival rates of 40–50% in patients ≤60 years of age [152]; another such study in adults showed that both high-dose daunorubicin and standard-dose idarubicin were superior to standard-dose daunorubicin in achieving complete response and long-term survival [153].

Dose intensification of daunorubicin during induction is not a new idea. Greene et al. [154] studied daunorubicin as a single dose of 180 mg/m^2 in 1972. Only a 25% complete response rate was obtained in 16 previously untreated patients aged 26–73 years. Seven of the 16 patients died during induction therapy and the rest suffered unacceptable toxicity.

Taken together, these data indicate that daunorubicin, 90 mg/m^2/daily × 3, is superior induction therapy for AML patients <60 years of age, compared with 45 mg/m^2. What is not clear is whether the higher dose is better than daunorubicin 60 mg/m^2 or a standard dose of idarubicin [155].

Daunorubicin, standard dose, and cytarabine were prospectively compared in six major randomized studies with an identical regimen except for the substitution of idarubicin, standard dose, for daunorubicin [156–162]. There were no significant differences in toxicity between the two treatments in any of the studies. In three of the studies [157–159] the complete response rate was superior with idarubicin plus cytarabine and the differences were significant for patients under the age of 60 years, and disease-free and overall survivals were significantly greater in idarubicin-treated patients in three of the studies [157, 158, 161]. The idarubicin–cytarabine regimen was significantly more effective in remission induction in patients with hyperleukocytosis than the daunorubicin–cytarabine regimen in the two studies in which that question was examined [157, 158]. In an Italian study for patients over the age of 55 years no difference in response rate or duration or survival was noted between the two treatments, but a significantly greater number of complete responders achieved remission with one course of idarubicin and cytarabine than with daunorubicin and cytarabine [161] and in a Japanese study no differences in outcome were noted [162]. In the ECOG study [156] of 349 patients over the age of 55 years the complete response rates were 40%, 43%, and 43% with the daunorubicin, idarubicin, and mitoxantrone regimens, respectively, and the differences were not significant. The median disease-free survival was 5.7, 9.7, and 6.9 months, respectively, but again the differences were not significant. A recent meta-analysis reported that idarubicin in induction therapy prolonged overall survival and disease-free survival, increased the complete response rate, and reduced the relapse rate compared with daunorubicin, although toxicity was greater with the former [163]. For patients under the age of 70 years the differences in complete response rates were greater (46%, 53%, and 52%, respectively), but the differences were still not significant. These data taken together strongly suggest that idarubicin is a more effective anthracycline than daunorubicin in the treatment of adult AML, especially in younger patients, and this fact was confirmed by a meta-analysis of 1052 patients randomized to receive daunorubicin or idarubicin, both at standard dosing, with cytarabine [164]. These clinical observations are consistent with the more favorable clinical pharmacokinetics of idarubicin [165] compared with those of daunorubicin, and with the observation that the intracellular accumulation of idarubicin is decreased to a much lesser degree by P-glycoprotein than that of daunorubicin [166].

Many investigators interpret currently available data to suggest that idarubicin should replace daunorubicin in the treatment of adults with AML, and an appropriate treatment regimen is detailed in Table 20.1.

In three randomized, prospective large studies the combination of mitoxantrone and cytarabine was compared with daunorubicin and cytarabine for induction therapy in adults with AML [156, 167, 168]. The standard dose and schedule of cytarabine were employed and mitoxantrone 12 mg/m^2 given daily for 3 days was substituted for daunorubicin in one arm of each study. No significant difference in outcome with respect to complete response rate, disease-free or overall survival, or toxicity was observed in any of the studies.

The addition of etoposide to the standard daunorubicin and cytarabine regimen improved disease-free and overall survival without improving the response rate, especially in patients less than 50 years of age in one study but not in others [169, 170].

Holowiecki et al. [171] reported that the addition of cladribine to a standard daunorubicin and cytarabine induction regimen increased the complete remission rate and overall survival at 3 years compared with the two-drug regimen in 652 newly diagnosed patients with AML ≤60 years of age. The survival advantage for the three-drug regimen was noted in patients ≥50 years of age, those with hyperleukocytosis, and those with unfavorable cytogenetics. These results deserve confirmation.

Hills et al. [172] performed a meta-analysis of studies in which gemtuzumab ozogamicin 3 mg/m^2 or 6 mg/m^2 was added to standard induction therapy or not, for adults with AML, and found that the agent prolonged survival at 5 years in patients without unfavorable cytogenetics. Both doses resulted in the same outcome but the lower dose was less toxic, as found in other studies [173]. This agent is no longer available in the USA but it clearly deserves further study.

Zeidner et al. randomized 165 newly diagnosed patients aged 18–70 years with intermediate or poor cytogenetics to cytarabine, 100 mg/m^2/day, as a continuous intravenous 7-day infusion plus daunorubicin, 90 mg/m^2, or a cyclin-dependent kinase inhibitor, alvocidib (formerly known as flavopiridol), together with cytarabine and mitoxantrone (FLAM). The complete response rate with FLAM was 70% compared with 46% for high-dose daunorubicin and cytarabine [174]. Further study of alvocidib in AML is planned.

Ravandi et al. [175] studied 62 patients with previously untreated AML with a median age of 53 years with the FLT3-ITD inhibitor sorafenib, cytarabine, and idarubicin. FLT3 mutations were present in 23 patients and 10 had unfavorable cytogenetics. A complete remission was obtained by 79% and an additional 8% attained a complete remission with incomplete platelet recovery. Interestingly, a 95% complete response rate was achieved in the patients with FLT3-ITD mutations. With a median follow-up of 52 months, the median survival for all patients was 29 months. Although this was a small study, it clearly suggests that sorafenib in patients with FLT3-ITD mutations deserves further study. Other inhibitors of FLT3-ITD have yielded impressive results as well [176, 177].

High-dose cytarabine in induction therapy has been evaluated in a number of studies. In two early studies it was associated with greater toxicity than standard-dose cytarabine but there was no improvement in complete response rate or survival [178, 179] and a meta-analysis involving 5945 patients concluded that high-dose cytarabine led to a lower relapse rate than did standard-dose cytarabine but no improvement in complete response rate or overall survival [180]. In a more recent study, high-dose cytarabine produced a higher complete response rate and better overall survival especially in patients younger than 46 years and in patients up to 60 years of age with unfavorable cytogenetics or FLT3-ITD mutation [181]. In the most recent study [182] no advantage for high-dose cytarabine in induction was observed. High-dose cytarabine during induction is not recommended.

The addition of sorafenib, a tyrosine kinase inhibitor, to standard induction therapy led to significant improvement in event-free and overall survival after a median follow-up of 36 months, compared with placebo in one study of 267 evaluable patients ≤60 years [183]. Grade 3 or 4 toxicity was significantly higher in the sorafenib group, however.

Toxicity of Induction Therapy

Virtually all patients treated with the regimen recommended in Table 20.5 will develop total capital alopecia, which is often more disconcerting to young men than to others. Attempts to prevent alopecia with scalp tourniquets or hypothermia caps are ill advised during leukemia treatment since the scalp may become a pharmacologic sanctuary when such methods are employed.

Moderately severe nausea and vomiting accompanies induction therapy in approximately 80% of patients not premedicated with antiemetics. Older patients tend to have a lower incidence of emesis, perhaps due to poorer blood supply to the chemoreceptor trigger zone of the brain. Modern antiemetics, such as ondansetron [185] and granisetron [186], usually completely eliminate vomiting during induction therapy. It is not necessary to include dexamethasone in the antiemetic regimen, and it may indeed be unwise to do so since glucocorticoids inhibit anthracycline reductase activity, which may result in decreased anthracycline effectiveness.

Table 20.5 A standard remission induction regimen for adult AML

A.	Idarubicin (12 mg/m^2) is given daily on each of the first 3 days of treatment. The drug is given as an injection over 10–15 min into a central venous catheter. Severe paravenous tissue damage may result from extravasation. Consider daunorubicin 60 mg/m^2 on the same schedule as an alternative anthracycline for patients <60 years old. Consider oral hydroxyurea [184] or leukapheresis for patients with a WBC > 50,000/μL prior to initiation of induction therapy
B.	Cytosine arabinoside is given as a continuous 7-day intravenous infusion at the rate of 100 mg/m^2 per day beginning on the first day of idarubicin administration. The infusion must be controlled by an electronic device to ensure the proper rate of administration
C.	Consider adding a FLT3-ITD inhibitor for patients with that mutation and intermediate cytogenetics

Stomatitis, esophagitis, and diarrhea are usually only of grade 1–2 intensity and can be expected in approximately 65%, 15%, and 80% of patients, respectively [158]. Oral mucosal ulceration is usually well managed with viscous xylocaine or a paste of gelatin, pectin, and carboxymethyl cellulose. Hepatic toxicity manifested by serum liver enzyme elevations occurs in half of patients and is usually unaccompanied by clinically significant hepatic dysfunction and virtually always resolves with the completion of induction therapy.

A generalized mild-to-moderate erythroderma may result from cytarabine or idarubicin treatment, and a unique cutaneous eruption has been reported after etoposide administration [187].

Profound bone marrow hypoplasia and pancytopenia are expected and desirable after induction therapy since, except in patients with the M3 subtype, complete remission is virtually never achieved without these results of therapy. Pancytopenic patients will require platelet transfusion and, very likely, packed red cell transfusion until the bone marrow recovers, usually in 3–4 weeks after the end of treatment. Transfusion support is discussed in Chaps. 56 and 57.

Response to Induction Therapy

Approximately 90% of patients who achieve complete remission will do so within the month after completion of the first induction course. Another 10% of patients who ultimately obtain a complete remission will require a second induction course to do so. The second course should be given in the same doses and schedule as the first. Patients who fail induction therapy with two courses of idarubicin and cytarabine may be candidates for regimens employing mitoxantrone [188], carboplatin [189], 2-chlorodeoxyadenosine [136], fludarabine [137], high-dose cytarabine [138], gemtuzumab ozogamicin [190], an investigational agent, or bone marrow transplantation, all of which are discussed next. Unfortunately, patients who fail initial therapy are not likely to subsequently do well, and at the present time it is difficult to recommend a standard approach to such patients [194]. Clinical trials should always be made available to patients who fail standard induction therapy.

Often the first sign of complete remission after induction therapy is a spontaneous rise in the platelet count. If the marrow aspirate demonstrates repopulation with normal elements at that time, and leukemic cells are rare, blood counts should be observed until they are normal. At that time another marrow aspirate should be examined to diagnose complete remission or persistent leukemia. No additional induction therapy is necessary if the former pertains, whereas the second induction course should be administered if less than complete marrow remission has been achieved. If residual leukemia without any evidence of maturation in the granulocyte series appears to be present in the first postinduction marrow aspirate, another aspirate should be examined several days later, before reinstituting induction therapy. This is necessary because a marrow recovering from anthracycline drug administration may appear hypocellular and frankly leukemic, but normalize without further therapy. Indeed, an occasional blast may even be found in the blood after anthracycline therapy in a patient who subsequently manifests complete remission without further therapy. In such patients the platelet count may begin to rise, followed within a week by a rise in the granulocyte count. Progressive improvement in both to normal levels as indicated by daily blood counts is usually a harbinger of complete remission. A transient platelet count elevation, often without a concomitant rise in granulocyte count, usually indicates an incomplete response to induction therapy. This must be confirmed by bone marrow examination when the progressive platelet count improvement levels off or reverses. Almost always the marrow examination will confirm an incomplete response in that situation. However, rarely the marrow examination may lead to confusion due to the presence of a megaloblastic maturation arrest in the granulocyte and erythroid series and no evidence of leukemia. In such cases the patient may be folate depleted, especially if significant mucous membrane toxicity occurred during treatment. Such patients may have a dramatic response to daily physiologic doses of parenteral folate, with morphologically normal marrow and normal blood counts evident 10–14 days after initiation of folate therapy. In other cases, all criteria for the diagnosis of complete remission may be present except for the continuation of significant thrombocytopenia and a continuing need for platelet transfusion despite an adequate number of megakaryocytes in the marrow. Most such patients will respond with a normal platelet count to daily, oral low-dose cyclosporin A administration (100–200 mg per day) for unknown reasons [195]. In such patients, cyclosporin A may need to be continued indefinitely. Such patients are designated CRp in many studies [107, 108] and may have impaired long-term prognosis [109]. These guidelines for reassessing the marrow after induction therapy will reduce the number of patients who receive a second induction course needlessly. The common practice of reassessing the marrow at day 14 makes no sense at all [196–198] and has led to overtreatment of many patients.

Many prognostic factors influence induction therapy results. There is an inverse relationship between time to achieve complete remission after one course of chemotherapy, and disease-free and overall survival in patients with AML [199]. The patient's age has the most consistent influence on results. Elderly patients, especially those older than 70 years, are less likely to withstand the severity of treatment [200, 201]. It is not entirely clear why this is so, but other coincidental medical problems such as cardiopulmonary disease common in the elderly may make them less likely to sustain treatment without intolerable toxicity. Poor marrow reserve usually found in the aged may delay or disallow bone marrow recovery after treatment and facilitate infectious complications. In addition, poor-prognosis karyotypes are more frequent in the elderly, whereas good-prognosis karyotypes are more frequent in young adults [200]. For these reasons and others, some have advocated less intensive therapy for elderly patients [202]. Others disagree [203]. Clearly, elderly patients require the maximum in supportive care if intensive treatment is to be given. When intensive treatment is given in a setting of maximum supportive care it is likely to be successful in elderly patients and is likely to yield more benefit than less aggressive therapy without additional significant toxicity [203–205]. In the near future, peripheral blood testing for the absence of minimal residual disease by quantitating the level of molecular mutations that remain after therapy may become the accepted method of documenting response to therapy [198].

Although in many studies remission duration in the elderly treated with standard induction regimens has been poor [200], remission duration and survival have been prolonged in others [205]. Elevated blood urea nitrogen concentration, poor performance status, high peripheral blood blast count, and hepatomegaly have been reported to be particularly poor prognostic factors for survival in the elderly with AML [206]. The treatment of elderly patients is more fully discussed below.

Patients with secondary AML, discussed in Chap. 24, and AML developing after a preleukemic phase or myelodysplastic syndrome [207] have a poorer response rate, response duration, and survival than do patients with de novo AML.

The bone marrow and blood become normal morphologically and the quantities of various cellular elements normalize absolutely and relative to each other in the majority of patients when complete remission is achieved. Some complete responders, however, manifest myelodysplastic changes permanently after stem cell damage from chemotherapy but produce normal blood cells in normal numbers [208, 209]. Remission is usually explained by the premise that chemotherapy kills most of the abnormal cells and allows residual normal stem cells to repopulate the marrow and function normally. However, some evidence suggests that remission may result from maturation and differentiation of leukemia cells induced by standard chemotherapy [210–212]. Rarely, patients in remission are noted to have Auer rods in otherwise normal granulocytes [212, 213] and some patients have been noted to degranulate mature granulocytes before other evidence of relapse is apparent. In addition, the normal leukocytes of some patients in remission express reverse transcriptase activity characteristic of leukemic cells and uncharacteristic of normal leukocytes [214]. These observations, together with the fact that a large number of agents, including many chemotherapeutic agents, are known to cause differentiation and maturation of leukemic cells in vitro [215, 216], suggest that remission does not necessarily derive from the cytotoxicity of induction therapy alone.

Postremission Therapy

It is universally agreed that postremission therapy prolongs complete remission and enhances the cure rate in AML. From the mid-1960s until recently, myriad maintenance regimens were tested. These regimens were usually given for a finite period each month, were usually less intensive than induction regimens, and usually consisted of multiple drugs most of which were not given during the induction phase of treatment. These treatments may have had a minimal favorable effect on remission duration [217], but were largely unsuccessful. The value of such treatments became even more doubtful when it was demonstrated that the frequency of their administration had no effect on remission duration [136]. Furthermore, some studies during that period suggested that remission duration was not adversely affected by omitting maintenance therapy altogether [218, 219]. Confusion was further compounded by the fact that most studies initiated after 1979 gave better remission duration results than previous studies irrespective of postremission therapy schemes. Most of those studies have employed an intensive induction regimen with an anthracycline and cytosine arabinoside in a schedule and doses similar to the treatment in Table 20.5. Not only have those studies resulted in superior response rates and durations compared with previous ones, but also the number of disease-free long-term survivors resulting from them was significantly greater [136, 138]. These observations suggest that the efficacy of induction chemotherapy is one important determinant of remission duration. This concept is further supported by several idarubicin studies [157, 159]. Such has also proved to be the case in other highly treatable hematologic neoplasms such as advanced Hodgkin's disease. Some biochemical substantiation of that contention has been offered by Rustum and Preisler [220], who found that patients with the longest remission durations were those whose pretreatment leukemic cells best activated cytosine arabinoside to cytosine arabinoside triphosphate and retained the activated compound longest intracellularly.

It has been suggested that postremission schemes as described previously are ineffective not because the concept of postremission therapy is wrong, but because the treatments were less intensive than necessary for optimal results. Therefore, a number of studies employing postremission schemes for a finite period that were at least as intensive as induction therapy were instituted [138, 221–226]. The results of such studies have been very impressive. Median durations of complete remission on the order of 18–24 months have been obtained and 20–45% or more of complete responders so treated have remained disease free for at least 15 years [227] after achieving complete remission. The intensive postremission programs, in general, produce results superior to those obtained with previously employed lower dose postremission therapy.

Four types of successful postremission therapy have emerged from studies conducted over the last 25 years. Consolidation therapy, which is usually given as one or more courses of high-dose cytarabine with or without other agents, has become a standard form of treatment [221, 222, 224, 228]. Such programs appear to be most effective when the dose of cytarabine is 1–3 g/m^2 given every 12 h, and doses of 3 g/m^2 are commonly employed on that schedule in patients under 60 years of age [164] while doses of 1.0–1.5 g/m^2 are used for elderly patients [156]. However, the optimal dose between 400 mg/m^2 and 3 g/m^2 on such schedules remains to be determined. This is important, since cytarabine toxicity escalates steeply above doses of 500 mg/m^2 given twice daily [229]. Treatment with a high-dose consolidation program is outlined as option I in Table 20.6. Other more complicated regimens have been studied [223, 230], but results are similar or inferior to those obtained with the regimen in that table.

High-dose cytarabine-based consolidation programs that employ cytarabine doses of 3 g/m^2 are toxic and associated with a death rate during remission of approximately 10%. Patients with hepatic or renal dysfunction and older patients tolerate this treatment especially poorly. Older patients are especially prone to severe neurotoxicity from this treatment [222, 266]. Whether cytarabine 3 g/m^2 in multiple doses is more effective than lower doses, such as 1 g/m^2, as consolidation therapy is the subject of much debate [267]. Others have employed lower doses of cytarabine without apparent loss of efficacy, although the lower doses have never been prospectively compared with doses of 1 g/m^2 or higher. Neither GM-CSF [141] nor G-CSF [268] has been particularly useful during the consolidation phase of treatment.

A less toxic but effective approach to postremission therapy utilizes conventional doses of cytarabine and 6-thioguanine given on an open-ended schedule until marrow hypoplasia is achieved [138] and is summarized as option II in Table 20.6. This treatment is associated with only

Table 20.6 Postremission therapy options for adult AML patients in first remission [231]

I. High-dose consolidation therapy of short duration
Example: adapted from Mayer et al. [222]
Regimen: Cytarabine, 3 g/m^2, is given as a 3-h infusion every 12 h on days 1, 3, and 5 for a total of six doses per course, beginning within 1 month of complete remission. Courses are repeated every 28–35 days, depending on marrow recovery. A total of four courses are given
Comment: This regimen resulted in a 44% projected disease-free survival at 5 years for patients 60 years of age or less [222]. Results were significantly poorer and toxicity was prohibitive in older patients. Toxicity was significant in patients over the age of 45 years. Therefore, the regimen may only be generally applicable to patients <60 years old. Serious neurotoxicity (usually cerebellar ataxia) occurred in 12% of patients and was permanent in 40% of patients who experienced it. Other serious toxicity included confluent maculopapular rash and desquamation, conjunctivitis, pulmonary fibrosis, and gastrointestinal tract ulceration. Treatment-related death occurred in 5% of patients. Most effective in patients with favorable cytogenetics
II. Intensive recurring regimen given on an open schedule for 3 years
Example: Dutcher et al. [138]
Regimen: Cytarabine, 100 mg/m^2, as an i.v. bolus and oral 6-thioguanine, 100 mg/m^2, are both given every 12 h until severe marrow hypoplasia is achieved. The treatment is given every 3 months for 3 years beginning 1 month after complete remission is established
Comment: Approximately 10 days of treatment is required to achieve marrow hypoplasia with the first several courses, but only 5–7 days of treatment is necessary after 12–18 months. Results are equal in younger and older patients up to age 75. Toxicity is virtually limited to the bone marrow, and only 1% drug-related deaths during remission have been noted in recent years. An observed 20% disease-free survival at 15 years has been reported [227]
III. Allogeneic myeloablative stem cell transplantation
Examples: Young et al. [232], Clift et al. [233], Bortin et al. [234], Zittoun et al. [235], Cassileth et al. [236], Sakamaki et al. [237]
Regimens: The patient's marrow is ablated with high doses of chemotherapy (usually alkylating agents) with or without total-body irradiation. In some studies ablation with irradiation + alkylating agent resulted in superior relapse rate, disease-free survival, and overall survival compared with alkylating agent ablation only [238]. Marrow or peripheral blood stem cells from an HLA-identical sibling or other source are used in this procedure. Long-term results have been reported to be best in patients without ABCG2 overexpression with intermediate- or poor-risk cytogenetics and age ≤50 years [239, 240]. Long-term results are poor (67% relapse rate) in patients with molecular evidence of minimal residual disease despite morphologic remission at the time of transplant [241]. There is considerable disagreement in the literature as to which AML patients in remission should undergo this procedure [242–248]. Haploidentical donors and matched unrelated donors may give similar results [249, 250]
Comment: The probability of disease-free survival at 5 years has been estimated to be 45–60%, and treatment-related mortality in remission has been reported to be 25–40% in various studies. Results vary inversely with age, and patients over the age of 45 years do less well. For logistical and other reasons, some patients for which this therapy is planned may never receive it [251]
IV. Allogeneic reduced-intensity stem cell transplantation
Examples: McClune et al. [252], Hemmati et al. [253], Ringdén et al. [254], Pagel et al. [255]
Regimens: Less intensive chemotherapy, usually without radiation
Comment: Performed with related or unrelated donors with similar results. Less nonrelapse mortality than with myeloablative conditioning and similar disease-free survival. Three-year overall survival rates of 45% are reported [256]. This procedure is often recommended for elderly patients [257] and other poor-risk patients [240]. There are no studies comparing reduced-intensity stem cell transplantation with chemotherapy alone
V. Cord blood allogeneic stem cell transplantation
Examples: Sanz et al. [258],Verneris et al. [259], Ballen and Lazarus [260, 261]
Regimens: Cyclophosphamide plus TBI ± fludarabine, as an example
Comment: Leukemia-free survival of 40–50% at 2 years has been reported, but nonrelapse mortality has been high and as many as 1/3 of survivors have extensive chronic GVHD. Marrow recovery in the recipient may be delayed.
VI. Autologous bone marrow transplantation
Examples: Gorin et al. [262], Körbling et al. [263], Zittoun et al. [235], Cassileth et al. [236], Czerw et al [264], Mannis et al [265]
Regimens: Preparation of the patient is similar to that for allogeneic transplantation. Marrow must be harvested from the patient after complete remission is achieved and before high-dose postremission chemotherapy
Comment: Long-term disease-free survival comparable to that obtained with allogeneic marrow transplantation has been reported by various authors. Autologous transplantation is much safer than allogeneic transplantation, with only 3–5% treatment-related deaths during remission observed with the former. Autologous marrow transplantation may, therefore, be preferable for older patients. The relative merits of both major types of marrow transplantation and other high-dose cytarabine-based postremission options have been prospectively evaluated by several large cooperative group studies. Most such studies show no difference in overall survival rates. Whatever advantage in DFS is provided by stem cell transplantation is usually offset by toxic deaths

a 1% death in remission rate and can safely be given to patients up to the age of 75 years. Long-term results are excellent, but this approach has never been prospectively compared with a high-dose cytarabine-based regimen.

Allogeneic bone marrow transplantation after marrow-ablative therapy is described as option III in Table 20.6. Best results have been reported in young patients, and most reported series are heavily weighted with such patients. Preparative regimens usually consist of alkylating agents such as busulfan and cyclophosphamide or busulfan and total body irradiation. The latter was more effective than the former with respect to relapse rate, disease-free survival, and overall survival in a prospective, randomized study of patients with AML [238]. With currently available techniques, patients under the age of 60 years, who have an HLA-compatible sibling donor whose blood lymphocytes do not react with those of the potential recipient in mixed lymphocyte culture, are considered optimal candidates for the procedure. Postremission consolidation therapy with high-dose cytarabine before allogeneic marrow transplantation for AML in first complete remission does not improve outcome compared with proceeding directly to transplantation after recovery from induction therapy [269]. Allogeneic transplants are more successful when the donor is less than 40 years old [270]. Thus, only 20% or less of patients with AML who achieve complete remission can be considered optimal candidates for allogeneic marrow transplantation using a sibling donor at this time, and some of them actually are not transplanted due to logistical and other problems [251].

Allogeneic bone marrow transplantation utilizing an HLA-matched unrelated donor has been studied in patients who do not have a sibling donor. In one study of 161 patients [271] leukemia-free survival at 5 years was 50 ± 12% for patients transplanted during first complete remission, and the relapse rate was 19% after a median posttransplant follow-up of 2.9 years. There was a direct relationship between the duration of leukemia-free survival and the dose of marrow cells infused. These results closely approach those obtained with sibling allografts and represent significant improvement in the efficacy of this procedure.

Many transplant experts think that the future of allogeneic stem cell transplantation lies with cord blood and/or reduced-intensity allogeneic transplantation [272]. Early results are encouraging, but most studies are small, and no studies in which those procedures are compared with chemotherapy alone exist to date.

Relapse after allogeneic stem cell transplantation occurs at about the same rate as in non-transplanted patients. The median time to relapse after transplantation is approximately 7 months, and less than a quarter of relapsed patients survive 1 year [273].

Autologous bone marrow transplantation, option VI in Table 20.6, has been developed more recently than allogeneic transplantation as a postremission option for AML, and in some studies [235, 236, 274], but not all [275, 276], results have been equivalent to those obtained with allogeneic transplantation. Marrow recovery seems to be more rapid after transplantation with allogeneic peripheral blood stem cells compared with marrow cells [277, 278] but there may be a higher incidence of relapse with peripheral blood stem cells [279]. Autologous bone marrow transplantation with [280, 281] and without [235, 275] ex vivo purging appears to yield similar results.

Disease-free and overall survivals for AML patients transplanted with allogeneic stem cells during first remission have been reported by innumerable investigators from around the world. The 5-year disease-free survival rate projected from actuarial analysis in most studies has ranged from 30 to 50%, and relapse rates of 15–25% have been reported. Occasionally, relapses are extramedullary [282], late [283], and possibly due to induction of leukemia in the graft [284, 285]. Most adult long-term survivors of marrow transplantation have been reasonably, if not entirely, well. In one large study, patients with no recurrence of leukemia at 2 years had an overall 82% chance of being alive in complete remission at 9 years following transplantation regardless of the type of transplant. Patients allografted, however, experienced a lower frequency of late relapse than patients autografted [286]. Females had a lower relapse rate than males, an observation also reported after chemotherapy alone [100]. In another large similar study [287] of patients who were free of AML 2 years after allogeneic transplantation, mortality remained higher than in the normal population through the ninth year post-transplantation. Recurrent leukemia was the major cause of death. Haploidentical transplants may give the same results as matched sibling donor transplants [250].

There is no doubt that both allogeneic and autologous bone marrow transplantation can cure AML. The question is the relative frequency of cure from these and other methods. In an effort to answer the question, a number of prospective studies were performed in which allogeneic or autologous bone marrow transplantation and intensive consolidation chemotherapy alone were compared [197, 221, 224, 235, 288–290, 307]. The results have been quite similar in most of these trials. Allogeneic bone marrow transplantation results in fewer leukemic relapses than consolidation chemotherapy alone, but overall survival of the two groups of patients is similar, and results with autologous transplantation are often in the middle [235] with respect to relapse rate.

The high death rate during remission after allogeneic transplantation is primarily due to acute graft-versus-host disease (GvHD). Unfortunately, treatments that reduce the incidence of acute or chronic GvHD, with the possible exception of thalidomide [291], usually lead to an increased incidence of leukemic relapse [292], since the undesired GvHD effect cannot yet be fully separated from the desired graft-versus-leukemia effect of allogeneic transplantation. Some data suggest that patients with favorable cytogenetics have longer disease-free survival after either autologous or allogeneic bone marrow transplantation than with consolidation chemotherapy alone [293, 294] and that patients with unfavorable cytogenetics fare best with allogeneic bone marrow transplantation, but these data need to be confirmed in a larger series. Chronic GVHD can be a serious problem for responders to allogeneic transplantation and its incidence has increased in recent years [295]. Recent data suggest that donor EBV+ status significantly increases the risk of chronic GVHD in the transplant recipient [296], and that low-dose interleukin-2 is highly effective in controlling steroid-refractory GVHD [297]. See Chap. 50 for information on management of the transplant patient.

Treatment of Refractory and Relapsed AML

Although significant improvement has been made in the therapy of AML and the number of potentially cured patients has increased in recent years, most patients still relapse after complete remission and ultimately die of their disease [192]. However, many relapsed patients respond to reinduction therapy with durable remissions and some of them, especially those with favorable cytogenetics such as inv(16), appear to be cured after obtaining a second complete remission. Complete responses to reinduction therapy are much more common in patients who have relapsed after an initial complete response than in patients who were refractory to initial therapy [298], and more common and more durable in patients whose first remission was longer than 1 year. Drug resistance in AML may be partially due to increased glycolysis in resistant AML cells, and this abnormality may be actionable [299].

Patients with relapsed or refractory disease are candidates for further therapy unless serious comorbidities or residual toxicity from prior therapy prevents it. Relapsed patients whose first remission was >1 year are usually retreated with the same induction regimen to which they initially responded. Others are candidates for regimens that they have not previously received followed or not by stem cell transplantation, or stem cell transplantation alone. The longer the first remission and the younger the age of the patient, the better the results with any so-called salvage therapy. Combinations of agents such as mitoxantrone and etoposide are associated with a second complete response in 25% of patients in first relapse and a median overall survival of <8 months [300–302].

A large number of studies in relapsed or refractory disease have used various doses and schedules of cytarabine with and without mitoxantrone [303]. Most yielded a complete response rate between 30% and 50%, depending on patient age and other prognostic factors. No such regimen appears to be superior to another. Although these regimens are popular in various quarters, they leave much to be desired. Relapsed or refractory patients with AML should be seriously considered for clinical trials, since to date there is no standard approach to them.

The combination of fludarabine, cytarabine, and G-CSF has been found to be quite active in poor-prognosis AML. The combination of nucleosides results in enhanced intracellular accumulation of Ara-CTP, the intracellularly active form of cytarabine, and increased DNA damage. G-CSF was thought to enhance the cytotoxicity of cytarabine by recruiting cells into the S-phase of the cell cycle and render them more sensitive to cycle-specific drugs [191, 233], but it does not appear to do this sufficiently to improve clinical results [234]. Results appear to be excellent with this regimen, with or without G-CSF, although it is quite toxic. Opportunistic infections with unusual organisms are rare but severe neurotoxicity [304–306] detracts from its appeal. Furthermore, fludarabine-based induction therapy does not overcome the negative impact of multidrug resistance proteins' overexpression [307].

The addition of gemtuzumab ozogamicin [193] to intensive reinduction therapy may improve those results and allow more patients to survive long enough to receive a stem cell transplant [308]. Recently, high-dose cytarabine, mitoxantrone, all-*trans* retinoic acid, and gemtuzumab ozogamicin was studied in 93 patients aged 18–60 years who were refractory to one cycle of standard induction therapy. The complete response rate was 51% and for patients who responded to this regimen and went on to an allogeneic stem cell transplant the 4-year survival rate was 49% [309]. These results are excellent and deserve confirmation. Others have reported similar results with a fludarabine-containing regimen [310]

Therapeutic results for patients with core-binding factor AML in first relapse are more encouraging. Such patients appear to be more sensitive to gemtuzumab ozogamicin than others, and in one study of 48 patients aged 16–76 years, patients treated with regimens including that agent had a complete second remission rate of 88% and a 5-year overall survival of 51% [311]. Unfortunately, core-binding factor AML patients account for a minority of AML patients.

New agents with major activity against relapsed or refractory AML continue to be identified and recently the specificity of new antileukemic agents has improved greatly. There is renewed interest in azacitidine, which demonstrated significant activity against de novo AML in early phase II studies [312]. Recent studies in patients who relapse after stem cell transplantation [313–316] or elderly patients are encouraging [317] as are data with a similar agent, decitabine [318, 319].

Carboplatin yields complete or partial responses in approximately 30% of relapsed or refractory AML patients [320]. No combinations including this agent have been studied in this setting, however.

Selective ablation of the leukemic clone in AML is theoretically possible with an anti-CD33—calicheamicin immunoconjugate, since CD33 is expressed by most AML cells but not by normal hematopoietic stem cells [321]. Gemtuzumab ozogamicin (GO) was such a conjugate tested clinically. A complete response was reported in 30% of 142 elderly patients with AML in first relapse with that agent [322]. However, more recent studies have been very disappointing. Martin et al. [323] reported that the addition of GO to a fludarabine, cytarabine, and idarubicin regimen failed to improve the outcome of treatment for relapsed or refractory patients. Yamaguchi et al. [324] reported that GO alone had little single-agent activity in relapsed or refractory patients, and Litzow et al. [325] reported a 12% CR rate in a phase II study of cytarabine plus GO in refractory or relapsed patients.

No patients with an initial CR of <6 months or with multiple relapses responded. Löwenberg et al. [326] reported similar results in patients ≥60 years of age in first CR. It should be mentioned that the agent has occasionally been associated with veno-occlusive disease [327]. Balaian and Ball [328] observed that CD33 upon ligation with anti-CD33 downregulates cell growth in a Syk-dependent manner, and demonstrated in vitro a correlation between GO antileukemic activity and Syk expression. Blocking Syk expression rendered AML cells unresponsive to GO, but upregulating Syk by exposing the cells to azacitidine resulted in enhanced GO activity. If these results can be confirmed it would be extremely interesting to study the sequential combination of azacitidine and GO in the clinic.

FLT3 mutations occur in approximately 30% of patients with AML and are associated with shorter disease-free and overall survival after initial or relapse therapy [329] except in patients with acute promyelocytic leukemia. These findings apply especially to younger patients [330]. Pemmaraju et al. [331] reviewed the outcome of 128 patients (22 received first salvage therapy) who received FLT3 inhibitors as part of their treatment. Median overall survival was 3.1 months and 4.2 months for those without and with FLT3 mutations, respectively, and all who had FLT3 mutations achieved CR. Mori et al. [332] demonstrated that inhibition of both FLT3-wt and mutant FLT3 is necessary for maximal antileukemic effect against cells that express both types of FLT3.

Metzelder et al. [333] treated 18 FLT3-ITD + relapsed patients with sorafenib and all had a hematological response. Lee et al. [334] reported a CR of several months' duration in an elderly relapsed male with extensive leukemia cutis. Ravandi et al. [335] reported CR in all 15 FLT3-mutated relapsed patients with a combination of idarubicin, high-dose cytarabine, and sorafenib.

Sunitinib is synergistic with cytarabine against FLT3-ITD + AML cell lines, but not cell lines with FLT-wt [336], and clinical responses have been recorded in mutated FLT3 patients [337], but the agent has not been fully studied in the clinic.

Midostaurin (PK412) is a multi-targeted kinase inhibitor with activity against mutant and wt FLT3 AML. In a study by Stone et al. [338] newly diagnosed patients under the age of 61 were induced with daunorubicin, cytarabine, and midostaurin and consolidated with high-dose cytarabine. A complete response was induced in 74% of FLT3-wt and 92% of mutant FLT3 patients, and 2-year overall survival rates were 62% for the latter and 59% for the former. These positive results led to a placebo-controlled international study (CALGB 10603) of 717 patients with FLT3 mutation. In that study at a median follow-up of 57 months the midostaurin arm reduced the risk of death by 23% [177].

Lestaurtinib (CEP-701), another FLT3 inhibitor in clinical trial, was studied in AML patients in first relapse, but results were disappointing [339]. AC220 is a second-generation FLT3 inhibitor with low nanomolar potency and exceptional kinase selectivity [340] and is currently in clinical trial [341].

FLT3 inhibitors provide us with an entirely new, more specific approach to AML treatment. However, in most studies to date, FLT3-ITD inhibition has been transient and resistance has been noted early. Resistance may be due to inadequate dosing, ligand interference, presence of residual dormant FLT3-ITD+ cells, all of these, or as-yet undiscovered mechanisms. It is too early to discard any of these agents or others not discussed, and all merit further study alone and in combination with chemotherapy and/or other agents such as mTOR inhibitors.

There are few data on post-second remission therapy that suggest that one treatment is superior to another. Robles et al. [342] demonstrated that low-dose cytarabine, 10 mg/m^2 given subcutaneously every 12 h until relapse, may have resulted in a second remission duration longer than that expected from no maintenance therapy. If these data can be confirmed, postremission cytarabine will be the first agent demonstrated to prolong second remission. A surprising finding in that study was the fact that 18% of patients in the control group also had second remissions longer than the first [343], which suggests that reinduction therapy was a more effective antileukemic therapy than initial induction and postremission therapy in that group. Therefore, it is essential to perform prospectively controlled post-second remission studies if new active therapies are to be identified, rather than simply to determine "inversion" rates from uncontrolled studies.

Farnesyl transferase inhibitors such as tipifarnib and lonafarnib have entered clinical trial in AML, but to date, results have been disappointing [344–346]. The combination of simvastatin and tipifarnib may be more active than tipifarnib alone against CD34+ AML cells [347], but clinical trials have not yet been done.

A regimen of fludarabine, cytarabine, and liposomal daunorubicin was successful in refractory and relapsed patients and produced a 44% and 56% complete response rate in them, respectively [348]. Remissions were relatively short, and a more recent study demonstrated little or no activity for liposomal daunorubicin in similar patients [224].

There is no doubt that bone marrow transplantation can cure some patients with relapsed and/or refractory AML [349–352]. However, it has been suggested by some that a bone marrow-preparative regimen without stem cell support may yield results equivalent to those reported after transplantation [353]. In a study by Forman et al. [349], 12 adults with AML who failed induction therapy were treated with an allogeneic transplant from a matched sibling and 75% achieved a complete remission. One-third of the complete responders relapsed and two-thirds (ages 20–29) remained in continuous complete remission for approximately 18–108 months. In a larger Seattle study [350] that included some older patients, allogeneic transplantation was tested in AML patients in untreated first relapse and the 5-year disease-free survival was projected to be 23%. Only one of ten patients with AML given an allogeneic transplant in second complete remission in another study [351] survived in long-term complete remission. Ipilimumab, an immune checkpoint blockade monoclonal antibody, may restore antitumor activity through a graft-versus-tumor effect in patients who relapse after allogeneic transplantation and by this mechanism restore response in such patients. The agent is under clinical investigation [354].

Autologous bone marrow transplantation for patients in first relapse or in second complete remission was studied by Petersen et al. [352]. In all patients, marrow was harvested and cryopreserved during first complete remission. The actuarial probabilities of relapse-free survival at 2 years for patients transplanted in first relapse (21 patients) or second remission (26 patients) were 45% and 32%, respectively. The outcome in patients who were in first relapse was comparable to that of other studies in which remission was induced prior to transplantation, which suggests that there is no clinical disadvantage in proceeding directly to transplantation upon the diagnosis of relapse. Early data from the same institution suggested that the addition of IL-2 to the management of autologous transplant patients in first relapse or later stages may improve outcome [355]. However, recent data suggest no benefit for IL-2 for patients in first remission after autologous marrow transplantation [356, 357].

Some data suggest that autologous stem cell transplantation may actually be more effective than allogeneic transplantation in relapsed or refractory patients [358].

Infusion of lymphocytes from the original marrow donor is highly effective in treating chronic myelocytic leukemia patients who relapse after allogeneic marrow transplantation, but donor lymphocyte infusions are less effective in treating posttransplant relapsed patients with AML [359–361]. The major problem with this form of treatment is the frequent induction of serious GvHD, which can be fatal [362]. However, such infusions can be successful, even for relapse after unrelated donor marrow transplantation [359]. Porter et al. [363] treated 23 patients with AML who relapsed after an unrelated donor marrow transplantation and 42% obtained a complete response with an estimated 1-year disease-free survival rate of 23%. Donor lymphocyte infusions may also be able to eradicate persistent disease after allogeneic hematopoietic cell transplantation [364].

Elderly Patients

Röllig et al. [365] devised a prognostic model for elderly patients with newly diagnosed AML in which karyotype, age, NPM1 mutation status, WBC, LDH, and CD34 expression were of independent prognostic significance for overall survival. This model may be useful in other studies and may be used to stratify patients in future prospective trials. Older patients with CEBPA double mutation, NPM1 mutation, and FLT3-wild type may have significantly better survival after intensive treatment than others [366].

There is no standard treatment for relapsed or newly diagnosed elderly patients (>70 years of age) with AML. As a general rule, the same intensity of treatment used for younger patients should be considered for elderly patients because results tend to be better than with less aggressive therapy for induction. However, elderly patients do not tolerate consolidation with cytarabine 3 g/m^2 and doses half that large are commonly used. As in younger patients, for patients whose initial remission was >1 year, the same induction therapy used initially will likely yield the best results for reinduction. It should be noted that many patients with late relapse (>5 years after CR) relapse with different cytogenetics than they originally displayed [367, 368] and have a poor likelihood of long-term survival after relapse. All elderly patients should be seriously considered for a clinical trial. Some data suggest that elderly patients are less sensitive to anthracyclines than younger patients [369] and resveratrol may be helpful in overcoming this relative resistance [370].

A common approach to induction therapy of elderly patients is low-dose cytarabine (20 mg once or twice a day) by subcutaneous injection for 10 consecutive days every 4–6 weeks. Although the complete response rate with this regimen is <10%, survival is better than with no treatment other than supportive care [371]. Results with new drugs may make this approach completely obsolete. Low-dose cytarabine was studied with volasertib, a selective inhibitor of polo-like kinases, and compared with low-dose cytarabine alone in a randomized study. The combination was given to 87 patients with a median age of 75 years and the complete response rate (31%) and event-free survival rate were double that obtained with low-dose cytarabine alone. Cytogenetics did not influence response. Volasertib added to the marrow and gastrointestinal toxicity of treatment, but did not lead to more deaths.

Clofarabine, a deoxyadenosine analog, was evaluated in elderly patients with AML with good results in previously untreated patients. A complete response was obtained by Kantarjian et al. [372] in 46% of 112 patients aged 60–88 years with a median duration of response >1 year. In a study by Burnett et al. [373] of 106 elderly patients a similar response rate was observed. In both studies the drug was reasonably well tolerated. Kadia et al. [374] studied an induction regimen of clofarabine and low-dose cytarabine alternating with decitabine in 118 patients aged 60–81 years followed by consolidation and maintenance therapy with the same drugs. The complete response rate was 60% overall and 50% in those with adverse cytogenetics. Overall median survival in the complete responders was 18.5 months. They concluded that the treatment was well tolerated and highly effective in older patients with AML. Takahashi et al. [375] compared clofarabine alone to idarubicin plus cytarabine in elderly patients and found equivalent responses and survival with the two treatments, but less toxicity with clofarabine alone. In a recent study 84 patients aged 40–75 years were treated with clofarabine and cytarabine and 67% of them went on to an allogeneic stem cell transplant that was preceded by a clofarabine-based conditioning regimen. Complete remission was achieved in 60% of patients after transplantation and the 2-year disease-free survival rate was 52%. These results are encouraging, but this was a single-arm study [376] and it is unclear whether these results are better than those that would have been obtained with other treatments. The drug needs further evaluation in combination with others.

Vosaroxin is a first-in-class quinolone derivative that acts as a topoisomerase II inhibitor and does not have the cardiac toxicity of topoisomerase II inhibitors. Its toxicity is primarily hematologic. In a phase II study of 116 previously untreated patients aged 60 years or more, several doses and schedules were studied and in the best group a 35% complete response rate was obtained, with a 1-year overall survival of 38% [377]. In another study vosaroxin was found to give results no better than low-dose cytarabine [378]. Despite other trials showing some activity for this agent [379], it seems unlikely that it will have a role in the treatment of AML.

Decitabine, alone and with other agents [381–383], is currently under evaluation for the treatment of elderly patients with AML but results are too early to fully evaluate [380, 381] or disappointing [382].

Another hypomethylating agent, azacitidine, appears to be somewhat more promising in elderly patients with AML. In one study [383] azacitidine or decitabine alone yielded essentially similar results as intensive chemotherapy in elderly patients. Another study demonstrated that hematologic improvement with azacitidine short of complete response led to improved survival [384]. In a study of 149 previously untreated patients with AML and a median age of 74, including 51 patients with de novo AML considered ineligible for intensive chemotherapy, the complete response rate with azacitidine alone was 33% and the median overall survival was 9.4 months. The 2-year overall survival was 51% in responders in this single-arm study [385]. In a study of low-dose subcutaneously administered azacitidine as maintenance therapy in elderly patients in first remission after standard induction therapy [386] the median overall survival was 20.4 months. The treatment was well tolerated and seems to have been effective. Obviously further study is needed before that impression can be confirmed.

Dombret et al. [387] performed a study of 488 elderly newly diagnosed patients randomized to receive azacitidine or several conventional treatments. Azacitidine was associated with a 3.8-month improvement in median overall survival and was well tolerated. The 1-year survival rate with azacitidine was 46.5%, compared with 34.2% for the other patients. This study provides the greatest impetus for the further study of azacitidine in elderly patients with AML. Unfortunately, to date, studies of combinations of azacitidine with intensive therapy [388] or a histone deacetylase inhibitor [389] are disappointing. On the other hand, azacitidine plus sorafenib may be effective for elderly patients with FLT3-ITD mutations [390], and in patients with FLT3-ITD and NPM1 mutation, azacitidine combined with lenalidomide may be promising postremission therapy [391]. Further studies of azacitidine in AML should take into account that low miR-29c expression by leukemic cells correlates with response to azacitidine by elderly patients [392].

In an early study of the addition of gemtuzumab ozogamicin to standard induction therapy for elderly patients the combination was found to only add toxicity without any benefit [393]. However, as a single agent gemtuzumab ozogamicin significantly improved overall survival compared with best supportive care in patients over the age of 60 years [394]. The drug remains a treatment option for elderly patients who are not candidates for more aggressive treatment if it were available.

The addition of sorafenib to standard induction therapy did not improve outcome in elderly patients, even those with FLT3-ITD mutation [395], although it does so in younger patients with that mutation [396].

A very interesting compound under investigation in elderly patients with secondary AML is CPX-351, a liposomal preparation of daunorubicin and cytarabine in a 1:5 molar ratio. In a randomized study of 309 patients aged 60–75 years comparing that agent to standard administration of daunorubicin and cytarabine in a standard schedule with standard doses, the new agent proved superior in terms of overall survival, response rate, and 60-day mortality [397]. This compound is likely to become widely used for elderly patients with AML.

At least 60% of patients with AML are 65 years of age or older. They are more likely to have an antecedent hematologic disorder, unfavorable cytogenetics, and poorer performance status at diagnosis mainly due to assorted comorbidities. Many, if not most, are judged by their physician to not be a candidate for intensive chemotherapy. Those that are treated have a significantly improved overall survival [398]. On the other hand older patients have a lower complete response rate to standard induction regimens than do younger patients and remission duration is usually shorter as well. Relapsed elderly patients rarely have useful responses to reinduction therapy although this is not always the case. Newer treatments briefly described above have not had a major impact on the results of treatment in elderly patients.

Therefore, treatment of elderly patients remains a major challenge. Hopefully, some newer agents and concepts just entering clinical trial will improve results for them. In the meantime, all elderly patients judged not eligible for standard treatment should be considered for clinical trials.

It should be noted that older patients who achieve remission after intensive or other therapy achieve significant improvements in quality of life, fatigue, and physical function as do younger patients [399].

Central Nervous System Leukemia

The diagnosis and treatment of CNS leukemia are discussed earlier in this chapter. CNS leukemia is an uncommon type of presentation or relapse in adults with AML. The incidence of CNS leukemia has decreased in AML patients since the common usage of infusional cytarabine in induction regimens due to the attainment of therapeutic levels of cytarabine in the CSF with such induction therapy. Nevertheless, about 1–2% of patients who relapse will have CNS leukemia with or without marrow evidence of relapse. These are usually young patients. Intracerebral leukemia is much less common in AML than in ALL, and virtually all adults with AML with CNS leukemia demonstrate meningeal leukemia, or cranial nerve palsy or both. Irradiation of the course of an involved cranial nerve will preserve function of that nerve if done early. Cranial nerve palsy does not respond to intrathecal chemotherapy. Patients with meningeal leukemia with cerebrospinal fluid pleocytosis usually respond to intrathecal chemotherapy, usually cytarabine, and usually do not require cranial irradiation. For reasons that are not understood, patients with AML usually have longer remissions of CNS leukemia after treatment than do patients with ALL [400].

As is the case in ALL, rapid attainment of remission of meningeal leukemia, long duration of initial marrow remission, and absence of cranial nerve palsy are favorable factors for CNS leukemia remission duration after treatment.

Mixed-Phenotype Acute Leukemia

This is an uncommon form of acute leukemia accounting for perhaps 2–3% of all pediatric and adult acute leukemias. When the leukemic blast cells display cytochemical and/or immunophenotypic features of both myeloid and lymphoid blasts the leukemia is referred to as biphenotypic and when there are two populations of cells, one clearly myeloid and the other clearly lymphoid, the leukemia is referred to as bilineal. There are few data to guide treatment for these leukemias but, in general, they are treated with ALL treatment programs and therefore will not be considered further here. For a full discussion of this "entity," see Wolach and Stone [401].

Future Directions

There is considerable interest in developing molecular tests for the diagnosis of AML [402] and for the detection of minimal residual disease in patients who have achieved complete hematologic remission [403, 404]. Determining the presence or absence of minimal residual disease will allow for informed decisions about whether or not patients require further therapy to potentially achieve cure [405].

New drugs and new techniques are under investigation for the treatment of AML and some may improve therapeutics in the future. Arsenic trioxide and all-trans retinoic acid have been found to induce apoptosis in NPM1-mutated AML cells in the laboratory [406]. Whether this induction can be demonstrated in patients remains to be seen. An old drug, pyrimethamine, was found to have significant activity against human AML in two mice xenograft models [407]. This is an oral agent that could be tested in elderly patients not fit for intensive treatment. A dendritic cell vaccine is being developed for the potential elimination of minimal residual disease and may soon come to clinical trial [408]. Vaccination with polyvalent WT1 peptides in patients with WT1+ AML in remission has been carried out at several institutions and found to be safe and possibly effective [409]. Larger clinical trials will be required to fully evaluate the effectiveness of this promising approach. Blocking MNK kinase activity in an AML xenograft model with merestinib, an orally administered multikinase inhibitor, suppresses primitive leukemic progenitors from patients with AML [410]. Preclinical studies with the agent will continue and ultimately it may come to clinical trial. Another approach under investigation involves targeting miR-126 in leukemic stem cells with antagomiR-126 nanoparticles [411]. Higher expression of miR-126, a marker for leukemic stem cells, is associated with a poor prognosis in older patients with AML and a normal karyotype treated with conventional treatment. A similar approach has been demonstrated to be feasible against FLT3-ITD+ AML [412]. Although interesting, this concept is not yet ready for clinical exploration. Another novel concept, inhibition of certain mitochondrial proteases as a leukemia therapy, is under laboratory investigation and likely to undergo clinical study in the future [413]. In an intriguing study reported in abstract only to date, Hazenberg et al. [414] reported that AML patients cured after allogeneic stem cell transplant produce tumor-specific cytotoxic antibodies that kill AML blast cells in vitro and in mouse models. Perhaps such antibodies can be used to treat other AML patients. A trial in elderly patients would be of great interest.

New prognostic markers for the disease that may serve as therapeutic targets continue to be identified. CD11b expression in a meta-analysis of 2619 patients was shown to be associated with a poorer outcome in patients with AML [415]. CTNNA1 hypermethylation, found in 25% of patients with AML, is an independent predictor for poor relapse-free survival [416].

Recent data have confirmed that smoking may influence the onset and pathogenesis of AML [417]. Hopefully these observations will be more fully explored.

Survivors of AML have an incidence of oral and pharyngeal cancer significantly higher than that of the general population for unknown reasons [418]. Is there a common viral etiology to both diseases, such as HPV?

There is a high risk of hepatitis B reactivation among patients with acute myeloid leukemia and prophylaxis with anti-HVB vaccine has been recommended [419]. It should be noted that decades ago several studies indicated that chronic viral hepatitis had a *favorable* effect on AML prognosis [420–422]. Perhaps the relationship between viral hepatitis and AML should be reexamined.

References

1. Cheng CL, Li CC, Hou HA, et al. Risk factors and clinical outcomes of acute myeloid leukemia with central nervous system involvement in adults. BMC Cancer. 2015;15:344.
2. Grewal H, Guillem JG, Quan SHQ, et al. Anorectal disease in neutropenic leukemic patients. Dis Colon Rectum. 1994;37:1095.
3. Arber DA, Orazi A, Hasserjian R, et al. The 2016 revision to the World Health Orginazation classification of myeloid neoplasms and acute leukemia. Blood. 2016;127:2391–405.
4. Döhner H, Estey EH, Amadori S, et al. Diagnosis and management of acute myeloid leukemia in adults: recommendations from an international expert panel, on behalf of the European LeukemiaNet. Blood. 2010;115:453–74.
5. Döhner H, Weisdorf DJ, Bloomfield CD. Acute myeloid leukemia. N Engl J Med. 2015;373:1136–52.
6. Harris JW, Koscick R, Lazarus HM, et al. Leukemia arising out of paroxysmal nocturnal hemoglobinuria. Leuk Lymphoma. 1999;32:401.
7. Kiraly JF III, Wheby MS. Bone marrow necrosis. Am J Med. 1976;60:361.
8. Cassileth PA, Brooks SJ. The prognostic significance of myelonecrosis after induction therapy in acute leukemia. Cancer. 1987;60:2363.
9. Resnitzky P, Shaft D. Distinct lysozyme content in different subtypes of acute myeloid leukaemic cells: An ultrastructural immunogold study. Br J Haematol. 1994;88:357.
10. Wiernik PH, Serpick AA. Clinical significance of serum and urinary muramidase activity in leukemia and other hematologic malignancies. Am J Med. 1969;46:330.
11. Kaiserling E, Horny H-P, Geerts M-L, et al. Skin involvement in myelogenous leukemia: morphologic and immunophenotypic heterogeneity of skin infiltrates. Mod Pathol. 1994;7:771.
12. Sepp N, Radaszkiewicz T, Meijer CJLM, et al. Specific skin manifestations in acute leukemia with monocytic differentiation. Cancer. 1993;71:124.
13. Luskin MR, Huen AO, Brooks SA, et al. NPM1 mutation is associated with leukemia cutis in acute myeloid leukemia with monocytic features. Haematologica. 2015;100:e412–4.
14. Baden TJ, Gammon WR. Leukemia cutis in acute myelomonocytic leukemia. Preferential localization in a recent Hickman catheter scar. Arch Dermatol. 1987;123:88.
15. Harakati MS. Cutaneous granulocytic sarcoma at the exit site of Hickman indwelling venous catheter. Int J Hematol. 1993;57:39.
16. Schiffer CA, Sanel FT, Steckmiller BK, et al. Functional and morphologic characteristics of the leukemia cells of a patient with acute monocytic leukemia: correlation with clinical features. Blood. 1975;46:17.
17. Sreejith G, Gangadharan VP, Elizabath KA, et al. Primary granulocytic sarcoma of the ovary. Am J Clin Oncol. 2000;23:239.
18. Movassaghian M, Brunner AM, Blonquist TM, et al. Presentation and outcomes among patients with isolated myeloid sarcoma: a Surveillance, Epidemiology, and End Results database analysis. Leuk Lymphoma. 2015;56:1698–703.
19. Cavdar AO, Babacan E, Gözdasoglu S, et al. High-risk subgroup of acute myelomonocytic leukemia (AMML) with orbito-ocular granulocytic sarcoma (OOGS) in Turkish children. Retrospective analysis of clinical, hematological, ultrastructural and therapeutic findings of thirty-three OOGS. Acta Haematol. 1989;81:80.
20. Lane DM, Birdwell RL. Ovarian leukemia detected by pelvic sonography. Cancer. 1986;58:2338.
21. Harris NL, Scully RE. Malignant lymphoma and granulocytic sarcoma of the uterus and vagina. Cancer. 1984;53:2530.
22. Antunez de Mayolo J, Ahn YS, Temple JD, et al. Spontaneous remission of acute leukemia after the termination of pregnancy. Cancer. 1989;63:1621.
23. Wodzinski MA, Collin R, Winfield DA, et al. Epidural granulocytic sarcoma in acute myeloid leukemia with 8;21 translocation. Cancer. 1988;62:1299.
24. Rottenberg GT, Thomas BM. Case report: granulocytic sarcoma of the small bowel—a rare presentation of leukaemia. Clin Radiol. 1994;49:501.
25. Norsworthy KJ, Bhatnagar B, Singh ZN, Gojo I. Myeloid sarcoma of the hepatobiliary system: a case series and review of the literature. Acta Haematol. 2016;135:241–51.
26. Wong KF, Chan JKC, Chan JCW, et al. Acute myeloid leukemia presenting as granulocytic sarcoma of the lung. Am J Hematol. 1993;43:77.
27. McCluggage WG, Boyd HK, Jones FG, et al. Mediastinal granulocytic sarcoma: a report of two cases. Arch Pathol Lab Med. 1998;122:545.
28. Thalhammer F, Gisslinger H, Chott A, et al. Granulocytic sarcoma of the prostate as the first manifestation of a late relapse of acute myelogenous leukemia. Acta Hematol. 1994;68:97.
29. Yilmaz AF, Saydam G, Sahin F, Baran Y. Granulocytic sarcoma: a systematic review. Am J Blood Res. 2013;3:265–70.
30. Solh M, Solmon S. Morris L, et al. Blood Rev: Extramedullary acute myelogenous leukemia. 2016;22:1403–9.
31. Hudock J, Chatten J, Miettinen M. Immunohistochemical evaluation of myeloid leukemia infiltrates (granulocytic sarcomas) in formaldehyde-fixed, paraffin-embedded tissue. Am J Clin Pathol. 1994;102:55.
32. Goldstein NS, Ritter JH, Argenyi ZB, et al. Granulocytic sarcoma. Int J Surg Pathol. 1995;2:177.
33. Yang WC, Yao M, Chen YH, Kuo SH. Complete response of myeloid sarcoma with cardiac involvement to radiotherapy. J Thorac Dis. 2016;8:1323–8.
34. Byrd JC, Edenfield J, Shields DJ, Dawson NA. Extramedullary myeloid cell tumors in acute nonlymphocytic leukemia: a clinical review. J Clin Oncol. 1995;13:1800.
35. Abe R, Umezu H, Uchida T, et al. Myeloblastoma with an 8;21 chromosome translocation in acute myeloblastic leukemia. Cancer. 1986;58:1260.
36. Tallman MS, Hakimian D, Shaw JM, et al. Granulocytic sarcoma is associated with the 8;21 translocation in acute myeloid leukemia. J Clin Oncol. 1993;11:690.
37. Heimann P, Vamos E, Ferster A, et al. Granulocytic sarcoma showing chromosomal changes other than the t(8;21). Cancer Genet Cytogenet. 1994;74:59.

38. Krishnan K, Ross CW, Adams PT, et al. Neural cell-adhesion molecule (CD 56)-positive, t(8;21) acute myeloid leukemia (AML, M-2) and granulocytic sarcoma. Ann Hematol. 1994;69:321.
39. Kazmi SM, Pemmaraju N, Patel KP, et al. Characteristics of Sweet syndrome in patients with acute myeloid leukemia. Clin Lymphoma Myeloma Leuk. 2015;15:358–63.
40. Soppi E, Nousiainen T, Seppa A, Lahtinen R. Acute febrile neutrophilic dermatosis (Sweet's syndrome) in association with myelodysplastic syndromes: a report of three cases and a review of the literature. Br J Haematol. 1989;73:43.
41. Cohen PR, Talpaz M, Kurzock R. Malignancy associated Sweet's syndrome: review of the world literature. J Clin Oncol. 1988;6:1887.
42. Cohen PR. Neutrophilic dermatoses: a review of current treatment options. Am J Clin Dermatol. 2009;10:301.
43. Schachat AP, Markowitz JA, Guyer DR, et al. Ophthalmic manifestations of leukemia. Arch Ophthalmol. 1989;107:697.
44. Karesh JW, Golgman EJ, Reck K, et al. A prospective ophthalmic evaluation of patients with acute myeloid leukemia: correlation of ocular hematologic findings. J Clin Oncol. 1989;7:1528.
45. Ritch PS, Hansen RM, Heuer DK. Ocular toxicity from high-dose cytosine arabinoside. Cancer. 1983;51:430.
46. Lass JH, Lazarus HM, Reed MD, Herzig RH. Topical corticosteroid therapy for corneal toxicity from systemically administered cytarabine. Am J Ophthalmol. 1982;94:617.
47. Soares FA, Landell GAM, Cardoso MCM. Pulmonary leukostasis without hyperleukocytosis: a clinicopathologic study of 16 cases. Am J Hematol. 1992;40:28.
48. Dombret H, Hunault M, Faucher C, et al. Acute lysis pneumopathy after chemotherapy for acute myelomonocytic leukemia with abnormal marrow eosinophils. Cancer. 1992;69:1356.
49. Wurthner JU, Kohler G, Behringer D, et al. Leukostasis followed by hemorrhage complicating the initiation of chemotherapy in patients with acute myeloid leukemia and hyperleukocytosis. Cancer. 1999;85:368.
50. van Buchem MA, Wondergem JH, Kool LJS, et al. Pulmonary leukostasis: radiologic-pathologic study. Radiology. 1987;165:739.
51. Doran HM, Sheppard MN, Collins PW, et al. Pathology of the lung in leukaemia and lymphoma: a study of 87 autopsies. Histopathology. 1991;18:211.
52. Mangal AK, Growe GH. Extensive pulmonary infiltration by leukemic blast cells treated with irradiation. Can Med Assoc J. 1983;128:424.
53. Von Eyben FE, Siddiqui MZ, Spanos G. High-voltage irradiation and hydroxyurea for pulmonary leukostasis in acute myelomonocytic leukemia. Acta Haematol. 1987;77:180.
54. Flasshove M, Schuette J, Sauerwein W, et al. Pulmonary and cerebral irradiation for hyperleukocytosis in acute myelomonocytic leukemia. Leukemia. 1994;8:1792.
55. Smith LJ, Katzenstein ALA. Pathogenesis of massive pulmonary hemorrhage in acute leukemia. Arch Intern Med. 1982;142:2149.
56. Andersson BS, Luna MA, Yee C, et al. Fatal pulmonary failure complicating high-dose cytosine arabinoside therapy in acute leukemia. Cancer. 1990;65:1079.
57. Vansteenkiste JF, Boogaerts MA. Adult respiratory distress syndrome in neutropenic leukemia patients. Blut. 1989;58:287.
58. Wiernik PH, Sutherland JC, Steckmiller BK, et al. Clinically significant cardiac infiltration in acute leukemia, lymphocytic lymphoma and plasma cell myeloma. Med Pediatr Oncol. 1976;2:75.
59. McAdams HP, Schaefer PS, Ghaed VN. Leukemic infiltrates of the heart: CT findings. J Comput Assist Tomogr. 1989;13:525.
60. Allen DC, Alderdice JM, Morton P, et al. Pathology of the heart and conduction system in lymphoma and leukaemia. J Clin Pathol. 1987;40:746.
61. Foucar K, Foucar E, Willman C, et al. Nonleukemic granulocytic sarcoma of the heart: a report of a fatal case. Am J Hematol. 1987;25:325.
62. Williford SK, Salisbury PL III, Peacock JE Jr, et al. The safety of dental extractions in patients with hematologic malignancies. J Clin Oncol. 1989;7:798.
63. Toljanic JA, Bedard J-F, Larson RA, Fox JP. A prospective pilot study to evaluate a new dental assessment and treatment paradigm for patients scheduled to undergo intensive chemotherapy for cancer. Cancer. 1999;85:1843.
64. Sklansky BD, Jafek BW, Wiernik PH. Otolaryngologic manifestations of acute leukemia. Laryngoscope. 1974;84:210.
65. Fulp SR, Nestok BR, Powell BL, et al. Leukemic infiltration of the esophagus. Cancer. 1993;71:112.
66. Tan SN, Gendeh HS, Sani A, Mat-Baki M. Myeloid sarcoma: an unusual and rare laryngeal presentation. Int J Surg Case Rep. 2016;21:99–103.
67. Almadori G, Del Ninno M, Cadoni G, et al. Facial nerve paralysis in acute otomastoiditis as presenting symptom of FAB M2, T8;21 leukemic relapse. Case report and review of the literature. Int J Pediatr Otorhinolaryngol. 1996;36:45.
68. Stankovic KM, Juliano AF, Hasserjian RP. Case records of the Massachusetts General Hospital. Case 36-2010. A 50-year old-woman with pain and loss of hearing in the left ear. N Engl J Med. 2010;363:2146–56.
69. Schimpff SC, Wiernik PH, Block JB. Rectal abscesses in cancer patients. Lancet. 1972;2:844.
70. Cartoni C, Dragoni F, Micozzi A, et al. Neutropenic enterocolitis in patients with acute leukemia: prognostic significance of bowel wall thickening detected by ultrasonography. J Clin Oncol. 2001;19:756.
71. O'Brien S, Kantarjian HM, Anaissie E, et al. Successful medical management of neutropenic enterocolitis in adults with acute leukemia. South Med J. 1987;80:1233.
72. Bishop JF, Schiffer CA, Aisner J, et al. Surgery in acute leukemia: a review of 167 operations in thrombocytopenic patients. Am J Hematol. 1987;26:147.
73. Thalhammer F, Gisslinger H, Chott A, et al. Granulocytic sarcoma of the prostate as the first manifestation of a late relapse of acute myelogenous leukemia. Ann Hematol. 1994;68:97.
74. Ferry JA, Snigley JR, Young RH. Granulocytic sarcoma of the testis: a report of two cases of a neoplasm prone to misinterpretation. Mod Pathol. 1997;10:320.
75. Wainer RA, Wiernik PH, Thompson WL. Metabolic and therapeutic studies of a patient with acute leukemia and severe lactic acidosis of prolonged duration. Am J Med. 1973;55:255.
76. Gewirtz AM, Stewart AF, Vignery A, et al. Hypercalcemia complicating acute myelogenous leukemia: a syndrome of multiple aetiologies. Br J Haematol. 1983;54:133.
77. Koeppler H, Pflueger KH, Knapp W, et al. Establishment of three permanent human leukaemia cell lines producing immunoreactive calcitonin. Br J Haematol. 1987;65:405.
78. Schenkein DP, O'Neill C, Shapiro J, et al. Accelerated bone formation causing profound hypocalcemia in acute leukemia. Ann Intern Med. 1986;105:375.
79. Budd D, Ginsberg H. Hypocholesterolemia and acute myelogenous leukemia. Cancer. 1986;58:1361.
80. Fritz RD, Forkner CD Jr, Freireich EJ. The association of fatal intracranial hemorrhage and "blastic crisis" in patients with acute leukemia. N Engl J Med. 1959;261:59.
81. Dutcher JP, Schiffer CA, Wiernik PH. Hyperleukocytosis in adult acute nonlymphocytic leukemia: impact on remission rate and duration, and survival. J Clin Oncol. 1987;5:1364.
82. van Buchem MA, te Velde J, Willemze R, et al. Leucostasis, an underestimated cause of death in leukaemia. Blut. 1988;56:39.
83. Ventura GJ, Hestar JP, Smith TL, et al. Acute myeloblastic leukemia with hyperleukocytosis: risk factors for early mortality in induction. Am J Hematol. 1988;27:34.

84. VanCamp B, Reynaerts PH, Naets JP, et al. Transient IgA1-paraprotein during treatment of acute myelomonocytic leukemia. Blood. 1980;55:21.
85. Atkins H, Drouin J, Izahuirre CA, et al. Acute promyelocytic leukemia associated with a paraprotein that reacts with leukemic cells. Cancer. 1989;63:1750.
86. Schiffer CA, Lichtenfeld JL, Wiernik PH, et al. Antibody response in patients with acute nonlymphocytic leukemia. Cancer. 1976;37:2177.
87. Spickermann D, Gause A, Pfreundschuh M, et al. Impaired antibody levels to tetanus toxoid and pneumococcal polysaccharides in acute leukemias. Leuk Lymphoma. 1994;16:89.
88. Hansen PB, Kjeldsen L, Dalhoff K, Olesen B. Cerebrospinal fluid beta-2-microglobulin in adult patients with acute leukemia or lymphoma: a useful marker in early diagnosis and monitoring of CNS-involvement. Acta Neurol Scand. 1992;85:324.
89. Furno P, Dionisi MS, Bucaneve G, et al. Ceftriaxone versus beta-lactams with antipseudomonal activity for empirical, combined antibiotic therapy in febrile neutropenia: a meta-analysis. Support Care Cancer. 2000;8:293.
90. Sickles EA, Young VM, Greene WH, Wiernik PH. Pneumonia in acute leukemia. Ann Intern Med. 1973;79:528.
91. Lichtman MA, Rowe JM. Hyperleukocytic leukemias: rheological, clinical, and therapeutic considerations. Blood. 1982;60:279.
92. Cuttner J, Holland JF, Norton L, et al. Therapeutic leukapheresis for hyperleukocytosis in acute myelocytic leukemia. Med Pediatr Oncol. 1983;11:76.
93. Nelson SC, Bruggers CS, Kurtzberg J, et al. Management of leukemic hyperleukocytosis with hydration, urinary alkalinization, and allopurinol. Am J Pediatr Hematol Oncol. 1993;15:351.
94. Fernandez G, Garcia JE, Ahijado F, et al. Allopurinol and bone marrow aplasia. Nephron. 1993;64:322.
95. Pui CH, Mahmoud HH, Wiley JM, et al. Recombinant urate oxidase for the prophylaxis or treatment of hyperuricemia in patients with leukemia or lymphoma. J Clin Oncol. 2001;19:697.
96. Giraldez M, Puto K. A single, fixed dose of rasburicase (6 mg maximum) for treatment of tumor lysis syndrome in adults. Eur J Haematol. 2010;85(2):177–9.
97. Lishner M, Avivi I, Apperley JF, et al. Hematologic malignancies in pregnancy: Management guidelines from an international consensus meeting. J Clin Oncol. 2016;34:501–8.
98. Reynoso EE, Sheperd FA, Messner HA, et al. Acute leukemia during pregnancy: the Toronto Leukemia Study Group experience with long-term follow-up of children exposed in utero to chemotherapeutic agents. J Clin Oncol. 1987;5:1098.
99. Feliu J, Juarez S, Ordonez A, et al. Acute leukemia and pregnancy. Cancer. 1988;61:580.
100. Thomas X. Acute myeloid leukemia in the pregnant patient. Eur J Haematol. 2015;95:124–36.
101. Ali S, Jones GL, Culligan DJ, et al. Guidelines for the diagnosis and management of acute myeloid leukaemia in pregnancy. Br J Haematol. 2015;170:487–95.
102. Aviles A, Niz J. Long-term follow-up of children born to mothers with acute leukemia during pregnancy. Med Pediatr Oncol. 1988;16:3.
103. Sanz GF, Sanz MA. Remision completa espontanea en leucemia mieloblastica aguda. Rev Clin Esp. 1986;178:229.
104. Krug U, Lübbert M, Büchner T. Maintenance therapy in acute myeloid leukemia revisited: will new agents rekindle an old interest? Curr Opin Hematol. 2010;17:85.
105. Canaani J, Luger SM. Revisiting maintenance therapy in acute myeloid leukemia with novel agents. Curr Opin Hematol. 2016;23:175–80.
106. Wei A, Tan P, Perruzza S, et al. Maintenance lenalidomide in combination with 5-azacitidine as post-remission therapy for acute myeloid leukaemia. Br J Haematol. 2015;169:199–210.
107. de Greef GE, van Putten WL, Boogaerts M, et al. Criteria for defining a complete remission in acute myeloid leukaemia revisited. An analysis of patients treated in HOVON-SAKK co-operative group studies. Br J Haematol. 2005;128:184.
108. Walter RB, Kantarjian HM, Huang X, et al. Effect of complete remission and responses less than complete remission on survival in acute myeloid leukemia: a combined Eastern Cooperative Group, Southwest Oncology Group, and M.D. Anderson Cancer Center study. J Clin Oncol. 2010;28:1766.
109. Chen X, Xie H, Wood BL, et al. Relation of clinical response and minimal residual disease and their prognostic impact on outcome in acute myeloid leukemia. J Clin Oncol. 2015;33:1258–64.
110. Pettit K, Stock W, Walter RB. Incorporating measurable ('minimal') residual disease-directed treatment strategies to optimize outcomes in adults with acute myeloid leukemia. Leuk Lymphoma. 2016;57:1527–33.
111. Ivey A, Hills RK, Simpson MA, et al. Assessment of minimal residual disease in standard-risk AML. N Engl J Med. 2016;374:422–33.
112. Paietta E. Should minimal residual disease guide therapy in AML? Best Pract Res Clin Haematol. 2015;28:98–105.
113. Zeijlemaker W, Kelder A, Oussoren-Brockhoff YJ, et al. Peripheral blood minimal residual disease may replace bone marrow minimal residual disease as an immunophenotypic biomarker for impending relapse in acute myeloid leukemia. Leukemia. 2016;30:708–15.
114. Bishop JF, Lowenthal RM, Joshua D, et al. Etoposide in acute nonlymphocytic leukemia. Blood. 1990;75:27.
115. Byrd JC, Dodge RK, Carroll A, et al. Patients with t(8;21)(q22;q22) and acute myeloid leukemia have superior failure-free and overall survival when repetitive cycles of high-dose cytarabine are administered. J Clin Oncol. 1999;17:3767.
116. Papaemmanuil E, Gerstung M, Bullinger L, et al. Genomic classification and prognosis in acute myeloid leukemia. N Engl J Med. 2016;374:2209–21.
117. Uras IZ, Walter GJ, Scheicher R, Bellutti F, et al. Palbociclib treatment of FLT3-ITD+ AML cells uncovers a kinase-dependent transcriptional regulation of FLT3 and PIM1 by CDK6. Blood. 2016;127:2890–902.
118. Minson KA, Smith CC, DeRyckere D, et al. The MERTK/FLT3 inhibitor MRX-2843 overcomes resistance-conferring FLT3 mutations in acute myeloid leukemia. JCI Insight. 2016;1:e85630.
119. De Freitas T, Marktel S, Piemontese S, et al. High rate of hematological responses to sorafenib in FLT3-ITD acute myeloid leukemia relapsed after allogeneic hematopoietic stem cell transplantation. Eur J Haematol. 2016;96:629–36.
120. Gallogly MM, Lazarus HM. Midostaurin: an emerging treatment for acute myeloid leukemia patients. J Blood Med. 2016;7:73–83.
121. Wu H, Hu C, Wang A, et al. Ibrutinib electively targets FLT3-ITD in mutant FLT3-positive AML. Leukemia. 2016;30:754–7.
122. El Hajj H, Dassouki Z, Berthier C, et al. Retinoic acid and arsenic trioxide trigger degradation of mutated NPM1, resulting in apoptosis of AML cells. Blood. 2015;125:3447–54.
123. Becker H, Marcucci G, Maharry K, et al. Favorable prognostic impact of NPM1 mutations in older patients with cytogenetically normal de novo acute myeloid leukemia and associated gene and microRNA-expression signatures: a Cancer and Leukemia Group B study. J Clin Oncol. 2010;28:596.
124. Ferrara F, Izzo T, Criscuolo C, et al. Favorable outcome in patients with acute myeloid leukemia with NPM1 mutation autografted after conditioning with high dose continuous infusion idarubicin and busulphan. Biol Blood Marrow Transplant. 2010;16(7):1018–24.
125. Damm F, Heuser M, Morgan M, et al. Single nucleotide polymorphism in the mutational hotspot of WT1 predicts a favorable

outcome in patients with cytogenetically normal acute myeloid leukemia. J Clin Oncol. 2010;28:578.

126. Dufour A, Schneider F, Metzeler KH, et al. Acute myeloid leukemia with biallelic CEBPA gene mutations and normal karyotype represents a distinct genetic entity associated with a favorable clinical outcome. J Clin Oncol. 2010;28:570.
127. Kornblau SM, Singh N, Qiu Y, et al. Highly phosphorylated FOXO3A is an adverse prognostic factor in acute myeloid leukemia. Clin Cancer Res. 2010;16(6):1865–74.
128. Schiller G, Gajewski J, Territo M, et al. Long-term outcome of high-dose cytarabine-based consolidation chemotherapy for adults with acute myelogenous leukemia. Blood. 1992;80:2977.
129. Grimwade D, Ivey A, Huntly BJP. Molecular landscape of acute myeloid leukemia in younger adults and its clinical relevance. Blood. 2016;127:29–39.
130. Kico JM, Miller CA, Griffith M, et al. Association between mutation clearance after induction therapy and outcomes in acute myeloid leukemia. JAMA. 2015;314:811–22.
131. Rose D, Haferlach T, Schnittger S, et al. Subtype-specific patterns of molecular mutations in acute myeloid leukemia. Leukemia. 2017;31:11–17.
132. Verhagen HJMP, Smit MA, Rutten A, et al. Primary acute myeloid leukemia cells with overexpression of EVI-1 are sensitive to all-*trans* retinoic acid. Blood. 2016;127:458–63.
133. Yamazaki J, Taby R, Jelinek J, et al. Hypomethylation of TET2 target genes identifies a curable subset of acute myeloid leukemia. J Natl Cancer Inst. 2015;13:108.
134. Tawana K, Wang J, Renneville A, et al. Disease evolution and outcomes in familial AML with germline CEBPA mutations. Blood. 2015;126:1214–23.
135. Megias-Vericat JE, Herrero MJ, Rojas L, et al. A systematic review and meta-analysis of the impact of WT1 polymorphism rs16754 in the effectiveness of standard chemotherapy in patients with acute myeloid leukemia. Pharmacogenomics J. 2016;16:30–40.
136. Yates G, Glidewell OH, Wiernik PH, et al. Cytosine arabinoside with daunorubicin or adriamycin for therapy of acute myelocytic leukemia. A CALGB study. Blood. 1982;60:454.
137. Van Sloten K, Wiernik PH, Schimpff SC. Evaluation of levamisole as an adjuvant to chemotherapy for treatment of acute nonlymphocytic leukemia. Cancer. 1983;51:1576.
138. Dutcher JP, Wiernik PH, Markus S, et al. Intensive maintenance therapy improves survival in adult acute nonlymphocytic leukemia: an eight-year follow-up. Leukemia. 1988;2:413.
139. Rai KR, Holland JF, Glidewell OH, et al. Treatment of acute myelocytic leukemia: a study by Cancer and Leukemia Group B. Blood. 1981;58:1203.
140. Preisler H, Davis RB, Kirshner J, et al. Comparison of three remission induction regimens and two postinduction strategies for the treatment of acute nonlymphocytic leukemia: a Cancer and Acute Leukemia Group B study. Blood. 1987;69:1441.
141. Rowe JM, Andersen JW, Mazza JJ, et al. A randomized placebo controlled phase III study of granulocyte macrophage colony stimulating factor in adult patients (>55–70 years of age) with acute myelogenous leukemia: a study of the Eastern Cooperative Oncology Group (E1490). Blood. 1995;86:457.
142. Stone RM, Berg DT, George SL, et al. Granulocyte-macrophage colony-stimulating factor after initial chemotherapy for elderly patients with primary acute myelogenous leukemia. Cancer and Leukemia Group B N Engl J Med. 1995;332:1671.
143. Fernandez HF, Sun Z, Yao X, et al. Anthracycline dose intensification in acute myeloid leukemia. N Engl J Med. 2009;361:1249.
144. Luskin MR, Lee J-W, Fernandez HF, et al. Benefit of high=dose daunorubicin in AML induction extends across cytogenetic and molecular groups. Blood. 2016;127:1551–8.
145. Löwenberg B, Ossenkoppeie GJ, van Putten W, et al. High-dose daunorubicin in older patients with acute myeloid leukemia. N Engl J Med. 2009;361:1235.
146. Lee JH, Joo YD, Kim H, et al. A randomized trial comparing standard versus high-dose daunorubicin induction in patients with acute myeloid leukemia. Blood. 2011;118:3832–41.
147. Burnett AK, Russell NH, Hills RK, et al. A randomized comparison of daunorubicin 90 mg/m^2 vs 60 mg/m^2 in AML induction: results from the UK NCRI AML 17 trial in 1206 patients. Blood. 2015;125:3978–85.
148. Prebet T, Bertoli S, Delaunay J, et al. Anthracycline dose intensification improves molecular response and outcome of patients treated for core binding factor acute myeloid leukemia. Haematologica. 2014;99:e185–7.
149. Reagan JL, Sullivan MR, Winer ES, et al. Potential for improved survival with intensification of daunorubicin based induction chemotherapy in acute myeloid leukemia patients who do not receive transplant: a multicenter retrospective study. Leuk Res. 2015;39:812–7.
150. Pautas C, Merabet F, Thomas X, et al. Randomized study of intensified anthracycline doses for induction and recombinant interleukin-2 for maintenance in patients with acute myeloid leukemia age 50 to 70 years: results of the ALFA-9801 study. J Clin Oncol. 2010;28:808–14.
151. Gong Q, Zhou L, Xu S, et al. High doses of daunorubicin during induction therapy of newly diagnosed acute myeloid leukemia: a systematic review and meta-analysis of prospective clinical trials. PLoS One. 2015;10:e0125612.
152. Teuffel O, Leibundgut K, Lehrnbecher T, et al. Anthracyclines during induction therapy in acute myeloid keukaemia: a systematic review and meta-analysis. Br J Haematol. 2013;161:192–203.
153. Sekine L, Morais VD, Lima KM, et al. Conventional and high-dose daunorubicin and idarubicin in acute myeloid leukaemia remission induction treatment: a mixed treatment comparison meta-analysis of 7258 patients. Hematol Oncol. 2015;33:21–9.
154. Greene W, Huffman D, Wiernik PH, et al. High-dose daunorubicin therapy for acute nonlymphocytic leukemia: correlation of response and toxicity with pharmacokinetics and intracellular daunorubicin reductase activity. Cancer. 1972;30:1419–27.
155. Dombret H, Gardin C. An update of current treatments for adult acute myeloid leukemia. Blood. 127:53–61.
156. Rowe JM, Neuberg D, Friedenberg W, et al. A phase III study of daunorubicin vs idarubicin vs mitoxantrone for older adult patients (>55 yrs) with acute myelogenous leukemia (AML): a study of the Eastern Cooperative Oncology Group (E3993). Blood. 1998;92(Suppl 1):2517a.
157. Berman E, Heller G, Santorsa J, et al. Results of a randomized trial comparing idarubicin and cytosine arabinoside with daunorubicin and cytosine arabinoside in adult patients with newly diagnosed acute myelogenous leukemia. Blood. 1991;77:1666.
158. Wiernik PH, Banks PLC, Case DC Jr, et al. Cytarabine plus idarubicin or daunorubicin as induction and consolidation therapy for previously untreated adult patients with acute myeloid leukemia. Blood. 1992;79:313.
159. Vogler WR, Velez-Garcia E, Weiner RS, et al. A phase III trial comparing idarubicin and daunorubicin in combination with cytarabine in acute myelogenous leukemia: a Southeastern Cancer Study Group study. J Clin Oncol. 1992;10:1.
160. Mandelli F, Petti MC, Ardia A, et al. A randomised clinical trial comparing idarubicin and cytarabine to daunorubicin and cytarabine in the treatment of acute non-lymphoid leukaemia. Eur J Cancer. 1991;27:750.
161. Mandelli F, Vignetti M, Suciu S, et al. Daunorubicin versus mitoxantrone versus idarubicin as induction and consolidation chemotherapy for adults with acute myeloid leukemia: the EORTC and GIMEMA Groups study AML-10. J Clin Oncol. 2009;27:5397.

162. Ohtake S, Miyawaki S, Fujita H, et al. Randomized study of induction therapy comparing standard-dose idarubicin with high-dose daunorubicin in adult patients with previously untreated acute myeloid leukemia: the JALSG AML201 study. Blood. 2011;117:2358–65.
163. Li X, Xu S, Tan Y, Chen J. The effects of idarubicin versus other anthracyclines for induction therapy of patients with newly diagnosed leukaemia. Cochrane Database Syst Rev. 2015;3:CD010432.
164. AML Collaborative Group. A systematic collaborative overview of randomized trials comparing idarubicin with daunorubicin (or other anthracyclines) as induction therapy for acute myeloid leukaemia. Br J Haematol. 1998;103:100.
165. Robert J, Rigal-Huguet F, Hurteloup P. Comparative pharmacokinetic study of idarubicin and daunorubicin in leukemia patients. Hematol Oncol. 1992;10:111.
166. Berman E, McBride M. Comparative cellular pharmacology of daunorubicin and idarubicin in human multidrug-resistant leukemia cells. Blood. 1992;79:3267.
167. Arlin Z, Case DC Jr, Moore J, et al. Randomized multicenter trial of cytosine arabinoside with mitoxantrone or daunorubicin in previously untreated adult patients with acute nonlymphocytic leukemia (ANLL). Leukemia. 1990;4:177.
168. Pavlovsky S, Gonzalez Llaven J, Garcia Martinez MA, et al. A randomized study of mitoxantrone plus cytarabine versus daunomycin plus cytarabine in the treatment of previously untreated adult
169. Hann IM, Stevens RF, Goldstone AH, et al. Randomized comparison of DAT versus ADE as induction chemotherapy in children and younger adults with acute myeloid leukaemia. Results of the Medical Research Council's 10th AML trial (MRC AML10). Adult and childhood leukaemia working parties of the Medical Research Council. Blood. 1997;89:2311.
170. Miyawaki S, Tanimoto M, Kobayashi T, et al. No beneficial effect from addition of etoposide to daunorubicin, cytarabine, and 6- mercaptopurine in individualized induction therapy of acute myeloid leukemia: the JALSG-AML92 study. Japan Adult Leukemia Study Group. Int J Hematol. 1999;70:97.
171. Holowiecki J, Grosicki S, Giebel S, et al. Cladribine, but not fludarabine, added to daunorubicin and cytarabine during induction prolongs survival of patients with acute myeloid leukemia: a multicenter, randomized phase III study. J Clin Oncol. 2012;30:2441–8.
172. Hills RK, Castaigne S, Appelbaum FR, et al. Addition of gemtuzumab ozogamicin to induction chemotherapy in adult patients with acute myeloid leukaemia: a meta-analysis of individual patient data from randomized controlled trials. Lancet Oncol. 2014;15:986–96.
173. Burnett A, Cavenagh J, Russell N, et al. Defining the dose of gemtuzumab ozogamicin in combination with induction chemotherapy in acute myeloid leukemia: a comparison of 3 mg/m^2 with 6 mg/m^2 in the NCRI AML 17 trial. Haematologica. 2016;101:724–31.
174. Zeidner JF, Foster MC, Blackford AL, et al. Randomized multicenter phase II study of flavopiridol (alvocidib), cytarabine, and mitoxantrone (FLAM) versus cytarabine/daunorubicin (7+3) in newly diagnosed acute myeloid leukemia. Haematologica. 2015;100:1172–9.
175. Ravandi F, Arana C, Cortes JE, et al. Final report of phase II study of sorafenib, cytarabine, and idarubicin for initial therapy in younger patients with acute myeloid leukemia. Leukemia. 2014;8:1543–5.
176. Hills RK, Gammon G, Trone D, Burnett AK. Quizartinib significantly improves overall survival in FLT3-ITD positive AML patients relapsed after stem cell transplantation or after failure of salvage chemotherapy: a comparison with historical AML database (UK NCRI data). Blood. 2015;126:2557.
177. Stone RM, Mandrekar S, Sanford BL, et al. The multi-kinase inhibitor midostaurin (M) prolongs survival compared with placebo (P) in combination with daunorubicin (D)/cytarabine (C) induction (ind), high-dose C consolidation (consol), and as maintenance (maint) therapy in newly diagnosed acute myeloid leukemia (AML) patients (pts) age 18-60 with FLT3 mutations (muts): an international prospective randomized (rand) P-controlled double-blind trial (CALGB 10603/RATIFY [Alliance]). Blood. 2015.; Plenary SessionAbstract #6
178. Weick JK, Kopecky KJ, Appelbaum FR, et al. A randomized investigation of high-dose versus standard-dose cytosine arabinoside with daunorubicin in patients with previously untreated acute myeloid leukemia: a Southwest Oncology Group study. Blood. 1996;88:2441–51.
179. Löwenberg B, Pabst T, Vellenga E, et al. Cytarabine dose for acute myeloid leukemia. N Engl J Med. 2011;364:1027–36.
180. Li W, Gong X, Sun M, et al. High-dose cytarabine in acute myeloid leukemia treatment: a systematic review and meta-analysis. PLoS One. 2014;9:e110153.
181. Willemze R, Suciu S, Meloni G, et al. High-dose cytarabine in induction treatment improves the outcome of adult patients younger than age 45 years with acute myeloid leukemia: results of the EORTC-GIMEMA AML-12 trial. J Clin Oncol. 2014;32:219–28.
182. Krug U, Berdel WE, Gale RP, et al. Increasing intensity of therapies assigned at diagnosis does not improve survival of adults with acute myeloid leukemia. Leukemia. 2016;30:1230–6.
183. Röllig C, Serve H, Hüttmann A, et al. Addition of sorafenib versus placebo to standard therapy in patients aged 60 years or younger with newly diagnosed acute myeloid leukaemia (SORAML): a multicentre, phase 2, randomized controlled trial. Lancet Oncol. 2015;16:1691–9.
184. Mamez AC, Raffoux E, Chevret S, et al. Pre-treatment with oral hydroxyurea prior to intensive chemotherapy improves early survival of patients with hyperleukocytosis in acute myeloid leukemia. Leuk Lymphoma. 2016;57:2281–8.
185. Carden PA, Mitchell SL, Waters KD, et al. Prevention of cyclophosphamide/cytarabine-induced emesis with ondansetron in children with leukemia. J Clin Oncol. 1990;8:1531.
186. Italian Group for Antiemetic Research. Dexamethasone, granisetron, or both for the prevention of nausea and vomiting during chemotherapy for cancer. N Engl J Med. 1995;332:1.
187. Yokel BK, Friedman KJ, Farmer ER, et al. Cutaneous pathology following etoposide therapy. J Cutan Pathol. 1987;14:326.
188. Bezwoda WR, Bernasconi C, Hutchinson RM, et al. Mitoxantrone for refractory and relapsed acute leukemia. Cancer. 1990;66:418.
189. Vogler WR, Harrington DP, Winton EF, et al. Phase II clinical trial of carboplatin in relapsed and refractory leukemia. Leukemia. 1992;6:1072.
190. Santana VM, Mirro J Jr, Kearns C, et al. 2-Chlorodeoxyadenosine produces a high rate of complete hematologic remission in relapsed acute myeloid leukemia. J Clin Oncol. 1992;10:364.
191. Gandhi V, Estey E, Keating MJ, et al. Fludarabine potentiates metabolism of cytarabine in patients with acute myelogenous leukemia during therapy. J Clin Oncol. 1993;11:116.
192. Schiller G. Treatment of resistant acute myeloid leukemia. Blood Rev. 1991;5:220.
193. van Der Velden VH, te Marvelde JG, Hoogeveen PG, et al. Targeting of the CD33-calicheamicin immunoconjugate Mylotarg (CMA-676) in acute myeloid leukemia: in vivo and in vitro saturation and internalization by leukemic and normal myeloid cells. Blood. 2001;97:3197.
194. Welborn JL, Lewis JP, Meyers FJ. Impact of reinduction regimens on the clinical course of adult acute nonlymphocytic leukemia. Leukemia. 1988;2:711.

195. Novik Y, Oleksowicz L, Wiernik PH. Therapeutic effect of cyclosporin A in thrombocytopenia after myeloablative chemotherapy in acute myeloid leukaemia. Med Oncol. 1997;14:43.
196. Ofran Y, Leiba R, Ganzel C, et al. Prospective comparison of early bone marrow evaluation on day 5 versus day 14 of the "3+7" induction regimen for acute myeloid leukemia. Am J Hematol. 2015;90:1159–64.
197. Ofran Y. Is the D14 bone marrow in acute myeloid leukemia still the gold standard? Curr Opin Hematol. 2016;23:108–14.
198. Yezefski T, Xie H, Walter R. Value of routine "day 14" marrow exam in newly =-diagnosed AML. Leukemia. 2015;29:247–9.
199. Estey EH, Shen Y, Thall PF. Effect of time to complete remission on subsequent survival and disease-free survival time in AML, RAEB-t, and RAEB. Blood. 2000;95:72.
200. Estey EH. How I treat older patients with AML. Blood. 2000;6:1670.
201. Whitely R, Hannah P, Holmes F. Survival in acute leukemia in elderly patients. J Am Geriatr Soc. 1990;38:527.
202. Kanamori H, Maruta A, Miyashita H, et al. Low-dose cytosine arabinoside for treating hypocellular acute leukemia in the elderly. Am J Hematol. 1992;39:52.
203. Yin JAL, Johnson PRE, Davies JM, et al. Mitozantrone and cytosine arabinoside as first-line therapy in elderly patients with acute myeloid leukaemia. Br J Haematol. 1991;79:415.
204. Sebban C, Archimbaud E, Coiffier B, et al. Treatment of acute myeloid leukemia in elderly patients. A retrospective study. Cancer. 1988;61:227.
205. Löwenberg B, Zittoun R, Kerkhofs H, et al. On the value of intensive remission-induction chemotherapy in elderly patients of 65+ years with acute myeloid leukemia: a randomized phase III study of the European Organization for Research and Treatment of Cancer Leukemia Group. J Clin Oncol. 1989;7:1268.
206. Johnson PRE, Hunt LP, Yin JAL. Prognostic factors in elderly patients with acute myeloid leukaemia: development of a model to predict survival. Br J Haematol. 1993;85:300.
207. Gajewski JL, Ho WG, Nimer SD, et al. Efficacy of intensive chemotherapy for acute myelogenous leukemia associated with a preleukemic syndrome. J Clin Oncol. 1989;7:1637.
208. Chang J, Geary CG, Testa NG. Long-term bone marrow damage after chemotherapy for acute myeloid leukaemia does not improve with time. Br J Haematol. 1990;75:68.
209. Tamura S, Kanamaru A. De-novo acute myeloid leukemia with trilineage myelodysplasia (AML/TMDS) and myelodysplastic remission marrow (AML/MRM). Leuk Lymphoma. 1995;16:263.
210. Fearon ER, Burke PJ, Schiffer CA, et al. Differentiation of leukemia cells to polymorphonuclear leukocytes in patients with acute nonlymphocytic leukemia. N Engl J Med. 1986;315:15.
211. Fialkow PJ, Singer JW, Raskind WH, et al. Clonal development, stem-cell differentiation, and clinical remissions in acute nonlymphocytic leukemia. N Engl J Med. 1987;317:468.
212. Huang C, Deng M, Guo R, et al. A study of the induction of differentiation of human leukemic cells by harringtonine combined with cytarabine. Leukemia. 1988;2:518.
213. Davies AR. Auer bodies in mature neutrophils. JAMA. 1969;202:895.
214. Viola MV, Frazier M, Wiernik PH, et al. Reverse transcriptase in leukocytes of leukemic patients in remission. N Engl J Med. 1976;294:75.
215. Koeffler HP. Review: induction of differentiation of human acute myelogenous leukemic cells: therapeutic implications. Blood. 1983;62:709.
216. Schwartz EL, Wiernik PH. Differentiation of leukemic cells by chemotherapeutic agents. J Clin Pharmacol. 1988;28:779.
217. Preisler HD, Anderson K, Rai K, et al. The frequency of long-term remission in patients with acute myelogenous leukemia treated with conventional maintenance chemotherapy: a study of 760 patients with a minimal follow-up time of 6 years. Br J Haematol. 1989;71:189.
218. Embury SH, Elias L, Heller PM, et al. Remission maintenance therapy in acute myelogenous leukemia. West J Med. 1977;126:267.
219. Vaughan WP, Karp JE, Burke PJ. Long chemotherapy-free remissions after single-cycle timed sequential chemotherapy for acute myelocytic leukemia. Cancer. 1980;45:859.
220. Rustum YM, Preisler HD. Correlation between leukemic cell retention of 1-β-D-arabinofuranosyl-cytosine 5′-triphosphate and response to therapy. Cancer Res. 1979;39:42.
221. Cassileth PA, Lynch E, Hines JD, et al. Varying intensity of postremission therapy in acute myeloid leukemia. Blood. 1992;79:1924.
222. Mayer RJ, Davis RB, Schiffer CA, et al. Intensive postremission chemotherapy in adults with acute myeloid leukemia. N Engl J Med. 1994;331:896.
223. Zittoun R, Jehn U, Fiere D, et al. Alternative v repeated postremission treatment in adult acute myelogenous leukemia: a randomized phase III study (AML6) of the EORTC Leukemia Cooperative Group. Blood. 1989;73:896.
224. Schiller GJ, Nimer SD, Territo MC, et al. Bone marrow transplantation versus high-dose cytarabine-based consolidation chemotherapy for acute myelogenous leukemia in first remission. J Clin Oncol. 1992;10:41.
225. Harousseau JL, Milpied N, Briere J, et al. Double intensive consolidation chemotherapy in adult acute myeloid leukemia. J Clin Oncol. 1991;9:1432.
226. Giordano M, Riccardi A, Girino M, et al. Postremission chemotherapy in adult acute nonlymphoblastic leukaemia including intensive or non-intensive consolidation therapy. Eur J Cancer. 1991;27:437.
227. Dutcher JP, Wiernik PH, Markus S, et al. 15-year follow-up of adult patients with acute myeloid leukemia: Study BCRC 7802. Proc XXV Cong Int Soc Hematol. 1994.; abstract #48
228. Ranson MR, Scarffe JH, Morgenstern GR, et al. Post consolidation therapy for adult patients with acute myeloid leukaemia. Br J Haematol. 1991;79:162.
229. Weick JK, Kopecky KJ, Appelbaum FR, et al. A randomized investigation of high-dose versus standard-dose cytosine arabinoside with daunorubicin in patients with previously untreated acute myeloid leukemia: a Southwest Oncology Group study. Blood. 1996;88:2841.
230. Tallman MS, Appelbaum FR, Amos D, et al. Evaluation of intensive postremission chemotherapy for adults with acute nonlymphocytic leukemia using high-dose cytosine arabinoside with L-asparaginase and amsacrine with etoposide. J Clin Oncol. 1987;5:918.
231. Wiernik PH. Optimal therapy for adult patients with acute myeloid leukemia in first complete remission. Curr Treat Options Oncol. 2014;15:171–86.
232. Young JW, Papadopoulos EB, Cunningham I, et al. T-cell-depleted allogeneic bone marrow transplantation in adults with acute nonlymphocytic leukemia in first remission. Blood. 1992;79:3380.
233. Clift RA, Buckner CD, Appelbaum FR, et al. Allogeneic marrow transplantation in patients with acute myeloid leukemia in first remission: a randomized trial of two irradiation regimens. Blood. 1990;76:1867.
234. Bortin MM, Horowitz MM, Rowlings PA, et al. Progress report from the International Bone Marrow Transplant Registry. Bone Marrow Transplant. 1993;12:97.
235. Zittoun RA, Mandelli F, Willemze R, et al. Autologous or allogeneic bone marrow transplantation compared with intensive chemotherapy in acute myelogenous leukemia. N Engl J Med. 1995;332:217.

236. Cassileth PA, Harrington DP, Appelbaum FR, et al. Chemotherapy compared with autologous or allogeneic bone marrow transplantation in the management of acute myeloid leukemia in first remission. N Engl Med. 1998;339:1649.
237. Sakamaki H, Miyawaki S, Ohtake S, et al. Allogeneic stem cell transplantation versus chemotherapy as post-remission therapy for intermediate or poor risk adult acute myeloid leukemia: results of the JALSG AML97 study. Int J Hematol. 2010;91:284–92.
238. Blaise D, Maraninchi D, Michallet M, et al. Long-term follow-up of a randomized trial comparing the combination of cyclophosphamide with total body irradiation or busulfan as conditioning regimen for patients receiving HLA-identical marrow grafts for acute myeloblastic leukemia in first complete remission. Blood. 2001;97:3669.
239. Damiani D, Tiribelli M, Geromin A, et al. ABCG2, cytogenetics, and age predict relapse after allogeneic stem cell transplantation for acute myeloid leukemia in complete remission. Biol Blood Marrow Transplant. 2016;22:621–1626.
240. Cornelissen JJ, Blaise D. Hematopoietic stem cell transplantation for patients with AML in first complete remission. Blood. 2016;127:62–70.
241. Araki D, Wood BL, Othus M, et al. Allogeneic hematopoietic cell transplantation for acute myeloid leukemia: time to move toward a minimal residual disease-based definition of complete remission? J Clin Oncol. 2016;34:329–36.
242. Ho AD, Schetelig J, Bochtler T, et al. Allogeneic stem cell transplantation improves survival in patients with acute myeloid leukemia characterized by a high allelic ratio of mutant FLT3-ITD. Biol Blood Marrow Transplant. 2016;22:462–9.
243. Schetelig J, Schaich M, Schäfer-Eckart K, et al. Hematopoietic cell transplantation in patients with intermediate and high-risk AML: results from the randomized Study Alliance Leukemia (SAL) AML 2003 trial. Leukemia. 2015;29:1060–8.
244. Versluis J, Hazenberg CL, Passweg JR, et al. Post-remission treatment with allogeneic stem cell transplantation in patients aged 60 years and older with acute myeloid leukaemia: a time-dependent analysis. Lancet Hematol. 2015;2:e427–36.
245. Ma Y, Wu Y, Shen Z, et al. Is allogeneic transplantation really the best treatment for FLT3/ITD-positive acute myeloid leukemia? A systematic review. Clin Transplant. 2015;29:149–60.
246. Brissot E, Mohty M. Which acute myeloid leukemia patients should be offered transplantation? Semin Hematol. 2015;52:223–31.
247. Gale RP, Wiernik PH, Lazarus HM. Should persons with acute myeloid leukemia have a transplant in first remission? Leukemia. 2014;28:1949–52.
248. Cornelissen JJ, Versluis J, Passeg JR, et al. Comparative therapeutic value of post-remission approaches in patients with acute myeloid leukemia aged 40-60 years. Leukemia. 2015;29:1041–50.
249. Rashidi A, DiPersio JF, Westervelt P, et al. Comparison of outcomes after peripheral blood haploidentical versus matched unrelated donor allogeneic hematopoietic cell transplantation in patients with acute myeloid leukemia: A retrospective single-center review. Biol Blood Marrow Transplant. 2016;22:1696–1701.
250. Wang Y, Liu QF, Xu LP, et al. Haploidentical vs identical-sibling transplant for AML in remission: a multicenter, prospective study. Blood. 2015;125:3956–62.
251. Berman E, Little C, Gee T, et al. Reasons that patients with acute myelogenous leukemia do not undergo allogeneic bone marrow transplantation. N Engl J Med. 1992;326:156.
252. McClune BL, Weisdorf DJ, Pedersen TL, et al. Effect of age on outcome of reduced-intensity hematopoietic cell transplantation for older patients with acute myeloid leukemia in first complete remission or with myelodysplastic syndrome. J Clin Oncol. 2010;28:1878.
253. Hemmati PG, Terwey TH, Masssenkeil G, et al. Reduced intensity conditioning prior to allogeneic stem cell transplantation in first complete remission is effective in patients with acute myeloid leukemia and an intermediate-risk karyotype. Int J Hematol. 2010;91:436.
254. Ringdén O, Labopin M, Ehninger G, et al. Reduced intensity conditioning compared with myeloablative conditioning using unrelated donor transplants in patients with acute myeloid leukemia. J Clin Oncol. 2009;27:4570.
255. Pagel JM, Gooley TA, Rajendran J, et al. Allogeneic hematopoietic cell transplantation after conditioning with 131I-CD$% antibody plus fludarabine and low-dose total body irradiation for elderly patients with advanced acute myeloid leukemia or high-risk myelodysplastic syndrome. Blood. 2009;114:5444.
256. Rashidi A, Ebadi M, Colditz GA, DiPersio JF. Outcomes of allogeneic stem cell transplantation in elderly patients with acute myeloid leukemia: a systematic review and meta-analysis. Biol Blood Marrow Transplant. 2016;22:651–7.
257. Devine SM, Owzar K, Blum W, et al. Phase II study of allogeneic transplantation for older patients with acute myeloid leukemia in first complete remission using a reduced-intensity conditioning regimen: Results from Cancer and Leukemia Group B 100103 (Alliance for Clinical Trials in Oncology)/Blood and Marrow Transplant Clinical Trial Network 0502. J Clin Oncol. 2015;33:4167–75.
258. Sanz J, Sanz MA, Saavedra S, et al. Cord blood transplantation from unrelated donors in adults with high-risk acute myeloid leukemia. Biol Blood Marrow Transplant. 2010;16:86.
259. Verneris MR, Brunstein CG, Barker J, et al. Relapse risk after umbilical cord blood transplantation: enhanced graft-versus-leukemia effect in recipients of 2 units. Blood. 2009;114:4293.
260. Ballen KK, Lazarus H. Cord blood transplant for acute myeloid leukemia. Br J Haematol. 2016;173:25–36.
261. Eckfeldt CE, Randall N, Shanley RM, et al. Umbilical cord blood transplantation is a suitable option for consolidation of acute myeloid leukemia with FLT3-ITD. Haematologica. 2016;101:e348–e351.
262. Gorin NC, Labopin M, Meloni G, et al. Autologous bone marrow transplantation for acute myeloblastic leukemia in Europe: further evidence of the role of marrow purging by mafosfamide. Leukemia. 1991;5:896.
263. Körbling M, Hunstein W, Fliedner TM, et al. Disease-free survival after autologous bone marrow transplantation in patients with acute myelogenous leukemia. Blood. 1989;74:1898.
264. Czerw T, Labopin M, Gorin NC, et al. Long-term follow-up of patients with acute myeloid leukemia surviving and free of disease recurrence for at least 2 years after autologous stem cell transplantation: a report from the Acute Leukemia Working Party of the European Society for Blood and Marrow Transplantation. Cancer. 2016;122:1880–7.
265. Mannis GN, Martin TG III, Damon LE, et al. Long-term outcomes of patients with intermediate-risk acute myeloid leukemia treated with autologous hematopoietic cell transplant in first complete remission. Leuk Lymphoma. 2016;57:1560–6.
266. Rubin EH, Andersen JW, Berg DT, et al. Risk factors for high-dose cytarabine neurotoxicity: an analysis of a Cancer and Leukemia Group B trial in patients with acute myeloid leukemia. J Clin Oncol. 1992;10:948.
267. Berman E. Chemotherapy in acute myelogenous leukemia: high dose, higher expectations? J Clin Oncol. 1995;13:1.
268. Harousseau JL, Witz B, Lioure B, et al. Granulocyte colony-stimulating factor after intensive consolidation chemotherapy in acute myeloid leukemia: results of a randomized trial of the Groupie Oust-Est Leukemias Agues Myeloblastics. J Clin Oncol. 2000;18:780.
269. Tallman MS, Rowlings PA, Milone G, et al. Effect of postremission chemotherapy before human leukocyte antigen-identical sibling transplantation for acute myelogenous leukemia in first complete remission. Blood. 2000;96:1254.

270. Zwann FE, Herman J. Report of the E.M.B.T. leukemia working party. Exp Hematol. 1983;11:3.
271. Sierra J, Storer B, Hansen JA, et al. Unrelated donor marrow transplantation for acute myeloid leukemia: an update of the Seattle experience. Bone Marrow Transplant. 2000;26:397.
272. Storb R. Reduced-intensity conditioning transplantation in myeloid malignancies. Curr Opin Oncol. 2009;21(Suppl 1):S3.
273. Bejanyan N, Weisdorf DJ, Logan BR, et al. Survival of patients with acute myeloid leukemia relapsing after allogeneic hematopoietic cell transplantation: a center for international blood and marrow transplant research study. Biol Blood Marrow Transplant. 2015;21:454–9.
274. Jung AS, Holman PR, Castro JE, et al. Autologous hematopoietic stem cell transplantation as an intensive consolidation therapy for adult patients in remission from acute myelogenous leukemia. Biol Blood Marrow Transplant. 2009;15:1306.
275. Reiffers J, Gaspard MH, Maraninchi D, et al. Comparison of allogeneic or autologous bone marrow transplantation and chemotherapy in patients with acute myeloid leukaemia in first remission: a prospective controlled trial. Br J Haematol. 1989;72:57.
276. Woods WG, Neudorf S, Gold S, et al. A comparison of allogeneic bone marrow transplantation, autologous bone marrow transplantation, and aggressive chemotherapy in children with acute myeloid leukemia in remission. Blood. 2001;97:56.
277. Blaise D, Kuentz M, Fortanier C, et al. Randomized trial of bone marrow versus lenograstim-primed blood cell allogeneic transplantation in patients with early-stage leukemia: a report from the Societe Francaise de Greffe de Moelle. J Clin Oncol. 2000;18:537.
278. Champlin RE, Schmitz N, Horowitz MM, et al. Blood stem cells compared with bone marrow as a source of hematopoietic cells for allogeneic transplantation. IBMTR histocompatibility and stem cell sources working committee and the European group for blood and marrow transplantation (EBMT). Blood. 2000;95:3702.
279. Gorin NC, Labopin M, Blaise D, et al. Higher incidence of relapse with peripheral blood rather than marrow as a source of stem cells in adults with acute myelocytic leukemia autografted during the first remission. J Clin Oncol. 2009;27:3987.
280. Chao NJ, Stein AS, Long GD, et al. Busulfan/etoposide–initial experience with a new preparatory regimen for autologous bone marrow transplantation in patients with acute nonlymphocytic leukemia. Blood. 1993;81:319.
281. Laporte JP, Douay L, Lopez M, et al. One hundred twenty-five adult patients with primary acute leukemia autografted with marrow purged by mafosfamide: a 10-year single institution experience. Blood. 1994;84:3810.
282. To LB, Chin DKF, Blumberg PA, et al. Central nervous system relapse after bone marrow transplantation for acute myeloid leukemia. Cancer. 1983;52:2236.
283. Witherspoon R, Flournoy N, Thomas ED, et al. Recurrence of acute leukemia more than two years after allogeneic marrow grafting. Exp Hematol. 1986;14:178.
284. Stein J, Zimmerman PA, Kochera M, et al. Origin of leukemic relapse after bone marrow transplantation: comparison of cytogenetic and molecular analyses. Blood. 1989;73:2033.
285. Crow J, Youens K, Michalowski S, et al. Donor cell leukemia in umbilical cord blood transplant patients. A case study and literature review highlighting the importance of molecular engraftment analysis. J Mol Diagn. 2010;12(4):530–7.
286. Frassoni F, Labopin M, Gluckman E, et al. Are patients with acute leukemia, alive and well 2 years post bone marrow transplantation cured? A European survey. Leukemia. 1994;8:924.
287. Socie G, Stone JV, Wingard JR, et al. Long-term survival and late deaths after allogeneic bone marrow transplantation. N Engl J Med. 1999;341:14.
288. Conde E, Iriondo A, Rayon C, et al. Allogeneic bone marrow transplantation versus intensification chemotherapy for acute myelogenous leukaemia in first remission: a prospective controlled trial. Br J Haematol. 1988;68:219.
289. Zander AR, Keating M, Dicke C, et al. A comparison of marrow transplantation with chemotherapy for adults with acute leukemia of poor prognosis in first complete remission. J Clin Oncol. 1988;6:1548.
290. Appelbaum FR, Fisher LD, Thomas ED, et al. Chemotherapy v marrow transplantation for adults with acute nonlymphocytic leukemia: a five-year follow-up. Blood. 1988;72:179.
291. Vogelsang GB, Farmer ER, Hess AD, et al. Thalidomide for the treatment of chronic graft-versus-host disease. N Engl J Med. 1992;326:1055.
292. Bäckman L, Ringden O, Tollemar J, et al. An increased risk of relapse in cyclosporin-treated compared with methotrexate treated patients: long-term follow-up of a randomized trial. Bone Marrow Transplant. 1988;3:463.
293. Slovak ML, Kopecky KJ, Cassileth PA, et al. Karyotypic analysis predicts outcome of preremission and postremission therapy in adult acute myeloid leukemia: a Southwest Oncology Group/Eastern Cooperative Oncology Group study. Blood. 2000;96:4075.
294. Linker CA, Ries CA, Damon LE, et al. Autologous bone marrow transplantation for acute myeloid leukemia using busulfan plus etoposide as a preparative regimen. Blood. 1993;81:311.
295. Arai S, Aora M, Wang T, et al. Increasing incidence of chronic graft-versus-host disease in allogeneic transplantation: a report from the Center for Internantional Blood and Marrow Transplant Research. Biol Blood Marrow Transplant. 2015;21:266–74.
296. Styczynski J, Tridello G, Gil L, et al. Impact of donor Epstein-Barr virus serostatus on the incidence of graft-versus-host disease in patients with acute leukemia after hematopoietic stem-cell transplantation: a study from the Acute Leukemia and Infaectious Diseases Working Parties of the European Society for Blood and Marrow Transplantation. J Clin Oncol. 2016;34:2212–20.
297. Koreth J, Kim HT, Jones KT, et al. Efficacy, durability, and response predictors of low-dose interleukin-2 therapy for chronic graft-versus-host disease. Blood. 128:130–7.
298. Smits P, Schoots L, de Pauw BE, et al. Prognostic factors in adult patients with acute leukemia at first relapse. Cancer. 1987;59:1631.
299. Song K, Li M, Xu X, et al. Resistance to chemotherapy is associated with altered glucose metabolism in acute myeloid leukemia. Oncol Lett. 2016;12:334–42.
300. Ho AD, Lipp T, Ehninger G, et al. Combination of mitoxantrone and etoposide in refractory acute myelogenous leukemia-an active and well-tolerated regimen. J Clin Oncol. 1988;6:213.
301. McHayleh W, Sehgal R, Redner RL, et al. Mitoxantrone and etoposide in patients with newly diagnosed acute myeloid leukemia with persistent leukemia after a course of therapy with cytarabine and idarubicin. Leuk Lymphoma. 2009;50:1848.
302. Im A, Amjad A, Agha M, et al. Mitoxantrone and etoposide for the treatment of acute myeloid leukemia patients in first relapse. Oncol Res. 2016;24:73–80.
303. Thol F, Schlenk RF, Hauser M, Ganser A. How I treat refractory and early relapsed acute myeloid leukemia. Blood. 2015;126:319–25.
304. Tosi P, Visani G, Ottaviani E, et al. Fludarabine + Ara-C + G-CSF: cytotoxic effect and induction of apoptosis on fresh acute myeloid leukemia cells. Leukemia. 1994;8:2076.
305. Estey E, Thall P, Andreeff M, et al. Use of granulocyte colony-stimulating factor before, during, and after fludarabine plus cytarabine induction therapy of newly diagnosed acute myelogenous leukemia or myelodysplastic syndromes: comparison with fludarabine plus cytarabine without granulocyte colony-stimulating factor. J Clin Oncol. 1994;12:671.
306. Kornblau SM, Cortes-Franco J, Estey E. Neurotoxicity associated with fludarabine and cytosine arabinoside chemotherapy for acute leukemia and myelodysplasia. Leukemia. 1993;7:378.

307. Damiani D, Tiribelli M, Michelutti A, et al. Fludarabine-based induction therapy does not overcome the negative effect of ABCG2 (BCRP) over-expression in adult acute myeloid leukemia patients. Leuk Res. 2010;34(7):942–5.
308. Chantepie SP, Reboursiere E, Mear JB, et al. Gemtuzumab ozogamicin in combination with intensive chemotherapy in relapsed or refractory acute myeloid leukemia. Leuk Lymphoma. 2015;56:2326–30.
309. Hütter-Krönke ML, Benner A, Döhner K, et al. Salvage therapy with high-dose cytarabine and mitoxantrone in combination with all-trans retinoic acid and gemtuzumab ozogamicin in acute myeloid leukemia refractory to first induction therapy. Haematologica. 2016;101:839–45.
310. Thiel A, Schetelig J, Pönish W, et al. Mito-FLAG with Ara-C as bolus versus continuous infusion in recurrent or refractory AML-long term results of a prospective randomized intergroup study of the East German Study Group Hematology/Oncology (OSHO) and the Study Alliance Leukemia (SAL). Ann Oncol. 2015;26:1434–40.
311. Hospital MA, Prebet T, Bertoli S, et al. Core-binding factor acute myeloid leukemia in first relapse: a retrospective study from the French AML Intergroup. Blood. 2014;124:1312–9.
312. Levi JA, Wiernik PH. A comparative clinical trial of 5-azacytidine and guanazole in previously treated adults 187 with acute non-lymphocytic leukemia. Cancer. 1976;38:36.
313. Czibere A, Bruns I, Kröger N, et al. 5-azacytidine for the treatment of patients with acute myeloid leukemia or myelodysplastic syndrome who relapse after allo-SCT: a retrospective analysis. Bone Marrow Transplant. 2009;45:872–6.
314. Lűbbert M, Bertz H, Wäsch R, et al. Efficacy of a 3-day, low-dose treatment with 5-azacytidine followed by donor lymphocyte infusions in older patients with acute myeloid leukemia or chronic myelomonocytic leukemia relapsed after allografting. Bone Marrow Transplant. 2010;45(4):627–32.
315. Steinmann J, Bertz H, Wäsch R, et al. 5-azacitidine and DLI can induce long-term remissions in AML patients relapsed after allograft. Bone Marrow Transplant. 2015;50:690–5.
316. Craddock C, Labopin M, Robin M, et al. Clinical activity of azacitidine in patients who relapse after allogeneic stem cell transplantation for acute myeloid leukemia. Haematologica. 2016;101:879–83.
317. Fenaux P, Mufti GJ, Hellström-Lindberg E, et al. Azacitidine prolongs overall survival compared with conventional care regimens in elderly patients with low bone marrow blast count acute myeloid leukemia. J Clin Oncol. 2009;28:562.
318. Cashen AF, Schiller GJ, O'Donnell MR, DiPersio JF. Multicenter, phase II study of decitabine for the first-line treatment of older patients with acute myeloid leukemia. J Clin Oncol. 2010;28:556.
319. Chowdhury S, Seropian S, Marks PW. Decitabine combined with fractionated gemtuzumab ozogamicin therapy in patients with relapsed or refractory acute myeloid leukemia. Am J Hematol. 2009;84:599.
320. Delmer A, Bauduer F, Vekhoff A, et al. Evaluation of carboplatin as a single agent in highly refractory acute myeloid leukemia. Leuk Lymphoma. 1994;15:311.
321. Sievers EL, Appelbaum FR, Spielberger RT, et al. Selective ablation of acute myeloid leukemia using antibody-targeted chemotherapy: a phase I study of an anti-CD33 calicheamicin immunoconjugate. Blood. 1999;93:3678.
322. Sievers EL, Larson RA, Stadtmauer EA, et al. Efficacy and safety of gemtuzumab ozogamicin in patients with CD33-positive acute myeloid leukemia in first relapse. J Clin Oncol. 2001;19:3244.
323. Martin MG, Augustin KM, Uy GL, et al. Salvage therapy for acute myeloid leukemia with fludarabine, cytarabine, and idarubicin with or without gemtuzumab ozogamicin and with concurrent or sequential G-CSF. Am J Hematol. 2009;84:733.
324. Yamaguchi Y, Usul N, Dobashi N, et al. Gemtuzumab ozogamicin (GO) in relapsed/refractory patients with acute myeloid leukemia. Gan To Kagaku Ryoho. 2009;36:1105.
325. Litzow MR, Othus M, Cripe LD, et al. Failure of three novel regimen to improve outcome for patients with relapsed or refractory acute myeloid leukaemia: a report from the Eastern Cooperative Oncology Group. Br J Haematol. 2010;148:217.
326. Löwenberg B, Beck J, Graux C, et al. Gemtuzumab ozogamicin as postremission treatment in AML at 60 years of age or more: results of a multicenter phase 3 study. Blood. 2010;115:2586.
327. O'Boyle KP, Murigeppa A, Jain D, et al. Probable veno-occlusive disease after treatment with gemtuzumab ozogamicin in a patient with acute myeloid leukemia and a history of liver transplantation for familial hemochromatosis. Med Oncol. 2003;20:379.
328. Balaian L, Ball ED. Cytotoxic activity of gemtuzumab ozogamicin (Mylotarg) in acute myeloid leukemia correlates with the expression of protein kinase Syk. Leukemia. 2006;20:2093.
329. Ravandi F, Kantarjian H, Faderl S, et al. Outcome of patients with FLT3-mutated acute myeloid leukemia in first relapse. Leuk Res. 2010;34(6):752–6.
330. Voutsasakis IA. Flt 3 in acute myelogenous leukemia: biology, prognosis, and therapeutic implications. Med Oncol. 2003;20:311.
331. Pemmaraju N, Kantarjian HM, Ravandi F, et al. Flt3 inhibitor therapy for patients with myelodysplastic syndromes (MDS) and acute myeloid leukemia (AML): impact on survival according to FLT3 status. Blood. 2009;114:424. Abstract 1026
332. Mori Y, Kiyoi H, Ishikawa Y, et al. Fl-dependent wild-type FLT3 signals reduce the inhibitory effects of FLT3 inhibitors on wild-type and mutant FLT3 co-expressing cells. Blood. 2009;114:816. Abstract 2067
333. Metzelder S, Scholl S, Matthias K, et al. Compassionate use of sorafenib in relapsed and refractory FLT3-ITD positive acute myeloid leukemia. Blood. 2009;114:813. Abstract 2060
334. Lee SH, Paietta E, Racevskis J, Wiernik PH. Complete resolution of leukemia cutis with sorafenib in an acute myeloid leukemia patient with FLT3-ITD mutation. Am J Hematol. 2009;84:701.
335. Ravandi F, Cortes JE, Jones D, et al. Phase I/II study of combination therapy with sorafenib, idarubicin, and cytarabine in younger patients with acute myeloid leukemia. J Clin Oncol. 2010;28:1856.
336. Yee KW, Schittenhelm M, O'Farrell AM, et al. Synergistic effects of SU11248 with cytarabine or daunorubicin on FLT3-ITD-positive leukemia cells. Blood. 2004;104:4202.
337. Fiedler W, Serve H, Döhner H, et al. A phase I study of SU11248 in the treatment of patients with refractory or resistant acute myeloid leukemia (AML) or not amenable to conventional therapy for the disease. Blood. 2005;105:986.
338. Stone RM, Fischer T, Paquette R, et al. Phase 1b study of midostaurin (PKC412) in combination with daunorubicin and cytarabine induction and high-dose cytarabine consolidation in patients under age 61 with newly diagnosed de novo acute myeloid leukemia: overall survival of patients whose blasts have FLT3 mutations is similar to those with wild-type FLT3. Blood. 2009;114:263. Abstract 634
339. Levis M, Ravandi F, Wang ES, et al. Results from a randomized trial of salvage chemotherapy followed by lestaurtinib for FLT3 mutant AML patients in first relapse. Blood. 2009;114:325. Abstract 788
340. Zarrinkar PP, Gunawardane RN, Cramer MD, et al. AC220 is a uniquely potent and selective inhibitor of FLT3 for the treatment of acute myeloid leukemia (AML). Blood. 2009;114:2984.
341. Belli BA, Dao A, Bhagwat S, et al. AC220, a potent and specific FLT3 inhibitor, enhances the cytotoxic effects of chemotherapeutic agents in cell culture and in mouse tumor xenografts. Blood. 2009;114:810. Abstract 2052
342. Robles C, Kim KM, Oken MM, et al. Low-dose cytarabine maintenance therapy vs observation after remission induction

in advanced acute myeloid leukemia: an Eastern Cooperative Oncology Group Trial (E5483). Leukemia. 2000;14:1349.
343. Lee S, Tallman MS, Oken MM, et al. Duration of second complete remission compared with first complete remission in patients with acute myeloid leukemia. Eastern Cooperative Oncology Group. Leukemia. 2000;14:1345.
344. Braun T, Fenaux P. Farnesyltransferase inhibitors and their potential role in therapy for myelodysplastic syndromes and acute myeloid leukaemia. Br J Haematol. 2008;141:576.
345. Epling-Burnette PK, Loughran TP Jr. Suppression of farnesyltransferase activity in acute myeloid leukemia and myelodysplastic syndrome: current understanding and recommended use of tipifarnib. Expert Opin Investig Drugs. 2010;19:689.
346. Harousseau JL, Martinelli G, Jedrzejczak WWW, et al. A randomized phase 3 study of tipifarnib compared with best supportive care, including hydroxyurea, in the treatment of newly diagnosed acute myeloid leukemia in patients 70 years or older. Blood. 2009;114:1166.
347. Van der Weide K, de Jonge-Peeters SD, Kuipers F, et al. Combining simvastatin with the farnesyltransferase inhibitor tipifarnib results in an enhanced cytotoxic effect in a subset of primary CD34+ acute myeloid leukemia samples. Clin Cancer Res. 2009;15:3076.
348. Camera A, Rinaldi CR, Palmieri S, et al. Sequential continuous infusion of fludarabine and cytarabine associated with liposomal daunorubicin (DaunoXome) (FLAD) in primary refractory or relapsed adult acute myeloid leukemia patients. Ann Hematol. 2009;88:151.
349. Forman SJ, Schmidt GM, Nademanee AP, et al. Allogeneic bone marrow transplantation as therapy for primary induction failure for patients with acute leukemia. J Clin Oncol. 1991;9:1570.
350. Clift RA, Buckner CD, Appelbaum FR, et al. Allogeneic marrow transplantation during untreated first relapse of acute myeloid leukemia. J Clin Oncol. 1992;10:1723.
351. Blume KG, Kopecky KJ, Henslee-Downey JP, et al. A prospective randomized comparison of total body irradiation-etoposide versus busulfan-cyclophosphamide as preparatory regimens for bone marrow transplantation in patients with leukemia who were not in first remission: a Southwest Oncology Group study. Blood. 1993;81:2187.
352. Petersen FB, Lynch MHE, Clift RA, et al. Autologous marrow transplantation for patients with acute myeloid leukemia in untreated first relapse or in second complete remission. J Clin Oncol. 1993;11:1353.
353. Brown RA, Herzig RH, Wolff SN, et al. High-dose etoposide and cyclophosphamide without bone marrow transplantation for resistant hematologic malignancy. Blood. 1990;76:473.
354. Ipilimumab for patients with relapse after allogeneic transplantation. N Engl J Med. 2016;372:143–54.
355. Fefer A, Benyunes MC, Massumoto C, et al. Interleukin-2 therapy after autologous bone marrow transplantation for hematologic malignancies. Semin Oncol. 1993;20(Suppl 9):41.
356. Blaise D, Attal M, Pico JL, et al. The use of a sequential high dose recombinant interleukin 2 regimen after autologous bone marrow transplantation does not improve the disease free survival of patients with acute leukemia transplanted in first complete remission. Leuk Lymphoma. 1997;25:469.
357. Blaise D, Attal M, Reiffers J, et al. Randomized study of recombinant interleukin-2 after autologous bone marrow transplantation for acute leukemia in first complete remission. Eur Cytokine Netw. 2000;11:91.
358. Thomas X, Le Q, Botton S, et al. Autologous or allogeneic stem cell transplantation as post-remission therapy in refractory or relapsed acute myeloid leukemia after highly intensive chemotherapy. Leuk Lymphoma. 2005;46:1007.
359. Dazzi F, Goldman J. Donor lymphocyte infusions. Curr Opin Hematol. 1999;6:394.
360. Schmid C, Labopin M, Nagler A, et al. Donor lymphocyte infusion in the treatment of first hematological relapse after allogeneic stem-cell transplantation in adults with acute myeloid leukemia: a retrospective risk factors analysis and comparison with other strategies by the EBMT acute leukemia working party. J Clin Oncol. 2007;25:4938.
361. Deol A, Lum LG. Role of donor lymphocyte infusions in relapsed hematological malignancies after stem cell transplantation revisited. Cancer Treat Rev. 2010;36(7):528–38.
362. Imoto S, Muryama T, Gomyo H, et al. Long-term molecular remission induced by donor lymphocyte infusions for recurrent acute myeloblastic leukemia after allogeneic bone marrow transplantation. Bone Marrow Transplant. 2000;26:809.
363. Porter DL, Collins RH Jr, Hardy C, et al. Treatment of relapsed leukemia after unrelated donor marrow transplantation with unrelated donor leukocyte infusions. Blood. 2000;95:1214.
364. McSweeney PA, Niederwieser D, Shizuru JA, et al. Hematopoietic cell transplantation in older patients with hematologic malignancies: replacing high-dose cytotoxic therapy with graft-versus-tumor effects. Blood. 2001;97:3390.
365. Röllig C, Thiede C, Gramatzki M, et al. A novel prognostic model in elderly patients with acute myeloid leukemia-results of 909 patients entered into the prospective AML96 trial. Blood. 2010;116:971–8.
366. Dickson GJ, Bustraan S, Hills RK, et al. The value of molecular stratification for CEBPA (DM) and NPM1(MUT) FLT3(WT) genotypes in older patients with acute myeloid leukaemia. Br J Haematol. 2016;172:573–80.
367. Lee SH, Abebe L, Paietta E, et al. Reappearance of acute myeloid leukemia after almost 23 years of continuous complete remission. Am J Hematol. 2009;84:455.
368. Verma D, Kantarjian H, Faderl S, et al. Late relapses in acute myeloid leukemia: analysis of characteristics and outcome. Leuk Lymphoma. 2010;51:778.
369. Rao AV, Valk PJ, Metzeler KH, et al. Age-specific differences in oncogenic pathway dysregulation and anthracycline sensitivity in patients with acute myeloid leukemia. J Clin Oncol. 2009;27:5580.
370. Kweon SH, Song JH, Kim TS. Resveratrol-mediated reversal of doxorubicin resistance in acute myeloid leukemia cells via downregulation of MRP1 expression. Biochem Biophys Res Commun. 2010;395:104.
371. Heiblig M, Elhamri M, Tigaud I, et al. Treatment with low-dose cytarabine in elderly patients (age 70 years or older) with acute myeloid leukemia: A single institution experience. Mediterr J Hematol Infect Dis. 2016;8:e2016009.
372. Kantarjian HM, Erba HP, Claxton D, et al. Phase II study of clofarabine monotherapy in previously untreated older adults with acute myeloid leukemia and unfavorable prognostic factors. J Clin Oncol. 2010;28:549.
373. Burnett AK, Russell NH, Kell J, et al. European development of clofarabine as treatment for older patients with acute myeloid leukemia considered unsuitable for intensive therapy. J Clin Oncol. 2010;28:815.
374. Kadia TM, Faderl S, Ravandi F, et al. Final results of a phase 2 trial of clofarabine and low-dose cytarabine alternating with decitabine in older patients with newly diagnosed acute myeloid leukemia. Cancer. 2015;121:2375–82.
375. Takahashi K, Kantarjian H, Garcia-Manero G, et al. Clofarabine plus low-dose cytarabine is as effective as and less toxic than intensive chemotherapy in elderly AML patients. Clin Lymphoma Myeloma Leuk. 2016;16:163–8.
376. Middeke JM, Herbst R, Parmentier S, Bug G, et al. Clofarabine salvage therapy before allogeneic hematopoietic stem cell transplantation in patients with relapsed or refractory AML: results of the BRIDGE trial. Leukemia. 2016;30:261–7.
377. Stuart RK, Cripe LD, Maris MB, et al. REVEAL-1, a phase 2 dose regimen optimization study of vosaroxin in older poor-risk

patients with previously untreated acute myeloid leukaemia. Br J Haematol. 2015;168:796–805.
378. Dennis M, Russell N, Hills RK, et al. Vosaroxin and vosaroxin plus low-dose Ara-c (LDAC) vs low-dose Ara-c alone in older patients with acute myeloid leukemia. Blood. 2015;125:2923–32.
379. Ravandi F, Ritchie EK, Sayar H, et al. Vosaroxin plus cytarabine versus placebo plus cytarabine in patients with first relapsed or refractory acute myeloid leukaemia (VALOR): a randomized, controlled, double-blind, multinational, phase 3 study. Lancet Oncol. 2015;16:1025–36.
380. Mawad R, Becker PS, Hendrie P, et al. Phase II study of tosedostat with cytarabine or decitabine in newly diagnosed older patients with acute myeloid leukaemia or high-risk MDS. Br J Haematol. 2016;172:238–45.
381. Grishina O, Schmoor C, Döhner K, et al. DECIDER: prospective randomized multicenter phase II trial of low-dose decitabine (DAC) administered alone or in combination with the histone deacetylase inhibitor valproic acid (VPA) and all-trans retinoic acid (ATRA) in patients > 60 60 years with acute myeloid leukemia who are ineligible for induction therapy. BMC Cancer. 2015;15:430.
382. Daver N, Kantarjian H, Ravandi F, et al. A phase II study of decitabine and gemtuzumab ozogamicin in newly diagnosed and relapsed acute myeloid leukemia and high-risk myelodysplastic syndrome. Leukemia. 2016;30:268–73.
383. Gupta N, Miller A, Gandhi S, et al. Comparison of epigenetic versus standard induction chemotherapy for newly diagnosed acute myeloid leukemia patients ≥ 60 years old. Am J Hematol. 2015;90:639–46.
384. Pleyer L, Burgstaller S, Girchikofsky M, et al. Azacitidine in 302 patients with WHO-defined acute myeloid leukemia: results from the Austrian azacitidine registry of the AGMT-Study Group. Ann Hematol. 2014;93:1825–38.
385. Thépot S, Itzykson R, Seegers V, et al. Azacitidine in untreated acute myeloid leukemia: a report on 149 patients. Am J Hematol. 2014;89:410–6.
386. Griffin PT, Komrokji RS, De Castro CM, et al. A multicenter, phase II study of maintenance azacitidine in older patients with acute myeloid leukemia in complete remission after induction chemotherapy. Am J Hematol. 2015;90:796–9.
387. Dombret H, Seymour JF, Butrym A, et al. International phase 3 study of azacitidine vs conventional care regimens in older patients with newly diagnosed AML with >30% blasts. Blood. 2015;126:291–9.
388. Müller-Tidow C, Tschanter P, Röllig C, et al. Azacitidine in combination with intensive induction chemotherapy in older patients with acute myeloid leukemia: The AML-AZA trial of the Study Alliance Leukemia. Leukemia. 2016;30:555–61.
389. Prebet T, Sun Z, Ketterling RP, et al. Azacitidine with or without entinostat for treatment of therapy-related myeloid neoplasm: further results of the E1905 North American Leukemia Intergroup study. Br J Haematol. 2016;172:384–91.
390. Ravandi F, Alattar ML, Grunwald MR, et al. Phase 2 study of azacitidine plus sorafenib in patients with acute myeloid leukemia and FLT3 internal tandem duplication mutation. Blood. 2013;121:4655–62.
391. Wei A, Tan P, Perruzza S, et al. Maintenance lenalidomide in combination with 5-azacitidine as post-remission therapy for acute myeloid leukaemia. Br J Haematol. 2015;169:199–210.
392. Butrym A, Rybka J, Baczyńska D, et al. Clinical response to azacitidine therapy depends on microRNA-29c (miR-29c) expression in older acute myeloid leukemia (AML) patients. Oncotarget. 2016;7:30250–57.
393. Amadori S, Suciu S, Stasi R, et al. Sequential combination of gemtuzumab ozogamicin and standard chemotherapy in older patients with newly diagnosed acute myeloid leukemia: results of a randomized phase III trial by the EORTC and GIMEMA consortium (AML-17). J Clin Oncol. 2013;31:4424–30.
394. Amadori S, Suciu S, Sellslag D, et al. Gemtuzumab ozogamicin versus best supportive care in older patients with newly diagnosed acute myeloid leukemia unsuitable for intensive chemotherapy: results of the randomized phase III EORTC-GIMEMA AML-19 trial. J Clin Oncol. 34:972–9.
395. Serve H, Krug U, Wagner R, et al. Sorafenib in combination with intensive chemotherapy in elderly patients with acute myeloid leukemia: results from a randomized, placebo-controlled trial. J Clin Oncol. 2013;31:3110–8.
396. Sammons SL, Pratz KW, Douglas SSmith B, et al. Sorafenib is tolerable and improves clinical outcomes in patients with FLT3-ITD acute myeloid leukemia prior to stem cell transplant and after relspse post-transplant. Am J Hematol. 2014;89:936–8.
397. Lancet JE, et al. Final results of phase III randomized trial of CPX-351 versus 7+3 in older patients with newly diagnosed high risk (secondary) AML. J Clin Oncol. 2016;34(15S):375s. (Abstract 7000)
398. Medeiros BC, Satram-Hoang S, Hurst D, et al. Big data analysis of treatment patterns and outcomes among elderly acute myeloid leukemia patients in the United States. Ann Hematol. 2015;94:1127–38.
399. Alibhai SM, Breunis H, Timishina N, et al. Quality of life and physical function in adults treated with intensive chemotherapy for acute myeloid leukemia improve over time independent of age. J Geriatr Oncol. 2015;6:262–71.
400. Stewart DJ, Smith TL, Keating MJ, et al. Remission from central nervous system involvement in adults with acute leukemia. Cancer. 1985;56:632.
401. Wolach O, Stone RM. How I treat mixed-phenotype acute leukemia. Blood. 2015;125:2477–85.
402. McKerrell T, Moreno T, Ponstingl H, et al. Development and validation of a comprehensive genomic diagnostic tool for myeloid malignancies. Blood. 2016;128:e1–9.
403. Willekens C, Blanchet C, Renneville A, et al. Prospective long-term minimal residual disease monitoring using RQ-PCR in RUNX1-RUNX1T1-positive acute myeloid leukemia: results of the French CBF-2006 trial. Haematologica. 2016;101:328–35.
404. Malmberg EB, Ståhlman S, Rehammar A, et al. Patient-tailored analysis of minimal residual disease in acute myeloid leukemia using next generation sequencing. Eur J Haematol. 2017;98:26–37.
405. Klco JM, Miller CA, Griffith M, et al. Association between mutation clearance after induction therapy and outcomes in acute myeloid leukemia. JAMA. 2015;314:811–22.
406. Martelli MP, Gionfriddo I, Mezzasoma F, et al. Arsenic trioxide and all-trans retinoic acid target NPM1 mutant oncoprotein levels and induce apoptosis in NPM1-mutated AML cells. Blood. 2015;125:3455–65.
407. Murphy C, Blanchard J, Genser A, et al. High-throughput drug screening identifies pyrimethamine as a potent and selective inhibitor of acute myeloid leukemia. Curr Cancer Drug Targets. 2016.; (In Press)
408. Subklewe M, Geiger C, Lichtenegger FS, et al. New generation dendritic cell vaccine for immunotherapy of acute myeloid leukemia. Cancer Immunol Immunother. 2014;63:1093–103.
409. Di Stasi A, Jimenez AM, Minagawa K, et al. Review of the results of WT1 peptide vaccination strategies for myelodysplastic syndromes and acute myeloid leukemia from nine different studies. Front Immunol. 2015;6:36.
410. Kosciuczuk EM, Saleiro D, Kroczynska B, et al. Merestinib blocks MNK kinase activity in acute myeloid leukemia progenitors and exhibits antileukemic effects in vitro and in vivo. Blood. 2016;128:410–14.

411. Dorrance AM, Neviani P, Ferenchak GJ, et al. Targeting leukemia stem cells in vivo with antagomiR-126 nanoparticles in acute myeloid leukemia. Leukemia. 2015;29:2143–53.
412. Jiang X, Bugno J, Hu C, et al. Eradication of acute myeloid leukemia with FLT3 ligand-targeted miR-150 nanoparticles. Cancer Res. 2016;76:4470–80.
413. Cole A, Wang Z, Coyaud E, et al. Inhibition of the mitochondrial protease ClpP as a therapeutic strategy for human acute myeloid leukemia. Cancer Cell. 2015;27:864–76.
414. Hazenberg M, Gillissen M, Martijn Kedde M, et al. Acute myeloid leukemia (AML) patients cured after allogeneic hematopoietic stem cell transplantation generate tumor-specific cytotoxic antibodies that kill AML blasts. Eur Hematol Assoc Cong. 2016.; abstract S124
415. Xu S, Li X, Zhang J, Chen J. Prognostic value of CD11b expression level for acute myeloid leukemia patients: a meta-analysis. PLoS One. 2015;10:e0135981.
416. Li M, Gao L, Li Z, et al. CTNNA1 hypermethylation, a frequent event in acute myeloid leukemia, is independently associated with an adverse outcome. Oncotraget. 2016;7:31454–65.
417. Colamesta V, D'Aguanno S, Breccia M, et al. Do the smoking intensity and duration, the years since quitting, the methodological quality and the year of publication of the studies affect the results of the meta-analysis on cigarette smoking and acute myeloid leukemia (AML) in adults? Crit Rev Oncol Hematol. 2016;99:376–88.
418. Ghimire KB, Shah BK. Second primary malignancies in adult acute myeloid leukemia-A US population-based study. Anticancer Res. 2014;34:3855–9.
419. Chen CY, Huang SY, Cheng A, et al. High risk of hepatitis B reactivation among patients with acute myeloid leukemia. PLoS One. 2015;10:e0126037.
420. Barton JC, Conrad ME. Beneficial effects of hepatitis in patients with acute myelogenous leukemia. Ann Intern Med. 1979;90:185–90.
421. Wong KK Jr, Golomb HM, Rowley J, et al. Prognostic significance of posttransfusion hepatitis and chromosomal abnormalities in adult acute nonlymphocytic leukemia. Cancer Genet Cytogenet. 1982;5:281–92.
422. Wade JC, Gaffey M, Wiernik PH, et al. Hepatitis in patients with acute nonlymphocytic leukemia. Am J Med. 1983;75:413–22.

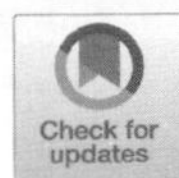

Acute Promyelocytic Leukemia

21

Peter H. Wiernik, Robert E. Gallagher, and Martin S. Tallman

Introduction

Acute promyelocytic leukemia (APL) is designated M3 in the French-American-British (FAB) classification. Because of its unique clinical features and unique response to certain differentiation inducing agents, and because of our advanced understanding of the molecular biology of this leukemia, APL deserves to be presented and discussed in detail, apart from the other acute myeloid leukemias.

APL was first described by Hillestad in 1957 [1, 2]. Three patients were described with the characteristic morphology of hypergranular APL, hypofibrinogenemia, and a hemorrhagic diathesis [1]. Caen et al. [3] established that the hemorrhagic syndrome was directly related to the proliferation of the leukemic cells in APL, and Bernard et al. [4] provided a precise description of the disease in a presentation that included 20 patients. Bernard et al. [5] subsequently discovered the unusual sensitivity of this AML variant to daunorubicin, an important observation revisited in the all-trans retinoic acid (ATRA) era discussed in detail next. Rowley et al. in 1976–1977 described the balanced cytogenetic translocation (15;17) in APL [6, 7] and found it to be present in virtually every patient (Fig. 21.1) [8]. Kantarjian et al. [9] reported that chemotherapy could induce complete remissions (CR) in APL without inducing marrow hypoplasia and that remission was often the result of a gradual morphologic evolution, an observation later confirmed by Stone et al. [10] who suggested that the mechanism of remission in APL may be leukemic cell differentiation. Breitman et al. [11] demonstrated that maturation and differentiation of leukemic cells thought to be human APL cells (HL-60 cell line) could be accomplished in vitro by several agents including retinoids. Huang et al. [12] reported the first large series of APL patients treated with oral ATRA and demonstrated a phenomenally high rate of relatively brief CR. Fenaux and colleagues [13] treated APL with ATRA and standard chemotherapy and reported results superior to those obtained with either treatment alone, and subsequently, arsenic trioxide was identified as the most active single agent in APL [14]. Coincident with these treatment advances, there has been an explosion of knowledge of APL at the molecular level. All of these events taken together have contributed to the fact that APL is now the most curable variant of acute myeloid leukemia in adults [15, 16]. For a more detailed history of APL, the reader is referred to Bernard [17].

Molecular Biological Aspects of APL

Overall Perspective

Perhaps more is known about the molecular biology of APL, both in terms of genetic mechanism and potential for tumor cell specific therapy, than for any other specific type of human cancer. The historical background underlying this statement derives from two distinct lines of investigation. One is genetic in nature, beginning with the discovery in 1977 that the APL phenotype of AML is consistently associated with a reciprocal translocation between chromosomes 15 and 17 [7]. The second is biological, stemming from the finding in 1981 that APL cells are unique in their property of undergoing terminal differentiation after exposure in short-term tissue culture to supraphysiological concentrations of the naturally occurring metabolite of vitamin A, all-*trans* retinoic acid (ATRA) [18]. The clinical relevance of the

P.H. Wiernik, M.D., D.hc., FASCO (✉)
Leukemia Program, Cancer Center, St. Lukes—Roosevelt and Beth Israel Hospitals, New York, NY 10019, USA
e-mail: pwiernik@aol.com

R.E. Gallagher, M.D.
Albert Einstein Cancer Center, 111 East 210th Street, Bronx, New York, NY 10467, USA
e-mail: robert.gallagher@einstein.yu.edu

M.S. Tallman, M.D.
Memorial Sloan Kettering Cancer Center, Weill Cornell Medical College, 1275 York Avenue, 380, New York, NY 10065, USA
e-mail: tallmanm@mskcc.org

P.H. Wiernik et al. (eds.), *Neoplastic Diseases of the Blood*, DOI 10.1007/978-3-319-64263-5_21

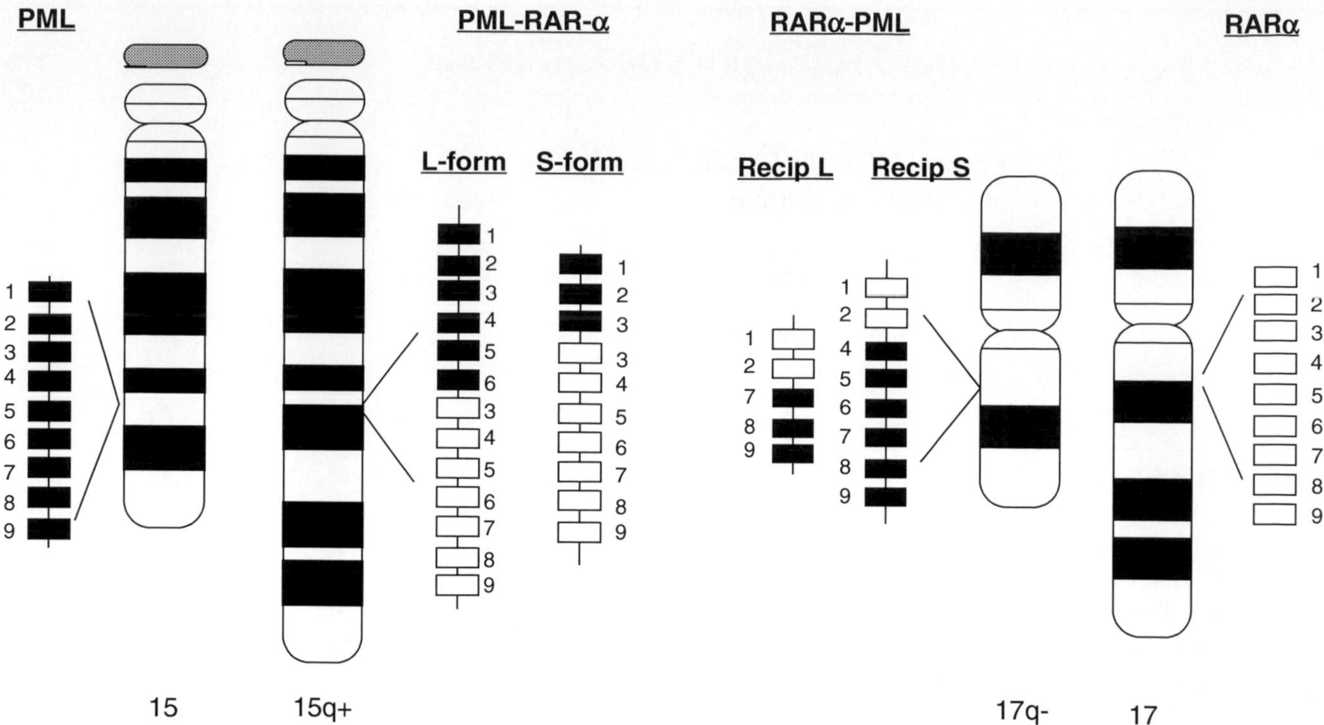

Fig. 21.1 Normal and translocated chromosomes 15 and 17 and the corresponding mRNA transcripts for the normal and hybrid forms of PML and RARα present in a typical case of APL. The vertical chains of *boxes* represent the 9 exons of both the PML (*filled boxes*) and RARα (*empty boxes*) gene transcripts. The short (S) and long (L) forms of PML-RARα result from break sites in PML introns 3 and 6, respectively, whereas RARa is uniformly broken in intron 2

in vitro findings was demonstrated in 1988 when Chinese investigators reported that ATRA produces complete remissions in a high percentage of APL patients [19]. In 1990, there was a remarkable confluence of these two investigative lines with the discovery that the t(15;17) consistently produced breakage of the retinoic acid receptor-alpha (RARα) gene on chromosome band 17q11–21 [20–22]. This seminal discovery provided instant access to a wealth of molecular information that had been developed related to the RARα gene since its discovery in 1987 [23, 24], which, as a ligand-dependent nuclear transcription factor that mediates cellular responses to ATRA, had obvious implications for the selective action of ATRA in APL cells. The following year, the fusion partner of the RARα gene from chromosome 15 was identified and was originally called myl but subsequently renamed PML (for ProMyeLocytes or ProMyelocytic Leukemia) [25–27]. Thus, the two hybrid gene products which result from the reciprocal t(15;17) in APL are PML-RARα and RARα-PML (Fig. 21.1).

In the intervening years, six alternative fusion gene partners of RARα have been discovered in rare cases of APL, each associated with a unique chromosome translocation (le 23.1; see discussion that follows) [28–33]. All of the fusion proteins include the same amino-truncated portion of RARα, indicating the central role of RARα in the pathogenesis of APL. The involvement of the PML gene in >98% of APL cases implies that it also contributes some essential function to pathogenesis, which has gained support from a variety of findings. Although the alternative fusion genes, generically referred to as X-RARαs, are rare and, hence are of limited clinical impact, they have provided useful information about the molecular pathogenesis of APL and about the effect of therapeutic agents on APL cells [34, 35].

Another milestone in the history of APL were mid-1990s Chinese reports that arsenic trioxide (ATO) was, like ATRA, selectively effective for the clinical treatment of APL but that the molecular biological response was different [14, 36]. These differences are presented in some detail in the succeeding sections as they relate both to the initial APL response to ATRA and ATO and to the development of resistance in the declining fraction of patients who experience disease relapse after treatment with these highly effective agents.

Studies of the molecular biology of APL have been markedly abetted by the establishment of the fusion gene-positive APL cell line NB4 in 1991 [37]. The derivation of this cell line importantly permitted more specific molecular evaluations than possible with the antecedent ATRA-sensitive prototype cell line HL-60 that had been isolated from a patient with APL features but lacked the PML-RARα fusion gene [38, 39].

Additionally, the development of transgenic mice (TM) bearing the fusion genes has provided an important resource for evaluating the role of the different fusion genes in APL pathogenesis and treatment [35, 40]. Recently, the TM models as well as studies with fusion gene-transduced hematopoietic progenitor cells have provided important insights into attributes of the so-called APL leukemia-initiating cell (LIC), which have important implications for treatment strategies [41–43]. However, detailed biological and molecular characterization of these LIC that are required for sustaining and propagating the disease must await their physical separation for analysis.

RARα and the Essentials of Nuclear Receptor Function

RARα is a member of the steroid/thyroid hormone receptor gene superfamily, which encodes proteins that function as ligand-dependent regulators of gene transcription [44]. Most essentially, these proteins contain two domains, a DNA binding domain (DBD) near the amino terminus and a ligand binding domain (LBD) near the carboxy terminus (Fig. 21.2). The DBD contains two characteristic zinc finger motifs that bind the receptors to specific oligonucleotide sequences, hormone response elements (HREs), in the promoter region of select genes, many of which have central effects on cell and tissue growth, differentiation, and homeostasis. RARs, which include separate genes for RARβ and RARγ in addition to RARα, belong to one major branch of the steroid/hormone receptor superfamily, along with the thyroid hormone receptors and vitamin D3 receptor. These nuclear receptors have the common property of residing in the nucleus in a bound state to their respective HREs, consisting of two direct repeats of the hexanucleotide (A/G)G(G/T) TCA (Figs. 21.2 and 21.3a). These receptors also share the property of binding to HREs as a heterodimer with common adapter proteins called retinoid X receptors (Figs. 21.2 and 21.3a), of which there are also three different genes (RXR-α, β, and γ). The discriminator for HRE specificity is the number of nucleotides between the two direct repeats, which is 2 or 5 for retinoic acid response elements (RAREs), 3 for vitamin D3 RE (VDRE), and 4 for thyroid hormone RE (TREs). Additionally, HRE spacers with one nucleotide have specificity for RXR homodimers or, in some cases, may heterodimerize with RAR in reverse polarity [45]. Through expression of different combinations of RXR/RAR heterodimers, variations in RAREs, competition between nuclear receptors and alternative transcription factors for limiting quantities of RXRs, and differences in retinoid ligand utilization, the retinoid receptor system can generate enormous heterogeneity which has been related to the discriminatory, instructive

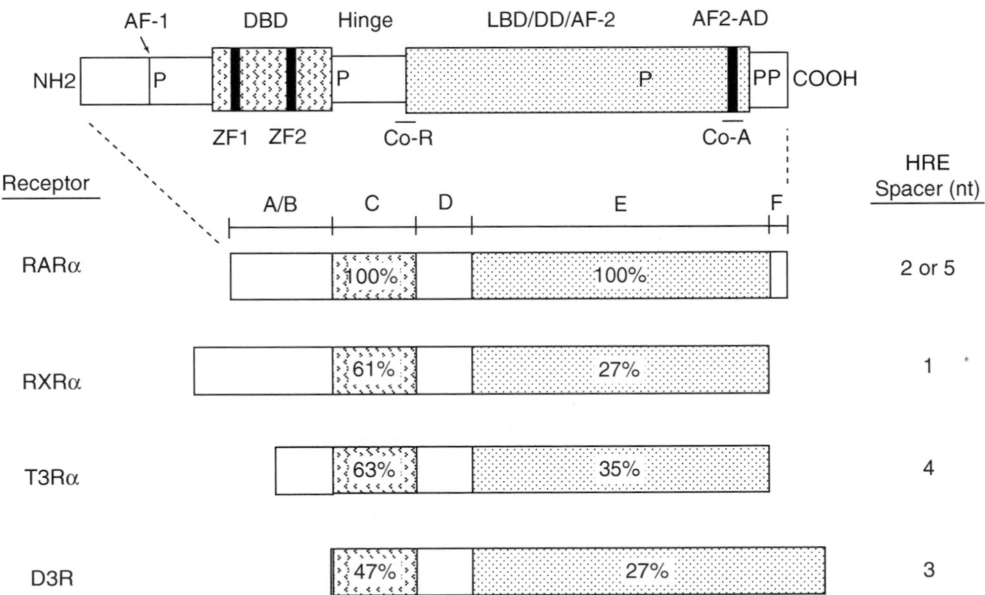

Fig. 21.2 Structure of RARα and its homology to related members of the RAR-RXR-T3R-D3R branch of the steroid-thyroid hormone receptor gene superfamily. AF1, activator function 1 (ligand-independent) domain; DBD, DNA-binding domain; LBD/DD/AF2, shared ligand binding, heterodimerization (RXR) and activator function 2 (ligand-dependent) domains; ZF1 and ZF2, zinc fingers 1 and 2; AF2-AD, AF2 activation core domain containing consensus sequence for binding coactivators (Co-A); CoR, corepressor-binding domain; P, phosphorylation sites. A through F are standard assigned regions/domains of these proteins. Vertical *arrow* indicates the universal break site in RARa between the A and B domains that occur in formation of the various fusion proteins. Percentage numbers indicate the degree of amino acid sequence homology of the DNA-binding (C-regions) and ligand-binding (E-regions) domains of each receptor protein to RARa. HRE, hormone response element; the numbers beneath indicate the number of nucleotides (nt) between the two one-half site direct repeats, PuG(G/T)TCA

a Co-repressor complex inhibits transcription by RXR/RARα heterodimer

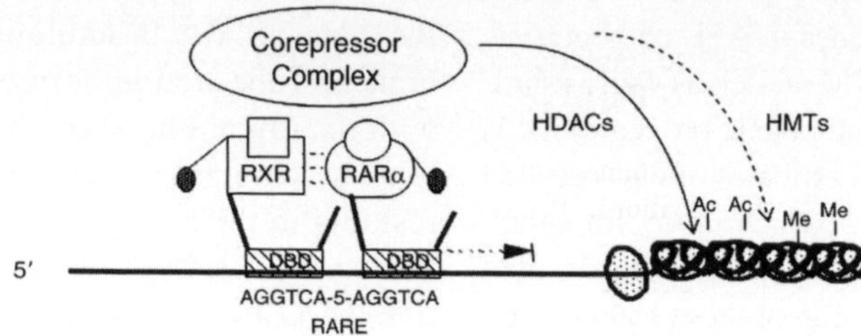

b Transcriptional activation by ligant-bound RXR/RARα heterodimer

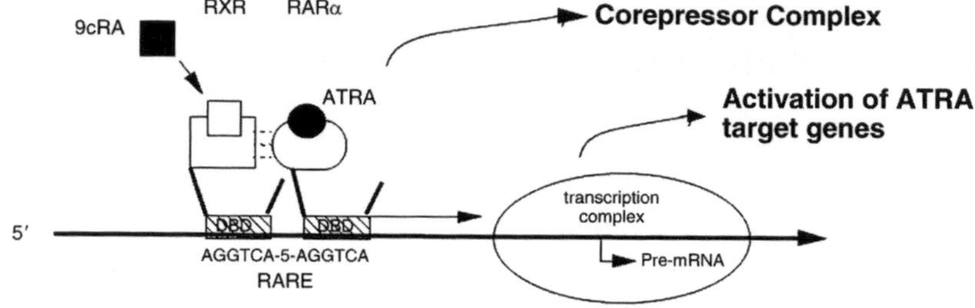

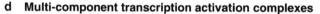

c Coactivator complex

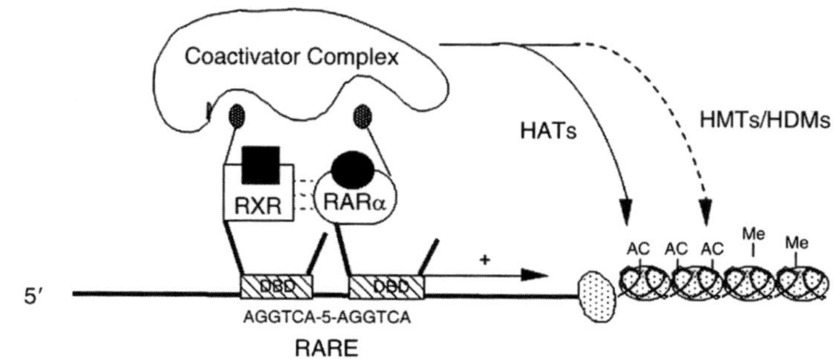

d Multi-component transcription activation complexes

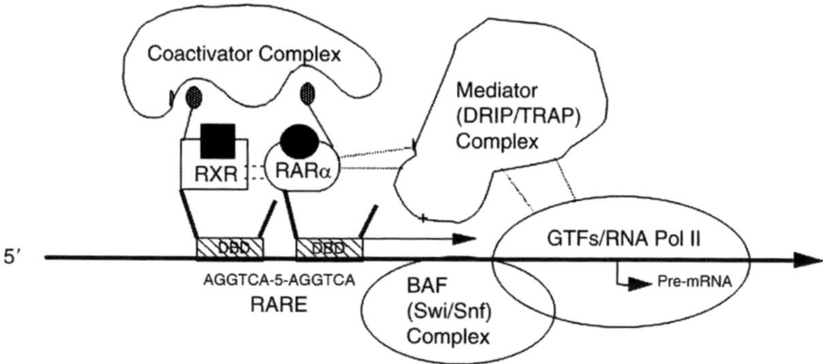

Fig. 21.3 Model for regulation of an ATRA-responsive gene promoter. (**a**) Native configuration of a RXR/RARα heterodimer bound to a canonical genomic retinoic acid response element (RARE) in the absence of ligand (ATRA). The carboxy-tail of the receptors containing the last of 12 helical motifs (*hatched oval*) is in an open position, and the receptors are engaged by a complex of corepressor proteins. A component of this complex is a histone deacetylase (HDAC) enzyme which removes acetyl (Ac) residues from the tails of select histone lysines, favoring a compact, repressed chromatin state that impedes gene transcription (*dotted arrow*). Histone methyl transferases (HMTs) directed to specific lysine residues can also contribute to the repressive effect. (**b**, **c**) Binding of ATRA to the RARα component of the heterodimer, Fig. 21.3 (continued), results in tightening of the receptor, including closure of the 12th helix over the bound ligand, associated with expulsion of the corepressor complex and recruitment of the alternative coactivator complex. This change also produces changes in the heterodimer such that the RXR component becomes permissive for binding its specific ligand 9-cis retinoic acid. The coactivator complex is nucleated by a p160/SRC family member and recruits other proteins, such as CREB-binding protein (CBP/300), with histone acetyltransferase (HAT) activity. Increased histone acetylation loosens chromatin structure, allowing access of transcription factors to promoter sites and fostering transcriptional activity. Highly site- and context-dependent methylation changes executed by specific HMTs and histone demethylases (HDMs) importantly modulate chromatin regulation of transcription. (**d**) Two additional multiprotein complexes complement or succeed the p160 coactivator complex to enhance access and functional activity of general transcription factors (GTFs) to transcribe RNA from active promoters, the mediator (DRIP/TRAP) and BAF (Swi/Snf-homologous) complexes (see text)

role of retinoids in different tissues and cells types during development [44].

In addition to the DBD and LBD domains, respectively, designated as the C and E regions, there are three other subregions of RARα (Fig. 21.2). The A/B-region has ligand-independent transcriptional activation function (AF-1). The D-region serves a rotational or "hinge" function related to heterodimer formation on RAREs. The function of the F-region, which is unique to RARs, is unknown. The E-region of RARα has been analyzed by many different methods, including site-directed mutagenesis and crystallographic analysis in the presence and absence of ligand [44, 46]. Such analysis has defined the three-dimensional structure of the region to consist of 12 α-helices and 2 β-strands linked by a series of loops. From this conformational model, it has been determined that key amino acids from various components of the LBD contribute to the formation of a binding pocket for ATRA, while those from a more restricted area stabilize a RXR/RAR dimerization interface through noncovalent bond interactions. In the absence of ligand, the apo-receptor forms a corepressor complex on RAREs in gene promoter regions, which impedes transcription of the associated gene (Fig. 21.3a). Central to this complex is the corepressor protein (SMRT or N-CoR) which directly interacts with each component of the apo-receptor and which recruits other proteins with histone deacetylase (HDAC) enzyme activity [47]. By removing negatively charged acetyl groups from lysine residues in the tails of histone proteins, HDACs increase the condensation of DNA-associated nucleosomal chromatin and inhibit gene transcriptional activity. The formation of the holoreceptor by entry of ATRA into the binding pocket produces tightening of the receptor, a prominent feature of which is a closing of the 12th, carboxy-terminal α-helix over the opening to the occupied binding site (Fig. 21.3a, b). This configurational shift results in displacement of the corepressor complex and recruitment of the coactivator complex (Fig. 21.3b, c). The core component of this complex is a p160 coactivator protein that recruits proteins with histone acetyl transferase (HAT) activity. By restoring acetyl groups on histone lysine residues in nucleosomes, these enzymes foster decondensation of chromatin and increased gene transcription. Thus, the essence of RARα function is as a sensitive switch to either repress or activate transcription from RARE-containing gene promoters in the absence or presence of ATRA, respectively.

The previously simply presented process is, in fact, highly complex and dynamic involving cell and gene promoter context-variable modifications of a multitude of molecular components that modulate transcriptional activity. At least eight classes of protein modifications have been identified that can affect the interactions and activities of these components [48]. Acetylation of histones, as described earlier, is one crucial representation of such modification. However, there is increasing documentation of the regulatory role of lysine acetylation of many nonhistone proteins, including RARα [49, 50]. Related to retinoid-mediated transcription, it has been proposed that acetylation of a p160 coactivator protein that results in disassociation of the coactivator complex from a nuclear hormone (estrogen) holoreceptor is likely commonly applicable to nuclear receptors and that this dissociation is required for engagement of the Mediator or DRIP/TRAP complex [51, 52]. The latter and another multicomponent complex, the ATP-dependent "chromatin remodeling machine" called SWI/SNF (yeast) or BAF (man), produces further chromatin decondensation essential for final engagement of the basal transcription apparatus and synthesis of mRNA by RNA polymerase II (Fig. 21.3d) [52–54]. Methylation of lysine and arginine residues in histone proteins in concert with methylation of DNA is considered to have an overall repressive effect on transcription. However, histone methylase enzymes have higher specificity than acetylases, and there is marked heterogeneity of effect depending on cellular context and the position and level of methylation (mono-, di-, or trimethylation). A defined set of histone lysine residues have been identified for which methylation or acetylation act reciprocally and in some instances in opposition to the more general effects of these protein modifications. These antagonizing "histone marks" for transcriptional repression or activation, referred to loosely as the "histone code," provide a reading guide for the chromatin modifiers involved in mediating the transcription process [55]. Protein modification by phosphorylation plays a major role in modulating retinoid-mediated transcription at all levels of the process [52]. There are at least four phosphorylation sites in RARα (Fig. 21.1), which are targeted by several different kinases, including the signaling kinases MSK1, PKA, and PKC. These and additional kinases also target RARα-associated cofactors and components of the intermediary and basal transcription complexes, most often with a stimulatory effect on transcription (but with many particular variations) [52].

PML and PML Nuclear Bodies

Structurally, PML is characterized by a conserved "tripartite motif" at the amino-terminus, which consists of a cysteine/histidine-rich (Cys3HisCys4) cluster called the RING domain, followed by two alternative cysteine/histidine clusters called B-boxes, succeeded by an α-helical coiled-coil domain (Fig. 21.4b) [56]. This RBCC structure is shared by eight other members of a large gene family, two of which in addition to PML can form oncogenic hybrid proteins as a result of tumor-associated chromosome translocations. Although all three of the cysteine/histidine clusters bind to zinc ions, which are characteristic of DNA-interacting zinc finger motifs, there is no evidence that PML directly interacts with DNA. Rather, the RING domain functions through protein–protein interactions facilitated by hydrophobic

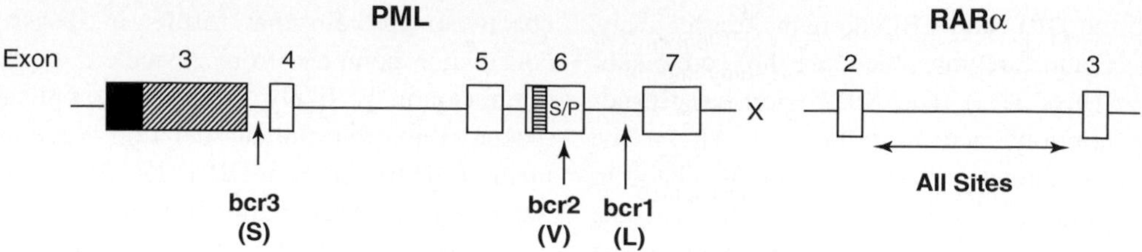

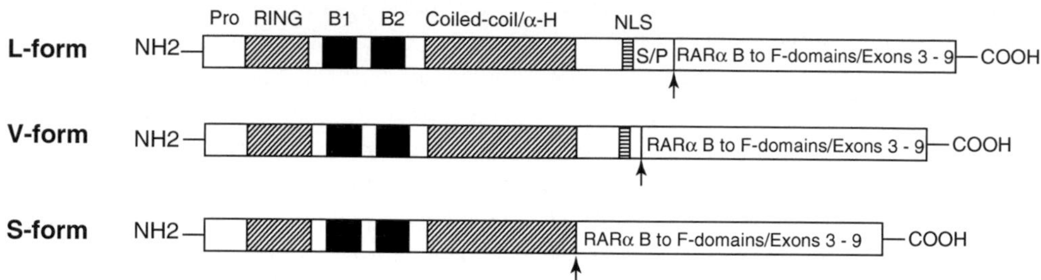

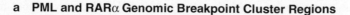

Fig. 21.4 Formation and PML region structure of PML-RARα isoforms. (**a**) DNA-level diagram is limited to the exons of PML and RARα involved in the formation of PML-RARα fusion transcript/protein. *Boxes*, numbered exons; lines, introns. Thin *arrows* indicate the intronic breakpoint cluster region (bcr) sites of DNA breakage that produce the L (bcr1), V (bcr2), and S (bcr3) isoforms of PML-RARα. (**b**) 5′-PML region linked to common RARα segment containing B–F domains shown in Fig. 21.2. The variably filled *rectangles* indicate the mRNA coding/protein regions for the proline-rich (Pro), RING, B-box (B1 and B2), coiled-coil, alpha-helical, and serine-proline-rich (S/P) domains. NLS indicates a nuclear localizing sequence in PML exon 6

amino acid heptad repeats in the coiled-coil region, which serves as a critical interface for the formation of PML homodimers and of heterodimers with PML-RARα in APL cells (see text to come). The RBCC motif, encoded by the first three exons of the PML gene, is present in all of the 18 isoforms generated by differential splicing of the succeeding 6 exons [56].

The physiological function of PML remains rather ill-defined despite many years of intensive investigation [57]. This is partly related to the lack of a compelling phenotype of PML knock-out (PML^{-}/PML^{-}) mice, which appear essentially normal under nonstressed conditions, and partly to the highly pleiotropic and complex functions that have been associated with PML. Massive experimental evidence indicates involvement in fundamental cellular processes, including proliferation, senescence, apoptosis, and differentiation and in pathological processes, including viral infections and oncogenesis. A cardinal early observation was that PML is expressed principally in nuclear structures called nuclear bodies (NB) in a wide variety of cell types [58, 59]. PML NB are quite heterogeneous ranging from 0.2 to 1 μM in size and in number from 1 to 30 per nucleus, where they often are nonrandomly distributed relative to other nuclear elements [57]. From studies using cells derived from PML^{-}/PML^{-} mice, it has been determined that PML expression is a central player in both NB structure and function [60], although there some evidence indicates that alternative NB proteins can also serve in this role [57]. An ever increasing number of proteins have been assigned to PML NBs, a recent review citing greater than 70 proteins and a recent bioinformatics study citing an interactome of 166 proteins [57, 61]. However, only a minority of the PML NB proteins have been demonstrated to directly interact with PML, importantly including a ubiquitin-related enzyme, SUMO-1 (small ubiquitin-related modifier), which produces posttranslational modification of PML required for the recruitment of many other PML NB proteins [62]. Based on the presence of several additional SUMOylation-involved proteins in PML-NBs and the presence of SUMO interaction motifs (SIMs) in the majority of PML interactome proteins, it was postulated that the on–off sumoylation status may provide a binary switch mechanism regulating the location, integrity, and activity of many PML NB components [61]. Recently, it was demonstrated that site-specific sumoylation is a prerequisite for recruitment of the ubiquitin E3 ligase RNF4, leading to degradation of PML by the proteosome [63, 64]. Several other posttranslational modifications, including phosphorylation, acetylation, and ISGylation among others have also been importantly related to PML protein biology [65]. Also, there has been a recent increased effort to dissect the specific activities of the multiple protein isoforms, including several present in the cytoplasm due to translation from mRNA splice forms lacking the nuclear localizing sequence (NLS) encoded by exon 6.

Pathologically, PML has been defined as a tumor suppressor gene based on many experiments demonstrating an inhibitory effect on cell proliferation and a stimulatory effect on apoptosis [66, 67]. Consistent with this designation, PML knock-out (PML^{-}/PML^{-}) mice have an increased incidence of skin papillomas and lymphomas, many of high grade, after treatment with a chemical mutagen, and cells from PML^{-}/PML^{-} mice are relatively resistant to different types of apoptogenic stimuli. Also consistent decreased levels of PML protein have been demonstrated in human cancer cells [68]. Conversely, an analysis of LIC in a human chronic myeloid leukemia (CML) model in PML^{+}/PML^{+} vs. PML^{-}/PML^{-} mice indicated that greater oncogenicity was associated with higher PML expression [69]. Further, this PML-associated effect was related to the preservation of stem cell/LIC function by inducing replicative quiescence, while PML deficiency was associated with continuous cell cycle entry, eventually leading to replicative exhaustion. Notably, older nonleukemic PML^{-}/PML^{-} mice developed hematopoietic insufficiency, suggesting that one physiological role of PML is to regulate stem cell replication to maintain a lifelong reservoir. These two differing scenarios related to tumor cell behavior are likely representative of the diversity and complexity of PML activity in different cell contexts [65, 67, 70].

Structure and Generation of PML-RARα and RARα-PML

The PML-RARα fusion gene derives in each APL case from breakage of the PML gene on chromosome 15 in one of three breakpoint cluster regions (bcrs) and from breakage of the RARα gene on chromosome 17 in the second intron (Fig. 21.4a, b). PML-RARα bcr1 cases result from genomic DNA breaks in PML intron 6, producing, after mRNA processing, the long(L)-form PML-RARα fusion transcript. In bcr3 cases, the breaksite occurs in PML intron 3, producing the short(S)-form of PML-RARα mRNA. Compared to L-form mRNA, the S-form transcript lacks PML exons 4–6 which primarily encode a proline/serine-rich region with several potential phosphorylation sites. Exon 6 also contains the PML nuclear localizing sequence (NLS) and an important proteolytic site. In bcr2 cases, the PML breaksite occurs at different sites in PML exon 6, which results in deletion of variable amounts of coding sequence from the resultant variable(V)-form PML-RARα fusion transcript. Frequently, additional nucleotides derived from RARα intron 2 are incorporated at the end of the deleted PML 6 exon, which preserves the translational open reading frame (ORF) in all PML-RARα V-form cases [71–73]. Among 221 PML-RARa-positive adult cases, the frequency of L-, S-, and V-form fusion transcripts were 55%, 37%, and 8%, respectively [74]. In pediatric cases, there is a higher frequency of V-form cases, up to 27%, and a proportionate reduction in S-form cases [75, 76].

The reciprocal product of t(15;17), RARα-PML is detected in about 75% of PML-RARα-positive APL cases [77–79]. A recent study demonstrated that a significant portion of the 25% RARα-PML-negative cases can be accounted for by complex rearrangements involving a third gene, by deletions and by alternative mRNA splicing [80].

In order to try to understand the genesis of PML-RARα/RARα-PML fusion gene products, detailed DNA sequence analyses have been performed to identify the precise genomic breaksites. The RARα breaksites can occur throughout the 17 kb-long intron 2, although a few favored microcluster sites were identified, only one of which had an identifiably significant consensus sequence—a high-stringency binding site for the DNA double-strand break repair enzyme topoisomerase II [72, 73]. A similar nondescript pattern prevailed for PML intron breaksites in random APL cases. However, in a subset of APL patients who relapsed after previous treatment with anthracycline topoisomerase II inhibitors for prior cancers or multiple sclerosis, agent-specific (mitoxantrone and epirubicin) strong hotspot breaksites were identified in PML intron 6, and similar but weaker breaksite clusters were found in RARα intron 2 [81–83]. In both PML and RARa, the breaksites contained short homologous sequences suggesting that the fusion gene was generated by means of the nonhomologous end-joining pathway. Of note in these treatment-related APL cases, the median time from drug exposure to leukemia development was about 2 years, which could be consistent with the latency period observed between initial PML-RARα exposure and leukemia development in preclinical models (see text to come). Interestingly, a longer latency period was documented in a spontaneous APL case in a 10-year-old boy by demonstrating the same DNA-level PML and RARα breaksites in the blood Guthrie card obtained at birth [84]. Further study is required to assess whether alternative consensus sequences with no known relationship to DNA break repair proteins found adjacent to RARα intron 2 breaksites in spontaneous APL cases may provide insight into alternative mechanisms of PML-RARα formation [72].

Role of PML-RARα in Leukemogenesis

An early and long-standing concept has been that the primary leukemogenic activity of PML-RARα is due to a dominant-negative inhibitory effect on normal RARα, which blocks RARα-mediated terminal granulocytic differentiation at physiological ATRA concentrations [85, 86]. One basis for this concept was the observation that over-expression of transduced RARα in lineage-negative mouse bone marrow progenitor cells could produce sustained self-renewal and arrest myeloid differentiation at the promyelocyte stage [87, 88]. These effects could also be produced by RARα with an inactivating mutation in the LBD [88], which had been demonstrated to inhibit ATRA-induced HL-60 cell differentiation by a dominant-negative mechanism [89]. Also supportive was the observation that transduction of PML-RARα into multipotential human hematopoietic progenitor/stem cells (HSC) co-opted the differentiation program, rapidly committing the transduced cells to the neutrophilic granulocyte pathway with arrest at the promyelocyte stage [90]. Two lines of experimentation provided a strong molecular rationale for the concept. First, ATRA exposure was shown to produce selective proteolytic degradation of PML-RARα, which would relieve the dominant-negative inhibition of still intact RARα, unblocking RARα-mediated differentiation [91, 92]. Second, PML-RARα was demonstrated to form a homodimer through the coiled–coiled dimerization interface of the PML region, which could usurp RARE binding sites and recruit a double dose of corepressor–HDAC complex compared to RXR:RAR heterodimers (Fig. 21.5a, b) [93–95]. This could explain the higher, pharmacological concentration of ATRA required to trigger differentiation of APL cells.

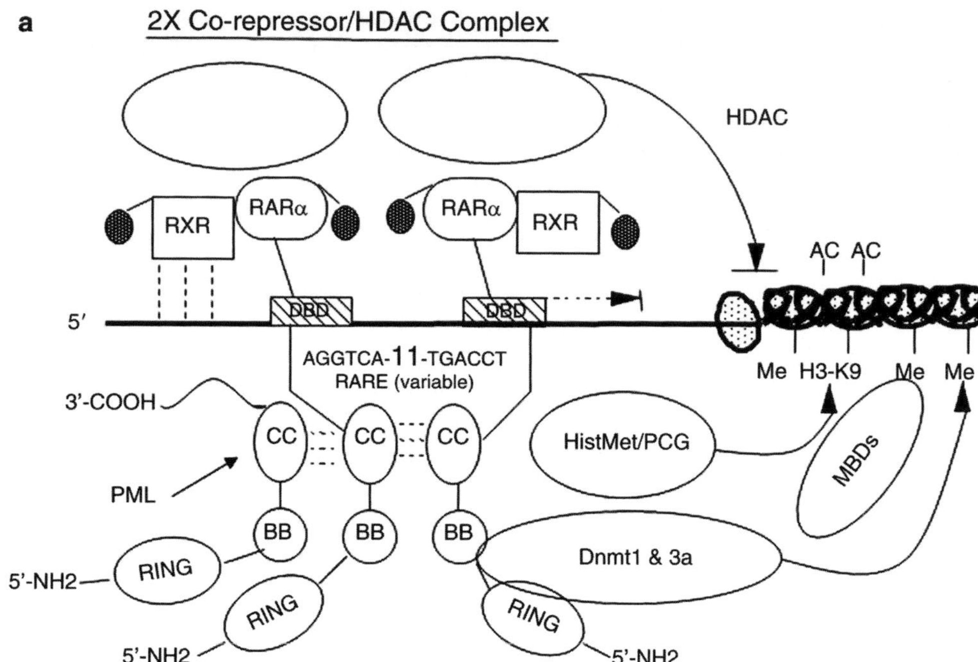

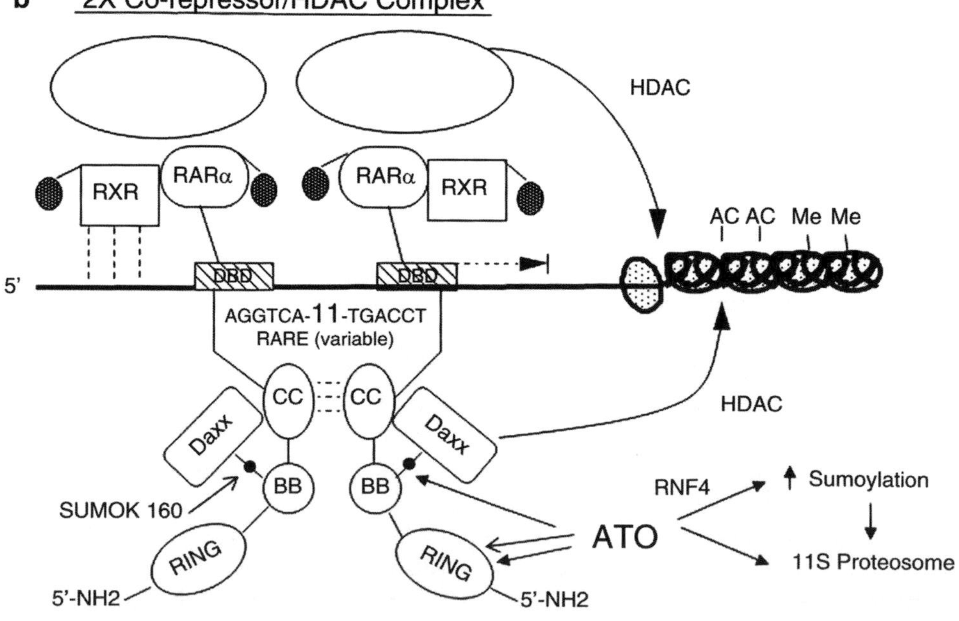

Fig. 21.5 Model illustration of the PML-RARα homodimer-nucleated hetero-oligomeric complex and action sites of arsenic trioxide (ATO). (**a**) PML-RARα homodimer situated on an atypical RARE (consisting of an inverted repeat of the right-side half-site separated from a canonical left-side half-site by 11 base pairs), stabilized by the noncovalent bonding between the two central coiled–coiled (cc) regions (*dashed lines*). Two RXR molecules form part of the complex by interacting with the interaction interface in the E-regions in the RARα portion of PML-RARα. On the lower *left side*, a normal PML molecule forms part of the complex also by interacting with the cc region of PML-RARα. On the *lower right*, several other repressor proteins have been recruited to the complex, including DNA methylases (Dnmt1 and 3a), histone methylases and demethylases (PCG, polycomb group proteins), and DNA methyl-binding proteins (MBDs). (**b**) *Lower left*: The suppressor gene Daxx is bound to the B-Box region (BB) of the PML portion of PML-RARα, which is dependent on sumoylation of lysine 160. *Lower right*: ATO degradation by the proteosome induces increased, polysumoylation of K160 by the ubiquitin E3 ligase RNF4 and also directly binds to and oxidizes vicinal cysteine residues in the PML RBCC region

It could, also, account for the effectiveness of HDAC inhibitors in complementing ATRA activity, which was particularly evident when ATRA-LBD interaction was compromised by an inactivating LBD mutation in PML-RARα [93]. A subsequent series of reports documented the staged recruitment of several additional components to PML-RARa-corepressor complex gene promoters, which are not usually evident or present at lower levels at RXR/RARα promoter sites, that can further modify chromatin structure and the level of transcriptional repression. Among these components are DNA methylases, DNA methyl-binding proteins, and histone methylases and demethylases (associated with polycomb group repressor proteins) [96–100].

This focus on the disruption of RARα-mediated transcriptional activity suggests that the PML region contribution to the fusion gene might be essentially facilitative related to homodimer formation. However, many experiments now indicate that the PML region has an active, even dominant, role in APL leukemogenesis. Most dramatically, in a TM model, a PML-RARα transgene with a mutation in the RARα-region LBD that prevented ATRA binding was equally leukemogenic compared to a nonmutant PML-RARα transgene, while a transgene with the same inactivating mutation in normal RARα was not leukemogenic [101]. These results demonstrate that PML-region activity but not RARα-region transcriptional regulatory activity is required for leukemogenesis. In accord, an artificial recombinant transgene in which an HDAC, the key effector of RARα-mediated corepressor activity (see RARα section), tethered to RARα was not leukemogenic [102]. In meticulous experiments with a variety of naturally occurring and artificially generated forms of X-RARα, it was demonstrated that homodimer formation is obligatory for leukemogenic activity and that PML-RARα homodimers were uniquely potent [103–105]. One way that PML-RARα homodimers have been considered to contribute to leukemogenicity is by interacting with the coiled–coiled region of normal PML, producing dominant-negative inhibition of this important cell regulatory molecule (Fig. 21.5a, b; see PML section) [106, 107]. In agreement, a PML-RARα transgene was more leukemogenic in PML^{-}/PML^{-} TM than PML^{+}/PML^{+}TM, while it had an intermediate effect in PML+/PML^{-} TM [108]. This interaction is also responsible for the signature cytological finding in PML-RARα-positive APL, as revealed by immunofluorescent staining: that PML is dispersed to myriad microspeckles throughout the nucleus in APL cells, rather than localized to discrete PML NBs as in normal cells [109]. Subsequent experiments demonstrated that a requirement for leukemogenesis in addition to the nucleating PML-RARα homodimer is the recruitment of RXR as part of a high molecular weight hetero-oligomeric complex [110–112]. Notably, the RARα region of PML-RARα is required for this interaction, since mutagenization of key amino acid sites in the LBD/E region of PML-RARα eliminates RXR recruitment and leukemogenicity [41]. Overall, these experiments indicate that the hetero-oligomeric complex can act as an inhibitor of both PML, as described previously, and of normal RARα by sequestering its heterodimerization partner RXR, as well as by competing for RARE DNA binding sites. Additional experimental evidence, however, indicates that this double dominant negative mode is still insufficient to explain the role of PML-RARα in the complex pathogenesis of APL.

A shortcoming of this presentation is that it does not consider the dynamics of the leukemogenic process. From several TM model studies a consensus conclusion is that PML-RARα is essential for the initiation of the disease process, but that additional complementary mutations are required for progression to full-blown APL-like leukemia [40]. The fundamental basis for this conclusion is a long latency period from PML-RARα initiation to leukemia development, which occurs in only a fraction of the at-risk mice (incidence, i.e., penetrance, <30%). In many molecular genetic experiments, the latency interval and penetrance fraction have been used as a measure of leukemogenic potency. A variety of evidence supports the presumption that secondary mutations required for disease progression occur during the latency interval, including cytogenetic changes indicative of clonal evolution and the divergence of gene expression patterns in leukemias arising in different TM models [113–115]. Genetic cross-breeding experiments to select TM with haploinsufficiency for genes affecting APL differentiation (*PU.1* and *CEBPA*) [43, 116] and/or other vital APL cell processes (PML; see earlier discussion) demonstrated markedly increased leukemia penetrance, suggesting that endogenous genetic or epigenetic changes that reduce the expression or activity of these molecules could be involved in disease progression. Finally, the co-expression of kinase genes with activating mutations that augment cell proliferation (*FLT3ITD* or oncogenic *RAS* mutations) had a potent effect, both decreasing latency and increasing penetrance [117, 118]. Based on these observations and evidence of cooperativity in human AML between activating kinase gene mutations that primarily affect cell proliferation and various transcription factor fusion gene mutations that primarily affect differentiation, it was proposed that these two types of mutations may be the minimal essential requirements for leukemogenesis [117], Overall, these observations indicate that the leukemogenic activity of PML-RARα must be considered on a temporal basis with respect to the disease process.

The primary leukemia initiating activity (LIA) of PML-RARα has been associated with little initial change in differentiation but, rather, with the acquisition of self-renewal capacity, a key property of LICs. Thus, during the preleukemic phase in TM, no differences in cell phenotype and very limited gene expression differences were noted between early myeloid cells or promyelocytes from PMR-RARα-expressing TM versus control wild-type mice [115]. Similarly, minimal early phenotypic changes were observed in a more natural "knock-in" mouse model in which a single copy of PML-RARα was inserted into the promoter region of the promyelocyte expression-specific gene cathepsin G (CG) [119]. Two remarkable observations were (1) that there was a marked increase in penetrance (≤20–90%) without a change in latency compared to the corresponding CG-promoted TM model and (2) that this was associated with a very low level of PML-RARα expression (only 3% of that observed in the corresponding TM). Since the expression level of PML-RARα was less than that of normal PML or RARα, it was importantly suggested that a gain of function rather than a dominant-negative mode of action might be involved in the establishment of initiated preleukemic cells (see text to come). Recently, it was demonstrated that the most essential change in PML-RARα-initiated cells from PML-RARα CG-knock-in mice was the acquisition of self-renewal capacity at all levels of the preleukemic myeloid differentiation hierarchy from HSCs up to the promyelocyte stage [42]. There was no expansion of myeloid cell precursors or promyelocytes with self-renewal capacity, only of postreplicative neutrophils, until the leukemic stage was reached, at which time there was a marked increase in granulocyte–monocyte progenitors and promyelocytes, accompanied by normalization of neutrophil levels. Additionally, it was demonstrated that 1 in 100 cells from the leukemic promyelocyte cell population was able to generate transplantable leukemias in syngeneic mice, certifying that these normally short-lived, effete cells had acquired the crucial in vivo self-renewal property of LICs. Similar observations were reported in a TM model [43]. These results lead to at least three important conclusions. First, they indicate that the self-renewal proliferation effect imparted by PML-RARα to initiate the disease process is insufficient to account for the expanded proliferative capacity of the fully developed leukemia cells, which must be complemented by the acquisition of secondary genetic or possibly epigenetic aberrations. Second, the variable levels of differentiation block at the promyelocyte stage in different mouse genetic APL models also indicate a requirement for the acquisition of secondary aberrations to complement the inherent differentiation inhibitory effects of PML-RARα. In this regard, a potential contributory factor might be variations in the level of PML-RARα expression during disease progression [120]. Alternatively, the complementary aberrations, e.g., in oncogenes with kinase activity, might affect PML-RARα transcription complexes in a manner that alters their activity on differentiation-modulating target genes. Third, the documentation in mouse genetic models that a significant subpopulation of leukemic promyelocytes (1:100) has LIC capability suggests that the disease, once established, can be maintained by this expanded cell population, as well as by any antecedent cell in the APL hierarchy targeted by PML-RARα to initiate the disease. If applicable to human disease, this has obvious treatment implications.

As introduced previously, there is now much experimental evidence to indicate that positive gain-of-function activity of PML-RARα is at least as important as its dominant-negative inhibitory activity particularly in disease initiation but also during disease progression. An experimental model that has been very useful in studying how PML-RARα produces gain-of-function activity has been a human myelomonocytic leukemia cell line harboring a transduced and conditionally inducible PML-RARα transgene (called U937PR9) [121]. Switching on this transgene, which mimics the initiation event in APL, results in many changes in the expression of gene transcripts, as measured by oligonucleotide gene expression (RNA) array analyses. Several genes of known importance for myeloid differentiation were downregulated, consistent with the dominant repressor effect of PML-RARα on differentiation. However, in accord with a gain-of-function mode, a number of genes were upregulated, including some critically associated with increased cell proliferation and self-renewal and with reduced DNA repair that might predispose to increased mutagenesis during disease progression [121–123]. Notably, the majority of the regulated genes are not known to have a canonical RARE in the gene promoter, which argues against direct regulation via the RARα region of PML-RARα in the absence or presence of ligand (ATRA). Extensive further investigation has implicated the PML component of the fusion gene in this aberrant gene regulation, essentially, by two different mechanisms. One is based on documentation that the hetero-oligomeric complex nucleated by the PML-RARα homodimer has a markedly relaxed specificity for the sequence, orientation, and spacing of the DNA promoter RARE (Fig. 21.5a, b) [124, 125]. Recent reports document that the expanded repertoire of PML-RARα target genes compared to normal RARα target genes is extensive and, furthermore, that most are associated with epigenetic alterations, including histone acetylation and methylation and DNA methylation, indicative of functional significance [126–129]. A second general mechanism is related to protein:protein interactions of the PML region with other transcription modulators. The precise mechanism has only been documented in only one instance in which two alternative transcription factors were rendered ATRA sensitive by tethering them to the PML region of the fusion gene [130]. However, some variation of this mechanism seems probably related to observations of ATRA-modulated gene expression by PML-RARα but not by normal RARα, which include observations in APL cells of the master myeloid differentiation regulatory genes PU.1 [129, 131], CEBPA [43], and CEBPB [132]. An alternative variation on this theme is that the dense corepressor complex formed by PML-RARα may indirectly affect the activity of alternative transcription factors by depleting modulating cofactors such as RXRs or HDACs [105]. This indirect mechanism may apply to the modulation of the AP-1 transcription factor composed of Fos and Jun [133, 134], which has been suggested to be of central importance in APL pathogenesis [135, 136].

Finally, based on evidence that sumoylation is critical for PML function (see PML section), a principal lysine sumoylation site (K160) in the B-box domain was mutagenized, and the mutant PML-RARα*K160R* was determined to retain most properties of wild-type PML-RARα but to lack the capacity to block terminal granulocytic differentiation [107]. Notably, PML-RARα*K160R* was able to form oligomeric complexes capable of binding a dense corepressor complex but, like artificial RARα homodimer fusions [103, 104], its "transforming capacity" was limited to hematopoietic cell immortalization in vitro and the generation of a expanded myeloproliferative disorder but not leukemia in an in vivo TM model. It was further demonstrated that full leukemogenic potential could be restored to PML-RARα*K160R* by linkage to the strong corepressor Daxx, previously demonstrated to require sumoylation for association with PML (Fig. 21.5a, b) [107]. Recently, Daxx was demonstrated to directly interact with and inhibit CEBPB [137] which is a key PML-RARα-specific early response gene required for differentiation after ATRA treatment [132]. Thus, the unique interaction of PML-RARα with the additional corepressor Daxx that has specific granulocyte differentiation inhibitory activity not provided by RARα-region-related corepressor complex may provide an explanation for the favored selection of PML-RARα rather than alternative RARα fusion gene partners in naturally occurring human APL [107].

Alternative RARα Genes

Six alternative RARα gene fusion gene partners in addition to PML have been reported in acute myeloid leukemia patients classified as APL by cytological criteria (Table 21.1). In all cases, the generically named X gene in the X-RARα fusion gene transcript is ligated to the beginning of the 5′-end of the third exon of RARα, as in PML-RARα. Thus, the 5′-truncated RARα segment lacks only a portion of the A/B-- region associated with ligand-independent activator function (although retaining the major phosphorylation site, Ser77). This consistent finding strongly implies that RARα is the critical factor in specification of the APL phenotype [34, 138]. As indicated in the previous section, genetic modification experiments surprisingly indicate that impairment of direct transcriptional regulatory activity of the RARα region of PML-RARα does not affect leukemogenic potency [101], but that, alternatively, this is related to mandatory recruitment of the RARα heterodimer partner RXR to the X-RARα high molecular weight hetero-oligomeric complex [110–112]. The mechanism by which recruitment of RXR contributes to the pathogenesis has not been fully determined, but it is a consistent requirement for leukemogenicity of all X-RARαs that have been tested. The recruitment of RXR enhances promoter DNA response element binding, suggesting that the constant finding of RARα in APL fusion genes is related to recruitment of RXR by X-RARα via the RARα region to aberrant RAREs selectively recognized by the X-component. The concept that the X-component adds a critical leukemogenic factor to the X-RARα-nucleated hetero-oligomeric complex is supported by the aforementioned finding that the mutagenization of a single amino acid site in the PML region of PML-RARα that did not disrupt the integrity of the hetero-oligomeric complex lost leukemogenic potential [107]. Nevertheless, the RXR sequestration effect posed by the hetero-oligomeric complex *vis-a-vis* normal RARα and alternative transcription factors, as described earlier, may provide an essential and common contribution to the transformed APL phenotype for all X-RARαs.

PLZF-RARα is the most common and most studied of the alternative X-RARαs (Table 21.1). Two studies indicate that the incidence of PLZF-RARα is <1% of APL cases: (1) in a European study of 611 cytogenetically characterized patients with a centrally evaluated consensus cytological diagnosis of APL, which included 18 PML-RARα-negative patients (2.9%), PLZF-RARα was detected in 11 patients (incidence,

Table 21.1 Alternative retinoic acid receptor-alpha fusion genes in APL

Fusion gene	X-partner name	Chromosome marker	Frequency	Reciprocal	ATRA sensitive	ATO sensitive
PLZF-RARA	Promyelocytic leukemia zinc finger	t(11;17)(q23;q21)	~0.5% of cases	Most	Weak; variable	No
NPM-RARA	Nucleophosmin	t(5;17)(q35;q21)	7 cases	Yes	Yes	Yes
STAT5b-RARA	Signal transducer and activator of transcription 5b	None or der(17)	4 cases	No	No	Not reported
NuMA-RARA	Nuclear mitotic apparatus	t(11;17)(q13;q21)	1 case	No	Yes	Not reported
PRKAR1A-RARA	cAMP-dependent protein kinase regulatory subunit R1alpha	None; FISH:del(17)(q21)	1 case	No	Not reported	Not reported
FIP1L1-RARA	Factor interacting with poly(A) polymerase	t(4;17)(q12;q21)	1 APL 1 JMML	Yes	Yes	Not reported

0.8%) [138], and (2) in 225 patients registered by the Eastern Cooperative Oncology Group (ECOG) to North American Intergroup APL trials with the clinical diagnosis of APL (no central review prior to registration), 22 patients were PML-RARα-negative (9.8%) and 1 patient was PLZF-RARα-positive (0.4%) [139]. In 10/12 of the cited cases, the PLZF-RARα fusion resulted from the reciprocal translocation t(11;17)(q23;q21), and in all cases tested, it was associated with the reciprocal fusion gene RARα-PLZF. In 1 of the 2t(11;17)-negative cases that could be tested, the PLZF-RARα fusion gene resulted from an RARα insertion in chromosome 11 and, accordingly, RARα-PLZF was absent [138, 140]. This distinction is clinically important, because the RARα-PLZF-negative case was responsive to ATRA-therapy, whereas patients with both PLZF-RARα and RARα-PLZF are relatively resistant to ATRA therapy (see clinical sections). More generally, PLZF-RARα APL is the only X-RARα reported to exhibit distinguishing cytological and immunophenotypic features—blasts with regular rather than indented nuclei, increased Pelger-like cells and expression of CD56—from those that can be common to X-RARα and PML-RARα cases [141]. Also, PLZF-RARα-positive APL is associated with a poorer prognosis than PML-RARα-positive APL. This has been ascribed both to insensitivity to ATO [142, 143] and to an inability of ATRA-containing therapy to eliminate APL LICs regardless of differentiation-inducing effect, which seems more profound than that for PML-RARα-positive APL [41, 144].

The molecular basis for the relative insensitivity of PLZF-RARα APL to ATRA therapy was initially linked to the binding of corepressor protein to the POZ domain of the PLZF region in a non-ATRA-releasable manner in addition to the common ATRA-sensitive corepressor binding to the RARα region [93–95, 145]. This conclusion was supported in these studies by in vitro and TM experiments indicating that the ATRA resistance of PLZF-RARα-positive APL cells could be at least partially overcome by co-treatment with inhibitors of HDACs recruited by the corepressors. Subsequent findings, however, have indicated that a more important factor is the absence or presence of the RARα-PLZF reciprocal gene product, as indicated previously. This relates to the structure and function of the PLZF gene, which belongs to a gene family homologous to the Droshophila transcription factor *Krüppel*. These proteins have a motif with nine zinc fingers near the carboxy-terminus that interacts with specific DNA response element sequences of select gene promoters. The PLZF intronic breaksites involved in formation of the reciprocal fusion genes usually provides seven, less frequently six, of the zinc fingers to RARα-PLZF [28, 146]. This protein was demonstrated to counter the repressive activity of normal PLZF on cell cycle progression, at least partly related to activation of the cyclin A2 gene promoter [147]. Similarly, RARα-PLZF countered the PLZF repressor activity on the promoter of CRABP1 producing a marked increase in the expression of this protein, which has been associated with increased retinoid metabolism and resistance [148]. Although it only contains two or three zinc fingers, PLZF-RARα was recently demonstrated to preferentially bind to an expanded repertoire of noncanonical RAREs that includes an APL-associated gene promoter set that is significantly overlapping with that described for PML-RARα binding [122, 125, 126, 144]. It was also demonstrated to specifically interfere with the transcriptional regulatory activity of its normal homolog PLZF [144], analogous to the interference of PML-RARα with normal PML function. A key specific effect was to increase cell proliferation in part by countering the repressive activity of PLZF to activate the cMYC gene promoter [144]. Thus, PLZF-RARα-positive APL resembles PML-RARα-positive APL by the critical contribution of the fusion gene product in countering the regulatory activity of the normal X-component, but it differs in the sense that the reciprocal PLZF-RARα and RARα-PLZF proteins are complementarily involved in the pathogenesis. These features likely account for the resistance of PLZF-RARα/RARα-PLZF APL to ATRA-induced differentiation (variably reported) and, particularly, for the ineffectiveness of ATRA in eliminating the self-renewal capacity of LICs [41, 144].

The other five X-RARαs that have been reported in APL are extremely rare, as listed in order of frequency and/or discovery in Table 21.1. Recurrent cases have been reported for NPM-RARα and STAT5β-RARα but only single cases for the other 3 X-RARαs. The FIP1L1-RARα fusion had previously been reported in a patient with juvenile monomyelocytic leukemia (JMML) [149], and, also, an alternative FIP1L1 fusion gene, FIP1L1-PDGFRA (platelet-derived growth factor receptor-alpha), has been associated with the hypereosinophilic syndrome and chronic eosinophilic leukemia [150]. Notably, the breaksite in FIP1L1 intron 15 in FIP1L1-RARα encoded a protein that could form homodimers, as characteristic of APL-associated fusion genes, while this was not so for FIP1L1-PDGFRA proteins in which the breaksite occurred in earlier introns [33]. Three of the fusion genes in which the X-partner was located outside chromosome 17 resulted from reciprocal translocations (NPM-RARα, NuMA-RARα, and FIP1L1-RARα) [33, 151, 152], while those located with RARα in chromosome 17q resulted from insertions and small deletions with (STAT5β) or without (PRKAR1A) microinversions [31, 32, 153]. Two of three translocation fusion genes were associated with the expression of the reciprocal fusions (RARα-NPM and RARα-FIP1L1); any functional role for each of these remains to be determined. Sensitivity to ATRA-induced differentiation has been established for APL cases derived from all three of the translocation-derived fusion genes [149, 152, 154, 155]. No evidence of ATRA sensitivity was observed in any of the four STAT5β-RARα APL cases, although only one of these patients was treated with ATRA as a single agent [153]. ATO sensitivity has only been tested in NPM-RARα APL, which, like PML-RARα APL, was reported to be sensitive in both a TM model and a relapse patient [156, 157]. No testing for ATRA or ATO sensitivity related to the PRKAR1A-RARα fusion has been performed, but it was speculated that sensitivity of both of these agents is likely since reduced function of the alpha regulatory subunit (PRKAR1A) would likely result in increased catalytic activity of PKA, which has been linked to increased sensitivity to both agents [32]. More generally, the finding of recurrent cases for NPM-RARα and STAT5β-RARα implies that the X-partners in these fusions, like PML and PLZF, have some important pathogenic role beyond the formation of homodimeric and hetero-oligomeric complexes, as described earlier. Indeed, it seems likely that all of the X-RARαs contribute by as yet undetermined diverse means to the increased self-renewal properties required for LIC activity in the context of the APL phenotype imposed by X-RARα/RXRα structural complexes on a shared subset of gene promoters. Finally, in this conglomerate consideration of alternative fusion genes, it is noted that one enigmatic APL case has been reported in which only RARα-PML and no PML-RARα could be detected at disease presentation [158]. Also, in a rigorously documented set of 611 patients with characteristic features of APL, five patients (0.8%) lacked any rearrangement of RARα [138]. Overall, the previous considerations suggest that additional pathogenic elements of this disease remain to be discovered.

Role of PML-RARα in the Response to Treatment

Both ATRA and ATO, two agents that have selectively potent therapeutic effects in APL compared to other types of leukemia, have the common property of inducing proteolytic degradation of PML-RARα [36, 91]. The simplest and most direct explanation for the therapeutic effect of these agents is that by removing the dominant-negative suppressor effect of PML-RARα, normal RARα and PML (produced by the non-translocated gene loci) can re-establish physiological pathways leading to granulocyte terminal differentiation and/or apoptosis [91, 159, 160]. Although this may provide a partial explanation, the experimental details indicate that the molecular response is more complex, as well as different, for the two agents.

Exposure of APL cells to ATRA is succeeded by changes in the regulation of many hundreds of genes, leading to discernible differentiation within 24–48 h associated with a temporary increase in resistance to apoptosis [121, 126, 161–165]. The "first wave" of these reported changes in gene transcript levels occurs within 6 h of ATRA exposure [126, 165], before there has been substantial degradation of PML-RARα [91, 92]. Among these early ATRA response genes, there is no enrichment of gene promoters containing canonical RAREs required for RARα-mediated transcription, while there is some enrichment of those with atypical RAREs that can be recognized by PML-RARα [126]. Further, there were many more genes regulated in response to ATRA in U937PR9 cells (defined earlier) previously induced to express PML-RARα than in control U937 cells containing endogenous RARα [126]. These observations provide incontrovertible evidence that at least the early transcription response to ATRA is mediated predominantly by PML-RARα, not RARα. The crucial importance of PML-RARα as the primary mediator of ATRA activity in APL is also supported by the observation that after clinical relapse from ATRA-containing therapy, inactivating mutations that develop in the RARα LBD in association with acquired ATRA resistance are invariably in PML-RARα, not RARα [166–168]. Many of the early ATRA response genes are regulated in the opposite direction from that observed after PML-RARα induction in U937PR9 cells with approximately equal numbers of genes being changed from downregulated by PML-RARα to upregulated by ATRA and vice versa [122, 126]. Several important functional classes of genes are selectively regulated, including the upregulation of several key transcription factors involved in terminal granulocyte differentiation (CEBPs, PU.1, ID1&2). PU.1 is a recognized master transcription regulator of differentiation processes in hematopoietic cells, and, when it is experimentally manipulated to be switched off or on in APL cells, it has the corresponding effects of inhibiting or promoting terminal granulocyte differentiation [131]. The transcription of the PU.1 gene is activated by the binding to its promoter region of two other transcription factors, CEBPB and OCT-1 [131]. CEBPB transcription is upregulated in APL cells within 1 h of ATRA exposure, and, as previously mentioned, is activated by PML-RARα but not RARα and is inhibited by the PML-associated gene Daxx [132, 137]. This suggests a cascade activation process involving CEBPB relief from Daxx-mediated repression at an early stage, which might then be propagated by activated PU.1, a possibility supported by the finding of coincident PU.1 binding sites and nearby PML-RARα potential binding half-sites in hundreds of gene loci [129]. A key PU.1 target gene in such a cascade may be CEBPE—which as a single upregulated gene can drive terminal granulocyte differentiation in TM APL cells—since a recent report suggests that PU.1 is its principal transcriptional regulator in response to ATRA despite the presence of a classical RARE in the CEPBE gene promoter [169, 170]. Although the exact mechanism of transcriptional regulation is not known, evidence is presented for the recruitment of the histone acetyltransferase p300 to the CEBPE promoter

[170]. This observation is consistent with another recent genome-wide assessment of early epigenetic changes after exposure of APL cells to ATRA (24 h), which demonstrated marked changes in histone acetylation but not in histone or DNA methylation [128]. Thus, these findings lead to the conclusion that the early response of APL cell response to ATRA does not occur by the long-held concept that it relieves dominant negative inhibition of direct RARα-regulated genes essential for terminal granulocyte differentiation. Rather, they indicate that the RARα region of the fusion gene provides ATRA sensitivity to PML-RARα via the PML region, which affects a wide array of target genes either directly or indirectly in a gain-of-function manner.

After 6 h of ATRA exposure there is progressive degradation of PML-RARα, and, although there is considerable variation in quantitative estimates between laboratories using the NB4 cell line, this is substantial by 12–24 h and virtually complete by 48–96 h [91, 92, 159, 171, 172]. This process has been attributed to both ubiquitin/proteosome and caspase proteolytic activities directed at the RARα region of the fusion protein, although neither is sufficient for complete degradation [92, 172]. Additionally, evidence has been presented for proteolysis directed at the PML region through an alternative process called ISGylation initiated by early ATRA activation of the ubiquitin-like E1 ligase UBE1L [173]. More global proteomic studies during this ATRA exposure interval have demonstrated the associated regulation of protein systems, particularly involving signal transduction (altered), ubiquitin/proteosome activity (increased), cell cycle progression (decreased), RNA metabolism (altered), and protein synthesis (decreased) [165, 174–176]. However, reported events during this post-ATRA interval are complex and sometimes apparently contradictory, e.g., a proteomics study reported the physical downregulation of protein translation initiation factors [174], while another study focusing on phosphorylation signaling reported an increase in translational initiation [177]. Notably, at the mRNA level PML-RARα and RARα transcripts are maintained, despite degradation at the protein level [92]. Concurrently, many continuing and new gene transcript level changes are observed between 6 and 48 h, several prominently affecting cell signaling involving calcium and interferon [165]. The complex gene networks involved in executing the steps to final terminal differentiation, including a "third wave" of gene transcription regulation involving terminal differentiation marker and functional genes [165], is poorly understood. This may partially involve regulation by RARα after relief of dominant negative suppression by degradation of PML-RARα, but it likely involves other regulatory mechanisms activated during the process as well [163, 178].

The molecular mechanisms that determine the clinical response of APL cells to ATO have been less precisely defined than for ATRA. This is partly related to the complex, pleiotropic activities of ATO that can vary depending on ambient conditions [179, 180] and partly to uncertainties about translating clinically effective ATO concentrations to in vitro studies. An initial study identified dual dose-dependent effects using both fresh APL cells in short-term culture and the NB4 cell line: at ≤0.5 μM ATO, the predominant effect was the induction of partial, atypical differentiation; at >0.5 μM, the predominant effect was the induction of apoptosis [14, 181]. The probable relevance of both types of activity was supported by pharmacokinetic (PK) analyses in ATO-treated APL patients demonstrating peak plasma concentrations of total arsenic >5 μM with a biphasic excretion profile over 24 h to near basal levels [182]. However, more recent studies using more advanced technologies capable of identifying the active trivalent arsenite form, as well as the oxidized, pentavalent arsenate form and methylated metabolites, indicate that very transient peak levels of total arsenic are almost always <1 μM and the arsenite form typically <0.5 μM after standard therapy with 0.15 mg/kg ATO intravenously over a 2-h period [183, 184]. During daily treatment, there is some enrichment of the methylated metabolites, which are not effective differentiation inducers but have a greater apoptotic effect than arsenite at 0.5 μM [185]. Of note, the highest concentration of arsenic is associated with the cellular fraction, primarily with erythrocytes bound to hemoglobin [186]. Also, there is substantial ATO concentration in some cell types, especially keratinized cells such as nails and hair [182], but the level in APL cells under clinical treatment conditions has not been defined. The clinical response of patients to standard ATO therapy strongly suggests that lower ATO concentrations (<0.5 μM) are most relevant and further suggests that in vitro studies conducted at much higher ATO concentrations, e.g., >1 μM, may have limited clinical relevance. As originally described, the typical clinical response consists of the appearance of partially differentiated myeloid cells admixed with apoptotic cells in the peripheral blood, frequently appearing at increased levels more than a week after initiating treatment [14, 187]. Whether the circulating apoptotic cells are derived from the differentiated cells, as occurs following ATRA-induced differentiation of APL cells [163], or by an independent process has not been determined.

As previously noted, a primary finding was the degradation of PML-RARα (and PML but not RARα) within a few hours after ATO exposure associated with the reformation of aggregated PML nuclear bodies [36, 160]. Degradation was noted at 0.1 μM ATO, but this occurs much more slowly at this low concentration than at 1 μM [160, 181]. A series of important discoveries have been made about the details of this process. First, it was demonstrated that ATO treatment results in the sumoylation of lysine residues in the PML region of PML-RARa [188], Second, it was demonstrated that sumoylation specifically of lysine-160 (K160) is required for recruitment along with sumoylated PML to reconstituted mature PML nuclear bodies where proteosome-dependent degradation occurs [189]. Third, it was found that polysumoylation of K160 via its SUMO interaction motifs (SIMs) recruits the RING finger ubiquitin E3 ligase RNF4, thus, defining a novel polySUMO-dependent ubiquitin-mediated proteolysis mechanism [63, 64]. Finally, it was demonstrated that within 10 min of exposure, ATO is bound to specific cysteine residues in two zinc finger motifs of the RBCC domain of the PML region [190]. Evidence was provided for the formation of octomer PML-RARα/PML complexes, including homodimers due to cross-linking between the RBCC regions of two PML-RARα/PML molecules, which could explain the rapid, aggregated PML nuclear body formation and enhanced polysumoylation required for proteosomal degradation [190].

Despite the informative detail, important questions remain about the relationship of PML-RARα degradation to the cell biological activity of ATO in APL. Is PML-RARα degradation *required* for the differentiation or apoptotic response of APL blasts to ATO? One set of experiments suggests that this could be so for differentiation: primary hematopoietic cells transduced either with the nondegradable K160-mutant PML-RARα or mutated dominant-negative RNF4 could not be induced to differentiate by 1 μM ATO, while this did occur with wild-type controls [63]. In this system, differentiation would presumably be mediated by physiological ATRA concentrations via normal RARα, which is not degraded by ATO [160], after the removal of PML-RARα dominant-negative inhibition. However, after treatment of NB4 cells with 0.1 μM ATO, the early postexposure (6 h) gene expression profile closely resembled, albeit at a lower level, that induced by ATRA [165, 181], which is primarily mediated by PML-RARα, as discussed previously. Notably, this low ATO concentration was surprisingly effective in dissociating corepressor protein (SMRT) from PML-RARα, which was attributed to SMRT phosphorylation secondary to ATO-mediated activation of the mitogen-activated protein (MAP) kinase MEK-1 [191]. Although the role of MEK-1 is controversial [192], dissociation of the corepressor in combination with delayed PML-RARα degradation at low ATO concentrations [181, 191] could result in the activation of aberrant PML-RARα-regulated gene promoters at endogenous ATRA levels [124, 125]. These results in different cell systems indicate that further studies are needed to understand how ATO mediates APL blast cell differentiation, particularly as observed in vivo. Assessment of the requirement of PML-RARα degradation for APL cell apoptosis is even more difficult, because at ≥1 μM concentrations ATO can induce apoptosis in many cell types that lack PML-RARα [193]. Thus, an alternative question is: does the presence of PML-RARα sensitize APL cells to ATO-induced apoptosis? Attempts to address this question have produced controversial results [188, 194], but a recent report suggests an intriguing mechanism by which this might occur (see text to come) [195]. Finally, is ATO-induced PML-RARα degradation *sufficient* to produce differentiation and/or apoptosis? The answer to this question is a definitive no, since studies of ATO-resistant NB4 cells effectively degrade PML-RARα without undergoing apoptosis or differentiation in response to ATO [194, 196].

Numerous studies have been performed to attempt to unravel how ATO produces apoptosis in APL cells regardless of PML-RARα contribution [179, 180]. Arsenite produces oxidative stress by binding to and decreasing the reducing capacity of the tripeptide GSH, the major intracellular buffer for reactive oxygen species (ROS), and by binding to vicinal, i.e., neighboring, sulfhydryl (thiol) groups in cysteine residues of redox-sensitive proteins [180, 197]. The relatively high sensitivity of APL cells to ATO-induced apoptosis has been attributed to low endogenous levels both of GSH and of enzymes (glutathione peroxidase, catalase, and glutathione-S-transferase) involved in regulating superoxide/free radical production from H_2O_2 [171, 198]. The importance of the GSH system in ATO sensitivity was experimentally demonstrated: increasing reduced GSH/sulfhydryl levels decreased ATO sensitivity and vice versa. Also, increased GSH levels were present in NB4 sublines selected for ATO resistance to which ATO sensitivity could be restored by depleting sulfhydryl levels [194, 198]. It was additionally proposed that postexposure ATO binding to vicinal thiols might inhibit H_2O_2-regulatory enzymes and augment endogenous APL sensitivity [171]. However, these enzymes apparently do not directly bind ATO at clinically relevant concentrations (≤1 μM), while this has been demonstrated for thioredoxin reductase (TrxR), a key regulatory enzyme in the alternative thioredoxin (Trx) ROS buffer system [199]. The oxidized (disulfide) forms of both GSH and Trx require NADPH as a reducing substrate (Fig. 21.6). Thus, it is of interest that after several days' exposure of NB4 cells to ATO at a concentration reported not to produce differentiation in these experiments (0.75 μM), gene expression analysis showed a remarkable selective increase in transcripts involved in neutrophil oxidant production, including several components of NADPH oxidase [200]. Further, this was identified as the main source of ROS. Subsequent studies found that NADPH-derived ROS are also increased in untreated NB4 cells and that aberrant regulation of NADPH oxidase is related to impairment of cyclic adenosine monophosphate (cAMP) signaling by PML-RARα [195, 201]. Although no mechanistic details about the impairment link were provided, this scenario seems a reasonable extension of the established inverse relationship of cAMP levels to NADPH oxidase activity in mature neutrophils, which is the principal source of superoxide generation in the antimicrobial response [202]. These studies implicating increased

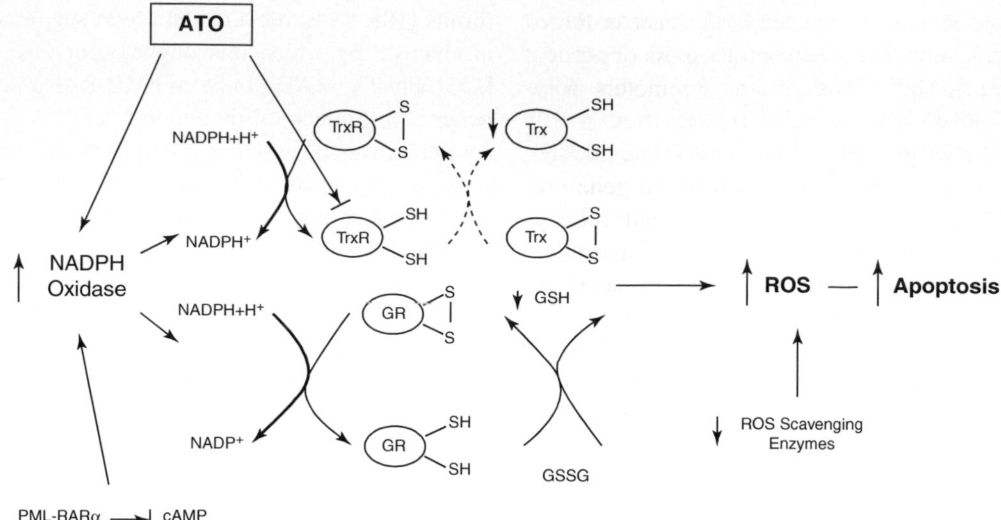

Fig. 21.6 Suggested pathways for the enhanced sensitivity of APL cells to ATO-induced apoptosis. APL promyelocytes, as committed neutrophilic lineage cells, have some increased basal levels of NADPH oxidase, a multicomponent enzyme complex involved in the antimicrobial activity of mature neutrophils. This may be enhanced by the inhibitory activity of PML-RARα on cAMP, which stimulates physiologic NADPH oxidase activity. Some studies also indicate that APL cells have constitutively diminished levels of glutathione (GSH) and reactive oxygen species (ROS) scavenging enzymes. Recent studies indicate that shortly after ATO exposure of APL cells, there are further increases in NADPH oxidase enzyme components associated with a demonstrable increase in the oxidative state. This has been related to depleted levels of NADPH, which is the principal substrate for maintaining the two main cellular antioxidant buffer molecules, GSH and thioredoxin (Trx), in an active, reduced state. ATO has also been demonstrated to strongly inhibit the key Trx system enzyme thioredoxin reductase (TrxR), further contributing to increased oxidative state that triggers the cascade of molecular events leading to apoptosis

ROS *production* due to NADPH depletion, principally after ATO treatment and specifically related to the neutrophilic lineage of APL cells, could supersede the importance of earlier-reported sources of ATO sensitization due to increased oxidative stress attributed to deficiencies in ROS scavenging with consequent decreased ROS *removal*. Regardless of attribution, the increased oxidative state generated by ATO has been linked to activation of a number of signaling pathways leading directly or indirectly to apoptosis mediated by a decrease in mitochondrial membrane potential and executed by activation of the classical caspase 3 pathway [171, 180]. Of particular note is a reportedly essential link of activation of the stress (SAPK/JNK) kinase pathway to apoptosis, possibly related to redox-sensitive conformational changes in glutathione-S-transferase pi [203, 204]. Many other potential effects due to direct interactions of ATO with vicinal sulfhydryl groups in redox sensitive proteins, e.g., with cysteines in zinc finger transcription factors, e.g., Sp1 [205], could be contributory to ATO activity, although this would presumably not be APL specific [180]. In summary, the mechanisms accounting for the high sensitivity of APL cells to ATO-induced apoptosis are complex, may involve complementary aberrations in ROS removing and producing systems, may have some PML-RARα-dependent component, can be modulated by ambient conditions that affect the APL cellular redox state—and, as mentioned before, are of uncertain importance to the clinical response of APL to ATO therapy.

Since the specific, high-sensitivity biological activities of ATRA and ATO in APL cells are dependent on differing interactions with the common target gene PML-RARα, these agents might reasonably be expected to have at least additive complementary activity. However, great variability in combined effects on differentiation and apoptosis in vitro have been experimentally demonstrated, including strong inhibitory interactions, using both sensitive and ATRA- or ATO-resistant APL cell lines and fresh APL cells [196, 206–208]. The variability is at least partly related to differing drug concentrations and schedule effects, as well as to variations in ambient conditions, each of which might affect the time-sensitive availability of PML-RARα and other protein mediators related to the differing activity kinetics of the two agents. In the only global gene transcript/protein expression study in which relatively low, differentiation-inducing concentrations of ATRA (0.1 μM) and ATO (0.5 μM) were concurrently applied to NB4 cells, the changes most closely resembled those of ATRA alone with synergistic upregulation of transcripts involved in protein degradation by the ubiquitin/proteosome system and downregulation of proteins involved in translation [165]. In contrast to the variability in vitro, in vivo studies of combined ATRA/ATO treatment in various mouse APL models have almost uniformly demonstrated positive, often strongly synergistic, antileukemia activity [143, 207, 209, 210]. A possible explanation for this difference with profound implications for the treatment of APL was recently published [41]. In this study, it was first shown in PML-RARα-transduced mixed hematopoietic progenitor cell assays that, although a relatively low concentration of ATRA (0.1 μM) induced terminal granulocytic differentiation, it did not eliminate a subpopulation of progenitor cells that retained clonogenic replating capability, i.e., replicative self-renewal capacity. This in vitro observation suggested that there might be a dissociation of the ability of ATRA to induce differentiation in the bulk of APL cells from an inability to extinguish APL LICs that maintain propagation of the disease. In a subsequent series of in vivo experiments using various APL mouse transplantation models and selected PML-RARα mutations and leukemia initiated by the alternative APL fusion gene PLZF-RARα, further strong evidence was developed in support of dissociation of the differentiation-inducing capacity of ATRA from its anti-LIC activity. Only the latter was able to produce disease cure in the mouse models, using ATRA alone at higher concentrations (≥1 μM) or, most effectively, in combination with ATO and/or cAMP analogs. Molecularly, curative anti-LIC treatment was linked to degradation of PML-RARα under various experimental conditions, including strong inhibition in vivo of synergistic combined ATRA/ATO activity by the proteosome inhibitor bortezomib [41]. The nature of the anti-LIC activity and exactly how it is linked to PML-RARα degradation could not be determined by the functional assays used in these experiments. This must await the identification and characterization of the APL LIC, which, as previously mentioned, appear to present at about a 1:100 level in isolated APL blasts with which they may share many phenotypic properties [42, 43]. Also, these experiments do not exclude a role for ATRA-mediated transcription or distinct ATRA or ATO anti-LIC activities, which could be heterogeneous in different APL cases, partly dependent on the level of hematopoietic progenitor initiated by PML-RARα [211, 212]. The results of these experiments are, however, quite consistent with clinical observations of the curative activity of sustained high-dose ATRA in liposomal form and of combined ATRA and ATO in human APL trials (see clinical sections).

Molecular Mechanisms of Treatment Resistance to ATRA and ATO

Excluding early death from advanced disease or treatment complications, failure to achieve initial clinical remission in patients with de novo PML-RARα-positive APL has rarely been reported after treatment with ATRA [168]. If this is observed, a possible explanation is leukemic chimerism, i.e., the co-existence of APL and a second type of non-ATRA-sensitive leukemia, most frequently t(8;21) AML [213]. The high sensitivity of molecular diagnostic assays for PML-RARα has the potential of masking such chimeras if confirmatory methods such as standard cytogenetics or FISH are not employed. Another documented cause of primary ATRA-resistant disease, reported in 2V-form PML-RARα cases, is a long in-frame insertion of a sequence from RARα intron 2 at the 3′-end of a markedly truncated PML exon 6 that encodes a binding site for additional corepressor protein [71, 72]. One of these cases, additionally, had a frame-shift mutation in the normal PML gene that encoded a truncated carboxy-terminus, deleting the nuclear localizing sequence, which may have also contributed to the ATRA resistance [214]. Combined treatment of ATRA with chemotherapy and/or ATO, as is now common practice, might either overcome or forestall the manifestation of less ATRA-sensitive disease.

The development of acquired ATRA resistance was virtually universal in early clinical studies using ATRA as a single, continuous agent or with low dose chemotherapy [19, 215, 216]. However, some repeat remissions could be secured with ATRA alone if relapse/re-treatment occurred several months after discontinuing ATRA, suggesting a partially reversible systemic mechanism of ATRA resistance [217]. This was substantiated by the pharmacokinetic finding of an ATRA-induced hypercatabolic state that could diminish achievable ATRA plasma levels by up to 80% [218]. The hypercatabolic response was attributed, at least in part, to an increase in liver enzymes that could principally account for the associated increase in oxidative metabolites of orally administered ATRA and, also, to an increase in cellular retinoic acid binding protein (CRABP) in skin that could sequester ATRA to reduce systemic levels. Subsequently, it was found that the hypercatabolic resistance mechanism can be largely avoided by administering ATRA intermittently rather than continuously [219], which has become the standard schedule for administering ATRA after remission induction. A logical deduction of this systemic ATRA resistance mechanism is that alternative agents not subject to its elements should be able to induce second remissions. However, three other retinoid formulations, each with some of these characteristics—oral 9-cis retinoic acid, oral Am80, and intravenous liposomal ATRA [220–222]—were unable to induce second remissions in the majority of ATRA-resistant patients. Overall, these results suggest that other resistance mechanisms are also operative.

By analogy to drug resistance mechanisms in other malignancies, the most probable alternative source of acquired ATRA resistance is an endogenous APL cell mechanism(s). Consistent with this hypothesis, variable loss of sensitivity to ATRA-induced differentiation of fresh APL blasts from patients who relapsed after ATRA treatment in short-term tissue culture has been demonstrated in a majority of cases [167]. Several potential mechanisms of APL cellular ATRA resistance have been proposed, primarily based on investigations of established APL cell lines selected for resistance to ATRA, the most frequent of which is the clonal emergence of cells with mutations in the LBD of the RARα region of PML-RARα [168, 223]. This is, indeed, the only mechanism of ATRA resistance so far demonstrated in APL patients who relapse after clinical ATRA therapy [166, 167]. Such mutations have been documented in 30–40% of patients at first relapse after ATRA-containing therapy, including cases of relapse long after the discontinuation of ATRA and after intervening chemotherapy [167, 224, 225]. A higher incidence of LBD mutations was observed after relapse from two or more treatment regimens containing ATRA [226]. Consistent with a functional role in ATRA resistance, the LBD mutations increase the transcriptional repressor activity of unliganded PML-RARα and diminish ATRA binding and/or its transcriptional activation [226, 227]. Although some of the mutations might be predicted to have an effect on the ability of ATRA to target PML-RARα for degradation, no specific information is available about this potential effect. Also, the downstream defects effected by the mutations in PML-RARα and their role in disease progression and relapse remain to be elucidated. Whatever, the exact mechanism, the high salvage therapy rate with ATO treatment suggests that this agent, in contrast to chemotherapy, can overcome the APL cellular resistance mechanism(s) associated with LBD mutations in many cases, although specific LBD mutations may be less ATO sensitive [225].

A second major hypothesis has been that ATRA resistance is related to altered metabolism of ATRA within APL cells (reviewed in [168]). An initial study suggested that an ATRA-triggered increase in CRABP2, which has an RARE in its gene promoter, could enhance intracellular sequestration and degradation of ATRA, reducing its effectiveness in inducing APL cell differentiation [228]. However, this result was not confirmed in a larger study, including relapse patients [229]. Further, in contrast to the negative effect of CRABP1 on ATRA activity by increasing ATRA catabolism [230], CRABP2 was subsequently determined to have a positive effect on ATRA activity by facilitating its delivery to nuclear receptors [231, 232]. To date, no evidence has been forthcoming in PML-RARα-positive APL to suggest a role of CRABP1 in ATRA resistance, as described earlier for PLZF-RARα/RARα-PLZF-positive APL [148]. Recently, however, a link was made between the ATRA-specific P450 catabolic enzyme, CYP26A1, and ATRA resistance [233]. Surprisingly, it was found that low sensitivity to ATRA-induced differentiation and to retinoid inhibition of NB4 clonal cell growth was associated with *decreased* levels of CYP26A1. It was postulated that the increased nuclear levels of ATRA found in low CYP26A1-expressing cells would increase selection pressure for ATRA-resistant cells, although the downstream resistance mechanism remained to be defined [233]. Notably, this conclusion seems at odds with the previously cited study indicating that high intracellular levels of ATRA are necessary to inhibit the self-renewal capacity of APL LIC and to effect disease cure [41]. In summary, although an attractive idea, a mechanistic role of variations in intracellular APL cell ATRA concentrations and metabolism in clinical ATRA resistance remains uncertain.

Two other potentially important mechanisms of ATRA resistance have been identified in two well-characterized sublines of the NB4 cell line after selection for ATRA resistance in vitro. In subline NB4.007/6, ATRA resistance was related to constitutive activation of the proteosome and resultant degradation of PML-RARα protein [234]. Sensitivity to ATRA could be partially restored by inhibition of proteosome activity and fully restored by forced expression of PML-RARα but not RARα, supporting other evidence that PML-RARα is required for the ATRA-mediated differentiation response. In NB4-MR2, a subcloned derivative of ATRA-resistant NB4 cells, an increased level of topoisomerase 2-beta (TOP2B) was demonstrated to decrease ATRA-mediated gene transcription and granulocytic differentiation by associating with and increasing suppression by the unliganded PML-RARα/corepressor complex [235]. The TOP2B suppressive activity was subsequently attributed to increased protein stability under regulation of protein kinase C-delta (PRKCD), the most abundant isoform of PRKC in hematopoietic cells [236]. Sensitivity to ATRA-induced differentiation could be restored in the NB4-MR2 cells by inhibiting PRKCD, an enzyme itself regulated by phosphorylation, suggesting the possible involvement of yet another upstream kinase in the pathway, possibly p38 MAP kinase. It is noted, however, that some apparently conflicting evidence regarding the role of PRKCD (and of p38 MAP kinase) in wild-type NB4 cell differentiation has been presented [237, 238]. Although neither of these in vitro ATRA-resistance mechanisms has been demonstrated in clinical circumstances, similarities to the second mechanism have been reported in other cancers. For example, ATRA resistance due to diminished ATRA-mediated RARα transcription has been linked to association with the corepressor complex by the suppressor proteins xeroderma pigmentosa-associated protein Xab2 and the tumor-associated protein Ski [239, 240]. Also, increased activation of protein kinases that can affect the activity of RARα or its transcriptional cofactors by phosphorylation, e.g., PI3K/Akt pathway enzyme components, has been implicated in ATRA resistance [241, 242].

In contrast to ATRA resistance, meager information exists about resistance to ATO under clinical conditions. From the single-agent ATO trials conducted in India, Iran, and China (see clinical sections), there is insufficient documentation to assess whether any of the patients who fail to achieve initial remission have primary refractory disease. The incidence of acquired resistance is, however, clearly much less frequent than for ATRA, since most patients with de novo disease sustain prolonged remissions with probable disease cure, even though optimal single-agent therapy has yet to be defined

[243–245]. Of these patients who relapse, almost all patients can achieve a second remission with ATO alone or in combination with other agents [246–248]. However, the second relapse rate is high associated with a significant incidence of ATO-refractory disease [243], implying the acquisition of ATO resistance. In the best documented trial with long-term follow-up, the great majority of patients who relapsed originally presented with a high APL blast count [244], which implies that acquired ATO resistance has an APL cellular basis rather than a systemic pharmacological basis. On the other hand, the observation in this study that patients with liver toxicity had superior disease-free survival raises the possibility that a pharmacogenetic factor could produce variability in ATO exposure and in the extent of response to treatment. Although no specific molecular mechanism of clinical ATO resistance has yet been identified, the recent finding of a high level of telomerase activity and telomere shortening in first relapse post-ATO treatment APL cells implies the presence of other acquired molecular abnormalities associated with disease progression [247].

In vitro studies, principally of ATO-resistant sublines of NB4 cells, have identified several molecular pathway abnormalities associated with resistance to ATO-induced apoptosis. Increased baseline levels of GSH, which can buffer the increased oxidative stress required for ATO-induced apoptosis, have been found in some ATO-resistant NB4 sublines [194, 249]. After the administration of ATO, however, the differential impact of GSH abnormalities in ATO-resistant cells was related to a more complex effect of the ratio of the reduced and oxidized forms (GSH::GSSG) on redox-sensitive proteins than control activation of JUN kinase-mediated apoptosis [204]. In another NB4 subline, ATO resistance was primarily related to increased activation of the MAP kinase ERK1/2-pathway with consequent inhibitory phosphorylation of the pro-apoptotic protein Bad [192]. In other studies, ATO resistance was related to activation of the PI3K/Akt pathway with secondary effects on the cellular redox state and modification of BCL-family proteins [250, 251]. ATO-sensitivity/resistance has also been related to the expression of the putative arsenic influx transporter aquaglyceroporin (AQP9; high expression with sensitivity) [252, 253], to the arsenic export transporter MRP1/ACBB1 (increase with resistance) [249], and of the metalloid-binding proteins, metallothioneins (increase with resistance) [254]. Detailed analysis in yeast has demonstrated ATO resistance to be a multifactorial complex process [253, 255, 256]. Overall, the in vitro results suggest that, if clinical ATO resistance in APL indeed involves reduced apoptosis, the mechanism is likely to be heterogeneous in different relapse cases and, not unlikely, multifactorial in individual relapse cases reflecting the pleiotropic nature of the agent.

APL Molecular Biology: Clinical Applications

The most essential clinical application of molecular biological knowledge in APL has been to provide a definitive diagnosis. Demonstration of the PML-RARα fusion gene (or one of the rare alternative X-RARα fusion genes) to make a genetic diagnosis is now the accepted standard requirement for certifying the diagnosis of APL [257]. The t(15;17) is also entirely specific for APL but this reciprocal translocation is not manifest by standard cytogenetic methods in up to 20% of PML-RARα-positive cases in which the gene rearrangement occurs either because insufficient APL cell metaphases are present or because more subtle intrachromosomal mechanisms are involved [138]. Fluorescence in situ hybridization (FISH) analysis using RARα- and PML-specific probes, which is not dependent on cell division, has a much lower incidence of false negative results and can provide useful supplementary information, particularly in cases with an atypical or complex derivation of PML-RARα. Another specific method, which is useful for rapidly confirming a suspected diagnosis of APL based on cytological evaluation, is a fluorescein-labeled anti-PML antibody to demonstrate the pathognomonic microspeckles in APL cells due to the displacement of PML from nuclear bodies by PML-RARα [258]. Although not entirely specific, immunophenotyping can also be valuable not only by providing early criteria for or against a suspected diagnosis but also for evaluating phenotypic variation among APL patients (see Chap. 17) [259].

A second clinical application of molecular biology relates to studies assessing the potential prognostic value of molecular markers. Most abundantly this has involved analyses of the three types of PML-RARα, the L, V, and S isoforms, which are revealed in the process of making the molecular genetic diagnosis of APL by reverse transcriptase-polymerase chain reaction (RT-PCR) procedure (Fig. 21.4a, b). Some studies have provided evidence that the minor V-form set of APL patients (3–10%) can be associated with potentially adverse risk or response factors, including higher WBC count and decreased ATRA sensitivity [72, 74, 260, 261], or with a high early relapse rate [71, 262]. However, the small number of these cases has prevented an adequate statistical assessment of potentially increased risk, which, in any event, has likely been eliminated by the increased efficacy of current treatment regimens. Much greater evidence has been presented for an association of the S-form patient set compared to the L (or combined L/V-form) patient set with adverse risk factors, including high WBC count, the microgranular (M3v) phenotype, and with internal tandem duplication mutations of the Fms-like tyrosine kinase-3 (FLT3/ITD; see text to come) [74, 261–264]. However, in most major clinical trial reports, the S isoform has not demonstrated statistical significance as a prognostic indicator of clinical outcome independently of its association with a high WBC count [74, 265–270]. With the advent of quantitative RT-PCR procedures (RQ-PCR; described next), prognostic significance has been associated with the level of the PML-RARα transcript but this has been quite variable: in two reports, an adverse prognosis was associated with high levels [268, 271], in a third study this was associated with low levels [269] and in a fourth study, the level had no prognostic significance [272]. Technical differences likely account for these variations, including differences in housekeeping genes controls and in the adjustments in raw data made to calculate the normalized PML-RARα copy number.

The only other specific gene structural variation recurrently tested for prognostic significance in APL clinical trials is mutation of the membrane receptor tyrosine kinase *FLT3* by the in-reading-frame insertion of variable numbers of internal tandem duplications of a juxtamembrane coding segment (FLT/ITD mutations). These mutations result in Flt3 ligand-independent, constitutive activation of Flt3 kinase activity and downstream activation of signaling pathways linked to increased myeloid leukemia cell growth (recently reviewed) [273]. FLT3/ITD mutations occur in 21–38% of occidental APL patients (median >30 vs 12–25% of oriental patients), and, as noted previously, have frequently been associated with increased WBC count, the M3v phenotype, and the S-isoform of PML-RARa (11 clinical trial data recently summarized) [274]. In a minority of studies, a trend toward an association of FLT3/ITD mutations with reduced disease-free or overall survival has been observed by univariate statistical analysis [261, 263, 274–276], however, after adjustment for the associated high WBC count, no study has shown a significant reduction in postremission disease outcome (ibid; 1 study showed a significant association with increased deaths during remission induction [269, 277, 278]. In other classes of AML, quantitative assessment of ITD mutations found that only those with a high ratio of the mutant to the normal FLT3 allele were associated with poor prognosis [279]. However, no such relationship was found in two recent APL studies in which the ITD mutation was quantitatively assessed [269, 278], although in one of these studies, a long insert sequence was independently associated with an increased incidence of disease relapse [269]. In the context of the studies cited earlier, several other mutations have been tested for a possible association with APL disease outcome, including alternative FLT3 activation mutations in the tyrosine kinase domain (FLT3/RTK mutations, most affecting aspartic acid residue 835) [263, 274, 277, 278], RAS gene mutations [261], and MLL gene partial tandem duplications and Kit [263], however, the low frequency of these mutations in APL has limited statistical assessment. Finally, one study found that transcripts for the tumor-testis antigen protein PRAME (preferentially expressed antigen of melanoma) were selectively expressed in APL cells and that a low level of PRAME expression was significantly associated with reduced relapse-free survival largely independent of WBC count [280].

In summary, many studies performed to assess potential molecular prognostic markers in APL find a significant association of high presenting WBC count, hypogranular (M3V) phenotype, S-form PML-RARα, and FLT3/ITD mutations. This is consistent with the proposal that at least a subgroup of patients with these characteristics have a disease variant that significantly differs from the predominant hypergranular disease, perhaps related to different levels of initial hematopoietic progenitor cell transformation [211]. In the context of the ATRA-chemotherapy clinical trials in which this data was developed, a high WBC count clearly takes precedence over the other three elements as a prognostic indicator, although some combined features may make some additional contribution [269, 270]. In at least three recent clinical trials, however, in which frontline arsenic trioxide (ATO) was added to ATRA/chemotherapy, neither a high WBC count nor any of the previously described molecular features of PML-RARα or FLT3 were differentially related to clinical outcome [278, 281–283]. These observations suggest that in the future an alternative set of prognostic indicators will be required to identify the minor fraction of patients (probably <5%), who remain at risk of relapse after the addition of ATO to ATRA/chemotherapy-based treatment.

A third clinical application of molecular biology in APL has been molecular monitoring of subclinical disease after achieving clinical remission (referred to as minimal residual disease; MRD), using the PML-RARα gene transcript as a disease-specific marker. Two RT-PCR methodologies have been applied: (1) a conventional procedure (cRT-PCR) that provides a positive vs negative read-out determined by the presence or absence of stained gel electrophoretic bands of the DNA product derived by terminal PCR amplification of complementary DNA (cDNA) after conversion from RNA by reverse transcriptase [284]; and (2) quantitative PCR (RQ-PCR) that provides a variable read-out depending on the number of PCR cycles that are required to detect the activation of a fluorescent dye indicating the initiation of cDNA amplification (the threshold cycle or C_T), which is dependent on the concentration of the PML-RARα transcript in total cellular RNA [285, 286]. In order to assure proper primer placement for PCR amplification, both of these methods require accurate assignment of the PML-RARα isoform type at the time of diagnosis when the fusion gene is abundantly present (Fig. 21.4a, b). cRT-PCR has a detection sensitivity between 1 in 10^3 and 10^4 (determined by the ability to detect PML-RARα transcript in a serially diluted RNA from a 100% APL cell source, usually an APL cell line), while RQ-PCR sensitivity can be up to ten times more sensitive [287, 288]. A major advantage of RQ-PCR, which has now largely supplanted cRT-PCR for MRD monitoring, is that it can be more accurately standardized. Importantly, this includes adjustment for RNA quality and efficiency of conversion to cDNA by normalization of the PML-RARα copies (calculated by comparison of the sample C_T to those for a plasmid standard curve with known copy numbers) to a constantly expressed housekeeping gene: thus, read-out is expressed as the normalized copy number (NCN) or normalized quotient (NQ).

Important lessons from the application of cRT-PCR to ATRA-chemotherapy clinical trials have included: persistence of MRD detection in the immediate postclinical remission induction period is not an indicator of long-term adverse outcome and is likely due to the slow clearance of terminally differentiated APL cells; detection of MRD after finishing consolidation therapy (molecular persistence) is a virtually certain prognostic indicator for subsequent clinical relapse if a repeat sample is also positive; and, the majority of eventual clinical relapse cases test negative at the postconsolidation checkpoint so that continued monitoring at relatively frequent intervals for 2–3 years is needed to identify most cases destined to clinically relapse [289, 290]. The clinical importance of MRD monitoring was supported by a report that the long-term outcome of patients initiated on salvage therapy based on the detection of MRD (molecular relapse) was superior to that of a historical control group in which salvage therapy was only initiated after clinical relapse [291]. This result was confirmed under internally controlled trial setting [292], and molecular relapse or persistence is now considered the equivalent of clinical relapse in calculating the relapse rate in clinical trial studies [257].

The application of RQ-PCR has confirmed the essential cRT-PCR MRD monitoring results with more accurate and refined criteria. Further, the quantitative NCN values have allowed an assessment of the kinetics of subclinical residual disease, e.g., not only whether a confirmatory, repeat test after a suspicious result is positive or negative but whether it is increasing or decreasing. From several RQ-PCR studies, it is apparent that low levels of MRD may remain detectable and yet not necessarily be a harbinger of inevitable clinical relapse, especially in the early postconsolidation treatment phase [272, 283, 287, 293, 294]. In these studies, it has been possible to define criteria—either threshold NCN values with a very high risk of subsequent clinical relapse [272, 287, 293] or compelling evidence of increasing MRD levels in serially collected samples [294]—that mandate immediate salvage therapy. In practice, prospective (rather than retrospective) RQ-PCR MRD monitoring with criteria for treatment change during the subclinical phase has only been realized in two clinical trial reports [283, 294]. In the first report, the principal clinical trial objective was to identify patients who were in subclinical relapse after ATRA-chemotherapy treatment in order to initiate early ATO salvage therapy [294]. Notable results of this study were: the clinical relapse rate after 3-years follow-up was reduced to 5% compared to 12% in an earlier similar clinical trial with no prospective MRD monitoring; there was no incidence of the differentiation syndrome when ATO salvage therapy was administered with subclinical disease which was sometimes present and problematic after hematological relapse; and MRD monitoring of bone marrow was more effective than peripheral blood. The latter is confirmation of earlier indications of this difference in studies with very limited case numbers [287, 293], although similar levels of MRD have been reported in simultaneously obtained bone marrow and blood samples, possibly related to disproportionate testing of early treatment samples [272, 287, 294]. Further, continued MRD monitoring during and after ATO salvage therapy was effective in detecting patients in incipient second relapse and in evaluating patients for transplant candidacy while the disease was still subclinical [294]. In the second report, intensive MRD monitoring was employed as a precautionary measure in an exploratory Phase II clinical trial in which frontline ATO therapy was administered with potentially insufficient, reduced-intensity chemotherapy in combination with ATRA [283]. However, among 37 patients (including 12 with high WBC counts) who completed consolidation therapy, there was only 1 relapse confined to the central nervous system and no hematological relapses (2.7% incidence of relapse with 2.7 years follow-up). Concordantly, after the completion of consolidation therapy, there were no RQ-PCR assays in bone marrow or peripheral blood that exceeded a high-risk NCN/NQ value ($>10^{-5}$; risk values defined in [272, 295]), a series of intermediate-risk values ($>10^{-6}$ but $<10^{-5}$; predominantly in blood) in the CNS relapse case, and only three assays (out of hundreds) that transiently exceeded an intermediate-risk NCN value in the remaining cases [283]. This study and other recent studies indicating that the relapse rate in APL is likely to be <5% after the addition of frontline ATO to ATRA chemotherapy even in high-risk, high WBC count patients [281, 282] bring into question the cost-to-benefit ratio of continuing to perform MRD monitoring in APL patients with primary disease. Consideration of this issue is sharpened by a recent study using mathematical modeling which concluded that to be highly effective in prospectively detecting MRD in time to implement preclinical relapse salvage therapy in APL, RQ-PCR testing would need to be performed on bone marrow samples every 2 months [296]. Thus, in the future it may be reasonable to limit MRD monitoring by RQ-PCR in primary disease to clinical trial settings in which the predicted incidence of relapse has not been established to be very low, e.g., in exploratory trials that attempt to further reduce exposure to cytotoxic chemotherapy. On the other hand, intensive application of this now highly validated method after the occurrence of increasingly rare first relapse seems indicated, since the long-term outcome of salvage therapy is less certain and molecular monitoring will likely be useful in making therapeutic adjustments to avoid secondary clinical relapses.

Clinical Features

APL accounts for about 10% of adult AML and the incidence appears to be approximately constant with respect to age [297], an observation not previously reported for any other neoplasm. The incidence in children is usually reported to be lower [298], although the incidence of APL in children diagnosed with AML and living in Italy seems to be about twice that of children living in Germany or the United States [299–301].

When Latinos develop AML they may be significantly more likely to develop APL than another AML subtype [302–305], and an investigation of the Eastern Cooperative Oncology Group database for leukemia studies E2491 and E3489 revealed that more APL patients are Latinos than are other AML patients ($P = 0.005$) [306]. Others have reported that blacks have a lower likelihood of APL than Hispanics, non-Hispanic whites, and Asians [307].

There is no difference in the incidence between the sexes [308] and the median age of patients with APL appears to be about 15 years younger than that of patients with other forms of AML (43 years vs. 59 years, $P < 0.00001$) [309]. Curiously, increasing body mass index was strongly associated with a diagnosis of APL among patients with AML ($P = 0.0003$) in one study [309] and associated with the differentiation syndrome (discussed in text to come) in another [310]. Some epidemiological studies have implicated exposure to electromagnetic fields [308] and radon exposure [308] in the etiology of APL. Therapy-related APL has been increasingly recognized [83, 311–313]. Exposure to drugs that target topoisomerase II may be especially likely to result in treatment-related APL [81]. An association with exposure to mitoxantrone for, among other diseases, multiple sclerosis, has been well established [82, 314, 315], and it has been suggested that gefitinib therapy for lung cancer may also result in secondary APL [316].

The most significant clinical feature of APL is a hemorrhagic diathesis manifested by ecchymoses, intracranial hemorrhage, or gastrointestinal bleeding, some evidence of which is present at diagnosis in the majority of patients [317, 318]. Sudden blindness due to sinus vein thrombosis has been reported [319] and other large vessel thromboses have been reported as well [320], although hemorrhage is much more common than thrombosis in APL. The most frequently documented laboratory evidence of the bleeding diathesis includes hypofibrinogenemia, increased fibrin degradation products in the serum, a prolonged prothrombin time, and, of course, thrombocytopenia [317, 318, 321]. The potential for bleeding is exacerbated by cytotoxic chemotherapy with consequent thrombocytopenia [318, 322]. The diagnosis and treatment of this important life-threatening manifestation of APL is fully discussed below.

The diagnostic hallmark of APL is the balanced cytogenetic translocation t(15;17)(q22;q11.2–12) [323] that has been discussed in detail above. However, approximately one-third of patients have additional cytogenetic abnormalities, most frequently trisomy 8 [324–326]. There may be a deleterious effect of additional cytogenetic abnormalities on the course of APL in general although the data available are conflicting. In a study of 47 APL patients, 17 with additional cytogenetic aberrations, Schoch et al. [327] found no influence of such abnormalities on prognosis. Some of their patients were treated with ATRA, others with chemotherapy. In a larger study of 161 patients treated with chemotherapy alone, Slack et al. [328] found that secondary cytogenetic changes were associated with significantly longer CR duration and event-free survival after treatment with anthracycline and cytarabine. They concluded that additional cytogenetic changes do not impair prognosis of patients with APL treated with chemotherapy. Pantic et al. [329] studied 43 APL patients treated with ATRA alone and found additional cytogenetic changes in 33%. The CR and early death rates were significantly different between those patients with and without additional abnormalities (36% vs. 76% $p = .0148$; 24 vs. 64%, $p = 0.0141$, respectively). They concluded that patients treated with ATRA who have additional cytogenetic abnormalities have a more aggressive disease than those with only t(15;17). We found this also to be true, and also that patients treated with ATRA with or without chemotherapy who had t(15;17) alone had a significantly better overall survival than did patients with additional cytogenetic abnormalities [330]. We concluded from a study of 140 patients that those with APL and t(15;17) alone were significantly more sensitive to ATRA than are patients with t(15;17) and additional cytogenetic abnormalities. Others have reported similar results in patients treated with ATRA and anthracyclines together [326] and concluded that additional cytogenetic changes may render patients less sensitive to ATRA, as suggested by the data of Pantic et al. [329] and Wiernik et al [330]. Consistent with these observations, Xu et al. [331] after a study of 284 patients with APL recently reported that relapse-free and overall survival are significantly poorer in patients with complex karyotypes compared with patients with only t(15;17). However, De Botton et al. [325] studied 292 patients treated with ATRA and chemotherapy. Additional cytogenetic abnormalities were present in 26% of cases and there was no difference in outcome between patients with and without additional cytogenetic aberrations. At present, because of conflicting data, there is no clear indication based on additional cytogenetic changes to alter what has become conventional therapy with ATRA and anthracycline-based chemotherapy [331] (discussed below). Secondary clonal cytogenetic abnormalities frequently appear in APL patients after treatment, but seem to be of no clinical importance [270, 332, 333]. Rarely, APL patients present with t(11;17) [138] as the only cytogenetic abnormality, and such patients are usually refractory to

ATRA treatment. Jansen et al. [334] induced a complete molecular remission in such a patient with the combination of ATRA plus G-CSF after demonstrating the efficacy of that regimen in vitro.

The immunophenotype of APL cells is unique among the myeloid leukemias, since they are characteristically HLA-DR-negative, CD34-negative, p-glycoprotein-negative, and CD33+ although the M3v (microgranular variant) subtype may be positive for either CD34, p-glycoprotein, or both (see Chap. 17). In addition, certain T-cell antigens, such as CD2, are frequently expressed by the FAB-M3v type of APL [318, 334, 335]. Rarely, APL cells express CD56, a neural-cell adhesion molecule. Such patients may have a poor prognosis for complete response and response duration [336].

The morphology of the leukemic cells in APL is unique and discussed in Chap. 16. Briefly, three morphological subtypes have been described. In the hypergranular type, which is the most common form of the disease, the cells appear to be abnormal promyelocytes with abundant cytoplasmic granulation that stains purple or pink with Wright's or similar stains. Auer rods are common, usually multiple, and frequently appear in bundles (haystacks) [337]. The nucleus is bilobed, folded, or reniform, suggestive of the nucleus of a monocyte [318, 337]. In the microgranular type [337], which accounts for approximately 25% of all APL cases [264, 338–340], cytoplasmic granules are difficult to see with the light microscope and Auer rods are rare. Occasional typical M3 cells are seen in the peripheral blood and are more numerous in the bone marrow. The nucleus in M3v appears similar to that of M3. M3v cells are much more commonly CD2+ than are M3 cells [335, 339] and the t(15;17) abnormality is almost always present [335, 339, 341]. A third, rare form of APL has been designated as the hyperbasophilic microgranular form [337, 342–344], by some authors. The cytoplasmic granules are intensely basophilic and prominent cytoplasmic budding is often evident in this as well as is in microgranular type. The morphology of those latter two types is reminiscent of that of micromegakaryocytes [321, 341]. Cytogenetic and immunophenotypic characteristics are typical for APL, except that in the hyperbasophilic microgranular type additional cytogenetic abnormalities such as 12p13 [344, 345], which has been described in AML with basophilic differentiation [338] may be found. At least one hyperbasophilic microgarnular patient developed hyperhistaminemia after treatment, presumably secondary to release of histamine from the basophilic granules of killed cells [346]. Both APL variants seem to have more severe bleeding at diagnosis than typical APL patients [264, 338, 342] despite higher platelet counts [339], and both are much more common in non-Whites [264, 318, 339–341, 347–349] and in females [339, 341, 343]. The determination of APL type must be made prior to therapy since arsenic trioxide therapy may induce basophilic differentiation of APL cells [350].

Histochemically, M3 cells are strongly peroxidase- and Sudan black-positive and, on occasion, strong α-naphthylacetate esterase activity sensitive to sodium fluoride may be demonstrated [337, 351–353], similar to that often observed in FAB-M4 or M5 AML. This finding is not observed in normal promyelocytes. Microgranular APL cells are less frequently peroxidase or esterase positive than typical APL cells [339, 340]. Microgranular APL may have had a poorer response to treatment and a poorer prognosis than typical APL with chemotherapy alone in the past [339], but this is no longer true when treatment includes ATRA [264].

Typically, patients with APL present with lower white blood cell counts (WBC) than do other patients with AML and counts of less than 1000 cells/μL are common [318]. Patients with microgranular APL generally present with higher WBC and leukocytosis is frequent [298, 334, 343]. Anemia is common at presentation [318] and may be severe in bleeding patients. Organomegaly, lymphadenopathy, and central nervous system (CNS) leukemia are rare in APL in the United States [298, 318], but may be more common in other countries for unknown reasons [343].

Approximately 3–5% of APL patients relapse at extramedullary sites. In the ATRA era, central nervous system (CNS) relapse appears be more common than in the pre-ATRA era and is more frequent among patients who present with a high white blood cell count [354–358]. An initial serum lactate dehydrogenase level of >3000 IU/L was recently found to be more strongly associated with CNS relapse than is an initial WBC of >10,000/μL [359]. Other factors associated with a higher incidence of CNS relapse include elderly patients, and CNS hemorrhage during induction therapy. CNS relapse is the most common form of extramedullary disease in APL [360] and usually occurs within 10 months of diagnosis. It may also rarely be diagnosed at initial presentation [361]. Other sites of extramedullary relapse include skin infiltration, [322, 349], and bone [362] after treatment with chemotherapy or ATRA [363–365], particularly among those patients who present with high a WBC. Rarely, isolated extramedullary relapse may occur after more than a decade of complete remission [362].

Most patients with APL do not have an antecedent hematologic or neoplastic disease. However, therapy-related APL with the typical t(15;17) has been reported after treatment for other neoplasms, including breast cancer, prostate cancer, non-Hodgkin's lymphoma [366], papillary thyroid carcinoma [367], and other neoplasms. In fact, most reported cases of therapy-related APL occurred in patients previously treated for breast cancer [367, 368]. This is curious because BRCA1 is located on chromosome 17 near the breakpoint involved in the formation of t(15;17) [369]. Wei et al [370] reported that ATRA inhibits a key regulator of oncogenic signaling pathways, the unique isomerase Pin1 in APL and breast cancer cells. This observation suggests some common pathways in the etiology of both diseases.The incidence of therapy-related APL may be increasing [371]. It occurs primarily in middle-aged adults with a peak incidence at 2 years post treatment for the initial neoplasm and is more common in women [371]. Topoisomerase II inhibitors, radiation, and mitoxantrone are the most common treatments prior to the development of APL. The complete response rate and prognosis after treatment of treatment-related APL is similar to that of de novo APL [371, 372]. Prostate cancer is being recognized more frequently recently as a tumor associated with an increasing incidence of treatment-related APL [372]. In addition, karyotypically confirmed promyelocytic blast crisis of chronic myelogenous leukemia (CML) has been occasionally reported [373–376], and promyelocytic blast crisis of CML with cytogenetic abnormalities other than t(15;17), but involving chromosome 17 has been documented [377]. In fact, such a patient was the first patient with leukemia in the United States to respond to ATRA [369]. Rarely, patients with APL relapse with a cytogenetically different AML or myelodysplasia following treatment of the original leukemia [378–382]. Most such patients to date have received prior anthracycline therapy.

On rare occasion APL may be diagnosed upon relapse of other types of acute myeloid leukemia (AML) [383], and in other rare instances APL may relapse as another type of AML or myelodysplastic syndrome [384]. APL has even been reported to develop in donor cells after an allogeneic stem cell transplant [385].

Three risk groups of patients with APL have been generally recognized: low-risk, intermediate-risk, and high-risk. Low-risk patients are those with an initial WBC <10,000/μL and a platelet count >40/000/μL, intermediate risk patients are those with a WBC <10,000/μL and a platelet count <40,000/μL; high-risk patients are those with a WBC >10,000/μL irrespective of platelet count. Low-risk and intermediate-risk patients have classically been considered together for treatment purposes but therapy is usually intensified for the 10–15% of patients that are at high-risk (see below) since they are at higher risk for relapse, hemorrhage [386] and death (but usually not for lower complete response to induction therapy). Elderly patients often fall into the high-risk category [387]. Leukapheresis does not improve the prognosis for patients with hyperleukocytosis [388].

More recently, additional factors associated with therapeutic response have been identified. Patients whose leukemic blasts are CD34+, CD56+ or CD2+ are at higher risk of relapse. These antigen expressions are often associated with leukocytosis [386]. Patients with the short PML/RARα isoform as well as those with FLT3-ITD mutations (also associated with leukocytosis) are at increased risk for relapse as well in some studies [386, 389], and FLT3-ITD mutations were associated with impaired survival after treatment with ATRA and chemotherapy in one study and event-free survival in another [390]. However, importantly, FLT3-ITD mutations had no effect on outcome after treatment with ATRA plus arsenic trioxide [390]. Another study identified by multivariate analysis that the quantity of RARα transcripts in blood prior to induction therapy as the sole independent prognostic factor for relapse. At 5 years after treatment patients with >209.6 PML-RARα/ng had a cumulative incidence of relapse of >50% compared with 7.5% for those with less molecular burden of transcript [391]. Low transcript levels of KMT2E (MLL5), a gene involved in the positive control of genes involved in hematopoiesis, results in lower remission rate and shorter overall survival in patients with APL treated with ATRA and an anthracycline [392], and WT1 expression was shown to be an independent prognostic factor for overall survival of complete responders to induction therapy [393].

The TP73 gene transcript is translated into an active TAp73) and inactive (ΔNp73) isoforms. Higher inactive form/active form RNA ratios are associated with a higher risk of relapse and poorer survival of patients treated with ATRA plus anthracycline [394]. Lastly, data suggesting that ETV6 rearrangement may be an independent unfavorable prognostic factors for overall survival in patients with APL [395].

Most of the prognostic factors described above have been identified in patients treated with ATRA and anthracycline chemotherapy. Since arsenic trioxide is playing an increasingly important role in the treatment of APL it will be important to verify which, if any, of these factors still are reliable prognostic indicators that can be used to stratify patients among various therapeutic approaches. Recently, Lou et al. [396] addressed this question in 184 patients treated with arsenic trioxide-base therapy. They found no significant association between 3-year relapse-free survival and initial WBC count, FLT3-ITD status or type of PML-RARα isoform. Only CD56 in their study retained prognostic value with respect to relapse-free survival. These data suggest that arsenic trioxide-based therapy is superior to ATRA plus anthracycline treatment and that some previously important prognostic factors are no longer relevant. Further studies of this kind are needed. It may be necessary in the near future to revise commonly used risk assessment schemes for patients with APL.

The primary cause of treatment failure for patients with APL is death caused by the coagulopathy characteristic of this disease [397]. The early death rate is approximately 10% in patients <50 years of age and 30% in older patients. It is higher in patients not enrolled in clinical trials than in patients enrolled in such trials [398, 399]. Death from this cause may even occur before treatment is begun. Early death rates may be higher in uninsured patients and among minority populations [400]. Therefore, it is imperative to remove the societal obstacles to early, competent care for these subpopulations.

Treatment of APL

APL patients must be prepared for induction therapy as described for other FAB types in Chap. 22 whenever possible, but time is of the essence in APL more so than in other FAB types in that the diagnosis of APL is a medical emergency that requires immediate intervention. Once the diagnosis is suspected and while it is being confirmed by polymerase chain reaction or by immunofluorescence staining with an antipromyelocytic leukemia antibody [401], aggressive supportive care measures with blood product support should be instituted, and ATRA should be started. If the diagnosis of APL is not confirmed, ATRA should be discontinued. Concurrent with initiation of induction therapy, the hemorrhagic diathesis, which clinically or subclinically is present in virtually every patient, must be brought under control since such therapy may exacerbate the bleeding problem, particularly in patients with leukocytosis. Specific recommendations for controlling hemorrhage are given next [402, 403].

Induction Therapy

The response of APL to appropriate induction therapy is unique among the acute leukemias. As initially pointed out by Kantarjian et al. [9] and by Daly et al. [317], hematologic recovery from induction chemotherapy in at least 85% of patients is accompanied by an increase rather than a decrease of promyelocytes in the bone marrow, which spontaneously mature over several or more weeks. Postinduction therapy bone marrow specimens with increased promyelocytes have frequently been erroneously interpreted as indicative of treatment failure and retreatment has led to the death of patients. Virtually no patients who survive induction therapy will require a second course because primary resistance of leukemic promyelocytes to commonly used agents, such as ATRA and arsenic trioxide is extremely rare. Resistance to ATRA when it occurs is associated with mutations in the RARα moiety of PML-RARα and resistance to arsenic trioxide is associated with mutations in the PML moiety. Both mutation types interfere with degradation of PML-RARα, the gene that drives the disease [404]. Both agents synergistically degrade mutated NPM1 genes which results in apoptosis [405].

History of Specific Induction Chemotherapy

Anthracyclines have been the cornerstone of chemotherapy for APL since the landmark observation of Bernard et al. that daunorubicin induced a high percentage of complete responses in this leukemia [5] and that CRs were of unusually long duration, compared with those in other morphologic subtypes of AML. Since that discovery, the most common treatment reported for APL has been the standard daunorubicin and cytarabine regimen originally described by Yates and colleagues [411] and recommended by them for all FAB types. There is, however, little evidence that cytarabine is actually necessary as an induction agent in APL [407, 408]. At least 350 patients with APL treated with daunorubicin alone can be gleaned from the literature, with an overall CR rate >70% [317, 342, 345, 409–413]. This result compares very favorably with the 67% CR rate published from 1990 to 2010 for 537 patients induced with daunorubicin and cytarabine with or without other chemotherapy [318, 406–421].

In a trial of idarubicin and cytarabine compared with historical controls treated with daunorubicin and cytarabine [422, 423], the former yielded significantly greater disease-free and overall survival compared with the latter. This result may be valid, since the same advantage for idarubicin and cytarabine over standard therapy has been reported for AML in general [424, 425], and others [426] have reported an unusually high complete response rate with idarubicin alone in APL. Newer strategies have included lower doses of idarubicin in children combined with ATRA [427]. The Italian GIMEMA group and Spanish PETHEMA group have reported high complete response rates with ATRA and anthracycline, and the combination became a standard induction regimen for APL [266, 408, 428–434].

ATRA Induction Therapy

Orally administered ATRA induces complete, albeit relatively brief remissions in the vast majority of patients with APL. Unfortunately, relapse usually occurs within months if no postremission therapy is given. Complete remission with ATRA is accomplished by induction of differentiation and maturation of leukemic cells, and not by a cytotoxic mechanism [431]. Clinical evidence of this fact includes the occasional observation of mature neutrophils in responding patients that contain Auer rods, suggesting that these neutrophils are matured leukemic cells [432].

Pharmacology of ATRA

Orally administered ATRA, 45 mg/m^2, results in a peak plasma concentration in 1–2 h [433] and is rapidly eliminated from humans, with a terminal half-life of approximately 45 min after an initial dose [434]. Following long-term daily administration of the agent, plasma concentrations of ATRA decrease significantly over time [218]. The only known metabolite is 4-oxo-all-*trans* retinoic acid, which is found in plasma and urine, but accounts for only about 10% of administered ATRA [433, 435]. ATRA does not enter the cerebrospinal fluid [433]. The mean area under the curve for plasma drug concentration of ATRA varies considerably from patient to patient [433, 434]. It was suggested that relapse on continuous administration of ATRA may be due to the progressive reduction of plasma concentration described previously to levels below those that effect leukemic cell differentiation, since leukemic cells from patients who relapsed on ATRA usually continued to be sensitive to the agent in vitro at ATRA concentrations that resulted in differentiation initially. However, it is now known that marked decreases in plasma concentration occur within days of initial administration, long before relapse occurs in virtually all patients [433]. Induction of accelerated catabolism by a cytochrome P-450-like enzyme system has been suggested as a mechanism for these peculiar aspects of ATRA catabolism [433]. This suggestion has merit, since inhibitors of oxidation by cytochrome P-450 enzymes such as ketoconazole, fluconazole [436], and liarozole [437] significantly increase plasma concentrations of ATRA and decrease concentrations of the oxo-metabolite when administered with ATRA. A recently offered possible alternative explanation for the accelerated ATRA catabolism observed after its continuous administration is that ATRA administration appears to result in increased levels of plasma lipid hydroperoxides, which accelerate the oxidative catabolism of ATRA in human microsomes in vitro [438]. And, of course, it is quite possible that ATRA blood levels correlate poorly with ATRA activity because they are irrelevant. Intracellular ATRA concentrations are much more determinant of ATRA activity [439].

Clinical Results with ATRA

Huang et al. [12] first reported on the clinical usefulness of ATRA in APL in 1988. They treated 16 previously untreated and eight previously treated patients with oral ATRA, 45–100 mg/m^2/day. All patients achieved a hematologic and clinical CR without developing bone marrow hypoplasia. Eight patients experienced early relapses within 5 months while still receiving ATRA, but the others remained in remission at the time of their publication for as long as 11+ months. This landmark observation that ATRA could induce remissions in the vast majority of patients with APL presumably by differentiation induction attracted little attention initially in the United States, but French collaborators of the Chinese investigators immediately recognized the importance of this observation and initiated their own trials, which proved to be confirmatory [440].

Chen et al. [215] observed that patients who were induced into remission with ATRA and then maintained with conventional chemotherapy could usually be successfully reinduced into second remission with ATRA after relapse, whereas patients who received both ATRA and chemotherapy as postremission treatment usually could not be induced into second remission with ATRA alone. Based on these observations, they suggested that ATRA should be discontinued upon the achievement of CR.

Subsequent studies by a large number of investigators demonstrated that, while the vast majority of patients with APL achieved CR with ATRA, some patients, perhaps 10–20%, did not respond well, primarily due to early death. In addition, a serious problem with ATRA therapy, initially termed the retinoic acid syndrome [441, 442] but now referred to as the APL differentiation syndrome, became evident (see below). This occasionally fatal, rapidly developing pulmonary distress syndrome is not related to pulmonary leukostasis, but is often but not always associated with a rapidly rising peripheral WBC count consisting of predominantly maturing cells. In initial studies, the differentiation syndrome developed in as many as one-quarter of patients within days or weeks of starting ATRA therapy. This observation, and those of Chen et al. [215] discussed earlier, led Fenaux et al. [443] to combine ATRA induction therapy with postremission chemotherapy on a flexible schedule. Their plan was to begin treatment with ATRA and switch to anthracycline-based chemotherapy after remission was achieved unless a rising WBC occurred with ATRA, a dangerous harbinger of the differentiation syndrome, in which case chemotherapy was administered early along with ATRA until CR was documented, after which chemotherapy was continued. A CR in 96% of patients was achieved with this approach in a pilot study of 26 patients and the actuarial disease-free survival of 87% at 18 months was significantly better than the 59% rate observed in their previous chemotherapy-alone study [443]. This pilot study led to a larger multi-institutional study in which 101 patients under the age of 65 years were randomized to receive daunorubicin and cytarabine alone, or those drugs preceded by ATRA treatment [444]. Both groups received two courses of daunorubicin and cytarabine as consolidation therapy after complete remission was achieved. The three-drug induction regimen yielded a 91% CR rate and a 9% death during induction rate, compared with an 81% complete response rate and an 8% death during induction rate for the two-drug regimen. Neither of the differences is significant. However, the estimated 4-year event-free survival in the ATRA plus chemotherapy induction group was 63% compared with 17% in the chemotherapy-alone group, which is a highly statistically significantly different outcome. Overall survival at 4 years for the combined modality and chemotherapy-alone groups was 76% and 49%, respectively, which is also a highly significant difference [445]. Therefore, although the addition of ATRA to standard induction chemotherapy did not result in a significantly higher CR rate or reduced early death rate, disease-free survival of complete responders was greatly enhanced.

In addition, ATRA therapy rapidly resolved the coagulopathy in most patients, an observation subsequently confirmed by others [446]. This approach to APL treatment was validated by Kanamaru et al. [447], who obtained results virtually identical to those of Fenaux et al. [444]. In that study [447], approximately 89% of 110 patients achieved CR with ATRA alone or ATRA and early chemotherapy and 6.3% developed the differentiation syndrome. With a median follow-up of 21 months, 81% of the complete responders were projected to be disease free at 23 months, which was significantly greater than the disease-free survival rate observed in a prior chemotherapy-alone study. Unlike the study reported by Fenaux et al. [445], the Japanese study demonstrated a significantly lower early mortality rate than observed in the chemotherapy-alone historical control [447]. Burnett et al. [267] demonstrated that prolonged ATRA administration starting simultaneously with chemotherapy and continuing throughout the induction period until complete response is diagnosed gave superior results compared with a short course of ATRA prior to chemotherapy. Patients in the former group had a significantly higher CR rate and fewer induction deaths, as well as superior survival at 4 years, compared with those treated with a short course of ATRA.

Liposomal ATRA given intravenously may be more active than orally administered ATRA [222, 448, 449]. When administered every other day at a dose of 90 mg/m^2, blood levels are maintained, rather than observed to decline as is the case with orally administered ATRA. Results are similar with the two formulations, but liposomal ATRA may be more likely to yield a molecular remission as determined by PCR than is oral ATRA [448]. However, liposome-encapsulated ATRA is no longer available, but a new preparation of ATRA loaded in cholesteryl butyrate solid lipid nanoparticles appears to be superior to ATRA alone against APL cell lines and may eventually come to clinical trial [450].

ATRA in conjunction with anthracycline chemotherapy or arsenic trioxide is superior to either approach alone for initial treatment of APL. The combined approach may not reduce the early death rate associated with APL therapy, however. Furthermore, CR rates with chemotherapy, ATRA, or a sequential combination of both appear to be quite similar. The major advantage for combined modality treatment with ATRA and chemotherapy is the significantly greater disease-free and overall survival achieved with the combination in virtually all controlled trials [451]. Yet another benefit appears to be a reduction in the incidence of the differentiation syndrome with concurrent therapy [452]. In addition, patients treated with ATRA prior to chemotherapy may have more rapid recovery of the peripheral granulocyte count compared with patients treated with chemotherapy alone [453].

More than 90% of newly diagnosed patients with APL initially treated with ATRA and idarubicin achieve a complete remission with that therapy. Almost all induction failures are due to death during induction from hemorrhage, infection, or differentiation syndrome which result in 5%, 2–3%, and 1–2% deaths of all treated patients, respectively. Elevated serum creatinine, increased peripheral blast count, and presence of coagulopathy correlate with an increased incidence of death from hemorrhage. Age >60 years, male sex, and fever at presentation correlate with an increased likelihood of death from infection, and poor performance score as well as hypoalbuminemia correlates with an increased likelihood of developing a fatal differentiation syndrome [454].

Whether other retinoids [221, 455–459] are superior to ATRA in the treatment of APL needs to be determined as well. Observations on the potentiation of megakaryocytopoiesis by ATRA [460, 461] and on the inhibition of marrow angiogenesis by ATRA [462] require further study, as does the observation that imatinib [463] and statins [464, 465] may potentiate ATRA activity against APL.

Retinoic Acid Toxicity

Differentiation Syndrome

The most serious toxicity associated with ATRA therapy is the APL differentiation syndrome [466] which occurs in 25% or more of patients treated with ATRA alone [467], or in combination with anthracycline chemotherapy [468]. Differentiation syndrome may also be induced by arsenic trioxide [469]. Half the patients who develop the syndrome have a severe form which can be fatal, and the others have a moderate form from which recovery is the rule [468]. Severe, life-threatening differentiation syndrome usually occurs in the first 2 weeks of treatment, while a milder form may occur later [470]. Fever and respiratory distress with or without pulmonary infiltrates on chest radiograph are the hallmarks of the syndrome. Weight gain, pedal edema, pleural and pericardial effusion, and hypotension may also occur. A bimodal incidence of the syndrome is reported with peaks occurring in the first and third weeks after the initiation of ATRA therapy [471]. Rarely, a patient may develop the syndrome during both peak incidence periods [471]. Autopsy reveals massive pulmonary parenchymal tissue infiltration with maturing myeloid cells [467]. A white blood cell count >5000/μL and a serum creatinine concentration above normal correlate with an increased risk for severe differentiation syndrome [472]. In most, but not all patients the syndrome is preceded by a rapidly rising white blood cell count. ATRA must be discontinued at once when the manifestations of the syndrome are severe and dexamethasone, 10 mg intravenously every 12 h should be administered until complete clinical resolution of the syndrome is obtained, usually in several days. Some evidence suggests that prophylactic dexamethasone can reduce the incidence of the syndrome [472]. If the manifestations are mild, ATRA can be continued with the institution of dexamethasone. Most patients so treated will survive and, once the syndrome has resolved, ATRA therapy can usually be safely reinstituted, but it is recommended that resumption of ATRA be carried out under the coverage of steroids [467]. The syndrome rarely, if ever, occurs in patients receiving ATRA as postremission therapy [467]. Curiously, there are no data on hydroxyurea as treatment for this syndrome.

The early (concurrent) administration of chemotherapy with ATRA for induction appears to have a benefit with respect to reduction in the incidence of this syndrome [468]. Diffuse pulmonary hemorrhage may mimic the syndrome or may be a manifestation of it [473, 474].

The pathogenesis of the ATRA syndrome is not entirely known. Expression of CD13 by APL cells obtained at diagnosis significantly correlated with the development of the ATRA syndrome in one study [473, 474], which is interesting since expression of that antigen (aminopeptidase N) has previously been associated with a poor prognosis in AML and with tumor invasive capacity in some human tumor cell lines. It has been suggested that bestatin [466], a specific inhibitor of aminopeptidase N, should be tested as a possible prophylactic agent against the ATRA syndrome. It has also been demonstrated that ATRA upregulates CD54, CD11b, and CD18 on APL cells, which facilitates adhesion of them to pulmonary microvasculature, which can be reversed in vitro by anti-CD54 and anti-CD18 antibodies [475]. Furthermore, ATRA may induce chemokine production in the lung and in APL cells which enhance migration of the leukemic cells out of the vascular system [476–478].

Other ATRA Toxicity

Other toxicities associated with ATRA therapy are usually mild and include dry mucous membranes, bone pain, headache, hypertriglyceridemia, hepatic enzyme elevation, and skin rash, which may rarely evolve into erythema nodosum [479]. Pseudotumor cerebri has been reported in approximately 2% of patients receiving ATRA. The incidence is higher in children and young adults than in older patients [480, 481]. The cause is entirely unclear, but recently thrombophilic factor dysmetabolism has been implicated [482]. Treatment in APL patients usually only requires diuretics. Sweet syndrome [483, 484] has rarely been reported after ATRA administration, presumably due to a mechanism similar to that of the ATRA syndrome. Occasionally, serious thrombotic episodes may occur with ATRA therapy even when thrombocytopenia is present [485]. ATRA-induced thrombocytosis has also been observed [486, 487].

Patients treated with ATRA and anthracycline-based chemotherapy have approximately a 2% incidence of an acute myeloid leukemia or myelodysplastic syndrome developing in a median of 4 years after completing treatment for APL. The treatment-related myeloid disorder is associated with deletions of chromosomes 5 and/or 7, or 11q23 rearrangements. Patients over the age of 35 years have a higher incidence of this complication than others (approximately 5%) [488].

Clinical Results with Arsenic Trioxide

The most important new development in the treatment of APL in recent years is the introduction of arsenic trioxide (ATO) as a therapeutic agent. The drug was used in the late 1800s in the treatment of CML with some success [489]. Shen et al. [182] reported the activity of this agent in APL 2 decades ago. They administered ATO, 10 mg daily as a continuous intravenous infusion to ten patients who relapsed after ATRA induction and chemotherapy maintenance and achieved a clinical CR in 90% [17] without significant toxicity. Soignet et al. [187] subsequently treated 12 patients with APL who had relapsed after extensive prior therapy with ATO doses ranging from 0.06 to 0.2 mg/kg/day until bone marrow remission could be documented morphologically. Eleven patients achieved a complete remission after 12–39 days of treatment and a total dose of 160–515 mg. Eight of 11 patients who initially had a positive RT-PCR assay for the PML-RARα fusion transcript tested negative during remission. Three other patients remained PCR positive and relapsed early. This is an important observation, since ATRA therapy alone rarely results in a negative test. Side effects were also reported to be minimal in this study.

Investigators at the Shanghai Institute of Hematology [490] reported on 47 relapsed and 11 newly diagnosed patients with APL treated with ATO; 8 of the newly diagnosed patients (73%) and 40 of the relapsed patients (85%) achieved a CR with a median disease-free survival of 17 months. Patients received a variety of postremission treatments and those that received postremission chemotherapy plus ATO had significantly longer remissions (P = 0.01). Unlike previous studies, however, serious ATO toxicity was reported in this study. Seven cases of significant hepatic toxicity, including two deaths, were observed, and in other recent studies other toxic effects of ATO such as renal failure, cardiac dysfunction, and chronic neuromuscular degeneration have been observed [491]. Furthermore, the frequent occurrence of leukocytosis (58% of patients in one study [492]) and the differentiation syndrome (31% of patients in the same study [493]) after treatment with ATO is now well documented [493].

In an effort to limit exposure to ATO, Kwong et al. [494] treated eight patients with relapsed APL with ATO, 10 mg daily dose intravenously until remission was achieved and then gave three monthly cycles of idarubicin. All patients were in molecular remission after idarubicin treatment, and six have remained so after a median follow-up of 13 months. Jing et al. [207] reported that the combination of ATO and ATRA may be more effective therapy than either drug alone. Others have reported that ATO plus GM-CSF may be more effective therapy than ATO alone [495].

Recently, there has been an evolution in the induction and consolidation therapy in newly diagnosed patients with APL (including treatment-related APL) [283] with less chemotherapy and the introduction of the combination of oral ATRA and intravenous ATO [244, 245, 281, 282, 496–498], or ATO alone [499]. Results appear to be at least comparable to those obtained with ATRA and an anthracycline, and in many comparative studies of ATRA plus arsenic trioxide compared with ATRA plus anthracycline chemotherapy results have been better with the former, especially in low- and intermediate risk patients [500–506]. The North American Leukemia Intergroup study C9710 [283] randomized 481 newly diagnosed adult APL patients to either ATRA plus daunorubicin and cytarabine followed by two courses of consolidation therapy with ATRA plus daunorubicin, or the same treatment plus two 25-day courses of ATO. After that treatment patients were randomized to receive 1 year of maintenance therapy with either ATRA alone or in combination with methotrexate and 6-mercaptopurine. A complete remission was obtained in 90% of patients with each treatment and patients were eligible for postremission therapy. Event-free survival was significantly better for patients who received ATO compared with those who did not (80% and 63%, respectively at 3 years, $P \leq 0.0001$). Overall survival was also better for patients who received ATO (86 vs. 81% at 3 years, $P = 0.059$) as was disease-free survival (90% vs. 70% at 3 years) ($P < 0.0001$). The study demonstrated a significantly better outcome for patients who received ATO in addition to standard induction and consolidation therapy. Whether postremission methotrexate and 6-mercaptopurine had any influence on results is unclear. In a more recent prospective, randomized study of 263 low or intermediate-risk patients [507], ATRA plus arsenic trioxide or ATRA plus chemotherapy was given. The complete response rate (100% vs. 97%), event-free survival (97.3% vs. 80%), cumulative incidence of relapse (1.9% vs. 13.9%) and overall survival at 50 months (99.2% vs. 92.6%) all favored the ATRA plus arsenic trioxide regimen. These studies demonstrate major activity for ATO plus ATRA in newly diagnosed patients with APL.

Results with ATRA plus ATO have led some experts to recommend that that regimen be adopted as standard of care for patients with low- or intermediate-risk disease as currently defined, and that the addition of an anthracycline to induction therapy should only be considered for high-risk patients [508]. Others have reported better quality of life for patients treated without an anthracycline [509], and that the omission of chemotherapy improves the cost- effectiveness of treatment in the USA in some studies [510].

Recently, oral preparations of arsenic have been developed and early clinical trials demonstrate that oral arsenic is as effective and no more toxic than intravenous arsenic trioxide [511–513]. These results have led to a proposal that low- and –intermediate-risk APL patients could be treated entirely as outpatients with the oral combination of ATRA and arsenic [514]. However, others have wisely cautioned that treating APL patients during induction without hospitalization could be dangerous in the first few weeks, when coagulopathy and differentiation syndrome may have sudden onset and lead to early death [515].

Toxicity of Arsenic Trioxide

Long-term complications of ATO plus ATRA treatment were reported by Zhu et al. [516] in 265 patients who received arsenic trioxide plus ATRA for APL with or without chemotherapy. They compared quality of life and a number of potential long-term problems with those of 112 age and gender matched healthy controls. Signs of chronic arsenic toxicity such as cardiovascular events, chronic renal insufficiency, diabetes and neurological dysfunction were not observed in the patients at a higher rate than in the controls. Only mild liver dysfunction (15.2%) and hepatic steatosis (42.9%) were observed more frequently in patients than controls. Acute liver dysfunction occurred in 42.9% of patients during treatment and was managed primarily by suspending ATO treatment until liver function normalized. The estimated 12-year survival rate for patients with low- and intermediate-risk APL was 87.4%, compared with the high-risk group survival rate of 77.5%. No increased incidence of second malignancies was observed in treated patients in this study. Quality of life for long-term survivors in general was impaired somewhat, with more than half of patients reporting mild to moderate weakness and 41.1% reporting memory problems. The accumulation of arsenic in hair or nails was similar in patients and controls. Liver damage has been observed in other studies of ATRA plus ATO as well [517].

Of some concern is the reported serious cardiac toxicity that can be associated with ATO treatment. Ohnishi et al. [518] treated eight patients with APL with ATO, 0.15 mg/kg administered as daily 2-h infusions for a maximum of 60 days. Five patients achieved CR. Prolonged QT intervals were observed in all patients during treatment and ventricular premature contractions occurred during 75% of treatment courses. Four patients required treatment for unsustained ventricular tachycardia. Unnikrishnan et al. [519, 520] and Naito et al. [521] reported patients who developed torsades de pointes (a form of ventricular tachycardia that has been observed in arsenic poisoning) after treatment with ATO, 10 mg total daily dose as a continuous intravenous infusion. Westervelt et al. [522] reported three sudden deaths among ten patients with relapsed APL who received ATO, 0.1 mg/kg/day intravenously. One of the patients became asystolic and died while being continuously monitored with cardiac telemetry, and the cause of death was unknown in the other two. It seems clear from these reports that the cardiac toxicity of therapeutic doses of ATO is greater than initially appreciated, and that fact must be taken into account in future studies, which must include careful cardiac monitoring [493, 523] and correction of hypokaemia and hypomagnesemia, if present, prior to ATO treatment [524].

More data need to be accumulated before we can be confident that we know the full story of arsenic short- and long-term toxicity. For instance, ATO may delay hematopoietic recovery after autologous stem cell transplantation [525], and accumulation of arsenic in thyroid tissue may have led to at least one late thyroid carcinoma [526]. Although patients who receive ATO seem to have a lower death during induction rate in some studies, it does not appear to resolve the coagulopathy associated with APL more quickly than treatments that do not contain ATO [527].

The observation that ascorbic acid can potentiate the activity of ATO in vitro [528] deserves clinical evaluation [529] in patients with APL, and the observation that ATO inhibits hepatitis C virus RNA replication deserves further exploration as well [530].

Postremission Therapy in APL

There is no question that consolidation therapy after successful induction therapy is necessary for optimal long-term results in APL, but the need for maintenance therapy after consolidation therapy is less clear. Initial studies from the Italian cooperative oncology group GIMEMA administered three courses of chemotherapy with intermittent-dose cytarabine plus idarubicin, mitoxantrone plus etoposide, and standard-dose cytarabine plus idarubicin plus 6-thioguanine [531]. Subsequently, it became apparent that cytarabine might not be important in induction and consolidation [266, 407, 532]. The Spanish cooperative oncology group PETHEMA treated patients with three courses of chemotherapy without cytarabine with excellent results [408, 429]. However, recent studies have shown that intermediate-dose or high-dose cytarabine appears effective in patients who present with high-risk disease [533–536]. The North American Intergroup, as indicated earlier, reported a prospective randomized trial showing that two cycles of early consolidation with ATO improves disease-free, event-free, and overall survival [282].

Maintenance therapy has fallen into disfavor, in general, in subtypes of AML other than APL although some studies strongly support its use [537]. Methotrexate and 6-mercaptopurine were reported to be particularly useful maintenance agents in APL years ago by Kantarjian et al. [538]. The North American Intergroup Study [539, 540] conclusively demonstrated the value of postremission ATRA therapy in one of the first large studies using ATRA. In that study, 350 patients were randomly assigned to induction therapy with standard doses of daunorubicin and cytarabine, or ATRA. Patients who achieved complete remission received another course of the successful induction regimen followed by a course of high-dose cytarabine plus standard-dose daunorubicin and were then randomized to maintenance therapy with ATRA, 45 mg/m^2 daily orally for a year, or observation. With a median follow-up of more than 6 years, the 5-year disease-free and overall survival rates for all patients induced with ATRA were substantially better than those for patients induced with chemotherapy (64% vs. 30%, $P < 0.0001$; 69% vs. 45%, $P = 0.0001$, respectively) although complete response rates were similar (73% vs. 70%, respectively). The 5-year disease-free survival was highest, 74%, in the subgroup of patients induced with ATRA and maintained with ATRA, which compared favorably to the 55% disease-free survival rate observed in those induced with ATRA who did not receive postconsolidation ATRA. Furthermore, providing ATRA maintenance to chemotherapy-induced complete responders improved the disease-free survival rate threefold, compared with observation alone. These data strongly indicate the value of ATRA therapy during remission. That study also demonstrated a low late relapse rate. With a median of almost 12 years of follow-up, only 4.6% of patients in complete remission for more than 3 years subsequently relapsed [541]. Equally compelling data on the value of maintenance therapy in APL come from Fenaux et al. [445]. In a study of 413 patients, those investigators randomized patients in complete remission to observation, intermittent ATRA (15 days every 3 months for 2 years), 6-mercaptopurine and methotrexate for 2 years, or that therapy plus intermittent ATRA for 2 years. The relapse rate at 2 years was 25% for patients who received no ATRA during remission and approximately half that for patients who did, 27% for patients who received no chemotherapy and less than half that for patients who did. The highest relapse rate (approximately 30%) was in the group that received no maintenance therapy at all. The study, therefore, confirms the value of maintenance therapy in APL with either ATRA or 6-mercaptopurine and methotrexate, and suggests that both are effective alone, but not additive. Long-term follow-up of this trial continued to show a benefit for maintenance therapy which significantly reduced the 10-year cumulative incidence of relapse from 42.3 to 33%, 23.4%, and 13.4% with no maintenance, maintenance with intermittent ATRA, continuous 6-mercaptopurine and methotrexate, and both treatments, respectively ($P < 0.001$). However, some trials have suggested that maintenance with neither ATRA nor low-dose chemotherapy as discussed earlier nor the combination nor intensive chemotherapy [542] is effective in improving outcome among patients who are molecularly negative after intensive anthracycline-based chemotherapy.

In one large study ATO consolidation improved event-free and disease-free survival, compared with patients who did not receive ATO consolidation, but it was not clear from that study whether arsenic trioxide was better than other consolidation approaches [282, 543]. Couutre et al concluded from a study of 105 patients in molecular remission post-consolidation therapy that maintenance therapy is not helpful if ATO is included in the consolidation regimen [544]. Leech et al. demonstrated that a 4 month ATO-based consolidation program was equally effective in high-risk and lower risk APL patients [507]. Liu et al. [545] reported on a retrospective study of 18 patients that is clearly in need of confirmation, but interesting nonetheless. They induced low-risk patients with ATRA plus ATO while high-risk patients received the same plus an anthracycline. After hematologic complete remission occurred arsenic alternating with chemotherapy was given as consolidation therapy and no maintenance therapy was employed. All patients achieved a molecular complete remission and no patients died during treatment, and no patients have relapsed with a median follow-up of 5 years. All 18 remain alive and can be considered cured [541]. Other recent studies have also suggested that maintenance therapy after consolidation therapy is unnecessary for low- and intermediate-risk patients with APL [546].

In a randomized study of 344 patients reported by Shinagawa et al. [458] results of maintenance therapy with ATRA or tamibarotene, a retinoic acid derivative also known as AM80, were compared. There was no difference in relapse-free survival for low-risk patients between the treatments, but for the 52 high-risk patients the relapse-free survival rates for ATRA and tmibarotene maintenance were 58% and 87%, respectively, which was significant. These data do not help determine whether *any* maintenance therapy is necessary for low-risk patients, but they do suggest that it is necessary for high-risk patients and that tamibarotene may be a better maintenance agent than ATRA for those patients.

It is important to monitor all patients with APL in clinical remission after treatment with molecular techniques such as real-time quantitative polymerase chain reaction to detect leukemia-specific transcripts, should they reappear. Patients who are PCR negative after treatment should be retreated if such transcripts reappear and before there is clinical hematologic or cytogenetic evidence of relapse in order to have the best opportunity of achieving a second molecular remission [294, 547, 548]. Patients who do not obtain a molecular remission after planned therapy should continue treatment with a different agent, such as ATO with or without other agents. Institution of salvage therapy at molecular relapse before hematological relapse leads to a better outcome of salvage therapy [292, 547].

Hematopoietic stem cell transplantation is not recommended for patients with APL in first molecular remission.

Recommended treatment for newly diagnosed patients with APL is detailed in Table 21.2.

Table 21.2 Recommended treatment: newly diagnosed and treatment-related APL

Induction therapy
Low-, intermediate-, and high-risk patients
ATRA[a], 45 mg/m^2/day orally in two divided doses until marrow hematologic remission
Idarubicin, I.V., 12 mg/m^2/day × 4 on alternate days
OR
ATRA[a], same oral dose and schedule until hematologic remission
ATO[b], 0.15 mg/kg IV daily until hematologic remission
Perform PCR for PML/RARα before starting therapy and when bone marrow morphologic remission is achieved. Monitor for coagulation abnormalities, arsenic toxicity, and differentiation syndrome as described in the text. Consider steroid prophylaxis for differentiation syndrome for high-risk patients.
Consolidation therapy
Low- and intermediate-risk patients
ATRA[a], orally, 45 mg/m^2/day in two divided doses X 45 days
Idarubicin, I.V. 5 mg/m^2/day, days 1–4
Idarubicin I.V. 12 mg/m^2 day 45
OR
ATO[b], I.V. 0.15 mg/kg/day 5 days/week × 4 weeks every 8 weeks for 4 cycles
ATRA[a], orally, 45 mg/m^2/day in two divided doses for 2 weeks every 4 weeks for 7 cycles
High-risk patients
ATRA[a], 45 mg/m^2/daily orally in two divided doses × 45 days
Idarubicin, 5 mg/m^2 I.V. day 1
Cytarabine, 1 g/m^2 I.V. daily, days 1–4
Idarubicin, 12 mg/m^2 I.V. day 30
Cytarabine, 150 mg/m^2 I.V. daily, days 30–33
OR
ATO[b] IV 0.15 mg/kg/day × 5 days for 10 weeks, then
ATRA[a] 45 mg/m^2 orally daily × 7 days plus
Idarubicin, 12 mg/m^2 I.V. daily × 3 days. Repeat same dose and schedule of idarubicin after counts recover
Perform PCR for PML/RARα after hematologic recovery and every 3 months for 2 years. If PCR becomes positive after being negative, repeat in 1 month. If positive again, the patient requires reinduction therapy for relapse. Consider a clinical trial. If PCR remains negative for 2 years, no further therapy is recommended.

[a]All-trans retinoic acid
[b]Arsenic trioxide

Treatment of Relapsed APL

Whether to begin treatment for relapsed APL early (molecular relapse, normal morphology) or late (morphologic relapse) is the subject of debate. No prospective, randomized trials have been reported, but an important historically controlled study suggests a major advantage for treatment of molecular relapse [547]. If the relapsed patient has had no exposure to ATO for at least 6 months reinduction therapy with ATO, 0.15 mg/kg IV daily plus ATRA, 45 mg/m^2 daily in two divided doses until marrow remission is documented should be given. A number of studies have now confirmed excellent activity of ATO, either alone or combined with ATRA, in patients with relapsed APL [248, 549–553].

Consider CNS prophylaxis with intrathecal cytarabine at this point. If the marrow is in molecular remission, consider an autologous stem cell transplant [554, 555, 557]. If the patient is not a candidate for a transplant, consider consolidation with arsenic trioxide, or a clinical trial. If a second morphologic remission is achieved, but not a second molecular remission, consider a clinical trial.

If the patient relapsed within 6 months of treatment with ATRA and/or ATO without an anthracycline, reinduction with ATRA, idarubicin and arsenic trioxide is recommended, followed by the same post-remission treatment outlined above. If the early relapsed patient did previously receive an anthracycline, only ATRA and arsenic trioxide should be given as reinduction therapy, again, followed by the above post remission recommendations. Patients who do not respond to reinduction therapy with a complete remission should be considered for a clinical trial [556].

Tamibarotene (Am-80) is a synthetic retinoid that is a more active inducer of differentiation in HL-60 and NB4 cells than is ATRA [558]. Of 24 evaluable patients with relapsed APL after ATRA-induced CR treated with Am-80, 6 mg/m^2 orally daily, 58% achieved CR [221]. Four patients relapsed within 6 months, but long-term responses (>49 months) were also observed. The same group recently updated that study but, curiously, no new patients had been entered in the trial for approximately 3 years [559]. A more recent small study of tamibarotene in relapsed patients initially successfully treated with ATRA and ATO achieved a complete molecular response in 21% of patients. Most patients relapsed with a few months and the median overall survival after treatment was only 9.5 months [459]. The drug should be studied in combination with idarubicin for patients relapsing after ATRA and ATO.

Liu et al. treated 31 patients with refractory APL with compound realgar natural indigo tablets (an oral arsenic compound based on Chinese herbal medicine) and chemotherapy. The complete response rate was 90.3% and the median response duration was over 42 months. The relapse rate was <10%, with 43 months median follow-up and the treatment was apparently very well tolerated. Patients received a variety of chemotherapy regimens and it is difficult to know exactly what role the oral arsenic compound played in the results. However, these results are excellent. Hopefully they will soon be explored by others.

Chendamarai et al. [560] found CD34 expression to be significantly increased in leukemic cells from relapsed patients compared with newly diagnosed patients, and that in relapsed patients there was significant microenvironment mediated resistance to ATO which was demonstrated in vitro.

Hematopoietic stem cell transplantation for APL patients in second complete molecular remission is recommended by many investigators. Autologous stem cell transplantation is recommended rather than allogeneic transplantation [561].

APL and Pregnancy

The treatment of AML in pregnancy is discussed in general in Chap. 22. Although retinoids are well known to be teratogenic and their use during pregnancy has been advised against, reports of successful use of ATRA during the second and third trimesters in more than 40 patients have appeared [562–564] and no cases of teratogenic effects were observed. At least one case of successful pregnancy after ATO treatment has been reported [565]. Since ATRA rapidly controls the coagulopathy associated with APL, it may be an attractive induction agent for the APL patient in late pregnancy. Most women with APL treated with standard chemotherapy in late pregnancy have also survived and delivered normal children [566]. However, APL in the first trimester is likely to be associated with obstetric and fetal complications [567, 568].

APL in Children

APL in children generally has the same features as in adults, except that the incidence of leukocytosis and the microgranular variant is greater in children than in adults [569]. Children under the age of 5 years have a worse prognosis than older ones. APL in children is generally treated as in adults. The same agents used for adult APL are used in children, although many successful studies have employed lower ATRA doses (25 mg/m^2 daily), lower total anthracycline dose, and cytarbine in consolidation [427, 570]. ATRA toxicity is more frequent in children [IIII], particularly pseudotumor cerebri.

The Coagulopathy Associated with APL

A major feature distinguishing APL from all other subtypes of AML is the very frequent association with a severe life-threatening coagulopathy. The pathogenesis of the coagulopathy is complex and includes disseminated intravascular coagulation (DIC), hyperfibrinolysis, proteolysis and exposure of tissue factor and annexin-II by leukemic blasts [571–573]. Historically, approximately 10–30% of patients with APL died of early fatal hemorrhage, often intracerebral hemorrhage [9, 409, 574–579]. Even in the modern era of therapy with *all-trans* retinoic acid (ATRA) plus idarubicin, hemorrhage remains the single most common cause of death before and after induction therapy [454]. This is particularly problematic since patients with APL historically [580–582] and now in the ATRA era are highly curable with ATRA plus anthracycline-based chemotherapy approaches or ATRA plus ATO regimens [506, 583]. Early death from coagulopathy has therefore emerged as the major obstacle to cure in APL [399, 584–590].

In every study to date, successful remission induction with ATRA has been accompanied by rapid resolution of clinical bleeding and generally, of biochemical evidence of the coagulopathy, although elevated plasma levels of sensitive markers of clotting activation may persist [446, 591, 592]. Studies of arsenic trioxide in patients with relapsed and refractory APL also show rapid correction of the clotting abnormality [182, 593]. The rapid resolution of coagulopathy in APL patients given ATRA and/or arsenic speaks to the importance of prompt treatment in order to prevent early death from coagulopathy [573, 584, 589].

Coagulopathy and Early Death in APL

Approximately 70–80% of patients with either previously untreated APL or relapsed disease have either laboratory or clinical evidence of a potentially life-threatening bleeding diathesis [9, 182, 354, 409, 415, 418, 574–578, 594]. Even in the modern era, the risk of hemorrhagic death during induction remains at about 5–9% in the controlled environment of clinical trials, and may be as high as 16–31% in population studies [399, 402, 454, 534, 542, 573, 585–587, 590, 595, 596] (Table 21.3). Clinical manifestations of coagulopathy in APL can include mucocutaneous bleeding in the form of ecchymoses, petechiae, epistaxis, and gastrointestinal hemorrhage, as well as increased bleeding at sites of minor trauma or catheter insertion [573]. Intracranial and pulmonary hemorrhages are the most feared manifestations of coagulopathy in APL, as these two sites of bleeding account for the majority of hemorrhagic deaths in most series [402, 454, 573, 584, 585, 588, 590, 597]. In the Spanish PETHEMA study, intracranial and pulmonary hemorrhage accounted for 65% and 32% of hemorrhagic deaths [454]. Similarly in the Japanese JALSG APL97 study, intracranial and pulmonary hemorrhages accounted for 66% and 22% of early deaths [597].

In addition to bleeding, some studies suggest that patients with APL are also more prone to thrombosis than patients with other leukemias [584]. Various thrombotic events have been documented in APL patients, including myocardial infarction, deep vein thromboses, pulmonary emboli, and CNS thromboses [584, 599–604]. The incidence of thrombo-embolic deaths in APL patients ranges from 5.1% to 9.6% in various studies [18, 42–44]. Thromboembolism in APL patients may be associated with procoagulant effects of ATRA and worsened by differentiation syndrome [584, 605, 606].

Pathophysiology of the Coagulopathy in APL

The etiology of coagulopathy in APL is complex, with multiple driving mechanisms including tissue factor-induced DIC and primary hyperfibrinolysis [573]. The characteristic pattern of laboratory abnormalities includes thrombocytopenia; prolongations of the prothrombin time (PT), partial thromboplastin time (PTT), and thrombin times; increased levels of fibrin degradation products; and hypofibrinogenemia [594, 607–610]. These findings are consistent with either DIC and hyperfibrinolysis or both. Notably, patients with APL can have potentially fatal bleeding even in the absence of abnormal PT and PTT. In addition, although APL patients classically experience profound hypofibrinogenemia, some individuals with APL do not have significantly decreased fibrinogen [573, 594]. Furthermore, levels of several anticoagulant proteins such as antithrombin III and protein C, often low in the setting of DIC, are usually not decreased in patients with APL [611]. Platelet survival in these patients is normal, reflecting a more complex process than DIC alone [612, 613].

Multiple procoagulant mediators have been described in patients with APL (Fig. 21.7) [622–624]. Tissue factor (TF) is the major procoagulant that initiates the extrinsic pathway of

Table 21.3 Early death rate and bleeding in APL in prospective cooperative group studies

Trial	*N*	Induction	CR%	ED%	ED from bleeding%	DFS%
PETHEMA [580, 598]	732	ATRA + Ida	91	9	56	84
JALSG [542]	283	ATRA/Ida/ara-C	94	5	69	69
GAMLCG [534]	142	ATRA/TAD/HAM	92	8	64	82
GIMEMA [596]	420	ATRA + Ida	94	6	32	87

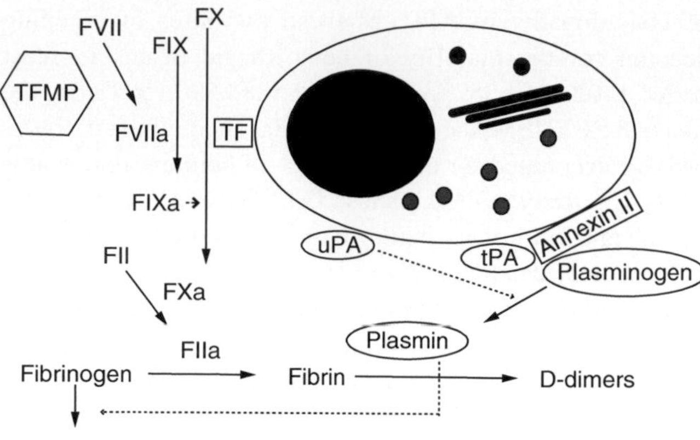

Fig. 21.7 Simplified schema of the coagulopathy associated with APL. Tissue factor present at the surface of leukemic blasts and microparticles binds to factor (F)VII, leading to activation of the latter. The TF-FVIIa complex activates FIX and FX. This leads to thrombin generation, which itself catalyzes fibrin formation. Parallel to this coagulation activation and factor consumption process, Annexin II present at the surface of malignant leukocytes binds tPA and plasminogen, resulting in the formation of plasmin, which goes on to cleave fibrin and fibrinogen. *APL* acute promyelocytic leukemia, *FII* coagulation factor II (prothrombin), *FIX* coagulation factor IX, *FVII* coagulation factor VII, *FX* coagulation factor X, *TF* tissue factor, *TFMP* tissue factor microparticle; *tPA* tissue plasminogen activator; *uPA* urokinase-type plasminogen activator. Reproduced with permission from Mantha S et al., Current Opinion in Hematology 2016 [573]

blood coagulation in vivo and is the membrane protein receptor for factor VII [614]. The resulting TF-factor VIIa complex activates factors IX and X, which leads to thrombin generation and fibrin formation. The TF gene is expressed in cells from patients with APL, and the TF promoter is activated by the PML/RARα fusion protein [615–618]. Recent work has also described tissue factor microparticles (TFMP) as potentially important for the pathogenesis of coagulopathy in APL [573, 619–621]. TFMP are cellular membrane fragments displaying TF derived from tumor cells, platelets, endothelial cells and monocytes. As in solid tumors, TFMP in APL manifest procoagulant activity as evidenced by measurements of thrombin generation [573, 619–621]. Increased expression of the cysteine proteinase cancer procoagulant (CP) protein by APL blasts has also been proposed as an additional mechanism of coagulopathy in APL [574–576]. Cytokines such as interleukin-1 (IL-1), tumor necrosis factor (TNF), and vascular permeability factor (VPF) are indirect procoagulants in APL by initiating coagulation through the induction of TF in endothelial cells and monocytes [625–627]. Interleukin-1 secreted by leukemic cells may induce DIC [628, 629]. Cytokines can generate plasminogen activator inhibitors that inhibit vessel wall fibrinolytic activity promoting coagulation [630, 631]. Interferon-γ and VPF-like mediators can induce endothelial cell procoagulant activity [632, 633].

Excessive fibrinolysis is also an important factor in the coagulopathy in APL [634, 635]. Plasminogen and alpha-2 antiplasmin levels are reduced in patients with APL [636, 637]. Furthermore, leukemic promyelocytes release plasminogen activators that cleave plasminogen and initiate fibrinolysis. Circulating tissue-type plasminogen activator can be found in the plasma of some patients with APL [638]. Decreased levels of circulating plasminogen-activator inhibitor type 1 (PAI-1) have been reported in some patients [639, 640]. APL cells contain elastases that inactivate alpha-2-plasmin inhibitor [641]. Annexin-VIII is one of a group of naturally occurring proteins that bind phospholipids and have both anticoagulant and phospholipase-A2 inhibitory properties [642]. The Annexin-VIII gene is expressed to a greater degree in cells from patients with APL compared to cells from patients with other subtypes of AML [643]. Annexin-VIII is highly expressed in the APL cell line NB4 and is significantly reduced after exposure to ATRA. Annexin-II is a cell surface receptor for plasminogen and its activator, tissue plasminogen activator (t-PA), which functions as a t-PA cofactor [644, 645]. Annexin-II is expressed in high levels on leukemic promyelocytes compared to leukemic cells from patients with other subtypes of AML [644, 645]. In APL, Annexin-II may play an important role in the formation of plasmin, serving as a driver for intense fibrinolytic activity [573, 644, 646, 647]. Studies suggest that plasmin- and elastase-induced degradation of von Willebrand factor also contributes to the hemostatic defect in APL [648].

Influence of ATRA on Coagulation Parameters

The effects of ATRA on APL coagulopathy are complex and incompletely understood. A number of studies have examined the specific changes in coagulation parameters before and after ATRA. Dombret and colleagues studied a small number of patients with APL treated with ATRA and reported that both DIC and proteolysis improved within 14 days [581]. Although proteolysis appeared to completely resolve, low-grade procoagulant activity persisted, even after patients achieved complete response, particularly in patients who developed hyperleukocytosis during treatment. Markers of thrombin generation such as thrombin–antithrombin complex (TAT), prothrombin fragment 1 + 2 (F1 + 2), and D-dimer did not completely normalize. These findings reflect a dissociation between the resolution of proteolysis (fibrinogenolysis) and DIC and may explain some reports of thromboembolic events during treatment with ATRA, particularly when ATRA is combined with antifibrinolytic therapy as prophylaxis against bleeding [584, 602, 605, 606, 649, 650].

Both TF-like and factor VII-independent (CP-like) procoagulant activity of APL blast cells is decreased after ATRA exposure [651, 652]. ATRA both upregulates thrombomodulin and downregulates TF expression in APL cells [654, 698]. However, several studies have demonstrated that retinoic acid also stimulates tissue-type plasminogen activator in human endothelial cells, which can initiate the fibrinolytic cascade and counterbalance the effects of a decrease in other procoagulant mediators [655, 656]. Levels of markers of coagulation activation including D-dimer, F1 + 2, TAT, and fibrinopeptide A have been shown to decline following exposure to chemotherapy or ATRA. Notably, plasma levels of D-dimer, F1 + 2, TAT, and fibrinopeptide-A decreased more rapidly among patients treated with ATRA compared to chemotherapy. D-dimer, TAT, and fibrinopeptide A levels also remain significantly elevated well above the upper limit of normal among the chemotherapy-treated patients [592]. Later in the course following ATRA and chemotherapy treatment, re-elevation of several molecular markers of coagulation may occur in some patients, potentially attributable to late effects of cytotoxic chemotherapy and infection [582]. Overall, most studies support the unifying hypothesis that as ATRA induces terminal differentiation of leukemic promyelocytes, markers of both procoagulant activity and fibrinolytic activity decrease with some evidence of persistent mild DIC.

Effect of the Improvement in the Bleeding Diathesis on Outcome of APL Patients Treated with ATRA or Arsenic

Nonrandomized and randomized prospective trials have examined the outcome of patients treated with ATRA alone or with ATRA and chemotherapy [267, 402, 430, 539, 657]. Before the ATRA era, the risk of early hemorrhagic death for APL patients ranged from 10 to 30% [9, 409, 574–579]. However, since the introduction of ATRA in 1988, the risk of early hemorrhagic death in prospective APL studies has decreased significantly to 5–10% [266, 402, 408, 430, 445, 539, 573, 658–661].

Arsenic trioxide also has emerged as an important agent in the treatment of APL, with recent studies demonstrating that ATRA plus arsenic trioxide is as at least noninferior and possibly superior to ATRA plus chemotherapy in the treatment of patients with low-to-intermediate-risk APL [506]. Unlike ATRA, arsenic trioxide binds the APL oncoprotein and leads to its degradation, resulting in decreased transcription of downstream target genes, suggesting that it could ameliorate the coagulopathy of APL early in its pathogenesis [63, 190, 573, 662]. Arsenic trioxide induces rapid loss of membrane procoagulant activity and TF mRNA [663]. Preliminary studies have shown that arsenic trioxide also has a beneficial effect on the coagulopathy in APL [605, 664]. Given the excellent outcomes in modern APL prospective clinical trials, it is difficult to assess the impact of arsenic in decreasing bleeding in contemporary studies. For example, there were no cases of early death in the ATRA + arsenic trioxide arm of the recent study comparing ATRA + arsenic and ATRA + chemotherapy in low-to-intermediate risk APL. However, there was only one death from hemorrhagic shock in the ATRA + chemotherapy group. Overall, patients with low-to-intermediate risk APL treated either with ATRA + arsenic or ATRA + chemotherapy had very good outcomes [506]. It is possible that there may be more room for improvement in reducing risk of early death from coagulopathy in high-risk APL. Since the mechanism of induction of remission of arsenic trioxide appears to be different from that of ATRA, new opportunities are present to explore the pathogenesis of the coagulopathy and the pathophysiologic basis for its improvement.

The Next Frontier: Management of Coagulopathy and Prevention of Early Death in APL

Despite the dramatic improvements in APL outcomes and reduced rates of hemorrhage in clinical trial settings, early death from hemorrhage remains a significant problem in population and community studies [399, 454, 573, 585, 587, 588, 590, 595] (Table 21.4). As early death in APL is driven significantly by coagulopathy, management of the coagulopathy of APL is therefore critical to ensuring high rates of cure [573, 584, 589] (Table 21.5). The most important initial step in managing the coagulopathy of APL involves suspecting the diagnosis of APL and prompt administration of ATRA. Given the rapid impact of ATRA in altering coagulation parameters

Table 21.4 Early death rate in APL in population studies

Study	N	ED%
Jeddi [595]	41	16
Lehmann [585]	99	31
McClellan [588]	70	26
Park [590]	1400	18

Table 21.5 Management of coagulopathy and prevention of early hemorrhagic death in APL

- Start ATRA at first suspicion of APL (based on clinical history and review of peripheral smear), BEFORE BONE MARROW AND BEFORE DIAGNOSIS CONFIRMED (in ER)
- Frequent platelet transfusion to >50,000/μL
- Cryoprecipitate to maintain fibrinogen >150 mg/dL
- No heparin, although not studied in ATRA era
- No antifibrinolytics

as noted above, ATRA should be given whenever APL is first suspected following review of the peripheral smear—without waiting for genetic confirmation of APL diagnosis and without waiting for bone marrow biopsy [257].

In addition to rapid administration of ATRA, vigilant monitoring of coagulation parameters and frequent administration of blood products are needed to prevent early hemorrhagic death in APL. Blood products serve as the cornerstone or prohemostatic treatments in APL, including platelet transfusions, fresh frozen plasma, as well as cryoprecipitate for repletion of fibrinogen [257, 573]. Guidelines support maintaining the platelet count above 30,000–50,000/μL and maintaining fibrinogen above 100–150 mg/dL (Table 21.5) [257]. Replacement therapy should be continued until all clinical and laboratory signs of coagulopathy have resolved. Although all patients presenting with APL are potentially at risk of hemorrhage, specific factors predicting high risk of fatal hemorrhage have been identified. In particular, patients with active bleeding, increased WBC or peripheral blast counts, abnormal renal function, poor performance status, hypofibrinogenemia (<100 mg/dL), or increased levels of fibrin degradation products combined with prolonged prothrombin or activated partial thromboplastin time are at increased risk of developing fatal hemorrhage [257, 267, 402, 454, 597, 660].

Beyond ATRA and blood products, there are no robust data to support the use of other prohemostatic modalities in APL. Intravenous heparin, antifibrinolytics, recombinant factor VIIa, and thrombomodulin have all been tested in APL patients, though none have been tested in randomized trials in the ATRA era [573]. Although heparin was advocated prior to the advent of ATRA, there are concerns as to the safety of heparin due to the possibility of worsening bleeding. Alternate concerns have been raised regarding the use of antifibrinolytics, due to the potential of thrombotic complications and the known predisposition of APL patients to thrombosis [584, 599–604]. Recombinant factor VIIa has been described in case reports of life-threatening hemorrhage in APL patients [665, 666]. However, the data for recombinant favor VIIa in this setting is highly limited, and recombinant factor VIIa presents similar safety concerns as antifibrinolytics in serving as a potential trigger for thrombosis. Recent retrospective postmarketing data from Japan suggests that the natural anticoagulant thrombomodulin may be useful in treating the coagulopathy of APL [667]. However, although the 3.5% rate of hemorrhagic death in APL patients who receive thrombomodulin is encouraging and lower than rates of hemorrhagic death in community studies, there are no randomized prospective trials of thrombomodulin that demonstrate clear efficacy in the treatment of coagulopathy in APL. Therefore, we would not recommend the use of thrombomodulin for treatment of APL coagulopathy outside of the context of clinical trials.

Management of coagulopathy in APL involves prompt suspicion of APL diagnosis, rapid administration of ATRA, and vigilant use of blood products. Given the disparity in rates of early hemorrhagic death between APL patients in population studies and in prospective academic clinical trials, education of community physicians in recognition and management of the coagulopathy of APL will be critical to improving overall rates of cure.

Future Treatment Research

Although tremendous progress has been made in the treatment of APL in the last two decades, problems remain. The coagulopathy characteristic of APL is not sufficiently addressed by the advent of ATRA or ATO. Mechanisms to interrupt the coagulopathy more rapidly need to be developed. Therapy, especially for high-risk patients needs to be improved. It is still unclear whether ATRA plus ATO or ATRA plus anthracycline is the best induction treatment for high-risk patients and experts have called for a randomized trial to address that issue [668]. A number of potential improvements in treatment are currently under investigation. Zoldronic acid was shown by Liu et al [669] to synergize with ATO in the inhibition of NB4 cells in vitro and should be explored clinically. Homoharringtonine [670] plus ATRA induction therapy followed by consolidation therapy and a 2-year maintenance program produced a 100% 9-year overall survival among patients with APL who were not overweight in one study, while obese patients had only a 73% 9-year survival rate. Other studies have shown that APL patients were more likely to be obese than other patients with AML. The effect of obesity on APL needs further study, and homoharringtonine as therapy for APL deserves further study as well. pVAX14DNA-mediated immunotherapy together with ATRA and ATO increased the survival of APL in mice [671]. This is an interesting observation that should also be explored further. AZD11512, a specific inhibitor of Aurora B which is overexpressed in APL, showed significant activity against NB4 cells and could lead to an entirely new approach to treatment of APL [672].

ATO degrades PML-RARα oncoprotein via the proteasome pathway. Ganesan et al. [673] demonstrated in the laboratory that ATO and bortezomib (a proteasome inhibitor) are synergistic against arsenic sensitive and resistant cell lines. They have begun a test of this finding in the clinic. A traditional Chinese agent, tanshinone, was shown to induce differentiation in APL cells and subsequently shown to significantly prolong survival of APL-bearing mice [674]. Clinical trials should be entertained. Fucoidan, a sulfated polysaccharide from brown algae, apparently enhanced the activity of ATRA or ATO in a mouse model of APL [675] and deserves further study.

These early studies are interesting and may lead to newer approaches to the treatment of APL in the future.

References

1. Hillestad L. Acute promyelocytic leukemia. Acta Med Scand. 1957;159:189.
2. Stavem P. Acute hypergranular promyelocytic leukemia. Priority of discovery. Scand J Haematol. 1978;20:287.
3. Caen J, Mathe G, Xuan Chat L, Bernard J. Etude de la fibrinolyse au cours des hémopathies malignes. In: Transactions of the 6th Congress of the European Society of Hématology. Basel: Karger; 1957. p. 502.
4. Bernard J, Mathe G, Boulay J, Ceoura B. La leucose aiguë à promyélocytes. Etude portant sur 20 observations. J Suisse Med. 1959;23:604.
5. Bernard J, Weil M, Boiron M, et al. Acute promyelocytic leukemia. Results with daunorubicin. Blood. 1973;41:489.
6. Golomb HM, Rowley JD, Vardiman J, et al. Partial deletion of long arm of chromosome 7. A specific abnormality in acute promyelocytic leukemia? Arch Intern Med. 1976;136:825.
7. Rowley J, Golomb H, Dougherty C. 15/17 translocation: a consistent chromosomal change in acute promyelocytic leukemia. Lancet. 1977;1:549.
8. Larson RA, Kondo K, Vardiman JW, et al. Evidence for a 15;17 translocation in every patient with acute promyelocytic leukemia. Am J Med. 1984;76:827.
9. Kantarjian HM, Keating MJ, Walters RS, et al. Acute promyelocytic leukemia. M.D. Anderson Hospital experience. Am J Med. 1986;80:789.
10. Stone RM, Maguire M, Goldberg MA, et al. Complete remission in acute promyelocytic leukemia despite persistence of abnormal bone marrow promyelocytes during induction therapy: expertonce in 34 patients. Blood. 1988;71:690.
11. Brittan T, Selznick S, Collins S. Induction of differentiation of the human promyelocytic leukemic cell line (HL-60) by retinoic acid. Proc Natl Acad Sci U S A. 1980;77:2936.
12. Huang M-E, Ye Y-C, Chen S-R, et al. Use of all-trans retinoic acid in the treatment of acute promyelocytic leukemia. Blood. 1988;72:567.
13. Fenaux P, Chas tang C, Degas L. Treatment of newly diagnosed acute promyelocytic leukemia (APL) by a combination of alltrans retinoic acid (ATRA) and chemotherapy. Leukemia. 1994;8(Suppl 2):S42.
14. Chen GQ, Shi XG, Tang W, et al. Use of arsenic trioxide (As_2O_3) in the treatment of acute promyelocytic leukemia (APL): I. As203 exerts dose-dependent dual effects on APL cells. Blood. 1997;89:3345.
15. Wiernik PH. Acute promyelocytic leukemia: another pseudoleukemia? Blood. 1990;76:1675.
16. Degos L. Is acute promyelocytic leukemia a curable disease? Treatment strategy for a long-term survival. Leukemia. 1994;8:S6.
17. Bernard J. History of promyelocytic leukemia. Leukemia. 1994;8(Suppl 2):1.
18. Breitman TR, Collins SJ, Keene BR. Terminal differentiation of human promyelocytic leukemic cells in primary culture in response to retinoic acid. Blood. 1981;57:1000–4.
19. Huang M-E, Ye Y-C, Chen S-R, Chai J-R, Lu J-X, Lin Z, et al. Use of all-*trans* retinoic acid in the treatment of acute promyelocytic leukemia. Blood. 1988;72:567–72.
20. Borrow J, Goddard AD, Sheer D, Solomon E. Molecular analysis of acute promyelocytic leukemia breakpoint cluster region on chromosome 17. Science. 1990;249:1577–80.
21. de The H, Chomienne C, Lanotte M, Degos L, Dejean A. The t(15;17) translocation of acute promyelocytic leukaemia fuses the retinoic acid receptor Ë gene to a novel transcribed locus. Nature. 1990;347:558–61.
22. Longo L, Pandolfi P, Biondi A, Rambaldi A, Mencarelli A, Lo Coco F, et al. Rearrangements and aberrant expression of the retinoic acid receptor Ï gene in acute promyelocytic leukemias. J Exp Med. 1990;172:1571–5.
23. Petkovich M, Brand NJ, Krust A, Chambon P. A human retinoic acid receptor which belongs to the family of nuclear receptors. Nature. 1987;330:444–50.
24. Giguere V, Ong ES, Segui P, Evans RM. Identification of a receptor for the morphogen retinoic acid. Nature. 1987;330:624–9.
25. de The H, Lavau C, Marchio A, Chomienne C, Degos L, Dejean A. The PML-RARa fusion mRNA generated by the t(15;17) translocation in acute promyelocytic leukemia encodes a functionally altered RAR. Cell. 1991;66:675–84.
26. Kakizuka A, Miller WH Jr, Umesono K, Warrell RP Jr, Frankel SR, Murty VVVS, et al. Chromosomal translocation t(15;17) in human acute promyelocytic leukemia fuses RARa with a novel putative transcription factor PML. Cell. 1991;66:663–74.
27. Pandolfi P, Grignani F, Alcalay M, Mencarelli A, Biondi A, LoCoco F, et al. Structure and origin of the acute promyelocytic leukemia myl/RARa cDNA and characterization of its retinoid-binding and transactivation properties. Oncogene. 1991;6:1285–92.
28. Chen Z, Brand N, Chen A, Chen S, Tong J, Wang Z, et al. Fusion between a novel Kruppel-like zinc finger gene and the retinoic acid receptor-a locus due to a variant t(11;17) translocation associated with acute promyelocytic leukemia. EMBO J. 1993;12:1161–72.
29. Redner RL, Chen JD, Rush EA, Li H, Pollock SL. The t(5;17) acute promyelocytic leukemia fusion protein NPM-RAR interacts with co-repressor and co-activator proteins and exhibits both positive and negative transcriptional properties. Blood. 2000;95:2683–90.
30. Wells RA, Catzavelos C, Kamel-Reid S. Fusion of retinoic acid receptor a to NuMA, the nuclear mitotic apparatus protein by a variant translocation in acute promyelocytic leukemia. Nat Genet. 1997;17:109–13.
31. Arnould C, Philippe C, Bourdon V, Gregoire MJ, Berger R, Jonveaux P. The signal transducer and activator of transcription STAT5b gene is a new partner of retinoic acid receptor a in acute promyelocytic-like leukaemia. Hum Mol Genet. 1999;8:1741–9.
32. Catalano A, Dawson MA, Somana K, Opat S, Schwarer A, Campbell LJ, et al. The PRKAR1A gene is fused to RARA in a new variant acute promyelocytic leukemia. Blood. 2007;110(12):4073–6.
33. Kondo T, Mori A, Darmanin S, Hashino S, Tanaka J, Asaka M. The seventh pathogenic fusion gene FIP1L1-RARA was isolated from a t(4;17)-positive acute promyelocytic leukemia. Haematologica. 2008;93(9):1414–6.
34. Zelent A, Guidez F, Melnick A, Waxman S, Licht JD. Translocations of the RARalpha gene in acute promyelocytic leukemia. Oncogene. 2001;20(49):7186–203.
35. Scaglioni PP, Pandolfi PP. The theory of APL revisited. Curr Top Microbiol Immunol. 2007;313:85–100.
36. Chen GQ, Zhu J, Shi XG, Zhong HJ, Ni JH, Si GY, et al. In vitro studies on cellular and molecular mechanisms of arsenic trioxide (As_2O_3) in the treatment of acute promyelocytic leukemia: As_2O_3 induces NB4 cell apoptosis with downregulation of bcl-2 expression and alteration of PML-RARa/PML protein localization. Blood. 1996;88:1052–61.
37. Lanotte M, Martin-Thouvenin B, Najman S, Balerini P, Valensi F, Berger R. NB4, a maturation inducible cell line with t(15;17) marker isolated from a human acute promyelocytic leukemia (M3). Blood. 1991;77(5):1080–6.
38. Gallagher R, Collins S, Trujillo J, McCredie K, Ahearn M, Tsai S, et al. Characterization of the continuous, differentiating myeloid leukemia cell line (HL-60) from a patient with acute promyelocytic leukemia. Blood. 1979;54:713–33.
39. Breitman T, Selonick S, Collins S. Induction of differentiation of the human promyelocytic leukemic cell line (HL-60) by retinoic acid. Proc Natl Acad Sci U S A. 1980;77:2936–40.
40. Kogan SC. Mouse models of acute promyelocytic leukemia. Curr Top Microbiol Immunol. 2007;313:3–29.

41. Nasr R, Guillemin MC, Ferhi O, Soilihi H, Peres L, Berthier C, et al. Eradication of acute promyelocytic leukemia-initiating cells through PML-RARA degradation. Nat Med. 2008;14(12):1333–42.
42. Wojiski S, Guibal FC, Kindler T, Lee BH, Jesneck JL, Fabian A, et al. PML-RARalpha initiates leukemia by conferring properties of self-renewal to committed promyelocytic progenitors. Leukemia. 2009;23(8):1462–71.
43. Guibal FC, Alberich-Jorda M, Hirai H, Ebralidze A, Levantini E, Di Ruscio A, et al. Identification of a myeloid committed progenitor as the cancer-initiating cell in acute promyelocytic leukemia. Blood. 2009;114(27):5415–25.
44. Chambon P. A decade of molecular biology of retinoic acid receptors. FASEB J. 1996;10:940–54.
45. Kurokawa R, DiRenzo J, Boehm M, Sugarman J, Gloss B, Rosenfeld M, et al. Regulation of retinoid signalling by receptor polarity and allosteric control of ligand binding. Nature. 1994;371:528–31.
46. Renaud J-P, Rochel N, Ruff M, Vivat V, Chambon P, Gronemeyer H, et al. Crystal structure of the RAR-g ligand binding domain bound to all-trans retinoic acid. Nature. 1995;378:681–9.
47. Perissi V, Staszewski LM, McInerney EM, Kurokawa R, Krones A, Rose DW, et al. Molecular determinants of nuclear receptor-corepressor interaction. Genes Dev. 1999;13:3198–208.
48. Kouzarides T. Chromatin modifications and their function. Cell. 2007;128(4):693–705.
49. Yang XJ, Seto E. Lysine acetylation: codified crosstalk with other posttranslational modifications. Mol Cell. 2008;31(4):449–61.
50. Huq MD, Tsai NP, Khan SA, Wei LN. Lysine trimethylation of retinoic acid receptor-alpha: a novel means to regulate receptor function. Mol Cell Proteomics. 2007;6(4):677–88.
51. Chen H, Lin RJ, Xie W, Wilpitz D, Evans RM. Regulation of hormone-induced histone hyperacetylation and gene activation via acetylation of an acetylase. Cell. 1999;98(5):675–86.
52. Bastien J, Rochette-Egly C. Nuclear retinoid receptors and the transcription of retinoid-target genes. Gene. 2004;328:1–16.
53. Narlikar GJ, Fan HY, Kingston RE. Cooperation between complexes that regulate chromatin structure and transcription. Cell. 2002;108(4):475–87.
54. Ho L, Crabtree GR. Chromatin remodelling during development. Nature. 2010;463(7280):474–84.
55. Strahl BD, Allis CD. The language of covalent histone modification. Nature. 1998;403:41–5.
56. Jensen K, Shiels C, Freemont PS. PML protein isoforms and the RBCC/TRIM motif. Oncogene. 2001;20(49):7223–33.
57. Borden KL. Pondering the puzzle of PML (promyelocytic leukemia) nuclear bodies: can we fit the pieces together using an RNA regulon? Biochim Biophys Acta. 2008;1783(11):2145–54.
58. Daniel M, Koken M, Romagne O, Barbey S, Bazarbachi A, Stadler M, et al. PML protein expression in hematopoietic and acute promyleocytic leukemia cells. Blood. 1993;82:1858–67.
59. Terris B, Baldin V, Dubois S, Degott C, Flejou J-F, Henin D, et al. PML nuclear bodies are general targets for inflammation and cell proliferation. Cancer Res. 1995;55:1590–7.
60. Bernardi R, Pandolfi PP. Structure, dynamics and functions of promyelocytic leukaemia nuclear bodies. Nat Rev Mol Cell Biol. 2007;8:1006–16.
61. Van Damme E, Laukens K, Dang TH, Van Ostade X. A manually curated network of the PML nuclear body interactome reveals an important role for PML-NBs in SUMOylation dynamics. Int J Biol Sci. 2010;6(1):51–67.
62. Zhong S, Muller S, Ronchetti S, Freemont PS, Dejean A, Pandolfi PP. Role of SUMO-1-modified PML in nuclear body formation. Blood. 2000;95:2748–52.
63. Lallemand-Breitenbach V, Jeanne M, Benhenda S, Nasr R, Lei M, Peres L, et al. Arsenic degrades PML or PML-RARalpha through a SUMO-triggered RNF4/ubiquitin-mediated pathway. Nat Cell Biol. 2008;10(5):547–55.
64. Tatham MH, Geoffroy MC, Shen L, Plechanovova A, Hattersley N, Jaffray EG, et al. RNF4 is a poly-SUMO-specific E3 ubiquitin ligase required for arsenic-induced PML degradation. Nat Cell Biol. 2008;10(5):538–46.
65. Reineke EL, Kao HY. Targeting promyelocytic leukemia protein: a means to regulating PML nuclear bodies. Int J Biol Sci. 2009;5(4):366–76.
66. Wang ZG, Delva L, Gaboli M, Rivi R, Giorgio M, Cordon-Cardo C, et al. Role of PML in cell growth and the retinoic acid pathway. Science. 1998;279:1547–51.
67. Bernardi R, Papa A, Pandolfi PP. Regulation of apoptosis by PML and the PML-NBs. Oncogene. 2008;27(48):6299–312.
68. Gurrieri C, Capodieci P, Bernardi R, Scaglioni PP, Nafa K, Rush LJ, et al. Loss of the tumor suppressor PML in human cancers of multiple histologic origins. J Natl Cancer Inst. 2004;96(4):269–79.
69. Ito K, Bernardi R, Morotti A, Matsuoka S, Saglio G, Ikeda Y, et al. PML targeting eradicates quiescent leukaemia-initiating cells. Nature. 2008;453(7198):1072–8.
70. Borden KLB, Boddy MN, Lally J, O'Reilly NJ, Martin S, Howe K, et al. The solution structure of the RING finger domain from the acute promyelocytic leukaemia proto-oncoprotein PML. EMBO J. 1995;14:1532–41.
71. Slack JL, Willman CL, Andersen JW, Li Y-P, Viswanatha DS, Bloomfield CD, et al. Molecular analysis and clinical outcome of adult APL patients with the type V PML-RARa isoform: results from Intergroup protocol 0129. Blood. 2000;95:398–403.
72. Gu BW, Xiong H, Zhou Y, Chen B, Dong S, Yu ZY, et al. Variant-type PML-RARa fusion transcript in acute promyelocytic leukemia: use of a cryptic coding sequence from intron 2 of the RARa gene and identification of a new clinical subtype of retinoic acid therapy. Proc Natl Acad Sci U S A. 2002;99:7640–5.
73. Reiter A, Saussele S, Grimwade D, Wiemels JL, Segal MR, Lafage-Pochitaloff M, et al. Genomic anatomy of the specific reciprocal translocation t(15;17) in acute promyelocytic leukemia. Genes Chromosomes Cancer. 2003;36(2):175–88.
74. Gallagher RE, Willman CL, Slack JL, Andersen JW, Li YP, Viswanatha D, et al. Association of PML-RARa fusion mRNA type with pretreatment hematologic characteristics but not treatment outcome in acute promyelocytic leukemia: an intergroup molecular study. Blood. 1997;90:1656–63.
75. Kane JR, Head DR, Balazs L, Hulshof MG, Motroni TA, Raimondi SC, et al. Molecular analysis of the PML/RAR alpha chimeric gene in pediatric acute promyelocytic leukemia. Leukemia. 1996;10(8):1296–302.
76. Guglielmi C, Martelli MP, Diverio D. Immunophenotype of adult and childhood acute promyelocytic leukaemia: correlation with morphology, type of PML gene breakpoint and clinical outcome: a cooperative Italian study on 196 cases. Br J Haematol. 1998;102:1035–10941.
77. Alcalay M, Zangrilli D, Fagioli M, Pandolfi P, Mencarelli A, Lo Coco F, et al. Expression pattern of the RARa-PML fusion gene in acute promyelocytic leukemia. Proc Natl Acad Sci U S A. 1992;89:4840–4.
78. Borrow J, Goddard AD, Gibbons B, Katz F, Swirsky D, Fioretos T, et al. Diagnosis of acute promyelocytic leukaemia by RT-PCR detection of PML-RARA and RARA-PML fusion transcripts. Br J Haematol. 1992;82:529–40.
79. Li YP, Andersen J, Zelent A, Rao S, Paietta E, Tallman MS, et al. RARa1/RARa2-PML mRNA expression in acute promyelocytic leukemia cells: a molecular and laboratory-clinical correlative study. Blood. 1997;90:306–12.
80. Walz C, Grimwade D, Saussele S, Lengfelder E, Hafelach C, Schnittger S, et al. Atypical mRNA fusions in PML-RARA positive, RARA-PML negative acute promyelocytic leukemia. Genes Chromosomes Cancer. 2010;49:471–9.
81. Mistry AR, Felix CA, Whitmarsh RJ, Mason A, Reiter A, Cassinat B, et al. DNA topoisomerase II in therapy-related acute promyelocytic leukemia. N Engl J Med. 2005;352(15):1529–38.

82. Hasan SK, Mays AN, Ottone T, Ledda A, La Nasa G, Cattaneo C, et al. Molecular analysis of t(15;17) genomic breakpoints in secondary acute promyelocytic leukemia arising after treatment of multiple sclerosis. Blood. 2008;112(8):3383–90.
83. Mays AN, Osheroff N, Xiao Y, Wiemels JL, Felix CA, Byl JA, et al. Evidence for direct involvement of epirubicin in the formation of chromosomal translocations in t(15;17) therapy-related acute promyelocytic leukemia. Blood. 2010;115(2):326–30.
84. McHale CM, Wiemels JL, Zhang L, Ma X, Buffler PA, Feusner J, et al. Prenatal origin of childhood acute myeloid leukemias harboring chromosomal rearrangements t(15;17) and inv(16). Blood. 2003;101(11):4640–1.
85. Collins SJ. Acute promyelocytic leukemia: relieving repression induces remission. Blood. 1998;91(8):2631–3.
86. Lin RJ, Evans RM. Acquisition of oncogenic potential by RAR chimeras in acute promyelocytic leukemia through formation of homodimers. Mol Cell. 2000;5:821–30.
87. Onodera M, Kunisada T, Nishikawa S, Sakiyama Y, Matsumoto S, Nishikawa S. Overexpression of retinoic acid receptor alpha suppresses myeloid cell differentiation at the promyelocyte stage. Oncogene. 1995;11:1291–8.
88. Du C, Redner RL, Cooke MP, Lavau C. Overexpression of wild-type retinoic acid receptor alpha (RARalpha) recapitulates retinoic acid-sensitive transformation of primary myeloid progenitors by acute promyelocytic leukemia RARalpha-fusion genes. Blood. 1999;94:793–802.
89. Robertson K, Emami B, Collins S. Retinoic acid-resistant HL-60R cells harbor a point mutation in the retinoic acid receptor ligand-binding domain that confers dominant negative activity. Blood. 1992;80:1885–8.
90. Grignani F, Valtieri M, Gabbianelli M, Gelmetti V, Botta R, Luchetti L, et al. PML/RARa fusion protein expression in normal human hematopoietic progenitors dictates myeloid commitment and the promyelocytic phenotype. Blood. 2000;96:1531–7.
91. Yoshida H, Kitamura K, Tanaka K, Omura S, Miyazaki T, Hachiya T, et al. Accelerated degradation of PML-retinoic acid receptor a (PML-RARA) oncoprotein by all-trans retinoic acid in acute promyelocytic leukemia: Possible role of the proteasome pathway. Cancer Res. 1996;56:2945–8.
92. Zhu J, Gianni M, Kopf E, Honore N, Chelbi-Alix M, Koken M, et al. Retinoic acid induces proteasome-dependent degradation of retinoic acid receptor a (RARa) and oncogenic RARa fusion proteins. Proc Natl Acad Sci U S A. 1999;96:14807–12.
93. Lin RJ, Nagy L, Inoue S, Shao W, Miller WH Jr, Evans RM. Role of the histone deacetylase complex in acute promyelocytic leukemia. Nature. 1998;391:811–4.
94. Grignani F, De Matteis S, Nervi C, Tomassoni L, Gelmetti V, Cioce M, et al. Fusion proteins of the retinoic acid receptor-a recruit histone deacetylase in promyelocytic leukemia. Nature. 1998;391:815–7.
95. Guidez F, Ivins S, Zhu J, Soderstrom M, Waxman S, Zelent A. Reduced retinoic acid-sensitivities of nuclear receptor corepressor binding to PML- and PLZF-RARa underlie molecular pathogenesis and treatment of acute promyelocytic leukemia. Blood. 1998;91:2634–42.
96. Di Croce L, Raker VA, Corsaro M, Faxi F, Fanelli M, Faretta M, et al. Methyltransferase recruitment and DNA hypermethylation of target promoters by an oncogenic transcription factor. Science. 2002;295:1079–82.
97. Carbone R, Botrugno OA, Ronzoni S, Insinga A, Di Croce L, Pelicci PG, et al. Recruitment of the histone methyltransferase SUV39H1 and its role in the oncogenic properties of the leukemia-associated PML-retinoic acid receptor fusion protein. Mol Cell Biol. 2006;26(4):1288–96.
98. Villa R, Morey L, Raker VA, Buschbeck M, Gutierrez A, De Santis F, et al. The methyl-CpG binding protein MBD1 is required for PML-RAR alpha function. Proc Natl Acad Sci U S A. 2006;103(5):1400–5.
99. Villa R, Pasini D, Gutierrez A, Morey L, Occhionorelli M, Vire E, et al. Role of the polycomb repressive complex 2 in acute promyelocytic leukemia. Cancer Cell. 2007;11(6):513–25.
100. Morey L, Brenner C, Fazi F, Villa R, Gutierrez A, Buschbeck M, et al. MBD3, a component of the NuRD complex, facilitates chromatin alteration and deposition of epigenetic marks. Mol Cell Biol. 2008;28(19):5912–23.
101. Kogan SC, Hong SH, Shultz DB, Privalsky ML, Bishop JM. Leukemia initiated by PMLRARa: the PML domain plays a critical role while retinoic acid-mediated transactivation is dispensable. Blood. 2000;95:1541–50.
102. Matsushita H, Scaglioni PP, Bhaumik M, Rego EM, Cai LF, Majid SM, et al. In vivo analysis of the role of aberrant histone deacetylase recruitment and RAR alpha blockade in the pathogenesis of acute promyelocytic leukemia. J Exp Med. 2006;203(4):821–8.
103. Sternsdorf T, Phan VT, Maunakea ML, Ocampo CB, Sohal J, Silletto A, et al. Forced retinoic acid receptor a homodimers prime mice for APL-like leukemia. Cancer Cell. 2006;9:81–94.
104. Kwok C, Zeisig BB, Dong S, So CW. Forced homo-oligomerization of RARalpha leads to transformation of primary hematopoietic cells. Cancer Cell. 2006;9(2):95–108.
105. Licht JD. Reconstructing a disease: what essential features of the retinoic acid receptor fusion oncoproteins generate actue promyelocytic leukemia? Cancer Cell. 2006;9:73–4.
106. Koken MHM, Reid A, Quignon F, Chelbi-Alix MK, Dong S, Chen S-J, et al. Leukaemia-associated RARa fusion partners, PML and PLZF, heterodimerize and co-localize onto nuclear bodies. Proc Natl Acad Sci U S A. 1997;94:10255–60.
107. Zhu J, Zhou J, Peres L, Riaucoux F, Honore N, Kogan SC, et al. A sumoylation site in PML/RARA is essential for leukemic transformation. Cancer Cell. 2005;7:143–53.
108. Rego EM, Wang ZG, Peruzzi D, He LZ, Cordon-Cardo C, Pandolfi PP. Role of promyelocytic leukemia (PML) protein in tumor suppression. J Exp Med. 2001;193:521–9.
109. Koken MHM, Puvion-Dutilleul F, Guillemin MC, Viron A, Linares-Cruz G, Stuurman N, et al. The t(15;17) translocation alters a nuclear body in a retinoic acid-reversible fashion. EMBO J. 1994;13:1073–83.
110. Zeisig BB, Kwok C, Zelent A, Shankaranarayanan P, Gronemeyer H, Dong S, et al. Recruitment of RXR by homotetrameric RARalpha fusion proteins is essential for transformation. Cancer Cell. 2007;12(1):36–51.
111. Zhu J, Nasr R, Peres L, Riaucoux-Lormiere F, Honore N, Berthier C, et al. RXR is an essential component of the oncogenic PML/RARA complex in vivo. Cancer Cell. 2007;12(1):23–35.
112. Minucci S, Pelicci PG. Determinants of oncogenic transformation in acute promyelocytic leukemia: the hetero-union makes the force. Cancer Cell. 2007;12(1):1–3.
113. Zimonjic DB, Pollock JL, Westervelt P, Popescu NC, Ley TJ. Acquired, nonrandom chromosomal abnormalities associated with the development of acute promyelocytic leukemia in transgenic mice. Proc Natl Acad Sci U S A. 2000;97(24):13306–11.
114. Le Beau MM, Bitts S, Davis EM, Kogan SC. Recurring chromosomal abnormalities in leukemia in PML-RARA transgenic mice parallel human acute promyelocytic leukemia. Blood. 2002;99(8):2985–91.
115. Walter MJ, Park JS, Lau SKM, Li X, Lane AA, Nagarajan R, et al. Expression profiling of murine acute promyelocytic leukemia cells reveals multiple model-dependent progression signatures. Mol Cell Biol. 2004;24:10882–93.
116. Walter MJ, Park JS, Ries RE, Lau SK, McLellan M, Jaeger S, et al. Reduced PU.1 expression causes myeloid progenitor expansion and increased leukemia penetrance in mice expressing PML-RARalpha. Proc Natl Acad Sci U S A. 2005;102(35):12513–8.
117. Kelly LM, Kutok JL, Williams IR, Boulton CL, Amarat SM, Curley DP, et al. PML/RARa and FLT3-ITD induce an APL-like disease in a mouse model. Proc Natl Acad Sci U S A. 2002;99:8283–8.

118. Chan IT, Kutok JL, Williams IR, Cohen S, Moore S, Shigematsu H, et al. Oncogenic K-ras cooperates with PML-RAR alpha to induce an acute promyelocytic leukemia-like disease. Blood. 2006;108(5):1708–15.
119. Westervelt P, Lane AA, Pollock JL, Oldfather K, Holt MS, Zimonjic DB, et al. High-penetrance mouse model of acute promyelocytic leukemia with very low levels of PML-RARa expression. Blood. 2003;102:1857–65.
120. Lane AA, Ley TJ. Neutrophil elastase is important for PML-retinoic acid receptor alpha activities in early myeloid cells. Mol Cell Biol. 2005;25(1):23–33.
121. Alcalay M, Meani N, Gelmetti V, Fantozzi A, Fagioli M, Orleth A, et al. Acute myeloid leukemia fusion proteins deregulate genes involved in stem cell maintenance and DNA repair. J Clin Invest. 2003;112(11):1751–61.
122. Park DJ, Vuong PT, de Vos S, Douer D, Koeffler HP. Comparative analysis of genes regulated by PML/RAR alpha and PLZF/RAR alpha in response to retinoic acid using oligonucleotide arrays. Blood. 2003;102(10):3727–36.
123. Muller-Tidow C, Steffen B, Cauvet T, Tickenbrock L, Ji P, Diederichs S, et al. Translocation products in acute myeloid leukemia activate the Wnt signaling pathway in hematopoietic cells. Mol Cell Biol. 2004;24(7):2890–904.
124. Perez A, Kastner P, Sethi S, Lutz Y, Reibel C, Chambon P. PMLRAR homodimers: distinct DNA binding properties and heterodimeric interactions with RXR. EMBO J. 1993;12:3171–82.
125. Kamashev D, Vitoux D, De The H. PML-RARA-RXR oligomers mediate retinoid and rexinoid/cAMP cross-talk in acute promyelocytic leukemia cell differentiation. J Exp Med. 2004;199(8):1163–74.
126. Meani N, Minardi S, Licciulli S, Gelmetti V, Coco FL, Nervi C, et al. Molecular signature of retinoic acid treatment in acute promyelocytic leukemia. Oncogene. 2005;24(20):3358–68.
127. Hoemme C, Peerzada A, Behre G, Wang Y, McClelland M, Nieselt K, et al. Chromatin modifications induced by PML-RARalpha repress critical targets in leukemogenesis as analyzed by ChIP-Chip. Blood. 2008;111(5):2887–95.
128. Martens JH, Brinkman AB, Simmer F, Francoijs KJ, Nebbioso A, Ferrara F, et al. PML-RARalpha/RXR alters the epigenetic landscape in acute promyelocytic leukemia. Cancer Cell. 2010;17(2):173–85.
129. Wang K, Wang P, Shi J, Zhu X, He M, Jia X, et al. PML/RARalpha targets promoter regions containing PU.1 consensus and RARE half sites in acute promyelocytic leukemia. Cancer Cell. 2010;17(2):186–97.
130. van Wageningen S, Breems-de Ridder MC, Nigten J, Nikoloski G, Erpelinck-Verschueren CA, Lowenberg B, et al. Gene transactivation without direct DNA binding defines a novel gain-of-function for PML-RARalpha. Blood. 2008;111(3):1634–43.
131. Mueller BU, Pabst T, Fos J, Petkovic V, Fey MF, Asou N, et al. ATRA resolves the differentiation block in t(15;17) acute myeloid leukemia by restoring PU.1 expression. Blood. 2006;107(8):3330–8.
132. Duprez E, Wagner K, Koch H, Tenen DG. C/EBPbeta: a major PML-RARA-responsive gene in retinoic acid-induced differentiation of APL cells. EMBO J. 2003;22(21):5806–16.
133. Doucas V, Brockes J, Yaniv M, de The H, Dejean A. The PML-retinoic acid receptor-a translocation converts the receptor from an inhibitor to a retinoic acid-dependent activator of transcription factor AP-1. Proc Natl Acad Sci U S A. 1993;90:9345–9.
134. Tussie-Luna MI, Rozo L, Roy AL. Pro-proliferative function of the long isoform of PML-RARalpha involved in acute promyelocytic leukemia. Oncogene. 2006;25(24):3375–86.
135. Yuan W, Payton JE, Holt MS, Link DC, Watson MA, DiPersio JF, et al. Commonly dysregulated genes in murine APL cells. Blood. 2007;109(3):961–70.
136. Chang LW, Payton JE, Yuan W, Ley TJ, Nagarajan R, Stormo GD. Computational identification of the normal and perturbed genetic networks involved in myeloid differentiation and acute promyelocytic leukemia. Genome Biol. 2008;9(2):R38.
137. Wethkamp N, Klempnauer KH. Daxx is a transcriptional repressor of CCAAT/enhancer-binding protein beta. J Biol Chem. 2009;284(42):28783–94.
138. Grimwade D, Biondi A, Mozziconacci MJ, Hagemeijer A, Berger R, Neat M, et al. Characterization of acute promyelocytic leukemia cases lacking the classic t(15;17): results of the European Working Party. Blood. 2000;96:1297–308.
139. Gallagher RE, Mak S, Paietta E, Cooper B, Ehmann C, Tallman MS. Identification of a second acute promyelocytic leukemia (APL) patient with the STAT-RARa fusion gene among PML-RARa-negative Eastern Cooperative Oncology Group (ECOG) APL protocol registrants. Blood. 2004;104:821a.
140. Petti MC, Fazi F, Gentile M, Diverio D, De Faritiis P, De Propris MS, et al. Complete remission through blast cell differentiation in PLZF/RARa-positive acute promyelocytic leukemia: in vitro and in vivo studies. Blood. 2002;100:1065–7.
141. Sainty D, Liso V, Cantu-Rajnoldi A, Head D, Mozziconacci MJ, Arnoulet C, et al. A new morphologic classification system for acute promyelocytic leukemia distinguishes cases with underlying PLZF/RARA gene rearrangements. Group Francais de Cytogenetique Hematologique, UK Cancer Cytogenetics Group and BIOMED 1 European Coomunity-Concerted Acion "Molecular Cytogenetic Diagnosis in Haematological Malignancies". Blood. 2000;96(4):1287–96.
142. Koken MH, Daniel MT, Gianni M, Zelent A, Licht J, Buzyn A, et al. Retinoic acid, but not arsenic trioxide, degrades the PLZF/RARalpha fusion protein, without inducing terminal differentiation or apoptosis, in a RA-therapy resistant t(11;17)(q23;q21) APL patient. Oncogene. 1999;18(4):1113–8.
143. Rego EM, He LZ, Warrell RP Jr, Wang ZG, Pandolfi PP. Retinoic acid (RA) and As2O3 treatment in transgenic models of acute promyelocytic leukemia (APL) unravel the distinct nature of the leukemogenic process induced by the PML-RARalpha and PLZF-RARalpha oncoproteins. Proc Natl Acad Sci U S A. 2000;97:10173–8.
144. Rice KL, Hormaeche I, Doulatov S, Flatow JM, Grimwade D, Mills KI, et al. Comprehensive genomic screens identify a role for PLZF-RARalpha as a positive regulator of cell proliferation via direct regulation of c-MYC. Blood. 2009;114(27):5499–511.
145. He LZ, Guidez F, Tribioli C, Peruzzi D, Ruthardt M, Zelent A, et al. Distinct interactions of PML-RARa and PLZF-RARa with co-repressors determine differential responses to RA in APL. Nat Genet. 1998;18:126–34.
146. Licht J, Chomienne C, Goy A, Chen A, Scott A, Head D, et al. Clinical and molecular characterization of a rare syndrome of acute promyelocytic leukemia associated with translocation (11;17). Blood. 1995;85:1083–94.
147. Yeyati PL, Shaknovich R, Boterashvili S, Li J, Ball HJ, Waxman S, et al. Leukemia translocation protein PLZF inhibits cell growth and expression of cyclin A. Oncogene. 1999;18:925.
148. Guidez F, Parks S, Wong H, Jovanovic JV, Mays A, Gilkes AF, et al. RARalpha-PLZF overcomes PLZF-mediated repression of CRABPI, contributing to retinoid resistance in t(11;17) acute promyelocytic leukemia. Proc Natl Acad Sci U S A. 2007;104(47):18694–9.
149. Buijs A, Bruin M. Fusion of FIP1L1 and RARA as a result of a novel t(4;17)(q12;q21) in a case of juvenile myelomonocytic leukemia. Leukemia. 2007;21(5):1104–8.
150. Cools J, Stover EH, Wlodarska I, Marynen P, Gilliland DG. The FIP1L1-PDGFRalpha kinase in hypereosinophilic syndrome and chronic eosinophilic leukemia. Curr Opin Hematol. 2004;11(1):51–7.

151. Redner RL, Rush EA, Faas S, Rudert WA, Corey SJ. The t(5;17) variant of acute promyelocytic leukemia expresses a nucleophosmin-retinoic acid receptor form. Blood. 1996;87:882–6.
152. Wells RA, Hummel JL, De Koven A, Zipursky A, Kirby M, Dube I, et al. A new variant translocation in acute promyelocytic leukaemia: molecular characterization and clinical consideration. Leukemia. 1996;10:735–40.
153. Kusakabe M, Suzukawa K, Nanmoku T, Obara N, Okoshi Y, Mukai HY, et al. Detection of the STAT5B-RARA fusion transcript in acute promyelocytic leukemia with the normal chromosome 17 on G-banding. Eur J Haematol. 2008;80(5):444–7.
154. Redner RL, Corey SL, Rush EA. Differentiation of t(5;17) variant acute promyelocytic leukemic blasts by all-trans retinoic acid. Leukemia. 1997;11:1014–6.
155. Okazuka K, Masuko M, Seki Y, Hama H, Honma N, Furukawa T, et al. Successful all-trans retinoic acid treatment of acute promyelocytic leukemia in a patient with NPM/RAR fusion. Int J Hematol. 2007;86(3):246–9.
156. Rego EM, Ruggero D, Tribioli C, Cattoretti G, Kogan S, Redner RL, et al. Leukemia with distinct phenotypes in transgenic mice expressing PML/RAR alpha, PLZF/RAR alpha or NPM/RAR alpha. Oncogene. 2006;25(13):1974–9.
157. Chen Y, Gu L, Zhou C, Wu X, Gao J, Li Q, et al. Relapsed APL patient with variant NPM-RARalpha fusion responded to arsenic trioxide-based therapy and achieved long-term survival. Int J Hematol. 2010;91(4):708–10.
158. Lafage-Pochitaloff M, Alcalay M, Brunel V, Longo L, Sainty D, Simonetti J, et al. Acute promyelocytic leukemia cases with nonreciprocal PML/RARa or RARa/PML fusion genes. Blood. 1995;85(5):1169–74.
159. Raelson JV, Nervi C, Rosenauer A, Benedetti L, Monczak Y, Pearson M, et al. The PML/RARa oncoprotein is a direct molecular target of retinoic acid in acute promyelocytic leukemia cells. Blood. 1996;88:2826–32.
160. Zhu J, Koken MHM, Quignon F, Chelbi-Alix MK, Degos L, Wang ZY, et al. Arsenic-induced PML targeting onto nuclear bodies: implications for the treatment of acute promyelocytic leukemia. Proc Natl Acad Sci U S A. 1997;94:3978–83.
161. Tamayo P, Slonim D, Mesirov J, Zhu Q, Kitareewan S, Dmitrovsky E, et al. Interpreting patterns of gene expression with self-organizing maps: methods and application to hematopoietic differentiation. Proc Natl Acad Sci U S A. 1999;96:2907–12.
162. Liu T-X, Zhang J-W, Tao J, Zhang R-B, Zhang Q-H, Zhao C-J, et al. Gene expression networks underlying retinoic acid-induced differentiation of acute promyelocytic leukemia cells. Blood. 2000;96:1496–504.
163. Altucci L, Rossin A, Raffelsberger W, Reitmair A, Chomienne C, Gronemeyer H. Retinoic acid-induced apoptosis in leukemia cells is mediated by paracrine action of tumor-selective death ligand TRAIL. Nat Med. 2001;6:680–6.
164. Park DJ, Chumakov AM, Vuong PT, Chih DY, Gombart AF, Miller WH Jr, et al. CCAAT/enhancer binding protein e is a potential retinoid target gene in acute promyelocytic leukemia treatment. J Clin Invest. 1999;103:1399–408.
165. Zheng PZ, Wang KK, Zhang QY, Huang QH, Du YZ, Zhang QH, et al. Systems analysis of transcriptome and proteome in retinoic acid/arsenic trioxide-induced cell differentiation/apoptosis of promyelocytic leukemia. Proc Natl Acad Sci U S A. 2005;102(21):7653–8.
166. Imaizumi M, Suzuki H, Yoshinari M, Sato A, Saito T, Sugawara A, et al. Mutations in the E-domain of RARa portion of the PML/RARa chimeric gene may confer clinical resistance to all-trans retinoic acid in acute promyelocytic leukemia. Blood. 1998;92:374–82.
167. Ding W, Li YP, Nobile LM, Grills G, Carrera I, Paietta E, et al. Leukemic cellular retinoic acid resistance and missense mutations in the PML-RARa fusion gene after relapse of acute promyelocytic leukemia from treatment with all-*trans* retinoic acid and intensive chemotherapy. Blood. 1998;92:1172–83.
168. Gallagher RE. Retinoic acid resistance in acute promyelocytic leukemia. Leukemia. 2002;16:1940–58.
169. Truong BT, Lee YJ, Lodie TA, Park DJ, Perrotti D, Watanabe N, et al. CCAAT/Enhancer binding proteins repress the leukemic phenotype of acute myeloid leukemia. Blood. 2003;101(3):1141–8.
170. Yoshida H, Ichikawa H, Tagata Y, Katsumoto T, Ohnishi K, Akao Y, et al. PML-retinoic acid receptor alpha inhibits PML IV enhancement of PU.1-induced C/EBPepsilon expression in myeloid differentiation. Mol Cell Biol. 2007;27(16):5819–34.
171. Jing Y, Dai J, Chalmers-Redman RME, Tatton WG, Waxman S. Arsenic trioxide selectively induces acute promyelocytic leukemia cell apoptosis via a hydrogen peroxide-dependent pathway. Blood. 1999;94:2102–11.
172. Nervi C, Ferrara FF, Fanelli M, Tippo MP, Tomassini B, Ferrucci PF, et al. Caspases mediate retinoic acid-induced degradation of the acute promyelocytic leukemia PML/RARa fusion protein. Blood. 1998;92:2244–51.
173. Shah SJ, Blumen S, Pitha-Rowe I, Kitareewan S, Freemantle SJ, Feng Q, et al. UBE1L represses PML/RAR{alpha} by targeting the PML domain for ISG15ylation. Mol Cancer Ther. 2008;7(4):905–14.
174. Harris MN, Ozpolat B, Abdi F, Gu S, Legler A, Mawuenyega KG, et al. Comparative proteomic analysis of all-trans-retinoic acid treatment reveals systematic posttranscriptional control mechanisms in acute promyelocytic leukemia. Blood. 2004;104(5):1314–23.
175. Hattori H, Zhang X, Jia Y, Subramanian KK, Jo H, Loison F, et al. RNAi screen identifies UBE2D3 as a mediator of all-trans retinoic acid-induced cell growth arrest in human acute promyelocytic NB4 cells. Blood. 2007;110(2):640–50.
176. Ozpolat B, Akar U, Steiner M, Zorrilla-Calancha I, Tirado-Gomez M, Colburn N, et al. Programmed cell death-4 tumor suppressor protein contributes to retinoic acid-induced terminal granulocytic differentiation of human myeloid leukemia cells. Mol Cancer Res. 2007;5(1):95–108.
177. Kannan-Thulasiraman P, Dolniak B, Kaur S, Sassano A, Kalvakolanu DV, Hay N, et al. Role of the translational repressor 4E-BP1 in the regulation of p21(Waf1/Cip1) expression by retinoids. Biochem Biophys Res Commun. 2008;368(4):983–9.
178. Witcher M, Ross DT, Rousseau C, Deluca L, Miller WH Jr. Synergy between all-trans retinoic acid and tumor necrosis factor pathways in acute leukemia cells. Blood. 2003;102(1):237–45.
179. Miller WH Jr, Schipper HM, Lee JS, Singer J, Waxman S. Mechanisms of action of arsenic trioxide. Cancer Res. 2002;62(14):3893–903.
180. Sumi D, Shinkai Y, Kumagai Y. Signal transduction pathways and transcription factors triggered by arsenic trioxide in leukemia cells. Toxicol Appl Pharmacol. 2010;244(3):385–92.
181. Cai X, Shen YL, Zhu Q, Jia PM, Yu Y, Zhou L, et al. Arsenic trioxide-induced apoptosis and differentiation are associated respectively with mitochondrial transmembrane potential collapse and retinoic acid signaling pathways in acute promyelocytic leukemia. Leukemia. 2000;14:262–70.
182. Shen ZX, Chen GQ, Ni JH, Li XS, Xiong SM, Qiu QY, et al. Use of arsenic trioxide (As2O3) in the treatment of acute promyelocytic leukemia (APL): II. Clinical efficacy and pharmacokinetics in relapsed patients. Blood. 1997;89:3354–60.
183. Fujisawa S, Ohno R, Shigeno K, Sahara N, Nakamura S, Naito K, et al. Pharmacokinetics of arsenic species in Japanese patients with relapsed or refractory acute promyelocytic leukemia treated with arsenic trioxide. Cancer Chemother Pharmacol. 2007;59(4):485–93.
184. Fox E, Razzouk BI, Widemann BC, Xiao S, O'Brien M, Goodspeed W, et al. Phase 1 trial and pharmacokinetic study of arsenic trioxide in children and adolescents with refractory or

relapsed acute leukemia, including acute promyelocytic leukemia or lymphoma. Blood. 2008;111(2):566–73.
185. Chen G-Q, Zhou L, Styblo M, Walton F, Jing Y, Weinberg R, et al. Methylated metabolites of arsenic trioxide are more potent than arsenic trioxide as apoptotic but not differentiation inducers in leukemia and lymphoma cells. Cancer Res. 2003;63:1853–9.
186. Yoshino Y, Yuan B, Miyashita SI, Iriyama N, Horikoshi A, Shikino O, et al. Speciation of arsenic trioxide metabolites in blood cells and plasma of a patient with acute promyelocytic leukemia. Anal Bioanal Chem. 2009;393(2):689–97.
187. Soignet SL, Maslak P, Wang ZG, Jhanwar S, Calleja E, Dardashti LJ, et al. Complete remission after treatment of acute promyelocytic leukemia with arsenic trioxide. N Engl J Med. 1998;339:1341–8.
188. Sternsdorf T, Puccetti E, Jensen K, Hoelzer D, Will H, Ottmann OG, et al. PIC-1/SUMO-1 modified PML-retinoic acid receptor a mediates arsenic trioxide-induced apoptosis in acute promyelocytic leukemia. Mol Cell Biol. 1999;19:5170–8.
189. Lallemand-Breitenbach V, Zhu J, Puvion F, Koken M, Honore N, Doubeikovsky A, et al. Role of promyelocytic leukemia (PML) sumolation in nuclear body formation, 11S proteasome recruitment, and As_2O_3-induced PML or PML/retinoic acid receptor alpha degradation. J Exp Med. 2001;193(12):1361–71.
190. Zhang XW, Yan XJ, Zhou ZR, Yang FF, Wu ZY, Sun HB, et al. Arsenic trioxide controls the fate of the PML-RARalpha oncoprotein by directly binding PML. Science. 2010;328(5975):240–3.
191. Hong SH, Yang Z, Privalsky ML. Arsenic trioxide is a potent inhibitor of the interaction of SMRT corepressor with Its transcription factor partners, including the PML-retinoic acid receptor alpha oncoprotein found in human acute promyelocytic leukemia. Mol Cell Biol. 2001;21(21):7172–82.
192. Lunghi P, Tabilio A, Lo-Coco F, Pelicci PG, Bonati A. Arsenic trioxide (ATO) and MEK1 inhibition synergize to induce apoptosis in acute promyelocytic leukemia cells. Leukemia. 2005;19(2):234–44.
193. Zhu X-H, Shen Y-L, Y-k J, Cai X, Jia P-M, Huang Y, et al. Apoptosis and growth inhibition in malignant lymphocytes after treatment with arsenic trioxide at clinically achievable concentrations. J Natl Cancer Inst. 1999;91:772–8.
194. Davison K, Cote S, Mader S, Miller WH. Glutathione depletion overcomes resistance to arsenic trioxide in arsenic-resistant cell lines. Leukemia. 2003;17(5):931–40.
195. Li L, Wang J, Ye RD, Shi G, Jin H, Tang X, et al. PML/RARalpha fusion protein mediates the unique sensitivity to arsenic cytotoxicity in acute promyelocytic leukemia cells: Mechanisms involve the impairment of cAMP signaling and the aberrant regulation of NADPH oxidase. J Cell Physiol. 2008;217(2):486–93.
196. Gianni M, Koken MHM, Chelbi-Alix MK, Benoit G, Lanotte M, Chen Z, et al. Combined arsenic and retinoic acid treatment enhances differentiation and apoptosis in arsenic-resistant NB4 cells. Blood. 1998;91:4300–10.
197. Sen CK. Redox signaling and the emerging therapeutic potential of thiol antioxidants. Biochem Pharmacol. 1998;55(11):1747–58.
198. Dai J, Weinberg RS, Waxman S, Jing Y. Malignant cell can be sensitized to undergo growth inhibition and apoptosis by arsenic trioxide through modulation of the glutathione redox system. Blood. 1999;93:268–77.
199. Lu J, Chew EH, Holmgren A. Targeting thioredoxin reductase is a basis for cancer therapy by arsenic trioxide. Proc Natl Acad Sci U S A. 2007;104(30):12288–93.
200. Chou WC, Jie C, Kenedy AA, Jones RJ, Trush MA, Dang CV. Role of NADPH oxidase in arsenic-induced reactive oxygen species formation and cytotoxicity in myeloid leukemia cells. Proc Natl Acad Sci U S A. 2004;101(13):4578–83.
201. Wang J, Li L, Cang H, Shi G, Yi J. NADPH oxidase-derived reactive oxygen species are responsible for the high susceptibility to arsenic cytotoxicity in acute promyelocytic leukemia cells. Leuk Res. 2008;32(3):429–36.
202. Lin P, Welch EJ, Gao XP, Malik AB, Ye RD. Lysophosphatidylcholine modulates neutrophil oxidant production through elevation of cyclic AMP. J Immunol. 2005;174(5):2981–9.
203. Davison K, Mann KK, Waxman S, Miller WH Jr. JNK activation is a mediator of arsenic trioxide-induced apoptosis in acute promyelocytic leukemia cells. Blood. 2004;103(9):3496–502.
204. Bernardini S, Nuccetelli M, Noguera NI, Bellincampi L, Lunghi P, Bonati A, et al. Role of GSTP1-1 in mediating the effect of As_2O_3 in the acute promyelocytic leukemia cell line NB4. Ann Hematol. 2006;85(10):681–7.
205. Chou WC, Chen HY, Yu SL, Cheng L, Yang PC, Dang CV. Arsenic suppresses gene expression in promyelocytic leukemia cells partly through Sp1 oxidation. Blood. 2005;106(1):304–10.
206. Shao W, Fanelli M, Ferrara FF, Riccioni R, Rosenauer A, Davison K, et al. As_2O_3 induced apoptosis and loss of PML/RARa protein in both retinoid sensitive and resistant APL cells. J Natl Cancer Inst. 1998;90:124–33.
207. Jing Y, Wang L, Xia L, Chen G-Q, Chen Z, Miller WH Jr, et al. Combined effect of all-*trans* retinoic acid and arsenic trioxide in acute promyelocytic leukemia cells in vitro and in vivo. Blood. 2001;97:264–9.
208. Sun Y, Kim SH, Zhou DC, Ding W, Paietta E, Guidez F, et al. Acute promyeloctyic leukemia cell line AP-1060 established as a cytokine-dependent culture from a patient clinically-resistant to all-*trans* retinoic acid and arsenic trioxide. Leukemia. 2004;18:1258–69.
209. Lallemand-Breitenbach V, Guillemin MC, Janin A, Daniel MT, Degos L, Kogan SC, et al. Retinoic acid and arsenic synergize to eradicate leukemic cells in a mouse model of acute promyelocytic leukemia. J Exp Med. 1999;189:1043–52.
210. Westervelt P, Pollock JL, Oldfather KM, Walter MJ, Ma MK, Williams A, et al. Adaptive immunity cooperates with liposomal all-trans-retinoic acid (ATRA) to facilitate long-term molecular remissions in mice with acute promyelocytic leukemia. Proc Natl Acad Sci U S A. 2002;99(14):9468–73.
211. Grimwade D, Enver T. Acute promyelocytic leukemia: where does it stem from? Leukemia. 2004;18(3):375–84.
212. Zheng X, Seshire A, Ruster B, Bug G, Beissert T, Puccetti E, et al. Arsenic but not all-trans retinoic acid overcomes the aberrant stem cell capacity of PML/RARa-positive leukemic stem cells. Haematologica. 2007;92:323–31.
213. Bonomi R, Giordano H, del Pilar MM, Bodega E, Gallagher R, et al. Simultaneous PML/RARalpha and AML1/ETO expression with t(15;17) at onset and relapse with only t(8;21) in an acute promyelocytic leukemia patient. Cancer Genet Cytogenet. 2000;123(1):41–3.
214. Gurrieri C, Nafa K, Merghoub T, Bernardi R, Capodieci P, Biondi A, et al. Mutations of the PML tumor suppressor gene in acute promyelocytic leukemia. Blood. 2004;103(6):2358–62.
215. Chen Z-X, Xue Y-Q, Zhang R, Tao R-F, Xia X-M, Li C, et al. A clinical and experimental study on all-*trans* retinoic acid-treated acute promyelocytic leukemia patients. Blood. 1991;78:1413–9.
216. Frankel SR, Eardley A, Heller G, Berman E, Miller WH Jr, Dmitrovsky E, et al. All-*trans*-retinoic acid for acute promyelocytic leukemia: results of the New York study. Ann Intern Med. 1994;120:278–86.
217. Warrell RP Jr. Retinoid resistance in acute promyelocytic leukemia: new mechanisms, strategies and implications. Blood. 1993;82:1949–53.
218. Muindi J, Frankel S, Miller WH Jr, Jakubowski A, Scheinberg D, Young C, et al. Continuous treatment with all-trans-retinoic acid causes a progressive reduction in plasma drug concentrations: implications for relapse and retinoid "resistance" in patients with acute promyelocytic leukemia. Blood. 1992;79:299–303.

219. Adamson PC, Bailey J, Pluda J, Poplack DG, Bauza S, Murphy RF, et al. Pharmacokinetics of all-*trans*-retinoic acid administered on an intermittent schedule. J Clin Oncol. 1995;13(4):1238–41.
220. Miller WH Jr, Jakubowski A, Tong WP, Miller VA, Rigas JR, Benedetti F, et al. 9-*cis* retinoic acid induces complete remission but does not reverse clinically acquired retinoid resistance in acute promyelocytic leukemia. Blood. 1995;85:3021–7.
221. Tobita T, Takeshita A, Kitamura K, Ohnishi K, Yanagi M, Hiraoka A, et al. Treatment with a new synthetic retinoid, Am80, of acute promyelocytic leukemia relapsed from complete remission induced by all-*trans* retinoic acid. Blood. 1997;90:967–73.
222. Douer D, Estey E, Santillana S, Bennett JM, Lopez-Berestein G, Boehm K, et al. Treatment of newly diagnosed and relapsed acute promyelocytic leukemia with intravenous liposomal *all-trans* retinoic acid. Blood. 2001;97:73–80.
223. Cote S, Rosenauer A, Bianchini A, Seiter K, Vandewiele J, Nervi C, et al. Response to histone deacetylase inhibition of novel PML/RARalpha mutant detected in retinoic acid-resistant APL cells. Blood. 2002;100:261–70.
224. Gallagher RE, Schachter-Tokarz EL, Zhou D-C, Ding W, Kim SH, Bi W, et al. Relapse of acute promyelocytic leukemia with PML-RARa mutant subclones independent of proximate all-*trans* retinoic acid selection pressure. Leukemia. 2006;20:556–62.
225. Schachter-Tokarz E, Kelaidi C, Cassinat B, Chomienne C, Gardin C, Raffoux E, et al. PML-RARalpha ligand-binding domain deletion mutations associated with reduced disease control and outcome after first relapse of APL. Leukemia. 2010;24:473–6.
226. Zhou D-C, Kim S, Ding W, Schulz C, Warrell RP Jr, Gallagher RE. Frequent mutations in the ligand binding domain of PML-RARa after multiple relapses of acute promyelocytic leukemia: analysis for functional relationship to response to all-*trans* retinoic acid and histone deacetylase inhibitors in vitro and in vivo. Blood. 2002;99:1356–63.
227. Cote S, Zhou D, Bianchini A, Nervi C, Gallagher RE, Miller WH Jr. Altered ligand binding and transcriptional regulation by mutations in the PML/RARa ligand-binding domain arising in retinoic acid-resistant patients with acute promyelocytic leukemia. Blood. 2000;96:3200–8.
228. Cornic M, Delva L, Guidez F, Balitrand N, Degos L, Chomienne C. Induction of retinoic acid-binding protein in normal and malignant human myeloid cells by retinoic acid in acute promyelocytic leukemia patients. Cancer Res. 1992;52:3329–34.
229. Zhou D-C, Hallam SJ, Klein RS, Wiernik PH, Tallman MS, Gallagher RE. Constitutive expression of cellular retinoic acid binding protein II and lack of correlation with sensitivity to all-*trans* retinoic acid in acute promyelocytic leukemia cells. Cancer Res. 1998;58:5770–6.
230. Napoli J. Retinoic acid biosynthesis and metabolism. FASEB J. 1996;10:993–1001.
231. Dong D, Ruuska SE, Levinthal DJ, Noy N. Distinct roles for cellular retinoic acid-binding proteins I and II in regulating signaling by retinoic acid. J Biol Chem. 1999;274:23695–8.
232. Delva L, Bastie J-N, Rochette-Egly C, Kraiba R, Balitrand N, Despauy G, et al. Physical and functional interactions between cellular retinoic acid binding protein II and the retinoic acid-dependent nuclear complex. Mol Cell Biol. 1999;19:7158–67.
233. Quere R, Baudet A, Cassinat B, Bertrand G, Marti J, Manchon L, et al. Pharmacogenomic analysis of acute promyelocytic leukemia cells highlights CYP26 cytochrome metabolism in differential all-trans retinoic acid sensitivity. Blood. 2007;109(10):4450–60.
234. Fanelli M, Minucci S, Gelmetti V, Nervi C, Gambacorti-Passerini C, Pelicci PG. Constitutive degradation of PML/RARa through the proteasome pathway mediates retinoic acid resistance. Blood. 1999;93:1477–81.
235. McNamara S, Wang H, Hanna N, Miller WH Jr. Topoisomerase IIbeta negatively modulates retinoic acid receptor alpha function: a novel mechanism of retinoic acid resistance. Mol Cell Biol. 2008;28(6):2066–77.
236. McNamara S, Nichol JN, Wang H, Miller WH Jr. Targeting PKC delta-mediated topoisomerase II beta overexpression subverts the differentiation block in a retinoic acid-resistant APL cell line. Leukemia. 2010;24(4):729–39.
237. Kambhampati S, Li Y, Verma A, Sassano A, Majchrzak B, Deb DK, et al. Activation of protein kinase C delta by all-trans-retinoic acid. J Biol Chem. 2003;278(35):32544–51.
238. Alsayed Y, Uddin S, Mahmud N, Lekmine F, Kalvakolanu DV, Minucci S, et al. Activation of Rac1 and the p38 mitogen-activated protein kinase pathway in response to all-trans-retinoic acid. J Biol Chem. 2001;276(6):4012–9.
239. Ohnuma-Ishikawa K, Morio T, Yamada T, Sugawara Y, Ono M, Nagasawa M, et al. Knockdown of XAB2 enhances all-trans retinoic acid-induced cellular differentiation in all-trans retinoic acid-sensitive and -resistant cancer cells. Cancer Res. 2007;67(3):1019–29.
240. Zhao HL, Ueki N, Marcelain K, Hayman MJ. The Ski protein can inhibit ligand induced RARalpha and HDAC3 degradation in the retinoic acid signaling pathway. Biochem Biophys Res Commun. 2009;383(1):119–24.
241. Neri LM, Borgatti P, Tazzari PL, Bortul R, Cappellini A, Tabellini G, et al. The phosphoinositide 3-kinase/AKT1 pathway involvement in drug and all-trans-retinoic acid resistance of leukemia cells. Mol Cancer Res. 2003;1(3):234–46.
242. Srinivas H, Xia D, Moore NL, Uray IP, Kim H, Ma L, et al. Akt phosphorylates and suppresses the transactivation of retinoic acid receptor alpha. Biochem J. 2006;395(3):653–62.
243. Ghavamzadeh A, Alimoghaddam K, Ghaffari SH, Rostami S, Jahani M, Hosseini R, et al. Treatment of acute promyelocytic leukemia with arsenic trioxide without ATRA and/or chemotherapy. Ann Oncol. 2006;17(1):131–4.
244. Mathews V, George B, Chendamarai E, Lakshmi KM, Desire S, Balasubramanian P, et al. Single-agent arsenic trioxide in the treatment of newly diagnosed acute promyelocytic leukemia: long-term follow-up data. J Clin Oncol. 2010;28(24):3866–71.
245. Zhou J, Zhang Y, Li J, Li X, Hou J, Zhao Y, et al. Single-agent arsenic trioxide in the treatment of children with newly diagnosed acute promyelocytic leukemia. Blood. 2010;115(9):1697–702.
246. Ghaffari SH, Rostami S, Bashash D, Alimoghaddam K, Ghavamzadeh A. Real-time PCR analysis of PML-RAR alpha in newly diagnosed acute promyelocytic leukaemia patients treated with arsenic trioxide as a front-line therapy. Ann Oncol. 2006;17(10):1553–9.
247. Ghaffari SH, Shayan-Asl N, Jamialahmadi AH, Alimoghaddam K, Ghavamzadeh A. Telomerase activity and telomere length in patients with acute promyelocytic leukemia: indicative of proliferative activity, disease progression, and overall survival. Ann Oncol. 2008;19(11):1927–34.
248. Thirugnanam R, George B, Chendamarai E, Lakshmi KM, Balasubramanian P, Viswabandya A, et al. Comparison of clinical outcomes of patients with relapsed acute promyelocytic leukemia induced with arsenic trioxide and consolidated with either an autologous stem cell transplant or an arsenic trioxide-based regimen. Biol Blood Marrow Transplant. 2009;15(11):1479–84.
249. Diaz Z, Mann KK, Marcoux S, Kourelis M, Colombo M, Komarnitsky PB, et al. A novel arsenical has antitumor activity toward As_2O3-resistant and MRP1/ABCC1-overexpressing cell lines. Leukemia. 2008;22(10):1853–63.
250. Tabellini G, Tazzari PL, Bortul R, Evangelisti C, Billi AM, Grafone T, et al. Phosphoinositide 3-kinase/Akt inhibition increases arsenic trioxide-induced apoptosis of acute promyelocytic and T-cell leukaemias. Br J Haematol. 2005;130(5):716–25.
251. Ramos AM, Fernandez C, Amran D, Sancho P, de Blas E, Aller P. Pharmacologic inhibitors of PI3K/Akt potentiate the apoptotic

action of the antileukemic drug arsenic trioxide via glutathione depletion and increased peroxide accumulation in myeloid leukemia cells. Blood. 2005;105(10):4013–20.

252. Leung J, Pang A, Yuen WH, Kwong YL, Tse EW. Relationship of expression of aquaglyceroporin 9 with arsenic uptake and sensitivity in leukemia cells. Blood. 2007;109(2):740–6.

253. Dilda PJ, Perrone GG, Philp A, Lock RB, Dawes IW, Hogg PJ. Insight into the selectivity of arsenic trioxide for acute promyelocytic leukemia cells by characterizing *Saccharomyces cerevisiae* deletion strains that are sensitive or resistant to the metalloid. Int J Biochem Cell Biol. 2008;40:1016–29.

254. Zhou P, Kalakonda N, Comenzo RL. Changes in gene expression profiles of multiple myeloma cells induced by arsenic trioxide (ATO): possible mechanisms to explain ATO resistance in vivo. Br J Haematol. 2005;128(5):636–44.

255. Thorsen M, Di Y, Tangemo C, Morillas M, Ahmadpour D, Van der Does C, et al. The MAPK Hog1p modulates Fps1p-dependent arsenite uptake and tolerance in yeast. Mol Biol Cell. 2006;17(10):4400–10.

256. Maciaszczyk-Dziubinska E, Migdal I, Migocka M, Bocer T, Wysocki R. The yeast aquaglyceroporin Fps1p is a bidirectional arsenite channel. FEBS Lett. 2010;584(4):726–32.

257. Sanz MA, Grimwade D, Tallman MS, Lowenberg B, Fenaux P, Estey EH, et al. Management of acute promyelocytic leukemia: recommendations from an expert panel on behalf of the European LeukemiaNet. Blood. 2009;113(9):1875–91.

258. Falini B, Flenghi L, Fagioli M, Lo Coco F, Cordone I, Diverio D, et al. Immunocytochemical diagnosis of acute promyelocytic leukemia (M3) with the monoclonal antibody PG-M3 (anti-PML). Blood. 1997;90(10):4046–53.

259. Paietta E, Goloubeva O, Neuberg D, Bennett JM, Gallagher RE, Racevskis J, et al. A surrogate marker profile for PML-RARa-expressing acute promyelocytic leukemia and the association of immunophenotypic markers with morphologic and molecular subtypes. Cytometry B Clin Cytom. 2004;59:1–9.

260. Gallagher RE, Li Y-P, Rao S, Paietta E, Andersen J, Etkind P, et al. Characterization of acute promyelocytic leukemia cases with PML-RARa break/fusion sites in PML exon 6: Identification of a subgroup with decreased in vitro responsiveness to all-trans-retinoic acid. Blood. 1995;86:1540–7.

261. Callens C, Chevret S, Cayuela JM, Cassinat B, Raffoux E, de Botton S, et al. Prognostic implication of FLT3 and Ras gene mutations in patients with acute promyelocytic leukemia (APL): a retrospective study from the European APL Group. Leukemia. 2005;19(7):1153–60.

262. Gonzalez M, Barragan E, Bolufer P, Chillon C, Colomer D, Borstein R, et al. Pretreatment characteristics and clinical outcome of acute promyelocytic leukaemia patients according to the PML-RARa isoforms: a study of the PETHEMA group. Br J Haematol. 2001;114:99–103.

263. Kuchenbauer F, Schoch C, Kern W, Hiddemann W, Haferlach T, Schnittger S. Impact of FLT3 mutations and promyelocytic leukaemia-breakpoint on clinical characteristics and prognosis in acute promyelocytic leukaemia. Br J Haematol. 2005;130(2):196–202.

264. Tallman MS, Kim HT, Montesinos P, Appelbaum FR, de la Serna J, Bennett JM, et al. Does microgranular variant morphology of acute promyelocytic leukemia independently predict for a less favorable outcome compared with classical M3 APL? A joint study of the North American Intergroup and the PETHEMA Group. Blood. 2010;116(25):5650–9.

265. Fukutani H, Naoe T, Ohno R, Yoshida H, Miyawaki S, Shimazaki C, et al. Prognostic significance of the RT-PCR assay of PML-RARA transcripts in acute promyelocytic leukemia. Leukemia. 1995;9:588–93.

266. Mandelli F, Diverio D, Avvisati G, Luciano A, Barbui T, Bernasconi C, et al. Molecular remission in PML/RARa-positive acute promyelocytic leukemia by combined all-*trans* retinoic acid and idarubicin (AIDA) therapy. Blood. 1997;90:1014–21.

267. Burnett AK, Grimwade D, Solomon E, Wheatley K, Goldstone AH. Presenting white blood cell count and kinetics of molecular remission predict prognosis in acute promyelocytic leukemia treated with all-*trans* retinoic acid: result of the randomized MRC trial. Blood. 1999;93:4131–43.

268. Stock W, Moser B, Powell BL, Appelbaum FR, Tallman MS, Larson RA, et al. Prognostic significance of initial clincial and molecular genetic features of actue promeylocytic leukemia (APL): results from the North American Intergroup Trial C9710 (Abstract #7016). J Clin Oncol. 2007;25(Suppl. 18):361s.

269. Chillon MC, Santamaria C, Garcia-Sanz R, Balanzategui A, Maria Eugenia S, Alcoceba M, et al. Long FLT3 internal tandem duplications and reduced PML-RARalpha expression at diagnosis characterize a high-risk subgroup of acute promyelocytic leukemia patients. Haematologica. 2010;95(5):745–51.

270. Cervera J, Montesinos P, Hernandez-Rivas JM, Calasanz MJ, Aventin A, Ferro MT, et al. Additional chromosome abnormalities in patients with acute promyelocytic leukemia treated with all-trans retinoic acid and chemotherapy. Haematologica. 2010;95(3):424–31.

271. Schnittger S, Weisser M, Schoch C, Hiddemann W, Haferlach T, Kern W. New score predicting for prognosis in PML-RARA-, AML1-ETO-, or CBFB-MYH11-positive acute myeloid leukemia based on quantification of fusion transcripts. Blood. 2003;102:2746–55.

272. Gallagher RE, Yeap BY, Bi W, Livak KJ, Beaubier N, Rao S, et al. Quantitative real-time RT-PCR analysis of PML-RARa mRNA in adult acute promyelocytic leukemia: assessment of prognostic significance in adult patients from intergroup protocol 0129. Blood. 2003;101:2521–8.

273. Weisberg E, Sattler M, Ray A, Griffin JD. Drug resistance in mutant FLT3-positive AML. Oncogene. 2010;29(37):5120–34.

274. Beitinjaneh A, Jang S, Roukoz H, Majhail NS. Prognostic significance of FLT3 internal tandem duplication and tyrosine kinase domain mutations in acute promyelocytic leukemia: a systematic review. Leuk Res. 2010;34(7):831–6.

275. Noguera N, Breccia M, Divona M, Diverio D, Costa V, Avvisati G, et al. Alterations of the FLT3 gene in acute promyelocytic leukemia: association with diagnostic characteristics and analysis of clinical outcome in patients treated with the Italian AIDA protocol. Leukemia. 2002;16:2185–9.

276. Au WY, Fung A, Chim CS, Lie AK, Liang R, Ma ES, et al. FLT-3 aberrations in acute promyelocytic leukaemia: clinicopathological associations and prognostic impact. Br J Haematol. 2004;125(4):463–9.

277. Gale RE, Hills R, Pizzey AR, Kottaridis PD, Swirsky D, Gilkes AF, et al. Relationship between FLT3 mutation status, biologic characteristics, and response to targeted therapy in acute promyelocytic leukemia. Blood. 2005;106(12):3768–76.

278. Stock W, Moser B, Najib K, Powell B, Gulati K, Holowka N, et al. High incidence of *FLT3* mutations in adults with acute promyelocytic leukemia (APL): correlation with diagnostic features and treatment outcome (C-9710) [abstract]. J Clin Oncol. 2008;26(Suppl. 15):7002.

279. Whitman SP, Archer KJ, Feng L, Baldus C, Becknell B, Carlson BD, et al. Absence of the wild-type allele predicts poor prognosis in adult de novo acute myeloid leukemia with normal cytogenetics and the internal tandem duplication of FLT3: a cancer and leukemia group B study. Cancer Res. 2001;61(19):7233–9.

280. Santamaria C, Chillon MC, Garcia-Sanz R, Balanzategui A, Sarasquete ME, Alcoceba M, et al. The relevance of preferentially expressed antigen of melanoma (PRAME) as a marker of

disease activity and prognosis in acute promyelocytic leukemia. Haematologica. 2008;93(12):1797–805.

281. Hu J, Liu YF, Wu CF, Xu F, Shen ZX, Zhu YM, et al. Long-term efficacy and safety of all-trans retinoic acid/arsenic trioxide-based therapy in newly diagnosed acute promyelocytic leukemia. Proc Natl Acad Sci U S A. 2009;106(9):3342–7.
282. Powell BL, Moser B, Stock W, Gallagher RE, Willman CL, Stone RM, et al. Arsenic trioxide improves event-free and over-all survival for adults with acute promyelocytic leukemia: North American Leukemia Intergroup Study C9710. Blood. 2010;116:3751–7.
283. Gore SD, Gojo I, Sekeres MA, Morris L, Devetten MP, Jamieson K, et al. A single cycle of arsenic trioxide-based consolidation chemotherapy spares anthracycline exposure in the primary management of acute promyelocytic leukemia. J Clin Oncol. 2010;28:1047–53.
284. van Dongen JJM, Macintyre EA, Gabert JA, Delabesse E, Rossi V, Saglio G, et al. Standardized RT-PCR analysis of fusion gene transcripts from chromosome aberrations in acute leukemia for detection of minimal residual disease. Leukemia. 1999;13:1901–28.
285. Livak KJ, Flood SJ, Marmaro J, Giusti W, Deetz K. Oligonucleotides with fluorescent dyes at opposite ends provide a quenched probe system useful for detecting PCR product and nucleic acid hybridization. PCR Methods Appl. 1995;4(6):357–62.
286. Gabert J, Beillard E, van der Velden V, Bi W, Grimwade D, Pallisgaard N. Standardization and quality control studies of 'real-time' quantitative reverse transcriptase polymerase chain reaction (RQ-PCR) of fusion gene transcripts for residual disease detection in leukemia—A Europe Against Cancer Program. Leukemia. 2003;17:2318–57.
287. Santamaria C, Chillon MC, Fernandez C, Martin-Jimenenz P, Balanzategui A, Sanz RG, et al. Using quantification of the PML-RARa transcript to stratify the risk of relapse in patients with acute promyelocytic leukemia. Haematologica. 2007;92:315–22.
288. Gallagher R, Schachter-Tokarz E, Zhou D-C, Liao K, Jones D, Estey E. MRD monitoring in acute promyelocytic leukemia: unresolved issues in 2005. Hematol Rep. 2005;1:76–9.
289. Diverio D, Rossi V, Avvisati G, De Santis S, Pistilli A, Pane F, et al. Early detection of relapse by prospective reverse transcriptase-polymerase chain reaction analysis of the PML/RARa fusion gene in patient with acute promyelocytic leukemia enrolled in the GIMEMA-AIEOP multicenter "AIDA" trial. Blood. 1998;92:784–9.
290. Grimwade D, Lo CF. Acute promyelocytic leukemia: a model for the role of molecular diagnosis and residual disease monitoring in directing treatment approach in acute myeloid leukemia. Leukemia. 2002;16:1959–73.
291. LoCoco F, Diverio D, Avvisati G, Petti MC, Meloni G, Pogliani EM, et al. Therapy of molecular relapse in acute promyelocytic leukemia. Blood. 1999;94:2225–9.
292. Esteve J, Escoda L, Martin G, Rubio V, Diaz-Mediavilla J, Gonzalez M, et al. Outcome of patients with acute promyelocytic leukemia failing to front-line treatment with all-trans retinoic acid and anthracycline-based chemotherapy (PETHEMA protocols LPA96 and LPA99): benefit of an early intervention. Leukemia. 2007;21(3):446–52.
293. Cassinat B, de Botton S, Kelaidi C, Ades L, Zassadowski F, Guillemot I, et al. When can real-time quantitative RT-PCR effectively define molecular relapse in acute promyelocytic leukemia patients? (Results of the French Belgian Swiss APL Group). Leuk Res. 2009;33(9):1178.
294. Grimwade D, Jovanovic JV, Hills RK, Nugent EA, Patel Y, Flora R, et al. Prospective minimal residual disease monitoring to predict relapse of acute promyelocytic leukemia and to direct pre-emptive arsenic trioxide therapy. J Clin Oncol. 2009;27(22):3650–8.
295. Gallagher RE. Real-time consensus on relapse risk in acute promyelocytic leukemia. Leuk Res. 2009;33(9):1170.
296. Ommen HB, Schnittger S, Jovanovic JV, Ommen IB, Hasle H, Ostergaard M, et al. Strikingly different molecular relapse kinetics in NPM1c, PML-RARA, RUNX1-RUNX1T1, and CBFB-MYH11 acute myeloid leukemias. Blood. 2010;115(2):198–205.
297. Vickers M, Jackson G, Taylor P. The incidence of cute promyelocytic leukemia appears constant over most of a human lifespan, implying only one rate limiting mutation. Leukemia. 2000;14:72.
298. Carter M, Kalwinsky DK, Dahl GV, et al. Childhood acute promyelocytic leukemia: a rare variant of nonlymphoid leukemia with distinctive clinical and biologic features. Leukemia. 1989;3:298.
299. Biondi A, Rovelli A, Cantù-Rajnoldi A, et al. Acute promyelocytic leukemia in children: Experience of the Italian Pediatric Hematology and Oncology Group (AIEOP). Leukemia. 1994;8(Suppl 2):S66.
300. Maule MM, Damma E, Mosso ML, et al. High incidence of acute promyelocytic leukemia in children in northwest Italy, 1980–2003: a report from the childhood cancer registry of Piedmont. Leukemia. 2008;22:439–41.
301. Biondi A, Rovelli A, Cantŭ-Raynoldi A, et al. Acute promyelocytic leukemia in children: experience of the Italian pediatric hematology and oncology group (AIEOP). Leukemia. 1994;8:1264–8.
302. Malta-Corea A, Pacheco Espinoza C, Cantù-Rajnoldi A, et al. Childhood acute promyelocytic leukemia in Nicaragua. Ann Oncol. 1993;4:892.
303. Douer D, Preston-Martin S, Chang E, et al. High frequency of acute promyelocytic leukemia among Latinos with acute myeloid leukemia. Blood. 1996;87:308.
304. Hernández P, Milanés MT, Svarch E, et al. High relative proportion of acute promyelocytic leukemia in children: experience of a multicenter study in Cuba. Leuk Res. 2000;24:739–40.
305. Matasar MJ, Ritchie EK, Consedine N, et al. Incidence rates of acute promyelocytic leukemia among Hispanics, blacks, Asians and non-Hispanic whites in the United States. Eur J Cancer Prev. 2006;15:367–70.
306. Wiernik PH, Andersen JW. Unpublished observations; 1994.
307. Mele A, Stazi MA, Pulsoni A, et al. Epidemiology of acute promyelocytic leukemia. Haematologica. 1995;80:405.
308. Pulsoni A, Stazi A, Cotichini R, et al. Acute promyelocytic leukemia: epidemiology and risk factors. A report of the GIMEMA Italian archive of adult acute leukaemia. GIMEMA Cooperative Group. Eur J Haematol. 1998;61:327.
309. Estey E, Thall P, Kantarjian H, et al. Association between increased body mass index and a diagnosis of acute promyelocytic leukemia in patients with acute myeloid leukemia. Leukemia. 1997;12:1503.
310. Jeddi R, Ghédira H, Mnif S, et al. High body mass index is an independent predictor of differentiation syndrome in patients with acute promyelocytic leukemia. Leuk Res. 2010;34:545–7.
311. Yin CC, Glassman AP, Lin P, et al. Morphologic, cytogenetic and molecular abnormalities in therapy-related acute promyelocytic leukemia. Am J Clin Pathol. 2005;123:840–8.
312. Beaumont M, Sanz M, Carli PM, et al. Therapy-related acute promyelocytic leukemia. J Clin Oncol. 2003;21:2123–37.
313. Au WY, Ma SK, Chung LP, et al. Two cases of therapy-related acute promyelocytic leukemia (t-APL) after mantle cell lymphoma and gestational trophoblastic disease. Ann Hematol. 2002;81:659–71.
314. Bosca I, Pascual AM, Cassanova B, et al. Four new cases of therapy-related acute promyelocytic leukemia after mitoxantrone. Neurology. 2008;71:457–8.
315. Ramkumar B, Chadra MK, Barcos M, et al. Acute promyelocytic leukemia after mitoxantrone therapy for multiple sclerosis. Cancer Genet Cytogenet. 2008;182:126–9.

316. Matsuo K, Kiura K, Tahata M, et al. Clustered incidence of acute promyelocytic leukemia during gefitinib treatment of non-small cell lung cancer: experience at a single institution. Am J Hematol. 2006;81:349–54.
317. Daly PA, Schiffer CA, Wiernik PH. Acute promyelocytic leukemia—Clinical management of 15 patients. Am J Hematol. 1980;8:347.
318. Biondi A, Luciano A, Bassan R, et al. CD2 expression in acute promyelocytic leukemia is associated with microgranular morphology (FAB M3v) but not with any PML gene breakpoint. Leukemia. 1995;9:1461.
319. Hazani A, Weidenfeld Y, Tatarsky I, Bental E. Acute promyelocytic leukemia presenting as sudden blindness and sinus vein thrombosis. Am J Hematol. 1988;28:56.
320. Jetha N. Promyelocytic leukemia with multiorgan infarctions and large vessel thrombosis. Arch Pathol Lab Med. 1981;105:683.
321. Hoyle CF, Swirsky DM, Freedman L, Hayhoe FGJ. Beneficial effect of heparin in the management of patients with APL. Br J Haematol. 1988;68:283.
322. Avvisati G, LoCoco F, Mandelli F. Acute promyelocytic leukemia: clinical and morphologic features and prognostic factors. Semin Hematol. 2001;38:4–12.
323. Lavau C, Dejean A. The t(15;17) translocation in acute promyelocytic leukemia. Leukemia. 1994;8(Suppl 2):S9.
324. Sessarego M, Fugazza G, Balleari E, et al. High frequency of trisomy 8 in acute promyelocytic leukemia: a fluorescence in situ hybridization study. Cancer Genet Cytogenet. 1997;97:161.
325. De Botton S, Chevret S, Sanz M, et al. Additional chromosomal abnormalities in patients with acute promyelocytic leukaemia (APL) do not confer poor prognosis: Results of APL 93 trial. Br J Haematol. 2000;111:801.
326. Hernandez JM, Martin G, Gutierrez NC, et al. Additional cytogenetic changes do not influence the outcome of patients with newly diagnosed acute promyelocytic leukemia treated with ATRA plus anthracyclin based protocol. A report of the Spanish group PETHEMA. Haematologica. 2001;86:807.
327. Schoch C, Haase D, Haferlach T, et al. Incidence and implication of additional chromosome aberrations in acute promyelocytic leukaemia with translocation t(15;17)(q22;q21): a report on 50 patients. Br J Haematol. 1996;94:493.
328. Slack JL, Arthur DC, Lawrence D, et al. Secondary cytogenetic changes in acute promyelocytic leukemia—prognostic importance in patients treated with chemotherapy alone and association with the intron 3 breakpoint of the PML gene: A Cancer and Leukemia Group B study. J Clin Oncol. 1997;15:1786.
329. Pantic M, Novak A, Marislavljevic D, et al. Additional chromosome aberrations in acute promyelocytic leukemia: characteristics and prognostic influence. Med Oncol. 2000;17:307.
330. Wiernik PH, Sun Z, Gundacker H, et al. Prognostic implications of additional chromosome abnormalities among patients with de novo acute promyelocytic leukemia with t(15;17). Med Oncol. 2012;29:2095–101.
331. Xu L, Zhao WL, Xiong SM, et al. Molecular cytogenetic characterization and clinical relevance of additional complex and/or variant chromosome abnormalities in acute promyelocytic leukemia. Leukemia. 2001;15:1359–68.
332. Batzios C, Hayes LA, He SZ, et al. Secondary clonal cytogenetic abnormalities following successful treatment of acute promyelocytic leukemia. Am J Hematol. 2010;133:484–90.
333. Dimov ND, Medeiros LJ, Ravandi F, Bueso Ramos CE. Acute promyelocytic leukemia at time of relapse commonly demonstrates cytogenetic evidence of clonal evolution and variability in blast immunophenotypic features. Am J Clin Pathol. 2010;133:454–90.
334. Jansen JH, de Ridder MC, Geertsma WM, et al. Complete remission of t(11;17) positive acute promyelocytic leukemia induced by all-trans retinoic acid and granulocyte colony-stimulating factor. Blood. 1999;94:39.
335. Krause JR, Stolc V, Kaplan SS, Penchansky L. Microgranular promyelocytic leukemia: a multiparameter examination. Am J Hematol. 1989;30:158.
336. Murray CK, Estey E, Paietta E, et al. CD56 expression in acute promyelocytic leukemia: a possible indicator of poor treatment outcome? J Clin Oncol. 1999;17:293.
337. Castoldi GL, Liso V, Specchia G, Tomasi P. Acute promyelocytic leukemia: morphological aspects. Leukemia. 1994;8(Suppl 2):S27.
338. Bennett JM, Catovsky D, Daniel MT, et al. A variant form of hypergranular promyelocytic leukemia (M3). French-American-British (FAB) Co-operative Group. Br J Haematol. 1980;44:169.
339. Rovelli A, Biondi A, Cantù Rajnoldi A, et al. Microgranular variant of acute promyelocytic leukemia in children. J Clin Oncol. 1992;10:1413.
340. Davey FR, Davis RB, MacCallum JM, et al. Morphologic and cytochemical characteristics of acute promyelocytic leukemia. Am J Hematol. 1989;30:221.
341. Golomb HM, Rowley JD, Vardiman JW, et al. "Microgranular" acute promyelocytic leukemia: a distinct clinical, ultrastructural, and cytogenetic entity. Blood. 1980;55:253.
342. McKenna RW, Parkin J, Bloomfield CD, et al. Acute promyelocytic leukemia: a study of 39 cases with identification of a hyperbasophilic microgranular variant. Br J Haematol. 1982;50:201.
343. Invernizzi R, Iannone AM, Bernuzzi S, et al. Acute promyelocytic leukemia: morphological and clinical features. Haematologica. 1993;78:156.
344. Tallman MS, Hakimian D, Snower D, et al. Basophilic differentiation in acute promyelocytic leukemia. Leukemia. 1993;7:521.
345. Erber WN, Asbahr H, Rule SA, Scott CS. Unique immunophenotype of acute promyelocytic leukemia as defined by CD9 and CD68 antibodies. Br J Haematol. 1994;88:101.
346. Koike T, Tatewaki W, Aoki A, et al. Brief report: severe symptoms of hyperhistaminemia after the treatment of acute promyelocytic leukemia with tretinoin (all-trans-retinoic acid). N Engl J Med. 1992;327:385.
347. Gilbert RD, Karabus CD, Mills E. Acute promyelocytic leukemia: a childhood cluster. Cancer. 1987;59:933.
348. Williams CKO, Folani AO, Saditan AAO, et al. Childhood acute leukemia in a tropical population. Br J Cancer. 1982;42:89.
349. Scott RM, Mayer RJ. The unique aspects of acute promyelocytic leukemia. J Clin Oncol. 1990;8:1913.
350. Masamoto Y, Nannya Y, Arai S, et al. Evidence for basophilic differentiation of acute promyelocytic leukemia cells during arsenic trioxide therapy. Br J Hematol. 2009;144:798–9.
351. Das Gupta A, Sapre RS, Shah AS, et al. Cytochemical and immunophenotypic heterogeneity in acute promyelocytic leukemia. Acta Haematol. 1989;81:5.
352. Scott CS, Patel D, Drexler HG, et al. Immunophenotypic and enzymatic studies do not support the concept of mixed monocytic-granulocytic differentiation in acute promyelocytic leukemia (M3): a study of 44 cases. Br J Haematol. 1989;71:50.
353. Drexler HG. Classification of acute myeloid leukemia: a comparison of FAB and immunophenotyping. Leukemia. 1987;1:697.
354. Sanz MA, Jarque I, Martín G, et al. Acute promyelocytic leukemia. Therapy results and prognostic factors. Cancer. 1988;61:7.
355. Breccia M, Carmosino I, Diverio D, et al. Early detection of meningeal localization in acute promyelocytic leukemia patients with high presenting leucocyte count. Br J Haematol. 2003;120:266–70.
356. Nagai S, Nammya Y, Arai S, et al. Molecular and cytogenetic monitoring and preemptive therapy for central nervous system relapse of acute promyelocytic leukemia. Haematologica. 2010;95:169–71.

357. Kaspers G, Gibson B, Grimwade D, et al. Central nervous system involvement in relapsed acute promyelocytic leukemia. Pediatr Blood Cancer. 2009;53:235–6.
358. Montesinos P, Díaz-Mediavilla J, Debén G, et al. Central nervous involvement at first relapse in patients with acute promyelocytic leukemia treated with all-trans retinoic acid and anthracycline monotherapy without intrathecal prophyllaxis. Haematologica. 2009;94:1242–9.
359. Ohanian M, Rozovski U, Ravandi F, et al. Very high levels of lactate dehydrogenase at diagnosis predict central nervous system relapse in acute promyelocytic leukaemia. Br J Haematol. 2015;169:595–7.
360. Akoz AG, Dagdas S, Oget G, et al. Isolated central nervous system relapse during cytologic and molecular hematologic remission in two patients with acute promyelocytic leukemia. Hematology. 2007;12:419–22.
361. Mishra J, Gupta M. Cerebrospinal fluid involvement in acute promyelocytic leukaemia at presentation. BMJ Case Rep. 2015;9:2015.
362. He Z, Tao S, Deng Y, et al. Extramedullary relapse in lumbar spine of patient with acute promyelocytic leukemia after remission for 16 years: a case report and literature review. Int J Clin Exp Med. 2015;8:22430–4.
363. Vega-Ruíz A, Faderl S, Estrov Z, et al. Incidence of extrameullary disease in patients with acute promyelocytic leukemia: a single-institution experience. Int J Hematol. 2009;89:489–96.
364. Ko B-S, Tang J-L, Chen Y-C, et al. Extramedullary relapse after all-*trans* retinoic acid treatment in acute promyelocytic leukemia—the occurrence of retinoic acid syndrome is a risk factor. Leukemia. 1999;13:1406.
365. de Botton S, Sanz MA, Chevret S, et al. Extramedullary relapse in acute promyelocytic leukemia treated with all-trans retinoic acid and chemotherapy. Leukemia. 2006;20:35–41.
366. De Renzo A, Santoro LFE, Notaro R, et al. Acute promyelocytic leukemia after treatment for non-Hodgkin's lymphoma with drugs targeting topoisomerase II. Am J Hematol. 1999;60:300.
367. Kantarjian HM, Keating MJ, Walters RS, et al. The association of specific "favorable" cytogenetic abnormalities with secondary leukemia. Cancer. 1986;58:924.
368. Detourmignies L, Castaigne S, Stoppa AM, et al. Therapy-related acute promyelocytic leukemia: a report of 16 cases. J Clin Oncol. 1992;10:1430.
369. Hall MJ, Li L, Wiernik PH, Olopade OI. BRCA2 mutation and the risk of hematologic malignancy. Leuk Lymphoma. 2006;47:765–7.
370. Wei S, Kozono S, Kats L, et al. Active Pin1 is a key target of all-trans retinoic acid in acute promyelocytic leukemia and breast cancer. Nat Med. 2015;21:457–66.
371. Rashidi A, Fisher SI. Therapy-related acute promyelocytic leukemia: a systematic review. Med Oncol. 2013;30:625.
372. Braun T, Cereja S, Chevret S, et al. Evolving characteristics and outcome of secondary acute promyelocytic leukemia (APL): a prospective analysis by the French-Belgian-Swiss APL Group. Cancer. 2015;121:2393–9.
373. Castaigne S, Berger R, Jolly V, et al. Promyelocytic blast crisis of chronic myelocytic leukemia with both t(9;22) and t(15;17) in M3 cells. Cancer. 1984;54:2409.
374. Rosenthal NS, Knapp D, Farhi DC. Promyelocytic blast crisis of chronic myelogenous leukemia. A rare subtype associated with disseminated intravascular coagulation. Am J Clin Pathol. 1995;103:185.
375. Misawa S, Lee E, Schiffer CA, et al. Association of the translocation (15;17) with malignant proliferation of promyelocytes in acute leukemia and chronic myelogenous leukemia at blast crisis. Blood. 1986;67:270.
376. Hogge DE, Misawa S, Schiffer CA, Testa JR. Promyelocytic blast crisis in chronic granulocytic leukemia with 15;17 translocation. Leuk Res. 1984;6:1019.
377. Wiernik PH, Dutcher JP, Paietta E, et al. Treatment of promyelocytic blast crisis of chronic myelogenous leukemia with all transretinoic acid. Leukemia. 1991;5:504–9.
378. Hatzis T, Standen GR, Howell RT, et al. Acute promyelocytic leukaemia (M3): Relapse with acute myeloblastic leukaemia (M2) and dic(5;17)(q11;p11). Am J Hematol. 1995;48:40.
379. Bseiso AN, Kantarjian H, Estey E. Myelodysplastic syndrome following successful therapy of acute promyelocytic leukemia. Leukemia. 1977;11:168.
380. Felice MS, Rossi J, Gallego M, et al. Acute trilineage leukemia with monosomy of chromosome 7 following an acute promyelocytic leukemia. Leuk Lymphoma. 1999;34:409.
381. Zompi S, Legrand O, Bouscany D, et al. Therapy-related acute myeloid leukemia after successful therapy for acute promyelocytic leukaemia with t(15;17): a report of two cases and a review of the literature. Br J Haematol. 2000;110:610.
382. Park TS, Choi JR, Yoon SH, et al. Acute promyelocytic leukemia relapsing as secondary acute myelogenous leukemia with translocation t(3;21)(q26;q22) and RUNX1-MDS1-EV11 fision transcript. Cancer Genet Cytogenet. 2008;187:61–73.
383. Vitale C, Jabbour E, Lu X, et al. Acute promyelocytic leukemia presented as a relapse of acute myeloid leukemia. Am J Hematol. 2016;91:e274–6.
384. Eghtedar A, Rodriguez I, Kantarjian H, et al. Incidence of secondary neoplasms in patients with acute promyelocytic leukemia treated with all-trans retinoic acid plus chemotherapy or with all-trans retinoic acid plus arsenic trioxide. Leuk Lymphoma. 2015;56:1342–5.
385. Wang HC, Liu YC, Tsai YF, et al. Donor cell-derived acute promyelocytic leukemia after allogeneic hematopoietic stem cell transplant. Ann Hematol. 2015;94:887–8.
386. Testa U, Lo-Coco F. Prognostic factors in acute promyelocytic leukemia: strategies to define high-risk groups. Ann Hematol. 2016;95:673–80.
387. Lengfelder E, Hanfstein B, Haferlach C, et al. Outcome of elderly patients with acute promyelocytic leukemia: results of the German Acute Myeloid Leukemia Cooperative Group. Ann Hematol. 2013;92:41–52.
388. Daver N, Kantarjian H, Marcucci G, et al. Clinical characteristics and outcomes in patients with acute promyelocytic leukaemia and hyperleucocytosis. Br J Haematol. 2015;165:646–53.
389. Lucena-ALraujo AR, Kim HT, Jacomo RH, et al. Internal tandem duplication of the FLT3 gene confers poor overall survival in patients with acute promyelocytic leukemia treated with all-trans retinoic and anthracycline-based chemotherapy: an International Consortium on Acute Promyelocytic Leukemia study. Ann Hematol. 2014;93:2001–10.
390. Cicconi L, Divona M, Ciardi C, et al. PML-RARα kinetics and impact of FLT3-ITD mutations in newly diagnosed acute promyelocytic leukemia treated with ATRA and ATO or ATRA and chemotherapy. Leukemia. 2016;30:1987–92.
391. Albano F, Zagaria A, Anelli L, et al. Absolute quantification of the pretreatment PML-RARA transcript defines the relapse risk in acute promyelocytic leukemia. Oncotarget. 2015;6:13269–77.
392. Lucena-ALraujo AR, Kim HT, Jacomo RH, et al. Prognostic impact of KMT2E transcript levels on outcome of patients with acute promyelocytic leukaemia treated with all-trans retinoic acid and anthracycline-based chemotherapy: and International Consortium on Acute Promyelocyti Leukaemia study. Br J Haematol. 2014;166:540–9.
393. Hecht A, Nolte F, Nowak D, et al. Prognostic importance of expression of the Wilms' tumor 1 gene in newly diagnosed acute promyelocytic leukemia. Leuk Lymphoma. 2015;56:2289–95.
394. Lucena-ALraujo AR, Kim HT, Thomé C, et al. High ΔNp73/Tap73 ratio is associated with poor prognosis in acute promyelocytic leukemia. Blood. 2015;126:2302–6.

395. Gao NA, Yu WZ, Wang XX, et al. Significance of ETV6 rearrangement in acute promyelocytic leukemia with t(15;17) promyelocytic leukemia/retinoic acid receptor alpha. Oncol Lett. 2016;11:3953–60.
396. Lou Y, Ma Y, Suo S, et al. Prognostic factors of patients with newly diagnosed acute promyelocytic leukemia treated with arsenic trioxide-based frontline therapy. Leuk Res. 2015;39:938–44.
397. Seftel MD, Barnett MJ, Couban S, et al. A Canadian consensus on the management of newly diagnosed and relapsed acute promyelocytic leukemia in adults. Curr Oncol. 2014;21:234–50.
398. Micol JB, Raffoux E, Boissel N, et al. Management and treatment results in patients with acute promyelocytic leukaemia (APL) not enrolled in clinical trials. Eur J Cancer. 2014;50:1159–68.
399. Paulson K, Serebrin A, Lambert P, et al. Acute promyelocytic leukaemia is characterized by stable incidence and improved survival that is restricted to patients in leukaemia referral centres: a pan-Canadian epidemiological study. Br J Haematol. 2014;166:660–6.
400. Abrahão R, Ribeiro RC, Medeiros BC, et al. Disparities in early death and survival in children, adolescents and young adults with acute promyelocytic leukemia in California. Cancer. 2015;121:3960–7.
401. Alhuraiji A, Jain N. Immunofluorescence staining with an anti-promyelocytic leukemia antibody for a rapid diagnosis of acute promyelocytic leukemia. Hematol Oncol Stem Cell Ther. 2017;10:33–34.
402. Di Bona E, Avvisati G, Castaman G, et al. Early haemorrhagic morbidity and mortality during remission induction with or without all-*trans* retinoic acid in acute promyelocytic leukaemia. Br J Haematol. 2000;108:689.
403. Visani G, Gugliotta L, Tosi P, et al. All-*trans* retinoic acid significantly reduces the incidence of early hemorrhagic death during induction therapy of acute promyelocytic leukemia. Eur J Haematol. 2000;64:139.
404. Lehmann-Che J, Bally C, de Thé H. Resistance to therapy in acute promyelocytic leukemia. N Engl J Med. 2014;371:1170–2.
405. El Hajj H, Dassouki Z, Berthier C, et al. Retinoic acid and arsenic trioxide trigger degradation of mutated NPM1, resulting in apoptosis of AML cells. Blood. 2015;125:3447–54.
406. Yates JW, Wallace J Jr, Ellison RR, Holland JF. Cytosine arabinoside (NSC-63878) and daunorubicin (NSC-83142) therapy in acute nonlymphocytic leukemia. Cancer Chemother Rep. 1973;57:485.
407. Estey E, Thall PF, Pierce S, et al. Treatment of newly diagnosed acute promyelocytic leukemia without cytarabine. J Clin Oncol. 1997;15:483.
408. Sanz MA, Guillermo M, Rayon C, et al. A modified AIDA protocol with anthracycline-based consolidation results in high antileukemic efficacy and reduced toxicity in newly diagnosed PML/RARα-positive acute promyelocytic leukemia. Blood. 1999;94:3015.
409. Head DR, Kopecky KJ, Weick J, et al. Effect of aggressive daunomycin therapy on survival in acute promyelocytic leukemia. Blood. 1995;86:1717.
410. Pallavicini EB, Luliri P, Anselmetti L, et al. High-dose daunorubicin (DNR) for induction and treatment of relapse in acute promyelocytic leukemia (APL): report of 17 cases. Haematologica. 1988;73:49.
411. Carotenuto M, Greco M, Bavaro P, et al. Acute promyelocytic leukemia: results of treatment of 10 cases (Abstr). In: Proceedings of the 3rd International Symposium on Therapy of Acute Leukemias; 1982.
412. Salvaneschi L, Lazzarino M, Morra E, et al. Survival in adult acute myeloid leukemia under conventional chemotherapy (Abstr). In: Proceedings of the 3rd International Symposium on Therapy of Acute Leukemias, 1982.
413. Marty M, Ganem G, Fisher J, et al. Leucémie aiguë promyélocytaire. Étude rétrospective de 119 malades traités par daunorubicine. Novu Rev Fr Hématol. 1984;26:371.
414. Mandelli F, Petti MC, Avvisati G, Amadori S, et al. Acute promyelocytic leukemia: clinical aspects and results of treatment in 62 patients. Haematologica. 1987;72:151.
415. Petti MC, Avvisati G, Amadori S, et al. Acute promyelocytic leukemia: clinical aspects and results of treatment in 62 patients. Haematologica. 1987;72:151.
416. Bennett JM, Andersen JW, Cassileth PA. Long term survival in acute myeloid leukemia: The Eastern Cooperative Oncology Group. Leuk Res. 1991;15:223.
417. Clarkson B. Retinoic acid in acute promyelocytic leukemia: the promise and the paradox. Cancer Cells. 1991;3:211.
418. Fenaux P, Pollet JP, Vandenbossche-Simon L, et al. Treatment of acute promyelocytic leukemia: a report of 70 cases. Leuk Lymphoma. 1991;4:239.
419. Head DR, Kopecky K, Hewlett J, et al. Survival with cytotoxic therapy in acute promyelocytic leukemia, a SWOG report. Blood. 1991;78:268a.
420. Thomas X, Archimbaud E, Treille-Ritouet D, et al. Prognostic factors in acute promyelocytic leukemia: a retrospective study of 67 cases. Leuk Lymphoma. 1991;4:249.
421. Willemze R, Suciu S, Mandelli F, et al. Treatment of patients with acute promyelocytic leukemia. The EORTC-LCG experience. Leukemia. 1994;8(Suppl 2):S48.
422. Berman E. A review of idarubicin in acute leukemia. Oncology. 1993;7:91.
423. Sanz MA, Montesinos P, Kim HT, et al. All-trans retinoic acid with daunorubicin or idarubicin for risk-adapted treatment of acute promyelocytic leukaemia: a matched-pair analysis of the PETHEMA LPA-2005 and IC-APL studies. Ann Hematol. 2015;94:1347–56.
424. Berman E, Heller G, Santorsa J, et al. Results of a randomized trial comparing idarubicin and cytosine arabinoside with daunorubicin and cytosine arabinoside in adult patients with newly diagnosed acute myelogenous leukemia. Blood. 1991;77:1666.
425. Wiernik PH, Banks PLC, Case DC Jr, et al. Cytarabine plus idarubicin or daunorubicin as induction and consolidation therapy for previously untreated adult patients with acute myeloid leukemia. Blood. 1992;79:313.
426. Avvisati G, Mandelli F, Petti MC, et al. Idarubicin (4-demethoxy-daunorubicin) as a single agent for remission induction of previously untreated acute promyelocytic leukemia: a pilot study of the Italian cooperative group GIMEMA. Eur J Haematol. 1990;44:257.
427. Takahashi H, Watanabe T, Kinoshita A, et al. High event-free survival rate with minimum-dose-anthracyclines treatment in childhood acute promyelocytic leukaemia: a nationwide prospective study of the Japanese Paediatric Leukaemia/Lymphoma Study Group. Br J Haematol. 2016;174:437–43.
428. Avvisati G, LoCoco F, Diverio D, et al. AIDA (all-trans retinoic acid + idarubicin) in newly diagnosed acute promyelocytic leukemia: A Gruppo Italiano Malattie Ematologiche Maligne dell'Adulto (GIMEMA) pilot study. Blood. 1996;88:1390–8.
429. Sanz MA, LoCoco F, Martín G, et al. Definition of relapse risk and role of nonanthracycline drugs for consolidation in patients with acute promyelocytic leukemia: a joint study of the PETHEMA and GIMEMA Cooperative Groups. Blood. 2000;96:1247–53.
430. Sanz MA, Martín G, González M, et al. Risk-adapted treatment of acute promyelocytic leukemia with all-trans retinoic acid an anthracycline monotherapy: a multicenter study by the PETHEMA Group. Blood. 2004;103:1237–43.
431. Tallman MS, Rowe JM. Acute promyelocytic leukemia: a paradigm for differentiation therapy with retinoic acid. Blood Rev. 1994;8:70.
432. Luu HS, Raharman PA. Mature neutrophils with Auer rods following treatment with all-trans retinoic acid for acute promyelocytic leukemia. Blood. 2015;126:121.
433. Muindi J, Frankel S, Huselton C, et al. Clinical pharmacology of oral all-trans retinoic acid with acute promyelocytic leukemia. Cancer Res. 1992;52:2138.

434. Lefebvre P, Thomas G, Gourmel B, et al. Pharmacokinetics of oral all-trans retinoic acid with acute promyelocytic leukemia. Leukemia. 1991;5:1054.
435. Smith MA, Adamson PC, Balis FM, et al. Phase I trial and pharmacokinetic evaluation of all-*trans*-retinoic acid in pediatric patients. J Clin Oncol. 1992;10:1666.
436. Schwartz EL, Hallam S, Gallagher RE, Wiernik PH. Inhibition of all-trans retinoic acid metabolism by fluconazole in vitro and in patients with acute promyelocytic leukemia. Mol Pharmacol. 1995;50:923.
437. Miller VA, Rigas JR, Muindi JRF, et al. Modulation of all-*trans* retinoic acid pharmacokinetics by liarozole. Cancer Chemother Pharmacol. 1994;34:522.
438. Muindi JF, Scher HI, Rigas JR, et al. Elevated plasma lipid peroxide content correlates with rapid plasma clearance of all-*trans*-retinoic acid in patients with advanced cancer. Cancer Res. 1994;54:2125.
439. Agadir A, Cornic M, Lefebvre P, et al. All-*trans* retinoic acid pharmacokinetics and bioavailability in acute promyelocytic leukemia: Intracellular concentrations and biologic response relationship. J Clin Oncol. 1995;13:2517.
440. Degos L, Chomienne C, Daniel MT, et al. All-*trans*-retinoic acid treatment for patients with acute promyelocytic leukemia. In: Saurat J-H, editor. Retinoids: 10 years on. Basel: Karger; 1991. p. 121.
441. Vahdat L, Maslak P, Miller W Jr, et al. Early mortality and the retinoic acid syndrome in acute promyelocytic leukemia: impact of leukocytosis, low-dose chemotherapy, PML/RAR-α isoform, and CD13 expression in patients treated with all-*trans* retinoic acid. Blood. 1994;84:3843.
442. Fenaux P, Degos L. Treatment of acute promyelocytic leukemia with all trans retinoic acid. Leuk Res. 1991;8:655.
443. Fenaux P, Castaigne S, Dombret H, et al. All-trans retinoic acid followed by intensive chemotherapy gives a high complete remission rate and may prolong remissions in newly diagnosed acute promyelocytic leukemia: a pilot study on 26 cases. Blood. 1992;80:2176.
444. Fenaux P, Le Deley MC, Castaigne S, et al. Effect of all trans retinoic acid in newly diagnosed acute promyelocytic leukemia. Results of a multicenter randomized trial. Blood. 1993;82:3241.
445. Fenaux P, Chevret S, Guerci A, et al. Long-term follow-up confirms the benefit of all-*trans* retinoic acid in acute promyelocytic leukemia. Leukemia. 2000;14:1371.
446. Kawai Y, Watanabe K, Kizaki M, et al. Rapid improvement of coagulopathy by all-*trans* retinoic acid in acute promyelocytic leukemia. Am J Hematol. 1994;46:184.
447. Kanamaru A, Takemoto Y, Tanimoto M, et al. All-*trans* retinoic acid for the treatment of newly diagnosed acute promyelocytic leukemia. Blood. 1995;85:1202.
448. Estey E, Koller C, Cortes J, et al. Treatment of newly-diagnosed acute promyelocytic leukemia with liposomal all-trans retinoic acid. Leuk Lymphoma. 2001;42:309.
449. Preetesh J, Kantarjian H, Estey E, et al. Single agent liposomal all-trans-retinoic acid (ATRA) as initial therapy for acute promyelocytic leukemia (APL): 13 year follow-up data. Clin Lymphoma Myeloma Leuk. 2014;14:e47–9.
450. Silva EL, Lima FA, Carneiro G, et al. Improved in vitro antileukemic activity of all-trans retinoic acid loaded in Cholesteryl butyrate solid lipid nanoparticles. J Nanosci Nanotechnol. 2016;16:1291–300.
451. Warrell RP Jr, Maslak P, Eardley A, et al. Treatment of acute promyelocytic leukemia with all-trans retinoic acid: an update of the New York experience. Leukemia. 1994;8(Suppl 2):S33.
452. de Botton S, Chevret S, Coiteux V, et al. Early onset of chemotherapy can reduce the incidence of ATRA syndrome in newly diagnosed acute promyelocytic leukemia (APL) with low white blood cell counts: results from APL 93 trial. Leukemia. 2003;17:339–42.
453. Visani G, Tosi P, Cenacchi A, et al. Pre-treatment with all-trans retinoic acid accelerates polymorphonuclear recovery after chemotherapy in patients with acute promyelocytic leukemia. Leuk Lymphoma. 1994;15:143.
454. de la Serna J, Montesinos P, Vellenga E, et al. Causes and prognostic factors of remission induction failure in patients with acute promyelocytic leukemia treated with all-trans retinoic acid and idarubicin. Blood. 2008;111:3395–402.
455. Levin A, Sturzenbecker L, Kazmer S, et al. 9-cis retinoic acid stereoisomer binds and activates the nuclear receptor RXRα. Nature. 1992;355:359.
456. Shinjo K, Takeshita A, Ohnishi K, et al. Good prognosis of patients with acute promyelocytic leukemia who achieved second complete remission (CR) with a new retinoid, AM80, after relapse from CR induced by all-trans-retinoic acid. Int J Hematol. 2000;72:470–3.
457. Di Veroli A, Ramadan SM, Divona M, et al. Molecular remission in advanced acute promyelocytic leukaemia after treatment with the oral synthetic retinoid Tamibarotene. Br J Haematol. 2010;151(1):99–101.
458. Shinagawa K, Yenada M, Sakura T, et al. Tamibarotene as maintenance therapy for acute promyelocytic leukemia: results from a randomized controlled trial. J Clin Oncol. 2014;32:3729–35.
459. Sanford D, Lo-Coco F, Sanz MA, et al. Tamibarotene in patients with acute promyelocytic leukaemia relapsing after treatment with all-trans retinoic acid and arsenic trioxide. Br J Haematol. 2015;171:471–7.
460. Visani G, Zauli G, Ottaviani E, et al. All-trans retinoic acid potentiates megakaryocyte colony formation: In vitro and in vivo effects after administration to acute promyelocytic leukemia patients. Leukemia. 1994;8:2183.
461. Visani G, Ottaviani E, Zauli G, et al. All-*trans* retinoic acid at low concentration directly stimulates normal adult megakaryocytopoiesis in the presence of thrombopoietin or combined cytokines. Eur J Haematol. 1999;63:149.
462. Kini AR, Peterson LA, Tallman MS, Lingen MW. Angiogenesis in acute promyelocytic leukemia: induction by vascular endothelial growth factor and inhibition by all-trans retinoic acid. Blood. 2001;97:3919.
463. Gianni M, Kalac Y, Ponzanelli I, et al. Tyrosine kinase inhibitor STI571 potentiates the pharmacologic activity of retinoic acid in acute promyelocytic leukemia cells: Effects on the degradation of RARα and PML-RARα. Blood. 2001;97:3234.
464. Sassano A, Katsoilidis E, Antico G, et al. Suppressive effects of statins on acute promyelocytic leukemia cells. Cancer Res. 2007;67:4524–32.
465. Tomiyama N, Matzno S, Kitada C, et al. The possibility of simvastatin as a chemotherapeutic agent for all-trans retinoic acid-resistant promyelocytic leukemia. Biol Pharm Bull. 2008;31:369–74.
466. Frankel SR, Eardley A, Lauwers G, et al. The "retinoic acid syndrome" in acute promyelocytic leukemia. Ann Intern Med. 1992;117:292.
467. Tallman MS, Andersen JW, Schiffer CA, et al. Clinical description of 44 patients with acute promyelocytic leukemia who developed the retinoic acid syndrome. Blood. 2000;95:90–5.
468. Montesinos P, Bergua M, Vellenga E, et al. Differentiation syndrome in patients with acute promyelocytic leukemia treated with all-trans retinoic acid and anthracycline chemotherapy: characteristics, outcome, and prognostic factors. Blood. 2009;113:775–83.
469. Sanz MA, Montesinos P. How we treat differentiation syndrome in patients with acute promyelocytic leukemia. Blood. 2014;123:2777–82.
470. Cabral R, Caballero JC, Alonso S, et al. Late diddreentiation syndrome in acute promyelocytic leukemia: a challenging diagnosis. Hematol Res. 2014;6:5654.
471. Jeddi R, Ghédira H, Amor RB, et al. Recurrent differentiation syndrome or septic shock? Unresolved dilemma in a patient with acute promyelocytic leukemia. Med Oncol. 2011;28(1):279–81.

472. Wiley JS, Firkin FC. Reduction of pulmonary toxicity by prednisolone prophylaxis during all-trans retinoic acid treatment of acute promyelocytic leukemia. Australian Leukemia Study Group. Leukemia. 1995;9:774–8.
473. Raanani P, Segal E, Levi I, et al. Diffuse alveolar hemorrhage in acute promyelocytic leukemia patients treated with ATRA- a manifestation of the basic disease or the treatment. Leuk Lymphoma. 2000;37:605–10.
474. Saiki I, Fujii H, Yeneda J, et al. Role of aminopeptidase N (CD13) in tumor cell invasion and extracellular matrix degeneration. Int J Cancer. 1993;54:137.
475. Cunha de Santis G, Tamarozzi MB, Sousa RB, et al. Adhesion molecules and differentiation syndrome: phenotypic and functional analysis of the effect of ATRA, As_2O_3, phenylbutyrate, and G-CSF in acute promyelocytic leukemia. Haematologica. 2007;92:1615–22.
476. Luesink M, Pennings JL, Wissink WM, et al. Chemokine induction by all-trans retinoic acid and arsenic trioxide in acute promyelocytic leukemia: triggering the differentiation syndrome. Blood. 2009;114:5512–21.
477. Luesink M, Jansen JH. Advances in understanding the pulmonary infiltration in acute promyelocytic leukaemia. Br J Haematol. 2010;151(3):209–20.
478. Csomós K, Német I, Fésűs L, Balajithy Z. Tissue transglutaminase contributes to the all-trans retinoic acid induced differentiation syndrome phenotype in the NB4 model of acute promyelocytic leukemia. Blood. 2010;116(19):3933–43.
479. Hakimian D, Tallman MS, Zugerman C, et al. Erythema nodosum associated with all-trans retinoic acid in the treatment of acute promyelocytic leukemia. Leukemia. 1993;7:758.
480. Gallipoli P, Drummond MW. Pseudotumour cerebri as a manageable side effect of prolonged all-trans retinoic acid therapy in an adult patient with acute promyelocytic leukaemia. Eur J Haematol. 2009;82:242–3.
481. Coombs CC, DeAngelis LM, Feusner JH, et al. Pseudotumor cerebri in acute promyelocytic leukemia patients on intergroup protocol 0129: clinical description and recommendations for new diagnostic criteria. Clin Lymphoma Myeloma Leuk. 2016;16:146–51.
482. Kesler A, Kliper E, Assayag EB, et al. Thrombophilic factors in idiopathic intracranial hypertension: a report of 51 patients and a meta-analysis. Blood Coagul Fibrinolysis. 2010;21:328–33.
483. Shirono K, Kiyofuji C, Tsuda H. Sweet's syndrome in a patient with acute promyelocytic leukemia during treatment with all*trans* retinoic acid. Int J Hematol. 1995;62:183.
484. Christ E, Linka A, Jacky E, et al. Sweet's syndrome involving the musculoskeletal system during treatment of promyelocytic leukemia with all-*trans* retinoic acid. Leukemia. 1996;10:731.
485. Torromeo C, Latagliata R, Avvisati G, et al. Intraventricular thrombosis during all-*trans* retinoic acid treatment in acute promyelocytic leukemia. Leukemia. 2000;15:1311.
486. Losada R, Espinosa E, Hernandez C, et al. Thrombocytosis in patients with acute promyelocytic leukaemia during all-*trans* retinoic acid treatment. Br J Haematol. 1996;95:704.
487. Kentos A, Le Moine F, Crenier L, et al. All-*trans* retinoic acid induced thrombocytosis in a patient with acute promyelocytic leukaemia. Br J Haematol. 1997;97:685.
488. Montesinos P, Gozález JD, Gozález J, et al. Therapy-related myeloid neoplasms in patients with acute promyelocytic leukemia treated with all-trans-retinoic acid and anthracycline-based chemotherapy. J Clin Oncol. 2010;28:3872–9.
489. Aulde J. A study of the pharmacology and therapeutics of arsenic. NY Med J. 1891;53:390.
490. Niu C, Yan H, Yu T, et al. Studies on treatment of acute promyelocytic leukemia with arsenic trioxide: Remission induction, followup, and molecular monitoring in 11 newly diagnosed and 47 relapsed acute promyelocytic leukemia patients. Blood. 1999;94:3315.
491. Huang S-Y, Yang C-H, Chen Y-C. Arsenic trioxide therapy for relapsed acute promyelocytic leukemia: an (sic) useful salvage therapy. Leuk Lymphoma. 2000;38:283.
492. Camacho LH, Soignet SL, Chanel S, et al. Leukocytosis and the retinoic acid syndrome in patients with acute promyelocytic leukemia treated with arsenic trioxide. J Clin Oncol. 2000;18:2620.
493. Lin C-P, Huang M-J, Chang IY, et al. Retinoic acid syndrome induced by arsenic trioxide in treating recurrent all-trans retinoic acid resistant acute promyelocytic leukemia. Leuk Lymphoma. 2000;38:195.
494. Kwong YL, Au WY, Chim CS, et al. Arsenic trioxide- and idarubicin-induced remissions in relapsed acute promyelocytic leukemia: clinicopathological and molecular features of a pilot study. Am J Hematol. 2001;66:274.
495. Muto A, Kizaki M, Kawamura C, et al. A novel differentiation-inducing therapy for acute promyelocytic leukemia with a combination of arsenic trioxide and GM-CSF. Leukemia. 2001;15:1176.
496. Dai CW, Zhang GS, Shen JK, et al. Use of all-trans retinoic acid in combination with arsenic trioxide for remission induction in patients with newly diagnosed acute promyelocytic leukemia and for consolidation/maintenance in CR patients. Acta Haematol. 2009;121:1–8.
497. Rvandi F, Estey E, Jones D, et al. Effective treatment of acute promyelocytic leukemia with all-trans retinoic acid, arsenic trioxide, and gemtuzumab ozogamicin. J Clin Oncol. 2009;27:504–10.
498. Estey E, Garcia-Manero G, Ferrajoli A, et al. Use of all-trans retinoic acid plus arsenic trioxide as an alternative to chemotherapy in untreated acute promyelocytic leukemia. Blood. 2006;108:3469–73.
499. Aznab M, Rezaei M. Induction, consolidation, and maintenance therapies with arsenic as a single agent for acute promyelocytic leukaemia in a 11-year follow-up. Hematol Oncol. 2017;35:113–17.
500. Song X, Hu X, Lü S, et al. Incorporation of arsenic trioxide in induction therapy improves survival of patients with newly diagnosed acute promyelocytic leukaemia. Eur J Haematol. 2014;93:54–62.
501. Platzbecker U, Avvisati G, Cicconi L, et al. Improved outcomes with retinoic acid and arsenic trioxide compared with retinoic acid and chemotherapy in non-high risk acute promyelocytic leukemia. Final results of the randomized Italian-German APL0406 trial. J Clin Oncol. 2017;35:605–12.
502. Wu F, Wu D, Duan C, et al. Bayesian network meta-analysis comparing five contemporary treatment strategies for newly diagnosed acute promyelocytic leukaemia. Oncotarget. 2016;7:47319–31.
503. Zhu H, Hu J, Li X, et al. All-trans retinoic acid and arsenic combination therapy benefits low-to intermediate-risk patients with newly diagnosed acute promyelocytic leukaemia: a long-term follow-up based on multivariate analysis. Br J Haematol. 2015.; (In Press)
504. Iland HJ, Collins M, Bradstock K, et al. Use of arsenic trioxide in remission induction and consolidation therapy for acute promyelocytic leukaemia in the Australasian Leukaemia and Lymphoma Group (ALLG) APML 4 study: a non-randomised phase 2 trial. Lancet Hematol. 2015;2:e357–66.
505. Burnett AK, Russell NH, Hills RK, et al. Arsenic trioxide and all-trans retinoic acid treatment for acute promyelocytic leukaemia in all risk groups (AML17): results of a randomized controlled phase 3 trial. Lancet Oncol. 2015;16:1295–305.
506. Lo-Coco F, Avvisati M, Vignetti C, et al. Retinoic acid and arsenic trioxide for acute promyelocytic leukemia. N Engl J Med. 2013;369:111–21.
507. Leech M, Morris L, Stewart M, et al. Real-life experience of a brief arsenic trioxide-based consolidation chemotherapy in the management of acute promyelocytic leukemia: favorable out-

comes with limited anthracycline exposure and shorter consolidation therapy. Clin Lymphoma Myeloma Leuk. 2015;15:292–7.
508. Band HJ, Wei A, Seymour JF. Have all-trans retinoic acid and arsenic trioxide replaced all-trans retinoic acid and anthracycline in APL as standard of care. Best Prac Res Clin Hematol. 2014;27:39–52.
509. Efficace F, Mandelli F, Avvisati G, et al. Randomized phase III trial of retinoic acid and arsenic trioxide in patients with acute promyelocytic leukemia: health-related quality-of-life outcomes. J Clin Oncol. 2014;32:3406–12.
510. Tallman M, Lo-Cocco F, Barnes G, et al. Cost-effectiveness analysis of treating acute promyelocytic leukemia patients with arsenic trioxide and retinoic acid in the United States. Clin Lymphoma Myeloma Leuk. 2015;15:771–7.
511. Zhu HH, Wu DP, Jin J, et al. Oral tetra-arsenic tetra-sulfide formula versus intravenous arsenic trioxide as first-line treatment of acute promyelocytic leukemia: a multicenter randomized controlled trial. J Clin Oncol. 2013;31:4215–21.
512. Torka P, Al Ustwani O, Wetzler M, et al. Swallowing a bitter pill-oral arsenic trioxide for acute promyelocytic leukemia. Blood Rev. 2016;30:201–11.
513. Yanfeng L, Pencheng HE, Xiaoyan C, Mei Z. Long-term outcome of 31 cases of refractory acute promyelocytic leukemia treated with compound realgar natural indigo tablets administered alternately with chemotherapy. Oncol Lett. 2015;10:1184–90.
514. Zhu H-H, Huang X-J. Oral arsenic and retinoic acid for non-high-risk acute promyelocytic leukemia. N Engl J Med. 2014;371:2239–41.
515. Lo-Coco F. Outpatient oral treatment for acute promyelocytic leukemia. N Engl J Med. 2015;372:884–5.
516. Zhu H, Hu J, Chen L, et al. The 12 year follow-up of survival, chronic adverse effects and retention of arsenic in patients with acute promyelocytic leukemia. Blood. 2016;128:1525–8.
517. Ma H, Yang J. Insights into all-trans-retinoic acid and arsenic trioxide combination treatment in acute promyelocytic leukemia: a meta-analysis. Acta Haematol. 2015;134:101–8.
518. Ohnishi K, Yoshida H, Shigeno K, et al. Prolongation of the QT interval and ventricular tachycardia in patients treated with arsenic trioxide for acute promyelocytic leukemia. Ann Intern Med. 2000;133:881.
519. Unnikrishnan D, Dutcher JP, Varshneya N, et al. Torsades de pointes in 3 patients with leukemia treated with arsenic trioxide. Blood. 2001;97:1514.
520. Unnikrishnan D, Dutcher JP, Garl S, et al. Cardiac monitoring of patients receiving arsenic trioxide therapy. Br J Haematol. 2004;124:610–7.
521. Naito K, Kobayashi M, Sahara N, et al. Two cases of acute promyelocytic leukemia complicated by torsade de pointes during arsenic trioxide therapy. Int J Hematol. 2006;83:318–23.
522. Westervelt P, Brown RA, Adkins DR, et al. Sudden death among patients with acute promyelocytic leukemia treated with arsenic trioxide. Blood. 2001;98:266.
523. Roboz GJ, Ritchie EK, Carlin RF, et al. Prevalence, management, and clinical consequences of QT interval prolongation during treatment with arsenic trioxide. J Clin Oncol. 2014;32:3723–8.
524. Raghu KG, Yadav GK, Singh R, et al. Evaluation of adverse cardiac events induced by arsenic trioxide, a potent anti-APL drug. J Environ Pathol Toxicol Oncol. 2009;28:241–52.
525. Mannis GN, Logan AC, Leavitt AD, et al. Delayed hematopoietic recovery after auto-SCT in patients receiving arsenic trioxide-based therapy for acute promyelocytic leukemia: a multi-center analysis. Bone Marrow Transplant. 2015;50:40–4.
526. Au WY, Lang BH, Fong BM, et al. Thyrid arsenic content and papillary thyroid carcinoma 10 years after oral arsenic trioxide therapy for refractory acute promyelocytic leukemia. Leuk Lymphoma. 2014;55:1184–5.
527. Zhang Y, Wu S, Luo D, et al. Addition of arsenic trioxide into induction regimens could not accelerate recovery of abnormality of coagulation and fibrinolysis in patients with acute promyelocytic leukemia. PLoS One. 2016;11:e0147545.
528. Yedjou C, Thuisseu L, Tchounwou C, et al. Ascorbic acid potentiation of arsenic trioxide anticancer activity against acute promyelocytic leukemia. Arch Drug Inf. 2009;2:59–65.
529. Chang JE, Voorhees PM, Kolesar JM, et al. Phase II study of arsenic trioxide and ascorbic acid for relapsed or refractory lymphoid malignancies: Wisconsin Oncology Network study. Hematol Oncol. 2009;27:11–6.
530. Kuroki M, Ariumi Y, Ikeda M, et al. Arsenic trioxide inhibits hepatitis C virus RNA replication through modulation of the glutathione redox system and oxidative stress. J Virol. 2009;83:2338–48.
531. Avvisanti G, Lo Coco F, Diverio D, et al. AIDA (all-trans retinoic acid + idarubicin) in newly diagnosed acute promyelocytic leukemia: a Gruppo Italiano Malattie Ematologiche Maligne dell'Adulto (GIMEMA) pilot study. Blood. 1996;88:1390–8.
532. Avvisati G, Petti MC, Lo-Coco F, et al. Induction therapy with idarubicin alone significantly influences event-free survival duration in patients with newly diagnosed hypergranular acute promyelocytic leukemia: final results of the GIMEMA randomized study LAP 0389 with 7 years minimal follow-up. Blood. 2002;100:3141–6.
533. Lengfelder E, Reichert A, Schoch C, et al. Double induction strategy including high dose cytarabine in combination with all-*trans* retinoic acid: effects in patients with newly diagnosed acute promyelocytic leukemia. Leukemia. 2000;14:1362.
534. Lengfelder E, Haferlach C, Saussele S, et al. High dose ara-C in the treatment of newly diagnosed acute promyelocytic leukemia: long-term results of the German AMLCG. Leukemia. 2009;23:2248–58.
535. Adès L, Sanz MA, Chevret S, et al. Treatment of newly diagnosed acute promyelocytic leukemia (APL): a comparison of French-Belgian-Swiss and PETHEMA results. Blood. 2008;111:1078–84.
536. Kelaidi C, Chevret S, De Botton S, et al. Improved outcome of acute promyelocytic leukemia with high WBC counts over the last 15 years: the European APL Group experience. J Clin Oncol. 2009;27:2668–76.
537. Dutcher JP, Wiernik PH, Markus S, et al. Intensive maintenance therapy improves survival in adult acute nonlymphocytic leukemia: an eight-year follow-up. Leukemia. 1988;2:413.
538. Kantarjian HM, Keating MJ, Walters RS, et al. Role of maintenance chemotherapy in acute promyelocytic leukemia. Cancer. 1987;59:1258.
539. Tallman MS, Andersen JW, Schiffer CA, et al. All-trans retinoic acid in acute promyelocytic leukemia. N Engl J Med. 1997;337:1021.
540. Tallman MS, Andersen JW, Schiffer CA, et al. All-trans retinoic acid in acute promyelocytic leukemia: long-term outcome results and prognostic factor analysis from the North American Intergroup protocol. Blood. 2002;100:4298.
541. Douer D, Zixkl LN, Schiffer CA, et al. All-trans retinoic acid and late relapss in acute promyelocytic leukemia: very long-term follow-up of the North American Intergroup study 10129. Leuk Res. 2013;37:795–801.
542. Asou N, Kishimoto Y, Kiyoi H, et al. A randomized study with or without intensified maintenance chemotherapy in patients with acute promyelocytic leukemia who have become negative for PML-RARα transcript after consolidation therapy: Japan Adilt Leukemia Study Group (JALSG) APL97 study. Blood. 2007;110:59–66.
543. Lancet JE. Postremission therapy in acute promyelocytic leukemia: room for improvement? J Clin Oncol. 2014;32:3692–6.
544. Coutre SE, Othus M, Powell B, et al. Arsenic trioxide during consolidation for patients with previously untreated low/intermediate

risk acute promyelocytic leukaemia may eliminate the need for maintenance therapy. Br J Haematol. 2014;165:497–503.
545. Liu CC, Wang H, Wang WD, et al. Consolidation therapy of arsenic trioxide alternated with chemotherapy achieves remarkable efficacy in newly diagnosed acute promyelocytic leukemia. Onco Targets Ther. 2015;8:3297–303.
546. Yamamoto M, Okada K, Akiyama H, et al. Evaluation of the efficacy of maintenance therapy for low-to-intermediate-risk acute promyelocytic leukemia in molecular remission: a retrospective single –institution study. Mol Clin Oncol. 2015;3:449–53.
547. Lo Coco F, Diverio D, Avvisati G, et al. Therapy of molecular relapse in acute promyelocytic leukemia. Blood. 1999;94:2225.
548. Lengfelder E, Lo-Cocco F, Ades L, et al. Arsenic trioxide-based therapy of relapsed acute promyelocytic leukemia: registry results from the European LeukemiaNet. Leukemia. 2015;29:1084–91.
549. Thomas X, Pigneux A, Raffoux E, et al. Superiority of an arsenic trioxide-based regimen over a historic control combining all-trans retinoic acid plus intensive chemotherapy in the treatment of relapsed acute promyelocytic leukemia. Haematologica. 2006;91:996–7.
550. Shigeno K, Naito K, Sahara N, et al. Arsenic trioxide therapy in relapsed or refractory Japanese patients with acute promyelocytic leukemia: updated outcomes of the phase II study and postremission therapies. Int J Hematol. 2005;82:224–9.
551. Raffoux E, Rousselot P, Poupon J, et al. Combined treatment with arsenic trioxide and all-trans retinoic acid in patients with relapsed acute promyelocytic leukemia. J Clin Oncol. 2003;21:2326–34.
552. Lazo G, Kantarjian H, Estey E, et al. Use of arsenic trioxide (As_2O_3) in the treatment of patients with acute promyelocytic leukemia: the M.D. Anderson experience. Cancer. 2003;97:2218–24.
553. Visani G, Piccaluga PP, Martinelli G, et al. Sustained molecular remission in advanced acute promyelocytic leukemia with combined pulsed retinoic acid and arsenic trioxide. Clinical evidence of synergistic effect and real-time quantification of minimal residual disease. Haematologica. 2003;88:15.
554. de Botton S, Fawaz A, Chevret S, et al. Autologous and allogeneic stem-cell transplantation as salvage treatment of acute promyelocytic leukemia initially treated with all-trans-retinoic acid: a retrospective analysis of the European acute promyelocytic leukemia group. J Clin Oncol. 2005;23:120–6.
555. Termuhlen AM, Klopfenstein K, Olshefski R, et al. Mobilization of PML-RARA negative blood stem cells and salvage with autologous peripheral blood stem cell transplantation in children with relapsed acute promyelocytic leukemia. Pediatr Blood Cancer. 2008;51:521–4.
556. Fenaux P, Tertian G, Castaigne S, et al. A randomized trial of amsacrine and rubidazone in 39 patients with acute promyelocytic leukemia. J Clin Oncol. 1991;9:1556.
557. Ganzel C, Mathews V, Alimoghaddam K, et al. Autologous transplant remains the preferred therapy for relapsed APL in CR2. Bone Marrow Transplant. 2016;51:1180–3.
558. Takeshita A, Shibata Y, Shinjo K, et al. Successful treatment of relapse of acute promyelocytic leukemia with a new synthetic retinoid, Am80. Ann Intern Med. 1996;124:893.
559. Shinjo K, Takeshita A, Kitamura K, et al. Good prognosis of patients with acute promyelocytic leukemia who achieved second complete remission (CR) with a new retinoid AM80, after relapse from CR induced by all-trans-retinoic-acid. Int J Hematol. 2000;72:470–3.
560. Chendamarai E, Ganesan S, Alex AA, et al. Comparison of newly diagnosed and relapsed patients with acute promyelocytic leukemia treated with arsenic trioxide: insight into mechanisms of resistance. PLoS One. 2015;10:0121912.
561. Holter-Chakrabarty JL, Rubinger M, Le-Rademacher J, et al. Autologous is superior to allogeneic hematopoietic cell transplantation for acute promyelocytic leukemia in second complete remission. Biol Blood Marrow Transplant. 2014;20:1021–5.
562. Yang D, Hladnik L. Treatment of acute promyelocytic leukemia during pregnancy. Pharmacotherapy. 2009;29:709–24.
563. Ganzitti L, Fachechi G, Driul L, Marchesoni D. Acute promyelocytic leukemia during pregnancy. Fertil Steril. 2010;94(6):2330.
564. Valappil S, Kurkar M, Howell R. Outcome of pregnancy in women treated with all-trans retinoic acid; a case report and review of the literature. Hematology. 2007;12:415–8.
565. Ammatuna E, Cavaliere A, Divona M, et al. Successful pregnancy after arsenic trioxide therapy for relapsed acute promyelocytic leukaemia. Br J Haematol. 2009;146:341.
566. Hoffman MA, Wiernik PH, Kleiner GJ. Acute promyelocytic leukemia and pregnancy. A case report Cancer. 1995;76:2237.
567. Sanz MA, Montesinos P, Casale MF, et al. Maternal and fetal outcomes in pregnant women with acute promyelocytic leukemia. Ann Hematol. 2015;94:1357–61.
568. Verma V, Giri S, Manandhar S, et al. Acute promyelocytic leukemia during pregnancy: a systematic analysis of outcome. Leuk Lymphoma. 2016;57:616–22.
569. Abla O, Ribeiro RC. How I treat children and adolescents with acute promyelocytic leukaemia. Br J Haematol. 2014;164:24–38.
570. Stein EM, Tallman MS. Acute promyelocytic leukemia in children and adolescents. Acta Haematol. 2014;132:307–12.
571. Tallman MS, Kwaan HC. Reassessing the hemostatic disorder associated with acute promyelocytic leukemia. Blood. 1992;79(3):543–53.
572. Barbui T, Finazzi G, Falanga A. The impact of all-trans-retinoic acid on the coagulopathy of acute promyelocytic leukemia. Blood. 1998;91(9):3093–102.
573. Mantha S, Tallman MS, Soff GA. What's new in the pathogenesis of the coagulopathy in acute promyelocytic leukemia? Curr Opin Hematol. 2016;23(2):121–6.
574. Gralnick HR, Bagley J, Abrell E. Heparin treatment for the hemorrhagic diathesis of acute promyelocytic leukemia. Am J Med. 1972;52(2):167–74.
575. Jones ME, Saleem A. Acute promyelocytic leukemia. Am J Med. 1978;65(4):673–7.
576. Cordonnier C, Vernant JP, Brun B, Heilmann MG, Kuentz M, Bierling P, et al. Acute promyelocytic leukemia in 57 previously untreated patients. Cancer. 1985;55(1):18–25.
577. Cunningham I, Gee TS, Reich LM, Kempin SJ, Naval AN, Clarkson BD. Acute promyelocytic leukemia: treatment results during a decade at Memorial Hospital. Blood. 1989;73(5):1116–22.
578. Rodeghiero F, Avvisati G, Castaman G, Barbui T, Mandelli F. Early deaths and anti-hemorrhagic treatments in acute promyelocytic leukemia. A GIMEMA retrospective study in 268 consecutive patients. Blood. 1990;75(11):2112–7.
579. Goldberg MA, Ginsburg D, Mayer RJ, Stone RM, Maguire M, Rosenthal DS, et al. Is heparin administration necessary during induction chemotherapy for patients with acute promyelocytic leukemia? Blood. 1987;69(1):187–91.
580. Bennett JM, Young ML, Andersen JW, Cassileth PA, Tallman MS, Paietta E, et al. Long-term survival in acute myeloid leukemia: the Eastern Cooperative Oncology Group experience. Cancer. 1997;80(11 Suppl):2205–9.
581. Dombret H, Scrobohaci ML, Ghorra P, Zini JM, Daniel MT, Castaigne S, et al. Coagulation disorders associated with acute promyelocytic leukemia: corrective effect of all-trans retinoic acid treatment. Leukemia. 1993;7(1):2–9.
582. Watanabe R, Murata M, Takayama N, Tokuhira M, Kizaki M, Okamoto S, et al. Long-term follow-up of hemostatic molecular

markers during remission induction therapy with all-trans retinoic acid for acute promyelocytic leukemia. Keio Hematology-Oncology Cooperative Study Group (KHOCS). Thromb Haemost. 1997;77(4):641–5.
583. Iland HJ, Bradstock K, Supple SG, Catalano A, Collins M, Hertzberg M, et al. All-trans-retinoic acid, idarubicin, and IV arsenic trioxide as initial therapy in acute promyelocytic leukemia (APML4). Blood. 2012;120(8):1570–80. quiz 752
584. Breccia M, Lo CF. Thrombo-hemorrhagic deaths in acute promyelocytic leukemia. Thromb Res. 2014;133(Suppl 2):S112–6.
585. Lehmann S, Ravn A, Carlsson L, Antunovic P, Deneberg S, Mollgard L, et al. Continuing high early death rate in acute promyelocytic leukemia: a population-based report from the Swedish Adult Acute Leukemia Registry. Leukemia. 2011;25(7):1128–34.
586. Rahme R, Thomas X, Recher C, Vey N, Delaunay J, Deconinck E, et al. Early death in acute promyelocytic leukemia (APL) in French centers: a multicenter study in 399 patients. Leukemia. 2014;28(12):2422–4.
587. Altman JK, Rademaker A, Cull E, Weitner BB, Ofran Y, Rosenblat TL, et al. Administration of ATRA to newly diagnosed patients with acute promyelocytic leukemia is delayed contributing to early hemorrhagic death. Leuk Res. 2013;37(9):1004–9.
588. McClellan JS, Kohrt HE, Coutre S, Gotlib JR, Majeti R, Alizadeh AA, et al. Treatment advances have not improved the early death rate in acute promyelocytic leukemia. Haematologica. 2012;97(1):133–6.
589. Tallman M, Lo-Coco F, Kwaan H, Sanz M, Gore S. Clinical roundtable monograph. Early death in patients with acute promyelocytic leukemia. Clinical advances in hematology & oncology : H&O. 2011;9(2):1–16.
590. Park JH, Qiao B, Panageas KS, Schymura MJ, Jurcic JG, Rosenblat TL, et al. Early death rate in acute promyelocytic leukemia remains high despite all-trans retinoic acid. Blood. 2011;118(5):1248–54.
591. Dombret H, Scrobohaci ML, Daniel MT, Miclea JM, Castaigne S, Chomienne C, et al. In vivo thrombin and plasmin activities in patients with acute promyelocytic leukemia (APL): effect of all-trans retinoic acid (ATRA) therapy. Leukemia. 1995;9(1):19–24.
592. Tallman MS, Lefebvre P, Baine RM, Shoji M, Cohen I, Green D, et al. Effects of all-trans retinoic acid or chemotherapy on the molecular regulation of systemic blood coagulation and fibrinolysis in patients with acute promyelocytic leukemia. J Thromb Haemost. 2004;2(8):1341–50.
593. Zhang P, Wang S, Hu X, Shi F, Qiu F, Hong G, et al. Arsenic trioxide treated 72 cases of acute promyelocytic leukemia. Chin J Hematol. 1996;17(1):58–60.
594. Mitrovic M, Suvajdzic N, Bogdanovic A, Kurtovic NK, Sretenovic A, Elezovic I, et al. International Society of Thrombosis and Hemostasis Scoring System for disseminated intravascular coagulation >/= 6: a new predictor of hemorrhagic early death in acute promyelocytic leukemia. Med Oncol. 2013;30(1):478.
595. Jeddi R, Kacem K, Ben Neji H, Mnif S, Gouider E, Aissaoui L, et al. Predictive factors of all-trans-retinoic acid related complications during induction therapy for acute promyelocytic leukemia. Hematology. 2008;13(3):142–6.
596. Lo-Coco F, Avvisati G, Vignetti M, Breccia M, Gallo E, Rambaldi A, et al. Front-line treatment of acute promyelocytic leukemia with AIDA induction followed by risk-adapted consolidation for adults younger than 61 years: results of the AIDA-2000 trial of the GIMEMA Group. Blood. 2010;116(17):3171–9.
597. Yanada M, Matsushita T, Asou N, Kishimoto Y, Tsuzuki M, Maeda Y, et al. Severe hemorrhagic complications during remission induction therapy for acute promyelocytic leukemia: incidence, risk factors, and influence on outcome. Eur J Haematol. 2007;78(3):213–9.
598. Sanz MA, Montesinos P, Vellenga E, Rayon C, de la Serna J, Parody R, et al. Risk-adapted treatment of acute promyelocytic leukemia with all-trans retinoic acid and anthracycline monochemotherapy: long-term outcome of the LPA 99 multicenter study by the PETHEMA Group. Blood. 2008;112(8):3130–4.
599. Ziegler S, Sperr WR, Knobl P, Lehr S, Weltermann A, Jager U, et al. Symptomatic venous thromboembolism in acute leukemia. Incidence, risk factors, and impact on prognosis. Thromb Res. 2005;115(1-2):59–64.
600. De Stefano V, Sora F, Rossi E, Chiusolo P, Laurenti L, Fianchi L, et al. The risk of thrombosis in patients with acute leukemia: occurrence of thrombosis at diagnosis and during treatment. J Thromb Haemost. 2005;3(9):1985–92.
601. Breccia M, Avvisati G, Latagliata R, Carmosino I, Guarini A, De Propris MS, et al. Occurrence of thrombotic events in acute promyelocytic leukemia correlates with consistent immunophenotypic and molecular features. Leukemia. 2007;21(1):79–83.
602. Escudier SM, Kantarjian HM, Estey EH. Thrombosis in patients with acute promyelocytic leukemia treated with and without all-trans retinoic acid. Leuk Lymphoma. 1996;20(5-6):435–9.
603. Tsukada N, Wada K, Aoki S, Hashimoto S, Kishi K, Takahashi M, et al. Induction Therapy with All-Trans Retinoic Acid for Acute Promyelocytic Leukemia: A Clinical Study of 10 Cases, Including a Fetal Case with Thromboembolism. Intern Med. 1996;35(1):10–4.
604. Pogliani EM, Rossini F, Casaroli I, Maffe P, Corneo G. Thrombotic complications in acute promyelocytic leukemia during all-trans-retinoic acid therapy. Acta Haematol. 1997;97(4):228–30.
605. Sanz MA, Montesinos P. Open issues on bleeding and thrombosis in acute promyelocytic leukemia. Thromb Res. 2010;125:S51–S4.
606. Choudhry A, DeLoughery TG. Bleeding and thrombosis in acute promyelocytic leukemia. Am J Hematol. 2012;87(6):596–603.
607. Fenaux P, Tertian G, Castaigne S, Tilly H, Leverger G, Guy H, et al. A randomized trial of amsacrine and rubidazone in 39 patients with acute promyelocytic leukemia. Journal of clinical oncology : official journal of the American Society of Clinical Oncology. 1991;9(9):1556–61.
608. Gralnick HR, Sultan C. Acute promyelocytic leukaemia: haemorrhagic manifestation and morphologic criteria. Br J Haematol. 1975;29(3):373–6.
609. Groopman J, Ellman L. Acute promyelocytic leukemia. Am J Hematol. 1979;7(4):395–408.
610. Collins AJ, Bloomfield CD, Peterson BA, McKenna RW, Edson JR. Acute promyelocytic leukemia. Management of the coagulopathy during daunorubicin-prednisone remission induction. Arch Intern Med. 1978;138(11):1677–80.
611. Bennett B, Booth NA, Croll A, Dawson AA. The bleeding disorder in acute promyelocytic leukaemia: fibrinolysis due to u-PA rather than defibrination. Br J Haematol. 1989;71(4):511–7.
612. Bennett M, Parker AC, Ludlam CA. Platelet and fibrinogen survival in acute promyelocytic leukaemia. BMJ. 1976;2(6035):565-.
613. Breen KA, Grimwade D, Hunt BJ. The pathogenesis and management of the coagulopathy of acute promyelocytic leukaemia. Br J Haematol. 2012;156(1):24–36.
614. Nemerson Y. Tissue factor and hemostasis. Blood. 1988;71(1):1–8.
615. Bauer KA, Conway EM, Bach R, Konigsberg WH, Griffin JD, Demetri G. Tissue factor gene expression in acute myeloblastic leukemia. Thromb Res. 1989;56(3):425–30.
616. Andoh K, Sadakata H, Uchiyama T, Narahara N, Tanaka H, Kobayashi N, et al. One-stage method for assay of tissue factor activity of leukemic cell with special reference to disseminated intravascular coagulation. Am J Clin Pathol. 1990; 93(5):679–84.

617. Kubota T, Andoh K, Sadakata H, Tanaka H, Kobayashi N. Tissue factor released from leukemic cells. Thromb Haemost. 1991;65(1):59–63.
618. Yan J, Wang K, Dong L, Liu H, Chen W, Xi W, et al. PML/RARalpha fusion protein transactivates the tissue factor promoter through a GAGC-containing element without direct DNA association. Proc Natl Acad Sci U S A. 2010;107(8):3716–21.
619. Kwaan HC, Rego EM, McMachon B, Weiss I. Thrombin generation and fibrinolytic activity in microparticles in acute promyelocytic leukemia. Blood. 2013;122(21):3620.
620. Kwaan HC, Rego EM. Role of microparticles in the hemostatic dysfunction in acute promyelocytic leukemia. Semin Thromb Hemost. 2010;36(8):917–24.
621. Ma G, Liu F, Lv L, Gao Y, Su Y. Increased promyelocytic-derived microparticles: a novel potential factor for coagulopathy in acute promyelocytic leukemia. Ann Hematol. 2013;92(5):645–52.
622. Gordon SG, Franks JJ, Lewis B. Cancer procoagulant A: a factor X activating procoagulant from malignant tissue. Thromb Res. 1975;6(2):127–37.
623. Falanga A, Gordon SG. Isolation and characterization of cancer procoagulant: a cysteine proteinase from malignant tissue. Biochemistry. 1985;24(20):5558–67.
624. Donati MB, Falanga A, Consonni R, Alessio MG, Bassan R, Buelli M, et al. Cancer procoagulant in acute non lymphoid leukemia: relationship of enzyme detection to disease activity. Thromb Haemost. 1990;64(1):11–6.
625. Bevilacqua MP. Interleukin 1 (IL-1) induces biosynthesis and cell surface expression of procoagulant activity in human vascular endothelial cells. J Exp Med. 1984;160(2):618–23.
626. Bevilacqua MP, Pober JS, Majeau GR, Fiers W, Cotran RS, Gimbrone MA. Recombinant tumor necrosis factor induces procoagulant activity in cultured human vascular endothelium: characterization and comparison with the actions of interleukin 1. Proc Natl Acad Sci. 1986;83(12):4533–7.
627. Nawroth PP, Handley DA, Esmon CT, Stern DM. Interleukin 1 induces endothelial cell procoagulant while suppressing cell-surface anticoagulant activity. Proc Natl Acad Sci U S A. 1986;83(10):3460–4.
628. Nawroth PP. Modulation of endothelial cell hemostatic properties by tumor necrosis factor. J Exp Med. 1986;163(3):740–5.
629. Clauss M. Vascular permeability factor: a tumor-derived polypeptide that induces endothelial cell and monocyte procoagulant activity, and promotes monocyte migration. J Exp Med. 1990;172(6):1535–45.
630. Cozzolino F, Torcia M, Miliani A, Carossino AM, Giordani R, Cinotti S, et al. Potential role of interleukin-1 as the trigger for diffuse intravascular coagulation in acute nonlymphoblastic leukemia. Am J Med. 1988;84(2):240–50.
631. Emeis JJ. Interleukin 1 and lipopolysaccharide induce an inhibitor of tissue-type plasminogen activator in vivo and in cultured endothelial cells. J Exp Med. 1986;163(5):1260–6.
632. Nachman RL. Interleukin 1 induces endothelial cell synthesis of plasminogen activator inhibitor. J Exp Med. 1986;163(6):1595–600.
633. Miyauchi S, Moroyama T, Kyoizumi S, Asakawa J-I, Okamoto T, Takada K. Malignant tumor cell lines produce interleukin-1-like factor. In Vitro Cell Dev Biol. 1988;24(8):753–8.
634. Noguchi M, Sakai T, Kisiel W. Identification and partial purification of a novel tumor-derived protein that induces tissue factor on cultured human endothelial cells. Biochem Biophys Res Commun. 1989;160(1):222–7.
635. Chan TK, Chan GT, Chan V. Hypofibrinogenemia due to increased fibrinolysis in two patients with acute promyelocytic leukemia. Aust N Z J Med. 1984;14(3):245–9.
636. Sterrenberg L, Haak HL, Brommer EJP, Nieuwenhuizen W. Evidence of Fibrinogen Breakdown by Leukocyte Enzymes in a Patient with Acute Promyelocytic Leukemia. Pathophysiol Haemost Thromb. 1985;15(2):126–33.
637. Schwartz BS. Epsilon-Aminocaproic Acid in the Treatment of Patients with Acute Promyelocytic Leukemia and Acquired Alpha-2-Plasmin Inhibitor Deficiency. Ann Intern Med. 1986;105(6):873.
638. Velasco F, Torres A, Andres P, Martinez F, Gomez P. Changes in plasma levels of protease and fibrinolytic inhibitors induced by treatment in acute myeloid leukemia. Thromb Haemost. 1984;52(1):81–4.
639. Wilson EL, Jacobs P, Dowdle EB. The secretion of plasminogen activators by human myeloid leukemic cells in vitro. Blood. 1983;61(3):568–74.
640. Sakata Y, Murakami T, Noro A, Mori K, Matsuda M. The specific activity of plasminogen activator inhibitor-1 in disseminated intravascular coagulation with acute promyelocytic leukemia. Blood. 1991;77(9):1949–57.
641. Hirata F, Schiffmann E, Venkatasubramanian K, Salomon D, Axelrod J. A phospholipase A2 inhibitory protein in rabbit neutrophils induced by glucocorticoids. Proc Natl Acad Sci. 1980;77(5):2533–6.
642. Chang KS, Wang G, Freireich EJ, Daly M, Naylor SL, Trujillo JM, et al. Specific expression of the annexin VIII gene in acute promyelocytic leukemia. Blood. 1992;79(7):1802–10.
643. Hajjar KA, Jacovina AT, Chacko J. An endothelial cell receptor for plasminogen/tissue plasminogen activator. I. Identity with annexin II. J Biol Chem. 1994;269(33):21191–7.
644. Menell JS, Cesarman GM, Jacovina AT, McLaughlin MA, Lev EA, Hajjar KA. Annexin II and Bleeding in Acute Promyelocytic Leukemia. N Engl J Med. 1999;340(13):994–1004.
645. Cesarman GM, Guevara CA, Hajjar KA. An endothelial cell receptor for plasminogen/tissue plasminogen activator (t-PA). II. Annexin II-mediated enhancement of t-PA-dependent plasminogen activation. J Biol Chem. 1994;269(33):21198–203.
646. Liu Y, Wang Z, Jiang M, Dai L, Zhang W, Wu D, et al. The expression of annexin II and its role in the fibrinolytic activity in acute promyelocytic leukemia. Leuk Res. 2011;35(7):879–84.
647. Stein E, McMahon B, Kwaan H, Altman JK, Frankfurt O, Tallman MS. The coagulopathy of acute promyelocytic leukaemia revisited. Best Pract Res Clin Haematol. 2009;22(1):153–63.
648. Federici AB, D'Amicob EA. The Role of Von Willebrand Factor in the Hemostatic Defect of Acute Promyelocytic Leukemia. Leuk Lymphoma. 1998;31(5-6):491–9.
649. Runde V, Aul C, Heyll A, Schneider W. All-trans retinoic acid: not only a differentiating agent, but also an inducer of thromboembolic events in patients with M3 leukemia. Blood. 1992;79(2):534–5.
650. Hashimoto S, Koike T, Tatewaki W, Seki Y, Sato N, Azegami T, et al. Fatal thromboembolism in acute promyelocytic leukemia during all-trans retinoic acid therapy combined with antifibrinolytic therapy for prophylaxis of hemorrhage. Leukemia. 1994;8(7):1113–5.
651. Falanga A, Iacoviello L, Evangelista V, Belotti D, Consonni R, D'Orazio A, et al. Loss of blast cell procoagulant activity and improvement of hemostatic variables in patients with acute promyelocytic leukemia administered all-trans-retinoic acid. Blood. 1995;86(3):1072–81.
652. Falanga A, Consonni R, Marchetti M, Mielicki WP, Rambaldi A, Lanotte M, et al. Cancer procoagulant in the human promyelocytic cell line NB4 and its modulation by all-trans-retinoic acid. Leukemia. 1994;8(1):156–9.
698. Koyama T, Hirosawa S, Kawamata N, Tohda S, Aoki N. All-trans retinoic acid upregulates thrombomodulin and downregulates tissue-factor expression in acute promyelocytic leukemia cells: distinct expression of thrombomodulin and tissue factor in human leukemic cells. Blood. 1994;84(9):3001–9.
654. Ishii H, Horie S, Kizaki K, Kazama M. Retinoic acid counteracts both the downregulation of thrombomodulin and the induction of

tissue factor in cultured human endothelial cells exposed to tumor necrosis factor. Blood. 1992;80(10):2556–62.
655. Medh RD, Santell L, Levin EG. Stimulation of tissue plasminogen activator production by retinoic acid: synergistic effect on protein kinase C-mediated activation. Blood. 1992;80(4):981–7.
656. Lansink M, Kooistra T. Stimulation of tissue-type plasminogen activator expression by retinoic acid in human endothelial cells requires retinoic acid receptor beta 2 induction. Blood. 1996;88(2):531–41.
657. Fenaux P, Chastang C, Chomienne C, Castaigne S, Sanz M, Link H, et al. Treatment of Newly Diagnosed Acute Promyelocytic Leukemia (APL) by All Transretinoic Acid (ATRA) Combined with Chemotherapy: The European Experience. Leuk Lymphoma. 1995;16(5-6):431–7.
658. Avvisati G, Lo-Coco F, Paoloni FP, Petti MC, Diverio D, Vignetti M, et al. AIDA 0493 protocol for newly diagnosed acute promyelocytic leukemia: very long-term results and role of maintenance. Blood. 2011;117(18):4716–25.
659. Asou N, Adachi K, Tamura J, Kanamaru A, Kageyama S, Hiraoka A, et al. Analysis of prognostic factors in newly diagnosed acute promyelocytic leukemia treated with all-trans retinoic acid and chemotherapy. Japan Adult Leukemia Study Group. J Clin Oncol. 1998;16(1):78–85.
660. Fenaux P, Chastang C, Chevret S, Sanz M, Dombret H, Archimbaud E, et al. A randomized comparison of all transretinoic acid (ATRA) followed by chemotherapy and ATRA plus chemotherapy and the role of maintenance therapy in newly diagnosed acute promyelocytic leukemia. The European APL Group. Blood. 1999;94(4):1192–200.
661. Ades L, Guerci A, Raffoux E, Sanz M, Chevallier P, Lapusan S, et al. Very long-term outcome of acute promyelocytic leukemia after treatment with all-trans retinoic acid and chemotherapy: the European APL Group experience. Blood. 2010;115(9):1690–6.
662. de The H, Chen Z. Acute promyelocytic leukaemia: novel insights into the mechanisms of cure. Nat Rev Cancer. 2010;10(11):775–83.
663. Zhu J, Guo WM, Yao YY, Zhao WL, Pan L, Cai X, et al. Tissue factors on acute promyelocytic leukemia and endothelial cells are differently regulated by retinoic acid, arsenic trioxide and chemotherapeutic agents. Leukemia. 1999;13(7):1062–70.
664. Slack JL, Rusiniak ME. Current issues in the management of acute promyelocytic leukemia. Ann Hematol. 2000;79(5):227–38.
665. Alimoghaddam K, Ghavamzadeh A, Jahani M. Use of Novoseven for arsenic trioxide-induced bleeding in PML. Am J Hematol. 2006;81(9):720.
666. Zver S, Andoljsek D, Cernelc P. Effective treatment of life-threatening bleeding with recombinant activated factor VII in a patient with acute promyelocytic leukaemia. Eur J Haematol. 2004;72(6):455–6.
667. Matsushita T, Watanabe J, Honda G, Mimuro J, Takahashi H, Tsuji H, et al. Thrombomodulin alfa treatment in patients with acute promyelocytic leukemia and disseminated intravascular coagulation: a retrospective analysis of an open-label, multicenter, post-marketing surveillance study cohort. Thromb Res. 2014;133(5):772–81.
668. Lo-Cocco F, Di Donato L. Targeted therapy alone for acute promyelocytic leukemia. N Engl J Med. 2016;374:1197–8.
669. Liu SS, Wang XP, Li XB, et al. Zoledronic acid exerts antitumor effects in NB4 acute promyelocytic leukemia cells by inducing apoptosis and S phase arrest. Biomed Pharmacother. 2014;68:1031–6.
670. Wang Y, Lin D, Wei H, et al. Long-term follow-up of homoharringtonine plus all-trans retinoic acid-based induction and consolidation therapy in newly diagnosed acute promyelocytic leukemia. Int J Hematol. 2015;101:279–85.
671. Patel S, Guerenne L, Gorombei P, et al. pVAX14DNA-mediated add-on immunotherapy combined with arsenic trioxide and all-trans retinoic acid targeted therapy effectively increases the survival of acute promyelocytic leukemia mice. Blood Cancer J. 2015;5:e374.
672. Ghanizadeh-Vesali S, Zekri A, Zaker F, et al. Significnace of AZD1152 as apotential treatment against Aurora B overexpression in acute promyelocytic leukemia. Ann Hematol. 2016;95:1031–42.
673. Ganesan S, Alex AA, Chendamarai E, et al. Rationale and efficacy of proteasome inhibitor combined with arsenic trioxide in the treatment of acute promyelocytic leukemia. Leukemia. 2016;30:2169–78.
674. Zhang K, Li J, Meng W, et al. Tashinone IIA inhibits acute promyelocytic leukemia cell proliferation and induces apoptosis in vivo. Blood Cells Mol Dis. 2016;56:46–52.
675. Atashrazm F, Lowenthal RM, Dickinson JL, et al. Fucoidan enhances the therapeutic potential of arsenic trioxide and all-trans retinoic acid in acute promyelocytic leukemia in vitro and in vivo. Oncotarget. 2016;7:46028–41.

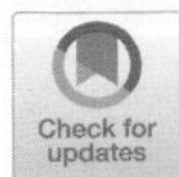

Therapy-Related Acute Myelogenous Leukemia

22

Hyung Chan Suh and H. Phillip Koeffler

Abbreviations

AD Autoimmune disease
ADC Antibody-drug conjugate
ALL Acute lymphoblastic leukemia
AlloHSCT Allogeneic hematopoietic stem cell transplant
AML Acute myelogenous leukemia
ATRA All-trans retinoic acid
AutoHSCT Autologous hematopoietic stem cell transplant
CLL Chronic lymphocytic leukemia
CR Complete remission
ECOG Eastern Cooperative Oncology Group
EGR-1 Early growth response-1
FLT3 fms-related tyrosine kinase 3
FPSG French Polycythemia Study Group
G-CSF Granulocyte colony-stimulating factor
GM-CSF Granulocyte-macrophage colony-stimulating factor
HDAC Histone deacetylation
HLA Human leukocyte antigen
HSC Hematopoietic stem and progenitor cells
IL Interleukins
LDH Lactate dehydrogenase
M-CSF Macrophage colony-stimulating factor
MDR Multiple drug resistance
MF Myelofibrosis
MLL Mixed-lineage leukemia
MPN Myleoproliferative neoplasia
MRI Magnetic resonance imaging
MUGA Multigated acquisition scan
NHL Non-Hodgkin lymphoma
OS Overall survival
PBSC Peripheral blood stem cells
PDGF Platelet-derived growth factor
PET Positron emission tomography
PLK Polo-like kinase
PML Promyelocytic leukemia protein
PVSG Polycythemia Vera Study Group
RAEB Refractory anemia with excess blasts
RAEB-t Refractory anemia with excess blasts in transformation
RARA Retinoic acid receptor alpha
RIC Reduced-intensity chemotherapy
SCN Severe congenital neutropenia
T-AML Therapy-related acute myelogenous leukemia
T-APL Therapy-related acute promyelocytic leukemia
T-MDS Therapy-related myelodysplastic syndrome
T-MN Therapy-related myeloid neoplasm
TNF Tumor necrosis factor
TP53 Tumor protein p53
TRM Treatment-related mortality
WBC White blood cell

Introduction

Individuals exposed to cytotoxic agents are at higher risk of developing myeloid disorders such as therapy-related myelodysplastic syndrome (t-MDS), therapy-related acute myeloid leukemia (t-AML), and therapy-related MDS/myeloproliferative neoplasms. However, all of these diseases are within the spectrum of a single disease entity, therapy-related myeloid neoplasms (t-MN), as categorized by the WHO classification system in 2008 [1]. WHO morphologic classification system defines t-MN as MDS and myeloid leukemia, which arise following the administration of chemotherapy and/or radiation for a prior malignancy. Patients who developed myeloid disorders by environmental toxins affecting hematopoiesis are not included in this disease category. Therapy-related MDS

H.C. Suh, M.D., Ph.D. (✉)
Division of Hematology Oncology, David Geffen School of Medicine at UCLA, Los Angeles, CA 90095, USA
e-mail: hcsuh@mednet.ucla.edu

H. Phillip Koeffler, M.D.
Department of Medicine/Hematology-Oncology, UCLA/Cedars-Sinai Medical Center, Los Angeles, CA 90048, USA
e-mail: H.Koeffler@cshs.org

P.H. Wiernik et al. (eds.), *Neoplastic Diseases of the Blood*, DOI 10.1007/978-3-319-64263-5_22

and AML comprise the vast majority of t-MN cases. The 2008 WHO classification did not consider t-MDS and t-AML sufficiently distinctively different. However, unlike secondary AML denoting AML did not develop spontaneously or *de novo*, t-AML has clear history of prior chemotherapy or radiation therapy.

T-MN has become increasingly common. The fast rising incidence can be attributed to a variety of factors including longer survival of patients after treatment of their primary malignancy, intensified chemotherapy, radiation therapy, and broaden awareness of this disease category. This is a heterogeneous and poorly defined group of patients who have a shorter median survival than patients with *de novo* AML, MDS, or MDS/myeloproliferative neoplasia (MPN). Retrospective studies have shown that their inferior outcomes are associated with poor-risk cytogenetics, present in 50–70% of t-MDS/AML compared with 15–25% in *de novo* disease. Other studies have identified additional risk factors, including comorbidities from primary malignancy and therapy of the disease. Because of the poor outcome, t-AML is among the most feared long-term complication of cancer therapy these days.

Epidemiology

Therapy-related myeloid neoplasms (t-MN) account for approximately 10–20% of all cases of AML, MDS, and MDS/MPN. US Surveillance, Epidemiology, and End Results data of approximately 426,000 adults treated for an initial primary malignancy between 1975 and 2008 showed a 4.7-fold increased risk of AML compared with the incidence of AML expected in the general population. With the increasingly successful management of malignancies overall and improved cancer survivorship, the overall incidence of t-MN is expected to increase. The estimated incidence after therapy for any single prior diagnosis varies from less than 1 to 20% depending on the agents administered, therapy intensity, and survival, since the overall median latency time varies 1–5 years.

Patients with t-AML are seen among survivors of both solid tumors and hematologic malignancies. Smith et al. studied 306 patients who developed therapy-related myelodysplasia and myeloid leukemia with cytogenetic analyses [2]. In the study population, 25% of the patients had Hodgkin disease, 23% had non-Hodgkin lymphoma, and 38% had a solid tumor as the primary malignancy. Breast cancer was the most common among the 38% patients. Interestingly, 6% of patients had undergone cytotoxic chemotherapy for the management of immune disorders. Kayser et al. also showed similar patient characteristics in their study with 200 patients having t-AML. The group found that 71% of t-MN patients had a prior solid tumor and 27.5% patients had a prior hematologic malignancy. Breast cancer and non-Hodgkin lymphoma were the largest subsets in these two groups [3].

T-AML patients can present at any age. The risk associated with alkylating agents and radiation appears to increase with age, while the risk associated with topoisomerase II inhibitors appears to be constant across all ages [1]. Among those treated for breast cancer, younger age at the time of exposure, higher dose intensity of cytotoxic treatments, concomitant treatment with radiation, and adjuvant use of hematopoietic growth factors with cytotoxic therapy for accelerated white blood cell recovery are factors associated with an increased risk of t-AML [4, 5]. However, some t-AML/MDS individuals may have a DNA repair apparatus that is not as robust as normal, which also might predispose them to develop t-AML.

Etiology

T-AML appears to be a direct consequence of mutational events by therapy-induced DNA double-strand breaks, with a subsequent genomic instability [6]. Frequency of the mutations may vary between individuals as a result of genetic susceptibility. This susceptibility is usually not measurable or very subtle; a few exceptions include Fanconi anemia, and mismatch repair abnormalities.

The effects of some cytotoxic agents in the development of abnormal cytogenetics are well documented (Table 22.1). The latency period between first exposure to an agent (cytotoxic chemotherapy, radiation) and development of t-AML ranges from 1 to 5 years and varies by etiologic agent. T-AML after exposure to alkylating agents or radiation therapy typically presents after a latency period of approximately 4 years [7–10]. Most of these patients initially present with MDS. The chromosomal abnormalities seen in this category of t-AML often involve complex abnormalities such as deletion of the long arm or the entire chromosome 5 and/or 7. Topoisomerase II inhibitors are another etiologic agent of t-AML. It causes t-AML with a relatively shorter latency of

Table 22.1 Risk factors for therapy-related leukemia

Alkylating agent therapy: May cause MDS (preleukemic phase), could take 4–10 years to develop AML 5q or 7q deletion, bad prognosis
DNA-topoisomerase II inhibitor therapy (epipodophyllotoxins and anthracyclines): May develop t-AML without preleukemic phase; short median latency (33 months) Frequent translocation of 11q23 (MLL) or 21q22 Morphologic phenotype often M4/M5 (by former FAB classification)
Ionizing radiation therapy: similar to alkylating-related AML
G-CSF in severe congenital neutropenia

1–3 years, and the patients present with overt leukemia rather than MDS or MDS/MPN [11–13]. The cytogenetic alterations in this category of t-AML occur frequently with translocations including the MLL gene located at 11q23 or AML1 (RUNX1) gene at 21q22 [e.g., t(9;11), t(8;21), or t(3;21)]. However, no reliable way exists to determine the duration of the "at-risk" period for developing t-AML. The latency periods with other agents are not as clear as these two drugs. Exposure to multiple agents also makes it difficult to determine the risk, etiology, and latency period.

Alkylating agents are frequently used chemotherapeutic agents; more than 85% of patients who developed chemotherapy-related leukemia had received an alkylator [14]. Melphalan, chlorambucil, or cyclophosphamide is the offending agent in nearly 65% of patients. Therefore, different alkylating agents may be associated with varying risks of leukemogenesis. For example, one study compared the rates of mutagen-related leukemia in ovarian cancer patients treated with either melphalan or cyclophosphamide, and found that melphalan may be a more potent leukemogen than cyclophosphamide. Thus, the mutagenic potential may differ between the antineoplastic agents [15].

Alkylating agents interact with DNA in a variety of ways: monoadduct formation, inter- and intra-strand cross-links, as well as alkylation of free DNA bases. This can lead to cell death, but also can cause termination of DNA replication and chromosome loss, leading to mutagenesis and resulting in development of leukemia. Alkylation events can also change the stereometric configuration of DNA bases, causing them to mispair resulting in single-base mutations. Many of the alkylating agents have been clearly implicated in leukemogenesis.

Topoisomerase II helps mediate the relaxation of the DNA supercoil by making double-strand breaks. The breaks are repaired when homologous chromosome fragments realign. Topoisomerase II inhibitors, such as epipodophyllotoxins (etoposide and teniposide), doxorubicin, 4-epodoxorubicin, mitoxantrone, razosane, and biomolane, induce incorrect DNA repair by crossover recombination with nonhomologous end joining between the two DNA strands, which may result in the development of a balanced chromosomal translocation (Fig. 22.1). Balanced chromosomal aberrations involving the MLL, RUNX1, RARA, or NUP98 genes characterize unique genetic pathways of t-AML. The rearrangements between these genes and other partners provide gain-of-function fusion proteins. These topoisomerase II inhibitors are important components of chemotherapy regimens for many tumors, such as testicular cancer, ALL, NHL, lung cancer, and many others. Razoxane and bimolane, used in the treatment of psoriasis, have also been demonstrated to be leukemogenic. Those patients in whom t-AML develops after therapy with DNA-topoisomerase II inhibitors often have acute leukemia with no t-MDS phase [16, 17], and a short latency period, in contrast to alkylating agent-induced AML.

In the Polycythemia Vera Study Group (PVSG), 431 polycythemia vera patients were randomized to one of the three treatment groups: phlebotomy alone, P32 and phlebotomy, or chlorambucil and phlebotomy [18]. Higher number of AML cases occurred in both the P32 (9.6%) and chlorambucil (13%) treatment groups compared to phlebotomy-only group (1.5%), indicating a role of radiation and a cytotoxic agent in the development of AML in these patient groups [19]. French Polycythemia Study Group (FPSG) reported a leukemia incidence in polycythemia vera patients of 5–15% after 10 years of observation [20]. In a randomized trial in patients >65 years of age, the FPSG reported 12% AML at 10 years in patients receiving P32 alone. Hydroxyurea

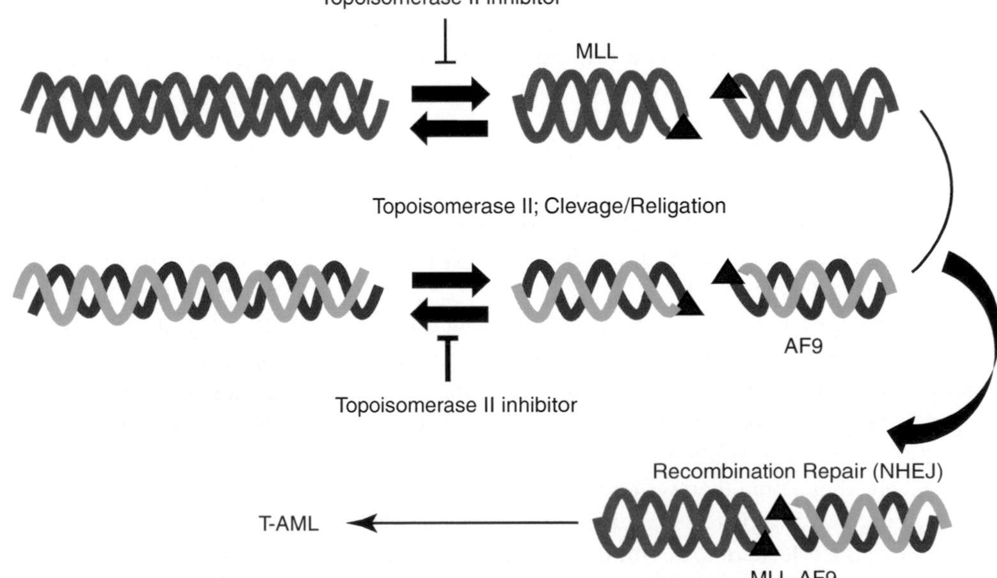

Fig. 22.1 Formation of topoisomerase II-DNA complex is necessary to perform critical cellular functions. If the amount of complexes is elevated as a result of topoisomerase II inhibitors, DNA repair/recombination process is activated, which subsequently generates chromosomal translocations or other DNA aberrations. If the fusion protein produced by chromosomal translocation results in the cells having a growth advantage, these cells may evolve and progress into t-AML

maintenance combined with initial P32 therapy also increased the risk of AML (21% at 10 years). In another case control study of MPN patients (68% of patients had polycythemia vera), the risk of AML/MDS development was significantly associated with high exposures of P32 and alkylators [21]. Taken together, a strong association exists of cytotoxic agents or radiation increasing the risk of development of AML in MPN patients.

Ionizing radiation clearly increases the risk of developing AML in humans and experimental animals. The incidence of leukemia after 400 cGy or less of radiation exposure from the Hiroshima nuclear explosion was approximately two cases of leukemia/10^6 persons/year/cGy [22]. Nearly the same incidence of leukemia was reported in patients who received 300–1500 cGy of spinal irradiation for ankylosing spondylitis. Likewise, increased rates of AML occurred in radiologists who practiced during the early years of clinical radiology before modern safety standards [23].

Animal studies confirmed the epidemiological observations in humans by showing that low-dose chronic irradiation induces leukemia in experimental animals. Half of dogs that received a daily low dose (5–10 cGy) of cobalt γ-irradiation developed AML after about 1000 days [24]. Single whole-body irradiation initiates leukemia in rodents. Myelogenous leukemia developed in 20% of mice after a single brief whole-body irradiation of 200 cGy [25]. The dose–response relationship was curvilinear; pulse irradiation of at least 300 cGy induced significantly fewer cases of leukemia than the 200 cGy dose; these doses produced marrow cell death, probably decreasing the number of cells that would otherwise have the potential to undergo malignant transformation.

Exposure to ionizing radiation can cause a DNA damage by a mechanism similar to alkylating agents. Radiation photon energy can directly lead to DNA strand breakage. Radiation is frequently used in conjunction with chemotherapy for cancer therapy, and only a few studies have specifically looked at the characteristics of myeloid neoplasms occurring after radiation alone. Recently, Nardi et al. showed that t-MDS occurring in the modern radiation therapy era, if alone, more nearly resembled *de novo* MDS/AML in cytogenetic characteristics and clinical behavior, and affected patients had better outcomes than patients with t-MDS secondary to chemotherapy [26].

Even though radiation therapy is leukemogenic [7, 27–29], studies in Hodgkin's disease suggest that the incidence of secondary leukemia in patients receiving radiation therapy alone was low compared with those receiving chemotherapy alone [30, 31]. In one study, a total of 957 patients exclusively received radiation therapy, and none developed leukemia. By contrast, 542 patients received only chemotherapy, and 12 developed leukemia. A similar finding was reported in ovarian cancer patients who received either chemotherapy or radiation therapy [32]. In most studies, the risk of AML in patients with either Hodgkin's disease or ovarian carcinoma treated exclusively with chemotherapy is not different from those treated with both chemotherapy and radiation therapy [7, 27–29, 32].

In a study of chromosomal abnormalities, only 37 of 344 patients with secondary leukemia had been treated with radiation therapy alone; the incidence of a normal karyotype was higher in patients who received only radiation than in patients who received chemotherapy either with or without radiation therapy (24.3 vs. 11.7%). Normal karyotype is associated with better response to antileukemic therapy, but with little improvement in overall survival (OS) [33]. Another study of 63 patients with either t-MDS or t-AML found that 11 of 63 had received only radiation, in most cases to ports including the pelvis or spinal bone marrow [34]. In this study, only two patients had a normal karyotype. The low risk of leukemia after currently used high-voltage irradiation may be analogous to the earlier mentioned murine model where high-dose irradiation has a lethal effect on marrow cells in contrast to lower dose exposure, which may be more likely to produce nonlethal marrow cell injury and mutations.

Although several studies examined secondary malignancies in patients with specific primary tumor types, few data have been published examining the long-term effect of pelvic radiation. Wright et al. analyzed patients with invasive tumors of the vulva, cervix, uterus, anus, and rectosigmoid treated with radiotherapy from 1973 to 2005 [35]. In a Cox proportional hazards model adjusting for other risk factors, posttreatment leukemia was increased by 72% (hazard ratio [HR], 1.72; 95% CI, 1.37–2.15) in the patients who received pelvic radiotherapy. The risk of secondary leukemia peaked at 5–10 years after primary treatment (HR, 1.85; 95% CI, 1.40–2.44) and remained elevated even 10–15 years after initial treatment (HR, 1.50; 95% CI, 1.03–2.18) [35].

Radioiodine (I-131) induces chromosomal aberrations, and theoretically can lead to leukemogenesis. However, the occurrence of t-AML after radioiodine treatment for thyrotoxicosis and thyroid cancer is infrequent. In a comprehensive meta-analysis of the currently available literature covering 16,502 patients with thyroid cancers, the relative risk of development of leukemia increased 2.5-fold in patients treated with radioiodine [36]. The latency period of t-AML associated with radiation was 5–7 years, similar to t-AML associated with alkylating agents [37].

The use of granulocyte colony-stimulating factor (G-CSF) in chemotherapy may be a risk factor for development of t-AML as shown in a meta-analysis examining data from 25 trials [38]. At a mean follow-up of 60 months, 43 t-MN cases were reported in G-CSF-treated patients, while 22 t-MN occurred in control group. G-CSF may accelerate damaged myeloid progenitors into cell cycling before repair of genetic injuries from cytotoxic therapy.

Cases of leukemic transformation in patients with severe congenital neutropenia (SCN) were prospectively studied [39]. A comprehensive analysis of the incidence of AML transformation showed that the annual risk of MDS/AML was 0.81% during the first 5 years, and 2.3% after 10 years among 374 SCN patients with G-CSF treatment. After 15 years on G-CSF, the cumulative incidence for MDS/AML was 22% in SCN, whereas none of the cyclic neutropenia patients who also received G-CSF developed MDS or AML [40]. Patients with SCN develop mutations of their G-CSF receptor, which affects the ability of the myeloid cells to differentiate.

T-MN occurring in patients with autoimmune diseases (AD) has been increasingly recognized. A large population-based study found that AD patients had significantly increased risk for AML and MDS [41], and this finding was subsequently confirmed by another study [42]. Immunosuppressive therapy may be another contributing factor for development of t-MN. Patients who received immune-suppressive agents including corticosteroids, antitumor necrosis factor (TNF) agents, sulfasalazine, and cytotoxic chemotherapeutics such as methotrexate, azathioprine, and cyclophosphamide had increased risk for hematological malignancies [43]. The development of t-APL in patients with multiple sclerosis has been reported [44, 45]. But patients receiving an antimetabolite as a single agent (e.g., fludarabine, azathioprine, and 6-thioguanine) for their autoimmune disease rarely develop t-AML [46–48]. Development of t-AML in AD patients who received immunosuppressive therapy other than cytotoxic agents could represent the importance of the immune-surveillance system in guarding against malignancies. Also, the underlying primary genetic defects in these individuals might increase susceptibility to AML.

Karyotypic Abnormalities in t-MDS/AML

Clonal chromosomal abnormalities can be detected in the blast cells of 80–95% of t-MDS/t-AML patients by routinely available techniques [7, 34, 49–53]. A hypodiploid modal number of chromosomes occur most frequently in t-MDS/t-AML patients. Hyperdiploidy, mainly trisomy 8, is rare and is often observed as an inconsistent aberration present in only a subclone of cells [52]. Chromosomes 5q and 7q probably contain critical myeloid tumor-suppressor genes in *de novo* and t-AML. The breakpoints for the deletions are variable, but a common chromosome region, the so-called critical region, is almost always deleted.

For chromosome 5, Le Beau et al. have narrowed down the critical region to 5q31.1, which includes the early growth response gene *(EGR-1)* [54]. Other genes located on the long arm of chromosome 5 include many growth factor genes, namely *granulocyte-macrophage colony-stimulating factor (GM-CSF*), and *interleukins-3, −4,* and *−5 (IL-3, −4, −5)* [34, 55–58], and the growth factor receptor genes known to be present on the long arm of chromosome 5, namely *macrophage colony-stimulating factor* (M-CSF or *FMS) receptor, platelet-derived growth factor (PDGF) receptor*, *glucocorticoid receptor, alpha1-adrenergic receptor, beta2-adrenergic receptor*, and *D1-dopamine receptor* [59, 60].

The breakpoints for the deletions of 7q are variable, but a common chromosome region, the so-called critical region, is located at band 7q22 proximally with the distal breakpoint varying from q31 to q36. Potentially important genes have been mapped to 7q, including genes for EZH2, erythropoietin, p glycoprotein 1/multiple drug resistance 1 (MDR-1), and MDR-3 [61]. Abnormalities of chromosome 7q are common in myeloid malignancies. Especially, homozygous EZH2 mutations were commonly found in MDS/MPN patients [61]. However, none has yet been shown to be involved in the development of t-AML [54, 59–62].

Although most of the chromosomal abnormalities reported in t-MDS/t-AML are either complete or partial deletion of chromosome 7 or 7q [del(−7/7q)], and/or 5, or 5q del(−5/5q)], in recent years recurring unbalanced translocations that also result in loss of the long arm of 7 and/or 5 have been reported with increasing frequency. These include t(1;7)(p11;q11), t(5;7)(q11.2;p11.2), and t(7;17)(p11;p11) for chromosome 7, and t(5;7)(q11.2;p11.2) and t(5;17)(p11;p11) for chromosome 5 [63]. While the loss of function of a single gene in each of these relatively large regions is possibly responsible for the development of t-MDS/t-AML, hemizygous loss of the function of several genes in each of these regions could also contribute to the disease phenotype. Another, not mutually exclusive hypothesis is that an unknown initiating abnormality causes genomic instability leading to the deletion and rearrangement of particularly susceptible chromosome regions, such as those on chromosome 5q and 7q.

A review of 431 cases of secondary leukemia found 16 nonrandom chromosomal changes involving chromosomes 3, 5, 7, 8, 9, 11, 14, 17, and 21. These changes were dependent on the type of primary disease, previous therapy, age, and gender [64]. In another single-institution study consisting of 63 patients, additional abnormalities involving chromosomes 1, 4, 5, 7, 12, 14, and 18 occurred, with significantly increased frequency of these changes in t-AML as compared to *de novo* AML [34]. Abnormalities in chromosome 17, especially translocations involving bands 17p11-p13 and 17q21, occasionally are observed in t-AML, for example, t(15;17)(q22;q11–21) [65, 66]. Other chromosomes often reported to be abnormal in t-MDS/t-AML are chromosomes 21 and 11, particularly involving balanced translocations of chromosome bands 11q23 and 21q22 in t-AML [i.e., t(4;11), t(6;11), t(9;11), t(11;19), t(3;21), and t(8;21)] [52, 59, 63, 64]. These translocations are associated with previous therapy targeting DNA-topoisomerase II, primarily the epipodophyllotoxins and the anthracyclines. The 11q23 reciprocal translocations and interstitial deletions structurally interrupt a small region of the *MLL* (also known as *HRX, ALL-1, HTRX1*) gene that codes for a human homolog of the *Drosophila trithorax* gene [67, 68]. A fragment of the *MLL* gene translocates to more than 200 other chromosomal regions, resulting in the creation of a fusion protein with the partner gene [69].

The t(9;11) that results in a fusion between *MLL* and *AF9* is a recurring chromosomal translocation in *de novo* AML and is one of the most common recurring chromosome translocations detected in about 50% of t-AML patients who have a *MLL* translocation [70]. In addition, involvement of the *AF9* gene in the development of t-AML is linked to the treatment with topoisomerase inhibitors [6]. Interestingly, the unbalanced rearrangements of the same two bands, 11q23 and 21q22, were most often associated with therapy with alkylating agents alone or in combination with radiation therapy [59]. In Chinese patients treated for psoriasis with bimolane, t(15;17) has been frequently reported. Also, therapy with doxorubicin has been associated with an increased incidence of t-AML with balanced translocations at chromosome band 21q22, in particular t(3;21) [52, 64]. In addition to balanced translocations involving chromosome bands 11q23 and 21q22, other balanced aberrations such as inv (16), t(8;16), t(15;17), and t(6;9) have been observed in t-AML after previous therapy with drugs targeting DNA topoisomerase II (Table 22.2) [52, 63].

In a study of 491 t-MDS/t-AML patients with at least one balanced translocation, Rowley and Olney reported that 149 of the patients were positive for the 11q23 translocation (30.3%), followed by the 21q22 rearrangement seen in 15%, inv (16) in 9%, and t(15;17) in 8% of the patients [70]. Interestingly, no significant difference occurred in the gender distribution of patients within the subgroups, and patients in the 11q23 subgroup were of the youngest age at their primary and secondary diagnosis. Moreover, the translocation 11q23, inv (16), and t(15;17) subgroups had the shortest latency, with a median latency of 25.9 months for translocation 11q23, 22.0 months for inv (16), and 28.9 months for t(15;17) [70].

Table 22.2 Thirty-eight HSC gene signatures predicting development of t-MDS/AML

Thirty-eight genes differentially expressed in CD34+ HSC of t-MDS/AML patients
NR4A2, FOS, EGR1, CARD6, PEX11B, EGR3, EGR4, MRPL15, SLC7111, REEP1, FOSB, GOLGA5, ACTL6A,
GOLPH3L, CCDC99, SMAD7, SHMT2, LRPPRC, CDCA4, PDIA4, GOT1, RTN3, KLF2, JUN, STK17B, PSMC2,
LRBA, XPOT, ZYG11B, ZNF137, GEM, PGRMC2, ARL6IP6, SLC2A3P1, NR4A3, RGS2, NROP3, SLC26A2

Chromosome studies have shown that when t-MDS becomes clinically diagnosable, the preleukemic clone represents a majority of the hematopoietic cells [7, 34, 49]. Additional chromosomal abnormalities occur in the original abnormal clone in 60–70% of cases as the disease evolves to frank leukemia [71, 72]. Karyotypic evolution usually involves further deletions or losses of chromosomes and a change to a lower modal chromosome number; rarely, the evolution is associated with a gain of chromosome 8. Evidence suggests that t-MDS patients who have a mixture of karyotypically normal and abnormal cells (AN) survive longer than those who have only abnormal cells (AA) [73]. Most individuals who are AN in the preleukemic phase become AA as the disease progresses [34]. Notably, Rowley and Olney observed in their study that patients presenting with a t-MDS had significantly more frequent abnormalities of chromosomes 5 and/or 7 (49%) than did patients presenting with a t-AML (16%), and that this subgroup also presented with the highest percentage of complex karyotypes (45% vs. ca. 20% for both 1 and 2 aberrations) [70].

Genetics of Therapy-Related AML

Patients who develop t-AML may be predisposed to develop AML because of defects in DNA repair or increased susceptibility to accumulation of genetic mutations [74]. Candidate single-nucleotide polymorphisms associated with either drug metabolism or DNA repair enzymes have been identified as a mechanism by which a subset of t-AML may develop [75]. The commonly found germline variants in t-AML patients are *NQ01*, glutathione S-transferase family of enzymes, *BRCA1/2*, *TP53*, and *MDM2* [76–78]. Li-Fraumeni syndrome and Fanconi anemia also predispose to acute leukemia [79]. Tumor protein 53 (*TP53*), *RUNX1*, V-Ki-ras2 Kirsten rat sarcoma viral oncogene homolog (*KRAS*), and neuroblastoma RAS viral (v-ras) oncogene homolog (*NRAS*) mutations are known mutations in the development of t-MDS/AML [80].

To understand the pathogenetic mechanisms underlying t-MDS/AML, Li et al. performed a prospective case-control study with patients undergoing autologous hematopoietic stem cell transplant for lymphoma. In the study, gene expression in CD34+ hematopoietic stem and progenitor cells (HSC) from patients who developed t-MDS/AML after autologous hematopoietic cell transplantation (autoHSCT) for lymphoma ($n = 30$) was compared with gene expression in CD34+ cells of control group. The authors demonstrated that the expression pattern of 38 genes was different long before the development of t-MDS/AML in the case group, and that this gene signature was involved in mitochondrial function, metabolism, and hematopoietic regulation in peripheral blood stem cells (PBSC) that could distinguish patients who developed t-MDS/AML post-autoHSCT from those who did not [81].

Table 22.3 Mutational profiles of therapy-related acute myeloid leukemia versus *de novo* AML [82, 83]

Group	More frequent in t-AML	Similar frequency in t-AML and *de novo* AML	More frequent in *de novo* AML
Genes mutated	*TP53*, ATP-binding cassette subfamily genes, *PTPN11*	*STAG2, DNMT3A, NRAS, KRAS, IDH1, IDH2, U2AF1, KIT, KHD1, PKDL2, TET2, RUNX1*	*FLT3, NPM1*

Another study assessed the bone marrow or peripheral blood samples of 70 t-MDS/AML (including 42 t-AML) patients using a next-generation sequencing of 53 targeted genes. The mutation profile of t-AML was different from those of 428 *de novo* MDS/AML patients [82]. TP53 was mutated at a significantly higher rate in t-AML than *de novo* AML (35.7% vs. 12.8%, $p = 0.002$). *PTPN11* mutations were observed in 11.9% of t-AML patients compared with 2.1% in *de novo* AML patients ($p = 0.008$). Mutations of *NPM1* and *FLT3* only occurred in 2.5% and 7.1% of t-AML patients, respectively, which was significantly lower than *de novo* AML patients (21.7% and 16.4%, respectively) (Table 22.3). Analysis of clonal evolution showed that *TP53* mutation often occurs early in the pathogenesis of t-AML, and mutations of other genes may provide a further evolution to t-AML [83].

Lindsley et al. reported the genetics of 101 t-AML patients [84]. The goal of the study was to find a distinct mutation profile of t-AML compared with secondary or *de novo* AML with comprehensive sequencing. Samples obtained from patients prior to treatment were analyzed for mutations in 82 genes and the results were compared to the genetic profiles in The Cancer Genome Atlas of *de novo* AML. The comparative analysis demonstrated three mutually exclusive patterns of mutations that were noted in the t-AML cohort. The first group had *TP53* mutations. The second group had mutations which were commonly associated with secondary AML. These "secondary" mutations at cohort included spliceosome genes (*SRSF2, SF3B1, U2AF1, ZRSR2*), chromatin remodeling genes (*ASXL1, EZH2, BCOR*), and cohesion gene (*STAG2*). The third group included those with *de novo*-type mutations (*NPM1*, CBF rearrangements, and MLL rearrangements). However, the authors did not find unique genetic profiles, associated with chemotherapy exposure other than the established link between exposure to topoisomerase II inhibitors and MLL rearrangements. The CR rate for t-AML patients with *de novo*-type mutations was less than in *de novo* AML patients with the same mutations, but t-AML with secondary-type mutations or *TP53* mutations had remission rates similar to the older *de novo* AML group with the same "secondary"-type mutations. But the t-AML cohort required more cycles of induction therapy for CR. Taken together, prior chemotherapy exposure may not produce a unique "therapy-related" genetic profile, but genetic profiles may help predict outcomes of t-AML patients [84].

Next-generation sequencing could identify mutations in the leukemic transformation of Severe Congenital Neutropenia (SCN). Mutations in *CSF3R*-T618I, *RUNX1*, and *ASXL1* were found only in the MDS/AML phase of SCN [85]. Another study revealed that 64.5% of patients of the study population had mutations in *RUNX1* and the mutation occurred in clones with earlier acquired *CSF3R* mutations [86]. A sequential analysis at stages prior to leukemia development demonstrated that the *RUNX1* mutations are late events in the AML development of SCN. The other mutations associated with leukemic transformation were *ASXL1*, *SUZ12*, and *EP300* in less frequent rate.

Several groups have tried to identify the major genetic mutations in progression of MPN to AML by performing genotypic analyses of AML cells evolved from MPN [87–92]. The process of AML transformation is considered to arise from additional mutations outside of the JAK-STAT pathway, which is supported by the findings that the canonical *JAK2*V617F mutation has not been correlated with leukemic transformation. Furthermore, this mutation can be absent in the leukemic clone [93]. In these analyses, mutations affecting epigenetic regulators and transcriptional factors (*ASXL1, TET2, EZH2, IDH1/IDH2, IKZF1*), splicing factors (*SRSF2, SF3B1, ZRSR2, U2AF1*), and *TP53* mutations were frequently observed in MPN-AML cells compared to MPN cells. While only 1.9% of PV patients had an *IDH1/2* mutation, MPN-AML patients had a high frequency (21.6%) of this mutation [94]. Among 22 patients with post-MPN AML, 45.5% of the patients had a P53-related defect. In a study of 29 post-MPN AML samples (including 162 chronic-phase PV) using SNP arrays, changes of chromosomes 1q, 7q, 5q, 6p, 7p, 19q, 22q, and 3q were associated with post-MPN AML [88].

Clinical Presentation and Diagnosis

No specific clinical presentation demarks t-AML, but most patients have symptoms similar to patients with *de novo* AML including cytopenias (i.e., anemia, neutropenia, and thrombocytopenia) associated with easy fatigue, generalized malaise, infections, and/or hemorrhagic symptoms as easy bruising, nose/gingival bleeding, menorrhagia, or petechiae. Patients may have clinical manifestations of hepatomegaly, splenomegaly, lymphadenopathy, gingival hypertrophy, skin infiltration, and neurological abnormalities.

A preleukemic or myelodysplastic phase occurs in over 70% of patients in whom AML develops following chemotherapy and/or radiation therapy for another disease [7, 27, 49–51, 95–98], whereas about 20% of patients with *de novo*

AML have a similar preleukemic phase. Indeed, the data suggest that a preleukemic period can be observed in nearly all patients with t-AML, when these patients are monitored closely. Exceptions are those individuals in whom t-AML develops after therapy with epipodophyllotoxins (VP16 and VM26) or other DNA-topoisomerase II inhibitors. In these patients, t-AML often develops with no preleukemic phase [16, 17]. The mean duration of the preleukemic phase is 11.2 months in typical t-AML. The preleukemic phase in individuals with *de novo* MDS who go on to develop AML is similar, about 14 months (Table 22.1) [95, 96, 98].

Prodromal symptoms of the emergence of t-AML may be similar. However, when a patient who has received cytotoxic agents has these symptoms, the appropriate workup to rule out t-AML should be done. The diagnostic evaluation includes a comprehensive medical history and physical examination with detailed information of exposure to cytotoxic agents (time, duration, cumulative doses). In addition, patient's age, comorbidities, performance status, organ dysfunction, and remission status of the primary disease are important for establishing management plan. A detailed family history is essential to rule out hereditary cancer syndrome. Peripheral blood smear is an important laboratory test to rule out dysplastic changes in myeloid cells. Complete blood differential counts, and metabolic panel, as well as lactate dehydrogenase and uric acid level are required for initial laboratory tests. The diagnosis of t-AML is eventually made when evaluation of the peripheral blood and bone marrow demonstrates circulating myeloblasts in peripheral blood and/or more than 20% of myeloblasts in bone marrow. This may be buttressed by typical immunophenotypic and cytogenetic changes.

The clinical manifestation of the preleukemic phase of t-AML is marked by ineffective hematopoiesis. The bone marrow morphology is characterized by trilineage dysplasia. The degree of dysplasia is usually very prominent. Interestingly, the RAEB and RAEB-t subgroups are more frequently linked to t-MDS (73%) than in *de novo* MDS (53%) [99]. Prominent abnormalities are observed in the red blood cells and their precursors. Most patients show decreased red cell production with low reticulocyte counts [27]. Oval macrocytosis and nucleated red cells are often the earliest recognizable changes observed in the peripheral blood in the preleukemic phase [100]. Macrocytosis after therapy for Hodgkin's disease was retrospectively found to be associated with a high risk of the development of leukemia [101]. Mild neutropenia is present in 75% of the individuals [27]. Neutrophils may be poorly granulated, and their nuclei can be hyposegmented (pseudo-Pelger-Hüet anomaly) [102]. Thrombocytopenia occurs in approximately 60% of patients [27], and they may be abnormally large and degranulated. Both the neutrophils and platelets can have a variety of qualitative defects. The bone marrow is often hypercellular, although hypo- and normocellular marrow can occur. Erythroid hyperplasia, megaloblastoid features, and occasionally ringed sideroblasts dominate the marrow picture [102–104]. Abnormalities of the marrow granulocytic and megakaryocytic series are usually more subtle. Micromegakaryocytes may be seen, particularly with monosomy 7. The percentage of immature granulocytic and megakaryocytic cells may be increased. The primary and specific granules of the granulocyte precursors occasionally are either deficient or abnormally large. Marrow fibrosis often is present during the preleukemic phase.

In summary, the development of unexplained pancytopenia and the finding of karyotypic abnormalities in the marrow cells of patients who received chemotherapy and/or radiation therapy for another disease are pathognomonic of preleukemia. Evolution to overt leukemia is universal if the preleukemic individual survives the complications of hemorrhage and infection. T-MDS can be viewed as an early phase of t-AML in which the malignant hematopoietic clone is established and becomes predominant.

Clinical manifestations of individuals with t-AML are typical of bone marrow failure, and their clinical course is rapidly fatal often from complications of bleeding and infection. The bone marrow morphology of t-AML has been difficult to classify according to FAB criteria for AML, as most of the leukemias demonstrate trilineage involvement and appear to bridge several subtypes. Nevertheless, the blast cells of patients with t-AML most often are myeloblastic in appearance according to AML without maturation or AML with minimal differentiation in agreement with the 2008 WHO classification. A lower frequency of acute monocytic forms of leukemia has been reported in several studies as compared to *de novo* AML [7, 105].

Auer rods are rarely observed in the blast cells in t-AML, but are seen in blast cells of 35% of patients with *de novo* AML. Many of the blast cells in t-AML lack myeloperoxidase and other granulocyte-specific enzymes. In one series, only one of ten patients with secondary AML had more than 10% peroxidase-positive blast cells compared with nearly 100% peroxidase-positive blast cells in 95% of patients with *de novo* AML [105]. In addition, less than 20% of the t-AML patients have either greater than or equal to 10% naphthol ASD chloroacetate esterase-positive blast cells compared with 47% of patients with *de novo* AML. These histochemical data suggest that the leukemic cells from secondary leukemia patients are blocked at an earlier stage of differentiation than the leukemic cells from most *de novo* AML patients.

A patient may develop t-AML after cytotoxic treatment for a *de novo* myeloid neoplasm. T-AML secondary to *de novo* myeloid neoplasm may be identified by performing cytogenetic testing and immunophenotype evaluation at

Table 22.4 Initial evaluation of a therapy-related acute myelogenous leukemia

History and physical examination	History of cytotoxic agent: cumulative doses Disease status of primary cancer Performance status Family history of cancer
Complete blood cell count, differential count	
Review of peripheral blood smear	
Serum chemistries	Liver/kidney function, LDH, uric acid
Bone marrow aspirate and biopsy	Immunophenotyping and cytogenetic analysis
HLA typing	
Organ function tests	Echocardiogram/MUGA for ejection fraction Pulmonary function tests

apparent t-AML development and by comparing with those at the time of primary disease diagnosis. The emergence of a distinctly different karyotype suggests, but does not prove, a therapy-related AML, rather than recurrence of the original leukemic clone.

For patients with good performance status, information about siblings is useful for establishing a management plan. HLA typing of patient can be done on final diagnosis and the identification of potential stem cell donor is the first step for matched related donor allogeneic transplant. To evaluate reserved organ function, echocardiogram, and pulmonary function tests is also required. Computed tomography/MRI or PET imaging can give information about the status of primary disease (Table 22.4).

Treatment

Effective treatment options for t-AML are often not available. The efficacy of various therapeutic modalities of t-AML has been difficult to assess because the number of reported cases is small. In addition, data for t-AML have been reported together with secondary leukemias following other hematological disorders such as MPN or *de novo* MDS, making the evaluation difficult. Daunorubicin in combination with cytarabine remains the standard induction chemotherapy combination for patients with AML for the last decades. All studies to date have shown that response rates, and OS, are significantly lower in whole t-AML patients compared with *de novo* AML. Complete remission rates in t-AML patients are reported in 40% of patients with median survivals of 6–8 months [106]. The treatment of patients with t-AML is a clinical challenge for multiple reasons. The patients have a greater number of comorbidities, decreased organ reserve from previous therapy or primary disease, and a higher incidence of unfavorable cytogenetic changes. The key prognostic factors in t-AML are patient age, performance status, and karyotype.

For all t-AML patients, the performance status is the first determinant for establishing a treatment plan. All medically fit patients should have HLA typing at initial diagnosis. Supportive care would be appropriate for patients with a poor performance status (ECOG PS >2) at initial diagnosis. Various attempts to improve survival in these patients have failed to change the course of the disease, with deaths due to infection, bleeding, or progression of the acute leukemia. Supportive therapy is, therefore, an important aspect of the medical care of these patients. No significant differences in survival have been shown between those patients who received chemotherapy and supportive care and those who received supportive care alone. Thus, supportive therapy with transfusions of red blood cells and platelets for symptomatic anemia or bleeding complications, or both, is often necessary as well as the treatment with antibiotics for infections. The goal of therapy in these individuals should be to maintain an acceptable quality of life. Clearly, innovative and radically novel approaches to this syndrome are required if these patients are to be cured.

Studies have suggested that no significant differences exist in clinical outcome between the t-AML and *de novo* AML in the same cytogenetic group. The therapy-related AML with favorable cytogenetic findings, such as t(8;21), t(15;17), and inv. (16), have a complete response rate, essentially the same as *de novo* AML with the same karyotype [63, 107, 108]. Similarly, patients who have secondary AML with unfavorable cytogenetic findings such as deletion of chromosomes 5 or 7 do poorly, similar to *de novo* AML individuals with the same abnormality. Therefore, though more single or complex clonal cytogenetic abnormalities are found in t-AML patients than *de novo* AML patients [3], the prognostic significance of karyotype in t-AML is similar to that in *de novo* AML.

No single form of post-remission therapy has been shown to be superior for t-AML. Post-remission therapy with high-dose cytarabine probably is appropriate in patients with favorable cytogenetic findings except for those t-APL patients with t(15;17). In contrast, because of their extremely poor outcome, patients with unfavorable cytogenetic findings should be encouraged to enter clinical trials. As part of the discussion of treatment options, t-AML patients with an extremely poor prognosis should probably be offered the spectrum of treatments from supportive care alone to intensive chemotherapy either with or without allogeneic hematopoietic stem cell transplantation.

Therapy-Related AML Patients with Favorable Cytogenetics

Therapy-related AML is a heterogeneous disease and cytogenetic profile remains prognostically relevant. Patients with t-AML and favorable cytogenetics including t(15;17), inv.(16), t(16;16), and t(8;21) generally have superior outcomes among patients with t-AML.

A European study identified 106 cases of t-APL in patients who received cytotoxic chemotherapy for breast cancer, non-Hodgkin's lymphoma, and other solid tumors over a period of 10 years [109]. These t-APL patients had a short latency time (2–3 years), and exposure to topoisomerase II inhibitors or prior radiation therapy, and shared similar clinical characteristics with *de novo* APL [110, 111]. Yin et al. demonstrated frequent dyserythropoiesis, dysmegakaryopoiesis, FLT3 mutation (43%), and frequent additional cytogenetic abnormalities (60%) in their report of 17 t-APL patients [112]. Mounting evidence supports the practice of treating t-AML with t(15;17) as *de novo* disease, even when accompanied by other karyotype abnormalities [110]. They have a good response to all-trans retinoic acid (ATRA) therapy. Induction response rates appear to be equivalent to *de novo* APL, but induction death was more common and was attributed to impaired physiologic reserves from prior therapy. Therefore, t-APL is currently treated as *de novo* APL. With the use of ATRA and arsenic trioxide (ATO) in up-front therapy, anthracyclines can be eliminated for low-risk APL, which would be particularly beneficial for patients with t-APL who have had a prior anthracycline therapy for their primary malignancy [113].

T-AML with t(8;21) is not a common type of t-AML. A review article noted 26 cases and concluded that these patients had very similar hematological characteristics and treatment response as *de novo* AML with t(8;21) [63]. The 2002 international workshop studied 72 cases of t-AML with 21q22 (RUNX1) rearrangement and found that 44 of these cases were t(8;21) [114]. In the study, patients with t(8;21) rearrangement had a more favorable outcome than patients with other rearrangements involving 21q22. Gustafson et al. observed 13 patients with t-AML having t(8;21) karyotype in a single institute and compared them to 38 patients with *de novo* AML with t(8;21) and found that patients with therapy-related t(8;21) AML were older, and had a higher frequency of *KIT* 816D mutations, and an inferior OS than their *de novo* counterparts [115]. Krauth et al. showed high frequencies of additional cytogenetic and molecular lesions in AML with t(8;21) [116]. Mutations in RAS pathway, *KIT* and *ASXL1* mutations, were the most frequent additional mutations in the study, and mutations in *KIT* D816 and *ASXL1* were strongly associated with adverse outcomes. At the chromosomal level, −Y appeared to be associated with a good prognosis whereas trisomy 8 had an inferior prognosis. In a large series of t(8;21), 22 t-AML patients showed no differences in secondary molecular genetic events from 117 *de novo* AML [116]. However, a study showed that the treatment outcomes of t(8;21) t-AML were inferior to those of *de novo* t(8;21) AML, possibly because the t-AML cohort was older and some patients had active primary cancer.

T-AML with inv (16) was often associated with prior therapy with topoisomerase II inhibitors [117]. Response rates to intensive chemotherapy in this study were comparable to those with *de novo* disease. However, t-AML with inv (16) showed a significantly shorter event-free survival than *de novo* AML. In general, secondary chromosomal aberrations as well as gene mutations are very frequent in AML with inv (16); 80–90% patients with inv (16) AML have at least one mutation involving *NRAS, KRAS, KIT*, or *FLT* [118–120]. In the German-Austrian AML Study Group (AMLSG) study, 12 patients out of 176 cases (7%) were considered to be therapy related and the secondary chromosomal abnormalities/mutations were not significantly different from *de novo* AML [120], suggesting that the additional mutation is not the reason for shorter event-free survival in t-AML patients after intensive chemotherapy.

In summary, t-AML with favorable cytogenetics shows similar response rate to their *de novo* counterpart when receiving a conventional AML treatment. However, compared to *de novo* counterparts, t-AML with favorable cytogenetics is associated with an inferior survival. This may relate to several factors such as the status of primary disease, toxicity from prior therapy, and additional genetic mutations. Considering that additional mutations in t-AML patients with favorable karyotypes may result in poor prognosis, comprehensive genetic tests may confer an appropriate decision making, especially in patients cured of the primary malignancy and who are good candidates for allogeneic HSCT.

Non-transplant Therapeutic Options for t-AML

Few retrospective studies have evaluated the efficacy of standard chemotherapy for t-AML. The German AML Cooperative Group analyzed outcomes after remission induction chemotherapy for 1511 *de novo* AML and 121 t-AML patients [121]. The study demonstrated that the survival of unfavorable and intermediate cytogenetic risk groups of t-AML was similar with the same risk groups of *de novo* AML (6 months vs. 7 months for unfavorable, 12 months vs. 16 months for intermediate-risk group, respectively). Another study, the German–Austrian AL Study Group assessed the clinical outcomes of 200 t-AML patients treated between 1993 and 2008 [3]. The survival of t-AML patients was compared with 2653 *de novo* AML patients. Although response rates to induction chemotherapy were similar, OS for t-AML patients was inferior to *de novo* AML patients.

In further analysis, patients less than 60 years old showed similar relapse rates, but their death in CR was greater, suggesting the higher toxicity of induction and post-remission therapy in this cohort. Patients older than 60 years had higher relapse rates, possibly due to lower intensity treatments, resulting in inferior survival. A retrospective study of 118 t-AML after treatment of breast cancer showed no significant difference in median OS compared with *de novo* AML (8.7 months vs. 10.2 months; $p = 0.17$) [122]. Multivariate analysis revealed cytogenetics, baseline white blood cell counts, age, and performance status as predictive factors for OS of t-AML patients.

In a prospective study of t-MDS/AML, 32 t-MDS/AML patients were treated with high-dose cytarabine and mitoxantrone induction followed by hematopoietic stem cell transplant [101]. A remarkable complete response rate of 66% was achieved. Thirteen patients who achieved CR were eventually treated with AlloHSCT for consolidation and the survival of the patients was 29% in 3 years. These studies show that patients with t-AML can achieve a comparable response with standard induction chemotherapy, and that cumulative toxicity/reserved function from prior therapy limit tolerance to induction and post-remission therapy.

T-AML patients have a higher risk of organ dysfunction due to chemotherapy and radiation-induced parenchymal and vascular toxicity, or primary malignancy. Even those with seemingly adequate organ reserves may have increased toxicity during t-AML therapy. Therefore, earlier diagnosis and treatment with less toxic therapy, while aggressively exploring transplant options, may be another critical factor in the trial of new therapeutics for t-AML. Emerging therapeutics in this area has focused on several approaches. These include novel delivery of chemotherapy as well as newer DNA-damaging agents delivered through antibody-drug conjugates, use of hypomethylating agents, and molecularly directed small molecules against specific mutations commonly occurring in t-AML.

CPX-351 is a liposomal formulation of daunorubicin and cytarabine at a fixed ratio of 5:1. The combination of these medications was developed based on in vitro data that demonstrated a synergistic effect of these two agents at the 5:1 ratio [123]. In a randomized phase II trial, CPX-351 was compared with standard daunorubicin/cytarabine in untreated patients older than the age of 60 years [124]. In a subset of secondary AML patients ($n = 52$), which included t-AML and AML evolving from myelodysplastic syndrome, patients treated with CPX-351 demonstrated a better OS (hazard ratio = 0.46, $p = 0.01$) at 24 months. Though the recovery from cytopenias was slower after CPX-351, the infection-related deaths (3.5% vs. 7.3%) or 60-day mortality (4.7% vs. 14.6%) was less than the conventional daunorubicin/cytarabine chemotherapy group. These data suggested a clinical benefit with CPX-351 in t-AML with better efficacy and tolerability.

A second approach to improving cytotoxic therapy for AML takes advantage of newer antibody-drug conjugate (ADC) technology. CD33 is a surface receptor found on more than 95% of AML cells except acute megakaryocytic leukemia. It has been a target for antibody-directed therapy. The treatment with a conjugated antibody targeting CD33 (gemtuzumab ozogamicin) as a single agent [125], and in combination with chemotherapy in untreated patients and those with relapsed AML, demonstrated clinical efficacy [126]. However, gemtuzumab ozogamicin failed to show the effectiveness in combination with standard daunorubicin/cytarabine regimen in high-risk AML patients [127]. A new ADC targeting CD33, SGN-CD33A, was developed using a novel antibody drug linkage system to a fully humanized anti-CD33 antibody. In contrast to gemtuzumab ozogamicin, SGN-CD33A exhibited a potent cytotoxicity against p53-mutated AML cells and leukemic cells with multidrug resistance-mediated drug efflux phenotypes in preclinical studies [128]. Therefore, careful clinical trials with this monoclonal antibody conjugate are appropriate for t-AML patients.

Since many cases of t-AML evolved from a preleukemic phase after being exposed to chemotherapeutics/radiation, hypomethylating agents have been evaluated as an alternative to traditional induction therapy [129]. Both azacitidine and decitabine are effective and well tolerated but the efficacy compared with cytotoxic chemotherapy is still under investigation. In a retrospective study conducted by Quintas-Cardama et al., 671 AML patients, older than 65 years, were treated with a hypomethylating agent and had a similar median survival rates with cytotoxic chemotherapy (6.5 months with hypomethylating agent and 6.7 months with chemotherapy, respectively) [130]. Moreover, a similar CR rate was observed in the subset of poor-risk cytogenetics patients carrying −5 and/or −7 (26% with hypomethylating agent vs. 28% with chemotherapy). Another retrospective study of 48 t-MDS/AML patients treated with hypomethylating agent showed 42% overall response rate including a complete response rate of 21% in a subset of patients with favorable cytogenetics, which is comparable with prospective hypomethylating agent studies for t-MDS group [131]. A phase 2 clinical trial, E1905 North American Leukemia Intergroup, studied 47 patients including 18 t-AML patients. A good response to azacitidine occurred with 46% complete hematologic response and 13 months of median OS [132]. Multivariate analyses comparing the t-MN patient with *de novo* MDS/AML patients treated with the same protocol showed no significant difference in complete hematologic response rate, and overall response rate between the two groups. However, another study of 54 t-MN patients (including 12 t-AML patients) treated with azacitidine demonstrated shorter 2-year OS (14%) compared with *de novo* MDS/AML patients (33.9%), though multivariate analysis showed that the survival was dependent on cytogenetic changes, not etiology of the AML [133].

Hypomethylating agents are frequently prescribed as an alternative to traditional AML induction chemotherapy for frail patients. They can support *de novo* and t-MDS/AML patients in order to receive a transplantation with less toxicity, and may be a safer option for low-blast-count t-AML. Response rates were equivalent to standard AML induction therapy in this population [131, 134], enhancing the likelihood of successful transplantations. A new hypomethylating agent, SGI-110, a metabolite of decitabine, is in clinical trials for treatment of MDS and AML [135].

An additional epigenetic modulator is the class of histone deacetylation (HDAC) inhibitors. They are often included in a combination regimen with a hypomethylating agent for MDS and AML patients. Valproic acid, vorinostat, pracinostat, and mocetinostat are the HDAC inhibitors being used in clinical trials in combination with hypomethylating agents [136–139].

P53 mutations and *MLL* rearrangements often occur in t-AML [140, 141]. Two agents targeting these mutations are in the drug pipeline. EPZ-5676 is a potent inhibitor of Dot1L, a histone methyl transferase which interacts with MLL oncogenic fusion protein products. In cell lines and in rat xenograft studies, EPZ-5676 significantly caused cell death and regression of MLL-rearranged leukemias [142]. It is currently in clinical trial in pediatric leukemias with MLL translocations.

Volasertib is an inhibitor of polo-like kinase (PLK). Preclinical studies demonstrated that p53-mutated cancer cells were more susceptible to PLK inhibition than p53 wild-type cancer cells [143]. In a randomized phase 2 study in untreated elderly patients with AML, volasertib, in combination with low-dose cytarabine, demonstrated a higher remission rate and improved survival compared with cytarabine alone, although median survival rates were still <1 year [144].

Hematopoietic Stem Cell Transplant for t-AML

Treatment of t-AML with conventional therapy is associated with a poor outcome. Response rate for t-AML induction therapy appears to be roughly equivalent to *de novo* AML when compared within their respective intermediate- and unfavorable-risk cytogenetic categories, but the responses on average are less durable, thereby justifying the use of transplantation in these patients.

A retrospective study of 545 t-AML patients transplanted between 1990 and 2004 found an OS of 22% at 5 years [145]. Inferior outcomes were associated with age greater than 35 years, poor-risk cytogenetics, uncontrolled disease, and use of a non-sibling-related or mismatched unrelated donor. Use of reduced-intensity chemotherapy (RIC) regimens did not decrease treatment-related mortality (TRM), which approached 50% at 5 years, but many of these patients had received a prior autologous transplant.

The European Group for Blood and Marrow Transplantation Group also reported on 461 t-MDS/AML patients, and noted an adverse impact of abnormal cytogenetics, age greater than 40 years, and uncontrolled disease [146]. Three-year relapse-free survival and OS rates were 33% and 35%, respectively. In contrast, a study of 24 breast cancer t-MN patients who underwent allogeneic stem cell transplantation for consolidation had nearly identical clinical results as female *de novo* MDS/AML patients regardless of cytogenetics [147]. In general, these studies show that transplantation can be used successfully in a fraction of t-AML patients, but it is clearly less effective than when used for *de novo* AML patients. A busulfan/cyclophosphamide conditioning regimen appears to offer one of the best 5-year relapse-free survival (43%) and lowest non-relapse mortality (28%). Relapse rates are lower with unrelated donor transplants [145, 146, 148]. After accounting for cytogenetic classification, t-AML patients have a similar outcome as *de novo* AML [149].

The Italian Network reported survival for transplant recipients of 58.8 months compared with 12.1 months for the non-transplant cohort [150]. A similar benefit was seen when the German Hodgkin Study Group reported clinical outcomes of 106 patients with t-MN after therapy for Hodgkin's lymphoma. Although the non-transplant median survival was dismal (7.2 months), the median survival for the transplanted t-MN had not been reached after a median follow-up of 41 months [151]. The survival of the patients after hematopoietic stem cell transplant at 2 years was 47% vs. 15% for the non-transplant group ($p = 0.03$). Although alloHSCT can provide a chance of long-term survival and cure in selected subgroups of patients with t-AML, major limitations of alloHSCT are availability of a donor and patients' age. Alternative treatment strategies including haploidentical donor alloHSCT or nonmyeloablative HSCT, especially for older patients, should be explored for t-AML patients.

Conclusion

Therapy-related AML (t-AML) is a recognizable subgroup of AML. Alkylating agents used in primary diseases are the most frequent etiology of t-AML. The disease arises from a series of mutations in hematopoietic stem cells, and these DNA changes provide a growth advantage to the progeny of the transformed cells. The abnormal clone of cells usually has a hypodiploid modal number of chromosomes and a deletion of part or all of chromosome 5 and/or 7. T-AML remains one of the most difficult subtypes of AML to treat. Once a patient who was treated with cytotoxic agents develops cytopenias, hematopoietic cell morphologic examination, immunophenotying, and cytogenetics should be done to detect t-AML in its early phase. The patients with t-AML have more comorbidities, decreased organ reserve, and a higher incidence of unfavorable cytogenetic phenotype than *de novo* AML. The key prognostic factors in t-AML are patient age, performance status, and karyotype. As *de novo* AML, t-AML patients can be stratified based on genetics. The performance status is the first determinant for establishing a treatment plan. Supportive care at initial diagnosis would be appropriate for patients with a poor performance status (ECOG PS >2). All medically fit patients should have HLA typing at initial diagnosis. The conventional cytotoxic chemotherapy or hypomethylating agents are being used as an initial therapy. For patients in complete remission, allogeneic transplantation is the best therapeutic modality for long-term survival for the younger patients. Emerging therapeutics for AML has focused on reduced toxicity, higher efficacy, and specificity. These include novel delivery of chemotherapy in liposome as well as newer DNA-damaging agents delivered through antibody-drug conjugates, use of hypomethylating agents, and molecularly directed small molecules against specific mutations commonly occurring in t-AML.

Acknowledgments H.C.S. is supported by John C. Hall Memorial Research Grant of Tower Cancer Research Foundation. H.P.K. is the holder of the Mark Goodson endowed Chair in Oncology Research at Cedars Sinai and a member of the Jonsson Comprehensive Cancer Center and Molecular Biology Institute at UCLA, as well as the Cancer Science Institute of Singapore, and is supported by the A*STaR award from the National University of Singapore and NIH RO-1 grant.

References

1. Vardiman JW, Thiele J, Arber DA, Brunning RD, Borowitz MJ, Porwit A, et al. The 2008 revision of the World Health Organization (WHO) classification of myeloid neoplasms and acute leukemia: rationale and important changes. Blood. 2009;114(5):937–51. PubMed PMID: 19357394
2. Smith SM, Le Beau MM, Huo D, Karrison T, Sobecks RM, Anastasi J, et al. Clinical-cytogenetic associations in 306 patients with therapy-related myelodysplasia and myeloid leukemia: the University of Chicago series. Blood. 2003;102(1):43–52. PubMed PMID: 12623843
3. Kayser S, Dohner K, Krauter J, Kohne CH, Horst HA, Held G, et al. The impact of therapy-related acute myeloid leukemia (AML) on outcome in 2853 adult patients with newly diagnosed AML. Blood. 2011;17(7):2137–45. PubMed PMID: 21127174
4. Le Deley MC, Suzan F, Cutuli B, Delaloge S, Shamsaldin A, Linassier C, et al. Anthracyclines, mitoxantrone, radiotherapy, and granulocyte colony-stimulating factor: risk factors for leukemia and myelodysplastic syndrome after breast cancer. J Clin Oncol. 2007;25(3):292–300. PubMed PMID: 17159192
5. Smith RE, Bryant J, DeCillis A, Anderson S, National Surgical Adjuvant B, Bowel Project E. Acute myeloid leukemia and myelodysplastic syndrome after doxorubicin-cyclophosphamide adjuvant therapy for operable breast cancer: the National Surgical Adjuvant Breast and Bowel Project Experience. J Clin Oncol. 2003;21(7):1195–204. PubMed PMID: 12663705
6. Allan JM, Travis LB. Mechanisms of therapy-related carcinogenesis. Nat Rev Cancer. 2005;5(12):943–55. PubMed PMID: 16294218
7. Rowley JD, Golomb HM, Vardiman JW. Nonrandom chromosome abnormalities in acute leukemia and dysmyelopoietic syndromes in patients with previously treated malignant disease. Blood. 1981;58(4):759–67. PubMed PMID: 7272506
8. Traweek ST, Slovak ML, Nademanee AP, Brynes RK, Niland JC, Forman SJ. Clonal karyotypic hematopoietic cell abnormalities occurring after autologous bone marrow transplantation for Hodgkin's disease and non-Hodgkin's lymphoma. Blood. 1994;84(3):957–63. PubMed PMID: 8043877
9. Kantarjian HM, Keating MJ, Walters RS, Smith TL, Cork A, McCredie KB, et al. Therapy-related leukemia and myelodysplastic syndrome: clinical, cytogenetic, and prognostic features. J Clin Oncol. 1986;4(12):1748–57. PubMed PMID: 3783201
10. Gundestrup M, Klarskov Andersen M, Sveinbjornsdottir E, Rafnsson V, Storm HH, Pedersen-Bjergaard J. Cytogenetics of myelodysplasia and acute myeloid leukaemia in aircrew and people treated with radiotherapy. Lancet. 2000;356(9248):2158. PubMed PMID: 11191547
11. Pedersen-Bjergaard J. Insights into leukemogenesis from therapy-related leukemia. N Engl J Med. 2005;352(15):1591–4. PubMed PMID: 15829541
12. Tebbi CK, London WB, Friedman D, Villaluna D, De Alarcon PA, Constine LS, et al. Dexrazoxane-associated risk for acute myeloid leukemia/myelodysplastic syndrome and other secondary malignancies in pediatric Hodgkin's disease. J Clin Oncol. 2007;25(5):493–500. PubMed PMID: 17290056
13. Pui CH, Relling MV. Topoisomerase II inhibitor-related acute myeloid leukaemia. Br J Haematol. 2000;109(1):13–23. PubMed PMID: 10848777
14. Casciato DA, Scott JL. Acute leukemia following prolonged cytotoxic agent therapy. Medicine. 1979;58(1):32–47. PubMed PMID: 105227
15. Greene MH, Harris EL, Gershenson DM, Malkasian GD Jr, Melton LJ 3rd, Dembo AJ, et al. Melphalan may be a more potent leukemogen than cyclophosphamide. Ann Intern Med. 1986;105(3):360–7. PubMed PMID: 3740675
16. Pui CH, Behm FG, Raimondi SC, Dodge RK, George SL, Rivera GK, et al. Secondary acute myeloid leukemia in children treated for acute lymphoid leukemia. N Engl J Med. 1989;321(3):136–42. PubMed PMID: 2787477
17. Ratain MJ, Kaminer LS, Bitran JD, Larson RA, Le Beau MM, Skosey C, et al. Acute nonlymphocytic leukemia following etoposide and cisplatin combination chemotherapy for advanced non-small-cell carcinoma of the lung. Blood. 1987;70(5):1412–7. PubMed PMID: 2822173
18. Berk PD, Goldberg JD, Donovan PB, Fruchtman SM, Berlin NI, Wasserman LR. Therapeutic recommendations in polycythemia Vera based on polycythemia Vera Study Group protocols. Semin Hematol. 1986;23(2):132–43. PubMed PMID: 3704665
19. Finazzi G, Caruso V, Marchioli R, Capnist G, Chisesi T, Finelli C, et al. Acute leukemia in polycythemia vera: an analysis of 1638 patients enrolled in a prospective observational study. Blood. 2005;105(7):2664–70. PubMed PMID: 15585653
20. Najean Y, Rain JD. Treatment of polycythemia vera: use of 32P alone or in combination with maintenance therapy using hydroxyurea in 461 patients greater than 65 years of age. The French Polycythemia Study Group. Blood. 1997;89(7):2319–27. PubMed PMID: 9116275
21. Bjorkholm M, Derolf AR, Hultcrantz M, Kristinsson SY, Ekstrand C, Goldin LR, et al. Treatment-related risk factors for transformation to acute myeloid leukemia and myelodysplastic syndromes in myeloproliferative neoplasms. J Clin Oncol. 2011;29(17):2410–5. PubMed PMID: 21537037. Pubmed Central PMCID: 3107755
22. Bizzozero OJ Jr, Johnson KG, Ciocco A. Radiation-related leukemia in Hiroshima and Nagasaki, 1946–1964. I. Distribution, incidence and appearance time. N Engl J Med. 1966;274(20):1095–101. PubMed PMID: 5932020

23. Ginevan ME. Nonlymphatic leukemias and adult exposure to diagnostic X-rays: the evidence reconsidered. Health Phys. 1980;38(2):129–38. PubMed PMID: 7372480
24. Seed TM, Tolle DV, Fritz TE, Devine RL, Poole CM, Norris WP. Irradiation-induced erythroleukemia and myelogenous leukemia in the beagle dog: hematology and ultrastructure. Blood. 1977;50(6):1061–79. PubMed PMID: 270374
25. Coltman CA Jr, Dixon DO. Second malignancies complicating Hodgkin's disease: a Southwest Oncology Group 10-year followup. Cancer Treat Rep. 1982;66(4):1023–33. PubMed PMID: 7074630
26. Nardi V, Winkfield KM, Ok CY, Niemierko A, Kluk MJ, Attar EC, et al. Acute myeloid leukemia and myelodysplastic syndromes after radiation therapy are similar to *de novo* disease and differ from other therapy-related myeloid neoplasms. J Clin Oncol. 2012;30(19):2340–7. PubMed PMID: 22585703
27. Pedersen-Bjergaard J, Philip P, Mortensen BT, Ersboll J, Jensen G, Panduro J, et al. Acute nonlymphocytic leukemia, preleukemia, and acute myeloproliferative syndrome secondary to treatment of other malignant diseases. Clinical and cytogenetic characteristics and results of in vitro culture of bone marrow and HLA typing. Blood. 1981;57(4):712–23. PubMed PMID: 7470622
28. Cadman EC, Capizzi RL, Bertino JR. Acute nonlymphocytic leukemia: a delayed complication of Hodgkin's disease therapy: analysis of 109 cases. Cancer. 1977;40(3):1280–96. PubMed PMID: 409479
29. Coleman CN, Williams CJ, Flint A, Glatstein EJ, Rosenberg SA, Kaplan HS. Hematologic neoplasia in patients treated for Hodgkin's disease. N Engl J Med. 1977;297(23):1249–52. PubMed PMID: 917069
30. Valagussa P, Santoro A, Fossati Bellani F, Franchi F, Banfi A, Bonadonna G. Absence of treatment-induced second neoplasms after ABVD in Hodgkin's disease. Blood. 1982;59(3):488–94. PubMed PMID: 6174160
31. Pedersen-Bjergaard J, Larsen SO. Incidence of acute nonlymphocytic leukemia, preleukemia, and acute myeloproliferative syndrome up to 10 years after treatment of Hodgkin's disease. N Engl J Med. 1982;307(16):965–71. PubMed PMID: 7110299
32. Greene MH, Boice JD Jr, Greer BE, Blessing JA, Dembo AJ. Acute nonlymphocytic leukemia after therapy with alkylating agents for ovarian cancer: a study of five randomized clinical trials. N Engl J Med. 1982;307(23):1416–21. PubMed PMID: 6752720
33. De Braekeleer M. Cytogenetic studies in secondary leukemia: statistical analysis. Oncology. 1986;43(6):358–63. PubMed PMID: 3808568
34. Le Beau MM, Albain KS, Larson RA, Vardiman JW, Davis EM, Blough RR, et al. Clinical and cytogenetic correlations in 63 patients with therapy-related myelodysplastic syndromes and acute nonlymphocytic leukemia: further evidence for characteristic abnormalities of chromosomes no. 5 and 7. J Clin Oncol. 1986;4(3):325–45. PubMed PMID: 3950675
35. Wright JD, St Clair CM, Deutsch I, Burke WM, Gorrochurn P, Sun X, et al. Pelvic radiotherapy and the risk of secondary leukemia and multiple myeloma. Cancer. 2010;116(10):2486–92. PubMed PMID: 20209618
36. Sawka AM, Thabane L, Parlea L, Ibrahim-Zada I, Tsang RW, Brierley JD, et al. Second primary malignancy risk after radioactive iodine treatment for thyroid cancer: a systematic review and meta-analysis. Thyroid. 2009;19(5):451–7. PubMed PMID: 19281429
37. Dohner H, Estey EH, Amadori S, Appelbaum FR, Buchner T, Burnett AK, et al. Diagnosis and management of acute myeloid leukemia in adults: recommendations from an international expert panel, on behalf of the European LeukemiaNet. Blood. 2010;115(3):453–74. PubMed PMID: 19880497
38. Lyman GH, Dale DC, Wolff DA, Culakova E, Poniewierski MS, Kuderer NM, et al. Acute myeloid leukemia or myelodysplastic syndrome in randomized controlled clinical trials of cancer chemotherapy with granulocyte colony-stimulating factor: a systematic review. J Clin Oncol. 2010;28(17):2914–24. PubMed PMID: 20385991
39. Rosenberg PS, Alter BP, Bolyard AA, Bonilla MA, Boxer LA, Cham B, et al. The incidence of leukemia and mortality from sepsis in patients with severe congenital neutropenia receiving long-term G-CSF therapy. Blood. 2006;107(12):4628–35. PubMed PMID: 16497969. Pubmed Central PMCID: 1895804
40. Rosenberg PS, Zeidler C, Bolyard AA, Alter BP, Bonilla MA, Boxer LA, et al. Stable long-term risk of leukaemia in patients with severe congenital neutropenia maintained on G-CSF therapy. Br J Haematol. 2010;150(2):196–9. PubMed PMID: 20456363. Pubmed Central PMCID: 2906693
41. Anderson LA, Pfeiffer RM, Landgren O, Gadalla S, Berndt SI, Engels EA. Risks of myeloid malignancies in patients with autoimmune conditions. Br J Cancer. 2009;100(5):822–8. PubMed PMID: 19259097. Pubmed Central PMCID: 2653768
42. Kristinsson SY, Bjorkholm M, Hultcrantz M, Derolf AR, Landgren O, Goldin LR. Chronic immune stimulation might act as a trigger for the development of acute myeloid leukemia or myelodysplastic syndromes. J Clin Oncol. 2011;29(21):2897–903. PubMed PMID: 21690473. Pubmed Central PMCID: 3138717
43. Bernatsky S, Clarke AE, Suissa S. Hematologic malignant neoplasms after drug exposure in rheumatoid arthritis. Arch Intern Med. 2008;168(4):378–81. PubMed PMID: 18299492
44. Ramkumar B, Chadha MK, Barcos M, Sait SN, Heyman MR, Baer MR. Acute promyelocytic leukemia after mitoxantrone therapy for multiple sclerosis. Cancer Genet Cytogenet. 2008;182(2):126–9. PubMed PMID: 18406875
45. Ammatuna E, Montesinos P, Hasan SK, Ramadan SM, Esteve J, Hubmann M, et al. Presenting features and treatment outcome of acute promyelocytic leukemia arising after multiple sclerosis. Haematologica. 2011;96(4):621–5. PubMed PMID: 21193421. Pubmed Central PMCID: 3069242
46. Leleu X, Soumerai J, Roccaro A, Hatjiharissi E, Hunter ZR, Manning R, et al. Increased incidence of transformation and myelodysplasia/acute leukemia in patients with Waldenstrom macroglobulinemia treated with nucleoside analogs. J Clin Oncol. 2009;27(2):250–5. PubMed PMID: 19064987
47. Coso D, Costello R, Cohen-Valensi R, Sainty D, Nezri M, Gastaut JA, et al. Acute myeloid leukemia and myelodysplasia in patients with chronic lymphocytic leukemia receiving fludarabine as initial therapy. Ann Oncol. 1999;10(3):362–3. PubMed PMID: 10355587
48. Morrison VA, Rai KR, Peterson BL, Kolitz JE, Elias L, Appelbaum FR, et al. Therapy-related myeloid leukemias are observed in patients with chronic lymphocytic leukemia after treatment with fludarabine and chlorambucil: results of an intergroup study, cancer and leukemia group B 9011. J Clin Oncol. 2002;20(18):3878–84. PubMed PMID: 12228208
49. Anderson RL, Bagby GC Jr, Richert-Boe K, Magenis RE, Koler RD. Therapy-related preleukemic syndrome. Cancer. 1981;47(7):1867–71. PubMed PMID: 7226081
50. Kapadia SB, Krause JR, Ellis LD, Pan SF, Wald N. Induced acute non-lymphocytic leukemia following long-term chemotherapy: a study of 20 cases. Cancer. 1980;45(6):1315–21. PubMed PMID: 6928396
51. Papa G, Alimena G, Annino L, Anselmo AP, Ciccone F, De Luca AM, et al. Acute non lymphoid leukaemia following Hodgkin's disease. Clinical, biological and cytogenetic aspects of 3 cases. Scand J Haematol. 1979;23(4):339–47. PubMed PMID: 295150
52. Pedersen-Bjergaard J, Rowley JD. The balanced and the unbalanced chromosome aberrations of acute myeloid leukemia may develop in different ways and may contribute differently to malignant transformation. Blood. 1994;83(10):2780–6. PubMed PMID: 8180374

53. Chromosomes in acute non-lymphocytic leukaemia. First International Workshop on Chromosomes in Leukaemia. Br J Haematol. 1978;39(3):311–6. PubMed PMID: 698112
54. Le Beau MM, Espinosa R 3rd, Neuman WL, Stock W, Roulston D, Larson RA, et al. Cytogenetic and molecular delineation of the smallest commonly deleted region of chromosome 5 in malignant myeloid diseases. Proc Natl Acad Sci U S A. 1993;90(12):5484–8. PubMed PMID: 8516290. Pubmed Central PMCID: 46745
55. Le Beau MM, Epstein ND, O'Brien SJ, Nienhuis AW, Yang YC, Clark SC, et al. The interleukin 3 gene is located on human chromosome 5 and is deleted in myeloid leukemias with a deletion of 5q. Proc Natl Acad Sci U S A. 1987;84(16):5913–7. PubMed PMID: 3497400. Pubmed Central PMCID: 298973
56. Le Beau MM, Lemons RS, Espinosa R 3rd, Larson RA, Arai N, Rowley JD. Interleukin-4 and interleukin-5 map to human chromosome 5 in a region encoding growth factors and receptors and are deleted in myeloid leukemias with a del(5q). Blood. 1989;73(3):647–50. PubMed PMID: 2783863
57. Nienhuis AW, Bunn HF, Turner PH, Gopal TV, Nash WG, O'Brien SJ, et al. Expression of the human c-fms proto-oncogene in hematopoietic cells and its deletion in the 5q- syndrome. Cell. 1985;42(2):421–8. PubMed PMID: 4028159
58. Le Beau MM, Westbrook CA, Diaz MO, Larson RA, Rowley JD, Gasson JC, et al. Evidence for the involvement of GM-CSF and FMS in the deletion (5q) in myeloid disorders. Science. 1986;231(4741):984–7. PubMed PMID: 3484837
59. Levine EG, Bloomfield CD. Leukemias and myelodysplastic syndromes secondary to drug, radiation, and environmental exposure. Semin Oncol. 1992;19(1):47–84. PubMed PMID: 1736370
60. List AF, Jacobs A. Biology and pathogenesis of the myelodysplastic syndromes. Semin Oncol. 1992;19(1):14–24. PubMed PMID: 1736366
61. Tsui LC, Farrall M, Donis-Keller H. Report of the committee on the genetic constitution of chromosomes 7 and 8. Cytogenet Cell Genet. 1989;51(1–4):166–201. PubMed PMID: 2676369
62. Kere J, Donis-Keller H, Ruutu T, de la Chapelle A. Chromosome 7 long-arm deletions in myeloid disorders: terminal DNA sequences are commonly conserved and breakpoints vary. Cytogenet Cell Genet. 1989;50(4):226–9. PubMed PMID: 2805820
63. Quesnel B, Kantarjian H, Bjergaard JP, Brault P, Estey E, Lai JL, et al. Therapy-related acute myeloid leukemia with t(8;21), inv (16), and t(8;16): a report on 25 cases and review of the literature. J Clin Oncol. 1993;11(12):2370–9. PubMed PMID: 8246025
64. Pedersen-Bjergaard J, Johansson B, Philip P. Translocation (3;21)(q26;q22) in therapy-related myelodysplasia following drugs targeting DNA-topoisomerase II combined with alkylating agents, and in myeloproliferative disorders undergoing spontaneous leukemic transformation. Cancer Genet Cytogenet. 1994;76(1):50–5. PubMed PMID: 8076352
65. Pedersen-Bjergaard J, Philip P, Larsen SO, Jensen G, Byrsting K. Chromosome aberrations and prognostic factors in therapy-related myelodysplasia and acute nonlymphocytic leukemia. Blood. 1990;76(6):1083–91. PubMed PMID: 2400804
66. Johansson B, Mertens F, Heim S, Kristoffersson U, Mitelman F. Cytogenetics of secondary myelodysplasia (sMDS) and acute nonlymphocytic leukemia (sANLL). Eur J Haematol. 1991;47(1):17–27. PubMed PMID: 1868912
67. Cimino G, Moir DT, Canaani O, Williams K, Crist WM, Katzav S, et al. Cloning of ALL-1, the locus involved in leukemias with the t(4;11)(q21;q23), t(9;11)(p22;q23), and t(11;19)(q23;p13) chromosome translocations. Cancer Res. 1991;51(24):6712–4. PubMed PMID: 1835902
68. Ziemin-van der Poel S, NR MC, Gill HJ, Espinosa R 3rd, Patel Y, Harden A, et al. Identification of a gene, MLL, that spans the breakpoint in 11q23 translocations associated with human leukemias. Proc Natl Acad Sci U S A. 1991;88(23):10735–9. PubMed PMID: 1720549. Pubmed Central PMCID: 53005
69. Marschalek R. Systematic classification of mixed-lineage leukemia fusion partners predicts additional cancer pathways. Ann Lab Med. 2016;36(2):85–100. PubMed PMID: 26709255. Pubmed Central PMCID: 4713862
70. Rowley JD, Olney HJ. International workshop on the relationship of prior therapy to balanced chromosome aberrations in therapy-related myelodysplastic syndromes and acute leukemia: overview report. Genes Chromosomes Cancer. 2002;33(4):331–45. PubMed PMID: 11921269
71. Baccarani M, Bosi A, Papa G. Second malignancy in patients treated by Hodgkin's disease. Cancer. 1980;46(8):1735–40. PubMed PMID: 6932997
72. Bernstein ML, Vekemans MJ. Chromosomal changes in secondary leukemias of childhood and young adulthood. Crit Rev Oncol Hematol. 1986;5(4):325–60. PubMed PMID: 3533293
73. Aksoy M, Erdem S. Followup study on the mortality and the development of leukemia in 44 pancytopenic patients with chronic exposure to benzene. Blood. 1978;52(2):285–92. PubMed PMID: 667356
74. Seedhouse C, Faulkner R, Ashraf N, Das-Gupta E, Russell N. Polymorphisms in genes involved in homologous recombination repair interact to increase the risk of developing acute myeloid leukemia. Clin Cancer Res. 2004;10(8):2675–80. PubMed PMID: 15102670
75. Knight JA, Skol AD, Shinde A, Hastings D, Walgren RA, Shao J, et al. Genome-wide association study to identify novel loci associated with therapy-related myeloid leukemia susceptibility. Blood. 2009;113(22):5575–82. PubMed PMID: 19299336. Pubmed Central PMCID: 2689055
76. Larson RA, Wang Y, Banerjee M, Wiemels J, Hartford C, Le Beau MM, et al. Prevalence of the inactivating 609C-->T polymorphism in the NAD(P)H:quinone oxidoreductase (NQO1) gene in patients with primary and therapy-related myeloid leukemia. Blood. 1999;94(2):803–7. PubMed PMID: 10397748
77. Allan JM, Wild CP, Rollinson S, Willett EV, Moorman AV, Dovey GJ, et al. Polymorphism in glutathione S-transferase P1 is associated with susceptibility to chemotherapy induced leukemia. Proc Natl Acad Sci U S A. 2001;98(20):11592–7. PubMed PMID: 11553769. Pubmed Central PMCID: 58774
78. Ellis NA, Huo D, Yildiz O, Worrillow LJ, Banerjee M, Le Beau MM, et al. MDM2 SNP309 and TP53 Arg72Pro interact to alter therapy-related acute myeloid leukemia susceptibility. Blood. 2008;112(3):741–9. PubMed PMID: 18426989. Pubmed Central PMCID: 2481552
79. Voso MT, Fabiani E, Zang Z, Fianchi L, Falconi G, Padella A, et al. Fanconi anemia gene variants in therapy-related myeloid neoplasms. Blood Cancer J. 2015;5:e323. PubMed PMID: 26140431. Pubmed Central PMCID: 4526773
80. Pedersen-Bjergaard J, Andersen MT, Andersen MK. Genetic pathways in the pathogenesis of therapy-related myelodysplasia and acute myeloid leukemia. Hematology. 2007:392–7. PubMed PMID: 18024656
81. Li L, Li M, Sun C, Francisco L, Chakraborty S, Sabado M, et al. Altered hematopoietic cell gene expression precedes development of therapy-related myelodysplasia/acute myeloid leukemia and identifies patients at risk. Cancer Cell. 2011;20(5):591–605. PubMed PMID: 22094254. Pubmed Central PMCID: 3220884
82. Ok CY, Patel KP, Garcia-Manero G, Routbort MJ, Fu B, Tang G, et al. Mutational profiling of therapy-related myelodysplastic syndromes and acute myeloid leukemia by next generation sequencing, a comparison with *de novo* diseases. Leuk Res. 2015;39(3):348–54. PubMed PMID: 25573287
83. Wong TN, Ramsingh G, Young AL, Miller CA, Touma W, Welch JS, et al. Role of TP53 mutations in the origin and evolution of therapy-related acute myeloid leukaemia. Nature.

2015;518(7540):552–5. PubMed PMID: 25487151. Pubmed Central PMCID: 4403236

84. Lindsley RC, Mar BG, Mazzola E, Grauman PV, Shareef S, Allen SL, et al. Acute myeloid leukemia ontogeny is defined by distinct somatic mutations. Blood. 2015;125(9):1367–76. PubMed PMID: 25550361. Pubmed Central PMCID: 4342352
85. Link DC, Kunter G, Kasai Y, Zhao Y, Miner T, McLellan MD, et al. Distinct patterns of mutations occurring in *de novo* AML versus AML arising in the setting of severe congenital neutropenia. Blood. 2007;110(5):1648–55. PubMed PMID: 17494858. Pubmed Central PMCID: 1975847
86. Skokowa J, Steinemann D, Katsman-Kuipers JE, Zeidler C, Klimenkova O, Klimiankou M, et al. Cooperativity of RUNX1 and CSF3R mutations in severe congenital neutropenia: a unique pathway in myeloid leukemogenesis. Blood. 2014;123(14):2229–37. PubMed PMID: 24523240
87. Vainchenker W, Delhommeau F, Constantinescu SN, Bernard OA. New mutations and pathogenesis of myeloproliferative neoplasms. Blood. 2011;118(7):1723–35. PubMed PMID: 21653328
88. Klampfl T, Harutyunyan A, Berg T, Gisslinger B, Schalling M, Bagienski K, et al. Genome integrity of myeloproliferative neoplasms in chronic phase and during disease progression. Blood. 2011;118(1):167–76. PubMed PMID: 21531982
89. Campbell PJ, Baxter EJ, Beer PA, Scott LM, Bench AJ, Huntly BJ, et al. Mutation of JAK2 in the myeloproliferative disorders: timing, clonality studies, cytogenetic associations, and role in leukemic transformation. Blood. 2006;108(10):3548–55. PubMed PMID: 16873677
90. Thoennissen NH, Krug UO, Lee DH, Kawamata N, Iwanski GB, Lasho T, et al. Prevalence and prognostic impact of allelic imbalances associated with leukemic transformation of Philadelphia chromosome-negative myeloproliferative neoplasms. Blood. 2010;115(14):2882–90. PubMed PMID: 20068225. Pubmed Central PMCID: 2854432
91. Vannucchi AM, Lasho TL, Guglielmelli P, Biamonte F, Pardanani A, Pereira A, et al. Mutations and prognosis in primary myelofibrosis. Leukemia. 2013;27(9):1861–9. PubMed PMID: 23619563
92. Zhang SJ, Rampal R, Manshouri T, Patel J, Mensah N, Kayserian A, et al. Genetic analysis of patients with leukemic transformation of myeloproliferative neoplasms shows recurrent SRSF2 mutations that are associated with adverse outcome. Blood. 2012;119(19):4480–5. PubMed PMID: 22431577. Pubmed Central PMCID: 3362363
93. Theocharides A, Boissinot M, Girodon F, Garand R, Teo SS, Lippert E, et al. Leukemic blasts in transformed JAK2-V617F-positive myeloproliferative disorders are frequently negative for the JAK2-V617F mutation. Blood. 2007;110(1):375–9. PubMed PMID: 17363731
94. Tefferi A, Lasho TL, Abdel-Wahab O, Guglielmelli P, Patel J, Caramazza D, et al. IDH1 and IDH2 mutation studies in 1473 patients with chronic-, fibrotic- or blast-phase essential thrombocythemia, polycythemia vera or myelofibrosis. Leukemia. 2010;24(7):1302–9. PubMed PMID: 20508616. Pubmed Central PMCID: 3035975
95. Dreyfus B. Preleukemic states. I. Definition and classification. II. Refractory anemia with an excess of myeloblasts in the bone marrow (smoldering acute leukemia). Nouvelle revue francaise d'hematologie. Blood Cells. 1976;17(1–2):33–55. PubMed PMID: 1005106
96. Koeffler HP, Golde DW. Human myeloid leukemia cell lines: a review. Blood. 1980;56(3):344–50. PubMed PMID: 6996765
97. Rowley JD, Alimena G, Garson OM, Hagemeijer A, Mitelman F, Prigogina EL. A collaborative study of the relationship of the morphological type of acute nonlymphocytic leukemia with patient age and karyotype. Blood. 1982;59(5):1013–22. PubMed PMID: 6951613
98. Saarni MI, Linman JW. Preleukemia. The hematologic syndrome preceding acute leukemia. Am J Med. 1973;55(1):38–48. PubMed PMID: 4515079
99. Kantarjian HM, Estey EH, Keating MJ. Treatment of therapy-related leukemia and myelodysplastic syndrome. Hematol Oncol Clin N Am. 1993;7(1):81–107. PubMed PMID: 7680643
100. Dohy H, Genot JY, Imbert M, D'Agay MF, Sultan C. Myelodysplasia and leukaemia related to chemotherapy and/or radiotherapy--a haematological study of 13 cases. Value of macrocytosis as an early sign of bone marrow injury. Clin Lab Haematol. 1980;2(2):111–9. PubMed PMID: 6931004
101. Ballen KK, Antin JH. Treatment of therapy-related acute myelogenous leukemia and myelodysplastic syndromes. Hematol Oncol Clin N Am. 1993;7(2):477–93. PubMed PMID: 8468276
102. Vardiman JW, Golomb HM, Rowley JD, Variakojis D. Acute nonlymphocytic leukemia in malignant lymphoma: a morphologic study. Cancer. 1978;42(1):229–42. PubMed PMID: 276415
103. Khaleeli M, Keane WM, Lee GR. Sideroblastic anemia in multiple myeloma: a preleukemic change. Blood. 1973;41(1):17–25. PubMed PMID: 4118108
104. Maldonado JE, Maigne J, Lecoq D. Comparative electron-microscopic study of the erythrocytic line in refractory anemia (preleukemia) and myelomonocytic leukemia. Nouvelle revue francaise d'hematologie. Blood Cells. 1976;17(1–2):167–85. PubMed PMID: 1069972
105. Vardiman JW, Coelho A, Golomb HM, Rowley J. Morphologic and cytochemical observations on the overt leukemic phase of therapy-related leukemia. Am J Clin Pathol. 1983;79(5):525–30. PubMed PMID: 6188364
106. Churpek JE, Larson RA. The evolving challenge of therapy-related myeloid neoplasms. Best Pract Res Clin Haematol. 2013;26(4):309–17. PubMed PMID: 24507808. Pubmed Central PMCID: 3920194
107. Fenaux P, Lucidarme D, Lai JL, Bauters F. Favorable cytogenetic abnormalities in secondary leukemia. Cancer. 1989;63(12):2505–8. PubMed PMID: 2720600
108. Lee EJ, George SL, Caligiuri M, Szatrowski TP, Powell BL, Lemke S, et al. Parallel phase I studies of daunorubicin given with cytarabine and etoposide with or without the multidrug resistance modulator PSC-833 in previously untreated patients 60 years of age or older with acute myeloid leukemia: results of cancer and leukemia group B study 9420. J Clin Oncol. 1999;17(9):2831–9. PubMed PMID: 10561359
109. Beaumont M, Sanz M, Carli PM, Maloisel F, Thomas X, Detourmignies L, et al. Therapy-related acute promyelocytic leukemia. J Clin Oncol. 2003;21(11):2123–37. PubMed PMID: 12775738
110. Duffield AS, Aoki J, Levis M, Cowan K, Gocke CD, Burns KH, et al. Clinical and pathologic features of secondary acute promyelocytic leukemia. Am J Clin Pathol. 2012;137(3):395–402. PubMed PMID: 22338051. Pubmed Central PMCID: 3578661
111. Ottone T, Cicconi L, Hasan SK, Lavorgna S, Divona M, Voso MT, et al. Comparative molecular analysis of therapy-related and *de novo* acute promyelocytic leukemia. Leuk Res. 2012;36(4):474–8. PubMed PMID: 22071137
112. Yin CC, Glassman AB, Lin P, Valbuena JR, Jones D, Luthra R, et al. Morphologic, cytogenetic, and molecular abnormalities in therapy-related acute promyelocytic leukemia. Am J Clin Pathol. 2005;123(6):840–8. PubMed PMID: 15899774
113. Elliott MA, Letendre L, Tefferi A, Hogan WJ, Hook C, Kaufmann SH, et al. Therapy-related acute promyelocytic leukemia: observations relating to APL pathogenesis and therapy. Eur J Haematol. 2012;88(3):237–43. PubMed PMID: 22023492
114. Slovak ML, Bedell V, Popplewell L, Arber DA, Schoch C, Slater R. 21q22 balanced chromosome aberrations in therapy-related hematopoietic disorders: report from an international workshop.

Genes Chromosomes Cancer. 2002;33(4):379–94. PubMed PMID: 11921272

115. Gustafson SA, Lin P, Chen SS, Chen L, Abruzzo LV, Luthra R, et al. Therapy-related acute myeloid leukemia with t(8;21)(q22;q22) shares many features with *de novo* acute myeloid leukemia with t(8;21)(q22;q22) but does not have a favorable outcome. Am J Clin Pathol. 2009;131(5):647–55. PubMed PMID: 19369623
116. Krauth MT, Eder C, Alpermann T, Bacher U, Nadarajah N, Kern W, et al. High number of additional genetic lesions in acute myeloid leukemia with t(8;21)/RUNX1-RUNX1T1: frequency and impact on clinical outcome. Leukemia. 2014;28(7):1449–58. PubMed PMID: 24402164
117. Andersen MK, Larson RA, Mauritzson N, Schnittger S, Jhanwar SC, Pedersen-Bjergaard J. Balanced chromosome abnormalities inv (16) and t(15;17) in therapy-related myelodysplastic syndromes and acute leukemia: report from an international workshop. Genes Chromosomes Cancer. 2002;33(4):395–400. PubMed PMID: 11921273
118. Goemans BF, Zwaan CM, Miller M, Zimmermann M, Harlow A, Meshinchi S, et al. Mutations in KIT and RAS are frequent events in pediatric core-binding factor acute myeloid leukemia. Leukemia. 2005;19(9):1536–42. PubMed PMID: 16015387
119. Haferlach C, Dicker F, Kohlmann A, Schindela S, Weiss T, Kern W, et al. AML with CBFB-MYH11 rearrangement demonstrate RAS pathway alterations in 92% of all cases including a high frequency of NF1 deletions. Leukemia. 2010;24(5):1065–9. PubMed PMID: 20164853
120. Paschka P, Du J, Schlenk RF, Gaidzik VI, Bullinger L, Corbacioglu A, et al. Secondary genetic lesions in acute myeloid leukemia with inv (16) or t(16;16): a study of the German-Austrian AML Study Group (AMLSG). Blood. 2013;121(1):170–7. PubMed PMID: 23115274
121. Kern W, Haferlach T, Schnittger S, Hiddemann W, Schoch C. Prognosis in therapy-related acute myeloid leukemia and impact of karyotype. J Clin Oncol. 2004;22(12):2510–1. PubMed PMID: 15197216
122. Chen Y, Estrov Z, Pierce S, Qiao W, Borthakur G, Ravandi F, et al. Myeloid neoplasms after breast cancer: "therapy-related" not an independent poor prognostic factor. Leuk Lymphoma. 2015;56(4):1012–9. PubMed PMID: 25048874. Pubmed Central PMCID: 4326620
123. Kim HP, Gerhard B, Harasym TO, Mayer LD, Hogge DE. Liposomal encapsulation of a synergistic molar ratio of cytarabine and daunorubicin enhances selective toxicity for acute myeloid leukemia progenitors as compared to analogous normal hematopoietic cells. Exp Hematol. 2011;39(7):741–50. PubMed PMID: 21530609
124. Lancet JE, Cortes JE, Hogge DE, Tallman MS, Kovacsovics TJ, Damon LE, et al. Phase 2 trial of CPX-351, a fixed 5:1 molar ratio of cytarabine/daunorubicin, vs cytarabine/daunorubicin in older adults with untreated AML. Blood. 2014;123(21):3239–46. PubMed PMID: 24687088. Pubmed Central PMCID: 4624448
125. Sievers EL, Larson RA, Stadtmauer EA, Estey E, Lowenberg B, Dombret H, et al. Efficacy and safety of gemtuzumab ozogamicin in patients with CD33-positive acute myeloid leukemia in first relapse. J Clin Oncol. 2001;19(13):3244–54. PubMed PMID: 11432892
126. Kharfan-Dabaja MA, Hamadani M, Reljic T, Pyngolil R, Komrokji RS, Lancet JE, et al. Gemtuzumab ozogamicin for treatment of newly diagnosed acute myeloid leukaemia: a systematic review and meta-analysis. Br J Haematol. 2013;163(3):315–25. PubMed PMID: 24033280
127. Burnett AK, Hills RK, Milligan D, Kjeldsen L, Kell J, Russell NH, et al. Identification of patients with acute myeloblastic leukemia who benefit from the addition of gemtuzumab ozogamicin: results of the MRC AML15 trial. J Clin Oncol. 2011;29(4):369–77. PubMed PMID: 21172891
128. Kung Sutherland MS, Walter RB, Jeffrey SC, Burke PJ, Yu C, Kostner H, et al. SGN-CD33A: a novel CD33-targeting antibody-drug conjugate using a pyrrolobenzodiazepine dimer is active in models of drug-resistant AML. Blood. 2013;122(8):1455–63. PubMed PMID: 23770776
129. Tawfik B, Sliesoraitis S, Lyerly S, Klepin HD, Lawrence J, Isom S, et al. Efficacy of the hypomethylating agents as frontline, salvage, or consolidation therapy in adults with acute myeloid leukemia (AML). Ann Hematol. 2014;93(1):47–55. PubMed PMID: 24149914. Pubmed Central PMCID: 3879720
130. Quintas-Cardama A, Ravandi F, Liu-Dumlao T, Brandt M, Faderl S, Pierce S, et al. Epigenetic therapy is associated with similar survival compared with intensive chemotherapy in older patients with newly diagnosed acute myeloid leukemia. Blood. 2012;120(24):4840–5. PubMed PMID: 23071272. Pubmed Central PMCID: 3952725
131. Fianchi L, Criscuolo M, Lunghi M, Gaidano G, Breccia M, Levis A, et al. Outcome of therapy-related myeloid neoplasms treated with azacitidine. J Hematol Oncol. 2012;5:44. PubMed PMID: 22853048. Pubmed Central PMCID: 3419605
132. Prebet T, Sun Z, Ketterling RP, Zeidan A, Greenberg P, Herman J, et al. Azacitidine with or without Entinostat for the treatment of therapy-related myeloid neoplasm: further results of the E1905 North American leukemia intergroup study. Br J Haematol. 2016;172(3):384–91. PubMed PMID: 26577691. Pubmed Central PMCID: 4794257
133. Bally C, Thepot S, Quesnel B, Vey N, Dreyfus F, Fadlallah J, et al. Azacitidine in the treatment of therapy related myelodysplastic syndrome and acute myeloid leukemia (tMDS/AML): a report on 54 patients by the Groupe francophone des Myelodysplasies (GFM). Leuk Res. 2013;37(6):637–40. PubMed PMID: 23499498
134. Klimek VM, Dolezal EK, Tees MT, Devlin SM, Stein K, Romero A, et al. Efficacy of hypomethylating agents in therapy-related myelodysplastic syndromes. Leuk Res. 2012;36(9):1093–7. PubMed PMID: 22608310
135. Montalban-Bravo G, Garcia-Manero G. Novel drugs for older patients with acute myeloid leukemia. Leukemia. 2015;29(4):760–9. PubMed PMID: 25142817
136. Kuendgen A, Bug G, Ottmann OG, Haase D, Schanz J, Hildebrandt B, et al. Treatment of poor-risk myelodysplastic syndromes and acute myeloid leukemia with a combination of 5-azacytidine and valproic acid. Clin Epigenetics. 2011;2(2):389–99. PubMed PMID: 22704349. Pubmed Central PMCID: 3365387
137. Gore SD, Hermes-DeSantis ER. Future directions in myelodysplastic syndrome: newer agents and the role of combination approaches. Cancer Control. 2008;15(Suppl):40–9. PubMed PMID: 18813208. Pubmed Central PMCID: 2727156
138. Bose P, Grant S. Orphan drug designation for pracinostat, volasertib and alvocidib in AML. Leuk Res. 2014;38(8):862–5. PubMed PMID: 24996975
139. Boumber Y, Younes A, Garcia-Manero G. Mocetinostat (MGCD0103): a review of an isotype-specific histone deacetylase inhibitor. Expert Opin Invest Drugs. 2011;20(6):823–9. PubMed PMID: 21554162
140. Shih AH, Chung SS, Dolezal EK, Zhang SJ, Abdel-Wahab OI, Park CY, et al. Mutational analysis of therapy-related myelodysplastic syndromes and acute myelogenous leukemia. Haematologica. 2013;98(6):908–12. PubMed PMID: 23349305. Pubmed Central PMCID: 3669447
141. Pedersen-Bjergaard J, Andersen MK, Andersen MT, Christiansen DH. Genetics of therapy-related myelodysplasia and acute myeloid leukemia. Leukemia. 2008;22(2):240–8. PubMed PMID: 18200041
142. Daigle SR, Olhava EJ, Therkelsen CA, Basavapathruni A, Jin L, Boriack-Sjodin PA, et al. Potent inhibition of DOT1L as treatment

of MLL-fusion leukemia. Blood. 2013;122(6):1017–25. PubMed PMID: 23801631. Pubmed Central PMCID: 3739029

143. Degenhardt Y, Greshock J, Laquerre S, Gilmartin AG, Jing J, Richter M, et al. Sensitivity of cancer cells to Plk1 inhibitor GSK461364A is associated with loss of p53 function and chromosome instability. Mol Cancer Ther. 2010;9(7):2079–89. PubMed PMID: 20571075

144. Dohner H, Lubbert M, Fiedler W, Fouillard L, Haaland A, Brandwein JM, et al. Randomized, phase 2 trial of low-dose cytarabine with or without volasertib in AML patients not suitable for induction therapy. Blood. 2014;124(9):1426–33. PubMed PMID: 25006120. Pubmed Central PMCID: 4148765

145. Litzow MR, Tarima S, Perez WS, Bolwell BJ, Cairo MS, Camitta BM, et al. Allogeneic transplantation for therapy-related myelodysplastic syndrome and acute myeloid leukemia. Blood. 2010;115(9):1850–7. PubMed PMID: 20032503. Pubmed Central PMCID: 2832815

146. Kroger N, Brand R, van Biezen A, Zander A, Dierlamm J, Niederwieser D, et al. Risk factors for therapy-related myelodysplastic syndrome and acute myeloid leukemia treated with allogeneic stem cell transplantation. Haematologica. 2009;94(4):542–9. PubMed PMID: 19278968. Pubmed Central PMCID: 2663618

147. Armand P, Kim HT, Mayer E, Cutler CS, Ho VT, Koreth J, et al. Outcome of allo-SCT for women with MDS or AML occurring after breast cancer therapy. Bone Marrow Transplant. 2010;45(11):1611–7. PubMed PMID: 20154738. Pubmed Central PMCID: 2889243

148. Witherspoon RP, Deeg HJ, Storer B, Anasetti C, Storb R, Appelbaum FR. Hematopoietic stem-cell transplantation for treatment-related leukemia or myelodysplasia. J Clin Oncol. 2001;19(8):2134–41. PubMed PMID: 11304765

149. Armand P, Kim HT, DeAngelo DJ, Ho VT, Cutler CS, Stone RM, et al. Impact of cytogenetics on outcome of *de novo* and therapy-related AML and MDS after allogeneic transplantation. Biol Blood Marrow Transplant. 2007;13(6):655–64. PubMed PMID: 17531775. Pubmed Central PMCID: 2743535

150. Fianchi L, Pagano L, Piciocchi A, Candoni A, Gaidano G, Breccia M, et al. Characteristics and outcome of therapy-related myeloid neoplasms: report from the Italian network on secondary leukemias. Am J Hematol. 2015;90(5):E80–5. PubMed PMID: 25653205

151. Eichenauer DA, Thielen I, Haverkamp H, Franklin J, Behringer K, Halbsguth T, et al. Therapy-related acute myeloid leukemia and myelodysplastic syndromes in patients with Hodgkin lymphoma: a report from the German Hodgkin Study Group. Blood. 2014;123(11):1658–64. PubMed PMID: 24478403

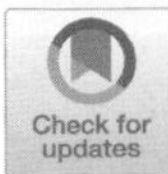

The Myelodysplastic Syndromes 23

Kenneth Miller and Monika Pilichowska

Introduction

The myelodysplastic syndromes (MDS) are a heterogeneous group of clonal stem cell disorders characterized by impaired, and/or ineffective, proliferation and maturation of hematopoietic progenitor cells resulting in symptomatic anemia, leukopenia, or thrombocytopenia. The clinical course is very variable, ranging from a chronic, stable, mildly symptomatic disorder to a malignancy that rapidly progresses to AML. Morphological and functional cellular abnormalities involving one or more cell lines are common resulting in infections and/or bleeding. The complications from MDS and its treatment remain the major cause of morbidity and mortality. MDS shares many clinical, cytogenetic, and laboratory features with aplastic anemia, hypoplastic anemias, the myeloproliferative neoplasms, and the acute leukemias. The updated WHO classification attempts to define the diagnosis of MDS and separate it from the myeloproliferative neoplasms, reactive and secondary causes of hypoproliferative disorders and the acute leukemias. Patients with MDS may present with clinical and laboratory features suggestive of a reactive, autoimmune or other malignant stem cell disorder. Therefore, in many instances, the diagnosis of MDS is based on the exclusion of other disorders associated with dysplasia and impaired or ineffective hematopoiesis.

MDS is a progressive clonal disorder and the diagnostic studies and the initial evaluations are similar to those used to define other neoplastic and non-neoplastic stem cell disorders. However, the clinical course, prognosis, and treatment approach for a patient with a MDS is different from the other neoplastic stem cell disorders. The bone marrow and peripheral blood abnormalities in MDS can be subtle and require the cooperative efforts of pathologists, cytogeneticists, and clinicians to diagnosis, classify and define prognosis. MDS is one of most common hematologic malignancies in older populations and treatments remain controversial and limited for many patients. Treatments for many patients should be individualized and tailored to the MDS subtype, patient's age, comorbidities, and other prognostic variables.

Myelodysplasia, derived from the Greek and meaning morphological abnormality of the bone marrow, is not a new disease but it has only recently been assigned as a separate category in the classification of malignant hematopoietic disorders based on specific diagnostic criteria. The initial reports identified elderly patients with progressive cytopenias, morphologically abnormal cells, and a propensity to progress to an acute leukemia. Terms such as smoldering leukemia, or preleukemia were used to describe this condition, reflecting that patients with MDS did not meet the usual criteria of acute leukemia but presented with a syndrome which included a hypercellular bone marrow with increased blast forms and dysplastic changes in one or more cell lines. In MDS, as in the myeloproliferative neoplasms and acute leukemias an oncogenic transforming event occurs at the level of the myeloid or pluripotential stem cell. Cytogenetic studies were first to identify the genetic alterations in MDS and are important in establishing the diagnosis and prognosis in MDS. More recently numerous specific gene mutations have been identified in MDS associated genes that may define prognosis and impact treatment. While many patients with MDS have features suggestive of an early, smoldering leukemia, and rapidly evolve into one of the myeloid leukemias, most patients do not evolve into AML but die as a result of the MDS or its treatment [1, 2]. MDS therefore should not be considered as a preleukemic disorder, but as a separate neoplastic disease of the hematopoietic pluripotential stem cells that is characterized by a progressive clonal proliferation of abnormal precursors that demonstrate both impaired maturation and ineffective proliferation. The separation of MDS from AML, myeloproliferative neoplasms,

K. Miller, M.D. (✉)
Department of Hematology/Oncology, Tufts Medical Center, 800 Washington Street, Boston, MA 02111, USA
e-mail: kbmiller@tuftsmedicalcenter.org

M. Pilichowska, M.D., Ph.D.
Department of Pathology, Tufts Medical Center, 800 Washington Street, Boston, MA 02111, USA
e-mail: mpilichowska@tuftsmedicalcenter.org

P.H. Wiernik et al. (eds.), *Neoplastic Diseases of the Blood*, DOI 10.1007/978-3-319-64263-5_23

aplastic anemia, and reactive disorders continues to be problematic, which is reflected in the evolving and at times inconsistent classification systems, prognostic models, and treatment options. A proposed revised 2016 WHO classification refines the morphologic interpretation and assessment of cytopenias addresses, and applies new diagnostic terminology for MDS. The WHO classification still relies mainly on the degree of dysplasia and the percent of blasts for disease classification and specific cytopenias now have only a minor impact on the MDS classification [3, 4]. Moreover the morphologic dysplasia may not correlate with the lineage specific cytopenias. Therefore the WHO has removed terms such a refractory anemia or refractory cytopenia and replaced it with the suffix Myelodysplastic Syndrome followed by the specific abnormality. The WHO also attempted to define and incorporate identified gene mutations associated with MDS and address the controversy and limitations of incorporating distinct mutations in the new proposed classification criteria. The WHO noted that that identification of dysplasia is subjective and may vary even among experienced hematopathologists [3]. Therefore when the dysplasia is subtle or limited to a single lineage it is important to consider other possible reactive and non-neoplastic causes of the dysplasia prior to making the diagnosis of MDS.

Pathogenesis and Etiology

MDS is one of the most common hematologic malignancies in western countries with an overall incidence of 3.5–12.6/100,000/year. The median age of MDS patients in western countries is 73 years, at the time of diagnosis, and the incidence increases with age. In individuals over the age of 70 years the incidence is between 15–50/100,000/year and is increasing with the aging population [5, 6]. However, the overall incidence of MDS is likely much higher due to difficulties in reporting, diagnosis, and classification [4]. The incidence of MDS is higher in men than women with the exception of the del (5q), which has a marked female predominance. In Asian countries, notably Japan and China, the median age of patients with MDS is between 40–50 years, some two decades earlier than in western countries [5, 7, 8]. The reason for the differences in the epidemiology of MDS in Japan and China is unclear but may, in part, reflect the variability and limitations of population-based databases. However, the role of environmental factors, industrial solvents and agricultural chemicals, and smoking may contribute to the observed 20-year differences in the epidemiology of MDS [9, 10].

Environmental agents have been implicated in the etiology of MDS. In case-controlled studies, there is an association between MDS and cigarette smoking, exposure to benzene, petroleum products, organic solvents, fertilizers, pesticides, and herbicides [10]. The associated between smoking and MDS may reflect that cigarette smoke contains benzene and other suspected carcinogens [9]. The MDS risk is related to the intensity and duration of smoking and may persist for up to 15 years after cessation of smoking [9, 10]. Ionizing radiation exposure is associated with a significant increase risk for the development of MDS. In the Nagasaki atomic bomb survivors risk for developing MDS was greater in individuals exposed at a younger age and occurred 40–60 years after exposure. In contrast to the reported radiation induced leukemia in Nagasaki which occurred 10–15 years after the exposure. The long latency may reflect the proposed multistep pathogenesis model for the development of MDS with age related changes and genetic instability associated with the prior radiation exposure [11]. In epidemiologic studies there was a linear radiation dose response for the development of MDS in Nagasaki atomic bomb survivors 40–60 years after exposure.

MDS is characterized by dysplastic, ineffective hematopoiesis. The bone marrow is typically hypercellular for the patient's age with peripheral cytopenias and an increase in hematopoietic precursors in the bone marrow and/or peripheral blood. The clonal origin of MDS has been confirmed by isozyme analysis of glucose 6 phosphate dehydrogenase (G6PD) in heterozygous females and more recently by molecular analysis of other loci such as the androgen receptor gene [8, 12]. Cytogenetic analysis has demonstrated recurrent genetic alterations that are prognostically important and next generation high throughput gene sequencing has defined a number of mutated genes in MDS [12] (Table 23.1). The appearance of clonal gene mutations arise

Table 23.1 Recurrent mutated genes in MDS

Mutated genes	Prognosis
Chromatin modification	
ASXL1	Unfavorable
EZH2	Unfavorable
UTX	Unfavorable
DNA methylation	
TET2	Neutral
DNMTA3A	Unfavorable
IDH1/	Unfavorable
RNA splicing	
SF3B1	Favorable
U2AF1/U2AF35	Unknown
SRSF2	Unfavorable
ZRSR2	Unfavorable
DNA repair	
p53(TP53)	Unfavorable
Transcription regulators	
RUNX1	Unfavoable
BCOR-L1	Unfavorable

Data from Ref. [23]

in hematopoietic stem cells and appear to be early events that are associated with clonal dominance. Specific gene mutations and the cytogenetic abnormalities can be demonstrated before the detections of morphological dysplasia or the clinical findings of MDS [13, 14]. The initial cytogenetic and somatic gene mutations are part of a multistep process that predisposes the pluripotential stem cell to secondary genetic events and the development of MDS [14]. Epigenetic alterations in one or more oncogenes including in the aberrant expression of specific tumor promotor, tumor suppressor, and transcription factor genes are associated with the progression of MDS [15, 16]. The diagnostic and prognostic role of specific gene mutations and aberrant methylation of epigenetic regulators, however, is still unclear. MDS progression is characterized by a progressive increase in chromosomal instability that leads to the development of aberrant clones and the emergence of complex karyotypes. Telomeres, noncoding repeated sequences at the ends of chromosomes, that function to stabilize chromosomes and prevent chromosomal breaks and aberrations critical in the maintaining normal hematopoiesis and are postulated to play a role in the progressive chromosomal instability in MDS [17]. Each somatic cell division is associated with loss of telomere length and the cumulative effects of telomere shortening leads to cell senescence. The shortening of telomeres is noted in patients with progressive, advanced MDS, with multiple complex karyotypic abnormalities. The genetic instability associated with shortening of telomeres may contribute, in part, to the leukemic transformation in some patients with MDS [17, 18]. Moreover, the alteration of telomere dynamics in hematopoietic stem cells may precede the clinical development of MDS [19]. However, the majority of patients that develop MDS are greater than 70 years old and loss of telomere length and function is part of the normal aging process [19].

The hematopoietic microenvironment may also play a role in the pathophysiology of MDS [20]. MDS is characterized by ineffective hematopoiesis and the increased susceptibility of hematopoietic progenitors to apoptosis. The bone marrow stroma responds to signals from the hematopoietic cells and is abnormal in some patients with MDS. Abnormalities of the bone marrow microenvironment and the hematopoietic stem cell niche may affect and promote apoptosis and telomere shortening in clonal hematopoietic cells [21]. The overexpression of TNF-a produced by MDS mononuclear cells can inhibit the growth of residual normal hematopoiesis and lead to increased cell death of normal precursors, and a growth advantage for the abnormal MDS precursors. The bone marrow in MDS patients has increased apoptotic cells which is most marked in the less proliferative, better prognosis, low risk subtypes of MDS.

Genetic, environmental, and exposure factors have been associated with an increased risk for the development of MDS [22]. Inherited constitutional genetic defects have been associated with up to 30% of children with MDS and related myeloproliferative disorders. Children with Shwachman–Diamond syndrome, Fanconi anemia, dyskeratosis congenital, and neurofibromatosis type 1 have constitutional genetic defects that are associated with the increased risk for the development of both MDS and AML [25, 26].

Mutations of specific genes mediating DNA repair appear to predispose to the acquisition of secondary cytogenetic abnormalities that can lead to the development of MDS [23]. Somatic mutations occur in the majority of patients and may be associated with specific clinical features. Specific point mutations were associated with the clinical phenotype, specific cytopenias, disease progression, and overall survival. Genes encoding runt-related transcription factor 1 (RUNX1), tumor protein p53 (TP53), and neuroblastoma RAS viral oncogene homologue (NRAS) are associated with thrombocytopenia and an increased percent of bone marrow blast forms [23, 24]. Point mutations resulting in the activation of the specific genes (TP53, EZH2, ETV6, RUNX1, and ASXL1) are independent markers of poor prognosis and may, in part, explain the clinical heterogeneity of MDS. The TET family of genes maps to chromosome 4q24 and modulate hypomethylation by catalyzing an intermediate of DNA methylation that block the formation of silencing proteins to methylated DNA [13]. Mutations of the TET2 gene are found in a number of myeloid neoplasms including AML, MPNs, and MDS. In MDS TET2 mutation is the most frequent gene mutation occurring 20–30% of patients. Mutations of TET2 associated with loss of function may result in increased methylation and silencing of genes that are normally expressed. However, the prognostic impact of TET2 mutations on survival in MDS is unclear. The TET2 mutation is associated with a number of additional gene mutations and therefore may be one of the initial mutational events MDS. Recurrent mutations of epigenetic regulators, genes encoding the splicing machinery, spliceosomal components, and transcription factors are not unique to MDS and are found in a number of other myeloid neoplasms and occur across a spectrum of cytogenetic subgroups. It is controversial if these gene mutations are the primary events in MDS and are diagnostic and prognostic markers that are independent of other abnormalities [23, 24]. The frequency of the recurrent somatic mutations in MDS patients increases with progression of the disease and the subsequent development of secondary cytogenetic events and AML [25]. However, the etiological role of each of the somatic point mutations in the development of and progression of MDS is controversial and it is unclear if these mutations just reflect the genetic instability of the abnormal clone and its propensity to develop random genetic mutations [26, 27]. Moreover, similar somatic mutations have been noted in older normal individuals without evidence of MDS [27–29]. Somatic mutations resulting in clonal hematopoietic cells are detected in greater than 10% of persons older than 70 years of age and the incidence of somatic mutations increases with age. These MDS associated acquired clonal mutations occur in hematopoietic cells of healthy older persons with normal blood counts and without evidence of dysplasia [29]. The presence of somatic mutations may confer an increased risk in the individual for the subsequent development of a hematological malignancy and are associated with an all cause-increased mortality [30–32]. The term "Clonal Hematopoiesis of Indeterminate Potential "(CHIP) is used describe these acquired clonal somatic mutations which are associated with hematologic malignancies in apparently healthy older individuals without any clinical features of a MDS or any myeloid malignancy. The natural history of individuals with CHIP is unclear and these persons should not be considered to have a malignancy. The revised 2016 WHO classifications addresses the controversy associated with somatic mutations and notes that the presence clonal somatic mutation alone, without other clinical manifestations of MDS, is not sufficient to make the diagnosis of MDS. While CHIP may represent a pre - malignant myeloid conditions, similar to monoclonal gammopathy of undetermined significance (MGUS) and multiple myeloma, the natural history of individuals with CHIP is not clearly defined. Testing for somatic mutations in healthy individuals should not part of routine clinical practice.

MDS patients have defects in a number of signal transduction pathways that appear to be related to the evolving ineffective hematopoiesis and epigenetic changes [33, 34]. These acquired abnormalities may contribute to the further dysregulation of progenitor cell cycle kinetics, response to cytokines, and the maintenance of DNA integrity, which results in progressive genetic instability. Abnormal regulation of microRNAs (miRNA) which function as epigenetic regulators of gene expression may play a role in the pathogenesis of MDS and alterations in miRNAs may be independent markers of prognosis [24].

MDS is associated with a number of immunoregulatory abnormalities including the development of autoantibodies and monoclonal gammopathies [35]. In subsets of patients with MDS, autoreactive T-cell clones are present that inhibit autologous erythroid and granulocytic colony growth. T-cell-mediated suppression of bone marrow growth and maturation is an important development of aplastic anemia and the hypoplastic variant of MDS [35, 36]. The incidence of MDS is increased in patients with autoimmune disorders and autoimmune disorders are more common in patients with MDS. The presence of autoimmune disorders is associated with a better overall survival and less frequent transformation to AML, The immunoregulatory abnormalities may also explain the response to immunosuppressive therapy in selected patients with MDS.

There are defined genetic predisposing factors in some MDS patients that relate to naturally occurring complex DNA polymorphisms in genes that mediate DNA repair and the metabolism of environmental carcinogens [37, 38]. In selected genetically predisposed individuals, MDS may arise as a result of cumulative environmental exposures and studies have linked the development of MDS and the nonfunction 609 C.T polymorphic allele of the NAD(P)Quinone oxidoreductase (NQO1) gene [40, 41]. These genes appear to play a critical role in detoxifying benzene and its metabolites. This association is controversial, but may explain the increased incidence of MDS in some patients exposed to organic solvents and benzene-containing compounds [39]. Similar controversial, but provocative results have been reported in the glutathione S-transferase (GST) genes that mediate the metabolism of cytotoxic and genotoxic agents [40].

A prior exposure to chemotherapy, especially alkylating agents and purine analogues is associated with an increased risk of MDS and AML (Table 23.2). The WHO identifies therapy-related MDS (t-MDS) as a separate category. Therapy related MDS represents approximately 10–20% of MDSs and MDS/MPNs [41]. The risk is, in part, related to the dose and duration of the cytotoxic therapy and generally occurs 3–7 years after the exposure. Patients who received combination radiation therapy and chemotherapy are at greater risk for the development of t-MDS [42]. Total body irradiation, administered as part of the preparative regimen for an autologous stem cell transplantation, is associated with an increased risk for MDS, and the combination of

Table 23.2 Cytotoxic drugs implicated in the development of MDS

Class/drug
Alkylating agents
Busulfan
Carboplatin
Cisplatin
Carmustine, Semustine, Lomustine
Chlorambucil
Cyclophosphamide
Dacarbazine
Mechlorethamine
Melphalan
Mitomycin C
Procarbazine
Thiotepa
Nucleoside analogs
Fludarabine
2-Chlorodexoyadenosine (Cladribine)
Antimetabolites
6-Mercaptopurine
Methotrexate
Azathioprine

Usually involving large fields, e.g., total body irradiation

Table 23.3 Cytogenetics in IPSS-R

Abnormality				
Prognostic subgroup/% of patients	Single	AML evolution/y	Median OS/months	Score
Very good (4%)	Del (11q)	NR	64	0
	−y			
Good (72%)	Normal	9.4	56	
	Del(5q)			
	Del(12p)			2
	Del(20q)			
Intermediate (13%)	Del (7q),+8,+19	2.5	31	
	i(17q)			4
	Any other			
	Independent clones			
Poor (4%)	Inv(3/t(3q)/de(3q)	1.7	18	6
	−7, double including			
	7/del7(7q), complex:3 abnormalities			
Very poor (7%)	Complex > 3 Abnormalities	0.7	8.4	8

OS overall survival, *NR* not reached
Data from Greenberg {L, Tuechler H, Sanz G, et al. Revised International Prognostic Scoring System for Myelodysplastic Syndromes. Blood 2012;120 (12): 2453–2465}

high-dose alkylator therapy and total body irradiation was associated with a 10–15% risk of t-MDS and secondary AML [41]. The MDS that occurs after chemotherapy, has a very poor prognosis [42]. Therapy-related MDS, is associated with deletions of chromosomes 5 and/or 7 and complex karyotypes. In contrast to the cytogenetic findings in AML, balanced cytogenetic abnormalities including translocations and inversions are rare in MDS. The cytogenetic abnormalities in MDS are important independent prognostic risk factors for overall survival and risk of the development of AML (Table 23.3). However, in the majority of patients with MDS there is no history of exposure to known mutagens, cytotoxic agents, or environmental agents and therefore the etiology of the syndrome remains idiopathic or unknown.

Diagnosis and Classification

The diagnosis and classification of MDS, similar to other myeloid malignancies, is evolving and incorporates new cytogenetic and molecular findings. The updated 2016 WHO classification attempts to addresses the heterogeneity of MDS and separates MDS from reactive processes and other malignant stem cell disorders. The revised classification refines the morphologic interpretations and addresses the influence of new genetic information in MDS diagnosis, classification and prognosis. The FAB (French–American–British) group was the first to define morphological criteria in the blood and bone marrow for the diagnosis and classification of MDS and was based only on morphology, and the percentage of blast forms in the blood and bone marrow. This classification system, although generally adopted at the time, was clinically and biologically inconsistent [43]. The separation of MDS from AML and other clonal disorders was based on an arbitrary number of blast forms. Moreover, many patients with MDS had clinical and laboratory features of AML, aplastic anemia, and myeloproliferative neoplasms which were not addressed in the FAB classification [44]. The FAB criteria also did not address the clinically important cytogenetic changes in MDS and were too variable to accurately predict prognosis, survival, or transformation to AML. The FAB classification remained as a widely accepted classification system for diagnosis of MDS for two decades. The FAB group defined five categories, of MDS based on morphologic dysplasia, cytochemical stains for iron to detect ring sideroblasts, and the percent of blast forms in the bone marrow and peripheral blood and included refractory anemia (RA), or refractory cytopenia, refractory anemia with ringed sideroblasts (RARS), refractory anemia with excess blasts (RAEB), chronic myelomonocytic leukemia (CMML), and refractory anemia with excess blasts in transformation (RAEB-T). The World Health Organization (WHO), in collaboration with the Society for Hematopathology and the European Association of Hematopathology in 2001, proposed a revision of the FAB morphological approach to the classification of MDS [45]. The WHO classification was updated in 2008 and most recently in 2016 [3, 46] (Table 23.4). The revised WHO classification attempts to combine clinical, morphologic, immunophenotypic, genetic and molecular features to define clinically and prognostically important subtypes. The current WHO classification is generally accepted and is incorporated in prognostic and treatment models of MDS.

Table 23.4 WHO 2008 and WHO 2016 classification of myelodysplastic syndromes

WHO 2008	Peripheral blood key features	WHO 2016 bone marrow key features
Refractory cytopenia with With unilineage dysplasia Dysplasia (RCUD) RA anemia (RA) Refractory neutropenia (RN) Refractory thrombocytopenia (RT)	<1% blasts	MDS with single lineage dysplasia (MDS-SLD)
Refractory anemia with ring sideroblasts (RARS)	Anemia no blasts	MDS with single lineage dysplasia and ring sideroblasts(MDS-RSSLD)
Refractory cytopenia with multilineage dysplasia (RCMD)	Cytopenia(s) <1% blasts No Auer rods	MDS with multilineage dysplasia and ring sideroblast(MDS-RSMLD)
Refractory anemia with excess blasts type 1 RAEB-1(RAEB1)	Cytopenia(s) <5% blasts No Auer rods	MDS with excess blasts-1(MDS-EB1)
Refractory anemia with excess blasts type 2 RAEB-2 (RAEB2)	Cytopenia(s) 5–19% blasts ± Auer rods	MDS with excess blasts-2(MDS-EB2)
MDS associated with isolated del(5q)	Anemia normal or high platelet count	MDS with isolated del(5q)
MDS, unclassifiable MDS-U	Cytopenias ≤ 1% blasts If no dysplasia, MDS-associated karyotype	MDS-U

The WHO classification included requirements for the type of specimens to be obtained, the assessment of blasts, assessment of blast lineage, and cytogenetic or mutational studies. The assessment of blasts in the peripheral blood (PB) and bone marrow (BM) should be obtained prior to any definitive therapy. Cytogenetic analysis and flow cytometry should be obtained, with additional material saved for later molecular genetic studies as needed [12]. The WHO lowered the threshold for percent of blasts to diagnose AML from 30% (FAB) to 20%. The percent of blasts should be derived from a 200-cell differential count of the peripheral blood smear and a 500-cell differential count of all nucleated bone marrow cells. The 2016 revised WHO classification changed the diagnostic criteria for myeloid neoplasms with erythroid dominance, defined as erythroid precursors ≥50% of all bone marrow cells. In the new classification the percent of blasts is based not on non-erythroid nucleated cells but on all nucleated bone marrow cells. This new criteria will result in cases previously diagnosed as the erythroid/myeloid subtype of acute erythroid leukemia to now being classified as MDS with excess blasts.

The FAB and the subsequent WHO classifications defined MDS as a clonal stem cell disorder characterized by ineffective, dysplastic hematopoiesis, with dysplasia in one or more hematopoietic cell lines and the dysplasia should be noted in >10% of cells in either the bone marrow or the blood. The WHO noted that morphological dysplasia is not specific or diagnostic of MDS and noted the difficulty in separating MDS from other disorders associated with cytopenias and dysplasia. The 2016 WHO classification recognized that dysplasia in excess of 10% may occur in some normal individuals and in other non-malignant hematologic disorders. The hematopathologist's identification of dysplasia is also variable and not always reproducible even by expert panels [47]. The WHO classifications like the original FAB classification is based on the degree of dysplasia and percent of blast forms in the blood and bone marrow. The WHO classification noted that the cell line demonstrating the most prominent dysplasia may not correlate with the cytopenia of the most affected lineage. The 2016 WHO classification therefore changed the descriptive terms such as refractory anemia and applied the new terminology Myelodysplastic syndrome followed by the "appropriate modifiers"; single or multilineage dysplasia, ring sideroblast, excess blast or the del(5q) cytogenetic abnormality (Table 23.4). There are, however, some of he morphological abnormalities that are more characteristic of MDS and are useful in confirming the diagnosis. The neutrophil and megakaryocytic dysplastic changes are the most specific and characteristic of MDS [3, 46, 48]. In the myeloid/neutrophilic dysmyelopoiesis the presence in the peripheral blood of the acquired, pseudo, Pelger–Huët anomaly is a frequent and useful characteristic finding in the MDS. This acquired abnormality resembles the inherited Pelger–Huët anomaly, therefore the designation of pseudo, and is characterized by mature neutrophils that are hypolobated with a single lobe or two joined by a thin band of chromatin [49]. Abnormal granulopoiesis is usually evident on the peripheral smear and includes hypersegmented neutrophils, with decreased or absent cytoplasmic granules The presence of dysmegakaryopoiesis including the presence of micromegakaryocytes in the bone marrow is also very suggestive of MDS rather than a reactive process [3, 45]. The finding of micromegakaryocytes and megakaryocytes that are the size of a myeloblast with one or two abnormal small nuclei in the bone marrow is one of the most characteristic, diagnostic and recognizable morphological features in MDS.

A majority of patients with MDS are asymptomatic at presentation and are usually diagnosed when they present with an unexplained macrocytic anemia (MCV > 102) with a absolute low reticulocyte count. Anemia is the most common presenting abnormality and patients may complain of the insidious onset fatigue and progressive dyspnea on exertion. Bone pain and weight loss are uncommon. While patients may be neutropenic and have dysplastic and impaired neutrophil function, infections are unusual at presentation. The physical examination is notable for the lack of adenopathy, cutaneous lesions, prominent splenomegaly, or hepatomegaly. The diagnosis of MDS relies largely on the morphological findings in the peripheral blood and the bone marrow (Table 23.5). MDS must be differentiated from other disorders that present with abnormalities of one or more cell line including aplastic anemia, myeloproliferative neoplasms, nutritional deficiencies, and autoimmune disorders (Table 23.6). AML in elderly patients may also present with progressive pancytopenia with rare circulating blast forms [56]. The differentiation of AML with dysplasia from MDS can be difficult. Patients with acute erythroleukemia may have prominent dysplastic erythroid precursors and may initially be diagnosed with one of the MDSs. Patients with hypoplastic AML can also be confused with one of the MDS subtypes. In prospective trials of MDS up to 15% of the patients with hypoplastic MDS were later reclassified as having AML [48, 50].

The finding of a clonal cytogenetic abnormality characteristic of MDS is important in establishing the diagnosis, assessing prognosis and differentiating it from other disorders [3]. The WHO defined specific cytogenetic abnormalities, even in the absence of diagnostic morphologic dysplasia, that where sufficient to make a diagnosis of MDS (Table 23.6). In these cases the cytogenetic abnormality must be demonstrated by conventional karyotyping and not by in fluorescence in situ hybridization (FISH) or sequencing technologies. FISH analysis has facilitated an accurate cytogenetic diagnostics and compliments karyotyping. FISH can be performed on the non-dividing cells and therefore can be performed on PB cells. FISH studies may be helpful in identifying specific rearrangements not recognized by banding studies alone. FISH also provides a convenient and sensitive method for monitoring patients with a specific cytogenetic abnormality. The WHO also defined some common MDS associated cytogenetic abnormalities as not sufficiently specific to diagnosis MDS in the absence of diagnostic morphologic findings. The presence of cytogenetic abnormalities +8, −Y, and del (20q) while frequently observed in patients with MDS was noted not to be diagnostic of MDS. In the updated 2016 WHO classification del(5q) remains the only cytogenetic or molecular genetic abnormality that defines a specific MDS subtype.

The patient's clinical findings and history are helpful in guiding the pathological evaluation. An analysis of the bone marrow is essential for the diagnosis of MDS. The bone marrow is typically hypercellular for the patient's age, confirming the ineffective hematopoiesis, and shows dysplastic features in one or several cell lines. A number of other disorders can present with finding similar to MDS (Table 23.7). A history of the patient receiving chemotherapy and or radiotherapy is important. Questions about environmental and occupational exposures should be noted, including the

Table 23.5 Morphologic features of dysplasia

Lineage	Peripheral blood	Bone marrow
Erythroid	Macrocytosis	Megaloblastic changes
	Elliptocytes	Nuclear budding
	Acanthocytes	Ringed sideroblasts
	Stomatocytes	Nuclear fragments
	Teardrops	Cytoplasmic vacuolization
	Basophilic stippling	Multinucleation
	Acquired thalassemia	
Myeloid	Pseudo-Pelger-Huet anomaly	Abnormal maturation
	Auer rods Blasts	Increase in monocytoid forms
	Hypogranulation	Abnormal localization of immature precursor (AILP)
	Hypersegmentation	
	Ring shaped nuclei-circle	Hypogranulation
	Cell blasts forms	Increased blasts
Megakaryocyte	Giant platelets,Megakaryocte fragments	Micromegakaryocyte
	Hypogranular or agranular	Hypogranulation
	Platelets	Multiple small nuclei
	Thrombocytopenia	Nuclear hypolobation
	Thrombocytosis	

Table 23.6 Recurring chromosomal abnormalities considered presumptive evidence of MDS in the absence of definitive morphological features

Abnormality	WHO-estimated frequency in MDS (%)
Unbalanced	
−7 or del(7q)	10
−5 or del(5q)	10
i(17q)or t(17p)	3–5
−13 or del(13q)	3
Del(11q)	3
Del(12q) or t(12q)	3
Del(9q)	1–2
idic(x)(q13)	1–2
Balanced	
t(11;16)	3 in t-MDS
t(3;21)	2 in t-MDS
t(1;3)	<1
t(2;11)(p21;q23)	<1
Inv(3)	
t(6;9)(p23;q34)	<1

Comments: Although +8, del(20q), and −y are common chromosomal abnormalities. In MDS, the presence of one of these three abnormalities as the sole cytogenetic abnormality in cases where morphological criteria for MDS are not met is not considered to be enough for presumptive diagnosis. t-MDS-Therapy related MDS [3]

Table 23.7 Differential diagnosis of myelodysplastic syndromes

Disorder	Comments
Congenital dyserythropoietic anemia	Inherited disorder characterized by marked dyspoiesis of mature and immature erythroid elements. Granulocytes and megakaryocytes unremarkable. Unstable hemoglobins normal karyotype.
Aplastic anemia	Both congenital (Fanconi) and acquired aplastic must be distinguished from hypocellular myelodysplasia. Karyotype normal in acquired aplastic anemia, rare cases with clonal abnormalities may actually represent hypocellular myelodysplasia. Severe malnutrition.
Hypocellular neoplasms	Hypocellular MDS must be distinguished from hypocellular AML. MDS with fibrosis may resemble primary myelofibrosis.
Megaloblastic anemia	Dyspoiesis restricted to megaloblastic changes. Normal karyotype. Use of antimetabolites need to confirm normal B_{12} level. Antimetabolites, chemotherapy.
Toxic exposure	Arsenic poisoning, alcohol, chemotherapy bone marrow cellularity normal; blasts are not increased. Normal karyotype; normal vitamin B_{12} and folate levels. Neurologic and gastrointestinal manifestations may dominate clinical picture.
Disorders with ringed sideroblasts	Chemotherapy, copper deficiency, hereditary sideroblastic anemia. Pyridoxine deficiency, zinc toxicity, alcohol toxicity, and in patients receiving Antituberculosis agents, chloramphenicol. Heavy metals.
Fibrotic disorders	Acute megakaryoblastic leukemia. Metastatic carcinoma with marked fibrosis, hairy cell leukemia, and primary myelofibrosis.
Viruses	Single, double or trilineage dyspoiesis common. HIV-1. Parvovirus. Karyotype normal
Autoimmune disorders	Myelodysplasia-like picture with dyspoiesis may be found in patients with underlying immune defects. May precede evolution to red cell aplasia. SLE, rheumatoid arthritis.
Paraneoplastic syndromes	Myelodysplasia-like picture (usually resembling chronic myelomonocytic leukemia). Occasionally noted at diagnosis in patients with solid tumors (lung, colon, prostate, and gastric carcinoma and lymphomas). Distinct from therapy-induced bone marrow neoplasms in carcinoma patients.
Bone marrow regeneration	Abnormal localization of immature precursors, dyspoiesis and increased immature myeloid cells may be transient phenomena after aggressive therapy. Increased blasts from recovering bone marrow after cytoxic chemotherapy, drug toxicity or bone marrow transplantation. Karyotype normal.
Colony-stimulation factor therapy	Transient increase in blasts in blood and bone marrow. Clusters of blasts on core biopsy. Hypolobated neutrophils and toxic granule in neutrophils may be seen.
Drugs	After purine analog therapy, Zidovudine and other antivirals Dilantin, methotrexate, valproic acid, sulfasalazine, mycophenolate, etc.

patient's smoking history. An occupation history is important because excess cases of MDS have been reported in agriculcultural and industrial workers.

Clonal cytogenetic abnormalities are found in 38–78% of patients with de novo MDS and greater than 80% of t-MDS patients [50]. Cytogenetics are critical in evaluating disease progression and prognosis. All of the currently used prognostic scoring system acknowledge the importance of specific cytogenetics abnormalities to define prognosis and plan therapy. In addition, the acquisition of new cytogenetic abnormalities is generally associated with progression of the disease and a poor prognosis. Although anemia is the most common presenting laboratory feature in patients with MDS, approximately 50% of patients will demonstrate an abnormality of more than one cell line [51]. The WHO thresholds for defining cytopenias remain the same in the new 2016 classification: hemoglobin <10 g/dL, platelets <100 × 10^9/L and a absolute neutrophil count of <1.8 × 10^9/L. Patients may be at risk for bacterial infection generally due to qualitative abnormalities of neutrophil function and platelet functional abnormalities are associated with increased risk for bleeding even with an adequate platelet count. Iron studies may demonstrate increased iron stores even in patients who have not received red cell transfusions. The use of flow cytometry to determine the percent of blasts, assessment of CD34+ cells, is not recommended by WHO criteria as a substitute for the visual inspection of the bone marrow, unless the aspirate was of poor quality. The percent of CD34+ cells generally correlates with morphologic examination of routine bone marrow aspirate and peripheral blood smear; however, the WHO noted that not all leukemic blasts express CD34 and hemodilution and processing artifacts can yield misleading results. Multiparameter flow cytometry was recommended to determine the blast lineage and to determine aberrant antigen expression. However, it remains unclear if these changes are specific for the diagnosis of MDS as they occur in other myeloid neoplasms [51].

Immunophenotyping combined with cytogenetics and morphology help in the diagnosis and assessing the possible evolution of MDS to AML [52]. An increase in the percentage of CD34+ cells or CD117+ positive cells may help in documenting the progression to AML in a low-grade MDSs. The WHO, however, while noting that aberrant antigen expression patterns are common in MDS did not consider the phenotypic abnormalities sufficient, in the absence of conclusive morphologic and/or cytogenetic abnormalities, for the diagnosis of MDS. The finding of three or more phenotypic abnormalities involving one or more of the myeloid lineages should be considering suggestive, but not diagnostic of MDS. Patients whose cells demonstrate aberrant immunophenotypic markers should be followed for morphologic features sufficient to diagnose MDS. The use of additional studies including FISH analysis and gene mutational analysis should be performed as clinically indicated. The myelodysplastic/myeloproliferative neoplasm (MDS/MPN) group is an overlap disorder reflecting that some patients have features of both MDS and MPN and patients present with a clinical picture that demonstrates both increased proliferation and dysplastic and ineffective maturation. The classification of MDS/MPN reflects difficulty-separating MDS from other myeloid neoplasms.

Patients with MDS/MPN usually present with a leukocytosis and hepatosplenomegaly. The MDS/MPN category includes four defined entities: chronic myelomonocytic leukemia (CMML), atypical chronic myelogenous leukemia (a CML-Philadelphia chromosome negative), juvenile myelomonocytic leukemia (JMML), and a more heterogenous group of unclassifiable MDS/MPN (U-MDS/MPN). The criteria for MDS/MPN with ring sideroblasts and thrombocytosis, MDS/MPN-RS-T, (previously known as RARS-T) is better defined and includes thrombocytosis, ≥450 × 10^9/L associated with anemia, erythroid dysplasia, with ring sideroblasts in ≥15% of erythroid precursors. Megakaryocytes with features of a chronic myeloproliferative neoplasm that are hyperlobulated and atypical and are increased in number with large or giant forms with lobated staghorn like nuclei and occur in lose clusters or found adjacent to the endosteum or within sinusoids and important pathologic finding [52]. The spliceosome gene mutation SF3B1, associated with ring sideroblast, is frequently present in cases of MDS/MPN-RS-T but the subtype still requires ≥15% ring sideroblasts. The JAK 2 V617F mutation has been noted in some of the cases of MPN/MDS but the proliferative potential of most cases appear to be related to aberration in the RAS/MAPK or other signaling pathways and the JAK 2 mutation is not the primary oncogenic event to explain the MPN [42, 66]. The prognosis of patients with MDS/MPN-RS-T is better than most of the MDS/MPN disorders. The transformation to AML is uncommon and unlike the MPN there does not appear to be an increase risk of thrombotic or bleeding complications associated with the elevated platelet count. The treatment options for this subtype are not clear and additional studies are needed to further define the clinical course. In addition to the JAK 2 mutation some patients demonstrate the MPL mutation and both mutations appear to correlate with the elevated platelet count. In general the MDS/MPN disorders have a variable clinical course but are generally associated with poorer prognosis than their myeloproliferative neoplastic counterpart and an increased incidence of leukemic transformation. In MDS/MPNs the karyotype is usually normal or demonstrates a typical MDS cytogenetic abnormality. Gene mutations are common in the MDS/MPNs and can be helpful in assessing difficult cases with a normal karyotype. The 2016 WHO classification, however, noted that gene mutations even of the most commonly mutated genes, SRSF2, TET2, ETV6 and ASXL1 is not sufficient proof of a neoplastic disorder because gene mutations occurs in healthy older persons with undetermined significance. While some of these mutations are prognostically important and define aggressive disease, and have been incorporated into new prognostic scoring systems they should not be the sole determinant of a neoplastic disorder [53].

The diagnosis of myelodysplastic/myeloproliferative neoplasm unclassifiable (MDS/MPN-U) includes patients with features of both myelodysplasia and myeloproliferation who cannot be assigned to a more specific category. Patients must meet the criteria of one of the categories of MDS and demonstrate prominent myeloproliferative features without a prior MPN or MDS. The WHO emphasizes that the diagnosis of MDS/MPN-U should not be made in patients who have recently recovered from cytotoxic chemotherapy or have received recent growth factor therapy.

A follow-up evaluation in these patients is essential to demonstrate that the changes in the PB and BM are independent of recent treatments or recovery from chemotherapy. The features that distinguish this subgroup include an elevated platelet count or WBC without evidence of BCR–ABL1 or rearrangement of PDGFRA, PDGFRB or FGFR1, del 5q, t (3; 3), or inv3. In most patients, the karyotype is normal and no abnormal mutational studies are noted but the JAK2 V617F mutation may be present [54].

MDS with Fibrosis and Hypocellular MDS

The WHO classifications did not define a number of MDS subtypes that are generally recognized as clinically distinct. The categories MDS with marrow fibrosis and hypocellularity MDS are distinct disorders but the WHO noted that because they lack a consensus on the precise definition or the importance of these findings as distinct entities they on not included in the current classification. A subset of patients with MDS present with a hypocellular bone marrow (less than 15% cellularity on bone marrow biopsy) and minimal dysplasia. Hypocellular MDS must be differentiated from aplastic anemia and hypocellular AML [55]. Hypocellular MDS and aplastic anemia may also be pathophysiologically related [54]. The similarity of both disorders is suggested by their response to immunosuppressive therapy. Hypocellular MDS may represent an intermediate stage in the evolution of aplastic anemia. However, hypocellular MDS in contrast to aplastic anemia tends to occur in older patients, with a more gradual onset and dysplasia involving more than one cell line. In contrast to aplastic anemia dysplastic megakaryocytes are more prominent in hypocellular MDS. Megaloblastic red cell precursors, pancytopenia, and the presence of a paroxysmal nocturnal hemoglobinuria clone (PNH)—occur in both hypoplastic MDS and aplastic anemia and are therefore not helpful diagnostic features A characteristic MDS cytogenetic abnormality sometimes helps to define hypocellular MDS but similar findings may also be present in aplastic anemia [48]. Patients with a PNH clone and hypocellular MDS respond better to immunosuppression.

MDS with fibrosis (MDS-F) can be difficult to differentiate from primary myelofibrosis (PMF), acute megakaryocytic leukemia or acute panmyelosis [55]. The bone marrow is usually not aspiratable (dry tap) and the morphological findings of dysplasia may be difficult to identify on the bone marrow biopsy. Splenomegaly and leukoerythroblastosis on peripheral smear are unusual in MDS-F and when present suggest the diagnosis of PMF. Staining the marrow biopsy and circulating blast forms with megakaryocytic lineage-specific antigens can identify abnormal megakaryoblasts [55]. The finding of diffuse fibrosis in MDS is associated with a poor prognosis and greater than 2+-reticulum fibrosis, as defined by the European consensus system, is an independent negative prognostic marker [52]. The diagnostic challenges that such cases present are discussed by the WHO with a recommendation that hematopathologists should specifically comment upon the hypocellularity or extensive fibrosis in interpretative reports. The WHO classification, however, does not recognize hypocellular MDS and MDS-F as distinct entities as the sub-classification of these cases can be problematic and there is no accepted agreement on the diagnostic features associated with these two disorders. Immunohistochemical stains for CD34 on the biopsy may demonstrate excess blasts and may help in identifying these patients. Bone marrow fibrosis is associated with a higher red cell transfusion requirement, multilineage dysplasia, pancytopenia, and a poor prognosis. The 2008 and 2016 WHO classification attempts to address these issues, about when to call a disorder a separate diagnostic entity, and raises the question of when sufficient clinical characteristics or morphologic findings are distinctive enough to warrant a separate diagnostic category.

The recognition and enumeration of blast cells is of critical importance for the diagnosis of AML, MDS and defining the subtypes of MDS and requires a differential blast count on 500 cells on the aspirate to be 20% or more for a diagnosis of AML (either de-novo or evolved from a prior MDS). If a concomitant non-myeloid neoplasm (i.e., plasma cells) is present those cells should be excluded from the count used to evaluate the percent of blast forms. If an aspirate is not available a touch preparation of the biopsy may yield valuable cytologic information, but differential counts from touch preparations may not be representative and should be confirmed on the bone marrow biopsy. The definition of a blast cell can be difficult in MDS. The WHO did not specifically define the definition of a blast, but noted that blasts can be granular or agranular [54]. Myeloblasts are defined by a high nuclear/cytoplasmic ratio, visible nucleoli and usually fine nuclear chromatin. Nuclear shape can be a variable with basophilic granule, or Auer rods, aggregates of lysozymes, may be noted but no Golgi zone is detected. Granular blast cells must be distinguished from promyelocytes and the principal distinguishing characteristic of the normal promyelocyte is the presence of a visible Golgi zone [54]. Dysplastic promyelocytes have the recognizable features of promyelocytes including round, oval or an indented nucleus that is often eccentric with decreased granules or irregular distributed granules and a poorly developed Golgi zone. Determining the overall percentage of blasts in the context of marked erythroid hyperplasia can be problematic. In the updated 2016 WHO classification the percent of blasts is based on all nucleated cells not just the non-erythroid cells. This new criteria will results in most cases previously diagnosed as the erythroid/myeloid subtype of acute erythroid leukemia in the 2008 WHO criteria now being classified as MDS with excess blasts. In the updated 2016 WHO classification the cytogenetic abnormalities that are MDS defining remain unchanged. While acknowledging the prognostic importance of genetic abnormalities in MDS, in the 2016 WHO criteria only the del(5q) cytogenetic or molecular genetic abnormality defines a specific MDS subtype even if an there is an additional cytogenetic abnormality [3].

The 2016 WHO criteria noted the association between ring sideroblasts and an SF3B1 mutation. The SF3B1 mutation appears to be a early initiating event in the development of MDS and manifests a distinct gene expression profile and correlates with a favorable and indolent course [56]. Patients with MDS carrying the SF3B1 mutation have a more homogeneous phenotype characterized by isolated erythroid dysplasia and the presence of ring sideroblasts. Moreover, the actual percent of cells with ring sideroblast does not affect the prognosis.

The 2008 WHO classification redefined a number of new subgroups [57, 58]. Three categories of refractory cytopenia with unilineage dysplasia (RCUD) are defined: Refractory anemia (RA), refractory neutropenia (RN) and refractory thrombocytopenia (RT). These subgroups do not have an increase in blasts and involve a single lineage. In the 2016 WHO classification these subgroups are part of MDS with Single lineage Dysplasia (MDS-SLD). Other causes of dysplasia need to be addressed and excluded before the diagnosis of single lineage MDS is established (Table 23.7). The expansion of the erythroid component can occur in non-neoplastic disorders, including hemolytic anemia, iron deficiency, and B12 or folate deficiency. Erythropoietin administration may also lead to a marked expansion of the erythroid precursors. Simultaneous or chronologically close administration of erythropoietin and granulocyte growth factors may lead to erythroid hyperplasia with an increase in pronormoblasts and myeloblasts. Therefore, the pathologist must have knowledge of the patient's clinical history, including the administration of recent chemotherapy or growth factors when evaluating the bone marrow. Other causes of erythroid dysplasia include alcohol abuse (vacuolated erythroid precursors and ring sideroblasts), anti-tuberculosis medications and chloramphenicol. Isolated unilineage dyspoiesis should raise suspicion for secondary causes, including disorders not associated with prescription medications as seen in zinc over consumption leading to copper deficiency. Zinc competes with copper for its carrier, ceruloplasmin. Primary copper deficiency can present with pancytopenia with marked vacuolation of erythroid and myeloid precursors, megaloblastoid changes in red cell precursors and ring sideroblasts [59, 60] (Table 23.6). The 2016 WHO classification notes that the prognostic importance of genetic finding in MDS and the expanding knowledge of the clinical importance of recurring mutations in MDS but notes that the finding of one or more somatic mutation is not considered diagnostic of MDS even in a patient with unexplained cytopenias where these mutation may be frequently found [3].

In patients with MDS who lack the appropriate finding of any defined MDS category diagnosed with subtype, MDS, unclassifiable (MDS-U). MDS-U has no specific morphological features but includes MDS with the presence of 1% blast forms in the peripheral blood and <5% blasts in the bone marrow. An occasional blast can be found in healthy individuals and to avoid over interpreting the rare blast form the WHO notes that blasts must be noted in the peripheral blood on two or more successive evaluations to confirm the diagnosis of MDS-U. In addition the diagnosis of MDS - U can be made in cases with 1% or fewer blasts in in the blood and <5% blasts in the bone marrow with unequivocal dysplasia in <10% of one or more myeloid lineages but have a diagnostic cytogenetic abnormality. MDS-U is a very heterogenous subtype and patients have a variable clinical course and should be reclassified if they develop findings characteristic of a specific MDS subtype. The MDS-U subtype may represent the early phase of one or more specific MDS subtypes but with nonspecific morphological features of MDS.

Idiopathic Cytopenia(s) of Undetermined Significance and Idiopathic Dysplasia of Uncertain Significance

Patients who present with cytopenias but lack the diagnostic criteria of MDS, but in whom the diagnosis of MDS is suspected, are classified with the diagnosis "Idiopathic Cytopenia(s) of Undetermined Significance" (ICUS) [61]. The criteria for this group of disorders reflects the diagnostic uncertainty in these patients. A key distinction of ICUS from other potential precursor conditions such as MGUS, monoclonal B-cell lymphocytosis (MBL) and T cell clonality of undetermined is that an ICUS designation does not necessarily imply a clonal disorder. Limited data are available about the frequency or natural history of ICUS and reflects that some patients present with persistent cytopenia but lack the diagnostic features of MDS. The term idiopathic dysplasia of uncertain significance (IDUS) was proposed to describe a group of patients with dysplasia but no or only mild cytopenias [61]. In contrast to ICUS, patients with IDUS demonstrate dysplasia in >10% of cells in one or more lineage with or without a MDS-related karyotype but without persistent cytopenias. ICUS and IDUS have very variable courses and it is unclear if all the patients will ultimately develop a defined subtype of MDS or another myeloid neoplastic disorder. Moreover, it is unclear if these disorders are mutually exclusive or if the classification of a potentially premalignant disorders will provide meaningful prognostic or diagnostic information for patients in whom no cause for the cytopenia

Table 23.8 New terms for patients who do not meet the criteria for MDS

ICUS	*Idiopathic Cytopenias of Undetermined Significance*. The natural history of patients with ICUS is unclear. May have clonal or nonclonal hematopoiesis (clonal ICUS vs nc ICUS) as defined by somatic mutations or non- diagnostic cytogenetic findings by karyotype or FISH. A proportion of patients with ICUS with develop MDS or another myeloid malignancy. Much more common than MDS and most patients will not develop a myeloid malignancy.
IDUS	*Idiopathic Dysplasia of Undetermined Significance*. Dysplasia without cytopenia. Need to confirm the dysplasia over a 3–6 month period. Unclear clinical course and prognosis and frequently associated with benign conditions.
CHIP	*Clonal Hematopoiesis of Indeterminant Potential*. Age dependent somatic mutations in persons without a known hematologic disorder. The prevalence of CHIP increases greatly with age over 10% in person over the age of 70 years. Most with never develop MDS but is associated with an increased incidence of myeloid malignancies and all-cause mortality. In most persons may be an incidental findings relating to aging.
CCUS	*Clonal Cytopenias of Underdetermined Significance*. Have one or more cell line decrease, hemoglobin <11 g/dL, absolute neutrophil count (ANC), 1.5 × 10^9/L, platelet count < 100 × 10^9/L. persons have an acquired chromosomal abnormality not diagnostic of a hematologic malignancy and/or the presence of a somatic mutation with a variable allele fraction ≥2% in hematologic malignancy—Associated gene in the peripheral blood or bone marrow. Most persons had somatic mutations fraction of >10% similar to lower risk MDS patients, including mutated genes associated with high risk MDS including TP53, ASXL1,RUNX1 and DNMT3A. More frequently diagnosed than MDS but less than ICUS. No evidence of dysplasia. The natural history for most persons in unknown unlikely that all will develop MDS or other myeloid malignancy.

is found. The proposed term Clonal Cytopenia of Undetermined Significance (CCUS) has been proposed for cases with somatic mutations, or a non-diagnostic chromosomal abnormality, defining a clonal population in the bone marrow, but without dysplasia and one or more cytopenia in the blood (Table 23.8) [62].

MDS Subtypes

MDS with Ring Sideroblasts (MDS-RS)

MDS with ring sideroblasts (MDS-RS) is characterized by anemia, erythroid dysplasia and >15% ring sideroblasts of bone marrow erythroid precursors. There is generally no or minimal dysplasia in the non-erythroid precursors. Myeloblasts comprise <5% of the nucleated BM cells and are not present in the PB. In the 2016 WHO criteria MDS-RS is associated with recurrent mutations of the spliceosome gene SF3B1. The classification of MDS-RS was changed to include MDS cases with ring sideroblasts and multilineage dysplasia. This change reflected the link between ring sideroblasts and an SF3B1 mutations. In the 2016 classification if the SF3B1 mutation is identified then the diagnosis of MDS—RS can be made even if the ring sideroblast comprise only 5% of nucleated erythroid cells. If the SF3B1 mutation is lacking then ≥15% ring sideroblasts of nucleated erythroid cells is still required. MDS-RS subtype is divided into two groups; a group with single lineage dysplasia (MDS-RS-SLD), previously classified as refractory anemia with ring sideroblasts, and second group with multilineage dysplasia (MDS-RS-MLD), previously classified as refractory cytopenia with multilineage dysplasia. Patients with MDS—RS who lack the SF3B1 mutation have a more heterogenous phenotype, a high prevalence of TP53 mutations and less favorable prognosis. The SF3B1 mutation is early event in the development of MDS and may be an important therapeutic target in MDS-RS [58]. MDS-RS constitutes approximately 10% of cases of MDS. A majority of patients present with a moderate normochromic or macrocytic anemia. The PB frequently reveals dimorphic red cells due to a small population of microcytic and hypochromic red cells. Basophilic stippling and Pappenheimer bodies may be noted in red cells. Dysplasia is present in <10% of neutrophils and platelets. The bone marrow is usually hypercellular for the patient's age and demonstrates erythroid hyperplasia. The iron stain, Prussian blue staining, reveals ring sideroblasts that surround at least a third of the nuclear circumference. Iron stores are generally increased even in the absence of red cell transfusions. The number of CD 34+ cells is normal and most patients do not demonstrate a cytogenetic abnormality. Ring sideroblasts may be seen in a number of other, non- MDS-related disorders including lead poisoning, drugs including isoniazid which inhibits delta aminolevulinic acid (ALA) dehydratase activity and block hemoglobin formation resulting in ring sideroblast formation [45]. A number of acquired and hereditary conditions are associated with ring sideroblast formation and should be excluded before a diagnosis of MDS-RS is established. In RARS the ring sideroblasts and increased iron stores reflect abnormal iron metabolism in the erythroid lineage resulting from the ineffective erythropoiesis. The overall prognosis for patients with MDS-RS is 69–108 months and less than 2% of cases transform into AML. Progressive anemia requiring transfusion support is frequent and in select patients iron chelation therapy should be considered early in the clinical course to prevent iron overload and end organ failure. However, the overall beneficial effects of early iron chelation has not been demonstrated to improve survival in prospective randomized studies and therefore remains controversial [63].

MDS with Single Lineage Dysplasia and MDS with Multilineage Dysplasia

This group of disorders was previously know as Refractory anemia and refractory anemia with multilineage dysplasia in the 2008 WHO classification and is now classified as MDS-SLD and MDS-MLD. The difference between these subtypes reflects either a single or 2 or more lineages demonstrate dysplasia. These groups constitute approximately 30% of MDS cases and are characterized by one or more cytopenias and dysplastic changes in one two or more of the myeloid lineages. Blasts are rare, <1%, in the PB and <5% in the BM. Auer rods are not present in either the PB or BM. The anemia is usually macrocytic or normocytic with prominent granulocytic dysplasia including hypo granularity, nuclear shape abnormalities including hypo-lobation, acquired pseudo Pelger-Huet anomaly, and abnormal nuclear clumping. The bone marrow is usually hypercellular for age of the patient with <5% blasts. Erythroid precursors may demonstrate cytoplasmic vacuoles and marked nuclear irregularity including internuclear bridging and nuclear budding. The BM may have variable number of ring sideroblasts but less than 15%. The previously described WHO category of refractory cytopenias with multilineage dysplasia with ring sideroblasts has been omitted and incorporated in MDS-RS-MLD. Megakaryocytic dysplasia includes hypolobated and non-lobated nuclei, multinucleated and micromegakaryocyte, megakaryocytes with non-lobated or bi-lobed nuclei. Clonal cytogenetic abnormalities are present in up to 50% of patients and are important in defining the prognosis. The prognosis is related to the degree of cytopenias and cytogenetic abnormalities.

MDS with Excess Blasts 1(MDS-EB1 and MDS-EB2)

MDS-EB1 and EB2 comprises 40% of cases of MDS and is divided into MDS-EB1 and MDS-EB2 on the basis of the number of blasts and the presence or absence of Auer rods. EB 1 is defined by 5–9% blasts in the BM or 2–4% blasts in the PB and no Auer rods and EB2 is defined by 10–19% blasts in the BM or 5–19% blasts in the PB. The presence of Auer rods confirms the diagnosis of EB2 irrespective of the percent of blast forms. Most patients present with symptoms of BM failure including anemia, bleeding or neutropenia. The PB generally shows dysplastic changes in all three-cell lines and is typically hypercellular for age of the patient. Erythroid precursors may be increased with megaloblastoid changes and ring sideroblasts. The excess blasts define these subtypes. Dysmegakaryopoiesis is a frequent finding including micromegakaryocytes and abnormal megakaryocytic clustering. Blasts may form abnormal aggregates or clusters that are located away from trabeculare and vascular structures, a histologic finding previously referred to an abnormal localization of immature precursors (ALIP). Immunohistochemical staining for CD34 may help in identifying blast forms. Clonal cytogenetic abnormalities are observed in 30–50% of cases including +8, -5, del(5q),−7, del(7q), del (20q) and complex karyotypes. Fibrosis may be present and results in a dry tap. The presence of fibrosis should be noted and the finding of extensive fibrosis is an independent negative prognostic marker in MDS [3]. MDS-EB1 and 2 frequently progress to AML, 25% and 33% respectively for MDS-EB1 and MDS-EB2 respectively. The median survival is approximately 16 months for MDS-EB1 and 9 months for MDS-EB2. The survival is dependent on the number of blast forms. Cases with >5% blasts and a complex karyotype have a median survival of ≤3 months similar to AML with myelodysplastic changes.

Myelodysplastic Syndrome with Isolated del (5q)

Heterozygous, interstitial deletions of the long arm of chromosome 5 (5q) are the most common cytogenetic abnormality in patients with MDS. Del 5q is associated with a consistent clinical phenotype previously known as the 5q- syndrome in a subset of patients. Abnormalities in chromosome 5 occur in approximately 25% of MDS patients, but the incidence of the originally described 5q- syndrome is much less frequent [63]. The 5q- syndrome was originally described in patients with a macrocytic anemia, dyserythropoiesis and erythroid hypoplasia in the bone marrow and a normal to elevated platelet count, hypolobated megakaryocytes and an intestinal deletion involving the long arm of chromosome 5. In addition the 5q- syndrome in characterized by the absence of circulating myeloblast and therapeutic sensitivity to treatment with lenalidomide. The deletion of 5q in MDS does not necessarily equate to the clinical 5q- syndrome. Both the original 5q-syndrome and del (5q) MDS respond to lenalidomide and the revised WHO changed its definitions to this cytogenetically defined subset from 5q- syndrome to MDS with abnormality del(5q) [64, 65]. The deletion occur on a single chromosome resulting in a heterozygous (haploinsufficient) with the unaffected chromosome 5 contains the normal allele of all the genes contained in deleted segment. None of the genes on the nondeleted chromosome 5q are mutated or undergo homozygous inactivation in MDS patients. The recurrent haploinsufficiency for critical genes within the common deleted regions (CDR) on chromosome 5q is the basis for the unique pathological phenotype that results in the MDS subtypes del (5q). Haploinsufficiency of the RPS 14 gene on the long arm of chromosome 5 (5q) leads to activation of the P53 pathways and the development of the characteristic macrocytic anemia. The CDR on chromosome 5 and the breakpoints and size of the deletions in the original 5q- syndrome patients and the del (5q) patients with advanced MDS and AML are variable. The CDR of the 5q–syndrome the interstitial deletion occurs in a 1.5 MB region at 5q32–33. The region contains genes for the ribosomal protein RPS14 and three micro RNAs mrR-143, miR-145, and mir-146. The non-allelic deletion of the RPS14 gene encodes for a component of the 40 s ribosome and is critical for the development of the macrocytic anemia. In contrast, patients with del (5q), and additional chromosomal abnormalities and excess blast have a different clinical course and response to treatment [85]. Patients with a deletion of 5q- and AML have large interstitial deletions that overlap the CDR of the 5q-syndrome and low risk del (5q) However, in high risk MDS and AML the deleted region was in a more distal CDR in the 5q32–33 region. Lenalidomide selectively inhibits the Del (5q) clone and results in RPS 14 inactivation of the p53 pathway. Lenalidomide exerts unique karyotype specific activity in Del (5q) MDS but does not eradicate the Del (5q) stem cell population in all patients. The inactivation RPS14 leads to defective erythropoiesis and increased apoptosis in erythroid progenitors. Moreover, in the congenital disorder Diamond- Blackfan anemia the down regulation of an another ribosomal gene (RPS19) is critical in the development of the erythroid hypoplasia and chronic anemia [65]. The down regulation of RPS14 may not be the sole genetic event underlying the del 5q- syndrome and alteration of other genes in the commonly deleted segment in 5q- may be required. The tumor suppressor SPARC (Secreted Protein Acidic and Rich in Cysteine) gene is located in the del 5q31 region. SPARC has tumor suppressor, antiproliferative, and anti angiogenesis properties and may also be important in this syndrome [64]. The loss of additional genes that code for these and other factors appear to contribute to the development of this syndrome and its unique response to the immune modulatory drug, lenalidomide. MDS with isolated del 5q syndrome is frequently associated with morphological features of MDS-SLD. Thrombocytosis and anemia is occasionally seen and when present is suggestive of the del 5q chromosomal abnormality. The bone marrow aspirate and biopsy are typically hypercellular for the patient's age with erythroid hypoplasia and dysplastic erythropoiesis. Ring sideroblasts may be present but <15% of erythroblasts. A del(5q) subtype should be suspected in patients who present with a refractory macrocytic anemia, with a normal or mildly low leukocyte counts, and thrombocytosis (a platelet count >400 × 10^9/L). In contrast to the other MDS subtypes, where the mononuclear megakaryocytes are smaller (micromegakaryocytes), in the MDS with del 5q the megakaryocytes are bilobed or non-lobulated but of normal size (mono lobulated). The MDS with del 5q has a marked female predominance (70%), and rarely transforms to AML. A majority of patients have progressive anemia and become red cell transfusion dependent and rarely respond to growth factors including erythropoietin. Lenalidomide is the treatment of choice and results in transfusion independence in over two thirds of cases with durable clinical and cytogenetics responses [42].

Clinical and Laboratory Features of MDS

Blood and Bone Marrow Findings

Red Cells/Anemia

Macrocytosis or a macrocytic anemia with a low reticulocyte count is common in MDS and reflects the ineffective erythropoiesis. Impaired red cell maturation has been associated with acquired abnormalities of globin chain synthesis, and red cell enzymes. PNH has been described in the setting of MDS, and these patients have many of the typical diagnostic features of PNH including a defect in the synthesis of the glycosylphosphatidylinositol (GPI)-linked surface protein, but lack the ongoing red cell hemolysis and thrombotic complications associated with PNH. Cases may have abnormalities in the size and shape of red cells including basophilic stippling (red cell inclusions composed of ribonucleoprotein and mitochondrial remnants), Pappenheimer bodies (basophilic iron-containing granules peripherally located in red cells), macro-ovalocytes, teardrop forms, and nucleated red cells. The bone marrow may reveal multinuclear fragments, inter-nuclear bridging, and nuclear cytoplasm asynchrony.

Neutrophils

Qualitative abnormalities of neutrophil function are a common feature of MDS and may explain the increased risk for bacterial infections. Morphological abnormalities include hypo-granular and hyposegmented neutrophils, which are associated with a negative peroxidase reaction and decreased myeloperoxidase activity. The neutrophils are hyposegmented and may be confused with band forms. Nuclear fragmentation and nuclear-cytoplasmic asynchrony in early myeloid precursors may be a prominent feature in the bone marrow. Dysplastic myeloid precursors can be difficult to distinguish from blast forms and therefore a pathologist experienced in the interpretation of MDS should review the bone marrow.

Platelets

Thrombocytopenia and abnormal platelet function occur in MDS. Thrombocytopenia is an adverse prognostic feature independent of other prognostic factors [66–68]. While thrombocytopenia is associated with poor performance status and other unfavorable prognostic variable bleeding complications are underreported. Thrombocytopenia (<100 × 10^9/L) has been reported in 66% of patients and was associated with a 24% incidence of deaths from hemorrhage. Impaired platelet function may also explain the increased risk of bleeding in patients with MDS. Spontaneous bruising and bleeding after surgery or mild trauma occurs in MDS patients with a normal or slightly depressed platelet counts. Dysplastic platelets and abnormal megakaryocytes are important diagnostic features and help in distinguishing MDS from other disorders. Giant platelets, and agranular (grey platelets) and megakaryocytic fragments in the peripheral blood film are important diagnostic features of MDS.

Bone Marrow Findings

A bone marrow aspirate and biopsy is essential for the making diagnosis of a MDS and to define the MDS subtype. Abnormal distribution of cells is often present; erythroid islands may be absent or very large. Granulocytic precursors may be clustered centrally rather than their normal paratrabecular distribution. Micromegakaryocyte, mononuclear megakaryocytes, and hyperlobulated megakaryocytes are important diagnostic features of MDS and are reliable morphological findings of dysplasia. In the bone marrow the megakaryocytes may be clustered or adjacent to the bony trabecula. The del 5q syndrome has mononuclear megakaryocytes that are of normal size but with a single eccentrically placed round non-lobulated nucleus [3]. Megaloblastic changes (nuclear cytoplasm asynchrony) can be seen in the myeloid and erythroid precursors. Dysgranulopoiesis and dyserythropoiesis are more readily noted in the bone marrow aspirate smear and not the biopsy. The bone marrow smear is necessary to identify ring sideroblasts that may not be apparent on the biopsy sample. Immunohistochemistry may be a useful supplement to histology. Small mononuclear megakaryocytes can be confused with myeloid precursors. A biopsy is necessary to access the degree of reticulin fibrosis and overall bone marrow cellularity. Immunophenotyping using flow cytometry on the bone marrow and/or peripheral blood may be helpful in the diagnosis and defining prognosis and response to treatment. However, while controversial there are currently no accepted standards for the diagnosis of MDS by flow cytometry.

The finding of aberrant immunophenotyping of myeloid blasts is helpful in corroborating the diagnosis of MDS, but is not diagnostic of MDS. The aberrant expression of the lymphoid antigen CD7 on myeloid blasts is a common phenotypic abnormality and correlates with a poor prognosis [42]. Increase and/or clustering of blasts favors MDS. Immunostaining for CD34 on core biopsy is very helpful to estimate blast numbers and possible clustering. In the absence of reliable aspirate smear, CD34 immunostaining on core biopsy and/or clot section can be used for estimating percentage of blasts. The use of flow cytometry on both the PB and BM is the focus of many studies and should be part of the initial evaluation of MDS [42].

Clinical and Prognostic Features

The initial evaluation of all patients with MDS should be performed before planning treatment and should include a detailed history of prior exposures to chemotherapy, radiation therapy or toxic exposures. The cellularity should be noted from the bone marrow biopsy. The percent of blasts and the iron stain and the presence of ring sideroblasts should be performed on the bone marrow aspirate. Iron studies including a ferritin and transferrin saturation should be obtained prior to starting growth factors and on patients who are receiving red cell transfusions. A serum erythropoietin should be determined in patients with symptomatic anemia. In patients who are candidates for an allogeneic hematopoietic stem cell transplant HLA typing should be performed on the patient and their siblings.

The WHO classification system attempts to offer general prognostic guidance for each subtype but additional information is usually needed to assign prognosis and plan therapy. In an effort to determine prognosis a number of prognostic scoring systems have been developed including the International Prognostic Scoring System (IPSS), the MD Anderson Prognostic Scoring System (MDAPSS), World Health Organization –based Prognostic Scoring System (WPSS) and others models have been developed to define the prognosis and guide therapy [69, 70]. The widely used and generally accepted International Prognostic Scoring System (IPSS) developed in 1997 and recently revised, IPSS-R, addresses clinical features not included in the WHO classification and attempts to define prognosis and leukemic progression. The IPSS-R included 5 cytogenetic subsets reflecting the importance of new prognostically important cytogenetic groupings (Table 23.9). The scoring system assigns a point score for each the following variables: the number of bone marrow blast forms, karyotypic abnormalities, and number of cell lines affected (cytopenias) (Table 23.10). The combined score determines the overall risk category: very low (risk score $\leq$ 1.50), Low (risk score > 1.5–3.0), Intermediate (risk score > 3–4.5), High (risk score > 4.5–6) and very high (risk score > 6). The IPSS-R risk category and score correlates with the overall survival and probability of transformation to AML (Table 23.9).

The other prognostic scoring systems include similar parameters but the IPSS-R scoring system continues to be widely used for stratification of patients enrolled in clinical trials [69, 70]. However, the IPPS-R system has a number of important limitations. The IPPS-R system is based in part on the FAB classification of MDS and includes MDS patients with 30% blasts. The threshold for AML in the WHO classification is 20% blasts which is not reflected in the IPSS–R blast scoring system. The IPSS also does not completely address the severity of the cytopenias or the need for transfusion support and does not take into account other prognostic

Table 23.9 MDS cytogenetic scoring system: IPSS-R

Prognostic subgroup	Cytogenetic abnormalities	Percent of patients	Survival (years median)	AML evolution[a]
Very good	−Y, del(11q)	4	5.4	NR
Good	Normal, del(5q), del(12p), del(20q), double including del(5q)	72	4.8	9.4
Intermediate	Del(7q), +8, +19, i(17q) any other single or double independent clones	13	2.7	2.5
Poor	−7, inv.(3)/t(3q)/del(3q), double including- 7/ del(7q),complex:3 abnormalities.	4	1.5	1.7
Very poor	Complex: >3 abnormalities	7	0.7	0.7

NR not reached
[a]AML evolution 25%—median time to 25% AML: median—years

Table 23.10 IPSS-R scoring system

Prog score variable	0	0.5	1.0	1.5	2.0	3.0	4.0
Cytogenetics	Very good		Good		Intermediate	Poor	Very poor
Bone marrow %blasts	≤2		>2–<5		5–10	>10	
Hemoglobin g/dL	≥10		8–<10	<8			
Platelets cmm	≥100	50–100	<50				
Absolute neutrophil counts/cmm	≥0.8	<0.8					

Very Good −7,del(11q), Good—Normal, del(5q),del(12p), del (20q), double including del(5q) Intermediate - del(7q), +8,+19,i(17q), any other single or double independentclones. Poor—7, inv.(3)/t3q)/del 3, double including −7/del(7q). Very Poor—Complex >3 abnormalities. See Table 23.3

variables. The IPSS-R acknowledged the prognostic importance of additional variable but did not assign a point score to these factors including LDH, serum ferritin, β2-microglobulin, marrow fibrosis, patient's age, performance status and comorbidities. Other prognostic factors including disease duration or prior treatments are not part of the IPSS-R. The IPPS and IPSS-R was intended to assign prognosis at the time of diagnosis and therefore is a static score that was not intended to change with time or treatments. The IPSS–R also includes a number of uncommon cytogenetic subsets does not address the expanding role of molecular genetic studies in MDS.

MDS is often broadly separated, for treatment decisions, into low risk and high-risk disease based on overall survival and risk of AML transformation. The lower risk subtypes include MDS with single lineage dysplasia, MDS with Multilineage dysplasia, MDS with ring sideroblasts, MDS with isolated del(5q). The IPSS-R low risk categories include the very low, low and intermediate risk categories. These groups are associated with a general survival of >3 years and a low risk for transformation to AML and generally correspond to a IPPS-R score of <3.5. In contrast the higher risk MDSs groups include MDS-EB 1 and 2 and IPSS-R groups high and very high and are associated with a greater risk for transformation to AML [70].

Treatment

The treatment of a patient with MDS should be individualized based on the patient's age, subtype, IPSS-R risk category, performance status, cytogenetics and co-morbid medical problems. The majority of patients with MDS are elderly and tolerate intensive chemotherapy poorly. Moreover, standard therapies do not result in a cure and their impact on survival for most patients is unclear. Therefore any potential benefits of treatment must be weighed against the side effects and the patient's overall prognosis. The alleviation of disease-related complications and improved quality of life are important goals for most patients. The most appropriate care for many patients still remains supportive care. Although there are a number of therapeutic options available for MDS patients, none, other than an allogeneic stem cell transplantation, offers the potential for cure. The therapeutic options for patients with MDS include the use of hematopoietic growth and trophic factors, immunosuppressive agents, low-intensity cytoreductive chemotherapy including the hypomethylating agents, and intensive chemotherapy. While advances in the diagnosis and risk stratification has refined the prognosis for patients and defined gene mutations that are potential targets in MDS, no new drugs s have been approved for the treatment of MDS in over a decade.

Guidelines for evaluating the response to treatment in patients with MDS have been updated and incorporated into the criteria by the International Working Group (IWG) [71]. These guidelines attempted to define standard, criteria for complete and partial responses to treatment. Moreover, the response criteria emphasized that the goals of treatment of MDS is to alter the natural history of the disease and alleviate the disease-related complications and improve the quality of life. Stable disease or minimal responses are difficult to interpret and make comparisons between trials difficult. In addition, the response rate in some Phase II trials did not translate into prolongation of survival, time to treatment failure, or improvement in the quality of life. The IWG criteria are a useful standard to use for comparing results across therapeutic trials and are now widely used for defining response to treatment.

Supportive Therapy

In many patients the diagnosis of MDS may require a period of observation and reevaluation. The WHO appropriately noted that in some patients reevaluating the peripheral blood and bone marrow after 3–6 months period was essential to exclude other causes of the dysplasia. In patients with indolent disease or who are asymptomatic, elderly, and frail or have co-morbidities, supportive therapy including transfusions represents a widely accepted standard of care. Patients should be followed for a change in their clinical pattern i.e., increase in red cell transfusion, declining platelet count, circulating blast forms, splenomegaly or decline in performance status. Red cell and platelet transfusions are administered for the symptomatic treatment of the anemia and thrombocytopenia. There is no one single hemoglobin cut off at which RBC transfusion should be offered to all patients but the use of transfusion support is increasing over the years in an effort to maintain a higher hemoglobin/hematocrit. Platelet transfusions are generally given when the platelet count is <10,000 × 10^9/L but should be adjusted on the basis of individual risk factors and bleeding history. Thrombocytopenia is common in MDS and bleeding complications are exacerbated by impaired platelet function [68]. Platelet dysfunction is common and patients may bleed even with an adequate platelet count. Therefore, platelet support may be required prior to surgery and procedures to prevent excess bleeding. Patients with a platelet count of ≤20,000 × 10^9/L are at higher risk for bleeding. Disease modifying agents such a lenalidomide and hypomethylating agents are associated with thrombocytopenia. The repeated use of platelet transfusions is associated with allo immunization and transfusion reactions. Danazol an attenuated synthetic androgen with immune modulating activity may be effect in some thrombocytopenic patients with MDS [72]. Thrombopoietin receptor agonist (TPO) are being tested in clinical trials as single agents in low-risk MDS patients and in combination therapy with disease modifying agents (lenalidomide) in high risk MDS. Romiplostim a Fc- peptide fusion protein with no sequence homology with endogenous TPO has been evaluated in low /intermediate risk MDS patients with thrombocytopenia [73, 74]. Romiplostim reduced overall bleeding events but the trial was stopped because of concerns regarding leukemic transformation. Eltrombopag and oral nonpeptide, noncompetitive TPO receptor agonist which is indicated for the treatment of ITP was evaluated in a phase 2 randomized trial in low/intermediate risk MDS patients, Eltrombopag increased the platelet count in a limited number of patients without a increase in leukemic risk. It was unclear in the limited studies that either TPO improved survival. The TPOs are not approved at this time for treatment of thrombocytopenia in MDS patients.

Neutropenia and impaired neutrophil function are also common in MDS patients. The use of prophylactic antibiotics, however, is not warranted for most patients. Neutropenia without a history of recurrent infection is not a justification for the initiation of therapy. Granulocyte colony stimulating factor or granulocyte macrophage colony stimulating factors can transiently increase the neutrophil and blast count in many patient with MDS. However, the clinical benefit of these growth factors is unclear. The use of G-CSF did decrease the incidence of serious infections but did not favorably impact survival in a prospective controlled trial. The use of these cytokines did increase the white blood count and the number of circulating blasts but did not appear to accelerate the progression to acute leukemia. Although in selected patients with active, serious infections there may be a role for the use of these cytokines in the MDS patient with neutropenia in combination with antibiotics, at present there is no evidence to support the general use of either G-CSF or GM-CSF [74].

Patients may require multiple transfusions over many years and the potential for iron overload should be addressed early in a patient's course. Each unit of RBC contains 200–250 mg of iron and iron overload from transfusions occurs when a patient has received 25 units of packed red cells [75–79]. The benefits of chelation therapy (ICT) in MDS remains controversial. Patients with transfusion dependent low risk MDS may benefit from the early introduction of iron chelation and chelation may reduce the effects of iron overload on cardiac and possibly prevent end organ damage due to tissue iron overload [77]. Iron chelation may also reduce the risk of infections and improve survival after allogeneic hematopoietic stem cell transplantation and may delay the leukemic progression and improve hematopoiesis [78]. Some observations suggest that cytopenias in iron-overloaded patients with MDS could be mitigated by ICT, possibly by a decrease in reactive oxygen species-mediated damage to hematopoietic cells [79]. In addition hematologic improvement was seen in some patients who received deferasirox including a normalization of labile plasma iron [79]. The use of ICT may suppress ineffective erythropoiesis by reducing iron and/or oxidative stress and modulating proliferation and differentiation. However, the risk of iron overload in transfusion dependent MDS patients is unclear. Iron toxicity in MDS patients may not only depend on tissue iron accumulation but also the extent of non-transferrin bound iron. Prospective studies evaluating the clinical benefit of iron chelation in MDS patients ongoing [77]. Iron chelation is a slow process and therefore it is important to view chelation as a preventive supportive measure. The use of deferoxamine is impractical for most patients with MDS. Deferoxamine has a short half-life and requires a prolonged parental, either subcutaneous or intravenous, infusion that is administered over 8–12 h. The rapid infusion of deferoxamine following a red cell transfusion has limited benefit and does not result effective chelation. The oral iron chelator deferasirox (Exjade, Jadenu) is administered daily and is effective in reducing the serum ferritin [79]. Deferasirox can cause reversible renal insufficiency and GI disturbances, including gastrointestinal bleeding. In a number of studies Deferasirox was poorly tolerated in MDS patients with serious renal and gastrointestinal side effects [76]. A number of guidelines on the use of chelation therapy in MDS have been reviewed and a consensus statement published recommending the use of oral chelation therapy in transfusion dependent patients with low risk MDS. Iron overload may contribute to increased morbidity and mortality in low risk MDS patients. However other studies did not demonstrate a direct correlation of the serum ferritin, numbers of transfusions and overall survival. The benefits of prolonged oral chelation therapy is low risk MDS patients remains controversial and in general the benefits should be weighed against the potential risks and its effect on quality of life. The beneficial effects of iron chelation therapy on organ function and survival in transfusion dependent MDS patients is currently lacking. But, in low risk transfusion dependent patients with a ferritin of >1000 mg/dL or patients considered eligible for an allogeneic stem cell transplant ICT should be considered and renal and hepatic function closely monitored.

Erythropoiesis Stimulating Agents (ESAs)

Recombinant hematopoietic growth factors have been used with varying degrees of success to treat the cytopenias in MDS. Recombinant human erythropoietin (rHuEPO, EPO and darbepoetin), granulocyte-colony-stimulating factor (G-CSF), and granulocyte-macrophage colony stimulating factor (GM-CSF) have a role in managing the anemia and neutropenia in selected patients with MDS. ESAs have been studied extensively and approximately 30% of anemic patients with MDS will respond to treatment [75]. The reported response rates in low risk MDS varies between 30 and 82% depending on patient selection and response criteria [80]. The best responses to erythropoiesis stimulating agents (ESA) are observed in patients with an endogenous erythropoietin level of <500 U, a transfusion requirement of less than two units of red cells a months and low risk MDS with <5% myeloblasts [81]. ESAs decrease red cell transfusion requirements and improved the quality of life (QOL). Higher doses of EPO appear to enhance the erythroid responses. The combination of EPO plus G-CSF appears to be synergistic and may optimize the response to EPO. The duration of response was 11–24 months and EPO with or without G-CSF did not increase the incidence of AML transformation. ESAs did improve the QOL but treatment did not impact on overall survival. The ESAs have been associated with an increased mortality, possible promotion of tumor growth in solid tumors and thromboembolic events in non-MDS patients. No increase in treatment related either cardiovascular or thrombotic events occurred in patients who received either EPO alone or combination cytokines EPO with G-CSF as compared to a control population. The FDA recently cited safety concerns from data in clinical studies with ESAs administered to patients with solid tumors [81]. In patients with various solid tumors the use of ESAs was associated with a shortened survival, and/or increased risk of tumor progression or recurrence as well as a increased risk for thrombotic events in patients with renal disease (http://www.fdagov/Drugs/DrugSafety/). MDS patients did not have a increase in disease progression or thrombotic complications associated with ESAs [80]. A predictive model for treatment with EPO and G-CSF demonstrated that patients with an EPO level of <500 mU/mL, and a pretreatment transfusion requirement of less than 2 units/month responded best to ESAs [81]. Best responses were noted in IPSS lower risk patients. Responses can take 8 or more weeks with most patients responding by 12 weeks and the recommended starting for the recombinant human erythropoietin alpha (rEPO) doses are 40–60,000 units administered once or twice a weekly, and increasing the dose up to 300,000 U/week depending on the response. The longer acting form, Darbepoetin, is administered starting at 50–300 mcg/weekly or every other week. Darpoetin administered every 2–3 weeks at a dose of 500 mcg is also effective. Adequate iron stores should be documented prior to starting EPO treatment and during therapy as the failure to respond or loss of response may be a manifestation of depleted iron stores. Low doses of G-CSF (1 μg/kg) with EPO can be added to patients who fail to respond and appeared to augment the response in selected patients [80]. The mechanism of the response to high doses of EPO is unclear but the growth factors may modulate apoptosis in MDS progenitors and enhance erythropoiesis. Moreover, the response to ESAs may define a more favorable group of MDS patients and in a Phase III trial MDS patients who responded to EPO had a longer overall survival versus those who did not respond [80].

Thrombocytopenia is an independent adverse prognostic factor for survival in MDS. Bleeding complications resulting from thrombocytopenia and MDS associated platelet dysfunction are major causes of morbidity and mortality in MDS. Treatments to increase the platelet count are limited. Danazol is an attenuated, synthetic androgen that has been used in the treatment of immune-mediated thrombocytopenia (ITP). Danazol may increase the platelet count in low-risk MDS patients who are thrombocytopenic [72]. The mechanism of action is unclear, but may reflect that some patients with MDS have immune-mediated thrombocytopenia that responds to the immunoregulatory effects of danazol. Danazol, 200 mg po tid, is generally well tolerated and associated with an increase in platelets in 10–46% of treated patients. The duration of response is variable, 2–26+ months, and maintained only while the drug is administered. Patients with platelet counts greater than 15×10^9/L appear to respond best, and the impact on survival or disease progression is unknown. Two thrombopoietin receptor agonists (TPO), eltrombopag and romiplostim, are currently available to treat patient with refractory ITP. Both agents are active in patients with ITP by increasing platelet production. However, safety concerns remain including the risk of marrow fibrosis and leukemic transformation [68]. A transient increase in blasts forms has been noted in patients treated with TPO. Eltrombopag is currently being studied in higher risk MDS patients. Ongoing studies are evaluating the role of these agents in the treatment of the thrombocytopenic patient with MDS. These early trials of TPOs suggest that they are well tolerated in MDS patients and increased the platelet count and decreased the need for platelet transfusions and clinical bleeding events. But their effect on survival and disease progression is unclear.

Immunosuppressive Therapy

Patients with MDS can present with a number of immune-mediating pancytopenias that potentially respond to immunosuppressive therapy [82]. Some patients with low risk and hypocellular MDS responded to immunosuppressive regimens used for the treatment of aplastic anemia. Selected patients with hypocellular or normal cellular bone marrows responded to the administration of anti-thymocyte globulin (ATG), cyclosporine A(CSA) and steroids [83]. Antithymocyte globulin (ATG) either rabbit or hoarse derived, administered at doses similar to those used in the treatment of aplastic anemia resulted in improvement of one or more cytopenia in 30–50% of selected patients [83]. Trilineage responses were observed in some patients and the median duration of response was 10+ months. Responses were more frequent with hypocellular MDS but were even noted in patients with normocellular bone marrows. Improvements were seen in patients with low-, intermediate-, and high-risk IPSS scores. Age, 60< years, HLA- DR15 positivity, low risk disease, shorter duration of transfusion dependency, and trisomy 8 cytogenetic abnormality correlated with the response to treatment [84]. The responses did not correlate with the loss of a previously noted cytogenetic abnormality, suggesting that the treatment was not affecting the MDS clone. A majority of the patients attained a partial response and treatment did not restore normal hematopoiesis. The mechanism of action is not clear but in vitro studies suggest that the response may be mediated by a loss of cytotoxic T-lymphocyte activity which correlated with changes in the T-cell receptor profiles [84]. The response to ATG appears greatest in low-risk patients. In some patients who initially responded to ATG and then relapsed, retreatment was effective. Toxicity of ATG therapy included fevers, infusion related side effects, and infections. Age was the most important predictor of response with patients >60 years of age having a poorer outcome and increased complications associated with immunosuppressive therapy. These studies suggested that older patients with MDS may have a decreased marrow reserve associated with a diminished response to immune-suppression. CSA, alone may also be effective in hypocellular MDS patients. The combination of CSA and ATG may enhance the response in selected patients. In addition the use of alemtuzumab, an antibody against CD52, has been used in selected patients. The reported studies of ATG and CSA treated a highly selected subset of patients that represent a minority of patients with MDS. Most of the responding patients presented with hypocellular marrows (<15% cellularity) with minimal dysplasia. The responses of MDS patients to immunosuppressive therapy reflect the heterogeneity of the disorder and the relationship between the immune system, marrow suppression and MDS remains controversial. In addition it is unclear if the use of ATG with or with CSA impacted overall survival. In at least one Phase 3 trial comparing ATG + CSA versus best supportive care found no difference in overall survival or transformation to AML in the ATG + CSA arm. The use of immunosuppressive therapy to modulate the abnormal clone represents a controversial but a potential treatment that needs to be further evaluated to define the optimal group of patients who are candidates for immunosuppression.

Lenalidomide

Lenalidomide is a second generation 4-amino-gluteramide analog of thalidomide. Lenalidomide has multiple modes of action including pro-apoptotic cytokine generation, T cell stimulation or inhibition, antiangiogenesis, altering cell adhesions to bone marrow stroma, direct antiproliferative activity and the inhibition of a pro-inflammatory cytokines [85]. Lenalidomide was active in patients with del (5q) by selectively inhibiting the del(5q) clone. Lenalidomide in a phase II trial was administered at 10 mg/day for a 28 cycle or 21/28 days cycle in transfusion dependent patients with del(5q) abnormality 67% of patients became transfusion independent and 45% obtained a complete cytogenetic; complete and partial responses occurred in 84% of patients with del (5q) [63]. The finding of additional cytogenetic abnormalities, with the exception of −7/del(7q), did not significantly affect the response to lenalidomide. All patients who had a cytogenetic response became transfusion independent which was associated with improvement in overall survival. Patients who did not response to lenalidomide had higher rate of progression to AML. The median duration of response was 2.2 years (range 0.1–4.4 years) and approximately 30% of patients remain transfusion independent after 3 years [63]. Most of the responding patients developed pancytopenia and the myelosuppression served as a surrogate marker of clonal suppression of the del(5q) clone and predictive of the response to lenalidomide. Greater than 70% of patients with the del(5q) developed thrombocytopenia within the first 4–8 weeks of treatment and the development of thrombocytopenia was significantly correlated with a favorable response and the development of transfusion independence and a cytogenetic response [63]. A platelet decline in the first 8 weeks of treatment correlated with the response to treatment and likely reflected a direct specific cytotoxic effect of lenalidomide on the MDS clone. Most patients needed dose reductions due to myelosuppression and/or thrombocytopenia and in phase III trial comparing 5 daily and 10 mg on days 1–21 on a 28-day cycle versus placebo, the 10 mg dose was superior. Long term follow up in patients treated with lenalidomide demonstrated a prolonged duration of response, with durable transfusion independence, cytogenetic responses and extended survival with improvement in quality of life [63]. In low risk, transfusion dependent MDS patient without the del (5q) cytogenetic abnormality the response rate to lenalidomide was much less and the mechanism of action appears to be very different. The overall response rate in this non del(5q) group was 33% but only 17% became transfusion independent. A majority of the responses were characterized as a decrease in RBC transfusions as compared to the baseline transfusion requirement. There were minimal or no changes in the bone marrow morphology and documented histological and cytogenetic responses were rare. Myelosuppression, grade 3/4, neutropenia and thrombocytopenia occurred only in 20–25% of patients. Moreover, the development of cytopenias including thrombocytopenia and neutropenia on lenalidomide for patients without the del(5q) was not associated with a response to treatment. The response duration of lenalidomide in the non-del (5q) patients ranged from 3 to 85 weeks with a median of 41 weeks. The median time to response was short at 4.8 weeks and response after 16 weeks of treatment were rare and alternate treatment was recommended for patients who fail to respond after 4 months of lenalidomide. Higher responses correlated with a baseline platelet count of >150 × 10^9/L and shorter duration of MDS. Lenalidomide mechanism of action in MDS is clearly karyotype dependent. In del(5q) patient's lenalidomide appears to have a direct cytotoxic effect on the dysplastic clone resulting in eradication of the malignant clone. In contrast in the lower risk transfusion dependent MDs patient without the del(5q) lenalidomide effects appear to be mediated indirectly perhaps by effecting the bone marrow microenvironment or cytokine modulation.

Low-Dose Chemotherapy

Potential Differentiating Agents

Cytarabine administered at low doses (low dose Ara-C: Lo DAC) has been the most extensively used chemotherapy for elderly patients with high-risk, symptomatic MDS [86]. Cytarabine is administered daily by either continuous infusion or bolus subcutaneous injections at doses of 10–20/mg/m^2 for 14–21 days. At low dose cytarabine may induce differentiation but most likely works by a direct cytotoxicity [86]. In a prospective controlled trial patients higher risk MDS patients had the highest response rates, 20–35% (complete remission partial response [CR] + PR). The median duration of response for all subtypes was 8–15 months, with a range of 6–24 months. The response to Lo DAC correlated with its cytoreductive effect on the bone marrow. In a Phase III trial treatment with low-dose cytarabine was not superior to supportive care with regards to overall survival or leukemic transformation [86]. The role of low-dose cytarabine in the treatment of patients with high-risk MDS is controversial. In high-risk patients it remains a widely used treatment that may be effective in inducing transient responses in a subset of patients with progressive disease who are not candidates for alternative treatments. Low doses of chemotherapy may have a supportive role in selected patients with MDS. A number of trials have addressed the use of low doses of oral chemotherapy that was well tolerated and administered over a prolonged period. Low-dose oral etoposide (VP-16) and hydroxyurea were effective in controlling symptoms in some patients [87]. The use of steroids alleviated some of the cytokine-mediated symptoms associated with MDS/MPN and produced transient hematological improvements. Low-dose melphalan (2 mg/day until response or progression) in high-risk, frail patients with MDS was well tolerated and responses were noted in both hypercellular and hypocellular MDS [88]. The overall response rate to a prolonged course of low-dose melphalan in Phase II studies was approximately 40%. The duration of the responses to low-dose melphalan is unclear and additional studies are needed to determine its role in treating high risk MDS.

Histone acetylation facilitates active gene transcription and highly regulated by histone deacylases (HDACs) and histone acetyltransferases (HATs). HDAC inhibition may restore normal acetylations of histone proteins and promote cell cycle arrest and induce apoptosis in malignant cells. Normal differentiation and cell death programs are influenced by histone modification. HDAC expression is frequently deregulated in high risk MDS and AML and is therefore a potential therapeutic target. A number of HDAC inhibitors have been developed including Valproic acid, Entinostat, Belinostat, Panobinostat, Romidepsin, Vorinostat and others in various stages of development. HDAC inhibitors have multiple potential mechanism of action leading to their pleiotropic activity and use in various disorders. The response rate for single agent HDACs is low and therefore they are combined with other agents including the DNA methyltransferase inhibitors including decitabine and azacitidine [88]. The potential synergism between demethylation and histone deacetylase inhibition made the use of combination therapy the focus of a number of ongoing trials.

DNA Methyltransferase Inhibitors

The DNA hypomethylating agents, 5-azacytidine (Azacitidine—Vidaza) and 2,5-deoxycytidine (Decitabine—Dacogen) are both analogs and the pyrimidine nucleoside cytidine. Both drugs inhibit DNA methyltransferase, reduce DNA methylation, and may induce re-expression of key tumor suppressor genes in MDS [89]. They are incorporated into the DNA of cells and result in hypomethylation of critical residues, cytosine prior to guanine sequences, (CpG) in the promoter regions in the DNA. At low doses they are believed to induce hypomethylation through depletion of cellular DNA methyltransferases and at higher doses both agents are cytotoxic by incorporation into RNA and/or DNA. The use of low doses in MDS is based on the principle that hypomethylation of DNA leads to reactivation of tumor suppressor genes expression which is passed down through subsequent generation of MDS cells.

The effect of azacitidine was evaluated in a randomized phase III trial. Azacitidine-treated patients showed a better overall response compared to those treated with supportive care only (60% versus 5%) and a longer time to progression to AML or death, but no overall survival advantage. A confirmatory international phase III trial evaluating the effects on long-term outcome with azacitidine versus conventional care (i.e., physician choice of low-dose cytarabine, standard chemotherapy, or best supportive care). Azacitidine was administered subcutaneously (75 g/m^2/day) for seven consecutive days every 28 days for patients with high risk MDS. Azacitidine treatment was associated with a significantly median overall survival 24.4 months compared to 15 months in the conventional care arm [89]. Most patients in the conventional treatment arm received low dose cytarabine. The 2 year survival was 50.8% in azacitidine as compared with 26.2% in the control, conventional treatment arm. This was the first randomized study to demonstrate a survival advantage for treatment with a hypomethylating agent. While some patients had a complete clinical response while receiving Azacitidine the durations of the complete response were short and not maintained when treatment was stopped. Myelosuppression was frequently observed in patients receiving Azacitidine and its role as a differentiating agent or de repressor of tumor suppressor genes in MDS was unclear. Responses were associated and improved quality of life in some patients. But in other trials the impact of treatment on survival was unclear. An oral formulation of 5-azacitidine is being studied in patients with low risk—intermediate risk MDS.

Decitabine (DAC) is a more potent inhibitor of DNA methyltransferase than azacitidine and is associated with greater myelosuppression. Decitabine has been effective in patients with high-risk MDS and may prolong the time to transformation to AML. The schedule of decitabine administration suggests that both the duration, dose and number of doses are important. Decitabine is given intravenously at various doses and dose schedules. The Phase I, II, and early Phase III trials DAC was administered the dose was 15 mg/m^2 over 3–4 h every 8 h for 3 days. The overall response rate in MDS was 49 and 64% in high-risk patients. The actuarial median survival time was 15 months and myelosuppression was common. In a randomized dose finding study, DAC was administered at 20 mg/m^2 IV over 1 h daily for 5 days; while not the FDA approved dosing, it is the standard of care at many institutions [89]. The CR rate in a dose finding trial was 39% and an overall response rate of 70%. The CR rate of 34% versus 9% when decitabine was given at a higher dose with fewer and less frequent cycles. Different dosing schedule have been associated with less myelosuppression and similar efficacy. Decitabine administered weekly, or 3 days a week was associated with a 60% trilineage response with minimal hematologic toxicity [90].

Phase III randomized studies however, did not demonstrate a survival benefit with DAC in a very high risk patient population. Azacitidine and decitabine generally require 3–6 treatment cycles to obtain an optimal therapeutic response, suggesting that the mechanism of action is more than just cytoreduction. For high-risk MDS, the hypomethylating agents either azacitidine and decitabine continue to be the treatments of choice [88]. MDS patients with monosomy 7(del 7) either alone or with other complex cytogenetic abnormalities may be particularly sensitive to treatment with DNMT inhibitors. High cytogenetic responses rates have been reported with both azacitidine and decitabine in retrospective analysis and both agents appear to alter the natural course of MDS and may be of benefit for selected patients. However, additional studies are needed to define the duration of therapy, dosing and their role as single agents or in combination for high risk patients with MDS. Some trials have shown a correlation between expression of methylated genes and clinical response but this finding remains controversial. Early trials using a combination of azacitidine and lenalidomide have reported acceptable toxicity and encouraging activity albeit in limited number of selected patients. In patients with low risk disease who have failed growth factors and/or lenalidomide the use of one of low dose azacitine or decitabine is associated with decrease in transfusion requirement with acceptable toxicity.

Intensive Chemotherapy

Combination, intensive cytoreductive induction chemotherapy regimens result in meaningful toxicity and modes responses in patients with high risk MDS. The complete remission rate with intensive AML regimens is 40–60% with a 20–30% induction related mortality [88]. High risk cytogenetics, advanced age, and performance status are associated with poor response to intensive chemotherapy. In a retrospective study evaluating 510 patients with high risk MDS who received intensive chemotherapy the induction related mortality was 17% and 5 year survival probability 8% [37]. However in selected younger patients who present with poor prognosis MDS and who may proceed to an allogeneic transplant are potential candidates for intensive combination chemotherapy. Newly diagnosed patients with high risk MDS without a prior history of MDS appear to respond to standard AML induction chemotherapy in a similar fashion to de novo AML. However, patients who present with an antecedent or evolving MDS generally respond poorly to intensive AML-type induction chemotherapy [88]. The complete remission rate is 13–40% with an incidence of toxic deaths during therapy of 1–53%. Moreover, the role of post induction chemotherapy is unclear in patients with MDS who respond to treatment. In selected younger patients with MDS intensive chemotherapy including an anthracycline and cytarabine has resulted in complete remission rates of 20–60% but with a relapse rate of 90%. The remission durations are typically 6–12 months with only rare instances of prolonged disease-free survival. The poor response of MDS patients to intensive induction chemotherapy reflects the biological differences between de novo AML that occurs in younger patients and MDS. Moreover, in patients who have poor risk cytogenetics and prior MDS treatment or a longer time to progression responded poorly to induction chemotherapy with a median overall survival of less than 4 months. Moreover a CR may not impact overall survival in patients with MDS and therefore may not be the best end point for evaluating studies. The use of AML intensive induction regimens should be reserved selected younger patients with high risk disease as a bridge to an allogeneic stem cell transplant or as part of a investigational trial.

Stem Cell Transplantation

Autologous and allogeneic stem cell transplantation has been used in patients with MDS or MDS-AML. The role of autologous transplantation remains very controversial. The 3-year disease-free survival in a selected group of patients ranges from 14 to 58% in single arm or single institution studies [90]. All patients were transplanted in first remission and adequate number of stem cells were harvested. The 2-year survival in selected patients reported to the EBMT for patients in first complete remission was 39%, with a disease-free survival of 34% and a relapse rate of 64% [90]. In patients over the age of 40 years the disease-free survival was 25%. Patients younger than 40 years of age, and in first complete remission, responded better. The transplant-related mortality was high: 39% and 17% for patients over and younger than the age of 40 years, respectively. The relapse rate is higher than in patients with AML. Larger prospective studies are needed to define the potential role, if any, of an autologous stem cell transplantation for patients with MDS. However it is possible, in selected patients, to harvest polyclonal and karyotypically normal progenitors from the peripheral blood in younger patients with MDS following intensive induction chemotherapy [90].

Allogeneic stem cell transplantation represents the only potential curative therapy for patients with MDS and should be considered for patients who have an HLA compatible donor. While there are no prospective randomized trials that have compared outcomes of HSCT versus no HSCT for patients with MDS who have eligible donors it is accepted as the standard of care and generally recommended for selected low risk and all clinical eligible high risk patients with MDS [91]. However, patients with MDS have an increased incidence of transplant-related mortality as compared to patients with AML undergoing similar HSCTs [91]. The non relapse morbidity and mortality in MDS patients is high and not solely explained by the older age of the patient population [91]. Younger patients with MDS also appear to have an increased incidence of transplant-related complications. Patients with advanced disease and unfavorable cytogenetics have a higher probability of relapse and lower overall survival. The outcome is better for patients with a lower risk IPSS-R score, who are less transfusion dependent and a good performance status. Moreover, the standard risk factors that predict overall survival in MDS appear to affect the post-transplant outcome [92]. Performance status, comorbidities and fragility scores predicted overall survival [93]. Age was not the most important factor relating to transplant related morbidity and mortality [93]. The timing of the transplant for most patients remains controversial [94]. The factors that determine the overall survival and rates of relapse of an allogenic stem cell transplant include the percent of blasts, transfusion dependence, serum ferritin, comorbidities and pre transplant genetic profiles. The IPSS-R does not consider the prognostic variables associated with transplant related complications or survival but the IPSS-R score correlates with the HSCT outcome. In the IPSS-R scoring system the very high risk MDS patients had a only 10–14 months survival from the time of diagnosis and derived limited benefit from standard treatments [95]. Patients with high risk MDS should therefore be referred early in their course for consideration of an hematopoietic allogeneic stem cell transplant (HSCT) [90]. The role of HSCT in low risk MDS, while a accepted standard of care is controversial [91]. Patients with (very) low and intermediated risk IPSS-R scores with good performance status and poor, high risk features should be considered for an allogeneic hematopoietic stem cell transplant. Low risk patients with poor risk cytogenectics, life threatening cytopenias and a transfusion requirement of ≥ units a month for 6 months should be considered for early referral to a transplant center. While the percent of bone marrow blasts did not significantly effect the overall survival cytoreductive therapy prior to HSCT is recommended for patients with ≥ bone marrow myeloblasts [96]. Patients with low risk disease have a better transplant related outcome than patients with more advanced disease [96]. However, treatment related complications is a major cause of morbidity and mortality after a HSCT transplant and must be considered in advising younger patients with low risk disease. Moreover older patients with multiple co-morbidities, very poor risk cytogenetic and mutational studies should not be offered a HSCT due to the very low chance of a successful HSCT. The patients pretransplant genetic profile and mutational findings are important predictors for overall survival and should be included in a decision to recommend a HSCT. TP 53, RAS and JAK 2 mutations were associated with a signigficantly shorter overall survival following a HSCT. Mutational studies are important predictors of overall response and should be obtained on all patients prior to performing a HSCT [96]. The use of reduced intensity regimens have decreased the early transplant related mortality and are generally recommended for patients with co morbid conditions or older age. The reduced intensity regimens are associated with a decrease in non relapse mortality but a higher risk of relapse. The reduced intensity transplant depend on the immune effects mediated by the donor derived cells and graft versus disease effect. Reduced intensity transplants, however, have not impacted the overall incidence of acute and chronic GVHD which remains the major cause of morbidity and mortality in older patients. Chronic GVHD remains a serious and life long complication of HSCTs. Studies have documented the decrease in quality of life in older patients with chronic GVHD [97]. Chronic GVHD is associated with an increase in cardiovascular disease, metabolic syndrome, diabetes, cognitive decline, fatigue, sexual dysfunction and endocrine abnormalities. However, for the younger patient with a good performance status and a suitable HLA matched donor an allogeneic stem cell transplant should be considered as it represents the only potential curative therapy and should be considered earlier in high risk patients. Determining the optimal timing of the HSCT remains a controversial issue and is the subject of a number of ongoing clinical trials [97, 98].

Future Directions and Evolving Role of Molecular Genetics

Advances in treatment will parallel our understanding of the molecular and immunological events involved in development and progression of MDS. Molecular genetic technolology may help in defining the prognosis of patients with MDS [99]. In AML the use of mutational analysis has helped define the prognosis of patients with favorable or normal cytogenetics [100]. Going forward molecular genetics, including DNA array technology and whole genome sequencing (WGS) studies are likely to play a significant role in defining more biologically based prognostic scoring system. The current MDS prognosis scoring systems stratify untreated patients at the time of diagnosis. The scoring systems do not account for changes in the prognostically important covariables over time. Currently used scoring models predict outcome at diagnosis but do not predict overall survival and transformation over time. The need for a biologically based model of MDS that can reflect the heterogenous course of high and low risk patients is needed to better define therapy and evaluate long term trials. A recent large study of patients with MDS undergoing stem-cell transplantation and evaluating the association of mutations with transplantation outcomes identified subgroups of patients with prognostic and therapeutic (conditioning regimen) implications. So for example TP53 mutations in patients with MDS were associated with sorter survival and shorter time to relapse and so was presence of RAS pathway and JAK2 mutations. Knowing mutational status of these key genes along with other biological parameters will help in clinical decision making [101] (Table 23.10).

Aberrations in gene mutations are still poorly characterized in MDS. The most common point mutations in MDS are still not specific for MDS but are associated with secondary, prognostically important mutations. In addition, most cases of MDS are genetically heterogenous with a dominant clone and many subclones and based on whole genome sequencing studies (WGS) no single gene is exclusively mutated in the funding clone [102]. The combined use of flow cytometry, mutational analysis and DNA arrays may identify the most appropriate therapy for patients with MDS. A recent Genomic classification of AML defined specific genomic categories that are biologically and prognostically important [99, 100]. Hopefully a similar classification system can be developed from the large MDS data bases. Incorporating molecular genetic studies into diagnostic and prognostic models for MDS with help in defining the role of newer agents with precise targets. A biologically based system will help evaluate studies of combination with immune based treatments for different subsets of patients. While it is till unclear how somatic mutations will be applied in cases of MDS. MDS associated genes, however not specific, appear to be relevant clinical markers for the diagnosis and prognosis but have yet to be incorporated in prognostic scoring systems. More dynamic scoring systems are needed to define biologically important subtype. A molecular diagnostic system will facilitate comparing the results of different trials and assessing treatments to specific subtypes. Newer prognostic models that incorporate molecular genetic studies are being developed and validated. The use of molecular genetic studies in a predictive model may provide for a more dynamic scoring system that evolves over the patient's course and may help in the developing targeted therapy and the timing of HSCTs [103].

Summary

The myelodysplastic syndromes are a heterogeneous group of disorders with a variable clinical course. The incidence of MDS is increasing with the aging population and now represents the most common hematologic malignancy in patients older than 60 years. A majority of MDS patients present with lower-risk MDS and do not progress to AML and die of infections or bleeding related to their MDS. The WHO classification system remains controversial but is currently accepted at the standard criteria for defining MDS and attempts to separate MDS from reactive disorders other clonal disorders. Defining and differentiating MDS from other clonal or reactive process is critical many disorders can result in dysplasia and cytopenias. Clonal cytogenetic abnormalities are helpful in establishing a diagnosis of MDS, particularly when morphologic findings are subtle. Multilineage dyspoiesis favors MDS; however, prominent dysplasia can be seen associated with chemotherapy, immunosuppressive medications, and nutritional deficiencies. The diagnosis and management of patients with MDS require the close cooperation of clinician, cytogenetist and pathologist. The application of newer molecular studies may aide in the diagnosis and planning therapy.

MDS diagnosis and classification is currently in a transitional phase from reliance almost entirely on cell morphology supplemented by cytochemistry and G-banded karyotyping, towards a new model in which molecular and perhaps immunophenotypic findings will be fully incorporated. The revised 2016 WHO MDS classification represents the new standard for the diagnosis of MDS and reflects the complexity and heterogeneity of MDS. The trend towards greater classification complexity seems likely as additional molecular and cytogenetic lesions in MDS are characterized and incorporated into the diagnosis and prognosis. It is hoped that with additional information unifying themes will emerge that will help in defining prognosis and address new therapies.

References

1. Santini V, Alessandrino PE, Angelucci E, et al. Clinical management of myelodysplastic syndromes: update of SIE, SIES, and GITMO practice guidelines. Leuk Res. 2010;34(12):1–13.
2. Dayyani F, Conley A, Strom SS, et al. Cause of death in patients with lower risk myelodysplastic syndrome. Cancer. 2010;116:2174–80.
3. Aber DA, Orazi A, Hasserijian R, et al. The 2016 revision to the World Health Organization classification of myeloid neoplasms and acute leukemia. Blood. 2016;127(20):2391–405.
4. Williamson PJ, Kruger AR, Reynolds PJ, Hamblin TJ, Oscier DG. Establishing the incidence of myelodysplastic syndrome. Br J Haematol. 2008;87:743–51.
5. Rollison DE, Howlader N, Smith MT, et al. Epidemiology of myelodysplastic syndromes and chronic myeloproliferative disorders in the United States, 2001–2004, using data from the NAACCR and SEER programs. Blood. 2008;112:45.
6. Nicolas B, Feller A, Rovo A, et al. Trends of classification, incidence, mortality and survival of MDS patients in Switzerland between 2001 and 2012. Cancer Epidemiology.2017;46:82–92.
7. Paydas S. Young age MDS: differences between western and eastern countries. Leuk Res. 2006;30:36–4.
8. Strom SS, Velez-Bravo V, Estey E. Epidemiology of myelodysplastic syndromes. Semin Hematol. 2008;45:8–13.
9. Du Y, Fryzek J, Sekeres MA, Taioli E. Smoking and alcohol intake as risk factors for myelodysplastic syndromes (MDS). Leuk Res. 2010;34:1–8.
10. Nisse C, Lorthois C, Dorp V, et al. Exposure to occupational and environmental factors in myelodysplastic syndromes. Preliminary results of a case control study. Leukemia. 1995;9:693.
11. Iwanaga M, Wan-Ling H, Soda M, et al. Risk of myelodysplastic syndromes in people exposed to ionizing radiation: a retrospective cohort study of Nagasaki atomic bomb survivors. J Clin Oncol. 2012;29:428–34.
12. Weimar IS, Bourhis J-H, de Gast GC, et al. Clonality in myelodysplastic syndromes. Leuk Lymphoma. 1994;13:215.
13. Busque L, Zhu J, Dehart D, et al. An expression based clonality assay at the human androgen receptor locus (HUMARA) on chromosome X. Nucleic Acids Res. 1994;2:697.
14. Ades LIR, Fanaux P. Myelodysplastic syndromes. Lancet. 2014;383:2239–52.
15. Chakraborty S, Sun C-L, Francisco L, et al. Accelerated telomere shortening precedes the development of therapy-related myelodysplasia or acute myelogenous leukemia after autologous transplantation for lymphoma. J Clin Onc. 2009;27:791.
16. Ohyashiki JH, Sasida G, Tauchi T, Ohyashiki K. Telomeres and telomerase in hematologic neoplasms. Oncogene. 2002;21:680.
17. Brummendorf TH, Balbanov S. Telomere length dynamics in normal hematopoiesis and in disease states characterized by increased stem cell turnover. Leukemia. 2006;20:1706.
18. Lange K, Vang Nielsen K, Hahn A, et al. Telomere shortening and chromosome instability in myelodysplastic syndromes. Genes Chromosomes Cancer. 2010;49:260.
19. Bejar R, Levine R, Ebert BL. Unraveling the molecular pathophysiology of myelodysplastic syndromes. J Clin Oncol. 2011;29:507–15.
20. Cogle RC, Saki N, Khodadi E, et al. Bone arrow niche in myelodysplastic syndromes. Leuk Res. 2015;39:1020–7.
21. Marcids AM, Ramakrishnan A, Deeg HJ. Myeloid malignancies and the microenvironment: some recent studies in patients with MDS. Curr Cancer Ther Rev. 2009;5(4):310.
22. Paul B, Reid MM, Davidson EV, et al. Familial myelodysplasia: progressive disease associated with emergence of monosomy 7. Br J Haematol. 1987;65:321.
23. Bejar R, Stevenson K, Abdel-Wahab O, et al. Clinical effect of point mutations in myelodysplastic syndromes. N Engl J Med. 2011;364:2496–506.
24. Zou Z, Calin GA, de Paula HM, et al. Circulating microRNAs let −7a and miR-16 predict progression—free survival and overall survival in patients with myelodysplastic syndome. Blood. 2011;118:413–5.
25. Steensma DP, List AF. Genetic testing in the myelodysplastic syndromes: molecular insights into hematologic diversity. Mayo Clin Proc. 2005;80:681–98.

26. Bejar R. Myelodysplastic syndrome diagnosis: what is the role of molecular testing? Curr Hematol Malig Rep. 2015;10(3):282–91.
27. Busque L, Patel JP, Figueroa ME, et al. Recurrent somatic TETS mutations in normal elderly individual with clonal hematopoiesis. Nat Genet. 2012;44:1179–81.
28. Welch JS, Ley TJ, Lin DC, et al. The origine and evolution of mutations in acute myeloid leukemia. Cell. 2012;150:264–74.
29. Jaiswal S, Fontanillas P, Flannick J, et al. Age related clonal hematopoiesis associated with adverse outcomes. NEJM. 2014;371:2488–98.
30. Steensma DP. Cytopenias + mutations-dysplasia=what? Blood. 2015;126(21):2349–51.
31. Steensma DP, Bejar R, Jaiswai S, et al. Clonal hematopoiesis of indeterminate potential and its distinction from myelodysplastic syndromes. Blood. 2015;126:9–16.
32. Xie M, Lu C, Wang J, et al. Age-related mutations associated with clonal hematopoiesis with adverse outcomes. N Engl J Med. 2014;371(26):1472–8.
33. Naiswal S, Fontanillas P, Flannick J, et al. Clonal hematopoiesis and blood –cancer risk inferred from blood DNA sequence. N Engl J Med. 2014;371(26):2488–98.
34. Bejar R. Myelodysplastic syndromes diagnosis: what is the role of molecular testing. Cur Hematol Malig Rep. 2015;10:282–91.
35. Barrett AJ, Sloand E. Autoimmune mechanisms in the pathophysiology of myelodysplastic syndromes and their clinical relevance. Haematolog. 2009;94:449–51.
36. West RR, Stafford DA, White AD, et al. Cytogenetic abnormalities in the myelodysplastic syndromes and occupational or environmental exposure. Blood. 2000;95:2093.
37. Bollag G, Clapp DW, Shih S, et al. Loss of NFI results in activation of the RAS pathway and leads to aberrant growth in hematopoietic cells. Nat Genet. 1996;12:144.
38. Rothman N, Smith MT, Hayes RB, et al. Benzene poisoning, a risk factor for hematological malignancy, is associated with the NQOI 609 C.T mutation and rapid fractional excretion of chlorzoxazone. Cancer Res. 1997;57:2839–44.
39. Larson RA, Wang Y, Banarjee M, et al. Prevalence of the inactivating 609 C.T polymorphism in the NAD(P)Quinone oxidoreductase (NQO1) gene in patients with primary and therapy-related myeloid leukemias. Blood. 1999;94:803.
40. Wiernals JL, Pagnamenta A, Taylor GM, et al. A lack of functional NAD(P)Quinone ox reductase allele is selectively associated with pediatric leukemias that have MLL fusions. Cancer Res. 1999;59:4095–9.
41. Larson RA, Le Beau MM. Therapy related myeloid leukemia: a model for leukemogenesis in humans. Chem Biol Interact. 2005;153–154:187–95.
42. Zeidan AM, Linhares Y, Gore SD. Current therapy of myelodysplastic syndromes. Blood Rev. 2013;27:243–50.
43. Bennett JM, Catovsky D, Daniel MT, et al. Proposals for the classification of the myelodysplastic syndromes. Br J Haematol. 1982;51:189.
44. Verhoef GE, Pittaluga S, De Wolf-Peters C, et al. FAB classification of myelodysplastic syndromes: merits and controversies. Ann Hematol. 1995;71:3.
45. Vardiman JW, Thiele J, Arber DA, et al. The 2008 revision of the WHO classification of myeloid neoplasms and acute leukemia: rationale and important changes. Blood. 2009;114:947.
46. Swerdlow SH, Campo E, Harris NL, Jaffe ES, Pileri SA, Stein H, Thiele J, Vardiman JW, editors. WHO classification of tumours of haematopoietic and lymphoid tissues. Lyon: International Agency for Research on Cancer; 2008. p. 88–107.
47. Font P, Loscertales J, Benavente C, et al. Inter-observer variance with the diagnosis of myelodysplastic syndromes (MDS) following the 2008 WHO classification. Ann Hematol. 2013;92(1):19–24.
48. Valent P, Horney HP, Bennett JM, et al. Definitions and standards in the diagnosis and treatment of the myelodysplastic syndromes: consensus statements and report from a working conference. Leuk Res. 2007;31:727.
49. Cunningham JM, Patnail MM, Hammerschmidt DE, Vercellotti GM. Historical perspective and clinical implications of the Pelger-Huet cell. Am J Hematol. 2009;84:116.
50. Haase D, Germing U, Schanz J, et al. New insights into the prognostic impact of the karyotype in MDS and correlation with subtypes: evidence from a core dataset of 2124 patients. Blood. 2007;110:4385–95.
51. Mughal TI, Cross NC, Padron E, et al. An international MDS/MPN working Group's perspective and recommendations on molecular pathogenesis, diagnosis and clinical characterization of myelodysplastic/myeloproliferative neoplasms. Haematologica. 2015;100(9):1117–30.
52. Foucar K. Myelodysplastic/myeloproliferative neoplasms. Am J Clin Pathol. 2009;132(2):282–92.
53. Kwork B, Hall JM, Witte JS, et al. MDS associated somatic mutations and clonal hematopoiesis are common in idiopathic cytopenias of indeterminant significance. Blood. 2015;126(21):2355–61.
54. Vardiman JW. The World Health Organization (WHO) classification of tumors of the hematopoietic and lymphoid tissue: an overview with emphasis on the myeloid neoplasm. Chem Biol Interact. 2010;184:16–23.
55. Della Porta MG, Malcovati L, Boveri E, et al. Clinical relevance of bone marrow fibrosis and CD34-positive cell clusters in primary myelodysplastic syndromes. J Clin Oncol. 2009;27:754.
56. MalcovatiL KM, Papaemmanuil E, et al. SF3B1 mutation identifies a distinct subset of myelodysplastic syndrome with ring sideroblasts. Blood. 2015;126:233–41.
57. Malcovati L, Karimi M, Papaemmanuil E, et al. SF3B1 mutation identifies a distinct subset of myelodysplastic syndrome with ring sideroblasts. Blood. 2015;126(2):233–1.
58. Apaemmanuil E, Cazzola M, Boultwood J, et al. Chronic myeloid disorders working group of the International Cancer Genone Consortium. Somatic SF3B1 mutation in myelodysplasia with ring sideroblasts. N Engl J Med. 2011;365(15):3376–82.
59. Gregg XT, Reddy V, Prchal J. Copper deficiency masquerading as myelodysplastic syndrome. Blood. 2002;100:1493–5.
60. Irving JA, Mattman A, Lockitcg G, Farrell K. Wadsworth. Element of caution: a case of reversible cytopenias associated with excessive zinc supplementation. CMAJ. 2003;169(2):129–31.
61. Valent P, Bain BJ, Bennett JM, et al. Idiopathic cytopenia of undetermined significance(ICUS) and idiopathic dysplasia of uncertain significance (IDUS) and their distinction from low risk MDS. Leuk Res. 2011;35:1016.
62. Kwok B, Hall JM, Witte JS, et al. MDS—associated somatic mutations and clonal hematopoiesis are common in idiopathic cytopenias of undetermined significance. Blood. 2015;126(21):2355–61.
63. Gaballa M, Basa E. Myelodysplastic syndromes with 5q deletion: pathophysiology and role of lenalidomide. Ann Hematol. 2014;93:723–33.
64. Komrokji RS, List AF. Short and long- term benefits of lenalidomide treatment in patients with lower-risk del (5q) myelodysplastic syndromes. Ann Oncol. 2016;27(1):62–8.
65. Komrokji RS, Padron E, Ebert BL, List AF. Deletion 5qMDS: molecular and therapeutic implications. Best Pract Res Clin Haematol. 2013;26:365–75.
66. Brierley CK, Steensma DP. Thrombopoiesis- stimulating agents and myelodysplastic syndromes. Br J Haematol. 2015;169:309–23.
67. Bussel JB. The new thrombopoietic agenda: impact on leukemias and MDS. Best Pract Res Clin Haematol. 2014;27:288–92.
68. Morrone WL, Kambhampati S, Will B, Steidl U, Verma A. Thrombocytopenia in MDS: epidemiology, mechanisms, clinical consequences and novel therapeutic strategies. Leuk. 2016;30:536–44.

69. Greenberg PL, Tuechier H, Schanz J, et al. Revised international prognostic scoring system for myelodysplastic syndromes. Blood. 2012;120:2454–65.
70. Zeidan AM, Sekeres MA, Garcia-Manero G, et al. Comparison of risk stratification tools in predicting outcomes of patients with higher—risk myelodysplastic syndromes treated with aza nucleosides. Leukemia. 2016;30(3):649–57.
71. Cheson BD, Greenberg PL, Bennett JM, et al. Clinical application and proposal for modification of the International Working Group (IWG) response criteria in myelodysplasia. Blood. 2006;108:419.
72. Chan G, DiVenuti MK. Danazol for the treatment of thrombocytopenia in patients with myelodysplastic syndromes. Am J Hemat. 2002;71:166–71.
73. Giagounidis A, Mufti GJ, Fenaux P, et al. Results of a randomized double blind study of romiplostim versus placebo in patients with low/intermediate −1-risk myelodysplastic syndrome and thrombocytopenia. Cancer. 2014;120:1838–46.
74. Negrin RS, Haeber DB, Nagler A, et al. Maintenance treatment of patients with myelodysplastic syndromes using recombinant human granulocyte colony—stimulating factor. Blood. 1990;76:36–43.
75. Steensma DP, Gattermann N. When is ion overload deleterious, and when and how should iron chelation therapy be administered in myelodysplastic syndromes. Best Pract Res Clin Haematol. 2013;26(4):431–44.
76. Pullark V. Objectives or iron chelation in myelodysplastic syndromes: more than meets the eye. Blood. 2009;114:5251–62.
77. Maurillo L, Breccia M, Voso MT, et al. Deferasirox chelation therapy in patients with transfusion—dependent MDS: a 'real-world' report from two Italian registries: Gruppo Romano Myelodysplasia and Registro Basilicata. Eur J Haematol. 2015;95(1):52–6.
78. Armand P, Kim HT, Cutler CS, et al. Prognostic impact of elevated pretransplant serum ferritin in patients undergoing myeloablative stem cell transplantation. Blood. 2007;114:5251–5.
79. Rachmilewitz E, Merkel D, Ghoti H, et al. Impovement of oxidative stress parameters in MDS patients with iron overload treated with deferasirox. Blood. 112:924–31.
80. Greenberg PL, Sun Z, Miller KB, et al. Treatment of myelodysplastic syndrome patients with erythropoietin with or without granulocyte colony stimulating factor: results of a prospective randomized phase 3 trial by the Eastern Cooperative Oncology Group (E1996). Blood. 2009;114:2393–400.
81. Steesnama DP. Myelodysplastic syndromes: diagnosis and treatment. Mayo Clin Proc. 2015;90(7):969–83.
82. Sloand EM, Wu CO, Greenberg P, et al. Factors affecting response and survival in patients with myelodysplasia treated with immunosuppression. J Clin Oncol. 2008;26:2505–11.
83. Calado RT. Immunologic aspects of hypoplastic myelodysplastic syndrome. Semin Oncol. 2011;38(5):667–72.
84. Passweg JR, Giagounidis AA, Simcock M, et al. Immunosuppressive therapy for patients with myelodysplastic syndrome: a prospective randomized multicenter phase III trial comparing antithymocyte globulin plus cyclosporine with best supportive care-SAKK 33/99. J Clin Oncol. 2011;29(3):303–9.
85. Fanaux P, Giagounidis A, Selleslag D, et al. A randomized phase 3 study of lenalidomide versus placebo in RBC transfusion dependent patients with low−/intermediate 1 risk myelodysplastic syndromes with del5q. Blood. 2011;118(14):3765–76.
86. Miller K, Kyungmann K, Morrison FS, et al. The evaluation of low dose cytarabine in the treatment of myelodysplastic syndromes: a phase III intergroup study. Ann Hematol. 1992;65:162–9.
87. Sekeres MA, Cutler C. How we treat higher–risk myelodysplastic syndromes. Blood. 2014;123(6):829–36.
88. Malcovati L, Hellstrom-Lindberg E, Bowen D, et al. Diagnosis and treatment of primary myelodysplastic syndromes in adults recommendations from the European leukemia net. Blood. 2013;122(17):2943–64.
89. Issa RF, Garcia-Manero G, Obrien S, et al. Superior outcome with hypomethylating therapy in patients with acute myeloid leukemia and high risk myelodysplastic syndrome and chromosome 5 and 7 abnormalities. Cancer. 2009;115:5746–51.
90. Majhail NS, Farnia SH, Carpenter PA, et al. Indications for autologous and allogeneic hematopoietic cell transplantation: guideline from the American Society for Blood Marrow Transplantation. Biol Blood Marrow Transplant. 2015;21(11):1863–9.
91. Michaelis LC, Hamadani DJ, Hari PN. Hematopoietic stem cell transplantation in older persons: respecting the heterogeneity of age. Exp Rev Hematol. 2014;7:321–4.
92. Garcia-Manero G, Jabbour E, Borthakur G, et al. Randomized open-label phase II study of decitabine in patients with low— or intermediate risk myelodysplastic syndromes. J Clin Oncol. 2013;31(20):2548–53.
93. Buckstein R, Wells RA, Zhu N, et al. Patient –related factors independently impact survival in patients with myelodysplastic syndrome: an MDS-CAN prospspective study. Br J Haematol. 2016;174:88–101.
94. Estey E. Acute myeloid leukemia and myelodysplastic syndromes in older patients. J Clin Oncol. 2007;25:1908–15.
95. Germing U, Kundgen A. Prognostic scoring systems in MDS. Leukemia Res. 2012;36:1463–9.
96. de Witte T, Bowen D, Robin M, et al. Allogeneic hematopoietic stem cell transplantation for MDS and CMML :recommendations from an international expert panel. Blood. 2017;129:1753–62.
97. Della Porta MG, Alessandrino EP, Bacigalupo A, et al. Predictive factors for he outcome of allogeneic transplantation in patients with MDS stratified according to the revised IPSS-R. Blood. 2014;123(15):2333–42.
98. El-Jawahri A, Pidala J, Inamoto Y, et al. Impact of age on quality of life, functional statusand survival with chronic graft versus host disease. Biol Blood Marrow Transplant. 2014;20(9):1341–8.
99. He R, Witkor AE, Durnick DK, et al. Bone marrow conventional karyotyping and fluorescence in situ hybridization. AM J Clin Path. 2016;146:86–94.
100. Papaemmauil E, Gerstung M, Bullinger L, et al. Genomic classification and prognosis in acute myeloid leukemia. N Engl J Med. 2016;374:2209–21.
101. Lindsley RC, Saber W, Mar BG, et al. Prognostic mutations in myelodysplastic syndrome after stem-cell transplantation. N Engl J Med. 2017;376:536–47.
102. Walter MJ, Shen D, Shao J, et al. Clonal diversity of recurrently mutated genes in myelodysplastic syndromes. Leukemia. 2013;27(6):1275–82. https://doi.org/10.1038/leu.2013.58.
103. Pfeilstocker M, Tuechler H, Sanz G, et al. Time dependent changes in mortality and transformation risk in MDS. Blood. 2016;128:902–10.

Part III

Myeloma and Related Diseases

History of Multiple Myeloma

24

David P. Steensma and Robert A. Kyle

The Peculiar Case of Thomas Alexander McBean

Saturday, Nov. 1st 1845

> *Dear Dr. Jones,*
> *–The tube contains urine of very high specific gravity. When boiled it becomes slightly opaque. On the addition of nitric acid, it effervesces, assumes a reddish hue, and becomes quite clear; but as it cools, assumes the consistence and appearance which you see. Heat reliquifies it. What is it?* [1]

This cryptic note and a urine sample were sent by a leading London general practitioner, Dr. Thomas Watson, to Dr. Henry Bence Jones, a 31-year-old physician at St. George's Hospital who had already established a reputation as a skilled chemical pathologist [2].

The patient, Thomas Alexander McBean, was a 45-year-old successful London grocer of "temperate habits and exemplary conduct," who had been married since 1825 and had numerous children [3, 4]. With the exception of two or three severe attacks of "frontal neuralgia," Mr. McBean enjoyed good health prior to his final illness. Over the course of the year 1844, Mr. McBean's family noted that he fatigued easily and appeared to stoop while walking. He also developed urinary frequency, and grew concerned that "his body-linen was stiffened by his urine" despite the absence of a urethral discharge [4]. He took a countryside holiday in September 1844 to try to regain his strength, which he felt had been impaired by overwork and a family illness.

While vaulting out of an underground cavern on his rustic vacation, Mr. McBean "instantly felt as if something had snapped or given way within the chest, and for some minutes he lay in intense agony, unable to stir" [4]. After the intense pain subsided, the patient made his way to a nearby inn where he rested for the night, and he felt considerably better the following day.

Upon his return to London, Mr. McBean saw Dr. William Macintyre, a 53-year-old Harley Street consultant and physician to the Metropolitan Convalescent Institution and to the Western General Dispensary in St. Marylebone, for an opinion regarding dyspepsia. During his consultation with Dr. Macintyre, Mr. McBean mentioned his recent accident, from which he was still somewhat sore. Dr. Macintyre applied a strengthening plaster to the patient's chest to try to reduce the pain produced by arm movement. The plaster and avoidance of exertion allowed the patient to recover enough to resume his work as a grocer, although pain and stiffness of the chest persisted. A month later, Mr. McBean consulted with a surgeon when acute chest pain and shortness of breath recurred; the surgeon removed a pound of blood (about 450 mL), and applied leeches and blistering agents. This treatment did not relieve the symptoms and was followed by several months of weakness.

In the Spring of 1845, Mr. McBean developed right-sided pleuritic pain, which was treated by cupping. Additional therapeutic bleeding induced further weakness. Wasting, pallor, and slight puffiness of his face and ankles led the patient to consult with Dr. Watson, who prescribed steel and quinine therapy, commonly used at the time for asthenic patients who had mysterious illnesses, especially if fever was present. The patient rapidly improved. By the middle of the Summer of 1845, Mr. McBean was able to travel to Scotland on holiday, where on the seacoast "he was capable of taking active exercise on foot during the greater part of the day, bounding over the hills, to use his own expression, as nimbly as any of his companions" [4]. His appetite became ravenous—so much so that he dreamed of eating dogs and cats, and ate great quantities of fish [1, 4]. His recovery was interrupted by the onset of diarrhea, "which proved obstinate, and reduced his strength considerably" [4].

In September 1845, Mr. McBean returned to London in a debilitated state, but free of pain. However, in October,

D.P. Steensma, M.D. (✉)
Department of Medical Oncology, Dana-Farber Cancer Institute, 450 Brookline Avenue, D2037, Boston, MA 02215, USA
e-mail: dsteensma@partners.org

R.A. Kyle, M.D.
Laboratory of Medicine and Pathology, Department of Hematology, Mayo Clinic, Rochester, MN, USA

P.H. Wiernik et al. (eds.), *Neoplastic Diseases of the Blood*, DOI 10.1007/978-3-319-64263-5_24

lumbar and sciatic pain developed and soon became severe. Warm baths, Dover's powder (ipecac and opium, as a purgative and for pain relief), tartrate of potash (frequently employed for rheumatism and for complex pain), acetate of ammonia (used in febrile and inflammatory conditions), camphor julep (frequently used for low-grade fevers, muscle spasms, and anxiety), and compound tincture of camphor did not help. The patient became confined to his home on Devonshire Street in the affluent Marylebone (Westminster) area of London. On October 30, 1845, Dr. Watson called in Dr. William Macintyre for a consultation.

Dr. Macintyre examined Mr. McBean's urine because of the patient's history of edema—a basic test that Dr. Watson had apparently neglected to perform. By 1845, urine examination was a well-established clinical practice, in large part because of the work of Richard Bright, a Guy's Hospital physician who linked proteinuria, "dropsy" (edema), and chronic kidney disease (thereafter known as "Bright's disease") in the 1820s [5]. Mr. McBean's urine specimen was opaque, acidic, and of high density, with a specific gravity of 1.035, but sugar was absent. When heated, the urine was found to "abound in animal matter"; with the addition of nitric acid, the turbid urine became clear, but a precipitate developed after an hour. Uniquely, this precipitate "underwent complete solution on the application of heat, but again consolidated on cooling" [1].

Upon receiving urine specimens sent by Drs. Watson and Macintyre on November 1, Bence Jones corroborated the finding that the addition of nitric acid produced a precipitate that was redissolved by heat and that formed again on cooling. He calculated that Mr. McBean was excreting more than 60 g/day of this proteinaceous material, and concluded that the protein was an oxide of albumin, specifically "hydrated deutoxide of albumen" [6]. Bence Jones calculated that there were 66.97 parts of "hydrated deutoxide of albumen" per 1000 parts of urine in the sample, and noted that this amount was equivalent to the proportion of albumin in healthy blood, so that every ounce of urine secreted was equivalent to the loss of protein from an equal volume of blood [1, 6].

Following Dr. Macintyre's visit, the patient continued to worsen. On November 3, 1845, the eminent clinical chemist Dr. William Prout (after whom Ernest Rutherford named the proton in 1920) joined Drs. Watson and Macintyre in consultation. Iron citrate and quinine were resumed, along with opiates, blistering agents, and counterirritants. Soon every movement of Mr. McBean's trunk produced excruciating pain. Great care and cautious maneuvering enabled the patient to "get in and out of bed on all fours," but he became weaker and eventually was confined to bed. He developed flatulence, and pronounced fullness and hardness in the region of the liver. He had phlegm in his chest and coughed fitfully, and suffered another episode of diarrhea.

On November 15, Dr. Bence Jones recommended treatment with alum, a substance used since ancient Egyptian times to clear turbid solutions, "with the view of checking the exhausting excretion of animal matter" [4]. The patient improved slightly in the following days and was able to sit up and enjoy his food, but on December 7 he "experienced a dreadful aggravation of lumbar pains" [4]. He had almost continual pain despite opiate treatment, became weaker, and died on January 1, 1846, exhausted but "in full possession of his mental faculties." The cause of death was listed as "atrophy from albuminuria" [3]. Involvement of the bones by the disease, aside from pain, was not recognized during the patient's illness.

Postmortem examination revealed emaciation. The ribs, which crumbled under the heel of the scalpel, were soft, brittle, readily broken, and easily cut by the knife. Their interior was filled with a soft "gelatiniform substance of a blood-red colour and unctuous feel" [4]. The sternum was soft and fragile and snapped when lifted. The heart and lungs were not remarkable. The liver was "voluminous, but of healthy structure." The kidneys appeared to be normal on both gross and microscopic examination, had "proved equal to the novel office assigned them," and were thought to have "discharged the task without sustaining, on their part, the slightest danger." The thoracic and lumbar vertebrae had the same degenerative changes as found in the ribs and sternum, but the humeri and femurs resisted "all efforts to bend or break them by manual force" [4].

John Dalrymple, surgeon to the Royal Ophthalmic Hospital, Moorfields (London), examined two lumbar vertebrae and a rib from Mr. McBean. In an 1846 paper on the "pathology of mollities ossium" (an obsolete general term for bony softness or fragility, analogous to the contemporary term "osteomalacia"), Mr. Dalrymple noted that the patient's lumbar vertebrae were markedly compressed and that they "scarcely exceed in thickness the intervertebral substance, and have lost nearly one-third of their normal bulk" [7]. The disease appeared to begin in the cancellous bone; it then grew and produced irregularly sized round dark red projections that were visible through the periosteum. Nucleated cells formed the bulk of the gelatiniform mass that filled the large cancellous cavities. Most of these cells were round or oval and about one-half to two times as large as an average blood cell. The cells contained one or two nuclei, each with a bright, distinct nucleolus. Wood engravings made from Mr. Dalrymple's drawings are consistent with the appearance of plasma cells (Fig. 24.1) [7]. Dalrymple postulated that these nucleated cells had a limited duration of life and then disintegrated, after which they were "carried out of the system by the circulation of the kidneys" [7].

In light of the autopsy findings, both Dalrymple and Macintyre believed that the disorder that Mr. McBean suffered from was a malignant disease of bone. Bright's disease

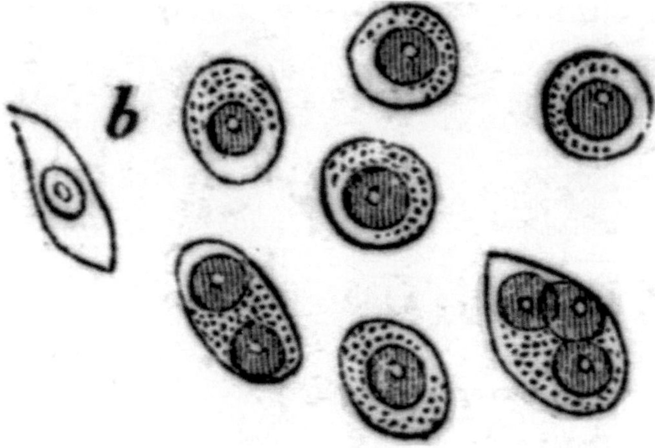

Fig. 24.1 Plasma cells obtained at the autopsy of Thomas Alexander McBean, January 1846 (wood engravings made from drawings by Mr. Dalrymple). https://commons.wikimedia.org/wiki/File:Plasmocytom-dalrymple.PNG; see also Dalrymple [7])

was considered in the differential diagnosis because of the albuminous matter in the urine, but there was no dropsy, and the kidneys appeared healthy. The diarrhea, weakness, emaciation, hepatic enlargement, flatulence, dyspepsia, edema of the ankles, puffiness of the face, and large amounts of Bence Jones proteinuria suggest to contemporary readers the possibility of amyloidosis in addition to myeloma. However, autopsy findings of a normal heart and kidneys and "voluminous liver of healthy structure" make the presence of amyloidosis less likely. Because the lardaceous or waxy changes of amyloidosis in the liver were commonly recognized during the 1840s (although not yet understood), it is unlikely that gross changes of amyloidosis would have been overlooked if present in Mr. McBean [8].

In 1967, Bristol experimental pathologist John Clamp located Mr. McBean's death certificate in the General Register Office in London, using dates and descriptions of the patient from the case reports of Drs. Macintyre and Bence Jones. Dr. Clamp suggested that the name *multiple myeloma* might instead have been *McBean's disease with Macintyre's proteinuria* [3]. However, although Dr. Macintyre first noticed the peculiar heat properties of Mr. McBean's urine, it was Bence Jones who emphasized its place in the diagnosis of myeloma—as he emphasized, "I need hardly remark on the importance of seeking for this oxide of albumen in other cases of mollities ossium"—and who can be credited with developing the first biochemical test for detection of cancer [1, 9]. The modest Dr. Macintyre stated that his "share in this part of the inquiry, it must have been seen, was very humble… I shall be content if I have succeeded in pointing out to future observers, gifted with the requisite qualifications for conducting researches of a higher order, certain definite and distinctive characters by which a peculiar and hitherto unrecorded pathological condition of the urine may be recognised and identified" [4].

Earlier Cases of Multiple Myeloma

Although the first clear description of multiple myeloma did not occur until the 1846–1850 chemical, clinical, and pathological reports of Bence Jones, Macintyre, and Dalrymple described above (all wrote single-authored publications describing the same individual patient), the disease has undoubtedly existed for centuries. It seems likely, for example, that some of the cases of "mollities ossium" reported in the eighteenth and early nineteenth centuries represent patients who had myeloma. However, without detailed microscopic description of plasma cells such as that provided by Mr. Dalrymple in Mr. McBean's case, or recognition of a unique disease-associated protein such as that first detected by Drs. Bence Jones and Macintyre, it is not possible to be certain.

When examining old skeletons, sharply demarcated spheroid skeletal lesions that are "purely lytic"—i.e., lacking gross evidence of sclerosis or formation of new bone—are suggestive of multiple myeloma, especially when such lesions are multiple and occur in the proximal long bones and axial skeleton [10]. Two male human skeletons with this bony lesion pattern, with estimated ages at death of between 40 and 60 years and dating from 3200 to 500 BCE, were identified from among 905 individuals excavated at Thebes-West and Abydos in Upper Egypt [11], while two similarly affected skeletons were found among 2547 individuals entombed in a rural South German ossuary between 1400 and 1800 AD [12].

Paleopathologists have identified additional ancient bones with features suggestive of multiple myeloma, such as the skeleton of a middle-aged Icelandic female from the eleventh to fifteenth century AD [13], two calvaria from medieval Britain [14], four American Indian skeletons from 200 to 1300 AD [15], and 14 pre-Columbian American skeletons dating back to 3300 BC [16]. The Hunterian Museum of the Royal College of Surgeons in London has in its collection the bones of an approximately 45-year-old Roman soldier with myeloma-like lesions. Suspicious rounded lytic lesions can also be seen in the remains of George Grenville (1712–1770), the Whig Prime Minister whose administration passed the notorious Stamp Act of 1765 that first alienated American colonists from England, and who was autopsied by pioneering Scottish surgeon John Hunter in 1770 [17].

Multiple myeloma with Bence Jones proteinuria occurs spontaneously in contemporary animals [18], raising the possibility that myelomatous lesions might be identifiable in prehistoric nonhuman fossils. Paleontologists have observed multiple lytic defects without evidence of bony remodeling in a few dinosaur skeletons from the Jurassic and Cretaceous periods, and these have been interpreted by some observers as evidence of an origin of multiple myeloma in the Mesozoic era or earlier [19]. However, caution is indicated in interpreting such ancient specimens.

In any case, it is almost certain that 39-year-old Sarah Newbury, a patient described by distinguished London surgeon Samuel Solly in 1844, had multiple myeloma [20]. Mrs. Newbury had experienced increasing fatigue and, 4 years before her death, was suddenly seized with a violent pain in her back when stooping. "Rheumatic pains" in her limbs occurred a year later, and these progressed to the point where her gait became unsteady. Her limb pain increased greatly after a fall in February 1842, which resulted in inability to lift her right leg, and she was confined to her room. Two months later, her femurs fractured "into a thousand pieces" when her husband, a policeman, lifted her from the fireside to carry her to her bed. Pathological fractures of the clavicles, right humerus, and right radius and ulna followed.

Mrs. Newbury first saw Solly in consultation in October 1843, but thereafter wrote him a letter asking him not to visit her again because she was vexed that he had prescribed a bitter infusion to try to improve her poor appetite. She was then lost to medical follow-up until she was admitted at the insistence of her husband to St. Thomas's Hospital in Southwark (South London) on April 15, 1844, in an extremely debilitated state. Over the next few days she was treated with an infusion of orange peel and a rhubarb pill, fed with bland foods including arrowroot, and given an opiate at night if required. Examination of the copious amount of urine she produced revealed a "large quantity of phosphate of lime," but blood tests could not be performed because Mrs. Newbury was "too suspicious and irritable" to allow them [20]. She died suddenly on April 20, 1844, of "asphyxia" [20].

At autopsy, Mrs. Newbury's thoracic cavity was reduced to just 4 in. in transverse diameter. The right lung was compressed to about one-fourth of its natural size, and the left lung was decreased to one-half the extent of the right lung because of skeletal changes. The cancellous portion of the sternum (Fig. 24.2) had been replaced by a red substance similar to that seen in Mr. McBean [4]. A peculiar red material had also replaced much of the femur; it ranged in color "from a deep Modena red to a bright scarlet crimson" (Fig. 24.3). Solly examined this red matter with John Birkett of Guy's Hospital, a surgeon and anatomist, who described the cells within as "very clear, their edge being remarkably distinct, and the clear *oval* outline enclosing *one* bright *central* nucleus, *rarely two, never more*" [italics Solly's] [20]. John Dalrymple noted that the microscopic appearance reported by Birkett "accords very nearly" with his description of Mr. McBean's marrow [7]. Solly postulated that the process affecting Mrs. Newbury was inflammatory and had begun with an abnormality of the blood vessels, in which the "earthy matter of the bone is absorbed and thrown out by the kidneys in the urine" [20].

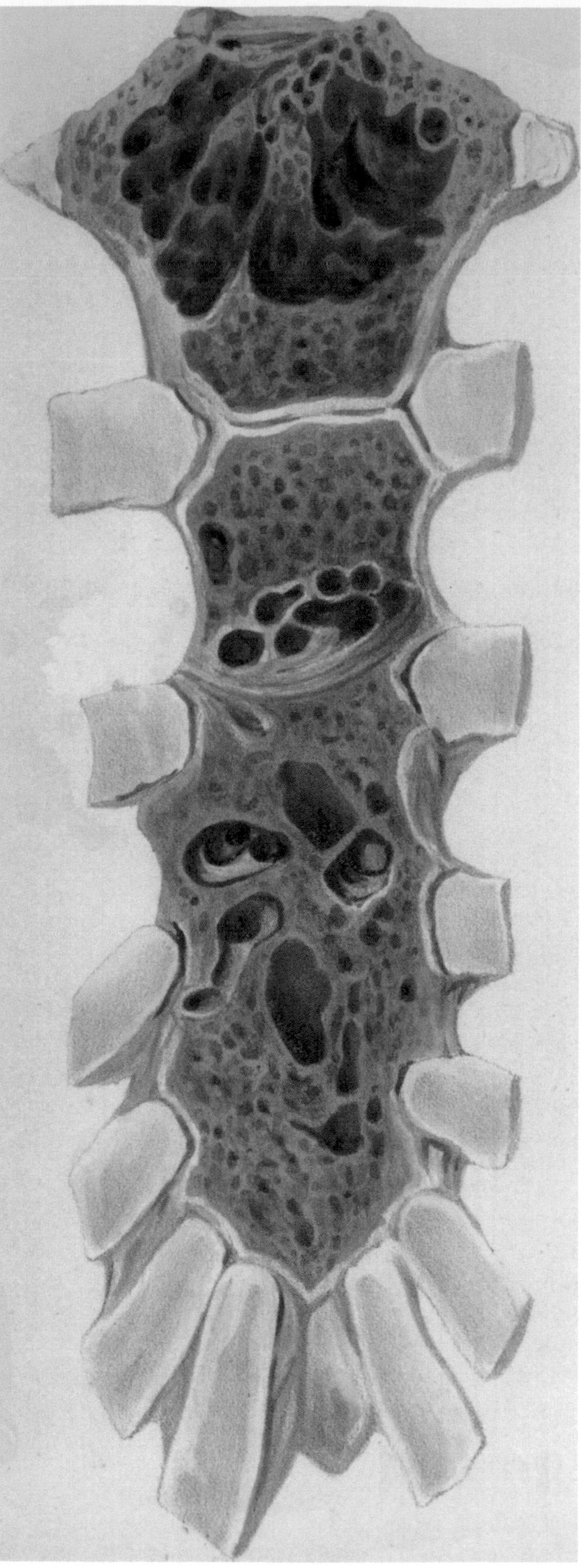

Fig. 24.2 Sternum of Sarah Newbury showing destruction of bone; drawn after her autopsy in April 1844 (from Solly [20])

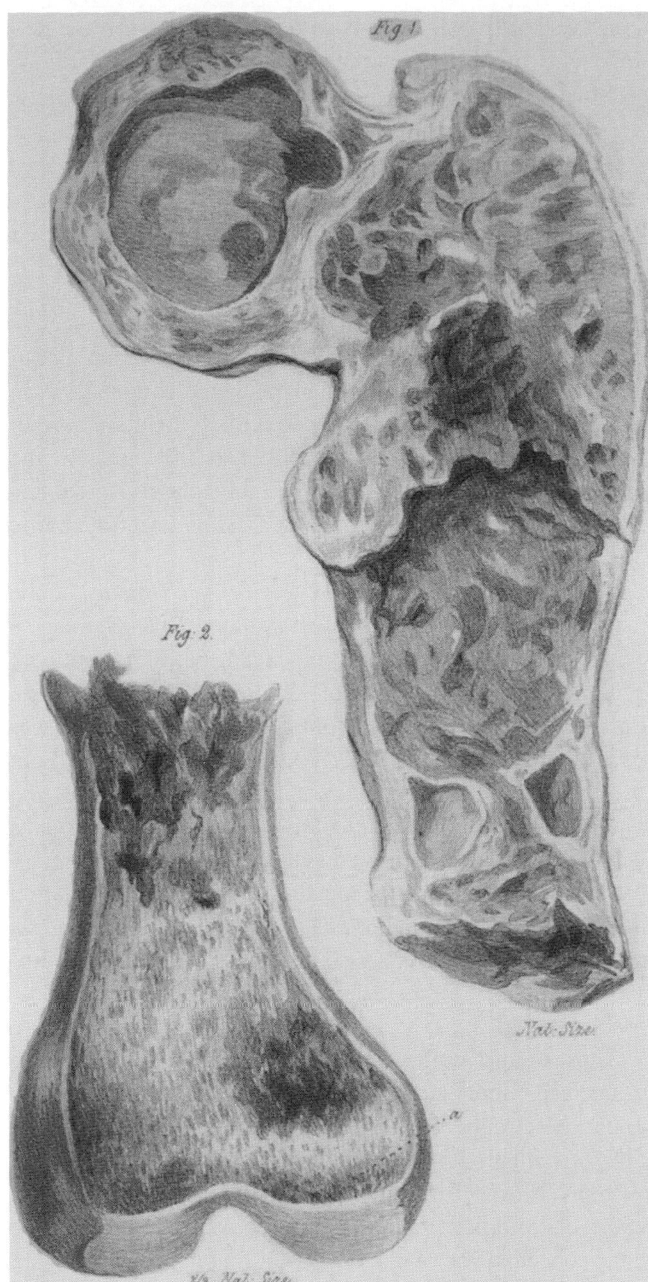

Fig. 24.3 Femur of Sarah Newbury showing destruction by myeloma tumor (from Solly [20])

Other Contributions to Bence Jones Proteinuria and Monoclonal Protein Detection

Although much has been written about the life and scientific work of Henry Bence Jones [2, 21–23], a number of other persons played a part in the evolving story of Bence Jones proteinuria.

In 1846, Johann Florian Heller, an Austrian chemist and physician working in Vienna, described a protein in the urine of a patient that precipitated when warmed a little above 50 °C and disappeared upon further heating [24]. Although Heller did not recognize the re-precipitation of the protein when the urine was cooled, it seems likely that he was observing a Bence Jones protein. Heller also distinguished this new protein from albumin and casein [24]. Richard Fleischer in Erlangen, Germany, was the first to use the term "Bence Jones protein" in writing, in an 1880 paper describing a substance with chemical characteristics of Bence Jones protein that he isolated from normal bone marrow [25].

In 1883, Wilhelm Friedrich Kühne, a prominent Berlin physiologist best known for coining the term "enzyme," described finding Bence Jones protein in the urine of a 40-year-old patient from Amsterdam who died in 1869 after an illness characterized by bone pain, spinal curvature, and cranial neuropathy, possibly from an extramedullary plasmacytoma [26]. Kühne isolated the protein and found that the carbon, hydrogen, and nitrogen levels were similar to those described by Bence Jones, and attributed any differences in results between his report and that of Bence Jones to the fact that his preparation was more pure than Bence Jones's preparation. He named the peculiar protein "albumosurie."

In 1898, Thomas R. Bradshaw of Liverpool observed that meals had little or no influence on the amount of Bence Jones proteinuria [27]. There was no nocturnal variation, and Bradshaw believed that the rate of protein excretion was "pretty constant throughout the 24 hours."

In 1899, Alexander Ellinger in Germany suggested that there might be an abnormal protein in the blood in patients with myeloma that was similar to the Bence Jones protein, but he was unable to prove this assertion [28].

Waltman Walters at Mayo Clinic in Minnesota described three carefully evaluated patients with multiple myeloma in 1921, and, like Bradshaw, reported that the quantity of Bence Jones proteinuria in these patients was independent of their oral protein intake and did not vary diurnally [29]. In one patient, intravenous injection of Bence Jones protein appeared to increase the amount of Bence Jones proteinuria. Walters also found Bence Jones protein in the blood of one patient and in the bronchial secretions of another. He concluded that Bence Jones proteins were of endogenous origin, and hypothesized that they were derived from blood proteins through some type of action of abnormal cells in the bone marrow [29].

The following year—1922—Stanhope Bayne-Jones and D.W. Wilson from Johns Hopkins made 12 preparations of Bence Jones proteins from five patients, two of whom had been included in Walters' report [30]. Bayne-Jones and Wilson immunized rabbits by intravenous injection of the Bence Jones protein, and performed precipitin tests with the Bence Jones protein preparations, concluding that Bence Jones proteins consisted of two groups of similar but not identical proteins.

Beginning in the 1930s, there was considerable debate between proponents of two schools of thought on the origin of Bence Jones protein. The first theory, championed by Adolf Magnus-Levy in Berlin, held that proteinaceous materials found in the urine were the result of overproduction of normal serum proteins by the bone marrow [31]. An alternative view was held by Maxwell Wintrobe and Mar Van Rensselaer Buell at Johns Hopkins in Baltimore. In a description of the phenomenon of cryoprecipitation in 1933, Wintrobe and Buell argued that pathologic proteins in plasma cell disorders were likely to be distinct from all normal serum components [32].

In the early 1950s, protein chemist Frank W. Putnam at the University of Chicago performed a series of experiments in myeloma patients using ^{13}C radioisotopes, which helped clarify the origin of Bence Jones proteins. Putnam first showed that the Bence Jones proteins from 18 different patients with myeloma were each biochemically unique, though as had been suggested by Bayne-Jones and Wilson they clustered into two antigenic groups. In 1955, Putnam and his coworker Sarah Hardy showed that Bence Jones proteins derived directly from the body's metabolic pool of nitrogen, rather than being a breakdown product of some sort of plasma precursor [33].

In 1956, Leonhard Korngold and Rose Lipari at New York's Sloan Kettering Institute for Cancer Research and Cornell Medical College Department of Biochemistry formally demonstrated a relationship between Bence Jones protein and the serum proteins of multiple myeloma [34]. As a tribute to Korngold and Lipari, the two major classes of Bence Jones proteins are designated by the Greek letters κ and λ.

One hundred and seventeen years after the initial description of the unique heat properties of Bence Jones protein—in 1962—Gerald Edelman and Joseph Gally at the Rockefeller Institute for Medical Research in New York demonstrated that the light chains prepared from a serum immunoglobulin G (IgG) myeloma protein and the Bence Jones protein from the same patient's urine were identical in all respects: the same amino acid sequence, similar spectrofluorometric behavior, the same molecular weight, identical appearance on chromatography with carboxymethylcellulose and on starch gel electrophoresis after reduction and alkylation, and the same ultracentrifugal pattern—as well as the same thermal solubility [35]. The light chains precipitated when heated to between 40 and 60 °C, dissolved on boiling, and reprecipitated when cooled to between 40 and 60 °C.

Shortly after Edelman and Gally's discovery, Norbert Hilschmann and Lyman Craig of the Rockefeller Institute [36] and Koiti Titani and colleagues in Putnam's laboratory [37] provided the first antibody amino acid sequences, and showed that Bence Jones proteins were not only related to the light chains of gamma globulin but also that each light chain was divided into a "variable" or V region, and a "constant" or C region. This structure accounts for the heterogeneity of normal gamma globulins and for antibody specificity and diversity.

Diagnostic Tests for Myeloma: Beyond Bence Jones Proteinuria

Arne Tiselius in Uppsala, Sweden, a 1948 Nobel Laureate in Chemistry, reported an improved method of serum electrophoresis in 1937, which allowed separation of serum globulins into three components: alpha, beta, and gamma [38]. In 1939, Tiselius isolated antibody activity to the gamma fraction [39], while Lewis Longsworth and colleagues at the Rockefeller Institute first noted the classic myeloma "M-spike" in that same year, using Tiselius' electrophoretic techniques [40].

In 1953, Pierre Grabar and Curtis A. Williams at the Institut Pasteur in Paris described immunoelectrophoresis, a technique that is infrequently practiced today but routinely facilitated the diagnosis of multiple myeloma [41]. Immunofixation or "direct immunoelectrophoresis" was reported by Armine T. Wilson from the Alfred I. duPont Institute in Wilmington, Delaware, in 1964 and is now the standard method for the recognition of monoclonal proteins [42]. Wilson applied antisera on the surface of the agar immediately after completion of electrophoresis. Immunofixation has proven useful when the results of immunoelectrophoresis are equivocal [43], and is also helpful in the recognition of small monoclonal light chains not detectable by immunoelectrophoresis [44].

Nonsecretory multiple myeloma is defined by the absence of detectable monoclonal proteins in serum and urine using immunoelectrophoresis or immunofixation; it accounts for <3% of patients with multiple myeloma. In 2001, Arthur J. Bradwell from Birmingham, England, and his colleagues reported an immunological method for detecting imbalance in the concentration of κ and λ serum free light chains, using specific antibodies that bind only to free light chains, not to light chains bound to immunoglobulin heavy chains [45]. Serum free light chain concentrations are now routinely measured in clinical practice.

Early Cases of Multiple Myeloma After Sarah Newbury and Thomas McBean

In 1867, Hermann Weber, a German physician working in London, described a 40-year-old man with mollities ossium and first linked this condition to the pathological finding of tissue deposition of amyloid [46]. The patient suffered severe sternal and lumbar pain, and movement of his head produced pain in his neck and arms. The patient died less than 4 months after the initial onset of pain. Postmortem examination revealed that the sternum was fractured in two places, and had been almost entirely replaced by a grayish-red substance that was thought to have the microscopic appearance of a sarcoma. Several round defects in the skull were also filled with the same morbid substance as that found in the sternum, and many of the ribs, several vertebrae, and parts of the pelvis were involved by the same process. The waxy changes of amyloid were found in the kidneys and spleen.

During a meeting of the Pathological Society of London in February 1872, William Adams exhibited (on behalf of Thomas Stretch Dowse of Highgate Infirmary) specimens from the body of a 62-year-old woman with "acute rheumatism" characterized by bone pain, fractures, and fever, who died 8 days after admission to the hospital for a humerus fracture. The left femur fractured while the body was being placed on the autopsy table. Lardaceous changes consistent with amyloid were found in the liver and kidneys, and the cancellous portions of the bones had been replaced by a homogeneous, soft, gelatinoid substance. When examined microscopically, the substance filling the hollowed bone was shown to consist of small spherical and oval cells that contained one eccentric oval nucleus (rarely two) [47].

The term "multiple myeloma" was introduced in 1873 by J. von Rusitzky from Kiev, of whom little is known other than that he had once worked in Friedrich von Recklinghausen's laboratory in Strasbourg. During an autopsy, von Rusitzky noted eight separate tumors of the bone marrow in a patient, which he called "multiple myelomas" [48]. The patient, a 47-year-old man, had presented with a gradually enlarging tumor in the right temple. Subsequently, thickening of the sternal manubrium and the seventh rib developed, followed by paraplegia. At autopsy, it was revealed that a fist-sized tumor in the right frontal region extended into the orbit and had produced ophthalmoplegia. Other postmortem findings included an apple-sized tumor in the right fifth rib, a tumor in the left seventh rib that produced a fracture, a tumor of the sternum, a tumor involving the sixth to the eighth thoracic vertebrae (the cause of the paraplegia), and three tumors of the right humerus. Although von Rusitzky's description of the tumor cells in this case is vague, he described round cells with a nucleus located in the periphery near the cell membrane, suggestive of plasma cells. The report did not comment on whether Bence Jones proteinuria was found during life. In Russia and Soviet-influenced regions, myeloma was called "von Rusitzky syndrome" for much of the twentieth century.

There were few further publications about the disease until 1889, when Otto Kahler, an internist from Prague working in Vienna, described the case of a 46-year-old physician named Dr. Loos [49]. In July 1879, Dr. Loos developed sudden severe pain in the right upper thorax, which was aggravated by taking a deep breath. Six months later, this pain recurred and became localized to the right third rib, which was tender to pressure. During the next 2 years, intermittent pain aggravated by exercise occurred in the ribs, spinal column, left shoulder, upper arm, and right clavicle. Albuminuria was first noticed in September 1881. Skeletal pain, made worse by movement, continued to occur intermittently. Pallor was noted in 1883 and pneumonia developed in February 1884. In December 1885, Dr. Loos was first seen by Kahler, who noted anemia and focal tenderness of many bones. Kyphosis was so severe that when Dr. Loos stood up, his lower ribs touched his anterior iliac crest. Dr. Loos subsequently suffered from recurrent bronchial infections and intermittent hemoptysis. During the following year, Dr. Loos' kyphosis increased and height decreased monthly, to the point where his chin pressed against the sternum, resulting in skin ulceration. On August 26, 1887, Dr. Loos died, a remarkable 8 years after his initial symptoms.

Kahler's autopsy report of Dr. Loos described hepatosplenomegaly, but lardaceous change was not mentioned. The ribs were soft and could be broken with minimal effort. Soft gray-reddish masses were noted in the ribs and thoracic vertebrae. Microscopic examination showed large round cells, consistent with myeloma. It is interesting to note that the patient had a high fluid intake and took sodium bicarbonate on a regular basis; this regimen may have helped prevent renal failure. Kahler recognized that the urinary protein obtained from Dr. Loos had the same characteristics that Bence Jones had described. For many years, the eponym "Kahler's disease" was widely used in Western Europe and the United States to describe the condition once known by "mollities ossium with Bence Jones proteinuria" and now called multiple myeloma.

Detailed examination of Dr. Loos' urine by Karl Hugo Huppert, professor of medicinal chemistry at the German University in Prague, showed that a protein in the urine precipitated at 53–59 °C, cleared with heating to boiling, and then reprecipitated during cooling [50]. The patient excreted 6.7 g of the protein daily, which Huppert noted was distinct from albumin.

It is likely that A.L., the 43-year-old engineer that Joseph Coats of Glasgow reported in 1891 as having "multiple sarcoma of bone," actually had multiple myeloma [51]. The patient developed a large tumor of the sternum 5 years before his final hospitalization and death, and later noticed tumors in the right clavicle, right humerus, and left hip. He experienced back pain radiating to the lower extremities, weakness of his legs, and a pathological fracture of the right humerus. Postmortem examination revealed multiple tumors with involvement of the ribs and vertebral bodies. Microscopic examination showed round or polygonal cells "about 1/2000 in. diameter" (~13 μm, a reasonably accurate estimate of the diameter of a neoplastic plasma cell) with oval nuclei constituting more than half the diameter of the cells [51].

An 1897 Italian description of Kahler's disease by Camillo Bozzolo, a Milanese physician and pathologist working in Torino, resulted in the dual eponym "*malattia di Kahler-Bozzolo*" gaining currency in Italy in the first part of the twentieth century [52].

Other Cases of Multiple Myeloma in the Nineteenth and Twentieth Centuries

In 1894, James Bryan Herrick and Ludvig Hektoen at Rush Medical College in Chicago reported what is probably the first recognized case of multiple myeloma in the United States, just a few years after the report of Kahler [53]. A 40-year-old woman complained of lumbar pain and a nodule on the lower end of the sternum. At autopsy, there were multiple nodules attached to the sternum, right clavicle, and ribs. The sternum was thickened, irregular, and covered with tumor masses, yet was soft and flexible. Multiple nodules were found on the ribs, which bent readily without cracking. Two of the dorsal vertebral bodies were largely replaced by soft tumor masses, and fungoid masses were seen in the skull. Microscopic examination of these lesions revealed round "lymphoid" cells with large nuclei. Herrick is also credited with the first clear description of sickle cell disease (initially recognized by one of his subordinates), as well as being the first to link angina with acute coronary syndromes [54, 55].

In 1898, Frederick Parkes Weber—honorary physician to the German Hospital in Queen's Square, London, and son of Hermann Weber mentioned above—reported a case of multiple myeloma, and suggested that radiographs (discovered by Würzburg physicist Wilhelm Conrad Röntgen in 1895) would greatly facilitate the diagnosis of such cases [56]. Weber also concluded in a report of another case that Bence Jones protein was produced by the bone marrow, and that the presence of Bence Jones protein was of "fatal significance" and nearly always indicated that the patient had multiple myeloma [57]. Weber and Lister Institute bacteriologist John Charles Grant Ledingham later suggested that Bence Jones protein derived from cytoplasmic residua of karyolyzed plasma cells [58].

In 1928, C.F. Geschickter and M.M. Copeland from Johns Hopkins reviewed all 425 cases of multiple myeloma reported since 1848 [59]. They called attention to six cardinal features of the disease: multiple tumors of the axial skeleton, pathological fractures, Bence Jones proteinuria, back pain, anemia, and chronic renal disease.

Sternal aspiration of bone marrow during life, described by Soviet physician Mikhail Arinkin in Leningrad in the late 1920s, greatly increased the recognition of multiple myeloma [60]. In 1938, hematologists Nathan Rosenthal and Peter Vogel at Mt. Sinai Hospital in New York reported that only 3 cases of multiple myeloma had been recognized at the Mt. Sinai Hospital from 1916 to 1935, but that 13 cases were found in the ensuing 2 1/2 years [61]. Rosenthal and Vogel attributed this marked increase in recognition to the use of sternal puncture in patients with obscure anemia or skeletal abnormalities, and suggested that many cases of myeloma had likely been missed in the past.

In 1947, Edwin (Ned) Bayrd and Frank Heck at Mayo Clinic in Minnesota described 83 patients with histological proof of myeloma seen at their institution through December 1945 [62]. The duration of survival in the Mayo series ranged from 1 to 84 months (median, 15 months). The median survival for myeloma would not increase much beyond this until the introduction of novel agents in the early twenty-first century [63].

Plasma Cells, Hyperproteinemia, Recognition of Monoclonality, and Prognosis

The term *plasma cell* was coined by German anatomist Heinrich Wilhelm Gottfried von Waldeyer-Hartz in 1875, but his description is not characteristic of plasma cells, and it is most likely that he was instead observing tissue mast cells [64]. Plasma cells were described accurately by Spanish neuroscientist Santiago Ramón y Cajal in 1890, during the study of syphilitic condylomas. Ramón y Cajal stated that the unstained perinuclear area ("hof," from a German term meaning yard or court) contained the Golgi apparatus. In 1891, German dermatologist Paul Gerson Unna used the term *plasma cell* while describing cells seen in the skin of patients with lupus erythematosus [65]. However, it is not known whether he actually saw plasma cells. In 1895, Hungarian pathologist Tamás Marschalkó outlined the essential characteristics of plasma cells, including blocked chromatin, eccentric position of the nucleus, a perinuclear pale area ("hof"), and a spherical or irregular cytoplasm [66].

In 1900, pathologist J.H. Wright of Johns Hopkins described a 54-year-old man with multiple myeloma, and pointed out that the tumor consisted of plasma cells, proposing the new term "plasma cell myeloma" [67]. Wright emphasized that the neoplasm originated not from red marrow cells collectively but from only one type of cell, the plasma cell. Interestingly, Wright's patient was probably the first in whom radiographs revealed changes in the ribs, thus contributing to the diagnosis.

Although Victor C. Jacobson of the Peter Bent Brigham Hospital in Boston reported Bence Jones protein in the serum in a patient with chronic nephritis in 1917 [68], it was not until 1928 that biochemist William A. Perlzweig and colleagues from Duke University reported hyperproteinemia when they described a patient with multiple myeloma who had 9–11 g of globulin in his serum [69]. The patient also had Bence Jones proteinuria and probably a small amount of Bence Jones protein in the plasma. Perlzweig and coworkers noted that it was almost impossible to obtain serum from the clotted blood because the clot failed to retract, even on prolonged centrifugation.

The concept of monoclonal versus polyclonal gammopathies was lucidly presented in the 1961 edition of the Harvey Society Lecture series (founded 1905) in New York by Jan Gösta Waldenström of Malmö General Hospital, Sweden [70]. Waldenström clearly described patients with a narrow band of hypergammaglobulinemia on electrophoresis as having a monoclonal protein. Although many of these patients had multiple myeloma, others had no evidence of malignancy and were considered to have idiopathic "essential hypergammaglobulinemia" or benign monoclonal gammopathy. Most physicians now use the term "monoclonal gammopathy of undetermined significance" (MGUS) instead, because in some of these patients, multiple myeloma, macroglobulinemia, or a related disorder will eventually develop [71–73]. Waldenström further correctly regarded the broad band in hypergammaglobulinemia as a polyclonal increase in proteins. This simple distinction is extremely important clinically because patients with a monoclonal gammopathy already have or may develop a neoplastic process, whereas patients with a polyclonal gammopathy have an inflammatory or a reactive cause of their hypergammaglobulinemia [70, 74].

In 1975, Brian G.M. Durie and Sydney Salmon proposed a three-tier myeloma staging system with prognostic value [75]. The Durie-Salmon staging system saw widespread clinical use for more than 30 years but had limitations, particularly with respect to categorization of bone lesions. In 2005, a multinational group chaired by Philip Greipp from Mayo Clinic used data from more than 11,000 patients to develop a simplified International Staging System, based on serum β (beta) 2-microglobulin and albumin levels [76]. Other important prognostic factors in myeloma defined in recent years include specific chromosomal abnormalities detectable by fluorescent in situ hybridization or conventional karyotyping, such as deletion of chromosomes 13 or 17p, abnormalities of chromosome 1, hyperdiploidy, or immunoglobulin heavy-chain translocations such as t(4;14), t(11;14), or t(14;16) [77]. A growing number of somatic mutations have been described in myeloma cells, including mutations in genes important in protein synthesis, histone modulation, coagulation, and NF-kappaB signaling [78].

Treatment of Multiple Myeloma

Treatment of multiple myeloma has progressed considerably since the nonspecific remedies attempted for Mr. McBean in 1845, especially with the introduction of highly active novel agents including immunomodulatory drugs and proteasome inhibitors [63]. Despite these novel drug therapies and the routine use of autologous stem cell transplantation for patients with myeloma [79], which have improved survival in recent years [64], the condition remains incurable.

The Urethane Distraction

In 1947, Nils Alwall, a Swedish dialysis pioneer, reported a patient with multiple myeloma who experienced a reduction in globulin levels from 5.9 to 2.2 g/dL, an increase in hemoglobin, disappearance of proteinuria, and reduction in bone marrow plasma cells from 33 to 0% when treated with urethane (ethyl carbamate) [80]. On the basis of this single report, for almost 20 years urethane was commonly used as a treatment of myeloma. The demise of urethane in myeloma therapy occurred in 1966, when James Holland and his colleagues reported results from a randomized trial of 83 patients with previously treated or untreated multiple myeloma who received either urethane or a placebo consisting of cherry- and cola-flavored syrup [81]. No difference was seen in objective improvement between the two treatment groups, and the urethane-treated patients died earlier on the average than those treated with placebo. This difference was ascribed to urethane-induced azotemia.

Alkylating Agents and Combination Chemotherapy

In 1958, a Soviet medical team led by Nikolai Blokhin reported benefit in three of six patients with multiple myeloma who were treated with "sarcolysin" (L-phenylalanine mustard, melphalan, Alkeran) [82]. Four years later, Daniel Bergsagel at the M.D. Anderson Cancer Center in Houston, Texas, and his colleagues observed improvement in 8 of 24 patients with multiple myeloma who were treated with melphalan [83].

In a 1964 report, cyclophosphamide-treated patients with myeloma had a median survival of 24.5 months, whereas a control myeloma group had a median survival of 9.5 months [84]. Objective improvement occurred in 81 of 207 cyclophosphamide-treated patients. Various combinations of alkylating agents with vinca alkaloids, anthracyclines, and corticosteroids (see below) were used for the treatment of multiple myeloma, but these combinations did not prove superior to melphalan and prednisone [85, 86].

Corticosteroids

Corticosteroids were first systematically tested in patients with myeloma by R.E. Mass in 1962, who reported the results of a placebo-controlled double-blind trial in which single-agent prednisone decreased serum globulin and increased hematocrit, but did not improve survival [87]. In 1967, Sydney Salmon and his colleagues reported that prednisone administered at a dose of 200 mg orally every other morning produced benefit in 8 of 10 patients with poor-risk myeloma, and adverse events were uncommon [88]. In two Cancer and Leukemia Group B myeloma treatment protocols, prednisone as a single agent produced a 44% objective response rate [89]. The combination of melphalan plus prednisone (MP) was established in a randomized trial of 183 myeloma patients led by Raymond Alexanian and colleagues; patients treated with MP lived 6 months longer than those who received melphalan alone [90]. Later dexamethasone became the corticosteroid of choice in myeloma therapy.

Stem Cell Transplantation

The first report of human hematopoietic stem cell transplantation was published in 1957 by E. Donnall Thomas and Joseph Ferrebee at the Mary Imogene Bassett Hospital in Cooperstown, New York, and their colleagues [91]. Thomas and Ferrebee treated six patients (one had multiple myeloma) with total-body irradiation and chemotherapy followed by an intravenous infusion of bone marrow cells from a healthy donor. Although none of the patients lived 100 days, and transient engraftment occurred in only two of the six patients, Thomas remained convinced of the procedure's potential and continued to purse it, in collaboration with immunologists who developed the concept of tissue (human leukocyte antigen) typing [92]. Thomas moved to Seattle in 1963, and his groundbreaking research on stem cell transplantation eventually led to a Nobel Prize in 1990.

The Seattle group reported a syngeneic bone marrow transplant in a patient with multiple myeloma in 1982; the patient's physician brother served as donor [93]. Four years later, Alexander Fefer from Seattle and his colleagues described five myeloma patients who received a syngeneic bone marrow transplant [94]. In 1987, a European group led by Gösta Gahrton of Sweden reported that 10 of 14 patients with multiple myeloma who received an allogeneic bone marrow transplant from an HLA-compatible sibling donor survived for at least 6 months (median, 12 months) [95].

The first autologous bone marrow transplantation for myeloma was reported in 1983 by Tim McElwain and Ray Powles from the Institute of Cancer Research and the Royal Marsden Hospital in the United Kingdom [96]. Four years later, Bart Barlogie and his colleagues at the University of Arkansas reported the use of melphalan 140 mg/m^2 and total-body irradiation (1.5 Gy) followed by autologous allogeneic bone marrow transplantation in multiple myeloma patients refractory to chemotherapy [97]. Subsequently, Barlogie developed intense treatment programs incorporating tandem autologous transplantation, which he called "total therapy"—a term and concept pioneered for childhood leukemia at St. Jude Children's Research Hospital in Memphis. Subsequent clinical trials of transplantation regimens played a major role in establishing high-dose therapy and stem cell rescue as a standard treatment for multiple myeloma.

Novel Agents

Since the late 1990s, several exciting new agents have emerged and achieved regulatory approval, which has improved outcomes for patients with myeloma [63].

Thalidomide, Lenalidomide, and "Immunomodulatory" Agents

The tragedy of thalidomide embryopathy is widely known outside of the medical profession, but the drug's rebirth as an immunomodulatory and antineoplastic agent is less well recognized.

In 1957, German pharmaceutical company Chemie Grünenthal began marketing thalidomide (α-N-[phthalimido] glutarimide) as a sedative. By 1960, thalidomide was sold in more than 40 countries, and achieved widespread use as a sedative that was thought to be safer than barbiturates, as well as a treatment for morning sickness of pregnancy [98].

On November 18, 1961, Widukind Lenz, a German pediatrician and geneticist, reported that thalidomide exposure during the first trimester of fetal development was associated with severe teratogenic malformations [99]. In December 1961, Lenz' findings were independently confirmed by an Australian obstetrician, William G. McBride [100]. By the end of 1961, thalidomide was removed from the market in most countries, but almost 10,000 infants had already been affected. The United States was largely spared because thalidomide had been denied approval by Frances Oldham Kelsey at the US Food and Drug Administration (FDA), due to a lack of safety data.

Thalidomide persisted as a therapeutic agent due to promising activity later seen in leprosy (1964), Behçet disease (1979), graft-versus-host disease (1988), and human immunodeficiency virus (HIV)-associated oral ulcers and wasting (1989) [98]. Under pressure from activists, the FDA approved thalidomide for the treatment of erythema nodosum leprosum in July 1998, with a risk-management system to control prescribing and prevent exposure of unborn infants to thalidomide.

In 1994, the antiangiogenic properties of thalidomide in a rabbit cornea micropocket assay were reported [101].

Based on the increasing awareness of angiogenesis in the pathobiology of cancer and the evidence of increased angiogenesis in myeloma, the spouse of an affected myeloma patient convinced Barlogie and his colleagues to initiate a compassionate-use trial of "antiangiogenic therapy" at the University of Arkansas in late 1997. The idea to use thalidomide in this setting came from Harvard's Judah Folkman, an angiogenesis researcher [102]. In an Arkansas study of 84 previously treated patients, 32% responded to thalidomide. Other investigators subsequently confirmed the Arkansas results and observed activity of thalidomide in newly diagnosed myeloma as well [103]. Although it was never clear whether the mechanism of action required inhibition of angiogenesis—various drug-associated changes in cytokines and immune cell subsets led to thalidomide and its derivatives also being called an "immunomodulatory agent" (iMid)—thalidomide soon became a therapy widely used in myeloma, including in combination with corticosteroids and other agents.

The sponsor of thalidomide subsequently synthesized several analogues to try to increase clinical activity and minimize adverse events such as neuropathy. The most successful of these analogs has been lenalidomide (formerly CC-5013), a 4-amino-substituted analog of thalidomide. A Phase 1 trial in 24 relapsed refractory myeloma patients was led by Paul G. Richardson at the Dana-Farber Cancer Institute; as reported in 2002, lenalidomide reduced paraprotein levels by at least 25% in 17 of 24 patients [104].

Richardson and colleagues then conducted a multicenter randomized Phase 2 trial that enrolled 102 patients with relapsed/refractory myeloma and confirmed the drug's activity [105]. In a Mayo Clinic study of lenalidomide and dexamethasone of 34 patients with newly diagnosed myeloma, 91% achieved an objective response with lenalidomide plus dexamethasone [106]. Lenalidomide plus dexamethasone was approved by the FDA in June 2006 for the treatment of myeloma in patients who failed one prior therapy; lenalidomide had previously been approved in 2005 for treatment of lower risk myelodysplastic syndromes associated with deletions of chromosome 5q. Numerous studies showed benefit of lenalidomide in combination regimens both as initial therapy and in relapsed/refractory disease. Lenalidomide was soon widely used in maintenance regimens for at least 2 years after stem cell transplant, which prolonged relapse-free survival in several studies [107]. Another immunomodulatory agent/thalidomide analogue, pomalidomide, received accelerated approval for patients with relapsed/refractory disease in 2013 [108].

The mechanism of thalidomide and lenalidomide in myeloma was only discovered in 2014, after both drugs had been in use for many years [109]. These drugs were found to bind to cereblon, a component of an E3 ubiquitin ligase complex, altering the affinity of this complex for various proteins and thereby changing their rate of degradation. In myeloma cells, increased ubiquitin ligase-mediated degradation of the transcription factors IKZF1 and IKZF3 results in cytotoxicity, since these factors are necessary for malignant plasma cell survival.

Proteasome Inhibitors

The ubiquitin-proteasome pathway contributes to the orderly degradation of unneeded eukaryotic cellular proteins [110]. Inhibition of the proteasome leads to cellular apoptosis, especially in neoplastic and rapidly proliferating cells [111].

Bortezomib (formerly PS-341), a derivative of boronic acid, was synthesized in 1995 and selected for preclinical and clinical testing in cancer [111]. In a Phase 1 study enrolling patients with relapsed and refractory hematological malignancies led by Robert Orlowski at the University of North Carolina and published in 2002, bortezomib demonstrated striking antimyeloma activity [112]. Kenneth Anderson at the Dana-Farber Cancer Institute in Boston and his colleagues also observed promising activity of bortezomib against myeloma cells in several preclinical models [113].

In the first Phase 2 trial of bortezomib in 202 patients with relapsed refractory myeloma, approximately one-third of patients responded to bortezomib therapy, with a median response duration of 1 year [114]. These results led the FDA to approve bortezomib for multiple myeloma in May 2003. Bortezomib has also been combined effectively with corticosteroids and with lenalidomide, and used in newly diagnosed patients. Subsequently several other proteasome inhibitors were developed, including carfilzomib (FDA approved for relapsed/refractory myeloma in mid-2012) and ixazomib (FDA approved in late 2015) [115, 116]. In 2015, in a cooperative group trial, a combination regimen of bortezomib, lenalidomide, and dexamethasone (VRd) was shown to improve overall survival compared with lenalidomide and dexamethasone (Rd) alone—the first time a "triplet" combination had shown benefit compared to a "doublet" [117].

Monoclonal Antibodies and Other Agents

Following the success of the anti-CD20 antibody rituximab in non-Hodgkin lymphoma, numerous monoclonal antibodies were developed for other hematological neoplasms. Antibodies used in myeloma include elotuzumab, a humanized antibody targeting signaling lymphocytic activation molecule F7 (SLAMF7), and daratumumab, a fully human antibody against CD38, which were both FDA approved in late 2015 [118, 119]. Panobinostat, a deacetylase inhibitor, also has activity in relapsed/refractory myeloma and was FDA approved in early 2015 [120]. Several other novel

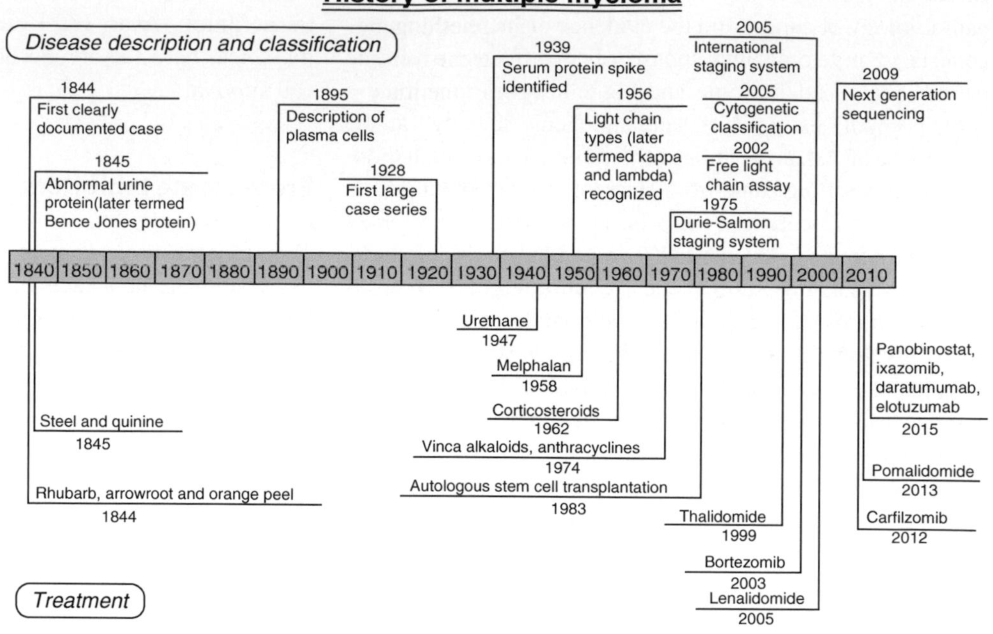

Fig. 24.4 Timeline of historical discoveries (*top*) and introduction of specific therapies (*bottom*) for multiple myeloma. For therapies approved in the twenty-first century, the date of initial FDA approval is given, rather than the first date these agents were used in humans (revised and updated from Kyle and Rajkumar [121])

agents are in various stages of development. After many years of limited therapeutic alternatives, the future looks brighter for patients with myeloma (Fig. 24.4).

References

1. Bence Jones H. Papers on chemical pathology; Prefaced by the Gulstonian Lectures, read at the Royal College of Physicians, 1846. Lecture III. Lancet. 1847;2:88–92.
2. Rosenfeld L. Henry Bence Jones (1813–1873): the best “chemical doctor” in London. Clin Chem. 1987;33:1687–92.
3. Clamp JR. Some aspects of the first recorded case of multiple myeloma. Lancet. 1967;2:1354–6.
4. Macintyre W. Case of mollities and fragilitas ossium, accompanied with urine strongly charged with animal matter. Med Chir Trans Lond. 1850;33:211–32.
5. Bright R. Reports of medical cases, selected with a view of illustrating the symptoms and cure of diseases by a reference to morbid anatomy. London: Longman, Rees, Orme, Browne and Green; 1827.
6. Bence Jones H. On the new substance occurring in the urine of a patient with mollities ossium. Philos Trans R Soc Lond. 1848;138:55–62.
7. Dalrymple J. On the microscopical character of mollities ossium. Dublin Q J Med Sci. 1846;2:85–95.
8. Kyle RA. Amyloidosis: a convoluted story. Br J Haematol. 2001;114:529–38.
9. Hajdu SI. A note from history: the first biochemical test for detection of cancer. Ann Clin Lab Sci. 2006;36:222–3.
10. Rothschild BM, Hershkovitz I, Dutour O. Clues potentially distinguishing lytic lesions of multiple myeloma from those of metastatic carcinoma. Am J Phys Anthropol. 1998;105:241–50.
11. Zink A, Rohrbach H, Szeimies U, et al. Malignant tumors in an ancient Egyptian population. Anticancer Res. 1999;19:4273–7.
12. Nerlich AG, Rohrbach H, Bachmeier B, Zink A. Malignant tumors in two ancient populations: an approach to historical tumor epidemiology. Oncol Rep. 2006;16:197–202.
13. Gestsdottir H, Eyjolfsson GI. Myeloma in an archaeological skeleton from Hofstadir in Myvatnssveit. Laeknabladid. 2005;91:505–9.
14. Wells C. Two mediaeval cases of malignant disease. Br Med J. 1964;1:1611–2.
15. Morse D, Dailey RC, Bunn J. Prehistoric multiple myeloma. Bull N Y Acad Med. 1974;50:447–58.
16. Steinbock T. Paleopathological diagnosis and interpretation. Springfield: CC Thomas; 1976.
17. Spigelman M, Berger L, Pinhasi R, Donoghue HD, Chaplin S. John Hunter’s post-mortem examination of George Grenville (1712–1770). Bull R Coll Surgeons Engl. 2008;90:338–9.
18. Hanna F. Multiple myelomas in cats. J Feline Med Surg. 2005;7:275–87.
19. Capasso LL. Antiquity of cancer. Int J Cancer. 2005;113:2–13.
20. Solly S. Remarks on the pathology of mollities ossium: with cases. Med Chir Trans Lond. 1844;27:435–61.
21. Kyle RA. Henry Bence Jones—physician, chemist, scientist and biographer: a man for all seasons. Br J Haematol. 2001;115:13–8.
22. Putnam FW. Henry Bence Jones: the best chemical doctor in London. Perspect Biol Med. 1993;36:565–79.
23. Obituary. Henry Bence Jones, M.D., F.R.C.P., F.R.S. Med Times Gaz. 1873;1:505.
24. Heller JF. Die Mikroscopisch-Chemisch-Pathologische Untersuchung. Vienna: Braumüller and Seidel; 1846.
25. Fleischer R. Ueber das Vorkemmen des sogenannten Bence Jones'schen Eiweisskörpers ím normalen Knochenmark. Arch Pathol Anatom Physiol Klin Med. 1880;80:842–9.
26. Kühne W. Ueber Hemialbumose im Harn. Z Biol. 1883;19:209–27.
27. Bradshaw TR. A case of albumosuria in which the albumose was spontaneously precipitated. Med Chir Trans Lond. 1898;81:259–71.
28. Ellinger A. Das Vorkommen des Bence-Jones’schen Korpers im Harn bei Tumoren des Knochenmarks und seine diagnostische Bedeutung. Deutsche Arch Klin Med. 1899;62:255–78.
29. Walters W. Bence Jones proteinuria: a report of three cases with metabolic studies. J Am Med Assoc. 1921;76:641–5.
30. Bayne-Jones S, Wilson DW. Immunological reactions of Bence Jones proteins. II. Differences between Bence Jones proteins from various sources. Bull Johns Hopkins Hosp. 1922;33:119–25.

31. Magnus-Levy A. Uber die Myelomakrankheit. III. vom Stoffwechsel: die Bence-Jones-Proteinurie. Z Klin Med. 1932;119:307–62.
32. Wintrobe MM, Buell MV. Hyperproteinemia associated with multiple myeloma: with report of a case in which an extraordinary hyperproteinemia was associated with thrombosis of the retinal veins and symptoms suggesting Raynaud's disease. Bull Johns Hopkins Hosp. 1933;52:156–65.
33. Putnam FW, Hardy S. Proteins in multiple myeloma. III. Origin of Bence-Jones protein. J Biol Chem. 1955;212:361–9.
34. Korngold L, Lipari R. Multiple myeloma proteins. III. The antigenic relationship of Bence Jones proteins to normal gammaglobulin and multiple myeloma serum proteins. Cancer. 1956;9:262–72.
35. Edelman GM, Gally JA. The nature of Bence-Jones proteins. Chemical similarities to polypetide chains of myeloma globulins and normal gamma-globulins. J Exp Med. 1962;116:207–27.
36. Hilschmann N, Craig LC. Amino acid sequence studies with Bence-Jones proteins. Proc Natl Acad Sci U S A. 1965;53:1403–9.
37. Titani K, Whitley E Jr, Putnam FW. Immunoglobulin structure: variation in the sequence of Bence Jones proteins. Science. 1966;152:1513–6.
38. Tiselius A. Electrophoresis of serum globulin. II. Electrophoretic analysis of normal and immune sera. Biochem J. 1937;31:1464–77.
39. Tiselius A, Kabat EA. An electrophoretic study of immune sera and purified antibody preparations. J Exp Med. 1939;69:119–31.
40. Longsworth LG, Shedlovsky T, MacInnes DA. Electrophoretic patterns of normal and pathological human blood serum and plasma. J Exp Med. 1939;70:399–413.
41. Grabar P, Williams CA. Method permitting the combined study of the electrophoretic and the immunochemical properties of protein mixtures; application to blood serum. Biochim Biophys Acta. 1953;10:193–4.
42. Wilson AT. Direct Immunoelectrophoresis. J Immunol. 1964;92:431–4.
43. Ritchie RF, Smith R. Immunofixation. I. General principles and application to agarose gel electrophoresis. Clin Chem. 1976;22:497–9.
44. Whicher JT, Hawkins L, Higginson J. Clinical applications of immunofixation: a more sensitive technique for the detection of Bence Jones protein. J Clin Pathol. 1980;33:779–80.
45. Bradwell AR, Carr-Smith HD, Mead GP, et al. Highly sensitive, automated immunoassay for immunoglobulin free light chains in serum and urine. Clin Chem. 2001;47:673–80.
46. Weber H. Molities ossium, doubtful whether carcinomatous or syphilitic. Trans Pathol Soc Lond. 1867;23:186–7.
47. Adams W. Mollities ossium. Trans Pathol Soc Lond. 1872;23:186–7.
48. von Rustizky J. Multiples myelom. Deutsch Z Chir. 1873;3:162–72.
49. Kahler O. Zur symptomatologie des multiplen myeloms: Beobachtung von Albumosurie. Prager Med Wochenschr. 1889;14:45.
50. Huppert KH. Ein Fall von Albumosurie. Prager Med Wochenschr. 1889;14:35–6.
51. Coats J. A case of multiple sarcoma of bone. Glasgow Med J. 1891;36:420–30.
52. Bozzolo C. Sulla malattia di Kahler. Clin. Med Ital. 1897;37:1–10.
53. Herrick JB, Hektoen L. Myeloma: report of a case. Med News. 1894;65:239–42.
54. Herrick JB. Peculiar elongated and sickle-shaped red corpuscles in a case of severe anemia. Arch Intern Med. 1910;6:517–21.
55. Herrick JB. Clinical features of sudden obstruction of the coronary arteries. J Am Med Assoc. 1912;59:2015–20.
56. Weber FP. General lymphadenomatosis of bones, one form of 'multiple myeloma'. J Pathol. 1898;5:59–64.
57. Weber FP, Hutchinson R, Macleod JJR. Multiple myeloma (myelomatosis), with Bence-Jones protein in the urine (myelopathic albumosuria of Bradhaw, Kahler's disease). Am J Med Sci. 1903;126:644–65.
58. Weber FL, JCG A. Note on the histology of a case of myelomatosis (multiple myeloma) with Bence-Jones protein in the urine (myelopathic albumosuria). Proc R Soc Med. 1909;2:193.
59. Geschickter CF, Copeland MM. Multiple myeloma. Arch Surg. 1928;16:807–63.
60. Arinkin MI. Die intravitale Untersuchungsmethodik des Knochenmarks. Folia Haematol. 1929;38:233–40.
61. Rosenthal N, Vogel P. Value of the sternal puncture in the diagnosis of multiple myeloma. J Mt Sinai Hosp. 1938;4:1001–19.
62. Bayrd ED, Heck FJ. Multiple myeloma: a review of eighty-three proved cases. J Am Med Assoc. 1947;133:147–57.
63. Kumar SK, Rajkumar SV, Dispenzieri A, et al. Improved survival in multiple myeloma and the impact of novel therapies. Blood. 2008;111:2516–20.
64. Waldeyer W. Über Bindegewebszellen. Arch Mikr Anat. 1875;11:176–94.
65. Unna PG. Über plasmazellen, insbesondere beim Lupus. Monatsschrift prak Dermatol. 1891;12:296.
66. Marschalkó T. Ueber die sogenannten plasmazellen, ein Beitrage zur Kenntniss der Herkunft der entzundlichen infiltrationszellen. Arch Dermatol Syphilol. 1895;30:241.
67. Wright JH. A case of multiple myeloma. Trans Assoc Am Phys. 1900;15:137–47.
68. Jacobson VC. A case of multiple myelomata with chronic nephritis showing Bence-Jones protein in urine and blood serum. J Urol. 1917;1:167.
69. Perlzweig WA, Delrue G, Geschicter C. Hyperproteinemia associated with multiple myelomas: report of an unusual case. J Am Med Assoc. 1928;90:755–7.
70. Waldenström J. Studies on conditions associated with disturbed gamma globulin formation (gammopathies). Harvey Lect. 1960–1961;56:211–31.
71. Kyle RA. Monoclonal gammopathy of undetermined significance. Natural history in 241 cases. Am J Med. 1978;64:814–26.
72. Kyle RA. "Benign" monoclonal gammopathy—after 20 to 35 years of follow-up. Mayo Clin Proc. 1993;68:26–36.
73. Kyle RA, Therneau TM, Rajkumar SV, et al. A long-term study of prognosis in monoclonal gammopathy of undetermined significance. N Engl J Med. 2002;346:564–9.
74. Kyle RA. Multiple myeloma: an odyssey of discovery. Br J Haematol. 2000;111:1035–44.
75. Durie BG, Salmon SE. A clinical staging system for multiple myeloma. Correlation of measured myeloma cell mass with presenting clinical features, response to treatment, and survival. Cancer. 1975;36:842–54.
76. Greipp PR, San Miguel J, Durie BGM, et al. International staging system for multiple myeloma. J Clin Oncol. 2005;23:3412–20.
77. Fonseca R, Bergsagel PL, Drach J, et al. International Myeloma Working Group molecular classification of multiple myeloma: spotlight review. Leukemia. 2009;23:2210–21.
78. Chapman MA, Lawrence MS, Keats JJ, et al. Initial genome sequencing and analysis of multiple myeloma. Nature. 2011;471:467–72.
79. Harousseau JL, Moreau P. Autologous hematopoietic stem-cell transplantation for multiple myeloma. N Engl J Med. 2009;360:2645–54.
80. Alwall N. Urethane and stilbamidine in multiple myeloma: report on two cases. Lancet. 1947;2:388–9.
81. Holland JR, Hosley H, Scharlau C, et al. A controlled trial of urethane treatment in multiple myeloma. Blood. 1966;27:328–42.
82. Blokhin N, Larionov L, Perevodchikova N, Chebotareva L, Merkulova N. Clinical experiences with sarcolysin in neoplastic diseases. Ann N Y Acad Sci. 1958;68:1128–32.
83. Bergsagel DE, Sprague CC, Austin C, Griffith KM. Evaluation of new chemotherapeutic agents in the treatment of multiple myeloma. IV. L-Phenylalanine mustard (NSC-8806). Cancer Chemother Rep. 1962;21:87–99.

84. Korst DR, Clifford GO, Fowler WM, Louis J, Will J, Wilson HE. Multiple myeloma. II. Analysis of cyclophosphamide therapy in 165 patients. JAMA. 1964;189:758–62.
85. Gregory WM, Richards MA, Malpas JS. Combination chemotherapy versus melphalan and prednisolone in the treatment of multiple myeloma: an overview of published trials. J Clin Oncol. 1992;10:334–42.
86. Myeloma Trialists' Collaborative Group. Combination chemotherapy versus melphalan plus prednisone as treatment for multiple myeloma: an overview of 6,633 patients from 27 randomized trials. J Clin Oncol. 1998;16:3832–42.
87. Mass RE. A comparison of the effect of prednisone and a placebo in the treatment of multiple myeloma. Cancer Chemother Rep. 1962;16:257–9.
88. Salmon SE, Shadduck RK, Schilling A. Intermittent high-dose prednisone (NSC-10023) therapy for multiple myeloma. Cancer Chemother Rep. 1967;51:179–87.
89. McIntyre OR, Pajak TF, Kyle RA, Cornwell GG 3rd, Leone L. Response rate and survival in myeloma patients receiving prednisone alone. Med Pediatr Oncol. 1985;13:239–43.
90. Alexanian R, Haut A, Khan AU, et al. Treatment for multiple myeloma. Combination chemotherapy with different melphalan dose regimens. JAMA. 1969;208:1680–5.
91. Thomas ED, Lochte HL Jr, Lu WC, Ferrebee JW. Intravenous infusion of bone marrow in patients receiving radiation and chemotherapy. N Engl J Med. 1957;257:491–6.
92. Appelbaum FR. Hematopoietic-cell transplantation at 50. N Engl J Med. 2007;357:1472–5.
93. Osserman EF, DiRe LB, DiRe J, Sherman WH, Hersman JA, Storb R. Identical twin marrow transplantation in multiple myeloma. Acta Haematol. 1982;68:215–23.
94. Fefer A, Cheever MA, Greenberg PD. Identical-twin (syngeneic) marrow transplantation for hematologic cancers. J Natl Cancer Inst. 1986;76:1269–73.
95. Gahrton G, Tura S, Flesch M, et al. Bone marrow transplantation in multiple myeloma: report from the European cooperative Group for Bone Marrow Transplantation. Blood. 1987;69:1262–4.
96. McElwain TJ, Powles RL. High-dose intravenous melphalan for plasma-cell leukaemia and myeloma. Lancet. 1983;2:822–4.
97. Barlogie B, Alexanian R, Dicke KA, et al. High-dose chemoradiotherapy and autologous bone marrow transplantation for resistant multiple myeloma. Blood. 1987;70:869–72.
98. Rajkumar SV. Thalidomide: tragic past and promising future. Mayo Clin Proc. 2004;79:899–903.
99. Lenz W. Thalidomide and congenital abnormalities. Lancet. 1962;1:45.
100. McBride WG. The teratogenic action of drugs. Med J Aust. 1963;2:689–92.
101. D'Amato RJ, Loughnan MS, Flynn E, Folkman J. Thalidomide is an inhibitor of angiogenesis. Proc Natl Acad Sci U S A. 1994;91:4082–5.
102. Singhal S, Mehta J, Desikan R, et al. Antitumor activity of thalidomide in refractory multiple myeloma [see comment] [erratum appears in N Engl J Med 2000;342(5):364]. N Engl J Med. 1999;341:1565–71.
103. Dimopoulos MA, Anagnostopoulos A, Weber D. Treatment of plasma cell dyscrasias with thalidomide and its derivatives. J Clin Oncol. 2003;21:4444–54.
104. Richardson PG, Schlossman RL, Weller E, et al. Immunomodulatory drug CC-5013 overcomes drug resistance and is well tolerated in patients with relapsed multiple myeloma. Blood. 2002;100:3063–7.
105. Richardson PG, Blood E, Mitsiades CS, et al. A randomized phase 2 study of lenalidomide therapy for patients with relapsed or relapsed and refractory multiple myeloma. Blood. 2006;108:3458–64.
106. Rajkumar SV, Hayman SR, Lacy MQ, et al. Combination therapy with lenalidomide plus dexamethasone (rev/Dex) for newly diagnosed myeloma. Blood. 2005;106:4050–3.
107. Palumbo A, Gay F, Falco P, et al. Bortezomib as induction before autologous transplantation, followed by lenalidomide as consolidation-maintenance in untreated multiple myeloma patients. J Clin Oncol. 2010;28:800 7.
108. San Miguel J, Weisel K, Moreau P, et al. Pomalidomide plus low-dose dexamethasone versus high-dose dexamethasone alone for patients with relapsed and refractory multiple myeloma (MM-003): a randomised, open-label, phase 3 trial. Lancet Oncol. 2013;14:1055–66.
109. Kronke J, Udeshi ND, Narla A, et al. Lenalidomide causes selective degradation of IKZF1 and IKZF3 in multiple myeloma cells. Science. 2014;343:301–5.
110. Ciechanover A. The ubiquitin-proteasome proteolytic pathway. Cell. 1994;79:13–21.
111. Adams J, Palombella VJ, Sausville EA, et al. Proteasome inhibitors: a novel class of potent and effective antitumor agents. Cancer Res. 1999;59:2615–22.
112. Orlowski RZ, Stinchcombe TE, Mitchell BS, et al. Phase I trial of the proteasome inhibitor PS-341 in patients with refractory hematologic malignancies. J Clin Oncol. 2002;20:4420–7.
113. Hideshima T, Richardson P, Chauhan D, et al. The proteasome inhibitor PS-341 inhibits growth, induces apoptosis, and overcomes drug resistance in human multiple myeloma cells. Cancer Res. 2001;61:3071–6.
114. Richardson PG, Barlogie B, Berenson J, et al. A phase 2 study of bortezomib in relapsed, refractory myeloma [see comment]. N Engl J Med. 2003;348:2609–17.
115. Dimopoulos MA, Moreau P, Palumbo A, et al. Carfilzomib and dexamethasone versus bortezomib and dexamethasone for patients with relapsed or refractory multiple myeloma (ENDEAVOR): a randomised, phase 3, open-label, multicentre study. Lancet Oncol. 2016;17:27–38.
116. Kumar SK, Berdeja JG, Niesvizky R, et al. Safety and tolerability of ixazomib, an oral proteasome inhibitor, in combination with lenalidomide and dexamethasone in patients with previously untreated multiple myeloma: an open-label phase 1/2 study. Lancet Oncol. 2014;15:1503–12.
117. Durie B, Hoering A, Rajkumar SV, et al. Bortezomib, Lenalidomide and dexamethasone vs. Lenalidomide and dexamethasone in patients (pts) with previously untreated multiple myeloma without an intent for immediate autologous stem cell transplant (ASCT): results of the randomized phase III trial S. Blood. 2015;126:25.
118. Lokhorst HM, Plesner T, Laubach JP, et al. Targeting CD38 with Daratumumab monotherapy in multiple myeloma. N Engl J Med. 2015;373:1207–19.
119. Lonial S, Dimopoulos M, Palumbo A, et al. Elotuzumab therapy for relapsed or refractory multiple myeloma. N Engl J Med. 2015;373:621–31.
120. San-Miguel JF, Richardson PG, Gunther A, et al. Phase Ib study of panobinostat and bortezomib in relapsed or relapsed and refractory multiple myeloma. J Clin Oncol. 2013;31:3696–703.
121. Kyle RA, Rajkumar SV. Multiple myeloma. Blood. 2008;111:2962–72.

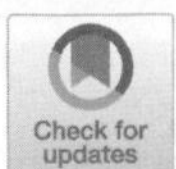

25 Monoclonal Gammopathy of Undetermined Significance

Malin Hultcrantz and Ola Landgren

Introduction

The presence of a monoclonal protein on serum electrophoresis in otherwise healthy individuals was first described by Prof. Jan Waldenström who named this condition "essential hypergammaglobulinemia" in 1960 [1]. Dr. Kyle et al. later observed that individuals with a monoclonal gammopathy were at a higher risk of developing multiple myeloma and therefore coined the term "monoclonal gammopathy of undermined significance" (MGUS) [2]. The diagnostic criteria for MGUS are presence of monoclonal protein <3.0 g/dL, <10% clonal plasma cells in the bone marrow, and absence of end-organ damage that can be attributed to a plasma cell disorder [3]. MGUS can be further classified into non-IgM MGUS, IgM MGUS, and light-chain MGUS (LC-MGUS) [3]. Typically, patients with non-IgM MGUS, IgM MGUS, and LC-MGUS progress to multiple myeloma, Waldenström's macroglobulinemia, and light-chain multiple myeloma, respectively. In addition, MGUS has been associated with comorbidities that are not necessarily caused by the plasma cell dyscrasia [4]. Several host factors, e.g., gender and ethnicity, as well as external factors, e.g., exposure to pesticides, are associated with an increased risk of MGUS [5, 6]. The rate of progression to multiple myeloma is approximately 0.5–1% per year and there is evidence that multiple myeloma is consistently preceded by MGUS [7]. A number of predictive factors as well as prognostic scoring systems have been developed to estimate the risk of progression to malignant disease [7–9]. In this review chapter, we discuss the diagnosis, risk of progression, as well as clinical implications for patients with MGUS.

M. Hultcrantz, M.D., Ph.D. (✉) • O. Landgren, M.D., Ph.D.
Myeloma Service, Department of Medicine,
Memorial Sloan Kettering Cancer Center,
1275 York Ave, New York, NY 10065, USA
e-mail: hultcram@mskcc.org

Diagnosis and Definition of MGUS

In the majority of patients, MGUS is diagnosed incidentally during workup for other various symptoms or disorders. The diagnostic criteria for MGUS, smoldering multiple myeloma, and multiple myeloma were updated in 2014 [3]. MGUS is defined as presence of a monoclonal protein (M-protein) <3.0 g/dL, <10% plasma cells in the bone marrow, and absence of events defining for myeloma or other plasma cell disorders; all three criteria must be met [3]. Myeloma-defining events are presence of end-organ damage that can be attributed to the plasma cell proliferation as defined by the CRAB criteria (hypercalcemia, renal failure, anemia, bone lesions, Table 25.1) or the recently added definitions of free light chain (FLC) ratio ≥100, >60% clonal plasma cells in the bone marrow, or >1 lytic bone lesion on whole-body MRI [3].

There are three different types of MGUS: *non-IgM MGUS, IgM MGUS,* and *light-chain MGUS* (Table 25.2). Non-IgM MGUS is the most common type and is diagnosed on serum electrophoresis. In non-IgM MGUS, most patients have M-proteins consisting of IgG or IgA while IgD is rare and there are only a few cases in the literature of IgE

Table 25.1 Definition of monoclonal gammopathy of undetermined significance (MGUS), smoldering multiple myeloma (SMM), and multiple myeloma (MM)

	MGUS	SMM	MM
Serum M-protein	<3.0 g/dL	≥3.0 g/dL	–
Clonal bone marrow plasma cells	<10%	≥10–60%	≥10%
Presence of myeloma-defining event[a]	No	No	Yes

[a]Myeloma-defining events are CRAB criteria (hypercalcemia [serum calcium >0.25 mmol/L (>1 mg/dL) higher than the upper limit of normal or >2.75 mmol/L (>11 mg/dL)], renal insufficiency [serum creatinine >177 μmol/L (2 mg/dL) or creatinine clearance <40 mL/min], anemia [hemoglobin value of >2 g/dL below the lower normal limit, or a hemoglobin value <10 g/dL], bone lesions [one or more osteolytic lesions revealed by skeletal radiography, CT, or PET-CT], or the presence of bone marrow plasma cells >60%, involved/uninvolved free-light chain ratio of ≥100, or >1 focal lesion on MRI [3]

P.H. Wiernik et al. (eds.), *Neoplastic Diseases of the Blood*, DOI 10.1007/978-3-319-64263-5_25

Table 25.2 Types of monoclonal gammopathy of undetermined significance (MGUS)

Type of MGUS	Definition
Non-IgM MGUS	M-protein <3.0 g/dL Clonal bone marrow plasma cells <10% No myeloma-defining event
IgM MGUS	IgM M-protein <3.0 g/dL Bone marrow lymphoplasmacytic cells <10% No myeloma or Waldenström's macroglobulinemia-defining event
Light chain MGUS	Abnormal free light chain ratio Elevated level of involved light chains No immunoglobulin heavy chain on serum electrophoresis or immunofixation Clonal bone marrow plasma cells <10% No myeloma-defining event No amyloidosis Urine M-protein <500 mg/24 h

MGUS. In the case of progression, non-IgM MGUS in the majority of cases transforms to smoldering myeloma and multiple myeloma [10].

IgM MGUS is less common than non-IgM MGUS and is defined as monoclonal IgM protein <3.0 g/L, <10% bone marrow lymphoplasmacytic cells, and absence of end-organ damage (anemia, hyperviscosity, lymphadenopathy, hepatosplenomegaly, constitutional symptoms) attributed to a lymphoproliferative disorder. Progression from IgM MGUS commonly means transition to smoldering Waldenström's macroglobulinemia or Waldenström's macroglobulinemia but also, although more rare, to IgM multiple myeloma, chronic lymphocytic leukemia or other lymphomas [11]. The *MYD88* mutation is present in the vast majority of Waldenström's macroglobulinemia patients and is found in ~50% of individuals with IgM MGUS [12–14]. IgM multiple myeloma on the other hand is rare, only 1% of all multiple myeloma cases, and is not associated with *MYD88* mutation [12, 15].

Light-chain MGUS (LC-MGUS) was described in 2010 by Dispezieri et al. and represent approximately 20% of all MGUS cases. LC-MGUS is defined as abnormal FLC ratio (<0.26 or >1.65) in combination with elevated concentration of the involved κ or λ light chains [16]. In addition, the definition includes no immunoglobulin heavy chain on serum electrophoresis or immunofixation, <10% clonal bone marrow plasma cells, and no sign of end-organ damage [16, 17]. LC-MGUS can progress to idiopathic Bence Jones proteinuria and light-chain multiple myeloma. Furthermore, LC-MGUS is associated with amyloidosis and renal impairment [16]. Due to the possibility that polyclonal light chains may be elevated in renal disease, Dispenzieri et al. discussed whether using the renal FLC reference range would be more optimal compared to the standard reference for the LC-MGUS definition. According to their estimation, this would affect the number of κ and λ LC-MGUS cases but would not have a major effect on the overall prevalence [16]. This issue was further highlighted by Hutchison et al. who suggested adjusted FLC ratio reference ranges for certain clinical settings [18]. Moreover, polyclonal increase in free light chains can be used as a biomarker for B-cell activation in a broader clinical context. Polyclonal free light chains have been associated with disease activity in autoimmune disease, risk of non-Hodgkin lymphoma, renal impairment, and overall survival in the general population [18]. Further studies are needed to fully elucidate the optimal LC-MGUS definition, polyclonal free light chain increase, and implications for progression to malignant disease.

Epidemiology

Recently, in a large population-based study of the US population, the overall prevalence of MGUS was 2.4% in individuals over the age of 50 years [5]. The study was based on the NHANES and NHANES III studies (2000–2004) which included screening of 12,482 individuals representative for the US population [5]. The highest prevalence of MGUS was found in African-American blacks (3.7%), followed by whites (2.3%), and the lowest prevalence was observed in Mexican-Americans (1.8%) [5]. IgA MGUS was more common among Mexican-Americans and there was a lower rate of IgM MGUS in blacks and Mexican-Americans compared to whites. African-American and African blacks were also more likely to have high-risk features including a higher median level of M-protein and had a higher risk of progression [5, 19]. The overall prevalence of MGUS was lower in the NHANES studies compared to the previous estimates from the Olmsted county studies where the reported prevalence of MGUS was 3.2–3.4% in individuals over 50 years [10, 16]. The difference in reported prevalence may be caused by differences in the patient population, i.e., screened population in the NHANES studies versus referral-based Mayo Clinic cohort [5, 10, 16].

IgM MGUS is less common than non-IgM MGUS but there is limited information on the overall prevalence of IgM MGUS. LC-MGUS comprises 20% of all MGUS cases and was found in 0.7–0.8% of the population over 50 years in studies from the Olmsted County and Germany [16, 20].

The prevalence of MGUS increases with increasing age across all studies. Reported prevalence of MGUS ranged from 1.2 to 2.8% in 50–59-year-olds to 4.6–8.7% in individuals 80 years or older [5, 16, 20]. Moreover, MGUS is consistently more common in men compared to women across all age groups [5].

Etiology

The etiology of both MGUS and multiple myeloma remains largely unknown. The prevalence has been associated with various host factors, e.g., gender, age, and ethnicity, and there was also a trend towards a higher prevalence of MGUS patients with elevated BMI [5, 19]. First-degree relatives of individuals with MGUS have an increased risk of developing MGUS and LC-MGUS [21–23]. Through genome-wide association studies, a number of single-nucleotide variants associated with an increased risk of multiple myeloma have been identified indicating a genetic susceptibility [24].

A higher risk of developing MGUS has also been reported in individuals exposed to pesticides and herbicides including Agent Orange [6, 25]. Constant immune stimulation may be a trigger of MGUS and an elevated prevalence of MGUS has been observed in patients with a prior autoimmune disorder [26].

Risk Assessment and Progression

Non-IgM MGUS typically progresses to IgG or IgA smoldering myeloma and later to multiple myeloma requiring therapy. The annual risk of progression from MGUS to multiple myeloma is 0.5–1% per year [7, 9]. Patterns of progression can vary from a steady increase in M-protein while others can have a stable M-protein level for many years and then suddenly increase [27]. On average, 75–90% of MGUS patients remain in the precursor stage and never develop malignant disease. However, the risk of progression does not decrease even after 25–35 years and hence lifelong follow-up of MGUS patients is necessary [9, 28]. Patients with smoldering myeloma have a 10% risk of progression per year during the first 5 years after diagnosis and the risk thereafter decreases to around 3% the next 5 years and then 1% per year for the 10 following years [29].

The risk assessment scores in MGUS rely largely on biomarkers. The most updated scoring system was published in 2014 by investigators from the National Cancer Institute and Nordic Myeloma Study Group (NCI/NMSG) [7]. In their population-based cohort followed up to 30 years, the overall risk of progression to multiple myeloma or other lymphoproliferative disorders was 0.5% per year [7]. The rate of progression to malignant disease was higher during the first 10 years after diagnosis, almost 1%/year, and those who remained in the precursor stage after more than 10 years had a lower progression rate. Additionally, by performing new assays on stored samples, they evaluated several biomarkers and the impact on disease progression. In the NCI/NMSG score, a higher risk of transformation to multiple myeloma and lymphoproliferative diseases was observed in patients who had an abnormal FLC ratio (<0.26 or >1.65), M-protein level >1.5 g/dL, and reduction of 1 or 2 noninvolved immunoglobulin isotype levels (immunoparesis) (Table 25.3). In MGUS patients who had all three risk factors, the 10-year risk of disease progression was 40% implying that this group of patients should be carefully monitored for disease progression [7].

Table 25.3 Comparison of the three scoring systems for risk of disease progression in MGUS from the Mayo Clinic, PETHEMA, and NCI/NMSG [7–9]

	NCI/NMSG[a]	Mayo Clinic[b]	PETHEMA[c]
Sample size (*n* MGUS patients)	728	1148	407
Risk factors	Non-IgG MGUS Abnormal FLC ratio M-protein >1.5 g/dL Immunoparesis	Non-IgG MGUS Abnormal FLC ratio M-protein >1.5 g/dL	≥95% aberrant plasma cells DNA aneuploidy
Overall risk of progression	0.5%	1%	~0.6%

FLC free light chain

[a]Population-based cohort with patients included 1964–2000. Score based on unanimously analyzed stored samples

[b]Referral center cohort with patients included between 1960 and 1994. Score based on retrospective laboratory results performed at the time of diagnosis

[c]Referral center cohort with patients included 1996–2003. Score based on flow cytometry performed at the time of diagnosis

Two additional risk scores were published in 2005 and 2007 by the Mayo Clinic and PETHEMA groups, respectively [8, 9]. The Mayo Clinic risk score is based on the type and size of M-protein as well as serum FLC ratio. High-risk criteria are defined as non-IgG M-protein, M-protein >1.5 g/dL, and an abnormal FLC ratio [9]. In this system, high-risk MGUS patients who have all the three risk factors had a cumulative risk of developing multiple myeloma of 58% during the first 20 years after the MGUS diagnosis. Patients with two, one, and no risk factors have a risk of progression of 37%, 21%, and 5%, respectively [10]. The PETHEMA group bases their prognostic system on aberrant plasma cells in the bone marrow and DNA aneuploidy both measured by flow cytometry. MGUS patients who had ≥95% aberrant plasma cells and DNA aneuploidy had a 5-year risk of progression of 46%, while individuals with one of the two risk factors had a 10% risk of progression and patients with no risk factor a 2% risk of progression at 5 years, respectively [8].

Additional markers associated with a higher risk of progression from MGUS to multiple myeloma are suppression of nonclonal bone marrow plasma cells, similar to the above-mentioned immunoparesis [7, 8, 30, 31]. A progressive increase in the M-protein level is also a prognostic marker of progression [32]. Different rates of progression were reported for IgG MGUS vs. non-IgG MGUS in the Mayo Clinic model while no such difference was seen in the NCI/NMSG and PETHEMA models. The underlying reason for this difference is not fully understood but may be related to the higher catabolic rate of IgA and IgM compared to IgG implying that at a given M-protein in serum, there may be more clonal plasma cells in the bone marrow in individuals with IgA and IgM isotype MGUS compared to those with IgG MGUS [7,

8]. Furthermore, gene expression profiling can additionally contribute to the risk assessment in MGUS and smoldering myeloma [33]. Presence of circulating plasma cells, abnormal metaphase cytogenetics, and cytoplasmic immunoglobulin measured by flow cytometry can also be valuable in predicting disease progression [34, 35]. It is on the other hand not clear if cytogenetic markers of poor risk in multiple myeloma, t(4;14) or del(17p), are associated with an increased risk of malignant transformation in MGUS patients [36].

The risk of progression from IgM MGUS to Waldenström's macroglobulinemia or other lymphoproliferative diseases is approximately 1.5% per year [37]. Risk factors for progression in IgM MGUS include M-protein size >1.5 g/dL and presence of *MYD88* mutation. Abnormal FLC ratio is not an established risk factor for progression and is not included in the recommended follow-up of patients with IgM MGUS [12, 14].

There is so far limited information on the risk of progression in LC-MGUS. Based on the two published studies so far, the risk of progression appeared to be lower than 1% per year but more information is needed in order to give an accurate estimate [16, 20]. In addition to light-chain multiple myeloma, patients with LC-MGUS are at an elevated risk of developing amyloidosis and renal disease. The latter was observed in 23% of patients and the majority of these had λ-restricted LC-MGUS [16].

The prognostic factors and existing scoring systems are valuable for risk stratification but there is a need to identify molecular markers to better predict the risks in the individual patient.

Genetic Background

Patients with multiple myeloma can be classified into two major cytogenetic groups: chromosome 14 translocations (*IGH* locus) and hyperdiploidy. In studies using fluorescent in situ hybridization (FISH), these cytogenetic aberrations were present already in MGUS and are thus considered early hits in myelomagenesis [38].

During recent years, knowledge of the genetic landscape in multiple myeloma has increased greatly through studies using modern sequencing techniques, i.e., whole-genome sequencing, whole-exome sequencing, and targeted sequencing. So far, no single disease-specific gene has been identified; the studies on the contrary revealed a complex genomic landscape including frequent somatic mutations in *KRAS*, *NRAS*, *FAM46C*, *BRAF*, *TP53*, *TRAF3*, *DIS3*, *CYLD*, and more [39–42]. There is so far limited information on driver mutations and changes in the genomic landscape during transition from precursor to malignant disease. Progression from MGUS to multiple myeloma may be caused by acquisition of additional genetic events or the expansion of preexisting clones already present at the MGUS stage. In both scenarios, interactions between the plasma cells and the bone marrow microenvironment as well as the immune system are likely to influence disease evolution [43].

Comorbidities

Through assessment of large clinical cohorts, MGUS has been associated with a number of comorbidities and mortality not only associated with the development of multiple myeloma. These include increased risk of infections, venous and arterial thrombosis, malignancies, and an inferior survival compared to the general population [21, 44, 45]. Furthermore, patients with MGUS have an increased bone turnover and an elevated risk of fractures [46, 47]. In screened cohorts, the rate of these complications tended to be lower indicating a possible role of other underlying comorbidities which may have led to the original clinical workup and diagnosis of MGUS [48, 49].

There is an increased risk of renal complications in patients with MGUS, especially LC-MGUS, and the term monoclonal gammopathy of renal significance has therefore been coined [50]. M-protein-related renal diseases include monoclonal immunoglobulin deposition disease, light-chain proximal tubulopathy, proliferative glomerulonephritis with monoclonal immunoglobulin deposits, and C3 glomerulopathy with monoclonal gammopathy. These renal diseases are characterized by deposition of monoclonal deposits in the kidney diagnosed on kidney biopsy [36, 50]. In addition, the M-protein can cause various systemic manifestations including neuropathy and skin disorders [36, 43].

Clinical Recommendations

The recommended workup for MGUS is aimed at detecting end-organ damage indicative of multiple myeloma, lymphoproliferative disorders, or amyloidosis. Workup recommended by the International Myeloma Working Group includes complete blood counts, electrolytes and renal function test, serum and urine electrophoresis, as well as serum FLC assay (Table 25.4) [3, 51]. Bone marrow biopsy and bone imaging are recommended to confirm the MGUS diagnosis and to rule out CRAB criteria of other findings of smoldering or multiple myeloma. In patients with low-risk MGUS, bone marrow biopsy and imaging can be deferred if there are no signs of high-risk MGUS, or end-organ damage indicating multiple myeloma, lymphoma, or amyloidosis [51, 52]. If amyloidosis is suspected, biopsy of the bone marrow or abdominal fat with Congo red staining should be performed [36].

Patients diagnosed with MGUS should be monitored every 4–6 months during the first year after initial diagnosis. Thereafter, evaluation every 6–12 months is recommended depending on the rate of M-protein increase. In patients with stable low-risk MGUS, evaluation every 24 months is sufficient while closer monitoring is recommended in high-risk MGUS patients [36, 52]. Patients with LC-MGUS should be evaluated regularly for development of kidney disease and amyloidosis with NT-pro-BNP and urine albumin.

Table 25.4 Clinical evaluation for newly diagnosed patients with monoclonal gammopathy of undetermined significance (MGUS)

• Complete blood count
• Chemistry including serum electrolytes, creatinine, beta-2 microglobulin, calcium, albumin, lactate dehydrogenase (LDH)
• Serum protein studies including total protein and serum electrophoresis
• Serum immunofixation
• Serum free light chain measurements
• 24-h urine collection for electrophoresis and immunofixation
• Bone marrow aspirate and biopsy for plasma cell infiltration, flow cytometry, and fluorescence in situ hybridization[a]
• Skeletal survey, low-dose CT, or PET-CT[a]

[a]These assessments can be excluded in patients who are considered low-risk MGUS (IgG MGUS, M-protein <1.5 g/dL, and normal free light chain ratio)

Recently, two independent studies have reported a better overall survival in multiple myeloma patients where the MGUS was previously known compared to multiple myeloma patients without prior knowledge of MGUS [53, 54]. This is likely an effect of earlier diagnosis and treatment and raises the question whether screening for MGUS would be beneficial. There are ongoing studies for earlier treatment of patients with smoldering myeloma, especially those with high risk, but so far treatment for patients with MGUS is not recommended.

Conclusion

MGUS is a premalignant disorder that in the majority of cases is asymptomatic and will not progress to malignant disease. The risk of progression to malignant disease persists throughout life and patients should therefore be monitored continuously. Thorough workup is needed to exclude more advanced disease stages and associated disorders. There are valuable risk-scoring systems for predicting the risk of transformation to multiple myeloma and there are ongoing research efforts to identify molecular markers that can better predict individual risk of progression.

References

1. Waldenstrom J. Studies on conditions associated with disturbed gamma globulin formation (gammopathies). Harvey Lect. 1960;56:211–31.
2. Kyle RA. Monoclonal gammopathy of undetermined significance. Natural history in 241 cases. Am J Med. 1978;64(5):814–26.
3. Rajkumar SV, Dimopoulos MA, Palumbo A, Blade J, Merlini G, Mateos MV, et al. International Myeloma Working Group updated criteria for the diagnosis of multiple myeloma. Lancet Oncol. 2014;15(12):e538–48.
4. Kristinsson SY, Bjorkholm M, Landgren O. Survival in monoclonal gammopathy of undetermined significance and Waldenstrom macroglobulinemia. Clin Lymphoma Myeloma Leuk. 2013;13(2):187–90.
5. Landgren O, Graubard BI, Katzmann JA, Kyle RA, Ahmadizadeh I, Clark R, et al. Racial disparities in the prevalence of monoclonal gammopathies: a population-based study of 12,482 persons from the National Health and Nutritional Examination Survey. Leukemia. 2014;28(7):1537–42.
6. Landgren O, Shim YK, Michalek J, Costello R, Burton D, Ketchum N, et al. Agent Orange exposure and monoclonal Gammopathy of undetermined significance: an Operation Ranch Hand veteran cohort study. JAMA Oncol. 2015;1(8):1061–8.
7. Turesson I, Kovalchik SA, Pfeiffer RM, Kristinsson SY, Goldin LR, Drayson MT, et al. Monoclonal gammopathy of undetermined significance and risk of lymphoid and myeloid malignancies: 728 cases followed up to 30 years in Sweden. Blood. 2014;123(3):338–45.
8. Perez-Persona E, Vidriales MB, Mateo G, Garcia-Sanz R, Mateos MV, de Coca AG, et al. New criteria to identify risk of progression in monoclonal gammopathy of uncertain significance and smoldering multiple myeloma based on multiparameter flow cytometry analysis of bone marrow plasma cells. Blood. 2007;110(7):2586–92.
9. Rajkumar SV, Kyle RA, Therneau TM, Melton LJ 3rd, Bradwell AR, Clark RJ, et al. Serum free light chain ratio is an independent risk factor for progression in monoclonal gammopathy of undetermined significance. Blood. 2005;106(3):812–7.
10. Kyle RA, Durie BG, Rajkumar SV, Landgren O, Blade J, Merlini G, et al. Monoclonal gammopathy of undetermined significance (MGUS) and smoldering (asymptomatic) multiple myeloma: IMWG consensus perspectives risk factors for progression and guidelines for monitoring and management. Leukemia. 2010;24(6):1121–7.
11. Kyle RA, Therneau TM, Dispenzieri A, Kumar S, Benson JT, Larson DR, et al. Immunoglobulin m monoclonal gammopathy of undetermined significance and smoldering Waldenstrom macroglobulinemia. Clin Lymphoma Myeloma Leuk. 2013;13(2):184–6.
12. Treon SP, Xu L, Yang G, Zhou Y, Liu X, Cao Y, et al. MYD88 L265P somatic mutation in Waldenstrom's macroglobulinemia. N Engl J Med. 2012;367(9):826–33.
13. Landgren O, Staudt L. MYD88 L265P somatic mutation in IgM MGUS. N Engl J Med. 2012;367(23):2255–6. author reply 6–7
14. Varettoni M, Arcaini L, Zibellini S, Boveri E, Rattotti S, Riboni R, et al. Prevalence and clinical significance of the MYD88 (L265P) somatic mutation in Waldenstrom's macroglobulinemia and related lymphoid neoplasms. Blood. 2013;121(13):2522–8.
15. Schuster SR, Rajkumar SV, Dispenzieri A, Morice W, Aspitia AM, Ansell S, et al. IgM multiple myeloma: disease definition, prognosis, and differentiation from Waldenstrom's macroglobulinemia. Am J Hematol. 2010;85(11):853–5.
16. Dispenzieri A, Katzmann JA, Kyle RA, Larson DR, Melton LJ 3rd, Colby CL, et al. Prevalence and risk of progression of light-chain monoclonal gammopathy of undetermined significance: a retrospective population-based cohort study. Lancet. 2010;375(9727):1721–8.
17. Landgren O, Kyle RA, Rajkumar SV. From myeloma precursor disease to multiple myeloma: new diagnostic concepts and opportunities for early intervention. Clin Cancer Res. 2011;17(6):1243–52.
18. Hutchison CA, Landgren O. Polyclonal immunoglobulin free light chains as a potential biomarker of immune stimulation and inflammation. Clin Chem. 2011;57(10):1387–9.
19. Landgren O, Katzmann JA, Hsing AW, Pfeiffer RM, Kyle RA, Yeboah ED, et al. Prevalence of monoclonal gammopathy of undetermined significance among men in Ghana. Mayo Clin Proc. 2007;82(12):1468–73.
20. Eisele L, Durig J, Huttmann A, Duhrsen U, Assert R, Bokhof B, et al. Prevalence and progression of monoclonal gammopathy of undetermined significance and light-chain MGUS in Germany. Ann Hematol. 2012;91(2):243–8.
21. Kristinsson SY, Bjorkholm M, Goldin LR, Blimark C, Mellqvist UH, Wahlin A, et al. Patterns of hematologic malignancies and solid tumors among 37,838 first-degree relatives of 13,896 patients with multiple myeloma in Sweden. Int J Cancer. 2009;125(9):2147–50.
22. Greenberg AJ, Rajkumar SV, Larson DR, Dispenzieri A, Therneau TM, Colby CL, et al. Increased prevalence of light chain monoclonal gammopathy of undetermined significance (LC-MGUS) in first-degree relatives of individuals with multiple myeloma. Br J Haematol. 2012;157(4):472–5.

23. Greenberg AJ, Rajkumar SV, Vachon CM. Familial monoclonal gammopathy of undetermined significance and multiple myeloma: epidemiology, risk factors, and biological characteristics. Blood. 2012;119(23):5359–66.
24. Morgan GJ, Johnson DC, Weinhold N, Goldschmidt H, Landgren O, Lynch HT, et al. Inherited genetic susceptibility to multiple myeloma. Leukemia. 2014;28(3):518–24.
25. Landgren O, Kyle RA, Hoppin JA, Beane Freeman LE, Cerhan JR, Katzmann JA, et al. Pesticide exposure and risk of monoclonal gammopathy of undetermined significance in the Agricultural Health Study. Blood. 2009;113(25):6386–91.
26. Lindqvist EK, Goldin LR, Landgren O, Blimark C, Mellqvist UH, Turesson I, et al. Personal and family history of immune-related conditions increase the risk of plasma cell disorders: a population-based study. Blood. 2011;118(24):6284–91.
27. Landgren O, Kyle RA, Pfeiffer RM, Katzmann JA, Caporaso NE, Hayes RB, et al. Monoclonal gammopathy of undetermined significance (MGUS) consistently precedes multiple myeloma: a prospective study. Blood. 2009;113(22):5412–7.
28. Kyle RA, Therneau TM, Rajkumar SV, Offord JR, Larson DR, Plevak MF, et al. A long-term study of prognosis in monoclonal gammopathy of undetermined significance. N Engl J Med. 2002;346(8):564–9.
29. Kyle RA, Remstein ED, Therneau TM, Dispenzieri A, Kurtin PJ, Hodnefield JM, et al. Clinical course and prognosis of smoldering (asymptomatic) multiple myeloma. N Engl J Med. 2007;356(25):2582–90.
30. Perez-Persona E, Mateo G, Garcia-Sanz R, Mateos MV, de Las Heras N, de Coca AG, et al. Risk of progression in smouldering myeloma and monoclonal gammopathies of unknown significance: comparative analysis of the evolution of monoclonal component and multiparameter flow cytometry of bone marrow plasma cells. Br J Haematol. 2010;148(1):110–4.
31. Katzmann JA, Clark R, Kyle RA, Larson DR, Therneau TM, Melton LJ 3rd, et al. Suppression of uninvolved immunoglobulins defined by heavy/light chain pair suppression is a risk factor for progression of MGUS. Leukemia. 2013;27(1):208–12.
32. Rosinol L, Cibeira MT, Montoto S, Rozman M, Esteve J, Filella X, et al. Monoclonal gammopathy of undetermined significance: predictors of malignant transformation and recognition of an evolving type characterized by a progressive increase in M protein size. Mayo Clin Proc. 2007;82(4):428–34.
33. Dhodapkar MV, Sexton R, Waheed S, Usmani S, Papanikolaou X, Nair B, et al. Clinical, genomic, and imaging predictors of myeloma progression from asymptomatic monoclonal gammopathies (SWOG S0120). Blood. 2014;123(1):78–85.
34. Kumar S, Rajkumar SV, Kyle RA, Lacy MQ, Dispenzieri A, Fonseca R, et al. Prognostic value of circulating plasma cells in monoclonal gammopathy of undetermined significance. J Clin Oncol. 2005;23(24):5668–74.
35. Papanikolaou X, Rosenthal A, Dhodapkar M, Epstein J, Khan R, van Rhee F, et al. Flow cytometry defined cytoplasmic immunoglobulin index is a major prognostic factor for progression of asymptomatic monoclonal gammopathies to multiple myeloma (subset analysis of SWOG S0120). Blood Cancer J. 2016;6:e410.
36. van de Donk NW, Mutis T, Poddighe PJ, Lokhorst HM, Zweegman S. Diagnosis, risk stratification and management of monoclonal gammopathy of undetermined significance and smoldering multiple myeloma. Int J Lab Hematol. 2016;38(Suppl 1):110–22.
37. Owen RG, Pratt G, Auer RL, Flatley R, Kyriakou C, Lunn MP, et al. Guidelines on the diagnosis and management of Waldenstrom macroglobulinaemia. Br J Haematol. 2014;165(3):316–33.
38. Fonseca R, Bailey RJ, Ahmann GJ, Rajkumar SV, Hoyer JD, Lust JA, et al. Genomic abnormalities in monoclonal gammopathy of undetermined significance. Blood. 2002;100(4):1417–24.
39. Bolli N, Avet-Loiseau H, Wedge DC, Van Loo P, Alexandrov LB, Martincorena I, et al. Heterogeneity of genomic evolution and mutational profiles in multiple myeloma. Nat Commun. 2014;5:2997.
40. Chapman MA, Lawrence MS, Keats JJ, Cibulskis K, Sougnez C, Schinzel AC, et al. Initial genome sequencing and analysis of multiple myeloma. Nature. 2011;471(7339):467–72.
41. Lohr JG, Stojanov P, Carter SL, Cruz-Gordillo P, Lawrence MS, Auclair D, et al. Widespread genetic heterogeneity in multiple myeloma: implications for targeted therapy. Cancer Cell. 2014;25(1):91–101.
42. Walker BA, Boyle EM, Wardell CP, Murison A, Begum DB, Dahir NM, et al. Mutational Spectrum, copy number changes, and outcome: results of a sequencing study of patients with newly diagnosed myeloma. J Clin Oncol. 2015;33(33):3911–20.
43. Dhodapkar MV. MGUS to myeloma: a mysterious gammopathy of underexplored significance. Blood. 2016. pii: blood-2016-09-692954 [Epub ahead of print].
44. Kristinsson SY, Fears TR, Gridley G, Turesson I, Mellqvist UH, Bjorkholm M, et al. Deep vein thrombosis after monoclonal gammopathy of undetermined significance and multiple myeloma. Blood. 2008;112(9):3582–6.
45. Kristinsson SY, Pfeiffer RM, Bjorkholm M, Goldin LR, Schulman S, Blimark C, et al. Arterial and venous thrombosis in monoclonal gammopathy of undetermined significance and multiple myeloma: a population-based study. Blood. 2010;115(24):4991–8.
46. Kristinsson SY, Tang M, Pfeiffer RM, Bjorkholm M, Blimark C, Mellqvist UH, et al. Monoclonal gammopathy of undetermined significance and risk of skeletal fractures: a population-based study. Blood. 2010;116(15):2651–5.
47. Ng AC, Khosla S, Charatcharoenwitthaya N, Kumar SK, Achenbach SJ, Holets MF, et al. Bone microstructural changes revealed by high-resolution peripheral quantitative computed tomography imaging and elevated DKK1 and MIP-1alpha levels in patients with MGUS. Blood. 2011;118(25):6529–34.
48. Lindqvist EK, Lund SH, Costello R, Burton D, Korde NS, Mailankody S, et al. No risk of arterial or venous thrombosis in monoclonal gammopathy of undetermined significance: results from a population-based study. Blood. 2015;126(23):4252.
49. Lindqvist EK, Lund SH, Costello R, Burton D, Korde N, Mailankody S, et al. Monoclonal Gammopathy of undetermined significance (Mgus) is associated with a 30% increased risk of dying at 8 years of follow-up: results from a screened cross-sectional population-based study. Haematologica. 2014;99:115.
50. Bridoux F, Leung N, Hutchison CA, Touchard G, Sethi S, Fermand JP, et al. Diagnosis of monoclonal gammopathy of renal significance. Kidney Int. 2015;87(4):698–711.
51. Mateos MV, Landgren O. MGUS and smoldering multiple myeloma: diagnosis and epidemiology. Cancer Treat Res. 2016;169:3–12.
52. van de Donk NW, Palumbo A, Johnsen HE, Engelhardt M, Gay F, Gregersen H, et al. The clinical relevance and management of monoclonal gammopathy of undetermined significance and related disorders: recommendations from the European Myeloma Network. Haematologica. 2014;99(6):984–96.
53. Sigurdardottir E, Turesson I, Lund S, et al. The role of diagnosis and clinical follow-up of monoclonal gammopathy of undetermined significance on survival in multiple myeloma. JAMA Oncol. 2015;1(2):168–74.
54. Go RS, Gundrum JD, Neuner JM. Determining the clinical significance of monoclonal gammopathy of undetermined significance: a SEER-Medicare population analysis. Clin Lymphoma Myeloma Leuk. 2015;15(3):177–186.e4.

Smoldering Multiple Myeloma

26

María-Victoria Mateos and Jesús F. San-Miguel

Introduction

Smoldering multiple myeloma (SMM) is an asymptomatic plasma cell disorder defined in 1980 by Kyle and Greipp on the basis of a series of six patients who met the criteria for multiple myeloma (MM) but whose disease did not have an aggressive course [1].

At the end of 2014, the International Myeloma Working Group (IMWG) updated the definition and SMM was defined as a plasma cell disorder characterized by the presence of ≥3 g/dL serum M-protein and/or 10–60% bone marrow plasma cells (BMPCs), but with no evidence of myeloma-related symptomatology (hypercalcemia, renal insufficiency, anemia, or bone lesions (CRAB)) or any other myeloma-defining event (MDE) [2]. According to these recent updated criteria, the definition of SMM excludes asymptomatic patients with BMPCs of 60% or more, serum free light chain (FLC) levels of ≥100, and those with two or more focal lesions in the skeleton as revealed by magnetic resonance imaging (MRI).

Kristinsson et al., based on the Swedish Myeloma Registry, have recently reported that 14% of patients diagnosed with myeloma had SMM and, accordingly, the age-standardized incidence of SMM would be 0.44 cases per 100,000 people [3].

Differential Diagnosis with Other Entities

SMM must be distinguished from other plasma cell disorders, such as monoclonal gammopathy of undetermined significance (MGUS) and symptomatic MM (Table 26.1). The MGUS entity is characterized by a level of serum M-protein of <3 g/dL plus <10% plasma cell infiltration in the bone marrow, with no CRAB and no MDE. Symptomatic MM must always have CRAB symptomatology or MDE, in conjunction with ≥10% clonal BMPC infiltration or biopsy-proven bony or extramedullary plasmacytoma [2].

End-organ damage often needs to be correctly evaluated to distinguish myeloma-related symptomatology from some signs or symptoms that could otherwise be attributed to comorbidities or concomitant diseases [4].

Due to the updated IMWG criteria for the diagnosis of MM, there are some specific assessments to which physicians have to pay attention in order to make a correct diagnosis of SMM [2].

1. For evaluation of bone disease, the IMWG recommends to perform in all patients with suspected SMM one of the following procedures: skeletal survey, ^{18}F-fluorodeoxyglucose

Table 26.1 Differential diagnosis of MGUS, SMM, and symptomatic MM

Feature	MGUS	SMM	MM
Serum-M protein	<3 g/dL and	≥3 g/dL and/or	
Clonal BMPC infiltration	<10%	10–60%	≥10% or biopsy-proven plasmacytoma
Symptomatology	Absence of CRAB[a]	Absence of MDE[b] or amyloidosis	Presence of MDE[b]

[a]CRAB includes (1) hypercalcemia: serum calcium >0.25 mmol/L (>1 mg/dL) higher than the upper limit of normal or >2.75 mmol/L (>11 mg/dL); (2) renal insufficiency: serum creatinine >177 μmol/L (2 mg/dL) or creatinine clearance <40 mL/min; (3) anemia: hemoglobin value of >2 g/dL below the lower normal limit, or a hemoglobin value <10 g/dL; (4) bone lesions: one or more osteolytic lesions revealed by skeletal radiography, CT, or PET-CT

[b]*MDE* Myeloma-defining events include CRAB symptoms (above) or any one or more of the following biomarkers of malignancy: clonal bone marrow plasma cell percentage ≥60%; involved/uninvolved serum free light chain ratio ≥100; >1 focal lesions revealed by MRI studies

M.-V. Mateos, M.D., Ph.D. (✉)
Department of Hematology, Complejo Asistencial Universitario de Salamanca/Instituto Biosanitario de Salamanca (CAUSA/IBSAL), Paseo San Vicente, 58-182, 37007 Salamanca, Spain
e-mail: mvmateos@usal.es

J.F. San-Miguel, M.D., Ph.D.
Clínica Universidad de Navarra, Navarra, Spain

P.H. Wiernik et al. (eds.), *Neoplastic Diseases of the Blood*, DOI 10.1007/978-3-319-64263-5_26

(FDG) positron emission tomography (PET)/computed tomography (CT), or low-dose whole-body CT, with the exact modality determined by availability and resources. The aim is to exclude the presence of osteolytic bone lesions, currently defined by the presence of at least one lesion (≥5 mm) revealed by X-ray, CT, or PET-CT. In addition, whole-body MRI of the spine and pelvis is a mandatory component of the initial workup. It provides detailed information about not only bone marrow involvement but also the presence of focal lesions that predict more rapid progression to symptomatic myeloma. Hillengass et al. reported in 2010 that the presence of more than one focal lesion in whole-body MRI was associated with a significantly shorter median time to progression (TTP) to active disease (13 months), as compared to patients without focal lesions [5]. Kastritis and colleagues reported similar results after the analysis of a subgroup of patients who underwent spinal MRI and were followed up for a minimum of 2.5 years. The median TTP to symptomatic disease was 14 months when more than one focal lesion was present [6]. Therefore, if more than one focal lesion in MRI is present in SMM patients, this entity should no longer be considered as SMM but as MM, according to the current IMWG criteria. It is important to emphasize that they should be unequivocal focal lesions of >5 mm.

2. With respect to bone marrow infiltration, the Mayo Clinic group evaluated BMPC infiltration in a cohort of 651 patients and found that 21 (3.2%) had an extreme infiltration (≥60%) [7]. This group of patients had a median TTP to active disease of 7.7 months, with a 95% risk of progression at 2 years. This finding was subsequently validated in a study of 96 patients with SMM, in whom a median TTP of 15 months was reported for the group of patients with this extreme infiltration [8]. In a third study, 6 of 121 patients (5%) with SMM were found to have ≥60% BMPC, and all progressed to MM within 2 years [9]. Therefore, if ≥60% of clonal plasma cell infiltration is present either in bone marrow aspirate or biopsy, the diagnosis of SMM should be replaced by MM. Additional assessments, for example, by flow cytometry or by identifying cytogenetic abnormalities in SMM patients, are not mandatory but can help to estimate the risk of progression to active disease.
3. With respect to the serum free light chain (FLC) assay, Larsen et al. studied 586 patients with SMM to determine whether there was a threshold FLC ratio that predicted 85% of progression risk at 2 years. They found a serum-involved/uninvolved FLC ratio of at least 100 in 15% of patients and their risk of progression to symptomatic disease was 72% [10]. Similar results were obtained in a study by Kastritis and colleagues from the Greek Myeloma Group. In their study of 96 SMM patients, 7% had an involved/uninvolved FLC ratio of ≥100 and almost all progressed within 18 months [8]. In a third study, the risk of progression within 2 years was 64% [9]. Therefore, physicians must perform the sFLC assay at the moment SMM is first suspected and, if the involved/uninvolved ratio is ≥100, a diagnosis of active MM instead of SMM should be established.

Table 26.2 Workup for newly diagnosed SMM patients

• Medical history and physical examination
• Hemogram
• Biochemical studies, including creatinine and calcium levels; beta-2 microglobulin, LDH, and albumin
• Protein studies
– Total serum protein and serum electrophoresis (serum M-protein)
– 24-h urine sample protein electrophoresis (urine M-protein)
– Serum and urine immunofixation
• Serum free light chain measurement (sFLC ratio)
• Bone marrow aspirate ± biopsy: infiltration by clonal plasma cells, flow cytometry, and fluorescence in situ hybridization analysis
• Skeletal survey, CT, or PET-CT
• MRI of thoracic and lumbar spine and pelvis; ideally, whole-body MRI

FLC free light chain, *CT* computed tomography, *PET-CT* ^{18}F-fluorodeoxyglucose (FDG) positron emission tomography (PET)/CT, *MRI* magnetic resonance imaging

If, after considering the specific assessments mentioned above (Table 26.2), a diagnosis of SMM is finally made, the serum and urine M-component, hemoglobin, calcium, and creatinine levels should be reevaluated 2–3 months later in order to confirm the stability of these parameters. The frequency of the subsequent follow-up exams should be adapted on the basis of risk factors for progression to symptomatic MM (see below).

How to Evaluate the Risk of Progression to MM?

The annual risk of progression from SMM to symptomatic MM is 10% per year for the first 5 years, 5% per year during the following 5 years, and only 1% per year after 10 years [11]. Though most patients diagnosed with SMM will progress to symptomatic MM and will need to start treatment, SMM is not a uniform disorder.

Several groups have reported possible predictors of progression to symptomatic MM, and this information could be useful for physicians and can help to explain to patients their risk of progression to active MM (Table 26.3).

– Size of serum M-protein and the extent of marrow involvement

Table 26.3 Smoldering MM: markers predicting progression to symptomatic MM

Features for identifying high-risk SMM patients: 50% at 2 years
• Tumor burden:
– ≥10% clonal plasma cell bone marrow infiltration plus
– ≥3 g/dL of serum M-protein and
– Serum free light chain ratio between 0.125 and 8
– Bence Jones proteinuria positive from 24-h urine sample
– Peripheral blood circulating plasma cells >5 × 10^6/L
– Peripheral blood circulating plasma cells ≥150 by flow cytometry
• Immunophenotyping characterization and immunoparesis:
– ≥95% of aberrant plasma cells by flow within the plasma cell bone marrow compartment plus
– Immunoparesis (>25% decrease in one or both uninvolved immunoglobulins relative to the lowest normal value)
• Cytogenetic abnormalities:
– Presence of t(4;14)
– Presence of del (17p)
– Gain of 1q21
– Hyperdiploidy
– Gene expression profiling risk score >–0.26
• Pattern of serum M-component or hemoglobin evolution:
– Evolving type: If M-protein ≥3 g/dL, increase of at least 10% within the first 6 months. If M-protein <3 g/dL, annual increase of M-protein for 3 years
– Increase in the M-protein to ≥3 g/dL over the 3 months since the previous determination
– Decrease of hemoglobin in ≥0.50 g/dL within 12 months of diagnosis
• Imaging assessments:
– MRI: Radiological progressive disease (MRI-PD) was defined as newly detected focal lesions (FLs) or increase in diameter of existing FL and a novel or progressive diffuse infiltration
– Positive PET/CT with no underlying osteolytic lesion

MRI magnetic resonance imaging, *PET-CT* ^{18}F-fluorodeoxyglucose (FDG) positron emission tomography (PET)/CT

– Mayo Clinic group [11] proposed three SMM subgroups according to BMPC infiltration and the size of the serum M-protein. Group 1 was characterized by ≥3 g/dL of M-protein and ≥10% of BMPCs, with a median TTP to symptomatic MM of 2 years. Group 2 featured ≤3 g/dL of M-protein and ≥10% BMPCs with a median TTP of 8 years. Group 3 had ≥3 g/dL of M-protein but <10% BMPC infiltration, resulting in a median TTP of 19 years.

– Serum free light chain ratio

– The Mayo Clinic group also evaluated the previously described patient population to identify the risk of progression to symptomatic myeloma on the basis of a free light chain (FLC) assay. A kappa/lambda FLC ratio between 0.125 and 8 was found to be associated with an increased risk of progression to symptomatic MM. This parameter was added to their previous score, which considered the size of serum M-protein and BMPC infiltration, to refine the Mayo risk stratification model. This yielded three groups, with a median TTP of 1.9 years for the high-risk group, whose members exhibited all three defined risk factors [12].

– The Danish Myeloma group did not found in the analysis of their registry any significant threshold for the serum free light chain ratio; therefore they do not support the recent IMWG proposal that identifies patients with a FLC ratio above 100 as having ultrahigh risk of transformation to MM [13].

– Immunophenotyping and immunoparesis

– Multiparameter flow cytometry (MFC) to identify the immunophenotypic profile of plasma cells in SMM has been evaluated by the Spanish Myeloma group. We reported that the presence of an aberrant BMPC phenotype in the vast majority of PC (≥95% phenotypically abnormal plasma cells from total PC), determined by MFC (defined as the overexpression of CD56 and CD19, CD45 negative, and/or decreased reactivity for CD38), was the most important predictor of early progression from SMM to active MM [14]. The presence of immunoparesis (i.e., a decrease in one or two of the uninvolved immunoglobulins to 25% below the lowest normal value) also emerged as a significant independent prognostic characteristic. Based on these two parameters, the Spanish group proposed a scoring system that stratified SMM patients into three categories with a median TTP of 23 months when the two risk factors were present, compared with 73 months when only one was present, and not reached when neither was present [15].

– The Danish Myeloma group has recently reported that both an M-protein ≥3 g/dL and immunoparesis significantly influenced TTP (HR 2.7 95% CI(1.5;4.7) $p = 0.001$ and HR 3.3 95%CI(1.4;7.8) $p = 0.002$, respectively) to myeloma [13].

– Peripheral blood circulating plasma cells

– The Mayo Clinic group has also evaluated the role of peripheral blood circulating PCs in 171 SMM patients, and in those (15%) who had high levels of circulating PCs (>5 × 10^6/L and/or >5% PCs per 100 cytoplasmic immunoglobulin (Ig)-positive mononuclear cells), the progression risk at 2 years was significantly higher than for patients with low levels of circulating PC (71% vs. 24%; $p = 0.001$) [16]. This group has recently improved the identification of peripheral blood circulating plasma cells in SMM using flow cytometry in 100 patients. The median TTP of patients with 150 or more circulating PCs was 9 months compared to not reached for patients with less than 150 circulating PCs ($P < 0.001$). In the future, this may allow reclassification of such patients as having MM requiring therapy prior to them enduring end-organ damage [17].

- Pattern of serum M-component evolution
- The pattern of evolution of the monoclonal component during the course of the disease enabled to identify two types of SMM: evolving and nonevolving. Based on the analysis of 207 SMM patients, the evolving type was defined by the following criteria: (1) if the concentration of M-protein was ≥3 g/dL at baseline, the evolving type featured an increase in M-protein of at least 10% within the first 6 months following diagnosis; (2) if the concentration of M-protein was <3 g/dL at baseline, the evolving type featured a progressive increase in M-protein in each consecutive annual measurement over a 3-year period [18]. The evolving pattern was recognized in 25% of patients, and was associated with a probability of progression of 45% at 2 years, with a median TTP to active MM of 3 years, compared with 19 years for those with the nonevolving type [19]. The Mayo Clinic group has recently validated the evolving change in the monoclonal protein (eMP) in a series of 191 patients with SMM, resulting in an odds ratio of 7.26 (2.89–18.26, $p < 0.001$); moreover, they found the BMPC infiltration >20% and the evolving change in hemoglobin (eHb), defined as ≥0.5 g/dL decrease within 12 months of diagnosis, as independent prognostic markers predicting progression and a new risk model comprising these variables was constructed, with median TTP of 12.3, 4.2, 2.8, and 1.0 years in patients with none, 1, 2, and 3 risk factors, respectively ($p < 0.001$). The 2-year risk of progression was 82.8% in patients with both eMP and eHb, and increased to 90.9% in those with all three risk factors. This new risk model would identify patients with SMM candidates to be considered in the future as MM [20]. The SWOG group also found that patients with an increase in the M-component ≥3 g/dL over the 3 months since their previous determination had an associated risk of progression of approximately 50% at 2 years [21].
- Bence Jones proteinuria
- One hundred and forty-seven SMM patients were examined for the presence of Bence Jones proteinuria at diagnosis, and its effect on progression to symptomatic disease was assessed. The study showed that in SMM patients in which the M-protein was defined by a complete immunoglobulin, but who were also positive for Bence Jones proteinuria, regardless of the amount, the risk of progression to active disease was significantly higher than in Bence Jones proteinuria-negative patients (22 vs. 83 months; $p < 0.001$). In addition, when Bence Jones proteinuria in the 24-h urine sample exceeded 500 mg, the risk was even higher, with a median TTP of 7 months indicating that this parameter would be a new biomarker to identify SMM patients that could be considered as MM [22].
- Novel imaging assessments
- The novel imaging assessments have contributed to the updated criteria for the definition of MM and SMM, as has been previously mentioned. However, the new imaging assessments can also help to predict progression risk in SMM. The first studies with spinal MRI were done in SMM patients and the presence of a focal pattern was associated with a shorter TTP as compared to that of a diffuse or variegated pattern (median 6 vs. 16 vs. 22 months). Hillengass et al. have recently evaluated the role of MRI during the follow-up of patients with SMM. Radiological progressive disease (MRI-PD), which they defined as the detection of new focal lesions or the increase in diameter of existing focal lesions, and a novel or progressive diffuse infiltration, was identified as a feature for classifying SMM patients at high risk of progression to symptomatic disease [23]. The role of PET/CT has also been evaluated in SMM. The Italian group has recently reported that approximately 10% of SMM patients from a series of 73 patients had a positive result with PET/CT with no underlying osteolytic lesion, and this predicted for high risk of progression to symptomatic disease (48% at 2 years compared with 32% for PET/CT-negative patients; $p = 0.007$) [24]. The Mayo Clinic group also identified a subgroup within a series of 132 SMM patients who showed a positive result with PET/CT in which the rate of progression to MM within 2 years was 56%, as compared to 28% among PET/CT-negative patients ($p = 0.001$). The rate of progression was even higher among patients on whom PET/CT was performed within 3 months of their diagnosis of SMM (74% vs. 27% in PET/CT-negative patients) [25].
- Cytogenetic abnormalities
- The Mayo Clinic group analyzed the cytogenetic abnormalities in a series of 351 SMM patients and identified a high-risk subgroup of patients with t(4;14) and/or del(17p) with a significantly shorter median TTP (24 months) as compared to the intermediate-, standard-, and low-risk patient subgroups [26]. The high risk of progression of SMM to MM with t(4;14) may be related to the fact that this abnormality is associated with markedly high FLC ratios. However, the mechanism by which a high FLC ratio is associated with a higher risk of progression is not clear and is only partly related to renal failure from cast nephropathy. Neben et al. have identified t(4;14), gain of 1q21, or hyperdiploidy as being independent prognostic factors for a shorter TTP. The median TTP for patients with del(17p) was 2.7 years (vs. 4.9 years for those without the translocation; $p = 0.019$), 2.9 years for patients

with t(4;14) (vs. 5.2 years for those without the translocation; $p = 0.021$), and 3.7 years for patients with gain of 1q21 (vs. 5.3 years for those without the gain; $p = 0.013$). In addition, hyperdiploidy was associated with a significantly shorter median TTP of 3.9 years (compared with 5.7 years for non-hyperdiploid patients; $p = 0.036$) [27].

Finally, the South West Oncology Group (SWOG) evaluated the Gene Expression Profiling 40 (GEP40) model in a group of 105 SMM patients. A gene signature derived from four genes, at an optimal binary cut point of 9.28, identified 14 patients (13%) with a 2-year progression risk of 85.7%. Conversely, a low four-gene score (< 9.28) combined with baseline monoclonal protein <3 g/dL and albumin ≥3.5 g/dL identified 61 patients with low-risk SMM with a 5.0% risk of progression at 2 years [28]. Landgren et al. have recently performed whole exome sequencing and RNA sequencing in 12 patients with high-risk SMM and 39 patients with newly diagnosed symptomatic MM. Despite having only a few high-risk SMM patients in this study, none of them had any mutations in the recurrently mutated genes found in the symptomatic MM group, indicating that the molecular profile of SMM could be different. Therefore, these findings might have some implications for risk assessment and initiation of therapy [29].

In summary, the diagnosis of SMM is associated with a variable risk of progression to active disease, and the presence of the aforementioned prognostic factors can discriminate subgroups of patients based on their degree of risk (Table 26.3).

Stratification and Management of SMM Patients

The first step in clinical practice is to identify the risk of progression to active disease for each newly diagnosed SMM patient. The key question is which risk model is better for evaluating the risk of progression to symptomatic disease for each individual SMM patient. Both the Mayo Clinic and Spanish models have been validated in a prospective trial. However, new risk models are emerging that incorporate novel clinical and biological features [9, 11, 13, 15, 18, 21, 27, 30, 31] (Table 26.4). The components of these models are not identical, and each patient's risk should probably be defined on the basis of all the available data rather than through the use of a restricted model (Table 26.3). These models identified their risk factors as independent variables in multivariate analysis. Some of the features evaluated in each risk model can overlap, but not all of them have to be present in a SMM patient to be defined as a high-risk SMM patient.

Table 26.4 Risk models for the stratification of SMM

Risk model	Risk of progression to MM	
Mayo Clinic		*Median TTP*
– ≥10% clonal PCBM infiltration – ≥3 g/dL of serum M-protein – Serum FLC ratio between <0.125 and >8	1 risk factor 2 risk factors 3 risk factors	10 years 5 years 1.9 years
Spanish myeloma		*Median TTP*
– ≥95% of aberrant PCs by MFC – Immunoparesis	No risk factor 1 risk factor 2 risk factors	NR 6 years 1.9 years
Heidelberg		*3-year TTP*
– Tumor mass using the Mayo model – t(4;14), del17p, or +1q	T-mass low + CA low risk T-mass low + CA high risk T-mass high + CA low risk T-mass high + CA high risk	15% 42% 64% 55%
SWOG		*2-year TTP*
– Serum M-protein ≥2 g/dL – Involved FLC >25 mg/dL – GEP risk score >–0.26	No risk factor 1 risk factor ≥2 risk factors	30% 29% 71%
Penn		*2-year TTP*
– ≥40% clonal PCBM infiltration – sFLC ratio ≥50 – Albumin ≤3.5 mg/dL	No risk factor 1 risk factor ≥2 risk factors	16% 44% 81%
Japanese		*2-year TTP*
– Beta-2 microglobulin ≥2.5 mg/L – M-protein increment rate >1 mg/dL/day	2 risk factors	67.5%
Czech and Heidelberg		*2-year TTP*
– Immunoparesis – Serum M-protein ≥2.3 g/dL – Involved/uninvolved sFLC >30	No risk factor 1 risk factor 2 risk factors 3 risk factors	5.3% 7.5% 44.8% 81.3%
Barcelona		*2-year TTP*
– Evolving pattern = 2 points – Serum M-protein ≥3 g/dL = 1 point – Immunoparesis = 1 point	0 points 1 point 2 points 3 points	2.4% 31% 52% 80%
Mayo Clinic evolving model		
– eMP – eHB – ≥20% plasma cells	0 points 1 point 2 points 3 points	12.3 years 4.2 years 2.8 years 1 year
Danish		*3-year TTP*
– Serum M-protein ≥3 g/dL – Immunoparesis	No risk factor 1 risk factor 2 risk factors	5% 21% 50%

SMM patients should be classified as follows:

1. Patients at low risk of progression who are characterized by the absence of the aforementioned high-risk factors (using the validated Mayo or the Spanish risk models), with a probability of progression at 5 years of only 8%. These patients behave similarly to MGUS-like patients and should be followed annually.
2. The second group includes patients at intermediate risk of progression and they only display some of the aforementioned high-risk factors. These are probably the true SMM patients. They have a risk of progression at 5 years of 42%, and they must be followed up every 6 months (except during the first year that should be followed every 3–4 months in order to exclude an SMM evolving form).
3. The third group includes high-risk patients classified on the basis of one of the risk models mentioned before. Half of them will progress during the 2 years following diagnosis. These group of patients need a close follow-up every 2–3 months. As there is not any treatment approved yet for these high-risk SMM patients, the best approach should be to refer them to specialized centers in MM therapy and to include them in clinical trials to better understand their biology and to confirm the survival benefit of early treatment in this cohort [32].

The Spanish myeloma group (GEM/Pethema) conducted a phase 3 randomized trial in 119 SMM patients at high risk of progression to active disease (according to the Mayo and/or Spanish criteria). This trial compared early treatment with lenalidomide plus dexamethasone as induction followed by lenalidomide alone as maintenance versus observation. The primary end point was TTP to symptomatic MM, and after a median follow-up of 40 months, the median TTP was significantly longer in patients in the early treatment group than in the observation arm (not reached vs. 21 months; hazard ratio, HR = 5.59; $p < 0.001$). This trial has been recently updated, and after a median follow-up of 75 months, lenalidomide plus dexamethasone continued to provide a benefit in terms of TTP compared with observation (median TTP not reached (95% CI 47 months–not reached) vs. 23 months (95% CI 16–31 months); hazard ratio (HR) 0.24 (95% CI (0.14–0.41); $p < 0.0001$)). Progression to multiple myeloma occurred in 53 (86%) of 62 patients in the observation group compared with 22 (39%) of 57 patients in the treatment group. At data cutoff, 10 (18%) patients had died in the treatment group and 22 (36%) patients had died in the observation group; median overall survival from the time of study entry had not been reached in either group (HR 0.43 (95% CI 0.21–0.92), $p = 0.024$)) [33]. The safety profile was acceptable and most of the adverse events reported were grade 1 or 2. This study showed for the first time the potential for changing the treatment paradigm for high-risk SMM patients based on the efficacy of early treatment in terms of TTP to active disease and of OS, confirmed after long-term follow-up. Moreover, several trials currently under way are investigating the role, on high-risk SMM patients, of novel agents such as lenalidomide alone, siltuximab (anti-IL6 monoclonal antibody), elotuzumab (anti-SLAMF7 monoclonal antibody), or lenalidomide-dexamethasone plus elotuzumab. Promising efficacy results have been reported for the combination of lenalidomide plus dexamethasone with the novel proteasome inhibitor carfilzomib in a series of 12 high-risk SMM patients. All patients achieved CR and most were in immunophenotypic CR [34]. The next step will be to develop a more intensive therapeutic approach for young high-risk SMM patients, similar to the treatment planned for young symptomatic MM patients, for whom "cure" should be the objective.

Conclusion and Future Directions

The treatment philosophy for MM patients has mainly focused on symptomatic patients. This approach is clearly different from those adopted to treat other malignancies, such as breast, colon, or prostate cancer, for which early intervention is not only appropriate, but also essential for success and cure. This difference in philosophy arose for several reasons: (1) in the past, only a few drugs, most of which were alkylating agents, were available to treat MM; (2) the trials conducted in asymptomatic MM patients failed to produce a significant benefit; and (3) the risk of progression to active disease in SMM patients is relatively low (10% per year).

However, significant advances are being made in the understanding and management of SMM patients. From the biological point of view, different subgroups of SMM patients have been identified, including those patients with >60% PC or FLC ratio >100 or two or more focal lesions, that are now considered as active MM patients in which treatment should be started before myeloma-related symptoms develop. In the near future, new biomarkers will be considered to expand the inclusion of SMM patients at imminent risk of progression to active disease in order to be considered as MM.

Moreover, we will soon have the results from several current trials conducted in high-risk SMM patients, which will enable us to offer early treatment for a selected group of asymptomatic myeloma patients with the confidence that some of them will be "cured." The cure-versus-control debate is particularly pertinent in asymptomatic myeloma patients. Some physicians argue in favor of controlling the disease through continuous oral therapy mainly based on immunomodulatory agents, while others support the intensive therapy approaches, including high-dose therapy and transplant, with the objective of eradicating the disease.

Ongoing biological studies will also help us to better understand the pathogenesis of the disease and to identify the key drivers of the transition from monoclonal gammopathy to smoldering and symptomatic disease. These drivers may represent optimal targets for new therapeutic approaches.

References

1. Kyle RA, Greipp PR. Smoldering multiple myeloma. N Engl J Med. 1980;302(24):1347–9.
2. Rajkumar SV, Dimopoulos MA, Palumbo A, Blade J, Merlini G, Mateos MV, et al. International Myeloma Working Group updated criteria for the diagnosis of multiple myeloma. Lancet Oncol. 2014;15(12):e538–48.
3. Kristinsson SY, Holmberg E, Blimark C. Treatment for high-risk smoldering myeloma. N Engl J Med. 2013;369(18):1762–3.
4. Blade J, Dimopoulos M, Rosinol L, Rajkumar SV, Kyle RA. Smoldering (asymptomatic) multiple myeloma: current diagnostic criteria, new predictors of outcome, and follow-up recommendations. J Clin Oncol. 2010;28(4):690–7.
5. Hillengass J, Fechtner K, Weber MA, Bauerle T, Ayyaz S, Heiss C, et al. Prognostic significance of focal lesions in whole-body magnetic resonance imaging in patients with asymptomatic multiple myeloma. J Clin Oncol. 2010;28(9):1606–10.
6. Kastritis E, Moulopoulos LA, Terpos E, Koutoulidis V, Dimopoulos MA. The prognostic importance of the presence of more than one focal lesion in spine MRI of patients with asymptomatic (smoldering) multiple myeloma. Leukemia. 2014;28(12):2402–3.
7. Rajkumar SV, Larson D, Kyle RA. Diagnosis of smoldering multiple myeloma. N Engl J Med. 2011;365(5):474–5.
8. Kastritis E, Terpos E, Moulopoulos L, Spyropoulou-Vlachou M, Kanellias N, Eleftherakis-Papaiakovou E, et al. Extensive bone marrow infiltration and abnormal free light chain ratio identifies patients with asymptomatic myeloma at high risk for progression to symptomatic disease. Leukemia. 2012;27:947.
9. Waxman AJ, Mick R, Garfall AL, Cohen A, Vogl DT, Stadtmauer EA, et al. Classifying ultra-high risk smoldering myeloma. Leukemia. 2014;29:751.
10. Larsen JT, Kumar SK, Dispenzieri A, Kyle RA, Katzmann JA, Rajkumar SV. Serum free light chain ratio as a biomarker for high-risk smoldering multiple myeloma. Leukemia. 2013;27(4):941–6.
11. Kyle RA, Remstein ED, Therneau TM, Dispenzieri A, Kurtin PJ, Hodnefield JM, et al. Clinical course and prognosis of smoldering (asymptomatic) multiple myeloma. N Engl J Med. 2007;356(25):2582–90.
12. Dispenzieri A, Kyle RA, Katzmann JA, Therneau TM, Larson D, Benson J, et al. Immunoglobulin free light chain ratio is an independent risk factor for progression of smoldering (asymptomatic) multiple myeloma. Blood. 2008;111(2):785–9.
13. Sorrig R, Klausen TW, Salomo M, Vangsted AJ, Ostergaard B, Gregersen H, et al. Smoldering multiple myeloma risk factors for progression: a Danish population-based cohort study. Eur J Haematol. 2016, 97(3):303–9.
14. Perez-Persona E, Vidriales MB, Mateo G, Garcia-Sanz R, Mateos MV, de Coca AG, et al. New criteria to identify risk of progression in monoclonal gammopathy of uncertain significance and smoldering multiple myeloma based on multiparameter flow cytometry analysis of bone marrow plasma cells. Blood. 2007;110(7):2586–92.
15. Perez-Persona E, Mateo G, Garcia-Sanz R, Mateos MV, de Las Heras N, de Coca AG, et al. Risk of progression in smouldering myeloma and monoclonal gammopathies of unknown significance: comparative analysis of the evolution of monoclonal component and multiparameter flow cytometry of bone marrow plasma cells. Br J Haematol. 2010;148(1):110–4.
16. Bianchi G, Kyle RA, Larson DR, Witzig TE, Kumar S, Dispenzieri A, et al. High levels of peripheral blood circulating plasma cells as a specific risk factor for progression of smoldering multiple myeloma. Leukemia. 2013;27(3):680–5.
17. Gonsalves WI, Rajkumar SV, Dispenzieri A, Dingli D, Timm MM, Morice WG, Lacy MQ, Buadi FK, Go RS, Leung N, Kapoor P, Hayman SR, Lust JA, Russell SJ, Zeldenrust SR, Hwa L, Kourelis TV, Kyle RA, Gertz MA, Kumar SK. Quantification of circulating clonal plasma cells (cPCs) via multiparametric flow cytometry (MFC) to identify patients with smoldering multiple myeloma (SMM) at high risk of progression. J Clin Oncol. 2016;34(Suppl.):Abstract 8015
18. Fernández de Larrea C, Isola I, Cibeira MT, Rosiñol L, Calvo X, Tovar N, et al. Smoldering multiple myeloma: impact of the evolving pattern on early progression. Blood. 2014;124(21):3363.
19. Rosinol L, Blade J, Esteve J, Aymerich M, Rozman M, Montoto S, et al. Smoldering multiple myeloma: natural history and recognition of an evolving type. Br J Haematol. 2003;123(4):631–6.
20. Ravi P, Kumar S, Larsen JT, Gonsalves W, Buadi F, Lacy MQ, Go R, Dispenzieri A, Kapoor P, Lust JA, Dingli D, Lin Y, Russell SJ, Leung N, Gertz MA, Kyle RA, Bergsagel PL, Rajkumar SV. Evolving changes in M-protein (M), quantitative involved immunoglobulin (Ig), and hemoglobin (Hb) to identify patients (pts) with ultra high-risk smoldering multiple myeloma (UHR-SMM). J Clin Oncol. 2016;34(Suppl.):Abstr 8004.
21. Dhodapkar MV, Sexton R, Waheed S, Usmani S, Papanikolaou X, Nair B, et al. Clinical, genomic, and imaging predictors of myeloma progression from asymptomatic monoclonal gammopathies (SWOG S0120). Blood. 2014;123(1):78–85.
22. Gonzalez-Calle V, Davila J, Escalante F, de Coca AG, Aguilera C, Lopez R, et al. Bence Jones proteinuria in smoldering multiple myeloma as a predictor marker of progression to symptomatic multiple myeloma. Leukemia. 2016;30:2026.
23. Merz M, Hielscher T, Wagner B, Sauer S, Shah S, Raab MS, et al. Predictive value of longitudinal whole-body magnetic resonance imaging in patients with smoldering multiple myeloma. Leukemia. 2014;28:1902.
24. Zamagni E, Nanni C, Gay F, Pezzi A, Patriarca F, Bello M, et al. 18F-FDG PET/CT focal, but not osteolytic, lesions predict the progression of smoldering myeloma to active disease. Leukemia. 2016;30(2):417–22.
25. Siontis B, Kumar S, Dispenzieri A, Drake MT, Lacy MQ, Buadi F, et al. Positron emission tomography-computed tomography in the diagnostic evaluation of smoldering multiple myeloma: identification of patients needing therapy. Blood Cancer J. 2015;5:e364.
26. Rajkumar SV, Gupta V, Fonseca R, Dispenzieri A, Gonsalves WI, Larson D, et al. Impact of primary molecular cytogenetic abnormalities and risk of progression in smoldering multiple myeloma. Leukemia. 2013;27:1738.
27. Neben K, Jauch A, Hielscher T, Hillengass J, Lehners N, Seckinger A, et al. Progression in smoldering myeloma is independently determined by the chromosomal abnormalities del(17p), t(4;14), gain 1q, hyperdiploidy, and tumor load. J Clin Oncol. 2013;31(34):4325–32.
28. Khan R, Dhodapkar M, Rosenthal A, Heuck C, Papanikolaou X, Qu P, et al. Four genes predict high risk of progression from smoldering to symptomatic multiple myeloma (SWOG S0120). Haematologica. 2015;100(9):1214–21.
29. Mailankody S, Korde N, Roschewski MJ, Christofferson A, Boateng M, Zhang Y, Manasanch EE, Kazandjian DG, Kwok M, Bhutani M, Tageja N, Zingone A, Costello R, Lamy L, Hultcrantz M, Papaemmanuil E, Stetler-Stevenson M, Figg WD, Keats JJ, Landgren O. Genetic plasma cell signatures in high-risk smoldering myeloma versus multiple myeloma patients. J Clin Oncol. 2016;34(Suppl.):Abstr 8003.
30. Muta T, Iida S, Matsue K, Sunami K, Isoda J, Harada N, et al. Predictive significance of serum beta 2-microglobulin levels and

M-protein velocity for symptomatic progression of smoldering multiple myeloma. Blood. 2014;124(21):3379.

31. Hajek R, Sandecka V, Seckinger A, Spicka I, Scudla V, Gregora E, et al. Prediction of progression of Smouldering into therapy requiring multiple myeloma by easily accessible clinical factors [in 527 patients]. Blood. 2014;124(21):2071.

32. Mateos MV, San Miguel JF. New approaches to smoldering myeloma. Curr Hematol Malig Rep. 2013;8:270.

33. Mateos MV, Hernández MT, Giraldo P, de la Rubia J, de Arriba F, Corral LL, Rosiñol L, Paiva B, Palomera L, Bargay J, Oriol A, Prosper F, López J, Arguiñano JM, Quintana N, García JL, Bladé J, Lahuerta JJ, Miguel JF. Lenalidomide plus dexamethasone versus observation in patients with high-risk smouldering multiple myeloma (QuiRedex): long-term follow-up a randomised, controlled, phase 3 trial. Lancet Oncol. 2016 [Epub ahead of print].

34. Korde N, Roschewski M, Zingone A, Kwok M, Manasanch EE, Bhutani M, et al. Treatment with Carfilzomib-Lenalidomide-dexamethasone with Lenalidomide extension in patients with smoldering or newly diagnosed multiple myeloma. JAMA Oncol. 2015;1(6):746–54.

Frail Patients with Newly Diagnosed Multiple Myeloma

27

Alessandra Larocca and Antonio Palumbo

Introduction

Multiple myeloma (MM) is a neoplastic disease deriving from an abnormal proliferation of monoclonal plasma cells in the bone marrow. MM is characterized by both intrinsic genetic alterations in the clonal plasma cells and microenvironmental changes [1].

This disease accounts for 13% of all hematological cancers, approximately 2% of all cancer deaths, and 20% of deaths caused by hematological malignancies. The annual age-adjusted incidence is 5.6 cases per 100,000 people in Western countries [1]. MM is typical of the elderly, median age at diagnosis is approximately 70 years, 37% of patients at diagnosis are less than 65 years, 27% are aged 66 to 75 years, and 37% of patients are over 75 years.

Of note, life expectancy is increasing worldwide. Indeed, the global population is rapidly aging, and the number of individuals aged ≥65 years is expected to double between 2000 and 2030. As a consequence, also the prevalence of myeloma is likely to increase [2].

The diagnosis of MM requires the presence of at least 10% of monoclonal plasma cells at the bone marrow biopsy. Myeloma is defined asymptomatic (smoldering), when no myeloma-related organ or tissue dysfunction is present, or symptomatic, when the so-called CRAB criteria are present: C: hypercalcemia (>11.5 mg/dL); R: renal failure (serum creatinine >1.73 mmol/L); A: anemia (hemoglobin <10 g/dL or >2 g/dL below the lower limit of normal); and B: bone disease (lytic lesions, severe osteopenia, or pathologic fractures) [3]. The diagnostic criteria have been recently updated, and the presence of more than 60% of monoclonal plasma cells in the bone marrow, or one or more focal lesions detected with magnetic resonance imaging (MRI), or an abnormal ratio of the serum free light chains have been added as a clinically relevant criteria to start treatment [4]. To date, treatment is started in patients with symptomatic disease, whereas only clinical observation is recommended in patients with asymptomatic myeloma. Yet, ongoing trials are evaluating the role of novel agents in delaying the progression from asymptomatic to active disease.

Treatment strategy for MM has long been based on patients' age. Patients aged 65–75 years are generally considered ineligible for autologous stem cell transplantation (ASCT). Biologic age does not always correspond to chronologic age, and this strict range may differ by approximately 5 years [5]. In Europe, current treatment for elderly patients older than 65 years or younger with significant comorbidities and ineligible for ASCT consists of the combinations of melphalan-prednisone plus either the immunomodulatory agent thalidomide (MPT) or the proteasome inhibitor bortezomib (VMP) [6, 7]. Recently the European and American regulatory authorities approved lenalidomide in combination with dexamethasone in the United States and in combination with dexamethasone or with melphalan and prednisone followed by lenalidomide monotherapy maintenance for ASCT-ineligible patients in Europe [8, 9]. In the United States, age is not the primary criterion to establish whether a patient is eligible for ASCT, and patients who are not candidates for ASCT can receive initial therapy with either bortezomib-lenalidomide-dexamethasone (VRD), bortezomib-cyclophosphamide-dexamethasone (VCD), or also Rd [10].

Usually, gentler approaches are used for patients older than 75 years, who may receive reduced-dose treatments based solely on their age [11].

Survival of MM patients varies greatly, from less than 6 months to more than 10 years, depending on both biological features of the disease at diagnosis (albumin,

A. Larocca, M.D. • A. Palumbo, M.D. (✉)
Dipartimento di Oncologia ed Ematologia, Azienda Ospedaliera Città della Salute e della Scienza di Torino, San Giovanni Battista, Via Genova, 3, 10126 Torino, Italy
e-mail: appalumbo@yahoo.com

P.H. Wiernik et al. (eds.), *Neoplastic Diseases of the Blood*, DOI 10.1007/978-3-319-64263-5_27

beta-2-microglobulin, and cytogenetics) and patient characteristics (age, performance status, comorbidities). In patients younger than 65 years eligible for ASCT, the current expected overall survival (OS) is 5–7 years; in patients ineligible for ASCT undergoing conventional chemotherapy it is 3–4 years [1].

The introduction of novel agents thalidomide, lenalidomide, and bortezomib in the twenty-first century has substantially changed the management of MM and markedly improved OS [12]. In particular, a significant 5-year OS improvement was seen in patients aged 45–64 years, while it was lower in patients aged 65–74, and absent in patients over 75 years of age [13]. The elderly population is highly heterogeneous and the well-known biologic and genetic prognostic factors, as well as age per se, are insufficient to explain this OS difference [14–17].

Indeed, aging is a complex process characterized by a gradual, progressive decrease in physiological reserve, changes in body composition, and clinically significant reductions in organ functions. It is commonly associated with the presence of comorbidity and an increased risk of developing disability, with physical and cognitive decline [18, 19], and frailty. Frailty is a state of increased vulnerability, with cumulative deficits in several physiological systems [11], which may result in a diminished resistance to stressors, such as MM and its treatment, negatively affecting patients' quality of life (QoL), treatment efficacy, and tolerability.

In MM, the term "frail" often improperly refers to a person >75 years, which sometimes leads to an inadequate under-treatment of patients based only on age. Of note, registrational trials are performed in selected patients, whereas frail patients usually do not meet eligibility criteria and thus are usually underrepresented in clinical studies [20].

Definition of Frailty

Older people are at high risk of cardio- and cerebrovascular diseases, type 2 diabetes, dementia, and cancer [21]. In particular, persons over 65 account for about 60% of newly diagnosed malignancies and about 70% of all cancer deaths. Elderly patients with cancer and comorbidities are also more likely to develop frailty, as well as physical and cognitive decline, with negative impact on lifestyle and treatment efficacy.

Indeed, the aging process is associated with a gradual, progressive decrease in physiological reserve, with changes in body composition and clinically significant reductions in renal function, gastric function, hepatic mass and blood flow, bone marrow status, and cardiovascular function [18, 22–24]. These changes affect the pharmacokinetics and pharmacodynamics of drugs, altering clinical efficacy and potentially increasing toxicity. Therefore, age-related organ function and metabolic changes can contribute to the poor tolerability of cancer treatments seen in elderly patients that can cause an increase in treatment-related adverse events. In these patients inadequate treatments can lead to excessive toxicities, unacceptable, unfavorable QoL, and increased healthcare costs.

In geriatric medicine, three terms are commonly used to characterize vulnerable adults: *frailty; comorbidity* (or multiple chronic conditions); and *disability* [25]. These are distinct clinical entities that occur individually and commonly in elderly patients. Moreover, they are interrelated and have a cumulative effect on health and prognosis of elderly patients. Of note, the use of score tables established in geriatric medicine provides additional information to performance status: in fact, 9–38% of elderly patients with good performance status (<2) were partially or fully dependent on others to carry out ordinary activities, such as household tasks and personal care [26, 27].

Frailty is a state of increased vulnerability to poor resolution of homoeostasis after a stressor event [28, 29]. It arises from cumulative deficits in several physiological systems and results in a diminished resistance to stressors. This is a condition more frequent in older individuals, as around 25% to 50% of people over 85 years of age are estimated to be frail. As yet, there is no consensus on the definition and assessment of frailty. The original definition of frailty focused on physical weakness and wasting, but many other definitions and criteria have been postulated, incorporating different aspects of aging that contribute to diminish physiological reserves. A phenotype of the clinically frail elderly adult was recently defined, based on the presence of a critical mass of ≥3 core elements of frailty: weakness; poor endurance; weight loss; low physical activity; and slow gait speed. *Comorbidity* is the concurrent presence of two or more medically diagnosed diseases in the same individual; it is associated with polymedication and increased risk of drug interactions [26]. Comorbidity is a significant concern among the elderly and 88% of the population aged over 65 years have at least one chronic condition. Many prognostic indices for the elderly that incorporate age and/or comorbidity are available. The Charlson comorbidity index is the one most frequently used in cancer patients [30, 31]. The Charlson index is a summary measure of 19 comorbid conditions weighted 1–6 corresponding to disease severity. This gives a total score ranging from 0 to 37. It can be adapted to account for increasing age, adding 1 point to the score for each decade over the age of 50 years. With this index, the relative risk of death that can be attributed to an increase of 1 point in the comorbidity score is equivalent to an additional decade of age. With aging, the incidence of comorbid conditions increases markedly, largely because the frequency of individual chronic conditions rises with age. As a result, 35% of men and 45% of women aged 60–69 years in the United States have ≥2 comorbid conditions; this percentage increases dramatically to 53% of men and 70% of women by age 80 years [32].

Disability (which can include both physical and mental impairments or limitations) can be defined as difficulty or dependency in carrying out activities essential to independent living, including both essential personal care and household tasks, and activities that are important to maintain an individual's quality of life [33, 34]. Physical disability is common among elderly adults and is more common in women than men. The major causes of physical disability in the elderly are chronic diseases, such as cardiovascular disease, stroke, and arthritis, highlighting the interrelationship between disability and comorbidity [35]. The incidence of disability rises steadily with age among people aged ≥65 years [34]. Of community-dwelling adults, 20–30% of those aged >70 years report some disability in mobility, tasks essential to household management (e.g., shopping, meal preparation, managing money), and basic self-care tasks (e.g., washing, dressing, eating). Disability is associated with a higher probability of hospitalization and risk of mortality [36]. In oncologic-hematologic patients, the performance status generally describes the overall fitness of patients by a systematic scoring system (KPS or Eastern Cooperative Oncology Group [ECOG]), but the use of scales established in geriatric medicine to screen for disability in self-care tasks (activities of daily living, ADL) and tasks of household management (instrumental activities of daily living, IADL) provides additional information to simpler performance status. Several organizations recommend that persons older than 70 years be screened with ADL and IADL scales on an annual basis [37].

Geriatric Assessment

Determining the optimal treatment for older patients according to their clinical characteristics and fitness is the modern challenge in geriatric onco-hematology. A personalized treatment, tailored not only to disease-specific parameters but also to patient's health status is fundamental.

To date, chronological age and performance status are the most frequently used instruments to stratify patients according to their fitness and consequently select therapy. However, geriatric impairments are highly prevalent in elderly patients with hematological malignancies (even in those with good performance status), they may not be easily detected, and may impact on the patient's ability to complete treatment [38, 39].

A comprehensive geriatric assessment (CGA)—commonly used in geriatric oncology—is a systematic procedure to objectively evaluate the health status of older people, focusing on somatic, functional, and psychosocial domains [40]. The CGA is a highly sensitive and specific tool, and it is more objective and reliable than clinical judgment. Alternatively, a brief assessment with screening tools may be adopted at diagnosis in order to help clinicians identify patients who need a deeper evaluation through a CGA [41, 42].

The International Society of Geriatric Oncology task force recommended that a CGA be implemented for older cancer patients [41]. A growing interest in the geriatric assessment has recently emerged to evaluate older patients with hematological malignancies. In particular, a geriatric assessment showed to predict survival in older AML patients [43]. A simplified geriatric assessment proved to be more accurate than the physicians' judgment to predict response, progression-free survival (PFS), and OS in older patients receiving chemo-immunotherapy in non-Hodgkin lymphomas [39].

Geriatric Assessment in Multiple Myeloma

Recently the International Myeloma Working group has conducted a pooled analysis of 869 individual newly diagnosed elderly patient data from three prospective trials and proposed a frailty score for the measurement of frailty in elderly myeloma patients [44]. At diagnosis, a geriatric assessment was performed and included three tools: the ADL and the IADL scales to assess self-care activities, tasks of household management, and independence status; and the CCI to evaluate number and severity of comorbidities (Tables 27.1 and 27.2) [31, 45]. An additive scoring system (range 0–5) based on these three tools and on patients' age was developed, and three groups of patients were identified: fit (score = 0, 39%), intermediate (score = 1, 31%), and frail (score ≥ 2, 30%). The 3-year OS was 84% in fit, 76% in intermediate (hazard ratio [HR], 1.61; $P = 0.042$), and 57% in frail (HR, 3.57; $P < 0.001$) patients. The cumulative incidence of grade ≥3 non-hematologic adverse events at 12 months was 22.2% in fit, 26.4% in intermediate (HR, 1.23; $P = 0.217$), and

34.0% in frail (HR, 1.74; $P < 0.001$) patients. The cumulative incidence of treatment discontinuation at 12 months was 16.5% in fit, 20.8% in intermediate (HR, 1.41; $P = 0.052$), and 31.2% in frail (HR, 2.21; $P < 0.001$) patients. Frailty was found to be associated with an increased risk of death, progression, non-hematologic toxicities, and treatment discontinuation, regardless of International Staging System stage, chromosome abnormalities, and treatment.

Because performing a geriatric assessment can be manpower and time consuming, a simple computer application was also created to support clinicians.

This geriatric score was also validated in the phase 3 FIRST trial [46, 47]. Patients were categorized into three severity groups as described by a proxy algorithm based on the IMWG frailty scale and including age, EQ-5D: Self Care score, EQ-5D: Usual Activities score, and CCI index. Of 1517 patients, 17% were classified as fit, 30% as intermediate, and 54% as frail. Similar breakdowns were observed across treatment arms. Frail patients were older and had higher International Staging System stage, higher Eastern Cooperative Oncology Group performance status scores, higher lactate dehydrogenase levels, and worse renal function than fit or intermediate patients. Of note, fit patients had a significantly longer OS: fit vs. intermediate (hazard ratio [HR] 0.66; $P = 0.004$), fit vs. frail (HR 0.42; $P < 0.0001$), and intermediate vs. frail (HR 0.62; $P < 0.0001$). This analysis of the FIRST trial population using a proxy of the IMWG frailty scale demonstrated predictive clinical outcomes in patients with newly diagnosed MM similar to the original scale. The majority of patients fell into the frail category, demonstrating that FIRST studied a high risk population with poor outcomes and unmet need.

Table 27.1 Scores used to perform a geriatric assessment: Activities of daily living (ADL), instrumental activities of daily living (IADL), and Charlson comorbidity index (CCI)

ADL			IADL		CCI	
Activity	Independent	Dependent	Activity	Related score	Comorbidity	Related score
BATHING Patient bathes completely autonomously or needs help in bathing only a single part of the body such as the back, genital area, or disabled extremity	1	0	**Ability to use telephone**		Myocardial infarct	1
			Patient can operate telephone on own initiative; looks up and dials numbers	1	Congestive heart failure	1
			Patient can dial a few well-known numbers	1	Peripheral vascular disease	1
			Patient answers telephone, but does not dial	1		
			Patient does not use telephone at all	0	Cerebrovascular disease	1
					Dementia	1
DRESSING Patient gets clothes from closets and drawers and puts on clothes. Patient my need help for tying shoes	1	0	**Shopping**		Chronic pulmonary disease	1
			Patient takes care of all shopping needs independently	1	Connective tissue disease	1
			Patient can do the shopping independently for small purchases	0	Mild liver disease	1
			They need to be accompanied on any shopping trip	0	Diabetes	1
			Completely unable to shop	0	Ulcer	1
TOILETING Patient goes to toilet, gets on and off, arranges clothes, cleans genital area without help (may use cane or walker for support and bedpan/urinal at night)	1	0	**Food preparation**		Diabetes with end-organ damage	2
			Patient plans, prepares, and serves adequate meals independently	1	Ictus	2
			They can prepare adequate meals if supplied with ingredients	0	Moderate-to-severe renal failure	2
			Patient heats and serves prepared meals or prepares meals but does not maintain adequate diet	0	Nonmetastatic solid tumor	2
			They need to have meals prepared and served	0	Leukemia	2

Table 27.1 (continued)

ADL			IADL		CCI	
Activity	Independent	Dependent	Activity	Related score	Comorbidity	Related score
TRANSFERRING Patient can move in and out of bed or chair unassisted. Mechanical transferring aides are acceptable	1	0	**Housekeeping**		Lymphoma, MM	2
			Patient maintains house alone with occasion assistance (heavy work)	1		
			They can perform light daily tasks such as dishwashing, bed making	1	Moderate-to-severe liver disease	3
			They can perform light daily tasks, but cannot maintain acceptable level of cleanliness	1	Metastatic solid tumor	6
			Patient needs help with all home maintenance tasks	1	AIDS	6
			Patient does not participate in any housekeeping tasks	0		
CONTINENCE Patient exercises complete self-control over urination and defecation	1	0	**Laundry**			
			They can do personal laundry completely	1		
			Patient launders small items, rinses socks, stockings, etc.	1		
			All laundry must be done by others	0		
FEEDING Patient gets food from plate into mouth without help. Preparation of food may be done by another person	1	0	**Mode of transportation**			
			They can travel independently on public transportation or drives own car	1		
			Patient arranges own travel via taxi, but does not otherwise use public transportation	1		
			Patient travels on public transportation when assisted or accompanied by another	1		
			Travel limited to taxi or automobile with assistance of another	0		
			They can not travel at all	0		
			Responsibility for own medications			
			Patient is responsible for taking medication in correct dosages at correct time	1		
			Patient takes responsibility if medication is prepared in advance in separate dosages	0		
			They are not capable of dispensing own medication	0		
			Ability to handle finances			
			Patient manages financial matters independently (budgets, writes checks, pays rent and bills, goes to bank); collects and keeps track of income	1		
			Patient manages day-to-day purchases, but needs help with banking, major purchases, etc.	1		
			Incapable of handling money	0		

ADL Activity of daily living, *IADL* instrumental activity of daily living, *CCI* Charlson comorbidity index

Table 27.2 Definition of frail patients with MM

	Frail patients can either be:		
Age	>80 years	76–80 years	≤75 years
Geriatric assessment	Independently of ADL, IADL, CCI	Plus at least one of the following: • ADL ≤ 4 • IADL ≤ 5 • CCI ≥ 2	Plus at least two of the following: • ADL ≤ 4 • IADL ≤ 5 • CCI ≥ 2

ADL Activity of daily living, *IADL* instrumental activity of daily living, *CCI* Charlson comorbidity index

The geriatric score can be calculated through the website http://www.myelomafrailtyscorecalculator.net/

Therapy at Diagnosis for Frail Patients

Start of Treatment

Particular attention is needed with frail patients and their comorbid conditions. Frail patients may present with CRAB-like symptoms that do not lead to actual organ dysfunction and do not require immediate anti-myeloma treatment, but only a close monitoring [3, 4, 48, 49]. Patients may have age-related osteopenia, or mild renal impairment due to hypertension or diabetes, or mild anemia secondary to iron or vitamin deficiency, renal failure, chronic inflammatory diseases, or concomitant dyserythropoietic/myelodysplastic syndrome [50]. Conversely, clear clinical manifestations of serious end-organ damage attributable to myeloma should be considered as CRAB, such as a progressive worsening of serum creatinine caused by light-chain cast nephropathy or a decrease in hemoglobin levels from baseline. Creatinine clearance should be considered with caution. The methods commonly used to estimate glomerular filtration rate have not been well validated at the extremes of age. In frail patients, a progressive renal impairment rather than a fixed concentration cutoff should be considered to confirm MM diagnosis.

According to the recently updated International Myeloma Working Group criteria, clonal bone marrow plasma cell percentage ≥60%, involved/uninvolved serum free light chain ratio ≥100, and >1 focal lesions on magnetic resonance imaging (MRI) studies are associated with near-inevitable development of CRAB features and should be included among the parameters for the diagnosis of MM [4]. Even if no data are present about frail patients, the assessment of these parameters may avoid serious organ damage that could inevitably worsen patients' condition.

The initial evaluation of MM frail patients includes the analysis of their medical history, physical examination, laboratory evaluation, bone marrow biopsy, and aspirate with conventional cytogenetics and fluorescence in situ hybridization for recurring chromosomal translocations and deletions/duplications seen in MM [11]. To assess bone disease, more complex investigations, such as MRI or positron emission tomography (PET), can be unnecessary on a routine basis in frail patients, and should be used only in selected cases, whereas skeletal survey and low-dose computed tomography scan are routine investigations.

Treatment Options

In the last decade, new effective treatments including novel agents thalidomide, bortezomib, and lenalidomide have replaced the former standard melphalan-prednisone [1]. Today, MPT and VMP are the standard treatments for elderly patients ineligible for ASCT [6, 7]. Recently, Rd continuously was shown to be more effective than MPT at diagnosis [46]. It should be noted that currently approved combinations were validated in studies that included selected elderly patients, and a geriatric evaluation was not performed [29].

The benefits obtained with new drug-based combinations were limited in older patients, mainly due to an increased treatment-related toxicity. Indeed, advanced age (≥75 years), occurrence of severe adverse events, and drug discontinuation predicted shorter survival in newly diagnosed MM patients treated with melphalan-prednisone alone or in combination with thalidomide and/or bortezomib [51, 52]. Therefore, avoiding treatment interruption and reducing the risk of side effects in the initial phase of therapy are fundamental, and low-dose intensity treatments are appropriate options for frail patients.

In patients with symptomatic myeloma, patient's age and a geriatric assessment should be considered to determine the most appropriate treatment. Based on the results of the geriatric assessment, patients can be stratified into fit patients suitable for full-dose therapy with three-drug combinations, or frail patients requiring dose-adjusted therapies. Treatment strategies for frail patients should have minimal cumulative toxicity and two-drug regimens showed similar efficacy and lower toxicity as compared to multidrug combinations [53].

A recent phase 3 trial compared the triplet melphalan-prednisone-lenalidomide (MPR) and cyclophosphamide-prednisone-lenalidomide versus the doublet Rd in newly diagnosed elderly MM. The three-drug alkylator-containing combinations were not superior to the two-drug combination Rd. In addition, grade ≥3 toxicity neutropenia was significantly higher with MPR (64%) than with Rd (25%; $P < 0.0001$) [54].

In another trial, the doublet bortezomib-dexamethasone (VD) was as effective as the triplets VMP and bortezomib-thalidomide-dexamethasone in elderly patients, and induced a lower rate of non-hematologic adverse events (22% compared with 33–37% with the three-drug combinations), and thus should be preferred in this patient population. Although all bortezomib-containing regimens produced good outcomes, VTD and VMP did not appear to offer an advantage over VD in patients with myeloma treated in US community practice [53].

A phase 2 trial evaluated three low-dose intensity subcutaneous bortezomib-based treatments in patients aged 75 years or older with newly diagnosed multiple myeloma (MM) [55]. Patients received subcutaneous bortezomib and oral prednisone (VP) or plus cyclophosphamide (VCP) or VP plus melphalan (VMP), followed by bortezomib maintenance, and half of the patients were frail. Response rate was 64% with VP, 67% with VCP, and 86% with VMP, and very good partial response rates or better were 26%, 28.5% and 49%, respectively. Median PFS was 14.0, 15.2, and 17.1 months, and 2-year OS was 60%, 70%, and 76% in VP, VCP, and VMP, respectively. At least one grade ≥3 nonhematologic adverse event occurred in 22% of VP, 37% of VCP, and 33% of VMP patients; discontinuation rates for AEs were 12%, 14%, and 20%, and the 6-month rates of toxicity-related deaths were 4%, 4%, and 8%, respectively. Yet, toxicity was higher with VMP, suggesting that a two-drug combination followed by maintenance should be preferred in frail patients [55].

These data underline the importance of avoiding treatment interruption and reducing the risk of side effects during the initial phase of therapy; thus low-dose intensity treatments should be preferred for frail patients.

Maintenance therapy showed to be effective also in elderly MM patients [1, 56]. Continuous Rd improved PFS compared with fixed-duration Rd for 18 cycles (Rd18) and significantly prolonged PFS and OS compared with MPT [46]. Continuous Rd caused a modest increase in toxicity compared with Rd18, and most of the toxicity occurred within the first 18 months and decreased over time. The superiority of continuous Rd over MPT for both PFS and OS was evident also in patients >75 years. Although toxicities were more common in patients >75 years, there was no marked difference in the rates of adverse events with continuous Rd and Rd18 within this age subgroup. Furthermore, Rd continuous resulted in PFS and OS benefits compared with MPT for patients of all frailty levels [47].

On the contrary, melphalan–prednisone–lenalidomide followed by lenalidomide maintenance (MPR-R) compared to MPR or melphalan-prednisone followed by placebo improved PFS in patients 65–75 years and not in patients >75 years [57]. This can be due to the higher toxicity of MPR and the need for more frequent dose modifications in patients >75 years. Of note, the major PFS benefit was achieved with lenalidomide maintenance therapy. In a landmark analysis, lenalidomide maintenance reduced the rate of progression by 66% as compared with placebo, regardless of age.

A main goal in frail patients is to maintain an asymptomatic disease status because older age and comorbidities may compromise subsequent salvage therapies. The benefits associated with continuous therapy should be balanced against the toxicity due to prolonged drug exposure, and this is particularly important in frail patients, who are more susceptible to treatment-related toxicities. Maintenance is a valuable option in frail patients who respond slowly to treatment and who tolerate it well. However, in case of significant adverse effects, dose reductions or treatment interruption should be considered.

Complete response has become an achievable aim also in elderly patients, yet toxicity may cancel the benefits derived from such a response [58]. Nevertheless, in frail patients the aim of therapy should not focus on the depth of response, but rather on controlling symptoms, maintaining an independence status and preserving quality of life. Therefore, the achievement of a stable disease without symptoms related to myeloma is an acceptable goal and keeping the balance between disease control and toxicity is crucial.

Dosing and Schedule

Dosing, schedule, and route of administration play a major role in the safety profile of therapy in frail patients. Once-weekly bortezomib significantly reduced the incidence of grade 3–4 adverse events (35% vs. 51%) and the rate of discontinuation due to toxicity (17% vs. 23%) compared with the twice-weekly schedule, in particular halving the rate of peripheral neuropathy. To overcome the limitations of bortezomib (intravenous administration and hospitalization), subcutaneous bortezomib is a valuable and equally effective strategy.

Lenalidomide has the advantage of the oral administration, which is more appealing in a frail patient population, and is preferable in subjects with preexisting neuropathy [46]. In particular, lenalidomide plus low-dose dexamethasone was better tolerated than lenalidomide plus high-dose dexamethasone [59]. Still, bortezomib-dexamethasone can be a valid option in case of aggressive disease, which needs a rapid cytoreduction and symptom control, and in case of acute renal dysfunction [53, 55].

In frail patients lower initial doses can be administered to minimize toxicity; dose escalation may be considered in the subsequent cycles if treatment is optimally tolerated or in case of inadequate response. The initial dose of lenalidomide should not exceed 10–15 mg/day and it can be adjusted based on renal function and blood counts to avoid profound and prolonged myelosuppression. Prophylactic growth factors and antimicrobial, at fixed dose and timing, can be used to prevent myelosuppression and infections, and thus treatment discontinuation. A previous history of cardiovascular disease or thromboembolism does not preclude the use of lenalidomide, if an adequate thromboprophylaxis is associated [11].

Corticosteroids may increase blood pressure and fluid retention; therefore they should be reduced, particularly in patients with cardiac diseases. Other adverse effects include hyperglycemia, gastritis, mood swings, insomnia, and increased risk of opportunistic infections. The dose of dexamethasone should be reduced to as little as 10 mg once a week. Alternatively, prednisone 25 mg every other day is a valid option in this setting [11].

Subcutaneous weekly bortezomib is a valid alternative option; it does not need dose reductions, although thrombocytopenia could be a concern [60–62]. This is a relevant strategy to improve tolerability, reduce treatment discontinuation, and increase the chance of disease control in frail patients. Bortezomib can cause peripheral neuropathy, differently from novel proteasome inhibitors [63, 64]. In frail patients, weekly carfilzomib, oral ixazomib, and oprozomib may be implemented in the future.

Finally, in patients with severe impairment of cognitive function or social dependency, a palliative treatment may be considered. In these cases, reduced-dose corticosteroids or melphalan-prednisone or cyclophosphamide-prednisone can be used to relieve disease symptoms.

Management of Complications

Despite the benefits associated with novel agents thalidomide, lenalidomide, and bortezomib, treatment-related toxicities are a major concern in frail patients. Full drug doses are difficult to be tolerated and side effects are frequent. In a retrospective analysis of 1435 elderly patients enrolled in four European phase III trials including thalidomide and/or bortezomib, the risk of death was increased in patients >75 years (HR 1.44, 95% CI: 1.20–1.72; $P < 0.001$); in patients with renal failure (HR 2.02, 95% CI: 1.51–2.70; $P < 0.001$); in those who had grade 3–4 infections, cardiac, or gastrointestinal adverse events during treatment (HR 2.53, 95% CI: 1.75–3.64; $P < 0.001$); and in those who discontinued therapy due to adverse events (HR 1.67, 95% CI; 1.12–2.51; $P = 0.01$). This increased risk was detected in the first 6 months after occurrence of adverse events or drug discontinuation and decreased over time [65]. More intensive approaches, such as the combination of bortezomib thalidomide, negatively affected outcome. Age 75 years or over or renal failure at presentation, occurrence of infections, and cardiac or gastrointestinal adverse events negatively affected survival.

Because frail patients are more susceptible to treatment-related side effects and treatment interruption, appropriate supportive care and an early identification of toxicities are fundamental [11].

Cytopenia is typical in hematologic patients treated with chemotherapy. It involves one or more cellular lineages of the bone marrow, due to both marrow invasion by neoplastic cells and chemotoxicity. Supportive care is essential to maintain an adequate quality of life and to enable the patient to stay on treatment [66].

Anemia is characterized by a hemoglobin level inferior to 13.5 g/dL for men and 12.0 g/dL for women. In elderly cancer patients anemia may be due to bone marrow invasion and chemotoxicity, but there are also other causes, such as renal insufficiency; iron, copper, and vitamin deficiency (folic acid, B12, and vitamin D); hypogonadism; relative erythropoietin system impairment; and possibly an underlying myelodysplasia or exhaustion of the hematopoietic progenitor. Approximately 50% of patients with anemia had two or more interconnected causes. Blood transfusions are recommended with hemoglobin levels below 7–8 g/dL. Erythropoietin-stimulating agents can improve fatigue and quality of life, and treatment could be continued until hemoglobin levels rise to 12 mg/dL [67].

Patients with neutropenia are also at risk of infections following chemotherapy, based on the severity and duration of neutropenia. Antibacterial prophylaxis can prevent febrile episodes, clinically or microbiologically documented bacterial infections including bacteremias, and hospitalization of outpatients [68]. Antibiotic prophylaxis should be started promptly when neutropenia occurs. Prophylaxis with antifungal agents (usually azoles) is recommended in cases of prolonged neutropenia. All patients undergoing chemotherapy or novel agent-based therapy should receive trimethoprim-cotrimoxazole as a prophylactic agent against the opportunistic infection of *Pneumocystis jiroveci* pneumonia.

Febrile neutropenia is characterized by an oral temperature higher than 38.5 °C or two consecutive measurements with a temperature higher than 38.0 °C for 2 h and an absolute neutrophil count of less than 0.5×10^9/L or one expected to fall below 0.5×10^9/L.

Chemotherapy-induced febrile neutropenia is a major risk factor for infection-related morbidity and death, as well as a significant dose-limiting toxicity in cancer treatment. Prognosis is worse in patients with bacteremia, with mortality rates of 18% in Gram-negative and 5% in Gram-positive bacteremia [69]. In elderly patients at high risk of developing febrile neutropenia, prophylactic granulocyte colony-stimulating factor (G-CSF) should be adopted based on age, medical history, disease characteristics, and myelotoxicity of their chemotherapy regimen. In patients with febrile neutropenia, the choice of initial antibiotic should be based on the patient's infectious disease history, prior antibiotic usage, and epidemiologic data of the area where the patient lives.

In patients receiving proteasome inhibitors, antiviral prophylaxis for herpes zoster reactivation is needed; immunomodulatory agents require an appropriate risk-based thromboprophylaxis. When corticosteroids are administered, gastrointestinal prophylaxis should be used. Antibacterial prophylaxis is recommended in case of severe myelosuppression, and growth factors should be used in patients experiencing neutropenia and anemia. In addition, a careful review of the patient's previous medications and attention to potential drug interactions are essential [11].

When an adverse event occurs in a frail patient, prompt action is required. Therapy should be stopped in case of grade 3–4 toxicity, and can be restarted at lower doses when toxicity decreases to at least grade 1 [1]. Lenalidomide dose may be decreased from 15 to 10 mg/day, or from 10 to 5 mg/day or, if required, to 5 mg every other day on days 1–21 every 4 weeks. Bortezomib may be reduced from 1.3 mg/m^2 weekly to 1.0 mg/m^2 once weekly or 0.7 mg/m^2 once weekly.

Conclusions

Treatment of elderly patients is particularly challenging today because of the complex phenomenon of aging. Aging is in fact associated with an increased incidence of tumors and of other comorbidities, and more than two-thirds of cancer diagnoses and of cancer deaths are reported among elderly people [21].

The presence of multiple diseases in elderly patients and the availability of newer and more targeted drugs require tailored treatments according to both the disease features and the patient's status. In this setting, cancer treatment decision should be based not only on age but a careful assessment of patients' frailty is crucial. To date there is no consensus about the definition and assessment of frailty, although recently the International Myeloma Working Group has proposed a valuable tool to better stratify patients according to age, CCI, ADL, and IADL. However, the most appropriate treatment in different subgroups of patients remains to be definitively determined and further studies are necessary.

References

1. Palumbo A, Anderson K. Multiple myeloma. N Engl J Med. 2011;364:1046–60.
2. Altekruse SF, Kosary CL, Krapcho M, Neyman N, Aminou R, Waldron W, Ruhl J, Howlader N, Tatalovich Z, Cho H, Mariotto A, Eisner MP, Lewis DR, Cronin K, Chen HS, Feuer EJ, Stinchcomb DG, Edwards BK, editors. SEER cancer statistics review, 1975–2007. Bethesda: National Cancer Institute. http://seer.Cancer.Gov/csr/1975_2007/, based on November 2009 SEER data submission, posted to the SEER web site, 2010.
3. Kyle RA, Rajkumar SV. Criteria for diagnosis, staging, risk stratification and response assessment of multiple myeloma. Leukemia. 2009;23:3–9.
4. Rajkumar SV, Dimopoulos MA, Palumbo A, Blade J, Merlini G, Mateos MV, et al. International Myeloma Working Group updated criteria for the diagnosis of multiple myeloma. Lancet Oncol. 2014;15:e538–48.
5. Palumbo A, Rajkumar SV, San Miguel JF, Larocca A, Niesvizky R, Morgan G, et al. International Myeloma Working Group consensus statement for the management, treatment, and supportive care of patients with myeloma not eligible for standard autologous stem-cell transplantation. J Clin Oncol. 2014;32(6):587–600.
6. Fayers PM, Palumbo A, Hulin C, Waage A, Wijermans P, Beksaç M, et al. Thalidomide for previously untreated elderly patients with multiple myeloma: meta-analysis of 1685 individual patient data from 6 randomized clinical trials. Blood. 2011;118(5):1239–47.
7. San Miguel JF, Schlag R, Khuageva NK, Dimopoulos MA, Shpilberg O, Kropff M, et al. Bortezomib plus melphalan and prednisone for initial treatment of multiple myeloma. N Engl J Med. 2008;359(9):906–17.
8. AnonymousRevlimid® (lenalidomide) [package insert]. Summit, NJ: Celgene Corporation; 2015.
9. Celgene E: Revlimid® (lenalidomide) [summary of product characteristics], 2015.
10. Rajkumar SV. Myeloma today: disease definitions and treatment advances. Am J Hematol. 2016;91(1):90–100.
11. Larocca A, Palumbo A. How I treat fragile myeloma patients. Blood. 2015;126(19):2179–85.
12. Brenner H, Gondos A, Pulte D. Expected long-term survival of patients diagnosed with multiple myeloma in 2006-2010. Haematologica. 2009;94(2):270–5.
13. Pulte D, Gondos A, Brenner H. Improvement in survival of older adults with multiple myeloma: results of an updated period analysis of SEER data. Oncologist. 2011;16:1600–3.
14. Chng WJ, Dispenzieri A, Chim CS, Fonseca R, Goldschmidt H, Lentzsch S, et al. IMWG consensus on risk stratification in multiple myeloma. Leukemia. 2014;28(2):269–77.
15. Kumar SK, Dispenzieri A, Gertz MA, Lacy MQ, Lust JA, Hayman SR, et al. Continued improvement in survival in multiple myeloma and the impact of novel agents [Abstract]. Blood. 2012;120:Abstract 3972.
16. Siegel DS, Desikan KR, Mehta J, Singhal S, Fassas A, Munshi N, et al. Age is not a prognostic variable with autotransplants for multiple myeloma. Blood. 1999;93(1):51–4.
17. Lenhoff S, Hjorth M, Westin J, Brinch L, Bäckström B, Carlson K, et al. Impact of age on survival after intensive therapy for multiple myeloma: a population-based study by the Nordic Myeloma Study Group. Br J Haematol. 2006;133(4):389–96.
18. Yuen GJ. Altered pharmacokinetics in the elderly. Clin Geriatr Med. 1990;6(2):257–67.
19. Fried LP, Ferrucci L, Darer J, Williamson JD, Anderson G. Untangling the concepts of disability, frailty, and comorbidity: implications for improved targeting and care. J Gerontol A Biol Sci Med Sci. 2004;59(3):255–63.
20. Hutchins LF, Unger JM, Crowley JJ, Coltman CA Jr, Albain KS. Underrepresentation of patients 65 years of age or older in cancer-treatment trials. N Engl J Med. 1999;341(27):2061–7.
21. Smith BD, Smith GL, Hurria A, Hortobagyi GN, Buchholz TA. Future of cancer incidence in the United States: burdens upon an aging, changing nation. J Clin Oncol. 2009;27(17):2758–65.
22. Vestal RE. Aging and pharmacology. Cancer. 1997;80:1302–10.
23. Baker SD, Grochow LB. Pharmacology of cancer chemotherapy in the older person. Clin Geriatr Med. 1997;13:169–83.
24. Sotaniemi EA, Arranto AJ, Pelkonen O, Pasanen M. Age and cytochrome P450-linked drug metabolism in humans: an analysis of 226 subjects with equal histopathologic conditions. Clin Pharmacol Ther. 1997;61(3):331–9.
25. Palumbo A, Bringhen S, Ludwig H, Dimopoulos MA, Bladé J, Mateos MV, et al. Personalized therapy in multiple myeloma according to patient age and vulnerability: a report of the European Myeloma Network (EMN). Blood. 2011;118(17):4519–29.
26. Repetto L, Fratino L, Audisio RA, Venturino A, Gianni W, Vercelli M, et al. Comprehensive geriatric assessment adds information to Eastern Cooperative Oncology Group performance status in elderly cancer patients: an Italian Group for Geriatric Oncology Study. J Clin Oncol. 2002;20(2):494–502.

27. Gironés R, Torregrosa D, Díaz-Beveridge R. Comorbidity, disability and geriatric syndromes in elderly breast cancer survivors. Results of a single-center experience. Crit Rev Oncol Hematol. 2010;73(3):236–45.
28. Fried LP, Tangen CM, Walston J, Newman AB, Hirsch C, Gottdiener J, et al. Frailty in older adults: evidence for a phenotype. J Gerontol A Biol Sci Med Sci. 2001;56(3):M146–57.
29. Clegg A, Young J, Iliffe S, Rikkert MO, Rockwood K. Frailty in elderly people. Lancet. 2013;381(9868):752–62.
30. Charlson M, Szatrowski TP, Peterson J, Gold J. Validation of a combined comorbidity index. J Clin Epidemiol. 1994;47(11):1245–51.
31. Charlson ME, Pompei P, Ales KL, MacKenzie CR. A new method of classifying prognostic comorbidity in longitudinal studies: development and validation. J Chronic Dis. 1987;40(5):373–83.
32. Guralnik JM, LaCroix AZ, Everett DF, Kovar MG. Aging in the eighties: the prevalence of comorbidity and its association with disability. National Center for Health Statistics; 1989. http://www.cdc.gov/nchs/data/ad/ad170.pdf
33. Pope AM, Tarlov AR. Disability in America. Toward a national agenda for prevention. Institute of Medicine; 1991. http://www.nap.edu/openbook.php?record_id=1579&page=R1
34. Adams PF, Hendershot GE, Marano MA. Current estimates from the National Health Interview Survey, 1996. Vital Health Stat. 1999;200:1–203.
35. Fried LP, Guralnik JM. Disability in older adults: evidence regarding significance, etiology, and risk. J Am Geriatr Soc. 1997;45(1):92–100.
36. Fried LP, Kronmal RA, Newman AB, Bild DE, Mittelmark MB, Polak JF, Robbins JA, et al. Risk factors for 5-year mortality in older adults: the Cardiovascular Health Study. JAMA. 1998;279(8):585–92.
37. Reuben DB. Guidelines, evidence-based medicine, and Glidepaths: talking the talk. J Am Geriatr Soc. 2002;50(11):1905–6.
38. Hamaker ME, Prins MC, Stauder R. The relevance of a geriatric assessment for elderly patients with a haematological malignancy—a systematic review. Leuk Res. 2014;38:275–83.
39. Tucci A, Ferrari S, Bottelli C, Borlenghi E, Drera M, Rossi G. A comprehensive geriatric assessment is more effective than clinical judgment to identify elderly diffuse large cell lymphoma patients who benefit from aggressive therapy. Cancer. 2009;115(19):4547–53.
40. Hamaker ME, Jonker JM, de Rooij SE, Vos AG, Smorenburg CH, van Munster BC. Frailty screening methods for predicting outcome of a comprehensive geriatric assessment in elderly patients with cancer: a systematic review. Lancet Oncol. 2012;13:e437–44.
41. Extermann M, Aapro M, Bernabei R, Cohen HJ, Droz JP, Lichtman S, et al. Use of comprehensive geriatric assessment in older cancer patients: recommendations from the task force on CGA of the International Society of Geriatric Oncology (SIOG). Crit Rev Oncol Hematol. 2005;55:241–52.
42. Kenis C, Bron D, Libert Y, Decoster L, Van Puyvelde K, Scalliet P, et al. Relevance of a systematic geriatric screening and assessment in older patients with cancer: results of a prospective multicentric study. Ann Oncol. 2013;24(5):1306–12.
43. Sherman AE, Motyckova G, Fega KR, Deangelo DJ, Abel GA, Steensma D, et al. Geriatric assessment in older patients with acute myeloid leukemia: a retrospective study of associated treatment and outcomes. Leuk Res. 2013;37(9):998–1003.
44. Palumbo A, Bringhen S, Mateos MV, Larocca A, Facon T, Kumar SK, et al. Geriatric assessment predicts survival and toxicities in elderly myeloma patients: an International Myeloma Working Group report. Blood. 2015;125(13):2068–74.
45. Lawton MP. Scales to measure competence in everyday activities. Psychopharmacol Bull. 1988;24(4):609–14.
46. Benboubker L, Dimopoulos MA, Dispenzieri A, Catalano J, Belch AR, Cavo M, et al. Lenalidomide and dexamethasone in transplant-ineligible patients with myeloma. N Engl J Med. 2014;371(10):906–17.
47. Facon T, Hulin C, Dimopoulos MA, Belch A, Meuleman N, Mohty M, et al. A frailty scale predicts outcomes of patients with newly diagnosed multiple myeloma who are ineligible for transplant treated with continuous lenalidomide plus low-dose dexamethasone on the first trial. ASH 2015; Abstract 4239.
48. Durie BG, Kyle RA, Belch A, Bensinger W, Blade J, Boccadoro M, et al. Myeloma management guidelines: a consensus report from the Scientific Advisors of the International Myeloma Foundation. Hematol J. 2003;4(6):379–98.
49. Durie BG, Harousseau JL, Miguel JS, Bladé J, Barlogie B, Anderson K, et al. International uniform response criteria for multiple myeloma. Leukemia. 2006;20(9):1467–73.
50. Mehta J, Cavo M, Singhal S. How I treat elderly patients with myeloma. Blood. 2010;116(13):2215–23.
51. Palumbo A, Bringhen S, Rossi D, Cavalli M, Larocca A, Ria R, et al. Bortezomib-melphalan-prednisone-thalidomide followed by maintenance with bortezomib-thalidomide compared with bortezomib-melphalan-prednisone for initial treatment of multiple myeloma: a randomized controlled trial. J Clin Oncol. 2010;28(34):5101–9.
52. Palumbo A, Bringhen S, Larocca A, Rossi D, Di Raimondo F, Magarotto V, et al. Bortezomib-melphalan-prednisone-thalidomide followed by maintenance with bortezomib-thalidomide compared with bortezomib-melphalan-prednisone for initial treatment of multiple myeloma: updated follow-up and improved survival. J Clin Oncol. 2014;32(7):634–40.
53. Niesvizky R, Flinn IW, Rifkin R, Gabrail N, Charu V, Clowney B, et al. Community-based phase IIIB trial of three UPFRONT Bortezomib-based myeloma regimens. J Clin Oncol. 2015;33(33):3921–9.
54. Magarotto V, Bringhen S, Offidani M, Benevolo G, Patriarca F, Mina R, et al. Triplet vs doublet lenalidomide-containing regimens for the treatment of elderly patients with newly diagnosed multiple myeloma. Blood. 2016;127(9):1102–8.
55. Larocca A, Bringhen S, Petrucci MT, Oliva S, Falcone AP, Caravita T, et al. A phase 2 study of three low-dose intensity subcutaneous bortezomib regimens in elderly frail patients with untreated multiple myeloma. Leukemia. 2016;30:1320. https://doi.org/10.1038/leu.2016.36. [Epub ahead of print]
56. Ludwig H, Durie BG, McCarthy P, Palumbo A, San Miguel J, Barlogie B, et al. IMWG consensus on maintenance therapy in multiple myeloma. Blood. 2012;119(13):3003–15.
57. Palumbo A, Hajek R, Delforge M, Kropff M, Petrucci MT, Catalano J, et al. Continuous lenalidomide treatment for newly diagnosed multiple myeloma. N Engl J Med. 2012;366(19):1759–69.
58. Gay F, Larocca A, Wijermans P, Cavallo F, Rossi D, Schaafsma R, et al. Complete response correlates with long-term progression-free and overall survival in elderly myeloma treated with novel agents: analysis of 1175 patients. Blood. 2011;117(11):3025–31.
59. Rajkumar SV, Jacobus S, Callander NS, Fonseca R, Vesole DH, Williams ME, et al. Lenalidomide plus high-dose dexamethasone versus lenalidomide plus low-dose dexamethasone as initial therapy for newly diagnosed multiple myeloma: an open-label randomised controlled trial. Lancet Oncol. 2010;11(1):29–37.
60. Moreau P, Pylypenko H, Grosicki S, Karamanesht I, Leleu X, Grishunina M, et al. Subcutaneous versus intravenous administration of bortezomib in patients with relapsed multiple myeloma: a randomised, phase 3, non-inferiority study. Lancet Oncol. 2011;12(5):431–40.
61. Petrucci MT, Finsinger P, Chisini M, Gentilini F. Subcutaneous bortezomib for multiple myeloma treatment: patients' benefits. Patient Prefer Adherence. 2014;8:939–46.
62. Mateos MV, San Miguel JF. Safety and efficacy of subcutaneous formulation of bortezomib versus the conventional intravenous formulation in multiple myeloma. Ther Adv Hematol. 2012;3(2):117–24.
63. Moreau P, Richardson PG, Cavo M, Orlowski RZ, San Miguel JF, Palumbo A, et al. Proteasome inhibitors in multiple myeloma: 10 years later. Blood. 2012;120(5):947–59.

64. Bringhen S, Gay F, Donato F, Troia R, Mina R, Palumbo A. Current Phase II investigational proteasome inhibitors for the treatment of multiple myeloma. Expert Opin Investig Drugs. 2014;23(9):1193–209.
65. Bringhen S, Mateos MV, Zweegman S, Larocca A, Falcone AP, Oriol A, et al. Age and organ damage correlate with poor survival in myeloma patients: meta-analysis of 1435 individual patient data from 4 randomized trials. Haematologica. 2013;98(6):980–7.
66. Gay F, Palumbo A. Multiple myeloma: management of adverse events. Med Oncol. 2010;27(3):646–53.
67. Tonelli M, Hemmelgarn B, Reiman T, Manns B, Reaume MN, Lloyd A, et al. Benefits and harms of erythropoiesis-stimulating agents for anemia related to cancer: a meta-analysis. CMAJ. 2009;180(11):E62–71.
68. Neumann S, Krause SW, Maschmeyer G, Schiel X, Lilienfeld-Toal v, Infectious Diseases M. Working Party (AGIHO); German Society of Hematology and Oncology (DGHO). Primary prophylaxis of bacterial infections and Pneumocystis jirovecii pneumonia in patients with hematological malignancies and solid tumors: guidelines of the Infectious Diseases Working Party (AGIHO) of the German Society of Hematology and Oncology (DGHO). Ann Hematol. 2013;92(4):433–42.
69. de Naurois J, Novitzky-Basso I, Gill MJ, Marti FM, Cullen MH, Roila F. Management of febrile neutropenia: ESMO Clinical Practice Guidelines. Ann Oncol. 2010;21(Suppl. 5):v252–6.

Newly Diagnosed Multiple Myeloma in Transplant-Eligible Patients

28

Rajshekhar Chakraborty and Morie A. Gertz

Introduction

Multiple myeloma (MM) is characterized by clonal proliferation of malignant plasma cells in the bone marrow. An estimated 30,280 new cases of MM will be diagnosed in the USA in 2017 [1]. The introduction of proteasome inhibitors (PIs) and immunomodulators (IMiDs) in conjunction with autologous stem cell transplantation (ASCT) has markedly improved the overall survival (OS) in MM, with the survival gap between MM patients and matched controls decreasing in the last decade [2]. The incorporation of ASCT into the frontline therapy of transplant-eligible (TE) patients in the late 1990s had shown a remarkable improvement in survival in younger myeloma patients between 2001 and 2005 [3]. Currently, PI and/or IMiD-based combinations are the standard of care for pretransplant induction therapy in TE newly diagnosed MM patients [4]. Furthermore, the addition of long-term maintenance therapy after ASCT has also led to improved progression-free and overall survival [5]. Hence, there has been a paradigm shift in the management of newly diagnosed MM, leading to the achievement of a deep and durable disease control and improved survival, with the current median OS being greater than 6 years [6].

Diagnosis and Risk Stratification

Traditionally, therapy for MM was initiated once patients developed signs of end-organ damage or *CRAB*, signifying _h_ypercalcemia, _r_enal failure, _a_nemia, and _b_one lesions. However, in 2014, the International Myeloma Working Group (IMWG) proposed an updated criteria for diagnosis of MM, so that early therapy can be initiated to prevent end-organ damage [7]. In addition to the traditional *CRAB* features as a requirement for diagnosis and initiation of therapy in MM, the new IMWG criteria added three biomarkers: bone marrow plasma cells (BMPCs) ≥60%, serum free light chain ratio (sFLCr; involved/uninvolved) ≥100, or ≥1 focal lesion on magnetic resonance imaging (MRI). Currently, the IMWG recommends initiating therapy in MM in the presence of either of the above-mentioned biomarkers even if the patient does not exhibit any of the *CRAB* features and is asymptomatic. The rationale behind early initiation of therapy in MM is twofold: firstly, there are currently multiple effective agents available for frontline therapy in MM, including PIs and IMiDs and, secondly, early therapy in asymptomatic high-risk patients could potentially reduce the risk of end-organ damage and prolong overall survival, as seen in patients with high-risk smoldering myeloma [8].

Once a diagnosis has been established, risk stratification should be performed using one of the prognostic models summarized in Table 28.1 [9–11], which are routinely used in clinical practice. In the revised International Staging System (rISS) for MM [10], chromosomal abnormalities by fluorescence in situ hybridization (FISH) and lactate dehydrogenase (LDH) have been incorporated into the ISS staging [12], which included albumin and β-2 microglobulin. Presence of deletion(17p), t(4;14), and t(14;16) by FISH has an independent negative prognostic impact on survival in MM [10]. The 5-year OS rate of patients with rISS stage I, II, and III are 82%, 62%, and 40%, respectively. Notably, the patient population in rISS staging received up-front novel agents in 95% and ASCT in 60% of cases. Other risk stratification tools like gene expression profiling [13] have also been used, but are not widely available.

R. Chakraborty, M.B.B.S. • M.A. Gertz, M.D., M.A.C.P. (✉)
Division of Hematology, Mayo Clinic,
200 First Street SW, Rochester, MN 55905, USA
e-mail: Gertz.morie@mayo.edu

P.H. Wiernik et al. (eds.), *Neoplastic Diseases of the Blood*, DOI 10.1007/978-3-319-64263-5_28

Table 28.1 Risk stratification systems in multiple myeloma

Prognostic model	Variables	Risk categories	Overall survival	Ref.
rISS	ISS staging, CA [deletion(17p), t(4;14), t(14;16)] and LDH	**rISS stage I:** ISS stage I, no high-risk CA and LDH ≤ UNL **rISS stage II**: All other combinations **rISS stage III:** ISS stage III *AND* high-risk CA or LDH > UNL	5-year OS rate: rISS-I: 82% rISS-II: 62% rISS-III: 40%	
mSMART	CA, GEP, and PCLI	**Standard risk**: All others including t(11;14) or t(6;14) on FISH **Intermediate risk**: t(4;14) on FISH, cytogenetic deletion 13, hypodiploidy or PCLI ≥3% **High risk**: Del(17p), t(14;16) or t(14;20) on FISH or high-risk signature on GEP	Median OS: Standard risk: 8–10 years Intermediate risk: 4–5 years High risk: 3 years	
IMWF	ISS staging and CA	**Low risk**: ISS stage I/II *AND* absence of t(4;14), deletion(17p) and +1q21 *AND* age <55 years **Standard risk**: Others **High risk**: ISS stage II/III *AND* t(4;14) or 17p13 deletion	Median OS: Low risk: 2 years Standard risk: 7 years High risk:>10 years	
IFM	LDH, ISS (III), and cytogenetics (FISH)	**Scores 0–3** (higher score indicating poor prognostic subgroup), with 1 point each for high LDH, ISS stage III, and high-risk CA [t(4;14) and/or del(17p)]	2-year OS rate: Score 0: 93% Score 1: 85% Score 2: 67% Score 3: 55%	

Optimal Induction Regimen for Transplant-Eligible Patients

The goal of induction therapy in MM is to rapidly reduce the tumor burden for minimizing the risk of end-organ damage with minimal toxicities. Furthermore, in TE patients, stem cell toxic drugs like alkylating agents should be avoided due to the risk of inadequate stem cell mobilization. Fortunately, with the introduction of PIs and IMiDs in the treatment armamentarium of MM, a wide variety of non-stem cell toxic induction regimens with high anti-myeloma activity are available in the current era. In TE patients, the combination of bortezomib and dexamethasone (VD) was shown to be superior to alkylating agent-based vincristine-adriamycin-dexamethasone (VAD) induction regimen in terms of response rate and progression-free survival (PFS) in the phase III IFM trial, with less toxicity [14]. Subsequently, a meta-analysis of three phase III RCTs on bortezomib- versus non-bortezomib-containing induction regimen prior to ASCT showed a superior PFS and OS with bortezomib-containing induction regimens [15], the comparator being alkylating agent in two and thalidomide-based induction regimen in one trial. These studies have paved the way for several combination regimens on a backbone of VD to be widely used as induction therapy in newly diagnosed TE-MM patients [4, 16, 17]. However, with a wide variety of available induction regimens, the optimal choice for frontline induction therapy is becoming increasingly complex. The 2017 NCCN guideline recommends using a three-drug over two-drug regimen for frontline therapy in MM based on the evidence of improved response rates and survival [4]. A study on serial genomic analysis of MM has shown that the tumor can exhibit either genomic stability, linear evolution, or clonal heterogeneity with shifting clonal predominance over time [18]. Furthermore, the genome of patients with standard-risk cytogenetics showed minimal changes over time, unlike those with high-risk cytogenetics which was characterized by clonal evolution. This study provides the biological rationale for preferentially using three-drug over two-drug regimens since a suboptimal frontline therapy especially in high-risk patients may fail to eradicate the aggressive clones and lead to future relapse due to clonal evolution. In patients with high-risk cytogenetic abnormalities like deletion (17p), three-drug regimens incorporating a PI and IMiD like bortezomib-lenalidomide-dexamethasone (VRD) or carfilzomib-lenalidomide-dexamethasone (KRD) should be used for induction therapy. Bortezomib-based regimens should be used in those presenting with renal insufficiency at diagnosis [19]. Medical comorbidities, including preexisting peripheral neuropathy should also be taken into consideration while choosing the induction regimen. Intensive induction therapy with bortezomib and/or alkylating agents followed by ASCT is recommended for patients presenting with primary plasma cell leukemia (PCL) [20].

The commonly used induction regimens along with the evidence supporting their use are summarized below and the important phase II and III clinical trials on induction regimens in TE patients are shown in Table 28.2 (three-drug combinations) and Table 28.3 (two-drug combinations).

Table 28.2 Induction regimens with three-drug combinations in transplant-eligible patients

Author	Phase	No.	Regimen used	Response rate		Long-term outcomes		Ref.
				Post-induction	Posttransplant	PFS	OS	
VRD (bortezomib-lenalidomide-dexamethasone)								
Kumar et al.	II	VRD:42 VCD:33 VCRD: 48	***VRD***: V 1.3 mg/m² days 1, 4, 8 and 11; R 25 mg days 1–14; D 40 mg days 1, 8, and 15 (21-day cycle) ***VCD***: V and D as above, C 500 mg/m² days 1 and 8 (21-day cycle) ***VCRD***: V, D, R, and C as above (21-day cycle) *Schema:* 8 cycles of induction [ASCT any time after 4 cycles in TE patients] → V*m* × 4 cycles	≥VGPR rate: VRD: 51% VCD: 41% VCRD: 58%	NR	1-year PFS rate: VRD: 83% VCD: 93% VCRD: 86%	1-year OS rate: VRD: 100% VCD: 100% VCRD: 92%	
Roussel et al.	II	31	***VRD***: V 1.3 mg/m² days 1, 4, 8 and 11; R 25 mg days 1–14; D 40 mg days 1, 8, and 15 (21-day cycle) *Schema:* VRD × 3 cycles → ASCT (Mel200) → VRD × 2 cycles → R*m* × 1 year	≥VGPR rate: 58%	≥VGPR rate: 70%	3-year PFS rate: 77%	3-year OS rate: 100%	
VTD (bortezomib-thalidomide-dexamethasone)								
Cavo et al.	III	480	***VTD:*** V 1.3 mg/m² days 1, 4, 8, and 11; T 100 mg days 1–14 and 200 mg days 15–21; D 40 mg on 8 of first 12 days (21-day cycle) ***TD:*** T and D as above (21-day cycle) VTD arm: VTD × 3 cycles → ASCT × 2 (Mel200) → VTD*c* × 2 cycles TD arm: TD × 3 cycles → ASCT × 2 (Mel200) → TD*c* × 2 cycles	≥VGPR rate: VTD: 62% Td: 28% ($P < 0.001$)	≥VGPR rate: VTD: 82% Td: 64% ($P < 0.001$)	3-year PFS rate: VTD: 68% Td: 56% ($P = 0.006$)	3-year OS rate: VTD: 86% Td: 84% ($P = 0.30$)	
Rosiñol et al.	III	386	***VTD:*** V 1.3 mg/m² days 1, 4, 8 and 11; T 200 mg days 1–28; D 40 mg on days 1–4 and 9–12 (28-day cycle) ***TD:*** T and D as above (28-day cycle) ***QT-V:*** Alkylating agent-based chemotherapy; V as above (5-week cycle) VTD arm: VTD × 6 cycles → ASCT (Mel 200) → IFN*m or* T*m or* VT*m* TD arm: VTD arm: VTD × 6 cycles → ASCT (Mel 200) → IFN*m or* T*m or* VT*m*	CR rate: VTD: 35% Td: 14% ≥VGPR rate: VTD: 60% Td: 29% ($P < 0.001$)	CR rate: VTD: 46% Td: 24% ($P = 0.004$)	Median PFS: VTD: 56 months TD: 28 months ($P = 0.01$)	4-year OS rate: VTD: 74% Td: 65% (P = NS)	
Moreau et al.	III	340	***VTD:*** V 1.3 mg/m² days 1, 4, 8, and 11; T 100 mg days 1–21; D 40 mg on days 1–4 and 9–12 (21-day cycle) ***VCD:*** V and D as above; C 500 mg/m² on days 1, 8, and 15 (21-day cycle) VTD arm: VTD × 4 cycles → ASCT ± *c/m* VCD arm: VTD × 4 cycles → ASCT ± *c/m*	≥VGPR rate: VTD: 66% VCD: 56% ($P = 0.05$)	NR	NR	NR	
VCD (bortezomib-cyclophosphamide-dexamethasone)								
Reeder et al.	II	33	***VCD***: V 1.3 mg/m² on days 1, 4, 8, and 11; D 40 mg on days 1–4, 9–12, and 17–20; C 300 mg/m² days 1, 8, 15, and 22 (28-day cycle) *Schema:* VCD × 4 cycles → ASCT	≥PR rate: 88% ≥VGPR rate: 61%	NR	NR	NR	
Einsele et al.	II/III	300	***VCD:*** V 1.3 mg/m² on days 1, 4, 8, and 11; C 900 mg/m² day 1; D 40 mg on days 1–2, 4–5, 8–9, and 11–12 (21-day cycle) *Schema:* VCD × 3 cycles → ASCT (Mel 200)	≥PR rate: 74% ≥CR rate: 10%	NR	NR	NR	

(continued)

Table 28.2 (continued)

Author	Phase	No.	Regimen used	Response rate		Long-term outcomes		Ref.
				Post-induction	Posttransplant	PFS	OS	
Mai et al.	III	504	***VCD***: V 1.3 mg/m² daily on days 1, 4, 8, and 11; C 900 mg/m² day 1; D 40 mg on days 1–2, 4–5, 8–9, and 11–12 (21-day cycle) ***PAD:*** P as above; A 9 mg/m² on days 1–4; D 20 mg on days 1–4, 9–12, and 17–20 (28-day cycle) VCD arm: VCD × 3 cycles → ASCT (Mel 200) × 1 or 2 → R*m* × 2 years *or* until CR PAD arm: PAD × 3 cycles → ASCT (Mel 200) × 1 or 2 → R*m* × 2 years *or* until CR	≥VGPR rate: VCD: 37% PAD: 34.3%	NR	NR	NR	
Bortezomib-doxorubicin-dexamethasone (PAD)								
Sonneveld et al.	III	827	***VAD***: V 0.4 mg daily on days 1–4; A 9 mg/m² daily on days 1–4; D 40 mg daily on days 1–4, 9–12, and 17–20 (28-day cycle) ***PAD:*** P 1.3 mg/m² daily on days 1, 4, 8, and 11; A and D as above (28-day cycle) VAD arm: VAD × 3 cycles → ASCT (Mel 200) × 1 or 2 → T*m* × 2 years PAD arm: PAD × 3 cycles → ASCT (Mel 200) × 1 or 2 → V*m* × 2 years	≥VGPR rate: VAD: 14% PAD: 42%	≥VGPR rate: VAD: 36% PAD: 62%	Median PFS (month): VAD: 28 PAD: 35 ($P = 0.002$)	5-year OS rate: VAD: 55% PAD: 61% ($P = 0.07$)	
Carfilzomib-lenalidomide-dexamethasone (KRD)								
Jakubowiak et al.	I/II	53	***KRD:*** K 20, 27 or 36 mg/m² on days, 1, 2, 8, 9, 15, 16 and days 1, 2, 8, 9 after cycle 8; R 25 mg daily on days 1–21; D 40 mg in cycles 1–4 and 20 mg in cycles 5+ on days 1, 8, 15 and 22 (28-day cycle) *Schema:* KRD × 4 cycles → SCC and ASCT (for TE patients) or 4 more cycles for non-TE patients → KRD*m* cycles 9–24	≥VGPR rate: 81% ≥nCR rate: 62% sCR rate: 42%	NR	PFS rates: 1-year: 97% 2-year: 92%	NR	
Korde et al.	II	41	***KRD:*** K 20/36 mg/m² on days, 1, 2, 8, 9, 15, 16; R 25 mg daily on days 1–21; D 20/10 mg on days 1, 2, 8, 9, 15, 16, 22, and 23 (28-day cycle) *Schema:* KRD × 4 cycles → SCC → KRD × 4 cycles → R × 24 cycles for patients ≥SD	≥VGPR rate: 89% ≥nCR rate: 63% sCR rate: 41%	NR	NR	NR	
Gay et al.	II	281						
Ixazomib-lenalidomide-dexamethasone (IRD)								
Kumar et al.	I/II	65	***IRD:*** I 1.68–3.95 mg/m² on days, 1, 8 and 15; R 25 mg daily on days 1–21; D 40 mg weekly (28-day cycle) *Schema:* IRD × 12–28 cycles (SCC after 4 cycles in TE-patients) → I*m*	≥VGPR rate: 58% ≥CR rate: 27%	NR	1-year PFS rate: 88%	1-year OS rate: 94%	

Table 28.3 Induction regimens with two-drug combinations in transplant-eligible patients

Author	Phase	No	Regimen used	Response rate		Long-term outcomes		Ref.
				Post-induction	Posttransplant	PFS	OS	
VD (bortezomib-dexamethasone)								
Harrousseau et al.	III	482	***VD:*** V 1.3 mg/m^2 on days 1, 4, 8, and 11; D 40 mg days 1–4 (all cycles) and days 9–12 (cycles 1–2) [21-day cycles] ***VAD:*** Vincristine 0.4 mg/day and A 9 mg/m^2/day on days 1–4; D 40 mg daily days 1–4 (all cycles) and days 9–12 and 17–20 (cycles 1–2) [28-day cycles] VD or VAD × 4 cycles → ASCT (Mel200) × 1 or 2 → L*c* × 2 months → L*m* or placebo per IFM 2005-02 protocol	≥VGPR rate: VD: 54 VAD: 37 ($P < 0.001$)	NR	Median PFS: VD: 36 VAD: 30 ($P = 0.064$)	3-year OS rates: VD: 81.4% VAD: 77.4% ($P = 0.508$)	
Moreau et al.	III	199	***VD:*** V 1.3 mg/m^2 on days 1, 4, 8, and 11; D 40 mg days 1–4 (all cycles) and days 9–12 (cycles 1–2) [21-day cycles] ***rVTD:*** V 1 mg/m^2 on days 1, 4, 8, and 11; T 100 mg daily; D as above (21-day cycles) VD or rVTD × 4 cycles → ASCT (Mel200)	≥VGPR rate: VD: 49 rVTD: 36 ($P = 0.05$)	≥VGPR rate: VD: 74 rVTD: 58 ($P = 0.02$)	Median PFS: VD: 30 months rVTD: 26 months ($P = 0.22$)	No difference in OS between the two groups	
TD (thalidomide-dexamethasone)								
Rajkumar et al.	III	470	***TD:*** T 50 mg daily days 1–14, 100 mg daily days 15–28 and 200 mg from day 1 of cycle 2 (28-day cycle) ***D***: D 40 mg days 1–4, 9–12, 17–20 in cycles 1–4 and days 1–4 from cycle 5 onwards *Schema:* TD or D until progression	ORR: TD: 63 D: 46 ($P < 0.001$) ≥VGPR rate: TD: 44 D: 16 ($P < 0.001$)	NR	Median PFS: TD: 14.9 months D: 6.5 months	No significant difference in the two arms	
RD (lenalidomide-dexamethasone)								
Zonder et al.	III	198	***RD:*** R 25 mg daily in 28 of 35 days for induction and 12 of 28 days for maintenance; D 40 mg days 1–4, 9–12, and 17–20 for induction and days 1–4, 15–18 for maintenance (35-day cycles) ***D***: D as above *Schema:* RD or D × 3 cycles → R*m or Dm*	CR rate: RD: 22% D: 4% ($P = 0.001$)	NR	1-year PFS rate: RD: 77% D: 55% ($P = 0.002$)	1-year OS rate: RD: 93% D: 91% (P = NS)	
Rajkumar et al.	III	445	***RD:*** R 25 mg daily days 1–21; D 40 mg days 1–4, 9–12, 17–20 (28-day cycle) ***RlowD:*** R as above; lowD: D 40 mg on days 1, 8, 15, and 22 (28-day cycle) *Schema:* RD or RlowD for 4 cycles until ASCT or until progression	≥PR rate: RD: 79% RlowD: 68% ($P = 0.008$)	NR	Median PFS: RD: 19 months RlowD: 25 months ($P = 0.026$)	1-year OS rate: RD: 87% RlowD: 96% ($P = 0.0002$)	

Three-Drug Combinations

Bortezomib-Lenalidomide-Dexamethasone (VRD)

VRD was initially evaluated as a frontline induction therapy in the phase I/II study by Richardson et al. [21]. The regimen was shown to be highly effective with an unprecedented post-induction partial response (PR) rate of 100% and a VGPR rate of 67%. The most common grade 2/3 AEs were sensory neuropathy and fatigue and grade 3/4 hematologic toxicities included thrombocytopenia, neutropenia, and lymphopenia. The 18-month PFS and OS rates were 75% and 97%, respectively, at a median follow-up of 21 months. Subsequently, a phase II study by the French group on VRD induction followed by frontline ASCT in newly diagnosed MM patients demonstrated a post-induction VGPR rate of 58% [22]. Notably, 16% of patients in this trial achieved post-induction MRD negativity by flow cytometry at a sensitivity level of 10^{-4}. The 3-year PFS and OS rates were 77% and 100%, respectively, at a median follow-up of 39 months. No treatment-related mortality was reported. Discontinuation due to AEs was noted in only 3% of patients during induction or consolidation phase. The most common grade 3/4 adverse events (AEs) were neutropenia and thrombocytopenia. The randomized phase II EVOLUTION study compared VRD with bortezomib-cyclophosphamide-dexamethasone (VCD) and VRCD in newly diagnosed MM patients, majority of whom were TE [23]. There was no significant difference in the incidence of post-induction VGPR and 1-year PFS rate in the either arms. AEs leading to discontinuation of therapy were seen in 19% of patients in the VRD and 12% in the VCD arm.

Currently, VRD remains the preferred induction regimen in both TE and non-TE MM patients. Although there is no data on OS benefit with VRD in TE patients, it has been shown to have a superior OS over RD in non-TE patients in the SWOG S0777 trial [24].

Bortezomib-Thalidomide-Dexamethasone (VTD)

VTD was found to be superior to TD as a pretransplant induction regimen in the phase III GIMEMA trial [25]. In this trial, 480 patients were randomized to either VTD or TD induction and consolidation therapy in the setting of tandem ASCT. The post-induction VGPR rates in VTD and TD arms were 62% and 28%, respectively ($P < 0.001$). Patients in the VTD arm had a significantly superior 3-year PFS rate compare to those receiving TD (68% vs. 56%, respectively; $P = 0.006$). However, there was no significant difference in the 3-year OS rates at a median follow-up of 36 months. Of note, VTD was shown to abrogate the negative prognostic impact of t(4; 14) cytogenetic abnormality. The incidence of grade 3/4 AEs was 56% in the VTD arm and 33% in the TD arm, with no significant difference in treatment-related mortality. Notably, the incidence of grade 3/4 peripheral neuropathy (PN) was higher in the VTD (10%) compared to TD arm (2%). However, treatment discontinuation in the VTD arm was seen in only 9% of patients developing PN, with 78% experiencing improvement or resolution of symptoms over time.

Another phase III trial by the PETHEMA/GEM group randomized 386 TE patients to receive either VTD, TD, or multiple alkylating agent-based chemotherapy with bortezomib, followed by ASCT and maintenance therapy [26]. The post-induction complete response (CR) rate was 35% in the VTD arm, compared to 14% in the TD arm ($P = 0.001$). In patients with extramedullary soft-tissue plasmacytomas, the post-induction CR rates in VTD and TD arms were 42% and 14%, respectively ($P = 0.02$). The incidence of grade 2–4 PN with VTD was 60% compared to 13% with TD. Dose reduction of bortezomib due to PN was needed in 25% of patients in the VTD arm and 2% had to discontinue therapy. Although patients in the VTD arm had a superior PFS compared to TD (median, 56 vs. 28 months; $P = 0.01$), there was no significant difference in the 4-year OS rate at a median follow-up of 35 months. Patients with high-risk cytogenetics had an inferior PFS and OS irrespective of the treatment arm.

VTD has also been compared with VCD as an induction regimen prior to ASCT in a phase III randomized trial by the IFM group [27]. The post-induction VGPR rate was higher with VTD compared to VCD (66% vs. 56%, respectively; $P = 0.05$). The posttransplant response and survival were not reported in this trial. The incidence of grade 2–4 PN was higher in the VTD compared to VCD arm and grade 3/4 hematologic toxicity was higher in the VCD arm.

VTD remains an active induction regimen in TE patients, with the potential limitation being high rates of PN. Notably, it does not need any dose modification in patients with renal dysfunction and is less expensive compared to other novel agent-based triplet regimens like VRD or KRD.

Bortezomib-Cyclophosphamide-Dexamethasone (VCD)

A phase II trial of VCD induction in newly diagnosed TE-MM patients showed a post-induction PR rate of 88%, with a VGPR rate of 61% [28]. Common grade 3/4 toxicities included hematologic toxicity, hyperglycemia, diarrhea, neuropathy, and thrombosis. Another phase II trial comparing once- versus twice-weekly bortezomib in VCD induction found similar VGPR rates of 60% and 61%, respectively in the two cohorts [29]. However, grade 3/4 AEs, including PN, were lower in the once-weekly compared to the twice-weekly cohort, favoring the use of once-weekly bortezomib with similar efficacy and improved tolerability. Long-term follow-up of VCD induction therapy followed by ASCT has shown 5-year PFS and OS rates of 42% and 70%, respectively [30]. A phase II/III German study on VCD induction in 300 TE patients showed 84% achieving a PR or better after induction, with 10% achieving a CR [31]. Serious AEs were observed in 26% of patients, with grade 3 PN in only 2.3%. Furthermore, VCD was shown to abrogate the negative prognostic impact of t(4; 14) abnormality. The phase II EVOLUTION study showed no significant difference in the post-induction response and 1-year PFS rates between VCD and VRD, as mentioned earlier [23]. The head-to-head comparison between VCD and VTD has shown higher post-induction VGPR rate in the latter but survival outcomes have not been reported thus far [27].

A phase III randomized trial comparing VCD with bortezomib-doxorubicin-dexamethasone (PAD) in 504 newly diagnosed TE-MM patients showed similar post-induction VGPR rates in the two arms (37% and 34% in VCD and PAD arms, respectively; P value for non-inferiority <0.001) [32]. The incidence of grade 2–4 neuropathy was higher in the PAD arm (15%) compared to the VCD arm (8%) [$P = 0.003$]. Similarly, severe AEs due to thromboembolic events were also higher in the PAD compared to the VCD arm (2.8% vs. 0.4%, respectively; $P = 0.04$). Stem cells were adequately collected for at least one transplant in both arms in close to 90% of patients. This study confirmed the non-inferiority in terms of efficacy and a superior safety profile of VCD compared to PAD as an induction regimen in TE-MM patients.

VCD is a highly effective induction regimen in TE patients. Further studies should aim at comparison of VCD with current standard-of-care regimens like VRD and VTD in terms of PFS and OS, as frontline VCD administration is cost effective and reserves the use of IMiDs later in the disease course [9].

Bortezomib-Doxorubicin-Dexamethasone (PAD)

PAD was compared head to head with VAD as a pretransplant induction regimen in the phase III HOVON/GMMG trial [33]. In this trial 827 patients were randomly assigned to receive three cycles of either PAD or VAD followed by a single or tandem ASCT. Patients in the PAD arm received 2 years of bortezomib maintenance after ASCT and those in the VAD arm received 2 years of thalidomide maintenance. The post-induction VGPR rates in the PAD and VAD arms were 42% and 14%, respectively ($P < 0.001$). Patients randomized to the PAD arm had a superior PFS compared to those in the VAD arm (median PFS, 35 vs. 28 months, respectively; $P = 0.002$) and the 5-year OS rates were 61% and 55%, respectively ($P = 0.07$), at a median follow-up of 41 months. Notably, in the subgroup of patients with deletion (17p) cytogenetic abnormality by FISH, the median PFS was 36 months in the PAD compared to 18 months in the VAD arm ($P < 0.001$) [34]. Similarly, the 3-year OS rates in the deletion (17p) subgroup was 83% and 36% in the PAD and VAD arms, respectively (HR 2.4 for VAD; $P < 0.001$). Furthermore, administration of bortezomib both before and after ASCT (as in the PAD arm) abrogated the negative prognostic impact of deletion (17p) [34]. Patients with renal failure also had a superior PFS and OS in the PAD arm [33]. Grade 2–4 PN was observed in 18% of patients receiving VAD and 40% receiving PAD. SCC was successful in close to 90% of patients in either arm.

Since patients with deletion (17p) have poor outcomes, administration of three-drug combinations including bortezomib or carfilzomib as pretransplant induction therapy and bortezomib maintenance after ASCT is recommended in this subgroup.

Carfilzomib-Lenalidomide-Dexamethasone (KRD)

Carfilzomib is a highly selective and irreversible next-generation PI with robust anti-myeloma activity [35, 36]. It has been shown to have a single-agent activity in relapsed/refractory (R/R) MM [37] and also in combination with RD in the phase III ASPIRE trial [38]. A phase I/II study of KRD in 53 patients with newly diagnosed MM showed an ORR of 98%, with 42% achieving a stringent CR (sCR) after induction [39]. At a median follow-up of 13 months, the 1- and 2-year PFS rates were 97% and 92%, respectively. Thirty-five patients in this trial underwent successful stem cell collection and seven eventually proceeded to ASCT. Common grade 3/4 AEs included hyperglycemia (23%), hypophosphatemia (25%), anemia (21%), thrombocytopenia (17%), and neutropenia (17%). PN was observed in 12% of patients, all being grades 1–2. There was no treatment-related mortality. Another phase II study of KRD induction followed by extended lenalidomide administration in 41 newly diagnosed TE and non-TE patients showed a post-induction VGPR rate of 89%, with a sCR rate of 41% [40]. Among 17 patients with at least a near CR (nCR) who underwent MRD testing at a sensitivity level of 10^{-5}, all were found to be MRD negative. Common non-hematologic grade 3/4 AEs included electrolyte disturbances (18%), abnormal liver function tests (13%), rash or pruritus (11%), fatigue (11%), cardiovascular toxicity (8%), and dyspnea (8%). The phase II FORTE trial has compared KRD and KCD (carfilzomib-cyclophosphamide-dexamethasone) in 281 TE-MM patients [41]. The post-induction rate of achieving VGPR or better response after four cycles of induction therapy was 74% with KRD and 61% with KCD ($P = 0.05$). The incidence of grade 3/4 AEs was higher in the KCD compared to KRD arm. On the other hand, grade 3/4 dermatological AEs and elevated liver function tests were common in the KRD arm. Stem cell mobilization was successful in more than 95% of patients in both arms.

KRD is emerging as a highly effective induction regimen in MM, with a high rate of sCR and MRD negativity post-induction. However, to the best of our knowledge, there is no phase III data on frontline therapy in TE-MM patients thus far. Although the incidence of PN is lesser with carfilzomib compared to bortezomib, cardiotoxicity observed in the clinical trials of carfilzomib is concerning. A meta-analysis of phase I/II, II, and III clinical trials on carfilzomib including 2594 patients has shown the risk of all grade and grade 3/4 cardiotoxicity (including arrhythmias, systolic congestive heart failure, and acute coronary syndrome) to be 18% and 8%, respectively [42]. Furthermore, the cardiotoxicity was dose dependent, with patients receiving carfilzomib dose ≥45 mg/m^2 having a twofold higher incidence of grade ≥3 cardiac AEs, compared to those receiving <45 mg/m^2. Hence, caution should be exercised in patients at a high risk of cardiovascular complications.

Ixazomib-Lenalidomide-Dexamethasone (IRD)

The combination of oral PI ixazomib with RD has been shown to be safe and effective in 65 TE and non-TE patients in an open-label phase I/II trial [43]. Grade 3–4 AEs were observed in 63% of patients, including disorders of skin and subcutaneous tissue (17%), neutropenia (12%), thrombocytopenia (8%), and PN (6%). The post-induction ORR was 92%, including a VGPR rate of 58% and a CR rate of 27%. At a median follow-up of 14 months, the 1-year PFS and OS rates were 88% and 94%, respectively. SCC was attempted in 45% of patients after a median of four cycles of induction therapy. Although the activity of IRD seems promising in newly diagnosed MM, further data from phase II and III clinical trials on head-to-head comparison with currently used regimens is needed prior to its incorporation in the frontline therapy for TE patients.

Two-Drug Combinations

Bortezomib-Dexamethasone (VD)

VD was the first novel agent-based induction regimen which was shown to be superior to alkylating agent-based induction prior to ASCT in newly diagnosed MM [14]. In this phase III IFM trial, 482 patients were randomized to receive VD, VAD, VD followed by consolidation with multiple alkylating agents, or VAD followed by a similar consolidation. Subsequently, all patients would proceed to a single ASCT, with tandem ASCT reserved for those achieving less than a VGPR after the first ASCT. Post-induction VGPR rate was significantly higher with VD compared to VAD (54% vs. 37%, respectively; $P < 0.001$). Patients receiving VD had a superior PFS; however, they did not reach statistical significance (median PFS, 36 months with VD vs. 30 months with VAD; $P = 0.064$). Consolidation with alkylating agents did not improve post-induction response rate. Adequate SCC was achieved in more than 95% of patients in both arms. The incidence of grade 3/4 anemia, neutropenia, and thrombosis was significantly higher in the VAD arm, as was the incidence of toxicity-related deaths. On the other hand, grade 2/3 PN was significantly higher in the VD arm. Analysis of patients with high-risk FISH cytogenetics either enrolled or treated according to the above protocol showed that induction with VD abrogated the negative prognostic impact of t(4;14) but not deletion (17p) [44]. Another phase III trial by the French group randomized patients to receive VD or reduced-dose VTD (rVTD). The post-induction VGPR rate was significantly higher in the rVTD arm compared to the VD arm (49% vs. 36%; $P = 0.05$). However, there was no significant difference in PFS or OS. Notably, the incidence of grade 2–4 PN was 34% in the VD and 14% in the rVTD arm ($P = 0.001$).

Thalidomide-Dexamethasone (TD)

Thalidomide is a first-generation IMiD and is not widely used in the USA due to the availability of lenalidomide, which has a superior safety profile and a higher potency compared to thalidomide. The 2017 NCCN guidelines have removed TD as a recommended induction regimen in TE patients [4]. However, due to low cost, it still remains valuable in resource-limited settings, where there is a lack of access to bortezomib and lenalidomide.

TD was shown to be superior to D alone as an induction therapy in newly diagnosed MM in a phase III trial. The post-induction ORR was significantly higher with TD compared to D, which translated into a superior PFS (median PFS, 14.9 months with TD vs. 6.5 months with D; $P < 0.001$) [45]. However, grade 3/4 AEs, especially thromboembolic complications (18%) and PN (3.4%), were significantly higher with TD. Of note, routine thromboprophylaxis was not administered in this trial, which is currently a standard of care in patients receiving IMiDs. VTD induction therapy has been shown to have a superior PFS compared to TD in two phase III trials, as mentioned earlier [15, 25, 26].

Lenalidomide-Dexamethasone (RD)

Lenalidomide is a second-generation IMiD with a better toxicity profile compared to thalidomide. In the randomized SWOG S0232 phase III trial, RD was shown to be superior to D alone for the treatment of newly diagnosed MM [46]. The CR rate was 22% in the RD arm and 4% in the D arm ($P = 0.001$), with the 1-year PFS rates being 77% and 55%, respectively ($P = 0.002$). The trial was halted after interim analysis due to ethical challenges with using D alone as the control arm and patients were allowed to cross over to RD. Thromboembolic events (TEE) were observed in 20% of patients receiving RD compared to 12% of those receiving D alone. However, thromboprophylaxis with aspirin 325 mg daily was added later in the trial after a high rate of TEE was noted in the RD arm.

Another phase III RCT evaluated whether RlowD (lenalidomide-low-dose dexamethasone) was non-inferior in terms of efficacy and safer compared to RD as an induction therapy for newly diagnosed MM [47]. Patients were randomized to receive dexamethasone 40 mg for 12 out of 28 days (RD) or 4 out of 28 days (RlowD) along with lenalidomide 25 mg daily from days 1 to 21. After four cycles, the cumulative rate of PR or better was 79% in the RD arm and 68% in the RlowD arm ($P = 0.008$). However, the 1-year respective OS rates in the two arms were 87% and 96% ($P = 0.0002$), mostly driven by the increased mortality during the first 4 months of therapy in the RD arm (5.4%) compared to the RlowD arm (0.45%). Notably, the incidence of grade ≥3 AEs was higher in the RD compared to RlowD arm (52% vs. 35%, respectively; $P < 0.001$), with the most common SAEs being DVT, infection, and fatigue.

In non-TE patients, RD has been shown to be inferior to VRD in terms of PFS and OS in the SWOG S0777 trial [24]. However, survival benefit of novel agent-based triplets over RD has not been shown in TE patients. Patients receiving RD should have stem cells collected after four cycles of therapy due to reports of impaired stem cell mobilization after prolonged exposure to lenalidomide [48, 49].

Stem Cell Transplantation

Stem cell transplantation is an integral part of the treatment backbone in eligible patients with newly diagnosed MM. Several RCTs, both in the context of conventional cytotoxic chemotherapy and novel agents like PIs and IMiDs, have shown ASCT to be an effective consolidative treatment. It improves the depth of response achieved by induction therapy with PIs and IMiDs [25, 50], with a negligible transplant-related mortality (TRM) of around 1% in most studies in the current era.

Transplant Eligibility

There is a lack of clear consensus on strict eligibility criteria for ASCT in MM. However, age and comorbidities are generally taken into consideration while determining transplant eligibility. Age greater than 65 years is considered to be a contraindication for transplant in most countries. However, in the USA, ASCT is frequently offered to patients over 65 years of age in a good functional status and several retrospective studies have shown similar posttransplant PFS and OS in elderly patients who undergo transplantation [51, 52]. There was no significant difference in TRM noted in elderly patients [52]. A prospective French study on MM patients aged 64–74 years has established the feasibility of ASCT in this age group, with 89% of patients undergoing ASCT successfully [53]. Melphalan 200 mg/m^2 was used as a conditioning regimen in 64% and 140 mg/m^2 in 36% of transplanted patients. At 100 days posttransplant, there was no treatment-related mortality observed in this age group. Prior to ASCT, sufficient cardiac, renal, liver, and pulmonary function is also desirable [4]. However, in a CIBMTR study on 1492 patients undergoing ASCT, there was no difference in PFS and OS among patients with and without renal dysfunction. Furthermore, 85% of patients with severe renal insufficiency achieved dialysis independence after ASCT [54]. Hematopoietic cell transplant comorbidity index (HCT-CI) [55] has also been shown to be effective as a risk stratification tool prior to ASCT in MM, with higher HCT-CI scores indicating an inferior survival after transplant [56].

Studies on ASCT in Newly Diagnosed MM (Table 28.4)

The first RCT performing a head-to-head comparison of conventional therapy using alkylating agents with high-dose chemotherapy followed by ASCT (HDT-ASCT) was reported by the IFM group in 1996 [57]. In this study 200 patients were randomized to receive either 18 alternating cycles of VMCP/BVAP (vincristine, melphalan, cyclophosphamide, prednisone/vincristine, carmustine, doxorubicin, prednisone) or 4–6 alternating cycles of VMCP/BVAP immediately followed by HDT-ASCT, using melphalan 140 mg/m^2 and total-body irradiation (TBI; 8Gy) as a conditioning regimen. The ORR was significantly higher in the ASCT arm compared to the conventional therapy arm (81% vs. 57%, respectively; $P < 0.001$), as was the CR rate (22% vs. 5%, respectively; $P < 0.001$). The 5-year PFS rates in the ASCT and conventional therapy arms were 28% and 10% ($P = 0.01$), respectively, and the respective 5-year OS rates were 52% and 12% ($P = 0.03$). TRM was seen in 2% of patients. The MRC Myeloma VII trial also compared alkylating agent-based chemotherapy with ASCT showing similar results, with a significantly superior CR rate, PFS, and OS in the ASCT arm [58]. Death within 100 days of ASCT was seen in 3% of patients in the MRC trial, the cause being sepsis in all but one patient.

With the superiority of HDT-ASCT being established in newly diagnosed MM, the next strategic question was whether all eligible patients must undergo frontline ASCT after induction therapy or can wait for ASCT until their first relapse without compromising survival. To answer this question, Fermand et al. reported a multicenter RCT comparing patients who underwent up-front HDT-ASCT (ASCT arm) with those who had standard-dose therapy (SDT) with the option of salvage ASCT either at first relapse or in the case of primary resistance to SDT (SDT arm) [59]. With a median follow-up of around 6 years, the median PFS in the ASCT arm was 39 months, compared to 13 months in the SDT arm. However, there was no significant difference in OS, with the median OS being 64.6 months in the ASCT arm and

Table 28.4 Trials comparing high-dose therapy with standard-dose therapy in transplant-eligible patients

Author	No.	Treatment schema	Response rate	Long-term outcomes		Ref.
				PFS	OS	
Attal et al.	200	***SDT arm:*** Alternative 3-week cycles of VMCP and BVAP × 12 months (Total of 18 cycles) ***ASCT arm:*** Alternating 3-week cycles of VMCP and BVAP (4–6 cycles) → ASCT (Mel140 + TBI)	≥VGPR rate: SDT: 14% ASCT: 38% ($P < 0.001$)	5-year EFS: SDT: 10% ASCT: 28% ($P = 0.01$)	5-year OS: SDT: 12% ASCT: 52% ($P = 0.03$)	
Child et al.	407	***SDT arm:*** Doxorubicin-carmustine-cyclophosphamide-Melphalan × 4–12 cycles (6-week cycles) → IFN*m* 3× weekly ***ASCT arm:*** Doxorubicin-vincristine-methylprednisolone-cyclophosphamide × 3 cycles or until response attained (3-week cycles) → ASCT (Mel200) → IFN*m* 3× weekly	CR rate: SDT: 8% ASCT: 44% ($P < 0.001$)	Median PFS: SDT: 20 months ASCT: 32 months ($P < 0.001$)	Median OS: SDT: 42 months ASCT: 54 months ($P = 0.04$)	
Fermand et al.	185	***SDT arm:*** SCC by CHOP regimen → VMCP × 6 cycles → option of salvage ASCT for primary resistance or at first relapse ***ASCT arm:*** SCC by CHOP regimen → VAMP × 3–4 cycles → ASCT (lomustine, VP16, cyclophosphamide, Melphalan 140 and TBI)	ORR: SDT: 62% ASCT: 86% CR rate: SDT: 5% ASCT: 19%	Median PFS: SDT: 13 months HDT: 39 months	Median OS: SDT: 64 months HDT: 64.6 months ($P = 0.92$)	
Barlogie et al.	516	***SDT arm:*** VAD × 4 cycles → VBMCP*c* after SCC with high-dose CTX (5-week cycles × 1 year) → IFN*m* or observation × 4 years (option of salvage ASCT at relapse) ***ASCT arm:*** VAD × 4 cycles → SCC with high-dose CTX → ASCT (Mel140 + TBI 12Gy) → IFN*m* or observation	Similar cumulative response rates in both arms	7-year PFS rate: SDT: 16% ASCT: 17% $P = 0.16$	7-year OS rate: SDT: 42% ASCT: 37% $P = 0.78$	
Fermand et al.	190	***SDT arm:*** VMCP (1-month courses) until stable plateau in case of PR or until progression/resistance ***ASCT arm:*** SCC reinforced by cyclophosphamide, doxorubicin, vincristine, and prednisone → VAMP × 3–4 cycles → ASCT (Mel 200 or busulfan + Mel140)	ORR: SDT: 58% ASCT: 83%	Median PFS: SDT: 19 months ASCT: 25 months ($P = 0.07$)	Median OS: SDT: 47.6 months ASCT: 47.8 months ($P = 0.91$)	
Palumbo et al.	273	***SDT arm:*** RD × 4 cycles (28-day cycle) → MPR × 6 cycles (28-day cycle) → R*m* until progression or toxicity or observation ***ASCT arm:*** RD × 4 cycles (28-day cycle) → ASCT × 2 (Mel 200 total) → R*m* until progression or toxicity or observation	CR rate: SDT: 20% ASCT: 16%	Median PFS: SDT: 22 months ASCT: 43 months ($P < 0.001$)	4-year OS rate: SDT: 65% ASCT: 82% ($P = 0.02$)	
Attal et al.	700	***Arm A:*** VRD × 3 cycles → ASCT (Mel200) + VRD × 2 cycles → R*m* × 1 year ***Arm B:*** VRD × 5 cycles → R*m* × 1 year	≥VGPR rate: Arm A: 88% Arm B: 77% ($P = 0.02$)	Median PFS: Arm A: 50 months Arm B: 36 months ($P < 0.001$)	4-year OS rate: Arm A: 81% Arm B: 82% ($P = 0.87$)	

64 months in the SDT arm (P = 0.92). Around 90% of patients in the SDT arm who were TE per protocol had successfully received a salvage ASCT. Notably, the average time without symptoms, treatment, or treatment toxicity was higher in the ASCT arm compared to the SDT arm (28 vs. 22 months, respectively).

Subsequently, the phase III US Intergroup trial by Barlogie et al. randomized 516 patients to SDT or HDT-ASCT after induction with VAD and SCC with high-dose cyclophosphamide [60]. Patients in the SDT arm had received consolidation with multiple alkylating agents (VBMCP) for a total of 1 year before being randomized to interferon (IFN)-based maintenance therapy or observation. The conditioning regimen used in the ASCT arm was melphalan 140 mg/m^2 along with total-body irradiation (TBI). The cumulative response rates were identical in both arms. Furthermore, there was no significant difference in the 7-year PFS and OS rates in either arms. Notably, around 55% of patients relapsing in the SDT arm received HDT-ASCT in their first relapse. Treatment-related mortality in the SDT arm was 0.4%, compared to 1.7% in the ASCT arm. A plausible explanation proposed for the lack of superiority of ASCT seen in this study was the use of TBI as a conditioning regimen, which has been shown to be inferior to high-dose melphalan (200 mg/m^2) in MM [4, 61]. Another study comparing frontline ASCT and SDT with alkylating agents showed a nonsignificant trend towards superior PFS in the ASCT arm but no difference in OS in either arms at a median follow-up of 10 years [62]. However, the duration without symptoms, treatment, or toxicity related to treatment was significantly longer for the ASCT compared to the SDT arm (25 vs. 17 months, respectively; $P = 0.033$).

In the era of PIs and IMiDs, two phase III studies have addressed the question of early versus delayed ASCT thus far. In a study by the Italian group, 273 patients were randomized to receive consolidation with either six cycles of melphalan-prednisone-lenalidomide (MPR) [SDT arm] or tandem auto-transplantation with a total melphalan conditioning dose of 200 mg/m^2 (ASCT arm) [63]. All patients had received induction with four cycles of RD prior to randomization. The median PFS in the ASCT and SDT arms were 43 and 22 months, respectively ($P < 0.001$), and the 4-year OS rates in the respective arms were 82% and 65%, respectively ($P = 0.02$). Notably, 63% of patients in the SDT arm received salvage ASCT at relapse. Grade 3/4 hematologic, gastrointestinal, and infectious adverse events were more common in the ASCT arm. A similar question in the context of VRD induction and consolidation therapy has been answered by the phase III IFM study by Attal et al. [50]. In this study, 700 patients were randomized to receive three cycles of VRD induction followed by consolidation with ASCT and two cycles of VRD (Arm A) or five cycles of VRD alone (Arm B). All patients received 1 year of lenalidomide maintenance. A total of 323 out of 350 patients (92%) underwent up-front ASCT in Arm A. Patients undergoing up-front ASCT had a higher VGPR rate compared to those receiving VRD alone (88% vs. 77%, respectively; $P = 0.02$). The rate of MRD negativity by flow cytometry at a sensitivity level of 10^{-4} was also higher in patients receiving early ASCT (79% in Arm A vs. 65% in Arm B; $P = 0.001$). At a median follow-up of 43 months for Arm A and 44 months for Arm B, the median PFS in the respective arms were 50 and 36 months ($P < 0.001$), favoring frontline transplantation. There was no difference in OS at 4 years, which was more than 80% in both arms. Among patients in Arm B who experienced symptomatic relapse necessitating a second-line therapy, 79% were able to successfully undergo a salvage transplant. The rates of grade 3/4 neutropenia, gastrointestinal toxicity, and infections were significantly higher in the group receiving up-front ASCT. There was no significant difference in the overall incidence of second primary malignancies (SPMs) in either arm.

Hence, in the era of PIs and IMiDs, ASCT with high-dose melphalan as a conditioning regimen remains an integral part of treatment and should be offered up front to all eligible patients, based on PFS benefit in both studies [50, 63] and OS benefit in one study [63]. Furthermore, early ASCT has been shown to be cost effective [64] and prolongs the treatment-free interval [59, 62]. Patients with progressive disease after induction therapy also benefit from ASCT [65, 66]. In TE patients who do not undergo frontline ASCT, adequate stem cells should be collected for at least two transplants and ASCT should be offered at first relapse.

Role of Tandem Transplantation

Tandem ASCT is defined as a planned course of treatment with high-dose therapy followed by stem cell infusion within 6 months of the first transplant [4]. The rationale behind a second ASCT is to improve the depth of response and potentially prolong long-term outcomes like PFS and OS. A list of RCTs comparing single and double ASCT in newly diagnosed MM has been summarized in Table 28.5.

In the USA, tandem transplant for newly diagnosed MM was pioneered by the University of Arkansas group. Tandem ASCT was shown to be feasible and superior to historical controls receiving standard therapy in terms of response rate, PFS, and OS [67]. A multicenter randomized trial by the French group (IFM94) in the era of alkylating agent-based induction therapy has shown a superior PFS and OS with double ASCT compared to single ASCT, despite no significant difference in the depth of response [68]. The 7-year OS rates with single and double ASCT in the study were 21% and 42%, respectively ($P = 0.01$), at a median follow-up of over 6 years. Notably, the subgroup of patients who did not achieve at least a VGPR after the first ASCT derived the most benefit from a second ASCT. However, a limitation of this trial was the suboptimal conditioning regimen used in the single-transplant arm. The cumulative melphalan dose in the tandem arm was 280 mg/m^2 compared to 140 mg/m^2 in the single-transplant arm. Seventy-eight percent of patients in the tandem arm were successfully able to undergo two transplantations with no significant difference in hematologic toxicity or TRM compared to patients who received a single transplant. In the HOVON24 trial comparing single and double ASCT after VAD-based induction therapy, the CR rate was significantly higher in patients receiving double transplant [69]. However, there was a marginal difference in the median PFS between the two groups and no significant difference in OS at a median follow-up of 56 months. Similarly, in the Bologna96 randomized trial, there was no significant difference in OS between the single- and double-transplant arms, despite an increase in response rate and PFS duration by 18 months in the double-transplant arm [70]. The cumulative melphalan dose in this trial was 200 mg/m^2 in the single-transplant and 320 mg/m^2 in the double-transplant arm, with no significant difference in TRM in the two arms. Similar to the IFM94 trial [68], patients who did not achieve nCR after the first ASCT benefitted the most from a second transplant, with a trend towards OS benefit in this subgroup of patients.

Two randomized trials have compared single and double transplants in the context of PI and IMiD-based induction and maintenance therapy. The StaMINA trial randomized 758 TE patients who had received 2–12 months of induction therapy to receive either a single ASCT (Arm A), single ASCT followed by four cycles of VRD consolidation therapy (Arm B), or tandem ASCT (Arm C) [71]. The conditioning

Table 28.5 Studies comparing single- with double-autologous stem cell transplantation

Author	No.	Treatment schema	Response rate	Long-term outcomes		Ref.
				PFS	OS	
Attal et al.	399	***Induction:*** VAD × 3–4 cycles (3-week cycles) ***Transplant:*** S-ASCT (Mel140 + TBI 8Gy) or D-ASCT (Mel140 for 1st and Mel140 + TBI 8Gy for 2nd) ***Maintenance:*** IFN 3× weekly initiated after hematologic reconstitution	≥VGPR rate: S-ASCT: 42% D-ASCT: 50% ($P = 0.01$)	7-year PFS rate: S-ASCT: 10% D-ASCT: 20% ($P = 0.03$)	7-year OS rate: S-ASCT: 21% D-ASCT: 42% ($P = 0.01$)	
Sonneveld et al.	303	***Induction:*** VAD × 3–4 cycles (3-week cycles) ***Transplant:*** S-ASCT (Mel70 × 2) or D-ASCT (Mel70 × 2 + CTX 120 mg/kg + TBI) ***Maintenance:*** IFN*m* in both arms	CR rate: S-ASCT: 13% D-ASCT: 28% ($P = 0.002$)	Median PFS: S-ASCT: 23 months D-ASCT: 24 months ($P = 0.032$)	Median OS: S-ASCT: 55 months D-ASCT: 50 months ($P = 0.39$)	
Cavo et al.	321	***Induction:*** VAD × 4 cycles (28 day cycles) ***Transplant:*** S-ASCT (Mel200) or D-ASCT (Mel200 for first and Mel120 + busulfan 12 mg/kg for second) ***Maintenance:*** IFN*m* in both arms	≥nCR rate: S-ASCT: 33% D-ASCT: 47% ($P = 0.008$)	Median PFS: S-ASCT: 24 months D-ASCT: 42 months ($P < 0.001$)	7-year OS rate: S-ASCT: 46% D-ASCT: 43% ($P = 0.90$)	
Stadmauer et al.	758	***Induction:*** 2–12 months of induction therapy (regimen not specified) ***Arm A:*** ASCT (Mel200) → R*m* until progression ***Arm B:*** ASCT (Mel200) → VRD × 4 cycles → R*m* until progression ***Arm C:*** ASCT (Mel200 × 2) → R*m* until progression	NR	38-month PFS rate: Arm A: 52% Arm B: 57% Arm C: 56% (P = NS)	38-month OS rate: Arm A: 83% Arm B: 86% Arm C: 82% (P = NS)	
Cavo et al.	614	***Induction:*** VCD → 3–4 cycles ***Transplant:*** Single or double ASCT ***Maintenance:*** R*m* until progression or toxicity	NR	3-year PFS rate: S-ASCT: 60% D-ASCT: 73% ($P = 0.03$)	NR	

dose of melphalan was 200 mg/m^2 for each transplant. All arms received lenalidomide maintenance until progression. At a median follow-up of 38 months, there was no significant difference between the PFS and OS rates in the three arms. The 38-month probabilities of OS was 83%, 86%, and 82% in Arm A, Arm B, and Arm C, respectively. The cumulative incidences of first SPM were 4%, 6%, and 5.9%, respectively, in the three arms. The phase III EMN02/HO95 trial randomized 614 TE patients to either VMP (bortezomib-melphalan-prednisone) consolidation, single-ASCT, or double-ASCT arm after induction therapy with 3–4 cycles of VCD [72]. All patients received lenalidomide maintenance until progression or toxicity. At a median follow-up of 27 months, the 3-year PFS rates in patients receiving a single and double ASCT was 60% and 73%, respectively ($P = 0.03$). The PFS benefit of double ASCT was evident in all pre-defined subgroups, including those with high β-2 microglobulin, bone marrow plasma cells >60%, lactate dehydrogenase above upper normal limit, revised ISS-II, and high-risk cytogenetic abnormalities by FISH. OS data was not mature at the time the study was reported. Based on these studies, there is a lack of convincing evidence to perform tandem ASCT in the era of PI- and IMiD-based induction and post-transplantation therapies. Randomized trials are currently under way to determine whether patients achieving less than a VGPR after the first transplant can benefit from a second transplant in the novel agent era.

Optimal Conditioning Regimen

The IFM group had tested high-dose melphalan (200 mg/m^2) with low-dose melphalan (140 mg/m^2) plus 8 Gy total-body irradiation (TBI) as a conditioning regimen in 282 patients in the context of induction therapy with four cycles of VAD [61]. Patients receiving high-dose melphalan had a superior 45-month OS rate of 66%, compared to 46% in patients receiving low-dose melphalan plus TBI ($P = 0.05$). Furthermore, patients receiving high-dose melphalan had a faster hematologic recovery, shorter duration of hospitalization, and lower rates of severe oral mucositis. This study paved the way for high-dose melphalan to be the optimal conditioning regimen in MM.

Recently, there has been some evidence on the benefit of combining bortezomib with melphalan during the conditioning phase [73, 74]. Administration of bortezomib within 24 h following melphalan was shown to induce robust plasma cell apoptosis in pharmacodynamics studies, with 51% achieving VGPR or better [73]. A phase II IFM study on the combination of melphalan 200 mg/m^2 with bortezomib at a cumulative dose of 4 mg/m^2 (Mel-Vel) showed a post-ASCT VGPR rate of more than 70%, with no increase in hematologic toxicity [74]. A matched control analysis with patients receiving melphalan alone showed that Mel-Vel led to higher rates of CR after transplant. However, RCTs comparing melphalan alone or combined with novel agents are needed before incorporation of such strategies in practice. Other alkylating agents like busulfan in addition to melphalan have shown PFS benefit but no difference in OS, with a higher TRM [75, 76]. Hence, high-dose melphalan (200 mg/m^2) remains the standard of care currently, except in patients with renal dysfunction where lower dose (140 mg/m^2) should be used [19].

Stem Cell Mobilization

The three most common stem cell mobilization strategies include growth factor, growth factor plus plerixafor, and chemotherapy. Strategies for mobilization vary among different institutions. Growth factor (granulocyte-colony-stimulating factor [G-CSF]) is one of the most common mobilization strategies currently. Factors predicting suboptimal mobilization with G-CSF include advanced age, low platelet count at mobilization, use of filgrastim instead of pegfilgrastim, and longer duration of lenalidomide therapy prior to mobilization [77]. Plerixafor, when added to G-CSF, leads to adequate stem cell mobilization in patients receiving lenalidomide-based induction therapy [78]. However, the efficacy of added plerixafor is similar to adding low-dose cyclophosphamide (1.5 mg/m^2) to G-CSF in the novel agent era [79]. Hence, due to low cost of cyclophosphamide, it should be preferred over plerixafor for use in conjunction with G-CSF in patients with prior exposure to lenalidomide. The threshold of stem cell infusion dose for a single transplant in Mayo Clinic is 3×10^6 CD34+ cells/kg [80].

Role of Allogeneic Transplantation

With the advent of effective and well-tolerated anti-myeloma agents and excellent activity of ASCT as a consolidative therapy, allogeneic stem cell transplantation (Allo-SCT) is not routinely used in newly diagnosed MM. In the IFM trials comparing ASCT → Allo-SCT (auto-allo) with tandem ASCT after induction therapy with VAD, the median PFS was similar in both arms and there was a nonsignificant towards a superior OS in the tandem ASCT arm [81]. Notably, 24% of patients developed grade 2–4 acute graft-versus-host disease (GVHD) after allo-SCT and 36% of evaluable patients developed extensive chronic GVHD. Another study on 162 TE newly diagnosed MM patients biologically randomized to either a non-myeloablative allo-SCT or ASCT after induction therapy with VAD and a single ASCT showed a superior PFS and OS in the allo-SCT arm [82]. The BMT-CTN and PETHEMA trials have shown comparable survival between ASCT and Allo-SCT, with a higher rate of TRM in the allo-SCT arms [83, 84]. Due to a high treatment-related morbidity and mortality, allo-SCT in newly diagnosed MM should be restricted to clinical trials in high-risk patients and can be an option in certain situations, including primary refractory disease or lack of response to ASCT [4].

Post-transplantation Maintenance and Consolidation

Despite increasing the depth of response and the rate of MRD negativity, ASCT is not curative in MM and most patients eventually relapse. Hence, post-transplantation maintenance or consolidation therapy is administered with the intent of further improving the depth and prolonging the duration of response, to eventually improve long-term outcomes, including PFS and OS. A pooled analysis of studies involving head-to-head comparison of continuous and fixed-duration therapy in MM has shown a superior PFS and OS with continuous therapy, with the 4-year OS rate being 69% with continuous and 60% with fixed-duration therapy ($P = 0.003$) [85]. Maintenance therapy involves prolonged treatment with an anti-myeloma agent, usually until progression or unacceptable toxicity. Consolidation involves a short course of single agent or combination therapy for a fixed duration after ASCT [86].

Prior to the introduction of PIs and IMiDs, glucocorticoid [87] and interferon [88, 89] were used for posttransplant maintenance therapy. Two large meta-analysis of interferon maintenance showed an OS benefit ranging from 4 to 7 months [88, 89]. However, currently, there is no role of interferon-based maintenance therapy in MM due to the toxicity profile and its impact on quality of life. With the advent of novel agents, thalidomide was tested as a maintenance therapy in various randomized trials [90–97]. A meta-analysis however showed that thalidomide maintenance in the context of ASCT significantly improved PFS (HR 0.67, 95% CI, 0.61–0.74; $P < 0.001$), but not OS (HR 0.90, 95% CI, 0.73–1.11; $P = 0.343$) [98]. The toxicity profile of thalidomide is unfavorable for long-term maintenance therapy due to high rates of PN and poor health-related quality of life (HRQOL) [97]. Furthermore, the UK MRC IX trial has shown worse OS with thalidomide maintenance in patients with high-risk cytogenetic abnormalities by FISH ($P = 0.01$)

Table 28.6 Phase III studies on lenalidomide and bortezomib maintenance

Author	No.	Maintenance dose/regimen	Long-term outcomes		Ref.
			PFS	OS	
McCarthy et al.	460	Lenalidomide 10 mg daily (range, 5–15 mg) until progression	Median PFS (month): Lenalidomide: 46 Placebo: 27 ($P < 0.001$)	3-year OS rate (%): Lenalidomide: 88 Placebo: 80 ($P = 0.03$)	
Attal et al.	614	Lenalidomide 10 mg daily × 3 months → 15 mg thereafter if tolerated until progression	Median PFS (month): Lenalidomide: 41 Placebo: 23 ($P < 0.001$)	3-year OS rate (%): Lenalidomide: 80 Placebo: 84 ($P = 0.29$)	
Palumbo et al.	251	Lenalidomide 10 mg daily days 1–21 (28-day cycle) until progression	Median PFS (month): Lenalidomide: 42 Placebo: 22 ($P < 0.001$)	3-year OS rate (%): Lenalidomide: 88 Placebo: 79 ($P = 0.14$)	
Jackson et al.	828	Lenalidomide until progression	Median PFS (month): Lenalidomide: 50 Placebo: 28 ($P < 0.001$)	NR	
Sonneveld et al.	827	Bortezomib 1.3 mg/m^2 every other week or thalidomide 50 mg daily for 2 years	Median PFS (month): Bortezomib: 35 Thalidomide: 28 ($P = 0.002$)	5-year OS rate: Bortezomib: 61% Thalidomide: 55% ($P = 0.07$)	

[99]. Hence, lenalidomide has largely replaced thalidomide as a posttransplant maintenance therapy due to better tolerability and data on improved OS, which will be described below.

Here, we discuss the lenalidomide and bortezomib-based maintenance strategies in MM in the posttransplant setting. The phase III studies on lenalidomide and bortezomib maintenance have been summarized in Table 28.6.

Lenalidomide Maintenance

Lenalidomide has been shown to be an effective maintenance therapy in MM in the posttransplant setting in four independent phase III RCTs [63, 100, 101]. The CALGB100104 was the first US trial showing a survival advantage with lenalidomide maintenance [100]. In this trial, 460 patients who had a stable disease or better 100 days post-transplantation were randomized to receive lenalidomide or placebo at a starting dose of 10 mg/day (range, 5–15 mg). Induction regimen other than bortezomib, lenalidomide, or thalidomide prior to ASCT was used in only 6% of patients. Lenalidomide was administered until disease progression or unacceptable toxicity. At a median follow-up of 34 months, the median PFS of patients in the lenalidomide group was 46 months compared to 27 months for those in the placebo group ($P < 0.001$). Furthermore, the 3-year OS rate was also significantly superior in the lenalidomide compared to the placebo group (88% vs. 80%, respectively: $P = 0.03$). Grade 3/4 hematologic AEs were significantly higher in the lenalidomide compared to the placebo group as expected. The cumulative incidence of SPMs was 8% in the lenalidomide and 3% in the placebo group ($P = 0.008$). The simultaneously released IFM trial randomized 614 patients with nonprogressive disease after ASCT to lenalidomide maintenance or placebo [101]. The starting dose of lenalidomide was 10 mg daily for the first 3 months, with subsequent escalation to 15 mg if well tolerated. Approximately 50% of patients had received VAD induction therapy pre-ASCT and the other half received VD. Maintenance was continued until relapse. At a median follow-up of 30 months, the median PFS was higher in the lenalidomide compared to the placebo group (41 vs. 23 months, respectively; $P < 0.001$). However, there was no significant difference in the 3-year OS rates, which was more than 80% in both arms. The cumulative incidence of SPMs was 3.1 per 100 patient-years in the lenalidomide and 1.2 per 100 patient-years in the placebo group ($P = 0.002$). Grade 3/4 hematologic toxicity including thromboembolic events was more frequent in the lenalidomide group, with no difference observed in the rate of grade 3/4 PN. The GIMEMA trial randomized 251 patients to lenalidomide or no maintenance after induction therapy with four cycles of RD and consolidation with either six cycles of MPR or tandem ASCT [63]. At a median follow-up of 51 months, the median PFS was significantly longer with lenalidomide maintenance compared to no maintenance (42 vs. 22 months, respectively; $P < 0.001$). However, there was no significant difference in the 3-year OS rates in the two arms. Grade 3/4 hematologic and dermatologic toxic effects were significantly higher in the lenalidomide arm.

A prospectively planned individual patient-level meta-analysis of the three studies (CALGB, IFM, and GIMEMA) showed a significant OS benefit with lenalidomide maintenance compared to no-maintenance therapy [5]. The 7-year OS rate was 62% with lenalidomide maintenance versus 50% with no-maintenance therapy ($P = 0.001$) at an updated median follow-up of 80 months. The OS benefit was evident in most subgroups; however, patients with ISS stage III disease and high-risk cytogenetics did not derive survival benefit from lenalidomide maintenance. The cumulative incidence of both hematologic and solid SPMs was higher with lenalidomide maintenance therapy. Notably, the HRQoL score of patients receiving lenalidomide maintenance in the real world has been shown to be similar to those receiving no-maintenance therapy [102].

The Myeloma XI study from the UK had randomized patients to lenalidomide maintenance or observation after induction therapy with CRD (cyclophosphamide-lenalidomide-dexamethasone) or CTD (cyclophosphamide-thalidomide-dexamethasone) and consolidation with ASCT. At a median follow-up of 36 months, the median PFS was 50 months in patients receiving lenalidomide maintenance compared to 28 months in those on observation. Furthermore, the PFS benefit with lenalidomide maintenance was evident in all prespecified subgroups, including in those with high-risk cytogenetic abnormalities and ISS stage III disease. The most common grade 3/4 AE was neutropenia.

In summary, given the OS benefit noted in the meta-analysis including three large RCTs, lenalidomide maintenance is currently the standard of care in all patients posttransplant. However, OS benefit has not yet been demonstrated in patients with high-risk cytogenetic abnormalities, in whom bortezomib maintenance should be preferred based on data from the HOVON trial, which will be described below. Furthermore, it is unclear whether a fixed duration of lenalidomide maintenance after ASCT is as good as prolonged maintenance until disease progression, and it needs to be answered by future RCTs.

Bortezomib Maintenance

There is a lack of placebo-controlled randomized trials evaluating bortezomib maintenance after ASCT in literature. However, the HOVON-65/GMMG-HD4 trial performed a head-to-head comparison of bortezomib-based induction and maintenance therapy with VAD induction followed by posttransplant maintenance with thalidomide [33]. It should be noted that patients were not randomized to bortezomib or thalidomide maintenance after ASCT and the study was not designed for direct comparison between bortezomib and thalidomide. Nevertheless, patients receiving bortezomib-based induction and maintenance therapy had a superior OS in the entire cohort and also in the subgroups with deletion (17p) and renal failure. Notably, in patients with deletion (17p), the median PFS was 18 months without bortezomib and 36 months with bortezomib-based therapy, which also translated into a superior OS [3-year OS 83% with bortezomib and 36% without bortezomib in deletion (17p) subgroup; $P < 0.001$] [34]. An updated report of this trial at a median follow-up of more than 7 years showed that the negative prognostic impact of deletion (17p) was abrogated in the bortezomib arm but not in the standard arm [103]. The plausible explanation for the excellent activity of bortezomib in deletion (17p) patients is the induction of apoptosis in myeloma cells by altering the balance between proteasome load and proteasome capacity in a p53-independent fashion [104]. The median duration of bortezomib maintenance at a starting dose of 1.3 mg/m^2 every other week was 23 months, compared to 14 months for thalidomide, indicating that bortezomib was well tolerated and feasible for long-term posttransplant maintenance therapy. Emergence of grade 3/4 PN during bortezomib maintenance therapy was seen in 5% of patients, with the rate of treatment discontinuation due to any toxicity being 11%.

Hence, lenalidomide should be used for posttransplant maintenance in the vast majority of MM patients, except in those with high-risk cytogenetics especially deletion (17p) and t(4;14), where bortezomib maintenance should be considered.

Posttransplant Consolidation Therapy

The goal of consolidation therapy in MM is to improve the depth of response and possibly long-term outcomes. A phase III trial evaluating VTD versus TD consolidation after ASCT showed a significant increase in CR rates after consolidation with VTD, which translated into a superior PFS but not OS at a median follow-up of 30 months [105]. Grade 2/3 PN was more frequent with VTD compared to TD (8.1 vs. 2.4%, respectively). Notably, high-risk cytogenetic abnormalities, including deletion(17p) and/or t(4;14), retained their negative prognostic impact on PFS in the TD arm but not in the VTD arm. Another study by the Nordic myeloma group randomized 370 patients 3 months after ASCT to receive either 21 weeks of bortezomib or no-consolidation therapy [106]. Consolidation with bortezomib led to an improvement in PFS by 7 months ($P = 0.05$), but did not have any impact on OS. Pooled results from two phase III studies comparing bortezomib consolidation and observation after ASCT in MM also showed only PFS but no OS benefit, with a significant PFS benefit seen only in patients achieving less than a VGPR after ASCT [107]. Finally, the StaMINA trial on 758 TE patients in the era of novel agent-based induction and post-transplantation therapy did not show any PFS or OS benefit from four cycles of VRD consolidation after ASCT [71].

Based on the data presented above, there is a lack of convincing evidence for use of consolidation therapy after ASCT, especially in the context of PI- and/or IMiD-based induction therapy and lenalidomide maintenance until progression.

Supportive Care and Toxicities

Peripheral Neuropathy

Peripheral neuropathy is one of the most common serious AEs of PI bortezomib and is also seen with IMiDs thalidomide and lenalidomide. Drug-induced PN by bortezomib or thalidomide can present with sensory, motor, and autonomic symptoms, with the potential targets being small fibers, dorsal root ganglia, and afferent sensory and efferent motor fibers [108]. Important predisposing conditions for drug-induced neuropathy are preexisting PN and medical comorbidities, including diabetes mellitus, vitamin deficiencies, alcohol abuse, or viral infections [108]. Subcutaneous bortezomib has been shown to be non-inferior to intravenous bortezomib in terms of efficacy, with a lower incidence of grade 2–4 PN (24% with subcutaneous and 41% with intravenous formulation; $P = 0.012$) [109]. Changing the route of administration of bortezomib to subcutaneous and the frequency from twice weekly to once weekly have led to deceased rates of bortezomib-induced PN (BiPN) in clinical practice. For moderate BiPN (grade 2), dose should be reduced from 1.3 to 1 mg/m^2, and for severe PN (grade 3), dose should be temporarily withheld and can be resumed at a lower dose of 0.7 mg/m^2, once symptoms resolve. Bortezomib should be discontinued if patients develop a disabling PN (grade 4) [110]. BiPN has been shown to resolve or improve in about two-thirds to three-quarters of patients, with median time for reversal or improvement being 2–3 months. On the other hand, recovery in thalidomide-induced PN (TiPN) is limited to about a quarter of patients and takes around 4–6 years [108]. Hence, dose modification guidelines should be strictly followed in the setting of drug-induced PN to maximize the chances of reversal or improvement.

Infections

The 2017 NCCN guidelines state that prophylaxis for *Pneumocystis jirovecii* pneumonia (PJP) can be considered in myeloma patients [4]. Similarly, intravenous immunoglobulin should be considered in life-threatening infections [4]; however, routine use is not recommended [17]. In the phase III APEX study comparing bortezomib-dexamethasone with dexamethasone alone, the incidence of herpes zoster virus infections was significantly higher in the bortezomib arm [111], which led to the recommendation of using acyclovir or valacyclovir prophylaxis in all patients receiving PI-based therapies [17]. Immediate therapy with broad-spectrum antibiotics and supportive care is needed.

Thromboembolic Phenomenon

Patients with MM have a higher base rate of thromboembolic phenomena compared to general population, with the baseline risk of venous thromboembolic (VTE) events being 3–4% [17]. The rate of thrombosis has been shown to be higher in patients receiving high-dose dexamethasone and IMiDs. The ECOG trial comparing RD with RlowD in newly diagnosed MM showed greater than a twofold higher rate of thromboembolic phenomena in the high-dose dexamethasone compared to the low-dose dexamethasone arm (26% vs. 12%, respectively; $P = 0.0003$) [47]. This study led to the routine use of low-dose dexamethasone in combination regimens. Aspirin at a dose of 100 mg daily is currently recommended for VTE prophylaxis in myeloma patients on IMiDs [4, 17, 112]. Full-dose anticoagulation with warfarin or low-molecular-weight heparin should be initiated in the setting of a clot, without any urgent need to discontinue IMiDs.

Bone Disease

Osteolytic bone disease due to the activation of osteoclasts is one of the most common clinical manifestations of MM and also causes significant worsening of HRQoL [113]. Bisphosphonates are the mainstay of therapy for myeloma bone disease, with their mechanism of action being inhibition of osteoclasts and subsequently bone resorption. A double-blind placebo-controlled trial on 392 MM patients with at least one lytic bone lesion showed a significantly reduced incidence of skeletal events in patients receiving pamidronate compared to those receiving placebo (24% vs. 41%; $P < 0.001$) [114]. Furthermore, pamidronate was well tolerated and led to decrease in bone pain. Another double-blind RCT on patients with hypercalcemia of malignancy compared zoledronic acid and pamidronate head-to-head [115]. Zoledronic acid was superior to pamidronate in terms of the rate of normalization of serum calcium level by day 4 and duration of response. The UK MRC Myeloma IX trial comparing zoledronic acid with clodronic acid in both TE and non-TE newly diagnosed MM patients showed a significant improvement in the median OS by 5.5 months in the zoledronic acid arm [116]. Current NCCN guidelines recommend addition of bisphosphonates to the treatment regimen in all symptomatic MM patients, regardless of the evidence of bony lesions. Monitoring of renal function, baseline dental examination, and monitoring for osteonecrosis of jaw while on bisphosphonates are also recommended [4].

Miscellaneous

In patients with myeloma-associated anemia, erythropoietin therapy can be used [117, 118] to maintain a target hemoglobin around 12 gm/dl. Granulocyte colony-stimulating factor (G-CSF) may be administered in patients with severe neutropenia during therapy [17]. In patients with symptomatic hyperviscosity, plasmapheresis can be used to reduce the risk of end-organ damage [4, 119]. For impending spinal cord compression, high-dose dexamethasone and radiation therapy should be emergently initiated [17]. Orthopedic consultation should be sought for pathological fractures. Certain patients with symptomatic vertebral compression fractures might benefit from kyphoplasty or vertebroplasty [4].

Bortezomib-based therapy should be used initially in those with renal insufficiency since bortezomib does not need dose modification in renal dysfunction [19]. Furthermore, it leads to a rapid reduction of tumor burden, which decreases the nephrotoxic effects of paraproteins. In TE patients with renal dysfunction, melphalan should be used at a dose of 140 mg/m^2 [19]. A high-cutoff hemodialysis (HD) technique to remove free light chains has shown a higher rate of dialysis independence compared to HD with conventional high-flux dialyzers in MM patients presenting with myeloma cast nephropathy receiving initial therapy with bortezomib-dexamethasone [120].

Acknowledgement Conflicts of interest: The authors declare no relevant conflicts of interest.

References

1. Siegel RL, Miller KD, Jemal A. Cancer Statistics, 2017. CA Cancer J Clin. 2017;67(1):7–30.
2. Fonseca R, Abouzaid S, Bonafede M, Cai Q, Parikh K, Cosler L, Richardson P. Trends in overall survival and costs of multiple myeloma, 2000–2014. Leukemia. 2017;31(9):1915–21.
3. Schaapveld M, Visser O, Siesling S, Schaar CG, Zweegman S, Vellenga E. Improved survival among younger but not among older patients with multiple myeloma in the Netherlands, a population-based study since 1989. Eur J Cancer (Oxford, England: 1990). 2010;46(1):160–9.
4. Kumar SK, Callander NS, Alsina M, Atanackovic D, Biermann JS, Chandler JC, et al. Multiple myeloma, version 3.2017, NCCN clinical practice guidelines in oncology. J Natl Compr Cancer Netw. 2017;15(2):230–69.
5. Attal M, Palumbo A, Holstein SA, Lauwers-Cances V, Petrucci MT, Richardson PG, et al. Lenalidomide (LEN) maintenance (MNTC) after high-dose melphalan and autologous stem cell transplant (ASCT) in multiple myeloma (MM): a meta-analysis (MA) of overall survival (OS). J Clin Oncol. 2016;34(Suppl 15):8001.
6. Kumar SK, Dispenzieri A, Lacy MQ, Gertz MA, Buadi FK, Pandey S, et al. Continued improvement in survival in multiple myeloma: changes in early mortality and outcomes in older patients. Leukemia. 2014;28(5):1122–8.
7. Rajkumar SV, Dimopoulos MA, Palumbo A, Blade J, Merlini G, Mateos MV, et al. International Myeloma Working Group updated criteria for the diagnosis of multiple myeloma. Lancet Oncol. 2014;15(12):e538–48.
8. Mateos MV, Hernandez MT, Giraldo P, de la Rubia J, de Arriba F, Lopez Corral L, et al. Lenalidomide plus dexamethasone for high-risk smoldering multiple myeloma. N Engl J Med. 2013;369(5):438–47.
9. Mikhael JR, Dingli D, Roy V, Reeder CB, Buadi FK, Hayman SR, et al. Management of newly diagnosed symptomatic multiple myeloma: updated Mayo Stratification of Myeloma and Risk-Adapted Therapy (mSMART) consensus guidelines 2013. Mayo Clin Proc. 2013;88(4):360–76.
10. Palumbo A, Avet-Loiseau H, Oliva S, Lokhorst HM, Goldschmidt H, Rosinol L, et al. Revised international staging system for multiple myeloma: a report from international myeloma working group. J Clin Oncol. 2015;33(26):2863–9.
11. Chng WJ, Dispenzieri A, Chim CS, Fonseca R, Goldschmidt H, Lentzsch S, et al. IMWG consensus on risk stratification in multiple myeloma. Leukemia. 2014;28(2):269–77.
12. Greipp PR, Miguel JS, Durie BGM, Crowley JJ, Barlogie B, Bladé J, et al. International staging system for multiple myeloma. J Clin Oncol. 2005;23(15):3412–20.
13. Broyl A, Hose D, Lokhorst H, de Knegt Y, Peeters J, Jauch A, et al. Gene expression profiling for molecular classification of multiple myeloma in newly diagnosed patients. Blood. 2010;116(14):2543–53.
14. Harousseau JL, Attal M, Avet-Loiseau H, Marit G, Caillot D, Mohty M, et al. Bortezomib plus dexamethasone is superior to vincristine plus doxorubicin plus dexamethasone as induction treatment prior to autologous stem-cell transplantation in newly diagnosed multiple myeloma: results of the IFM 2005-01 phase III trial. J Clin Oncol. 2010;28(30):4621–9.
15. Sonneveld P, Goldschmidt H, Rosiñol L, Bladé J, Lahuerta JJ, Cavo M, et al. Bortezomib-based versus Nonbortezomib-based induction treatment before autologous stem-cell transplantation in patients with previously untreated multiple myeloma: a meta-analysis of phase III randomized, controlled trials. J Clin Oncol. 2013;31(26):3279–87.
16. Moreau P, Attal M, Facon T. Frontline therapy of multiple myeloma. Blood. 2015;125(20):3076–84.
17. Moreau P, San Miguel J, Sonneveld P, Mateos MV, Zamagni E, Avet-Loiseau H, et al. Multiple myeloma: ESMO clinical practice guidelines for diagnosis, treatment and follow-updagger. Ann Oncol. 2017;28(Suppl 4):iv52–61.
18. Keats JJ, Chesi M, Egan JB, Garbitt VM, Palmer SE, Braggio E, et al. Clonal competition with alternating dominance in multiple myeloma. Blood. 2012;120(5):1067–76.
19. Dimopoulos MA, Terpos E, Chanan-Khan A, Leung N, Ludwig H, Jagannath S, et al. Renal impairment in patients with multiple myeloma: a consensus statement on behalf of the international myeloma working group. J Clin Oncol. 2010;28(33):4976–84.
20. Fernandez de Larrea C, Kyle RA, Durie BG, Ludwig H, Usmani S, Vesole DH, et al. Plasma cell leukemia: consensus statement

on diagnostic requirements, response criteria and treatment recommendations by the international myeloma working group. Leukemia. 2013;27(4):780–91.

21. Richardson PG, Weller E, Lonial S, Jakubowiak AJ, Jagannath S, Raje NS, et al. Lenalidomide, bortezomib, and dexamethasone combination therapy in patients with newly diagnosed multiple myeloma. Blood. 2010;116(5):679–86.
22. Roussel M, Lauwers-Cances V, Robillard N, Hulin C, Leleu X, Benboubker L, et al. Front-line transplantation program with lenalidomide, bortezomib, and dexamethasone combination as induction and consolidation followed by lenalidomide maintenance in patients with multiple myeloma: a phase II study by the Intergroupe Francophone du Myelome. J Clin Oncol. 2014;32(25):2712–7.
23. Kumar S, Flinn I, Richardson PG, Hari P, Callander N, Noga SJ, et al. Randomized, multicenter, phase 2 study (EVOLUTION) of combinations of bortezomib, dexamethasone, cyclophosphamide, and lenalidomide in previously untreated multiple myeloma. Blood. 2012;119(19):4375–82.
24. Durie BG, Hoering A, Abidi MH, Rajkumar SV, Epstein J, Kahanic SP, et al. Bortezomib with lenalidomide and dexamethasone versus lenalidomide and dexamethasone alone in patients with newly diagnosed myeloma without intent for immediate autologous stem-cell transplant (SWOG S0777): a randomised, open-label, phase 3 trial. Lancet (London, England). 2017;389(10068):519–27.
25. Cavo M, Tacchetti P, Patriarca F, Petrucci MT, Pantani L, Galli M, et al. Bortezomib with thalidomide plus dexamethasone compared with thalidomide plus dexamethasone as induction therapy before, and consolidation therapy after, double autologous stem-cell transplantation in newly diagnosed multiple myeloma: a randomised phase 3 study. Lancet (London, England). 2010;376(9758):2075–85.
26. Rosinol L, Oriol A, Teruel AI, Hernandez D, Lopez-Jimenez J, de la Rubia J, et al. Superiority of bortezomib, thalidomide, and dexamethasone (VTD) as induction pretransplantation therapy in multiple myeloma: a randomized phase 3 PETHEMA/GEM study. Blood. 2012;120(8):1589–96.
27. Moreau P, Hulin C, Macro M, Caillot D, Chaleteix C, Roussel M, et al. VTD is superior to VCD prior to intensive therapy in multiple myeloma: results of the prospective IFM2013-04 trial. Blood. 2016;127(21):2569–74.
28. Reeder CB, Reece DE, Kukreti V, Chen C, Trudel S, Hentz J, et al. Cyclophosphamide, bortezomib and dexamethasone induction for newly diagnosed multiple myeloma: high response rates in a phase II clinical trial. Leukemia. 2009;23(7):1337–41.
29. Reeder CB, Reece DE, Kukreti V, Chen C, Trudel S, Laumann K, et al. Once- versus twice-weekly bortezomib induction therapy with CyBorD in newly diagnosed multiple myeloma. Blood. 2010;115(16):3416–7.
30. Reeder CB, Reece DE, Kukreti V, Mikhael JR, Chen C, Trudel S, et al. Long-term survival with cyclophosphamide, bortezomib and dexamethasone induction therapy in patients with newly diagnosed multiple myeloma. Br J Haematol. 2014;167(4):563–5.
31. Einsele H, Liebisch P, Langer C, Kropff M, Wandt H, Jung W, et al. Velcade, intravenous cyclophosphamide and dexamethasone (VCD) induction for previously untreated multiple myeloma (German DSMM XIa trial). Blood. 2009;114(22):131.
32. Mai EK, Bertsch U, Durig J, Kunz C, Haenel M, Blau IW, et al. Phase III trial of bortezomib, cyclophosphamide and dexamethasone (VCD) versus bortezomib, doxorubicin and dexamethasone (PAd) in newly diagnosed myeloma. Leukemia. 2015;29(8):1721–9.
33. Sonneveld P, Schmidt-Wolf IG, van der Holt B, El Jarari L, Bertsch U, Salwender H, et al. Bortezomib induction and maintenance treatment in patients with newly diagnosed multiple myeloma: results of the randomized phase III HOVON-65/ GMMG-HD4 trial. J Clin Oncol. 2012;30(24):2946–55.
34. Neben K, Lokhorst HM, Jauch A, Bertsch U, Hielscher T, van der Holt B, et al. Administration of bortezomib before and after autologous stem cell transplantation improves outcome in multiple myeloma patients with deletion 17p. Blood. 2012;119(4):940–8.
35. Demo SD, Kirk CJ, Aujay MA, Buchholz TJ, Dajee M, Ho MN, et al. Antitumor activity of PR-171, a novel irreversible inhibitor of the proteasome. Cancer Res. 2007;67(13):6383–91.
36. Kuhn DJ, Chen Q, Voorhees PM, Strader JS, Shenk KD, Sun CM, et al. Potent activity of carfilzomib, a novel, irreversible inhibitor of the ubiquitin-proteasome pathway, against preclinical models of multiple myeloma. Blood. 2007;110(9):3281–90.
37. Siegel DS, Martin T, Wang M, Vij R, Jakubowiak AJ, Lonial S, et al. A phase 2 study of single-agent carfilzomib (PX-171-003-A1) in patients with relapsed and refractory multiple myeloma. Blood. 2012;120(14):2817–25.
38. Stewart AK, Rajkumar SV, Dimopoulos MA, Masszi T, Spicka I, Oriol A, et al. Carfilzomib, lenalidomide, and dexamethasone for relapsed multiple myeloma. N Engl J Med. 2015;372(2):142–52.
39. Jakubowiak AJ, Dytfeld D, Griffith KA, Lebovic D, Vesole DH, Jagannath S, et al. A phase 1/2 study of carfilzomib in combination with lenalidomide and low-dose dexamethasone as a frontline treatment for multiple myeloma. Blood. 2012;120(9):1801–9.
40. Zingone A, Kwok ML, Manasanch EE, Bhutani M, Tageja N, Kazandjian D, et al. Phase II clinical and correlative study of carfilzomib, Lenalidomide, and dexamethasone followed by Lenalidomide extended dosing (CRD-R) induces high rates of MRD negativity in newly diagnosed multiple myeloma (MM) patients. Blood. 2013;122(21):538.
41. Gay FM, Scalabrini DR, Belotti A, Offidani M, Petrucci MT, Esma F, et al. Carfilzomib-lenalidomide-dexamethasone (KRd) vs carfilzomib-cyclophosphamide-dexamethasone (KCd) induction: Planned interim analysis of the randomized FORTE trial in newly diagnosed multiple myeloma (NDMM). J Clin Oncol. 2017;35(Suppl 15):8003.
42. Waxman AJ, Clasen SC, Garfall AL, Carver JR, Vogl DT, O'Quinn R, et al. Carfilzomib-associated cardiovascular adverse events: a systematic review and meta-analysis. J Clin Oncol. 2017;35(Suppl 15):8018.
43. Kumar SK, Berdeja JG, Niesvizky R, Lonial S, Laubach JP, Hamadani M, et al. Safety and tolerability of ixazomib, an oral proteasome inhibitor, in combination with lenalidomide and dexamethasone in patients with previously untreated multiple myeloma: an open-label phase 1/2 study. Lancet Oncol. 2014;15(13):1503–12.
44. Avet-Loiseau H, Leleu X, Roussel M, Moreau P, Guerin-Charbonnel C, Caillot D, et al. Bortezomib plus dexamethasone induction improves outcome of patients with t(4;14) myeloma but not outcome of patients with del(17p). J Clin Oncol. 2010;28(30):4630–4.
45. Rajkumar SV, Rosinol L, Hussein M, Catalano J, Jedrzejczak W, Lucy L, et al. Multicenter, randomized, double-blind, placebo-controlled study of thalidomide plus dexamethasone compared with dexamethasone as initial therapy for newly diagnosed multiple myeloma. J Clin Oncol. 2008;26(13):2171–7.
46. Zonder JA, Crowley J, Hussein MA, Bolejack V, Moore DF, Whittenberger BF, et al. Superiority of lenalidomide (Len) plus high-dose dexamethasone (HD) compared to HD alone as treatment of newly-diagnosed multiple myeloma (NDMM): results of

the randomized, double-blinded, placebo-controlled SWOG trial S0232. Blood. 2007;110(11):77.

47. Rajkumar SV, Jacobus S, Callander NS, Fonseca R, Vesole DH, Williams ME, et al. Lenalidomide plus high-dose dexamethasone versus lenalidomide plus low-dose dexamethasone as initial therapy for newly diagnosed multiple myeloma: an open-label randomised controlled trial. Lancet Oncol. 2010;11(1):29–37.
48. Kumar S, Giralt S, Stadtmauer EA, Harousseau JL, Palumbo A, Bensinger W, et al. Mobilization in myeloma revisited: IMWG consensus perspectives on stem cell collection following initial therapy with thalidomide-, lenalidomide-, or bortezomib-containing regimens. Blood. 2009;114(9):1729–35.
49. Kumar S, Dispenzieri A, Lacy MQ, Hayman SR, Buadi FK, Gastineau DA, et al. Impact of lenalidomide therapy on stem cell mobilization and engraftment post-peripheral blood stem cell transplantation in patients with newly diagnosed myeloma. Leukemia. 2007;21(9):2035–42.
50. Attal M, Lauwers-Cances V, Hulin C, Leleu X, Caillot D, Escoffre M, et al. Lenalidomide, Bortezomib, and dexamethasone with transplantation for myeloma. N Engl J Med. 2017;376(14):1311–20.
51. Dhakal B, Nelson A, Guru Murthy GS, Fraser R, Eastwood D, Hamadani M, et al. Autologous hematopoietic cell transplantation in patients with multiple myeloma: effect of age. Clin Lymphoma Myeloma Leuk. 2017;17(3):165–72.
52. Muchtar E, Dingli D, Kumar S, Buadi FK, Dispenzieri A, Hayman SR, et al. Autologous stem cell transplant for multiple myeloma patients 70 years or older. Bone Marrow Transplant. 2016;51(11):1449–55.
53. Garderet L, Beohou E, Caillot D, Stoppa AM, Touzeau C, Chretien ML, et al. Upfront autologous stem cell transplantation for newly diagnosed elderly multiple myeloma patients: a prospective multicenter study. Haematologica. 2016;101(11):1390–7.
54. Mahindra A, Hari P, Fraser R, Fei M, Mark T, Nieto Y, et al. Patients (pts) with renal insufficiency (RI) and multiple myeloma (MM) have similar outcomes after autologous hematopoietic cell transplantation (AHCT) as those without. Blood. 2016;128(22): 994.
55. Sorror ML, Maris MB, Storb R, Baron F, Sandmaier BM, Maloney DG, et al. Hematopoietic cell transplantation (HCT)-specific comorbidity index: a new tool for risk assessment before allogeneic HCT. Blood. 2005;106(8):2912–9.
56. Saad A, Mahindra A, Zhang MJ, Zhong X, Costa LJ, Dispenzieri A, et al. Hematopoietic cell transplant comorbidity index is predictive of survival after autologous hematopoietic cell transplantation in multiple myeloma. Biol Blood Marrow Transplant. 2014;20(3):402–8.e1.
57. Attal M, Harousseau JL, Stoppa AM, Sotto JJ, Fuzibet JG, Rossi JF, et al. A prospective, randomized trial of autologous bone marrow transplantation and chemotherapy in multiple myeloma. Intergroupe Francais du Myelome. N Engl J Med. 1996;335(2):91–7.
58. Child JA, Morgan GJ, Davies FE, Owen RG, Bell SE, Hawkins K, et al. High-dose chemotherapy with hematopoietic stem-cell rescue for multiple myeloma. N Engl J Med. 2003;348(19):1875–83.
59. Fermand JP, Ravaud P, Chevret S, Divine M, Leblond V, Belanger C, et al. High-dose therapy and autologous peripheral blood stem cell transplantation in multiple myeloma: up-front or rescue treatment? Results of a multicenter sequential randomized clinical trial. Blood. 1998;92(9):3131–6.
60. Barlogie B, Kyle RA, Anderson KC, Greipp PR, Lazarus HM, Hurd DD, et al. Standard chemotherapy compared with high-dose chemoradiotherapy for multiple myeloma: final results of phase III US Intergroup Trial S9321. J Clin Oncol. 2006;24(6):929–36.
61. Moreau P, Facon T, Attal M, Hulin C, Michallet M, Maloisel F, et al. Comparison of 200 mg/m² melphalan and 8 Gy total body irradiation plus 140 mg/m² melphalan as conditioning regimens for peripheral blood stem cell transplantation in patients with newly diagnosed multiple myeloma: final analysis of the Intergroupe Francophone du Myelome 9502 randomized trial. Blood. 2002;99(3):731–5.
62. Fermand JP, Katsahian S, Divine M, Leblond V, Dreyfus F, Macro M, et al. High-dose therapy and autologous blood stem-cell transplantation compared with conventional treatment in myeloma patients aged 55 to 65 years: long-term results of a randomized control trial from the Group Myelome-Autogreffe. J Clin Oncol. 2005;23(36):9227–33.
63. Palumbo A, Cavallo F, Gay F, Di Raimondo F, Ben Yehuda D, Petrucci MT, et al. Autologous transplantation and maintenance therapy in multiple myeloma. N Engl J Med. 2014;371(10):895–905.
64. Pandya C, Hashmi S, Khera N, Gertz MA, Dispenzieri A, Hogan W, et al. Cost-effectiveness analysis of early vs. late autologous stem cell transplantation in multiple myeloma. Clin Transpl. 2014;28(10):1084–91.
65. Hahn T, Wingard JR, Anderson KC, Bensinger WI, Berenson JR, Brozeit G, et al. The role of cytotoxic therapy with hematopoietic stem cell transplantation in the therapy of multiple myeloma: an evidence-based review. Biol Blood Marrow Transplant. 2003;9(1):4–37.
66. Kumar S, Lacy MQ, Dispenzieri A, Rajkumar SV, Fonseca R, Geyer S, et al. High-dose therapy and autologous stem cell transplantation for multiple myeloma poorly responsive to initial therapy. Bone Marrow Transplant. 2004;34(2):161–7.
67. Barlogie B, Jagannath S, Vesole DH, Naucke S, Cheson B, Mattox S, et al. Superiority of tandem autologous transplantation over standard therapy for previously untreated multiple myeloma. Blood. 1997;89(3):789–93.
68. Attal M, Harousseau JL, Facon T, Guilhot F, Doyen C, Fuzibet JG, et al. Single versus double autologous stem-cell transplantation for multiple myeloma. N Engl J Med. 2003;349(26):2495–502.
69. Sonneveld P, van der Holt B, Vellenga E, Croockewit S, Verhoef G, Segeren C, et al. Intensive versus double intensive therapy in untreated multiple myeloma: final analysis of the HOVON 24 trial. Blood. 2005;106(11):2545.
70. Cavo M, Tosi P, Zamagni E, Cellini C, Tacchetti P, Patriarca F, et al. Prospective, randomized study of single compared with double autologous stem-cell transplantation for multiple myeloma: bologna 96 clinical study. J Clin Oncol. 2007;25(17):2434–41.
71. Stadtmauer EA, Pasquini MC, Blackwell B, Knust K, Bashey A, Devine SM, et al. Comparison of autologous hematopoietic cell transplant (autoHCT), bortezomib, lenalidomide (Len) and dexamethasone (RVD) consolidation with len maintenance (ACM), tandem autohct with len maintenance (TAM) and autohct with len maintenance (AM) for up-front treatment of patients with multiple myeloma (MM): primary results from the randomized phase III trial of the blood and marrow transplant clinical trials network (BMT CTN 0702—StaMINA Trial). Blood. 2016;128(22):LBA-1.
72. Cavo M, Petrucci MT, Di Raimondo F, Zamagni E, Gamberi B, Crippa C, et al. Upfront single versus double autologous stem cell transplantation for newly diagnosed multiple myeloma: an intergroup, multicenter, phase III study of the European myeloma network (EMN02/HO95 MM trial). Blood. 2016;128(22):991.
73. Lonial S, Kaufman J, Tighiouart M, Nooka A, Langston AA, Heffner LT, et al. A phase I/II trial combining high-dose melphalan and autologous transplant with bortezomib for multiple myeloma: a dose- and schedule-finding study. Clin Cancer Res. 2010;16(20):5079–86.

74. Roussel M, Moreau P, Huynh A, Mary JY, Danho C, Caillot D, et al. Bortezomib and high-dose melphalan as conditioning regimen before autologous stem cell transplantation in patients with de novo multiple myeloma: a phase 2 study of the Intergroupe Francophone du Myelome (IFM). Blood. 2010;115(1):32–7.
75. Blanes M, Lahuerta JJ, Gonzalez JD, Ribas P, Solano C, Alegre A, et al. Intravenous busulfan and melphalan as a conditioning regimen for autologous stem cell transplantation in patients with newly diagnosed multiple myeloma: a matched comparison to a melphalan-only approach. Biol Blood Marrow Transplant. 2013;19(1):69–74.
76. Lahuerta JJ, Mateos MV, Martinez-Lopez J, Grande C, de la Rubia J, Rosinol L, et al. Busulfan 12 mg/kg plus melphalan 140 mg/m^2 versus melphalan 200 mg/m^2 as conditioning regimens for autologous transplantation in newly diagnosed multiple myeloma patients included in the PETHEMA/GEM2000 study. Haematologica. 2010;95(11):1913–20.
77. Costa LJ, Nista EJ, Buadi FK, Lacy MQ, Dispenzieri A, Kramer CP, et al. Prediction of poor mobilization of autologous CD34+ cells with growth factor in multiple myeloma patients: implications for risk-stratification. Biol Blood Marrow Transplant. 2014;20(2):222–8.
78. Kumar SK, Mikhael J, Laplant B, Lacy MQ, Buadi FK, Dingli D, et al. Phase 2 trial of intravenously administered plerixafor for stem cell mobilization in patients with multiple myeloma following lenalidomide-based initial therapy. Bone Marrow Transplant. 2014;49(2):201–5.
79. Chaudhary L, Awan F, Cumpston A, Leadmon S, Watkins K, Tse W, et al. Peripheral blood stem cell mobilization in multiple myeloma patients treat in the novel therapy-era with plerixafor and G-CSF has superior efficacy but significantly higher costs compared to mobilization with low-dose cyclophosphamide and G-CSF. J Clin Apher. 2013;28(5):359–67.
80. Gertz MA, Dingli D. How we manage autologous stem cell transplantation for patients with multiple myeloma. Blood. 2014;124(6):882–90.
81. Garban F, Attal M, Michallet M, Hulin C, Bourhis JH, Yakoub-Agha I, et al. Prospective comparison of autologous stem cell transplantation followed by dose-reduced allograft (IFM99-03 trial) with tandem autologous stem cell transplantation (IFM99-04 trial) in high-risk de novo multiple myeloma. Blood. 2006;107(9):3474–80.
82. Bruno B, Rotta M, Patriarca F, Mordini N, Allione B, Carnevale-Schianca F, et al. A comparison of allografting with autografting for newly diagnosed myeloma. N Engl J Med. 2007;356(11):1110–20.
83. Rosinol L, Perez-Simon JA, Sureda A, de la Rubia J, de Arriba F, Lahuerta JJ, et al. A prospective PETHEMA study of tandem autologous transplantation versus autograft followed by reduced-intensity conditioning allogeneic transplantation in newly diagnosed multiple myeloma. Blood. 2008;112(9):3591–3.
84. Krishnan A, Pasquini MC, Logan B, Stadtmauer EA, Vesole DH, Alyea E 3rd, et al. Autologous haemopoietic stem-cell transplantation followed by allogeneic or autologous haemopoietic stem-cell transplantation in patients with multiple myeloma (BMT CTN 0102): a phase 3 biological assignment trial. Lancet Oncol. 2011;12(13):1195–203.
85. Palumbo A, Gay F, Cavallo F, Raimondo FD, Larocca A, Hardan I, et al. Continuous therapy versus fixed duration of therapy in patients with newly diagnosed multiple myeloma. J Clin Oncol. 2015;33(30):3459–66.
86. McCarthy PL, Holstein SA. Role of stem cell transplant and maintenance therapy in plasma cell disorders. Hematology American Society of Hematology Education. Program. 2016;2016(1):504–11.
87. Berenson JR, Crowley JJ, Grogan TM, Zangmeister J, Briggs AD, Mills GM, et al. Maintenance therapy with alternate-day prednisone improves survival in multiple myeloma patients. Blood. 2002;99(9):3163–8.
88. Fritz E, Ludwig H. Interferon-alpha treatment in multiple myeloma: meta-analysis of 30 randomised trials among 3948 patients. Ann Oncol. 2000;11(11):1427–36.
89. Myeloma Trialists' Collaborative Group. Interferon as therapy for multiple myeloma: an individual patient data overview of 24 randomized trials and 4012 patients. Br J Haematol. 2001;113(4):1020–34.
90. Attal M, Harousseau JL, Leyvraz S, Doyen C, Hulin C, Benboubker L, et al. Maintenance therapy with thalidomide improves survival in patients with multiple myeloma. Blood. 2006;108(10):3289–94.
91. Barlogie B, Pineda-Roman M, van Rhee F, Haessler J, Anaissie E, Hollmig K, et al. Thalidomide arm of total therapy 2 improves complete remission duration and survival in myeloma patients with metaphase cytogenetic abnormalities. Blood. 2008;112(8):3115–21.
92. Palumbo A, Bringhen S, Liberati AM, Caravita T, Falcone A, Callea V, et al. Oral melphalan, prednisone, and thalidomide in elderly patients with multiple myeloma: updated results of a randomized controlled trial. Blood. 2008;112(8):3107–14.
93. Lokhorst HM, van der Holt B, Zweegman S, Vellenga E, Croockewit S, van Oers MH, et al. A randomized phase 3 study on the effect of thalidomide combined with adriamycin, dexamethasone, and high-dose melphalan, followed by thalidomide maintenance in patients with multiple myeloma. Blood. 2010;115(6):1113–20.
94. Ludwig H, Adam Z, Tothova E, Hajek R, Labar B, Egyed M, et al. Thalidomide maintenance treatment increases progression-free but not overall survival in elderly patients with myeloma. Haematologica. 2010;95(9):1548–54.
95. Maiolino A, Hungria VT, Garnica M, Oliveira-Duarte G, Oliveira LC, Mercante DR, et al. Thalidomide plus dexamethasone as a maintenance therapy after autologous hematopoietic stem cell transplantation improves progression-free survival in multiple myeloma. Am J Hematol. 2012;87(10):948–52.
96. Morgan GJ, Gregory WM, Davies FE, Bell SE, Szubert AJ, Brown JM, et al. The role of maintenance thalidomide therapy in multiple myeloma: MRC Myeloma IX results and meta-analysis. Blood. 2012;119(1):7–15.
97. Stewart AK, Trudel S, Bahlis NJ, White D, Sabry W, Belch A, et al. A randomized phase 3 trial of thalidomide and prednisone as maintenance therapy after ASCT in patients with MM with a quality-of-life assessment: the National Cancer Institute of Canada Clinicals trials group myeloma 10 trial. Blood. 2013;121(9):1517–23.
98. Wang Y, Yang F, Shen Y, Zhang W, Wang J, Chang VT, Andersson BS, Qazilbash MH, Champlin RE, Berenson JR, Guan X, Wang ML. Maintenance Therapy With Immunomodulatory Drugs in Multiple Myeloma: A Meta-Analysis and Systematic Review. J Natl Cancer Inst. 2015;108(3):pii:djv342. doi: https://doi.org/10.1093/jnci/djv342. Print 2016 Mar. Review. PubMed PMID: 26582244.
99. Morgan GJ, Davies FE, Gregory WM, Bell SE, Szubert AJ, Cook G, et al. Long-term follow-up of MRC myeloma IX trial: survival outcomes with bisphosphonate and thalidomide treatment. Clin Cancer Res. 2013;19(21):6030–8.
100. McCarthy PL, Owzar K, Hofmeister CC, Hurd DD, Hassoun H, Richardson PG, et al. Lenalidomide after stem-cell transplantation for multiple myeloma. N Engl J Med. 2012;366(19):1770–81.
101. Attal M, Lauwers-Cances V, Marit G, Caillot D, Moreau P, Facon T, et al. Lenalidomide maintenance after stem-cell transplantation for multiple myeloma. N Engl J Med. 2012;366(19):1782–91.
102. Abonour R, Durie BGM, Jagannath S, Shah JJ, Narang M, Terebelo HR, et al. Health-related quality of life of patients with newly diagnosed multiple myeloma receiving any or lenalidomide

maintenance after autologous stem cell transplant in the Connect® MM disease registry. Blood. 2016;128(22):537.

103. Sonneveld P, Salwender H-J, Van Der Holt B, el Jarari L, Bertsch U, Blau IW, et al. Bortezomib induction and maintenance in patients with newly diagnosed multiple myeloma: long-term follow-up of the HOVON-65/GMMG-HD4 trial. Blood. 2015;126(23):27.
104. Manasanch EE, Orlowski RZ. Proteasome inhibitors in cancer therapy. Nat Rev Clin Oncol. 2017;14:417.
105. Cavo M, Pantani L, Petrucci MT, Patriarca F, Zamagni E, Donnarumma D, et al. Bortezomib-thalidomide-dexamethasone is superior to thalidomide-dexamethasone as consolidation therapy after autologous hematopoietic stem cell transplantation in patients with newly diagnosed multiple myeloma. Blood. 2012;120(1):9–19.
106. Mellqvist UH, Gimsing P, Hjertner O, Lenhoff S, Laane E, Remes K, et al. Bortezomib consolidation after autologous stem cell transplantation in multiple myeloma: a Nordic myeloma study group randomized phase 3 trial. Blood. 2013;121(23):4647–54.
107. Straka C, Vogel M, Müller J, Kropff M, Metzner B, Langer C, et al. Results from two phase III studies of bortezomib (BTZ) consolidation vs observation (OBS) post-transplant in patients (pts) with newly diagnosed multiple myeloma (NDMM). J Clin Oncol. 2015;33(Suppl 15):8511.
108. Delforge M, Blade J, Dimopoulos MA, Facon T, Kropff M, Ludwig H, et al. Treatment-related peripheral neuropathy in multiple myeloma: the challenge continues. Lancet Oncol. 2010;11(11):1086–95.
109. Moreau P, Pylypenko H, Grosicki S, Karamanesht I, Leleu X, Grishunina M, et al. Subcutaneous versus intravenous administration of bortezomib in patients with relapsed multiple myeloma: a randomised, phase 3, non-inferiority study. Lancet Oncol. 2011;12(5):431–40.
110. Cavaletti G, Jakubowiak AJ. Peripheral neuropathy during bortezomib treatment of multiple myeloma: a review of recent studies. Leuk Lymphoma. 2010;51(7):1178–87.
111. Chanan-Khan A, Sonneveld P, Schuster MW, Stadtmauer EA, Facon T, Harousseau JL, et al. Analysis of herpes zoster events among bortezomib-treated patients in the phase III APEX study. J Clin Oncol. 2008;26(29):4784–90.
112. Palumbo A, Rajkumar SV, Dimopoulos MA, Richardson PG, San Miguel J, Barlogie B, et al. Prevention of thalidomide- and lenalidomide-associated thrombosis in myeloma. Leukemia. 2008;22(2):414–23.
113. Terpos E, Berenson J, Raje N, Roodman GD. Management of bone disease in multiple myeloma. Expert Rev Hematol. 2014;7(1):113–25.
114. Berenson JR, Lichtenstein A, Porter L, Dimopoulos MA, Bordoni R, George S, et al. Efficacy of pamidronate in reducing skeletal events in patients with advanced multiple myeloma. Myeloma Aredia Study Group. N Engl J Med. 1996;334(8):488–93.
115. Major P, Lortholary A, Hon J, Abdi E, Mills G, Menssen HD, et al. Zoledronic acid is superior to pamidronate in the treatment of hypercalcemia of malignancy: a pooled analysis of two randomized, controlled clinical trials. J Clin Oncol. 2001;19(2):558–67.
116. Morgan GJ, Davies FE, Gregory WM, Cocks K, Bell SE, Szubert AJ, et al. First-line treatment with zoledronic acid as compared with clodronic acid in multiple myeloma (MRC myeloma IX): a randomised controlled trial. Lancet (London, England). 2010;376(9757):1989–99.
117. Osterborg A, Boogaerts MA, Cimino R, Essers U, Holowiecki J, Juliusson G, et al. Recombinant human erythropoietin in transfusion-dependent anemic patients with multiple myeloma and non-Hodgkin's lymphoma—a randomized multicenter study. The European Study Group of Erythropoietin (Epoetin Beta) treatment in multiple myeloma and non-Hodgkin's lymphoma. Blood. 1996;87(7):2675–82.
118. Ludwig H, Fritz E, Kotzmann H, Hocker P, Gisslinger H, Barnas U. Erythropoietin treatment of anemia associated with multiple myeloma. N Engl J Med. 1990;322(24):1693–9.
119. Lindsley H, Teller D, Noonan B, Peterson M, Mannik M. Hyperviscosity syndrome in multiple myeloma. A reversible, concentration-dependent aggregation of the myeloma protein. Am J Med. 1973;54(5):682–8.
120. Bridoux F, Pegourie B, Augeul-Meunier K, Royer B, Joly B, Lamy T, et al. Treatment of myeloma cast nephropathy (MCN): a randomized trial comparing intensive Haemodialysis (HD) with high cut-off (HCO) or standard high-flux dialyzer in patients receiving a Bortezomib-based regimen (the MYRE study, by the Intergroupe francophone du Myélome (IFM) and the French Society of Nephrology (SFNDT)). Blood. 2016;128(22):978.

29 Role of Hematopoietic Cell Transplantation for Myeloma

Heather Landau and Sergio Giralt

Introduction and Historical Perspective

More than 30 years ago McElwain and Powles demonstrated that dose intensification of melphalan could result in significant responses in patients with relapsed and refractory multiple myeloma (MM) [1]. However, significant myelosuppression occurred which limited the utility of this treatment strategy [2]. Barlogie et al. demonstrated that high-dose melphalan therapy followed by infusion of autologous bone marrow was feasible and resulted in predictable hematologic recovery within 28 days [3]. Subsequent confirmatory trials in the setting of relapsed disease were followed by the use of high-dose therapy (HDT) with autologous hematopoietic cell transplantation (HCT) as consolidation of initial remissions in patients with newly diagnosed MM [4–14]. Randomized trials in the front-line setting compared treatment outcomes of patients receiving multiagent chemotherapy regimens (usually combinations of vinca alkaloids, anthracyclines, alkylators, nitrosoureas, and steroids) to patients who received consolidation with HDT and auto-HCT [7–14]. The preponderance of evidence showed that HDT was associated with improved outcomes including event-free (EFS), progression-free (PFS), and in some but not all studies overall survival (OS) [7–14]. Depth of response, particularly achievement of a complete response (CR), was associated with longer PFS and OS in MM and was likely responsible for the initial success of HDT and autologous HCT [15].

The advent of proteasome inhibitors (bortezomib and carfilzomib) and the immunomodulatory (IMID) drugs (thalidomide and lenalidomide) have rendered all prior randomized trials of HDT versus chemotherapy in MM less relevant since induction therapy with these agents has been shown to be associated with more frequent and deeper responses than the traditional vincristine, adriamycin, and dexamethasone (VAD) induction [16]. In this chapter we review the basics of HCT for myeloma, current results, and future direction of this important treatment modality.

Basics of Hematopoietic Cell Transplantation (HCT) for Myeloma [17]

HCT is a complex procedure. The patient receives a combination of chemical and physical agents to eliminate a malignant disorder or a poorly functioning bone marrow supported by reinfusion of HSC from the patient or a third-party source (related or unrelated). As with solid organ transplantation HCT candidates should meet a set of organ function and psychosocial criteria that may vary from transplant center to transplant center but are aimed at determining the risk-benefit ratio of HCT versus other treatment approaches.

Depending on the source of stem cells, HCT can be categorized as either autologous (hematopoietic stem cells (HSCs) are obtained from patient) or allogeneic (HSCs are obtained from a third party). HSCs can be obtained from the marrow cavity or can be mobilized in large quantities into the peripheral blood using medications such as filgrastim or plerixafor and collected through apheresis techniques.

Transplant Eligibility

MM is the most common indication for autologous HCT in the world today with more than 6000 procedures performed in the United States every year [18]. Which MM patient is an appropriate candidate for HCT has been a subject of continued discussion in the HCT and MM literature. Table 29.1 lists the current criteria being utilized to determine HCT eligibility for both autologous and allogeneic HCT in MM patients according to recently published guidelines from the American Society of Blood and Marrow Transplantation (ASBMT) [19].

H. Landau, M.D.
Adult BMT Service, Memorial Sloan Kettering Cancer Center, New York City, NY, USA

S. Giralt, M.D. (✉)
Chief, Adult Bone Marrow Transplant Service,
Memorial Sloan Kettering Cancer Center, New York, NY, USA
e-mail: giralts@mskcc.org

P.H. Wiernik et al. (eds.), *Neoplastic Diseases of the Blood*, DOI 10.1007/978-3-319-64263-5_29

Table 29.1 Criteria used to determine HCT eligibility for MM

Criteria	Autologous HCT	Allogeneic HCT	Comments and references
Age	No age limit but rarely performed over age 80	No age limit but rarely performed over age 70	[18–20]
Performance status	KPS $\geq$ 70	KPS $\geq$ 80	[18, 21]
HCT-CI	No limit	≤ 1	Patients with KPS < 80 and high HCT-CI should be considered for alternative therapies rather than autologous HCT
Response to therapy	At least a PR	At least a PR	Patients with "primary" refractory disease are an exception for autologous HCT
Social support	Required	Required	Older myeloma patients undergoing HCT may require help for activities of daily living during the early post-HCT period to ensure compliance with medications and adequate hydration and nutrition
Patient wishes	Required	Required	

Initially limited to younger patients (less than 65 years of age), multiple retrospective analyses have demonstrated that outcomes for patients over the age of 65 are not statistically significantly different than outcomes for younger patients and thus age alone should not be considered a contraindication for HCT [20–24]. Notwithstanding, few autografts are performed in patients over the age of 80 and few allografts for MM are performed in patients over 70 years of age.

The hematopoietic cell transplantation comorbidity index (HCT-CI) developed by Sorror et al. to predict nonrelapse mortality after allogeneic HCT incorporates various measurements of organ function (cardiac, pulmonary, renal, hepatic) together with existence of other comorbidities into one score. Patients with HCT-CI scores of 0 to 1 have significantly less NRM than those with scores of 2 or greater with either a myeloablative or reduced-intensity conditioning regimen (RIC) [25].

The HCT-CI has been validated in the setting of autologous HCT and is a valuable tool to determine the risk–benefit ratio of this procedure. The Center for International Blood and Marrow Transplant Research (CIBMTR) recently analyzed the outcomes of 1156 MM patients reported to the registry who underwent auto-HCT after high-dose melphalan. NRM rates were similar for patients with HCT-CI scores of 0 to 1 versus 2 or greater and were 2%. However, on multivariate analysis, OS was inferior in groups with HCT-CI score of 1 to 2 (relative risk, 1.37, [95% CI, 1.01 to 1.87]; $P = 0.04$) and HCT-CI score of greater than 2 (relative risk,1.5 [95% CI, 1.09–2.08]; $P = 0.01$). OS was also inferior with Karnofsky performance status <90 ($P < 0.001$) [26]. Patients with KPS of less than 80 and high HCT-CI had 100-day NRM rates after HDT with autologous HCT of approximately 10%. Therefore the risk–benefit ratio of HDT should be balanced against the benefits of continued nontransplant therapies. In general, for older patients with high HCT-CI and KPS of less than 80 we have recommended proceeding to autologous HCT only if they have failed to achieve at least a very good partial response (VGPR) to induction therapy. End-stage renal disease is not an absolute contraindication to HCT in MM with many centers routinely performing autografting for MM in patient dialysis [27, 28].

Although response to induction therapy has been associated with HCT outcomes most retrospective data suggests that patients with primary induction failure (i.e., less than a partial response to induction therapy) still benefit from HDT with autologous HCT [29–32]. Whether this still holds true for patients failing modern induction therapy is uncertain but retrospective analysis of CIBMTR data suggests that although additional lines of therapy may improve response prior to autologous HCT this did not result in improved outcomes over proceeding directly to HDT [33].

Stem Cell Procurement

Autologous HSCs for MM patients are most frequently obtained through peripheral blood stem cell mobilization utilizing either chemotherapy in combinations with cytokines or cytokines alone. In North America autologous HSC mobilization is most commonly performed with granulocyte colony-stimulating factor (GCSF-filgrastim) alone or in combination with the CXCR4 antagonist plerixafor [34, 35]. In a randomized trial the combination of plerixafor and GCSF resulted in significant improvement in stem cell collection yields a total of 106 of 148 (71.6%) patients in the plerixafor group and 53 of 154 (34.4%) patients in the placebo group met the primary endpoint ($P < 0.001$). A total of 54% of plerixafor-treated patients reached target after one apheresis, whereas 56% of the placebo-treated patients required four aphereses to reach target [36]. Because of cost considerations many centers only use plerixafor in the event that CD34 peripheral blood counts are low (usually less than 10 CD34 cells/microliter) after 4 days of filgrastim therapy. This "just-in-time" plerixafor strategy has been shown to be cost effective [37]. A number of risk factors for poor mobilization in MM patients have been described and are summarized in Table 29.2.

Conditioning Regimen

The conditioning regimen is the combination of agents given to eliminate malignant cells exploiting the dose–response phenomena that most cancer cells exhibit and in the setting of allogeneic SCT suppress the host immune system to allow engraftment of donor cells. For allogeneic HCT conditioning regimen intensity has been classified according to their myelosuppressive effects into myeloablative, reduced intensity, and non-myeloablative [17].

For MM the most commonly utilized conditioning regimen for autologous HCT is melphalan 200 mg/m^2 throughout the world. Moreau et al. performed the only randomized trial comparing melphalan 200 mg/m^2 to melphalan and total-body irradiation. A total of 282 evaluable patients were randomized. The median duration of event-free survival was similar in both arms (21 vs. 20.5 months, $P = 0.6$), but the 45-month survival was 65.8% for high-dose melphalan and 45.5% for melphalan and total-body irradiation (TBI) ($P = 0.05$) [38]. The addition of busulfan or bortezomib to the standard melphalan has in retrospective analysis been proposed as potentially superior than high-dose melphalan but prospective comparative trials need to be done [39–42].

For allogeneic HCT, RIC is the most frequently utilized unless in the context of a CD34 selected peripheral blood stem cell graft (PBSC) [43]. However, the role of myeloablative conditioning for allografting continues to be explored particularly in the context of CD34 selected allografts [44].

Table 29.2 Risk factors for poor mobilization in myeloma patient

Patient factors	Treatment factors	Procedure factors
Age—older age reduces mobilization yields	Treatment with melphalan or bendamustine	Poor catheter flow
Extent of marrow infiltration	More than four cycles of lenalidomide	Low apheresis volumes
Platelet count (measurement of marrow reserve)	Radiation to pelvis- or marrow-bearing bones	
	Extensive prior therapy	

Complications of High-Dose Therapy in Myeloma

HDT is associated with significant morbidity due to the effects of intense myelosuppression and the effects of the conditioning regimen on normal tissues. The HCT procedure can be divided into five phases [17]:

Phase I: Chemotherapy phase
Phase II: Cytopenic phase
Phase III: Early recovery phase
Phase IV: Early convalescence phase
Phase V: Late convalescence

Although considered the least intense and less toxic of all conditioning regimens high-dose melphalan is associated with a variety of complications that are summarized in Table 29.3.

Despite being associated with low mortality rates (less than 3%), high-dose melphalan is associated with significant morbidity and a high treatment-related symptom burden as documented by Campagnaro et al. Fatigue, insomnia, loss of appetite, weakness, and feeling sick were the most common described symptoms that interfered with patients' quality of life and activity level. The peak symptom burden

Table 29.3 Randomized trials of early vs. delayed HCT in up-front therapy for myeloma

Author (ref)	*N*	Median PFS	OS at 4 years	Comments
Palumbo (2014)	273	HDT 43.3 months No HDT 22.4 months	HDT 81.6% No HDT 65.3%	No proteosome inhibitor Second randomization to lenalidomide maintenance
Gay (2015)	389	HDT 43.3 months No HDT 28.6 months	HDT 77% No HDT 68%	No proteosome inhibitor exposure
Attal (2015)	700	HDT Not reached 61% at 3 years Delayed HDT 46% at 3 years	3-year OS 88% for both groups	
Sonneveld (2016)	1510	HDT Not reached No HDT 44 months	HDT Not reached No HDT Not reached No difference	Induction CyBorD Consolidation VMP All groups benefitted from HCT

occurred at the time of white blood cell count nadir and approximately a third of the patients had not recovered to baseline a month posttransplant [45]. Increased plasma levels of interleukin 6 have been correlated with increasing symptom burden and could be a potential target for reduction of symptom burden [46].

Current Controversies in HCT for Myeloma

Optimal Induction Regimen

The optimal induction regimen should be effective, well tolerated, spare hematopoietic stem cell, and not negatively impact HDT outcomes. A detailed discussion of optimal induction therapy for MM patients is addressed in other chapters of this book. In brief, randomized trials have demonstrated that for transplant-eligible patients optimal induction therapy will include a IMID (thalidomide or lenalidomide) and a proteosome inhibitor (bortezomib or carfilzomib). Deeper and quicker responses are typically achieved with three-drug regimens such as thalidomide-bortezomib-dexamethasone (VTD), cyclophosphamide-bortezomib-dexamethasone (CyBorD), bortezomib-adriamycin-dexamethasone (PAD), or lenalidomide-bortezomib-dexamethasone (VRD) versus two-drug regimens, thalidomide-dexamethasone (TD), lenalidomide-dexamethasone (RD), or bortezomib-dexamethasone (VD) although the impact on OS has not been established until recently. In the United States the most commonly used induction regimens are the combination of RVD or CyBorD [47].

Carfilzomib-based combinations are emerging as some of the most potent induction regimens in MM. Carfilzomib has been combined with lenalidomide-dexamethasone (CRD), and in 53 newly diagnosed patients with MM, 38% achieved at least a near-complete response (nCR) after four cycles [27]. Stem cells were successfully collected in 34/35 patients. CRD was well tolerated with minimal neuropathy, allowing for prolonged administration with deeper responses over time. After a median of 24 cycles and 47.5 months of follow-up the 4-year PFS was 64% with a 93% OS rate [48]. Subsequently 76 patients received the same induction for four cycles and underwent autologous HCT after high-dose melphalan consolidation followed by CRD consolidation and prolonged maintenance. Median age was 59 years (range 40–76), with 57% of patients with ISS stage II/III and 36% with high-risk cytogenetics. Response rates after four cycles of CRD consolidation post-auto-HCT were 96% VGPR, 73% CR, and 69% sCR. Among CR patients tested 82% of them were MRD negative by flow and 66% by next-generation sequencing (NGS). With a median follow-up of 17.5 months 2-year PFS was 97% and 2-year OS was 99% for all 76 patients. These excellent results need to be confirmed and compared head to head with bortezomib, lenalidomide, and dexamethasone before CRD can be considered standard of care. CRD was well tolerated with few grade 3 or 4 toxicities generally lymphopenia (28%), neutropenia (18%), and infections (8%). Only two patients were reported to have an asymptomatic decrease of ejection fraction to 45–50%.

Timing of HCT

The achievement of major responses (CR and VGPRs) to induction therapy with IMIDs and proteasome inhibitors, especially in combination, has called into question the role of HDT and HCT as consolidation of first remission for all patients with MM. Yet, even in the context of modern induction regimens where over 90% respond the quality of response continues to improve following HCT and PFS approaches or exceeds 3 years [15, 16]. Four large randomized trials have now been performed comparing early versus delayed HCT in the context of modern induction treatment and are summarized in Table 29.4.

Palumbo et al. randomized 273 newly diagnosed MM patients to receive an autologous HCT after melphalan at a

Table 29.4 Common toxicities associated with high-dose melphalan

Toxicity	Incidence	Time peak occurrence	Preventive measures
Cytopenias	100%	5–7 days post-HCT infusion	Filgrastim or Peg-filgrastim will reduce duration of neutropenia Transfusion support not universally required Cell dose of greater than 5 × 10^6 CD34+ cells not effective in reducing cytopenias
Mucositis	30%	5–7 days post-infusion	Cryotherapy effective in reducing incidence of severe mucositis Keratinocyte growth factor not effective nor indicated Incidence increases with prior exposure to cytotoxic chemotherapy
Infections	40–50%	During cytopenic fever	Neutropenic fever common Severe sepsis and life-threatening infections rare. HSV reactivation rare with acyclovir prophylaxis CMV reactivation rare (<5%), thus monitoring not indicated Fungal infection rare, but fluconazole prophylaxis during neutropenia required

dose of 200 mg/m^2 or continued treatment with melphalan-prednisone-lenalidomide (MPR) followed by a second randomization to lenalidomide maintenance therapy. After a median follow-up of 51.2 months the PFS was significantly longer with high-dose melphalan plus HCT compared to MPR (43.0 months vs. 22.4 months $P < 0.001$). Overall survival at 4 years was also superior for high-dose melphalan and auto-HCT (81.6% vs. 65.3%; $P = 0.02$). Median progression-free survival was significantly longer with lenalidomide maintenance than with no maintenance (41.9 months vs. 21.6 months; $P < 0.001$), but 3-year overall survival was not significantly prolonged (88.0% vs. 79.2%) [49].

Gay et al. recently reported on 389 newly diagnosed MM patients less than 65 years of age receiving induction with four 28-day cycles of lenalidomide (25 mg, days 1–21) and dexamethasone (40 mg, days 1, 8, 15, and 22). Patients were randomized to consolidation with either chemotherapy plus lenalidomide (six cycles of cyclophosphamide [300 mg/m^2, days 1, 8, and 15], dexamethasone [40 mg, days 1, 8, 15, and 22], and lenalidomide [25 mg, days 1–21]) or two courses of high-dose melphalan (200 mg/m^2) and auto-HCT with a second randomization to maintenance with lenalidomide (10 mg, days 1–21) plus prednisone (50 mg, every other day) or lenalidomide alone. With a median follow-up of 52 months PFS was significantly shorter with chemotherapy plus lenalidomide compared with high-dose melphalan and ASCT (median 28·6 months vs. 43·3 months $P < 0·0001$). Fewer grade 3 or 4 adverse events were recorded with chemotherapy plus lenalidomide than with high-dose melphalan and HCT. At 4 years, overall survival was 86% for autologous HCT with lenalidomide maintenance vs. 73% with chemotherapy plus lenalidomide maintenance [50].

The Intergroup Francophone du Myeloma-Dana-Farber Cancer Institute (IFM-DFCI) study of bortezomib, lenalidomide, and dexamethasone with or without high-dose melphalan consolidation and HCT was presented in December of 2015 at the American Society of Hematology meeting. A total of 700 patients were randomized to receive either eight cycles of RVD followed by lenalidomide maintenance or three cycles of the same induction followed by high-dose melphalan consolidation and followed by two cycles of the same chemo as consolidation with subsequent lenalidomide maintenance. With a median follow-up of 39 months HCT improved the complete response rate (58% vs. 46%) and 3-year PFS from 48% in the delayed HCT arm to 61% in the early HCT arm ($P < 0.0002$). The PFS benefit was observed in all subgroups. The 3-year post-randomization OS rate of overall survival was 88% in both groups [51].

Cavo et al. recently updated the results of EMN02/HO95 MM Trial in which patients were randomized to either four 42-day cycles of bortezomib-melphalan-prednisone (VMP) vs. either a single course or two sequential courses of melphalan at 200 mg/m^2 (HDM) with autologous stem cell support. All patients received induction therapy with CyBorD for 3–4 cycles. A second randomization to consolidation therapy with RVD vs. no consolidation was performed after intensification, to be followed by lenalidomide maintenance until progression or toxicity in both arms. From February 2011 to April 2014, 1510 patients 65 years or less were registered. Of these, 1192 were randomly assigned to receive either VMP ($n = 497$ patients) or HDM (1 ± 2 courses) ($n = 695$ patients). Median age was 58 years in both groups, ISS stage III was 21% in VMP and 20% in HDM, while revised ISS stage III was 9% in both groups. With a median follow-up from registration of 26 months median PFS was 44 months in the VMP arm and was not yet reached in the HDM arm; 3-year estimates of PFS were 57.5% and 66%, respectively ($P = 0.003$). PFS benefit with HDM was retained across predefined subgroups, including patients with ISS stage, cytogenetic risk category. The probability of achieving a very good partial response or higher quality response was 85.5% in the HDM group vs. 74% in the VMP group ($P < 0.001$). In a multivariate Cox regression analysis stratified by ISS, randomization to HDM and absence of high-risk cytogenetic abnormalities were the most important independent predictors of prolonged PFS. No difference in OS has been seen among the groups but the limited follow-up and small numbers of events make any conclusions difficult at this time [52].

Role of Tandem Transplants

Two studies have suggested that two courses of high-dose melphalan are superior to a single SCT, but the benefit appears to be limited to patients who had not achieved VGPR after the first transplant [53, 54]. Neither of these studies included induction therapies with either an IMID or a proteasome inhibitor and therefore may not be relevant today. More recently, patients who received bortezomib-based induction therapy and either single or double SCT on European phase III trials were analyzed. In comparison with patients for whom a single SCT was planned by study design, those who were assigned to receive tandem SCT had significantly longer PFS (median: 38 vs. 50 months, $P < 0.001$) and OS (5-year estimates: 63% vs. 75%, $P = 0.002$). From this dataset, the benefit of tandem ASCT was greatest for patients with high-risk cytogenetics defined as t(4;14) and/or del 17p and also for those who had not attained CR following bortezomib-based induction [55].

More recently, Cavo et al. presented the first interim analysis of the European Myeloma Network 02 (EMN02). Six hundred and fourteen eligible patients who received the diagnosis of MM in centers with a double-intensification policy were randomly assigned to either VMP ($n = 199$) or to a single ($n = 208$) or a tandem ($n = 207$). With similar patient and disease characteristics and a median follow-up of

27 months the median PFS was 45 months in the single-HCT group and has not been reached in the tandem HCT group. Three-year PFS were 60% and 73%, respectively ($P = 0.030$). Tandem HCT was found to be associated with an increased PFS in all predefined subgroups. In a multivariate Cox regression analysis stratified by ISS stage, randomization to tandem HCT and high-risk cytogenetics (any of the five pre-specified abnormalities) were the leading independent predictors of PFS. No difference in OS was seen between the two treatment groups [56].

In contrast the Blood and Marrow Transplant Clinical Trials Network (BMT-CTN) StAMINA Trial randomized 758 patients to one of the three consolidation strategies after an initial melphalan 200 mg/m^2 autologous HCT. A third of the patients ($n = 254$) received four cycles of consolidation with RVD, another third ($n = 247$) underwent a second autograft also with melphalan 200 mg/m^2, and the last third ($n = 257$) received no further consolidation. All three groups received lenalidomide maintenance 5–15 mg daily. At 38 months post-randomization the PFS was 52% for lenalidomide maintenance, 57% for RVD consolidation, and 56% for tandem transplant. OS at 38 months was excellent in all three groups (83, 86, and 82%). It is important to note that in the BMT CTN trial 32% of patients randomized to the tandem transplant arm did not received their "per-protocol" therapy which could explain some of the differences with the HOVON EMN trial of Cavo et al. [57].

Role of Allogeneic HCT

Although a graft-versus-MM effect has been well documented allogeneic HCT as frontline therapy for MM should be limited to younger patients with very-high-risk features due to high treatment-related mortality (TRM) and the risk of graft-versus-host disease even with non-myeloablative regimens. The European Group for Blood and Marrow Transplantation Non-Myeloablative allogeneic stem cell transplantation in MM 2000 study compared tandem HCT and reduced-intensity conditioning (RIC) allogeneic transplantation to HCT (single or tandem optional) alone in 357 patients that were biologically randomized based on the availability of an HLA-identical sibling. At a median of 96 months of follow-up, PFS and OS were 22% and 49% vs. 12% ($P = 0.027$) and 36% ($P = 0.030$) with HCT/RIC allogeneic HCT and autologous HCT, respectively [58]. The largest study including 625 patients performed through the BMT-CTN biologically assigned patients to tandem ASCT or RIC allogeneic and showed that at 36 months of follow-up there was no difference in PFS or OS [59].

Two other prospective studies, from the HOVON and Italian Study groups with somewhat different trial designs, have failed to conclusively show a benefit for allogeneic HCT in the up-front treatment of MM despite some suggestion of a better outcome with RIC allogeneic SCT in the Italian study [60, 61]. However, the tandem HCT arm of that study has a curiously short survival (median 48 months). Recent registry data assessing the role of allogeneic HCT in over 1200 patients with MM reported 5-year PFS and OS of 14% and 29%, respectively, with older age, longer interval from diagnosis to transplantation, and unrelated donor grafts adversely affecting OS [62].

Role of Salvage HCT

With the increasing number of patients opting for delayed HCT the optimal treatment for patients relapsing after primary therapy that did not include HCT, re-induction treatment with combination chemotherapy is the standard and most experts agreed that high-dose therapy consolidation should be considered the standard of care for this patient population. Data from both the CIBMTR and the EBMT show increasing use of salvage HCT, but prospective trials are urgently needed in this setting [63].

Cook et al. reported the first prospective randomized trial studying autologous HCT versus less intensive alkylating agent consolidation (weekly cyclophosphamide). Patients were eligible if they had relapsed after an initial autologous HCT and had at least an 18-month remission. Re-induction therapy included bortezomib, doxorubicin, and dexamethasone induction therapy. Eligible patients (with adequate stem cell harvest) were randomly assigned (1:1) to either high-dose melphalan 200 mg/m^2 plus salvage HCT or oral cyclophosphamide (400 mg/m^2 per week for 12 weeks). Time to progression was longer for patients who underwent salvage HCT (19 vs. 11 months ($P < 0.0001$) [64].

Salvage allogeneic HCT is being routinely performed particularly in younger patients with either multiply relapsed MM or short initial remission after autologous HCT. Freytes et al. performed a large registry analysis comparing the outcomes of a second autotransplant to those of a salvage allograft with a reduced-intensity conditioning regimen. NRM at 1 year after transplantation was higher in the allograft group 13% vs. 2%. Three-year PFS and OS were 6% and 20% for the allograft group and inferior to the outcomes for the autologous HCT 12% and 46%, respectively. [65]. In contrast, Patriarca et al. analyzed outcomes in patients relapsing after an initial autograft. The 2-year NRM was 22% among the 75 patients who had an identified HLA-compatible donor (donor group) versus 1% for those without a donor (no-donor group). The 2-year PFS was 42% in the donor group and 18% in the no-donor group ($P < 0.0001$) with similar 2-year OS of 54% and 53% for the donor and no donor groups, respectively [66].

De Lavallade et al. compared the outcomes of 32 relapsed MM patients. Nineteen had an HLA-identical sibling donor ("donor" group), while 13 patients had no donor ("no-donor" group). There were no significant differences between these two groups as for prognosis risk factors. With a median follow-up of 36 months, OS was similar between both groups; however, PFS was significantly higher in the "donor" group as compared to the "no-donor" group (46 vs. 8% at 3 years) [67].

Role of Maintenance Therapy and Consolidation Post-HCT

Post-HCT consolidation therapy was initially reported by Ladetto et al. who showed that four cycles of VTD consolidation following tandem HCT in patients with MM who achieved at least a VGPR ($N = 39$) increased the frequency of CR from 15 to 49% and molecular remissions from 3 to 18% [68].

Post-HCT consolidation has traditionally included similar drugs given during the induction phase. Cavo et al. reported on 480 newly diagnosed MM patients who received induction with VTD or TD that was followed by tandem HCT and two cycles of VTD or TD consolidation according to the induction arm [69]. Following HCT, the CR rate was 61% after VTD and 47% after TD consolidation ($P = 0.012$). To date, PFS but not OS is longer in the VTD arm.

The Nordic Myeloma Study Group randomized 370 bortezomib-naïve patients to 20 weekly doses of bortezomib or no consolidation at 3 months post-transplantation [70]. Again, response rates improved in patients who received consolidation with 71% vs. 57%, ($P < 0.01$) achieving at least VGPR and PFS was extended (27 vs. 20 months, $P = 0.05$), but the advantage was only seen in patients with <VGPR after HCT. There was no difference in OS between the groups. In contrast, the BMT-CTN StAMINA trial did not show a benefit for RVD consolidation followed by lenalidomide maintenance when compared to lenalidomide alone [57].

An extensive review of the different strategies and drugs tried as maintenance therapy after autologous HCT is beyond the scope of this chapter. Table 29.5 summarizes the three randomized trials demonstrating a PFS benefit for lenalidomide maintenance. The role of lenalidomide maintenance post-autologous HCT is fairly established [71–74]. The CALGB 100104 study examined 462 MM patients who were randomized to lenalidomide or placebo without consolidation until disease progression [71]. A significant increase in TTP was seen for patients in the lenalidomide arm compared with those receiving placebo (46 vs. 27 months, $P < 0.0001$). All patients benefitted from lenalidomide maintenance regardless of remission status or prior exposure to IMID therapy; at 48 months of follow-up despite crossover of 71% of placebo patients, the risk of death on lenalidomide maintenance is lower than on placebo (20% vs. 30%; $P = 0.008$) [71].

Table 29.5 Lenalidomide maintenance (versus placebo) following ASCT

	CALGB 100104 [71]	IFM 2005-02 [72]	RV-MMP 1209 [73]
N	460	614	200 (randomized to HCT)
Initial dosing	10 mg (5–15 mg) daily	10 mg (5–15 mg) daily	10 mg (5–15) 21/28 days
Duration	Until progression	24 months	Until progression
TTP/PFS	TTP: 46 vs. 27 months ($P < 0.001$)	PFS: 41 vs. 23 months ($P < 0.001$)	PFS 54.7 vs. 37.4 months
OS	3-year OS: 88% vs. 80% ($P = 0.028$)	5-year OS: 68% vs. 67%	5-year OS 78.4% vs. 66.6%
SPM total	18 vs. 6 cases	23 vs. 8 cases	11 cases (5 in lenalidomide)

The IFM 2005–02 trial reported on 614 patients who were randomized to lenalidomide or placebo after single (79%) or tandem (21%) and two cycles of lenalidomide consolidation [72]. Lenalidomide maintenance improved median PFS (41 months vs. 23 months) compared to placebo ($P < 0.001$). However, the 5 year post-randomization OS is similar (68% vs. 67%). A higher incidence of secondary primary malignancies (SPM) in the lenalidomide arm was detected in both studies.

Palumbo et al. randomized 200 patients who had been randomized to receive high-dose melphalan consolidation to lenalidomide maintenance given 21 out of 28 days. Similar to the other two trials a significant benefit on PFS was seen in patients randomized to the lenalidomide arm (54 vs. 37 months from diagnosis) but without an increase in SPM [73].

A recent meta-analysis of the three large randomized trials was recently presented at the American Society of Clinical Oncology Meeting in Chicago in July 2016. A total of 1209 patients were randomized from 2005 to 2009 to receive either lenalidomide or placebo. With a median follow-up of 6.6 years the median OS for lenalidomide maintenance had not been reached vs. 86 months for patients in the control arms ($p = 0.001$). All patients benefitted from lenalidomide maintenance regardless of response [74].

Future Directions

Despite doubling of the remission duration with post-autologous HCT lenalidomide maintenance, MM recurrence remains the most important cause of treatment failure. Depth of response has been shown to impact remission duration and survival; notwithstanding, even patients achieving a CR will relapse and progress [75, 76].

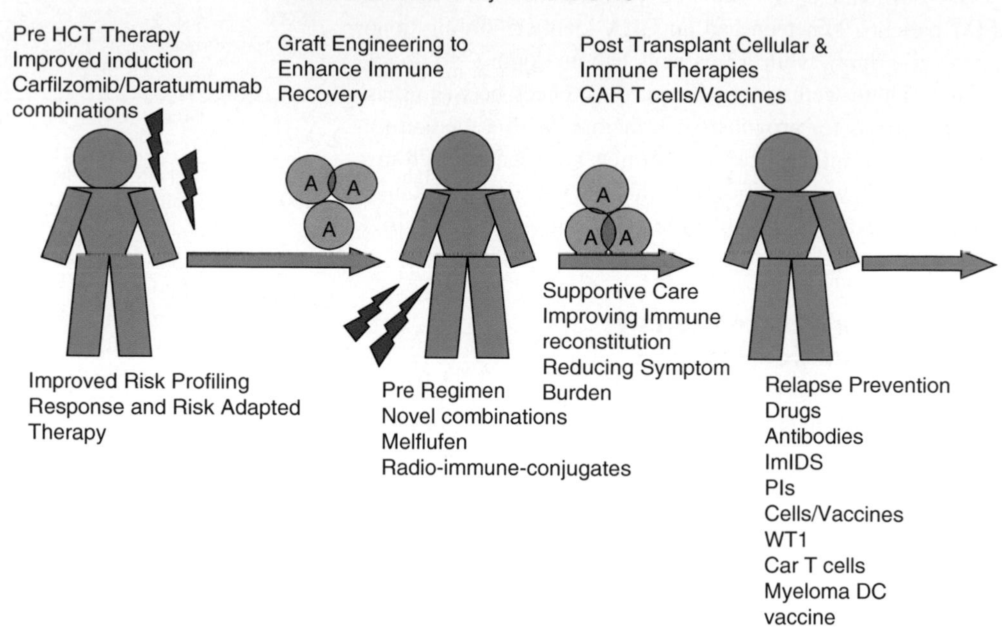

Fig. 29.1 Future directions in myeloma hematopoietic cell transplantation

Minimal residual disease detection (MRD) either by multiparameter flow cytometry (MFC) or next-generation sequencing (NGS) has been shown to be an important marker for long-term disease control in patients achieving a CR (reviewed in [77]).

Thus strategies aimed at increasing the proportion of patients that can attain an MRD-negative state are being actively explored and are summarized in Fig. 29.1. These include novel induction regimens incorporating carfilzomib and/or daratumumab as well as novel posttransplant immunotherapies such as CAR T cells, vaccines, and checkpoint blockade [78–81]. Likewise, incorporation of MRD assessment as part of a risk-adapted strategy was considered a "high-priority area to study" at the recent State of the Science Symposium of the BMT-CTN and will probably dictate treatment paradigms in the future [81–83].

As molecular techniques evolve, the goal is to individualize therapy based on predictive markers that provide insight into the likelihood of response and/or toxicity to certain drugs or regimens. Robust data already exists regarding the benefit of proteosome inhibition in the treatment of high-risk MM [84]. More recently, venetoclax a BCL 2 inhibitor has been shown to be extremely active in MM patients with the 11,14 translocation [85]. Thus the era of targeted therapies for specific MM subtypes has begun.

Finally, the burden of treatment both in regard to symptom burden cost of therapy will become a major issue in MM therapy and will be important endpoints to consider when choosing the treatment strategy that will provide patients with the longest life and the best quality of life with the least treatment burden.

References

1. McElwain TJ, Powles RL. High-dose intravenous melphalan for plasma-cell leukaemia and myeloma. Lancet. 1983;2(8354):822–4.
2. Selby PJ, McElwain TJ, Nandi AC, et al. Multiple myeloma treated with high dose intravenous melphalan. Br J Haematol. 1987;66(1):55–62.
3. Barlogie B, Hall R, Zander A, Dicke K, Alexanian R. High-dose melphalan with autologous bone marrow transplantation for multiple myeloma. Blood. 1986;67:1298–301.
4. Barlogie B, Alexanian R, Dicke KA, Zagars G, Spitzer G, Jagannath S, Horwitz L. High-dose chemoradiotherapy and autologous bone marrow transplantation for resistant multiple myeloma. Blood. 1987;70(3):869–72.
5. Jagannath S, Barlogie B, Dicke K, Alexanian R, Zagars G, Cheson B, Lemaistre FC, Smallwood L, Pruitt K, Dixon DO. Autologous bone marrow transplantation in multiple myeloma: identification of prognostic factors. Blood. 1990;76(9):1860–6.
6. Goldschmidt H, Hegenbart U, Wallmeier M, Moos M, Haas R. High-dose chemotherapy in multiple myeloma. Leukemia. 1997;11(Suppl 5):S27–31.
7. Fermand JP, et al. High-dose therapy and autologous peripheral blood stem cell transplantation in multiple myeloma: up-front or rescue treatment? Results of a multicenter sequential randomized clinical trial. Blood. 1998;92(9):3131–6.
8. Child JA, Morgan G, Davies F, et al. High-dose chemotherapy with hematopoietic stem-cell rescue for multiple myeloma. N Engl J Med. 2003;348(19):1875–83.
9. Blade J, Rosiñol L, Sureda A, et al. High-dose therapy intensification compared with continued standard chemotherapy in multiple myeloma patients responding to the initial chemotherapy: long-term results from a prospective randomized trial from the Spanish cooperative group PETHEMA. Blood. 2005;106(12):3755–9.
10. Fermand JP, Katsahian S, Divine M, et al. High-dose therapy and autologous blood stem-cell transplantation compared with conventional treatment in myeloma patients aged 55 to 65 years: long-term results of a randomized control trial from the Group Myelome-Autogreffe. J Clin Oncol. 2005;23(36):9227–33.

11. Attal M, Harrousseau JL, Stoppa AM, et al. A prospective, randomized trial of autologous bone marrow transplantation and chemotherapy in multiple myeloma. Intergroupe Francais du Myelome. N Engl J Med. 1996;335(2):91–7.
12. Barlogie B, et al. Superiority of tandem autologous transplantation over standard therapy for previously untreated multiple myeloma. Blood. 1997;89(3):789–93.
13. Lenhoff S, Hjorth M, Turesson I, et al. Impact on survival of high-dose therapy with autologous stem cell support in patients younger than 60 years with newly diagnosed multiple myeloma: a population-based study. Nordic Myeloma Study Group. Blood. 2000;95(1):7–11.
14. Koreth J, Cutler CS, Djulbegovic B, et al. High-dose therapy with single autologous transplantation versus chemotherapy for newly diagnosed multiple myeloma: a systematic review and meta-analysis of randomized controlled trials. Biol Blood Marrow Transplant. 2007;13(2):183–96. Review
15. Alexanian R, et al. Impact of complete remission with intensive therapy in patients with responsive multiple myeloma. Bone Marrow Transplant. 2001;27(10):1037–43.
16. Lane SW, Gill D, Mollee PN, Rajkumar SV. Role of VAD in the initial treatment of multiple myeloma. Blood. 2005;106(10):3674; author reply 3674–5. No abstract available.
17. Wiedewult M and Giralt S: Clinical Hematopoietic Cell Transplantation American Society of Hematology Self Assessment Program 6th Edition.
18. CIBMTR data.
19. Shah N, Callander N, Ganguly S, et al. Hematopoietic Stem Cell Transplantation for Multiple myeloma: guidelines from the american society for blood and marrow transplantation. Biol Blood Marrow Transplant. 2015;21:1155–66.
20. Ozaki S, Harada T, Saitoh T, et al. Survival of multiple myeloma patients aged 65–70 years in the era of novel agents and autologous stem cell transplantation. A multicenter retrospective collaborative study of the Japanese Society of Myeloma and the European Myeloma Network. Acta Haematol. 2014;132:211–9.
21. Bashir Q, Shah N, Parmar S, et al. Feasibility of autologous hematopoietic stem cell transplant in patients aged ≥70 years with multiple myeloma. Leuk Lymphoma. 2012;53:118–22.
22. Merz M, Neben K, Raab MS, et al. Autologous stem cell transplantation for elderly patients with newly diagnosed multiple myeloma in the era of novel agents. Ann Oncol. 2014;25:189–95.
23. Muchtar E, Dingli D, Kumar S, Buadi FK, et al. Autologous stem cell transplant for multiple myeloma patients 70 years or older. Bone Marrow Transplant. 2016 Nov;51(11):1449–55. https://doi.org/10.1038/bmt.2016.174.
24. Reece D, Bredeson C, Perez WS, et al. Autologous stem cell transplantation in multiple myeloma patients <60 vs. ≥60 years of age. Bone Marrow Transplant. 2003;32(12):1135–43.
25. Sorror ML, Maris MB, Storb R, et al. Hematopoietic cell transplantation (HCT)-specific comorbidity index: a new tool for risk assessment before allogeneic HCT. Blood. 2005;106:2912–9.
26. Saad A, Mahindra A, Zhang MJ, et al. Hematopoietic cell transplant comorbidity index is predictive of survival after autologous hematopoietic cell transplantation in multiple myeloma. Biol Blood Marrow Transplant. 2014;20(3):402–408.e1. https://doi.org/10.1016/j.bbmt.2013.12.557.
27. El Fakih R, Fox P, Popat U, et al. Autologous hematopoietic stem cell transplantation in dialysis-dependent myeloma patients. Clin Lymphoma Myeloma Leuk. 2015;15(8):472–6. https://doi.org/10.1016/j.clml.2015.03.003.
28. Parikh GC, Amjad AI, Saliba RM, et al. Autologous hematopoietic stem cell transplantation may reverse renal failure in patients with multiple myeloma. Biol Blood Marrow Transplant. 2009;15(7):812–6. https://doi.org/10.1016/j.bbmt.2009.03.021.
29. Singhal S, Powles R, Sirohi B, et al. Response to induction chemotherapy is not essential to obtain survival benefit from high-dose melphalan and autotransplantation in myeloma. Bone Marrow Transplant. 2002;30:673–9.
30. Kumar S, Lacy MQ, Dispenzieri A, et al. High-dose therapy and autologous stem cell transplantation for multiple myeloma poorly responsive to initial therapy. Bone Marrow Transplant. 2004;34:161–7.
31. Alexanian R, Weber D, Delasalle K, et al. Clinical outcomes with intensive therapy for patients with primary resistant multiple myeloma. Bone Marrow Transplant. 2004;34:229–34.
32. Rosinol L, Garcia-Sanz R, Lahuerta JJ, et al. Benefit from autologous stem cell transplantation in primary refractory myeloma? Different outcomes in progressive versus stable disease. Haematologica. 2012;97:616–21.
33. Vij R, Kumar S, Zhang MJ, et al. Impact of pretransplant therapy and depth of disease response before autologous transplantation for multiple myeloma. Biol Blood Marrow Transplant. 2015;21:335–41.
34. Kumar S, Giralt S, Stadtmauer EA, et al. Mobilization in myeloma revisited: IMWG consensus perspectives on stem cell collection following initial therapy with thalidomide, lenalidomide-, or bortezomib-containing regimens. Blood. 2009;114:1729–35.
35. Giralt S, Costa L, Schriber J, et al. Optimizing autologous stem cell mobilization strategies to improve patient outcomes: consensus guidelines and recommendations. Biol Blood Marrow Transplant. 2014;20:295–308.
36. DiPersio JF, Stadtmauer EA, Nademanee A, et al. Plerixafor and G-CSF versus placebo and G-CSF to mobilize hematopoietic stem cells for autologous stem cell transplantation in patients with multiple myeloma. Blood. 2009;113(23):5720–6. https://doi.org/10.1182/blood-2008-08-174946.
37. Kumar S, Giralt S, Stadtmauer EA. Mobilization in myeloma revisited: IMWG consensus perspectives on stem cell collection following initial therapy with thalidomide-, lenalidomide-, or bortezomib-containing regimens. Blood. 2009;114(9):1729–35. https://doi.org/10.1182/blood-2009-04-20501.
38. Moreau P, Facon T, Attal M, et al. Comparison of 200 mg/m^2 melphalan and 8 Gy total body irradiation plus 140 mg/m^2 melphalan as conditioning regimens for peripheral blood stem cell transplantation in patients with newly diagnosed multiple myeloma: final analysis of the Intergroupe Francophone du Myelome 9502 randomized trial. Blood. 2002;99:731–5.
39. Lahuerta JJ, Mateos MV, Martinez-Lopez J, et al. Busulfan 12 mg/kg plus melphalan 140 mg/m^2 versus melphalan 200 mg/m^2 as condition in regimens for autologous transplantation in newly diagnosed multiple myeloma patients included in the PETHEMA/GEM2000 study. Haematologica. 2010;95:1913–20.
40. Fenk R, Schneider P, Kropff M, et al. High-dose idarubicin, cyclophosphamide and melphalan as conditioning for autologous stem cell transplantation increases treatment-related mortality in patients with multiple myeloma: results of a randomised study. Br J Haematol. 2005;130:588–94.
41. Lonial S, Kaufman J, Tighiouart M, et al. A phase I/II trial combining high-dose melphalan and autologous transplant with bortezomib for multiple myeloma: a dose- and schedule-finding study. Clin Cancer Res. 2010;16:5079–86.
42. Sharma M, Khan H, Thall PF, et al. A randomized phase 2 trial of a preparative regimen of bortezomib, high-dose melphalan, arsenic trioxide, and ascorbic acid. Cancer. 2012;118:2507–15.
43. Sahebi F, Jacobelli S, Biezen AV, et al. Comparison of upfront tandem autologous–allogeneic transplantation versus reduced intensity allogeneic transplantation for multiple myeloma. Bone Marrow Transplant. 2015;50:802–7. https://doi.org/10.1038/bmt.2015.45; published online 23 March 2015.

44. Smith E, Devlin SM, Kosuri S, et al. cd34-selected allogeneic hematopoietic stem cell transplantation for patients with relapsed, high-risk multiple myeloma. Biol Blood Marrow Transplant. 2016;22(2):258–67. https://doi.org/10.1016/j.bbmt.2015.08.025.
45. Campagnaro E, Saliba R, Giralt S, et al. Symptom burden after autologous stem cell transplantation for multiple myeloma. Cancer. 2008;112:1617–24.
46. Wang XS, Giralt SA, Mendoza TR, et al. Clinical factors associated with cancer-related fatigue in patients being treated for leukemia and non-Hodgkin's lymphoma. J Clin Oncol. 2002;20(5):1319–28.
47. D'Souza A, Huang J, Fei M, Hari P. Trends in pre- and post-transplant therapies prior to first autologous hematopoietic cell transplantation among patients with multiple myeloma in the United States, 2004–2014. Blood. 2016; Abstract.
48. Jakubowiak AJ, et al. A phase 1/2 study of carfilzomib in combination with lenalidomide and low-dose dexamethasone as a frontline treatment for multiple myeloma. Blood. 2012;120(9):1801–9.
49. Palumbo A, Cavallo F, Gay F, et al. Autologous transplantation and maintenance therapy in multiple myeloma. N Engl J Med. 2014;371(10):895–905. https://doi.org/10.1056/ NEJMoa 1402888.
50. Gay F, Oliva S, Petrucci MT, et al. Chemotherapy plus lenalidomide versus autologous transplantation, followed by lenalidomide plus prednisone versus lenalidomide maintenance, in patients with multiple myeloma: a randomised, multicentre, phase 3 trial. Lancet Oncol. 2015;16(16):1617–29. https://doi.org/10.1016/S1470-2045(15)00389-7.
51. Attal M, Lauwers-Cances V, Hulin C, et al. Autologous transplantation for multiple myeloma in the era of new drugs: a Phase III Study of the Intergroupe Francophone Du Myelome (IFM/DFCI 2009 trial). Blood. 2015;126:391.
52. Cavo M, Beksac M, Dimopoulos M, et al Intensification therapy with Bortezomib-Melphalan-Prednisone versus autologous stem cell transplantation for newly diagnosed multiple myeloma: an intergroup, multicenter, Phase III Study of the European Myeloma Network (EMN02/HO95 MM Trial). Blood. 2016; Abstract.
53. Attal M, et al. Single versus double autologous stem-cell transplantation for multiple myeloma. N Engl J Med. 2003;349(26):2495–502.
54. Cavo M, et al. Prospective, randomized study of single compared with double autologous stem-cell transplantation for multiple myeloma: Bologna 96 clinical study. J Clin Oncol. 2007;25(17):2434–4.
55. Salwender H, et al. Double vs. single autologous stem cell transplantation after Bortezomib-based induction regimens for multiple myeloma: an integrated analysis of patient-level data from Phase European III studies. Blood. 2013;122(21):767.
56. Cavo M, Petrucci MT, Di Raimondi F, et al. Upfront single versus double autologous stem cell transplantation for newly diagnosed multiple myeloma: an intergroup, multicenter, Phase III study of the European Myeloma Network (EMN02/HO95 MM trial). Blood. 2016;128:991.
57. Stadtmauer E, Pasquini M, Blackwell B, et al. Comparison of autologous hematopoietic cell transplant (autoHCT), bortezomib, lenalidomide (Len) and dexamethasone (RVD) consolidation with len maintenance (ACM), tandem autohct with len maintenance (TAM) and autohct with len maintenance (AM) for up-front treatment of patients with multiple myeloma (MM): primary results from the randomized Phase III trial of the blood and marrow transplant clinical trials network (BMT CTN 0702—StaMINA trial) Blood. 2016;128.
58. Gahrton G, et al. Autologous/reduced-intensity allogeneic stem cell transplantation vs autologous transplantation in multiple myeloma: long-term results of the EBMT-NMAM2000 study. Blood. 2013;121(25):5055–63.
59. Krishnan A, Pasquini M, Logan B, et al. Autologous haemopoietic stem-cell transplantation followed by allogeneic or autologous haemopoietic stem-cell transplantation in patients with multiple myeloma (BMT CTN 0102): a phase 3 biological assignment trial. Lancet Oncol. 2011;12(13):1195–203.
60. Lokhorst HM, et al. Donor versus no-donor comparison of newly diagnosed myeloma patients included in the HOVON-50 multiple myeloma study. Blood. 2012;119(26):6219–25.
61. Bruno B, Rotta M, Patriarca F, et al. A comparison of allografting with autografting for newly diagnosed myeloma. N Engl J Med. 2007;356(11):1110–20.
62. Kumar S, et al. Trends in allogeneic stem cell transplantation for multiple myeloma: a CIBMTR analysis. Blood. 2011;118(7):1979–88.
63. Giralt S, Garderet L, Duric B, et al. American Society of Blood and Marrow Transplantation, European Society of Blood and Marrow Transplantation, Blood and Marrow Transplant Clinical Trials Network, and International Myeloma Working Group Consensus Conference on salvage hematopoietic cell transplantation in patients with relapsed multiple myeloma. Biol Blood Marrow Transplant. 2015;21:2039–51.
64. Cook G, Williams C, Brown JM, et al. High-dose chemotherapy plus autologous stem-cell transplantation as consolidation therapy in patients with relapsed multiple myeloma after previous autologous stem-cell transplantation (NCRI Myeloma X Relapse [intensive trial]): a randomised, open-label, phase 3 trial. Lancet Oncol. 2014;15:874–85.
65. Freytes CO, Vesole DH, LeRademacher L, et al. Second transplants for multiple myeloma relapsing after a previous autotransplant-reduced intensity allogeneic versus autologous transplantation. Bone Marrow Transplant. 2014;49:416–21.
66. Patriarca F, Einsele H, Spina F, et al. Allogeneic stem cell transplantation in multiple myeloma relapsed after autograft: a multicenter retrospective study based on donor availability. Biol Blood Marrow Transplant. 2012;18:617–26.
67. De Lavallade H, El-Cheikh J, Faucher C, et al. Reduced-intensity conditioning allogeneic SCT as a salvage treatment for relapsed multiple myeloma. Bone Marrow Transplant. 2008;41:953–60.
68. Ladetto M, et al. Major tumor shrinking and persistent molecular remissions after consolidation with bortezomib, thalidomide, and dexamethasone in patients with autografted myeloma. J Clin Oncol. 2010;28(12):2077–84.
69. Cavo M, et al. Bortezomib-thalidomide-dexamethasone is superior to thalidomide-dexamethasone as consolidation therapy after autologous hematopoietic stem cell transplantation in patients with newly diagnosed multiple myeloma. Blood. 2012;120(1):9–19.
70. Mellqvist UH, et al. Bortezomib consolidation after autologous stem cell transplantation in multiple myeloma: a Nordic Myeloma Study Group randomized phase 3 trial. Blood. 2013;121(23):4647–54.
71. McCarthy P, Owzar K, Hofmeister CC, et al. Lenalidomide after stem-cell transplantation for multiple myeloma. N Engl J Med. 2012;366(19):1770–81.
72. Attal M, Lauwers-Cances V, Marit G, et al. Lenalidomide maintenance after stem-cell transplantation for multiple myeloma. N Engl J Med. 2012;366(19):1782–91.
73. Palumbo A, Cavallo F, Gay F, et al. Autologous transplantation and maintenance therapy in multiple myeloma. N Engl J Med. 2014;371:895–905. https://doi.org/10.1056/NEJMoa1402888.
74. Attal M, Palumbo A, Holstein SA, et al. Lenalidomide (LEN) maintenance (MNTC) after high-dose melphalan and autologous stem cell transplant (ASCT) in multiple myeloma (MM): A meta-analysis (MA) of overall survival (OS). J Clin Oncol. 2016;34 (suppl; abstr 8001).
75. Chanan Khan A, Giralt S. Importance of achieving a complete response in multiple myeloma, and the impact of novel agents. J Clin Oncol. 2010;28(15):2612–24. https://doi.org/10.1200/JCO.2009.25.4250.
76. Lahuerta JJ, et al. Influence of pre- and post-transplantation responses on outcome of patients with multiple myeloma: sequential improvement of response and achievement of com-

plete response are associated with longer survival. J Clin Oncol. 2008;26(35):5775–82.

77. Mailankody S, Korde N, Lesokhin AM, et al. Minimal residual disease in multiple myeloma: bringing the bench to the bedside. Nat Rev Clin Oncol. 2015;12(5):286–95. https://doi.org/10.1038/nrclinonc.2014.239. Review
78. Garfall AL, Stadtmauer EA. Cellular and vaccine immunotherapy for multiple myeloma. Hematology Am Soc Hemtol Educ Program. 2016;2016(1):521–7.
79. Rosenblatt J, Avigan D Targeting the PD-1/PD-L1 axis in multiple myeloma: a dream or a reality .Blood. 2016. pii: blood-2016-08-731885 [Epub ahead of print].
80. Chung DJ, Pronschinske KB, Shyer JA, et al. T-cell exhaustion in multiple myeloma relapse after autotransplant: optimal timing of immunotherapy. Cancer Immunol Res. 2016;4:61–71.
81. Appelbaum FR, Anasetti C, Antin JH, et al. Blood and marrow transplant clinical trials network state of the Science Symposium 2014. Biol Blood Marrow Transplant. 2015;21(2):202–24. https://doi.org/10.1016/j.bbmt.2014.10.003.
82. Landgren O, Giralt S. MRD-driven treatment paradigm for newly diagnosed transplant eligible multiple myeloma patients. Bone Marrow Transplant. 2016;51(7):913–4. https://doi.org/10.1038/bmt.2016.24.
83. Dispenzieri A. Myeloma: management of the newly diagnosed high risk patient. Hematology Am Soc Hemtol Educ Program. 2016;1:485–94.
84. Moreau P, Chanan-Khan A, Roberts AW, et al. Venetoclax combined with bortezomib and dexamethasone for patients with relapsed/refractory multiple myeloma. Blood. 2016;128:975.
85. Zimmerman T, Raje NS, Vij R, et al. Final results of a Phase 2 trial of extended treatment (tx) with carfilzomib (CFZ), lenalidomide (LEN), and dexamethasone (KRd) plus autologous stem cell transplantation (ASCT) in newly diagnosed multiple myeloma (NDMM). Blood. 2016; Abstract 675.

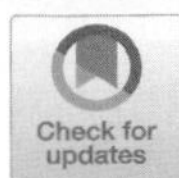

Solitary Plasmacytomas and Soft-Tissue Involvement in Multiple Myeloma

30

Joan Bladé and Laura Rosiñol

Localized Plasmacytomas

Localized plasmacytomas are plasma cell tumors, histologically indistinguishable on multiple myeloma that develop as single tumors either in bone (solitary plasmacytoma of bone—SPB) or in soft tissues (extramedullary—EMP) [1]. Both are uncommon disorders accounting for less than 5% of all plasma cell malignancies [2–15].

Solitary Plasmacytoma of Bone

Clinical Findings and Diagnostic Criteria

Solitary plasmacytoma of bone (SPB) was first recognized almost one century ago and since then single-case reports as well as a number of series have been reported [2–15]. The diagnostic requirements have been revised by the International Myeloma Working Group [1]. SPB consists of a single plasma cell tumor localized in bone and it is an uncommon disorder with a frequency ranging from 3 to 5% of all plasma cell neoplasms. Typically the histopathological pattern shows a diffuse involvement by mature plasma cells identical to those observed in multiple myeloma (MM). SPB is more frequent in males than in females (ratio 2:1) and the median age is about 10 years less than that observed in patients with MM. The most frequent complain at presentation is pain at the site of the skeletal lesion. The bones more commonly involved are vertebrae followed by sternum, pelvis, and proximal long bones. Thoracic vertebrae are more commonly involved than lumbar and cervical. Back pain or features of spinal cord compression are the most frequent presenting features. Soft tissue from a plasmacytoma, as in the sternum, may result in a palpable mass. The diagnostic criteria are shown in Table 30.1. To ensure that there are no other plasmacytomas radiological imaging techniques are necessary. Classically, it was required that a complete skeletal survey did not show other lesions. Today the skeletal survey must be completed with a PET/CT to exclude other lesions. The bone marrow aspirate must contain less than 10% bone marrow plasma cells. Theoretically, there should be no serum or urine M-protein. However, more than 50% of the patients have a small M-component. Of course, it should be no evidence of CRAB (i.e., hypercalcemia, renal function impairment, or anemia related to the plasma cell proliferation) features apart from those resulting from localized bony plasmacytoma [1].

Table 30.1 Solitary plasmacytoma of bone: diagnostic criteria

– Single area of bone destruction due to the plasma cell proliferation
– Bone marrow with <10% plasma cells
– Absence of other skeletal lesions on PET/CT
– No anemia, hypercalcemia, or renal impairment
– Absence of serum and urine M-protein[a]

[a]50% of patients have a small serum M-component

Prognostic Features

The prognosis of SPB depends on the risk of transformation to MM since progression to MM is observed in up to 75% of cases. The median time to progression is 2–4 years and the median overall survival ranges from 8 to 12 years [2–15]. The most frequent features associated with progression to MM are (1) involvement of the axial skeleton versus long bones, (2) older age, (3) persistence of the M-protein after treatment with radiation therapy, (4) plasmacytoma size larger than 5 cm, (5) low levels of uninvolved immunoglobulins, (6) abnormal free light chain (FLC) ratio at diagnosis, (7) presence of focal lesions at magnetic resonance imaging (MRI) or more than one

J. Bladé, M.D., Ph.D. (✉) • L. Rosiñol, M.D., Ph.D.
Amyloidosis and Myeloma Unit, Hematology Department, Hospital Clínic, IDIBAPS, Barcelona, Spain
e-mail: jblade@clinic.cat

P.H. Wiernik et al. (eds.), *Neoplastic Diseases of the Blood*, DOI 10.1007/978-3-319-64263-5_30

Table 30.2 Solitary plasmacytoma of bone. Adverse prognostic features

– Older age
– Involvement of axial skeletal versus long bones
– Plasmacytoma size ≥5 cm
– Immunoparesis
– Persistence of the M-protein after radiation therapy
– Abnormal free light chain ratio
– Presence of focal lesions on MRI or >1 metabolic lesion at PET
– Abnormal bone marrow flow cytometry

metabolic lesion at PET examination, and (8) abnormal bone marrow flow cytometry (Table 30.2). In a recent study, only immunoparesis emerged as negative predictor for progression to MM at the multivariate analysis [16]. In this study, classical prognostic factors such as age, disappearance of the M-protein after radiation therapy, location, or tumor size did not have impact on outcome. In an MD Anderson series of 60 patients, 45 (75%) had a serum M-protein at diagnosis. Most of the 32 in whom the M-protein persisted after radiation therapy evolved to MM while only 1 of the 13 patients in whom the M-protein disappeared with therapy developed MM [17]. Of note, in all these 13 patients the M-protein disappeared within the first year beyond radiation therapy was finalized and 7 of them were free from progression to myeloma between 16 and 25 years of follow-up [17]. The Mayo Clinic group reported the impact of serum FLC on the transformation rate to MM in a series of 116 patients diagnosed between 1960 and 1995 with SPB [18]. Forty-three patients progressed to MM after a median of 1.8 years. Fifty-four patients had an abnormal sFLC ratio and the progression rate at 5 years was 44% in patients with an abnormal sFLC ratio and 26% for those with normal sFLC ratio. The abnormal sFLC ratio at diagnosis had an adverse effect on both time to progression to MM and overall survival. The persistence beyond 1–2 years from diagnosis of a serum M-protein value of 5 g/L or higher was an additional factor associated with progression. Combining the FLC ratio at diagnosis and an M-protein of less than 5 g/L at 1 or 2 years beyond diagnosis a simple staging system with low (no features), intermediate (one risk factor), and high risk (both risk factors) was developed showing a 13, 26, and 62% rate of progression to MM at 5 years of follow-up [18]. In a recent study involving 43 patients, 48% had abnormal involved sFLC value and 64% an abnormal sFLC ratio while 33% had two or more hypermetabolic lesions at the PET/CT examination [19]. In a multivariate analysis, abnormal involved sFLC, and presence of at least two hypermetabolic lesions on PET/CT were the two predictors for early evolution to MM [19]. Finally, multiparameter flow cytometry (MFC) has recently been shown as a valuable biomarker to predict both high risk and low risk of progression. In this regard, Paiva et al. [20] studied 35 patients with SPB and 29 with EMP through MFC. Bone marrow clonal PCs were observed in 17 of the 35 (49%) patients with SPB and in 11 of the 29 (38%) of patients with EMP. Seventy-one percent of patients with positive flow versus only 8% of flow-negative SPB evolved to MM with a median time to progression of 26 months. In contrast, no significant differences in progression depending on the MFC findings were observed among patients with EMP. Of interest, MFC may also help to identify the so-called true SP characterized by flow-negative bone marrow and the absence of M-protein with an exceedingly rare rate of progression to MM [20]. Furthermore, almost identical results with MFC were reported by Hill et al. [21], in 50 patients with SPB. Aberrant PC phenotype was observed in 34 patients (68%). Progression to MM was observed in 72% of flow-positive patients versus in 12.5% for those flow negative, with a median time to progression of 26 months. In this study, the presence of urinary light chains was also highly predictive of the outcome with a progression rate of 91% for those with urine light-chain protein excretion versus 44% for those without. Using both parameters the authors identified a subset of patients (flow negative, no urine light chains) with a probability of progression as low as 7.7% and a high-risk subset with a bone marrow-positive flow and/or urine light-chain protein excretion with a progression rate of 75%. It is very likely that the patients with a bone marrow-positive MFC have in fact an "early myeloma" rather than a true SPB. In summary, the current most important predictors of progression to MM in patients with SPB are bone marrow MFC, serum FLC values, and finding of more than one hypermetabolic lesions on PET imaging [18–21].

Treatment Approach

In many instances patients have had surgery, with complete or partial tumor removal, as part of the diagnostic procedure. Apart from the diagnostic approach, the indications for surgery are internal fixation of fractures or as prevention of fractures, urgent decompressive laminectomy, or stabilization of spine using Harrington rods.

The treatment of choice is local radiation therapy involving the entire tumor volume with a margin of health tissue of at least 2 cm [2, 16, 22–24]. In case of vertebral plasmacytomas the irradiation field should include the proximal and distal uninvolved vertebrae. The recommended dose is between 40 and 50 Gy fractionated in over 4–5 weeks. It has been recommended that in plasmacytomas larger than 5 cm the radiation dose should be 50 Gy. However, the relationship between radiation therapy dose and tumor response is controversial when the radiation dose is higher than 35 Gy

[12, 13, 17, 23], since no clear relationship between the doses of local radiation therapy and the progression to MM has been clearly shown. It is considered that in the vast majority of cases adjuvant chemotherapy is of no benefit. The Greek group reported no improvement using either conventional chemotherapy or novel agents including bortezomib [16]. However, in this retrospective study, it might be a bias (i.e., poorer prognosis for the subset given adjuvant therapy versus radiation alone). In any event, the authors of this chapter strongly believe that in nonresponders to radiation therapy as well as in patients with bulky masses (i.e., >5 cm) located in pelvis, sternum, or a large bone such as humera or femora a multiple myeloma treatment approach should be considered, including high-dose melphalan followed by autologous hematopoietic stem cell rescue for younger patients. Currently, the response should be assessed by PET/CT imaging at least 3 months after radiation therapy is completed. For complete response all metabolic activity suggestive of active disease must have disappeared.

Multiple Solitary Plasmacytomas, Recurrent Plasmacytomas, and Macrofocal Myeloma

Among all patients diagnosed with "SPB," about 5% have more than one bone lesion with or without soft-tissue involvement and with no features consistent with MM [1]. Although patients with two or more "solitary" plasmacytomas can be treated with radiation therapy alone, we would favor a multiple myeloma treatment approach. In case of early recurrence (i.e., <2 years) either as a new lesion or as a local recurrence in an irradiated area a MM treatment approach is mandatory. In case of late recurrence (>2 years) as a new single lesion rechallenge with radiation therapy is reasonable.

The Greek group reported a variant of MM characterized by multiple lytic lesions with or without soft-tissue masses, less than 10% bone marrow plasma cells, and small M-protein in younger patients and associated with a favorable outcome [25]. This form of multiple myeloma had been previously recognized in patients younger than 30 years [26, 27]. The treatment approach is the same as for general multiple myeloma, including high-dose melphalan followed by autologous stem cell rescue whenever possible.

Extramedullary Plasmacytoma

Extramedullary plasmacytoma is an uncommon plasma cell disorder consisting of a plasma cell soft-tissue tumor. EMP may originate in many anatomical sites, although more than 90% developed in the head or neck area, particularly in the upper respiratory structures [2–4].

Clinical Findings and Diagnostic Criteria

The incidence of EMP is about 3% of all plasma cell malignancies. It is more frequent in males than in females (2:1) and the median age at diagnosis is 60 years [2–4]. The clinical features depend on the site and organ involved. As a result of the frequent locations in the upper respiratory tract patients usually present with symptoms such as nasal obstruction or discharge, epistaxis, hoarseness, or hemoptysis. Pain and tenderness at the plasmacytoma site may occur. EMP can develop in any organ including gastrointestinal tract, brain, thyroid, breast, testes, or lymph nodes [2, 4–6]. There is a predominance of IgA immunoglobulin type. The diagnosis is based on the finding of a plasma cell proliferation in an extramedullary site in the absence of MM (Table 30.3).

Treatment and Outcome

As in SPB, the treatment consists of fractionated radiation therapy at the total dose of 40–50 Gy over 4–5 weeks. Radiation therapy on local lymph nodes may be considered since up to 25% of patients with EMP of the head and neck may develop lymph node involvement. EMPs localized in the upper respiratory tract have a better outcome than those arising outside the head and neck area. Involvement of the adjacent bone has been reported as an adverse factor. Local relapses, including lymph node involvement, occur in up to 15% of cases. Progression to MM is uncommon with a reported frequency ranging from 8 to 30% [3, 4, 6–8, 10, 14, 16, 24]. The most prominent features of SPB and EMP are shown in Table 30.4.

Table 30.3 Extramedullary plasmacytoma: diagnostic criteria

– Single extramedullary tumor of clonal plasma cells
– Normal bone marrow
– Absence of other lesions on PET/CT
– No anemia, hypercalcemia, or renal impairment
– Absence of serum and urine M-protein[a]

[a]Some patients may have a small serum M-component

Table 30.4. Clinical features

	SBP	EMP
Median age (years)	55	55
M:F	2:1	3:1
Main location	Axial skeleton (vertebral)	Head and neck
M-protein (%)	50	<25
Progression to MM (%)	≥75	8–30
10-year survival (%)	40–50	70

Solitary plasmacytoma of bone (SPB) versus extramedullary plasmacytoma (EMP)

Soft-Tissue Plasmacytomas in Multiple Myeloma

Multiple myeloma (MM) is characterized by a proliferation of plasma cells (PCs) with a strong dependence on the bone marrow (BM) microenvironment. However, in up to one-third of the patients the plasma cells escape the microenvironment influences resulting in soft-tissue plasmacytomas [28]. The existence of soft-tissue involvement in MM is long-term known and old autopsy studies have shown an extra-skeletal involvement in up to 70% of patients [29–32]. In patients with multiple myeloma, the soft-tissue masses can have two different origins: (1) direct growth from skeletal lesions by disrupting the cortical bone and (2) plasma cell tumors resulting from hematogenous spread. The mechanisms involved in the extramedullary myeloma dissemination are not well understood. However, possible explanations are (1) decreased expression of adhesion molecules, (2) low expression of some cytokine receptors or downregulation of CXCR4 and its ligands, and/or (3) increased angiogenesis [33–42]. It is likely that the physiopathologic mechanisms of the two variants of plasmacytomas (hematogenous spread versus direct growth from lytic lesions) are different. Hopefully, future studies matching and comparing the characteristics of malignant BMPCs with those growing at soft tissues help to better understand the mechanisms of myeloma dissemination outside the bone marrow.

Definition

Pasmantier and Azar reported in 1969 the findings of 57 autopsy cases and proposed a classification in three stages according to the presence or absence of macroscopic tumor outside bones [43]. Stage I or intraskeletal: disease confined to the bone marrow or bone, stage II or paraskeletal: presence of soft-tissue masses arising directly from bones extending to paraskeletal areas, and stage III or extraskeletal resulting from metastatic or hematogenous spread. Of interest, in most patients in stage I and II the plasma cells were well differentiated (plasmacytic myeloma) whereas in the majority of patients in stage III the plasma cells were poorly differentiated (plasmablastic myeloma). However, the definition of extramedullary involvement in MM has not been uniform. Recently, the International Myeloma Working Group (IMWG) agreed on that two different types must be considered. (1) paraskeletal consisting of soft-tissue masses arising from skeletal lesions and (2) pure extramedullary resulting from hematogenous spread and involving only soft tissues with no contact with bone (Rosiñol et al., manuscript in preparation). Some patients develop simultaneously or successively the two types of plasmacytomas.

Incidence and Location

The reported incidence of paraskeletal plasmacytomas at diagnosis is from 7 to 34.4% [28, 44–48] while the reported rate of pure extramedullary involvement ranges between 1.7 and 4.5% [49, 50]. At relapse, the incidence of paraskeletal involvement remains similar to that observed at the time of diagnosis [44–48] while the frequency of extramedullary disease increases ranging up to 3.4–10% [49–53]. In two recent studies, 45 and 56% of patients with plasmacytomas at the time of diagnosis had paraskeletal or extramedullary disease at relapse [45, 54]. It has been suggested that patients undergoing allogeneic transplantation, particularly with dose-reduced intensity conditioning and those treated with novel antimyeloma agents, such as thalidomide, bortezomib, or lenalidomide, may have a higher incidence of plasmacytomas [55–57]. However, there is no evidence that the incidence of plasmacytomas increases at relapse after allogeneic transplantation or after exposure to novel antimyeloma agents [45, 48, 52, 54]. However, a better control of medullary disease with novel drugs can result in a more prolonged survival with a higher risk of extramedullary progression.

The extramedullary myeloma spread may consist of (1) single or multiple highly vascularized large red-purple subcutaneous nodules; (2) multiple small nodules located at any organ, particularly skin, liver, breast, or kidney; (3) pleura with myelomatous pleural effusion; (4) lymph nodes; and (5) central nervous system (CNS). Skin is the most frequent location at diagnosis whereas there is an increased incidence of liver, pleural, and CNS involvement at the time of relapse [49]. Leptomeningeal involvement occurs in about 1% of the patients [58–63]. The more common presenting features are confusion, paraparesis, and cranial nerve palsies. The cerebrospinal fluid (CSF) shows increased protein value and positive immunofixation for the myeloma M-protein as well as plasma cells usually with plasmablastic features. CNS involvement is associated with poor prognostic features such as high-risk cytogenetics, plasma cell leukemia, and high LDH serum levels. CNS involvement is usually seen in advanced phases of the disease along with the involvement of other extramedullary locations. However, in some instances CNS involvement can present at diagnosis or as isolated relapse in patients in complete remission. The prognosis is very poor with median survivals shorter than 3 months, even when novel agents are used [64]. Treatment of CNS involvement with intrathecal therapy with methotrexate, hydrocortisone, and cytosine arabinoside is unsatisfactory. Craniospinal radiation can be considered. It has been reported in a multicenter study that local plus systemic therapy can improve the prognosis [63].

Paraskeletal involvement is the most frequent cause of plasmacytomas in MM and, as previously mentioned, consists of soft-tissue masses arising from lytic skeletal lesions [28]. The most common locations are vertebrae, ribs, sternum, skull, and pelvis. Plasmacytomas arising from vertebrae can cause spinal cord compression, the most common neurological complication of MM occurring in up to 10% of the cases [65]. The dorsal spine is the most frequently involved with a clinical picture consisting of back pain and paraparesis that can evolve to paraplegia in a matter of hours or days. The complication is a medical emergency that requires confirmation by an immediate MRI. Treatment with high-dose dexamethasone at a loading dose of 100 mg followed by 25 mg every 6 h with subsequent progressive tapering plus radiation therapy should be immediately started [66]. Plasmacytomas can be triggered by surgical invasive procedures usually performed during the course of the disease [67–70]. They can originate from laparotomy scars or catheter insertions and can even precede systemic relapses. Extensive extramedullary involvement resulting from bone surgery or fractures has also been reported [68].

Plasma Cell Characteristics in Soft-Tissue Plasmacytomas

Plasma cells from extramedullary disease commonly show immature or plasmablastic features. In contrast, myeloma cells from paraskeletal masses arising from focal bony lesions are less undifferentiated and show a more mature or plasmacytic morphology [28, 43]. CD56 expression is usually downregulated in plasma cells at extramedullary sites [71, 72]. However, more studies are needed to establish the role of CD56 in the extramedullary myeloma dissemination. The information on genetic abnormalities in extramedullary myeloma is limited. The frequency of high-risk cytogenetics, particularly 17p deletion, at extramedullary sites is usually higher than that reported in BMPCs [73–78]. It also seems that the hematogenous spread is more frequent in patients with gene expression profile (GEP)-defined high-risk myeloma [49]. However, molecular genetic studies on paired samples from medullary and extramedullary sites in the same patients are required in order to identify potential extramedullary disease-associated genes and to understand the mechanisms of extramedullary myeloma dissemination [49].

Assessment of Plasmacytomas

In some patients plasmacytomas consist of palpable masses which can be assessed by physical examination. However, in many instances radiographic imaging techniques are needed [79, 80]. Magnetic resonance imaging (MRI) is useful when spinal cord or nerve root compression is suspected and it is the best imaging technique to assess leptomeningeal or cerebral involvement [81]. The typical findings are leptomeningeal enhancement and/or meningeal based lesions resembling intracerebral masses [81]. Fluorodeoxyglucose (FDG) positron emission combined with computed tomography (PET/CT) is the most valuable whole-body technique in patients in whom the presence of plasmacytomas is suspected [82–86]. The main limitation of the PET/CT is that it is not standardized and the potential lack of interobserver reproducibility. A PET/CT should be done when myeloma soft-tissue involvement is suspected on the basis of clinical manifestations and in patients at high risk such as in those with high LDH serum levels as well as at the time of relapse in patients with previous history of plasmacytomas given the high frequency of plasmacytomas at relapse in this population [45, 54]. It is crucial and mandatory to include the plasmacytoma assessment when evaluating the response to therapy in patients with MM. The IMWG criteria requires the disappearance of plasmacytomas for CR and a decrease equal or higher to 50% for PR. Progression is defined by either the increase in at least 25% of preexisting masses, recurrence of a plasmacytoma that had disappeared with therapy, or development of any new soft-tissue involvement [87]. Ideally, the same imaging technique should be used at baseline and during follow-up [88].

Prognosis

The presence of soft-tissue involvement in MM is associated with a shorter survival. Thus, the Pavia group showed that the presence of soft-tissue involvement at any time during the course of the disease was associated to shorter PFS and OS [45] and the Royal Marsden group reported that the presence of plasmacytomas was associated to worse prognosis in patients treated with conventional chemotherapy [44]. Of interest, in the above two series [44, 45] as well as in a recent South Korea study [89] the administration of high-dose therapy followed by autologous stem cell rescue was able to overcome the negative impact of the presence of plasmacytomas. In contrast, in a PETHEMA transplant trial the OS of patients with paraskeletal involvement was significantly shorter in those with plasmacytomas [90]. It must be taken into account that in all the above studies the majority of patients had paraskeletal disease and only few pure extramedullary disease. In fact, the Arkansas group reported that patients with extramedullary disease had a significantly shorter PFS and OS even in the era of novel agents and treated in the context of the total therapy approaches [49]. Pour et al. [51] reported that in relapsed patients the presence of plasmacytomas was associated with a poorer outcome. Of interest, the survival of patients with extramedullary disease was significantly shorter than that of those with paraskeletal involvement [51]. The prognosis of patients with CNS disease is ominous even in the era of novel agents [64].

Treatment

In the frontline setting, alkylating agents, particularly high-dose melphalan, are of benefit in patients with paraskeletal disease while their efficacy in patients with hematogenous extramedullary disease is doubtful [28, 44, 45]. Bortezomib seems to be of benefit in patients with paraskeletal involvement with less evidence for hematogenous dissemination [91–93]. There is no published data on the efficacy of other proteasome inhibitors such as carfilzomib or ixazomib. The efficacy of IMIDs seems limited. In this regard, thalidomide is not effective in any type of plasmacytomas [94–98]. There is no published data on the efficacy of lenalidomide. The Mayo Clinic reported that 31% (4 out of 13) patients with extramedullary involvement responded to pomalidomide plus low-dose dexamethasone [50]. However, the authors of this chapter have treated nine patients with advanced MM and plasmacytomas with pomalidomide and low-dose dexamethasone and no response in plasmacytomas was observed. It is of interest that a dissociation between paraproteinemic and plasmacytoma response has been reported in patients treated with both thalidomide and bortezomib [93–96, 98]. The small sample size and the absence of controlled studies are important limitations to draw durable conclusions on the efficacy of bortezomib and IMiDs on soft-tissue involvement in MM. There are no reports on the potential efficacy of monoclonal antibodies such as elotuzumab and daratumumab on paraskeletal or extramedullary myeloma.

Considering that alkylating agents and bortezomib seem the most effective agents in patients with soft-tissue masses, although the evidence is lower for extramedullary than for paraskeletal disease, the treatment of choice for patients non-eligible for ASCT would be a combination of melphalan and prednisone with bortezomib (MPV) [99, 100]. Taking into account that high-dose therapy, particularly high-dose melphalan, can overcome the poor prognosis of paraskeletal involvement, a triple bortezomib-based regimen (VTD, PAD, or VRD) followed by ASCT could be the treatment of choice for younger patients [101, 102]. For transplant-eligible patients with extramedullary disease a combined anti-myeloma/anti-lymphoma regimen such as VTD/PACE followed by an allogeneic stem cell transplantation in patients younger than 50 years or by a tandem ASCR followed by dose-reduced intensity conditioning allogeneic transplantation (Allo-RIC) in those aged 50–65 years should be considered [103].

The prognosis of patients with MM relapsing with soft-tissue involvement (i.e., paraskeletal or extramedullary) is very poor [48–53]. Since these patients have already received previous bortezomib and/or IMiD-based regimens, the most effective treatment consists of lymphoma-like regimens such as PACE, Dexa-BEAM, or HyperCVAD [28, 104, 105]. The response rate is about 50%; however, the median duration of response is of only 4 months [105]. For this reason, in patients who are eligible for ASCT the best approach would be the administration of two or three cycles immediately followed by the high-dose procedure.

Local radiation therapy should be urgently administered in case of spinal cord compression and also considered in patients with severe compressive pain, bulky plasmacytomas, and persistent local disease after systemic therapy. There are not yet data on the potential efficacy of monoclonal antibodies such as elotuzumab or daratumumab, the new proteasome inhibitors carfilzomib and ixazomib, or the new IMiDs or other drugs still in their early development.

Acknowledgements This work has been supported in part by Grants RD12/0036/0046 and PI12/1093 from Instituto de Salud Carlos III and Fondo Europeo de Desarrollo Regional (FEDER) and 2014SGR-552 from AGAUR (Generalitat de Catalunya).

References

1. International Myeloma Working Group. Criteria for classification of monoclonal gammopathies, multiple myeloma and related disorders: a report of the International Myeloma Working Group. Br J Haematol. 2003;121:749–57.
2. Wiltshaw E. The natural history of extramedullary plasmacytoma and its relation to solitary myeloma of bone and myelomatosis. Medicine. 1976;55:217–37.
3. Woodruff RK, Whittle JM, Malpas J. Solitary plasmacytoma. I. Extramedullary soft-tissue plasmacytoma. Cancer. 1979;43:2340–3.
4. Knowling MA, Harwood AR, Bergsagel DE. Comparing extramedullary plasmacytomas with solitary with solitary and multiple myeloma cell tumours of bone. J Clin Oncol. 1983;1:255–62.
5. Meiss JM, Butler JJ, Osborne BM, Ordoñez NG. Solitary plasmacytoma of bone and extramedullary plasmacytoma. A clinicopathologic and immunohistochemical study. Cancer. 1987;59:1475–85.
6. Mayr NA, Wen BC, Hussey DH, et al. The role of radiation therapy in the treatment of solitary plasmacytoma. Radiother Oncol. 1990;17:293–303.
7. Tong D, Griffien TW, Laramore GE, et al. Solitary plasmacytoma of bone and soft tissues. Radiology. 1980;135:195–8.
8. Corwin L, Lindberg RD. Solitary plasmacytoma of bone vs. extramedullary plasmacytoma and its relationship to multiple myeloma. Cancer. 1979;45:1007–13.
9. Bataille R, Sany J. Solitary plasmacytoma: clinical and prognostic features of a review of 114 cases. Cancer. 1981;48:845–51.
10. Chak LY, Cox RS, Bostwick DG, Hoppe RT. Solitary plasmacitoma of bone: treatment, progression and survival. J Clin Oncol. 1987;5:1811–5.
11. Frassica DA, Frassica FJ, Schray MF, Sim FH, Kyle RA. Solitary plasmacytoma of bone: Mayo Clinic experience. Int J Rad Oncol. 1989;16:43–8.
12. Dimopoulos MA, Moulopoulos LA, Maniatis A, Alexanian R. Solitary plasmacytoma of bone and asymptomatic multiple myeloma. Blood. 2000;96:2037–44.
13. Knobel D, Zouhair A, Tsang RW, et al. Prognostic factors in solitary plasmacytoma of the bone: a multicentric Rare Cancer Network study. BMC Cancer. 2006;6:118.

14. Dores GM, Landgren O, McGlynn KA, et al. Plasmacytoma of bone, extramedullary plasmacytoma, and multiple myeloma: incidence and survival in the United States, 1992–2004. Br J Haematol. 2008;144:86–94.
15. Warsame R, Gertz MA, Lacy MQ, et al. Trends and outcomes of modern staging of solitary plasmacytoma of bone. Am J Hematol. 2012;87:647–51.
16. Katidrotou I, Terpos E, Symeonidis AS, et al. Clinical features, outcome, and prognostic factors for survival and evolution to multiple myeloma of solitary plasmacytomas: a report of the Greek myeloma study group in 97 patients. Am J Hematol. 2014;89:803–8.
17. Wilder RB, Ha CS, Cox JD, Weber D, Delasalle K, Alexanian R. Persistence of myeloma protein for more than 1 year after radiotherapy is an adverse prognostic factor in solitary plasmacytoma of bone. Cancer. 2002;94:1532–7.
18. Dingli D, Kyle RA, Rajkumar SV, et al. Immunoglobulin free light chains and solitary plasmacytoma of bone. Blood. 2006;108:1979–83.
19. Fouquet G, Guidez S, Herbaux C, et al. Impact of initial FDG-PET/CT and serum free light chain on transformation of conventionally defined plasmacytoma to multiple myeloma. Clin Cancer Res. 2014;20:3254–60.
20. Paiva B, Chandia M, Vidriales MV, et al. Multiparameter flow cytometry for staging of solitary bone plasmacytoma: new criteria for risk progression to myeloma. Blood. 2014;124:1300–3.
21. Hill QA, Rawstron AC, de Tute RM, Owen RG. Outcome prediction in plasmacytoma of bone: a risk model utilizing bone marrow flow cytomtry and light-chain analysis. Blood. 2014;124:1296–9.
22. Holland J, Trenkner DA, Wasserman TH, Fineberg B. Plasmacytoma: treatment results and conversion to myeloma. Cancer. 1992;69:1513–7.
23. Tsang RW, Gospodarowicz MK, Pintilie M, et al. Solitary plasmacytoma treated with radiotherapy: impact of tumor size on outcome. Int J Radiat Oncol Biol Phys. 2001;50:113–20.
24. Reed V, Shah J, Medeiros LJ, et al. Solitary plasmacytomas. Outcome and prognostic factors after definitive radiation therapy. Cancer. 2011;117:4468–74.
25. Dimopoulos MA, Pouli A, Anagnastopoulos A, et al. Macrofocal multiple myeloma in young patients: a distinct entity with favourable prognosis. Leuk Lymphoma. 2006;47:1553–6.
26. Hewell GM, Alexanian R. Multiple myeloma in young patients. Arch Intern Med. 1976;84:441–3.
27. Bladé J, Kyle RA, Greipp PR. Multiple myeloma in patients younger than 30 years. Arch Intern Med. 1996;156:1463–8.
28. Bladé J, Fernández de Larrea C, Rosiñol L, Cibeira MT, Jiménez R, Powles R. Soft-tissue plasmacytomas in multiple myeloma: incidence, mechanisms of extramedullar spread, and treatment approach. J Clin Oncol. 2011;29:3805–12.
29. Azar HA. Pathology of multiple myeloma and related disorders. In: Azar HA, Potter M, editors. Multiple msyeloma and related disorders, vol. 1. Hagerstown: Harper and Row; 1973. p. 1–85.
30. Churg J, Gordon AJ. Multiple myeloma with unusual visceral involvement. Arch Pathol. 1942;34:546–56.
31. Churg J, Gordon AJ. Multiple myeloma: lesions of extra-osseous hematopoietic system. Am J Clin Pathol. 1950;20:934–45.
32. Hayes DW, Bennett WA, Heck FJ. Extramedullary lesions in multiple myeloma: review of the literature and pathologic studies. AMA Arch Pathol. 1952;53:262–72.
33. Ghobrial I. Myeloma as a model for the process of metastasis: implications for therapy. Blood. 2012;120:20–30.
34. Mitsiades CS, McMillin DW, Kippel S, et al. The role of bone marrow microenvironment in the pathpphysiology of myeloma and its significance in the development of more effective therapies. Hematol Oncol Clin North Am. 2007;21:1007–14.
35. Van de Broek I, Vanderkerken K, Van Camp B, Van Riet I. Extravassation and homing mechanisms in multiple myeloma. Clin Exp Metastasis. 2008;25:325–34.
36. Hideshima T, Chauban D, Havashi T, et al. Biological sequelae of stromal cell-derived factor-1alfa in multiple myeloma. Mol Cancer Ther. 2002;1:539–44.
37. Alsayed Y, Ngo H, Runnels J, et al. Mechanisms of regulation of CXCR4/SDF-1 (CXCL12)-dependent migration and homing in multiple myeloma. Blood. 2007;109:2708–17.
38. Menu E, Asosingh K, Indraccolo S, et al. Involvement of stromal derived factor-1alfa in homing and progression of multiple myeloma in 5TMM model. Haematologica. 2006;91:606–12.
39. Azab AK, Runnels JM, Pitsillides C, et al. CXCR4 inhibitor AMD3100 disrupts the interactivity of myeloma cells with the bone marrow microenvironment and enhances theirs sensitivity to therapy. Blood. 2006;113:4341–51.
40. Van den Broek I, Leleu X, Schots R, et al. Clinical significance of chemokine receptor (CCR3, CCR2 and CXCR4) expression in human myeloma cells: the association with disease activity and survival. Haematologica. 2006;91:200–6.
41. Azab KA, Sahin I, Azab F, et al. CXCR7-dependent angiogenic mononuclear cell trafficking regulates tumour progression in multiple myeloma. Blood. 2014;124:1905–14.
42. Nakayama T, Hideshima T, Izawa D, et al. Profile of chemokine receptor expression on human plasma cells accounts for their efficient recruitment to target tissues. J Immunol. 2003;170:1136–40.
43. Pasmantier MW, Azar HA. Extraskeletal spread in multiple plasma cell myeloma: a review of 57 autopsied cases. Cancer. 1969;23:167–74.
44. Wu P, Davies F, Boyd K, et al. The impact of extramedullary disease at presentation in the outcome of myeloma. Leuk Lymphoma. 2009;50:230–5.
45. Varettoni M, Corso A, Pica G, et al. Incidence, presenting features and outcome of extramedullary disease in multiple myeloma: a longitudinal study on 1,003 consecutive patients. Ann Oncol. 2009;21:325–30.
46. Bladé J, Lust JA, Kyle RA. Immunoglobulin D multiple myeloma: presenting features, response to therapy, and survival in a series of 53 patients. J Clin Oncol. 1994;12:2398–404.
47. Bladé J, Kyle RA, Greip PR. Presenting features and prognosis in 72 patients with multiple myeloma who were younger than 40 years. Br J Haematol. 1996;93:345–51.
48. Varga C, Xie W, Laubach J, et al. Development of extramedullary myeloma in the era of novel agents: no evidence of increased risk with lenalidomide-bortezomib combinations. Br J Haematol. 2015;169:843–50.
49. Usmani SZ, Heuck C, Mitchell A, et al. Extramedullary disease portends poor prognosis in multiple myeloma and is overexpressed in high-risk disease even in the era of novel agents. Haematologica. 2012;97:4761–7.
50. Short KD, Rajkumar SV, Larson D, et al. Incidence of extramedullary disease in patients with multiple myeloma in the era of novel therapy and activity of pomalidomide in extramedullary myeloma. Leukemia. 2011;25:906–8.
51. Pour L, Sevcikova S, Greslikova H, et al. Soft-tissue extramedullary multiple myeloma prognosis is significantly worse in comparison with bone-related extramedullary relapse. Haematologica. 2014;99:360–4.
52. Weinstock M, Aljawai Y, Morgan EA, et al. Incidence and clinical features of extramedullary multiple myeloma in patients who underwent stem cell transplantation. Br J Haematol. 2015;169:851–8.
53. Papanikolaou X, Repousis P, Tzenou T, et al. Incidence, clinical features, laboratory findings and outcome of patients with multiple myeloma presenting with extramedullary relapse. Leuk Lymphoma. 2013;54:1459.1464.

54. Fernández de Larrea C, Jimenez R, Rosiñol L, et al. Pattern of relapse and progression after autologous stem cell transplantation as upfront therapy in multiple myeloma. Bone Marrow Transplant. 2014;49:223–7.
55. Pérez-Simón JA, Sureda A, Fernández-Avilés F, et al. Reduced-intensity conditioning allogeneic transplantation is associated with a high incidence of extramedullary relapses in multiple myeloma patients. Leukemia. 2006;20:542–5.
56. Minnema MC, van de Donk NW, Zweegman S, et al. Extramedullary relapses after allogeneic non-myeloablative stem cell transplantation in multiple myeloma patients do not negatively affect treatment outcome. Bone Marrow Transplant. 2004;34:1057–65.
57. Zeiser R, Deschler B, Bertz H, et al. Extramedullary vs. medullary relapse after autologous or allogeneic hematopoietic stem cell transplantation (HSCT) in multiple myeloma (MM) and its correlation with clinical outcome. Bone Marrow Transplant. 2004;34:1057–65.
58. Fassas AB, Ward S, Muwalla F, et al. Myeloma of central nervous system: strong association with unfavourable chromosomal abnormalities and other high-risk disease features. Leuk Lymphoma. 2004;45:291–300.
59. Nieuwenhuizen L, Biesma DH. Central nervous system myelomatosis: review of the literature. Eur J Haematol. 2007;80:1–9.
60. Schluteman KO, Fassas AB, Van Hemert RL, et al. Multiple myeloma invasion of the central nervous system. Arch Neurol. 2004;61:1423–9.
61. Chamberlain MC, Glanz M. Myelomatous meningitis. Cancer. 2008;112:1562–7.
62. Gozzetti A, Cesare A, Lotti F, et al. Extramedullary intracranial localization of multiple myeloma and treatment with novel agents: a retrospective survey of 50 patients. Cancer. 2012;118:1574–84.
63. Jurczyszyn A, Grzasko N, Gozzetti A, et al. Central nervous system involvement by multiple myeloma: a multi-institutional retrospective study of 172 patients in daily clinical practice. Am J Hematol. 2016;91:575–80.
64. Katadritou E, Terpos E, Kastritis E, et al. Lack of survival improvement with novel anti-myeloma agents for patients with multiple myeloma and central nervous system involvement: the Greek Myeloma Study Group experience. Ann Hematol. 2015;94:2033–42.
65. Bladé J, Rosiñol L. Complications of multiple myeloma. Hematol Oncol Clin North Am. 2007;21:1231–46.
66. Posner JB. Back pain and epidural spinal cord compression. Med Clin North Am. 1987;71:185–201.
67. Reseblum MD, Bredeson CN, Chang CC, et al. Subcutaneous plasmacytomas with tropism to sites of previous trauma in a multiple myeloma patient treated with autologous bone marrow transplant. Am J Hematol. 2003;72:274–7.
68. Fernández de Larrea C, Rosiñol L, Cibeira MT, et al. Extensive soft-tissue involvement by plasmablastic myeloma arising from displaced humeral fractures. Eur J Haematol. 2010;85:448–51.
69. Muchtar E, Raanani P, Yeshurun M, Shpilberg O, Magen-Nativ M. Myeloma in scar tissue—an underreported phenomenon or an emerging entity in the novel agents' era? A single center series. Acta Haematol. 2014;132:39–44.
70. Rosiñol L, Fernández de Larrea C, Bladé J. Extramedullary myeloma spread triggered by surgical procedures: an emerging entity? Acta Haematol. 2014;132:36–8.
71. Katadritou E, Gastari V, Verrou E, et al. Extramedullary (EM) relapse in unusual locations in multiple mieloma: is there an association with precedent thalidomide administration and a correlation of special biological features with treatment and outcome? Leuk Res. 2009;33:1137–40.
72. Chang H, Barlett E, Patterson B, Chen I, Yi QL. The absence of CD56 on malignant plasma cells in the cerebrospinal fluid is the hallmark of multiple myeloma involving central nervous system. Br J Haematol. 2005;129:539–41.
73. Sheth N, Yeung L, Chang H. P53 nuclear accumulation is associated with extramedullary progression in multiple myeloma. Leuk Res. 2009;33:1357–60.
74. Chang H, Sloan S, Li D, Stewart K. Multiple myeloma involving central nervous system: high frequency of chromosome 17p13 (p53) deletions. Br J Haematol. 2004;127:280–4.
75. López-Anglada L, Gutiérrez NC, García JL, Mateos MV, Flores T, San Miguel JF. P53 deletion may drive the clinical evolution and treatment response in multiple myeloma. Eur J Haematol. 2010;84:359–61.
76. Billecke L, Murga Penas EM, May AM, et al. Similar incidence of TP53 deletions in extramedullary organ infiltrations, soft-tissue and osteolysis of patients with multiple myeloma. Anticancer Res. 2012;161:87–94.
77. Billecke L, Murga Penas EM, May AM, et al. Cytogenetics of extramedullary manifestations in multiple myeloma. Br J Haematol. 2013;161:87–94.
78. Rasche L, Benard C, Topp MS, et al. Features of extramedullary myeloma relapse: high proliferation, minimal marrow involvement, adverse cytogenetics. A retrospective single center study of 24 cases. Ann Hematol. 2012;91:1031–7.
79. Dimopoulos MA, Terpos E, Comenzo RL, et al. International Myeloma Working Group consensus statement and guidelines regarding the current role of imaging techniques in the diagnosis and monitoring of multiple myeloma. Leukemia. 2009;23:1545–56.
80. Dimopoulos MA, Kyle RA, Fermand JP, et al. Consensus recomendations for standard investigative work-up: report on the International Myeloma Workshop Consensus Panel 3. Blood. 2011;117:4701–5.
81. Dimopoulos MA, Hillengass J, Usmani S, et al. Role of magnetic resonance imaging in the management of multiple myeloma: a consensus statement. J Clin Oncol. 2015;33:657–64.
82. Zamagni E, Cavo M. The role of imaging techniques in the management of multiple myeloma. Br J Haematol. 2012;159:499–513.
83. Zamagni E, Nanni C, Tachetti P, et al. Positron emission tomography with computed tomography-based diagnosis of massive extramedullary progression in a patient with high-risk multiple mieloma. Clin Lymphoma Myeloma Leuk. 2014;14:101–4.
84. Nanni C, Zamagni E, Versari A, et al. Image interpretation criteria for FDG PET/CT in multiple myeloma: a new proposal from an Italian Expert Panel. IMPeTUs (Italian Myeloma criteria for PET use). Eur J Nucl Med Mol Imaging. 2016;43:414–21.
85. Lu YY, Chen JH, Lin WY, et al. FDG-PET or PET/CT for detecting intramedullary and extramedullay lesions in multiple myeloma: a systematic review and meta-analysis. Clin Nucl Med. 2012;37:833–7.
86. Van Lammeren-Venema D, Regelink JC, Riphagen II, Zweegman S, Hoekstra OS, Zijlstra JM. FDG positron emission tomography in assessment of mieloma-related bone disease. Cancer. 2012;118:1971–81.
87. Durie BGM, Harousseau JL, San Miguel JF, et al. International uniform response criteria for multiple myeloma. Leukemia. 2006;20:1467–73.
88. Mesguish C, Fardanesh R, Tanenbaum L, Chari A, Jaganath S, Kostakoglu L. State of the art imaging in multiple myeloma: comparative review of FDG PET/CT imaging in various clinical settings. Eur J Radiol. 2014;83:2203–23.
89. Lee SE, Kim JH, Jeon YW, et al. Impact of extramedullary plasmacytomas on outcomes according to treatment approach in

newly diagnosed symptomatic multiple myeloma. Ann Hematol. 2015;94:445–52.

90. Rosiñol L, Oriol A, Teruel AI, et al. Superiority of bortezomib, thalidomide, and dexamethasone (VTD) as induction pre-transplantation therapy in multiple myeloma: results of a randomized phase III PETHEMA/GEM study. Blood. 2012;120:1589–96.
91. Patriarca F, Prosdocimo S, Tomadini V, et al. Efficacy of bortezomib therapy for extramedullary relapse of myeloma after autologous and non-myeloablative allogeneic transplantation. Haematologica. 2005;90:278–9.
92. Paubelle E, Coppo P, Garderet L, et al. Complete remission with bortezomib on plasmacytoma in an end-stage patient with refractory multiple myeloma who failed all other therapies including haematopoietic stem cell transplantation: possible enhancement of graft-versus tumour effect. Leukemia. 2005;19:1702–4.
93. Rosiñol L, Cibeira MT, Uruburu C, et al. Bortezomib: an effective agent in extramedullary disease in multiple myeloma. Eur J Haematol. 2006;76:405–8.
94. Rosiñol L, Cibeira MT, Bladé J, et al. Extramedullary multiple myeloma escapes the effect of thalidomide. Haematologica. 2004;89:832–6.
95. Avigdor A, Raanani P, Levi I, et al. Extramedullary progression despite a good response in the bone marrow in patients treated with thalidomide for multiple myeloma. Leuk Lymphoma. 2001;42:683–7.
96. Juliusson G, Celsing F, Turesson I, et al. Frequent good partial remissions from thalidomide including best response ever in patients with advanced refractory and relapsed myeloma. Br J Haematol. 2000;109:89–96.
97. Muers B, Grimley C, Crouch D, et al. Lack of response to thalidomide in plasmacytomas. Br J Haematol. 2001;115:234.
98. Anagnostopoulos A, Gika D, Hamilos G, et al. Treatment of relapsed refractory multiple myeloma with thalidomide-based regimens: identification of prognostic factors. Leuk Lymphoma. 2004;45:2275–9.
99. San Miguel JF, Schlag R, Khuageva NK, et al. Bortezomib plus melphalan and prednisone for initial treatment of multiple myeloma. N Engl J Med. 2008;359:906–17.
100. Mateos MV, Oriol A, Martínez-López J, et al. Bortezomib plus melphalan and prednisone versus bortezomib, thalidomide and prednisone as induction therapy followed by maintenance treatment with bortezomib and thalidomide versus bortzomib and prednisone in elderly patients with untreated multiple myeloma: a randomized trial. Lancet Oncol. 2010;11:934–41.
101. Sonneveld P, Goldschmith H, Rosiñol L, et al. Bortezomib-based versus non-bortezomib-based induction treatment before autologous stem-cell transplantation in patients with previously untreated multiple myeloma: a meta-analysis of phase III randomized, controlled trials. J Clin Oncol. 2013;31:3279–87.
102. Barlogie B, Anaissie E, Rhee F, et al. The Arkansas approach to therapy in patients with multiple myeloma. Best Pract Clin Res. 2007;20:761–81.
103. Rosiñol L, Jimenez R, Rovira M, et al. Allogeneic hematopoietic SCT in multiple myeloma: long-term results from a single institution. Bone Marrow Transplant. 2015;15:658–62.
104. Srikanth M, Davies FE, Wu P, et al. Survival and outcome of blastoid variant myeloma following treatment with the novel thalidomide containing regimen DT-PACE. Eur J Haematol. 2008;81:432–6.
105. Rasche L, Strifler S, Duell J, et al. The lymphoma-like polychemotherapy regimen "Dexa BEAM" in advanced and extramedullary multiple myeloma. Ann Hematol. 2014;93:1207–14.

31 Supportive Care in Multiple Myeloma

Simit Mahesh Doshi, Tom T. Noff, and G. David Roodman

Myeloma Bone Disease

Multiple myeloma (MM) is the second most common hematologic malignancy, affecting more than 60,000 patients in the United States with 30,000 patients diagnosed in 2016 [1, 2]. Multiple myeloma (MM) is the most frequent cancer to involve bone with almost 70% of patients presenting with bone lesions at diagnosis [3]. Twenty percent of patients present with a pathologic fracture at diagnosis and until recently up to 60% of patients developed a pathologic fracture over the course of their disease [7]. This is extremely important since pathologic fractures increase mortality of MM patients by 20% [8]. In addition, MM bone disease can cause excruciating bone pain that remains undertreated in many patients, and hypercalcemia that can be life threatening, as well as require surgery and/or radiation to bone to control bone pain, treat impending or repair fractures, and relieve spinal cord compression. Further, in the vast majority of patients, MM bone lesions rarely heal even when patients are in long-term remission [10], and MM patients continue to suffer from the sequelae of their bone disease, even when their MM is under excellent control. Tremendous progress has been made in the treatment of MM, with a median survival of patients increasing to more than 6.1 years in the last decade and a much better overall survival for patients over the age of 65 [9]. Thus, treatment and repair of MM bone disease are increasingly important, both for enhancing the quality of life of patients, increasing their survival, prevention of hypercalcemia or fracture, and suppressing the growth of MM cells in the bone marrow.

S.M. Doshi, M.D., M.P.H.
Department of Nephrology, IUH University Hospital, 950 W Walnut Street, Indianapolis, IN 46202, USA

T.T. Noff, M.D.
Department of Neurology, University of Indiana School of Medicine, 355 W 16th Street, Indianapolis, IN 46202, USA

G. David Roodman, M.D., Ph.D. (✉)
Department of Hematology and Oncology, Indiana University School of Medicine, 980 W Walnut Street, Suite C312, Indianapolis, IN 46202, USA
e-mail: groodman@iu.edu

Pathophysiology of Myeloma Bone Disease

During the normal bone-remodeling process, osteoclastic bone resorption is coupled to osteoblastic bone formation, so that bone removal and formation are balanced (Fig. 31.1). However, in MM the normal bone-remodeling process is essentially uncoupled, with markedly increased bone resorption at sites of MM and absent or severely decreased bone formation. This is due to suppression of osteoblast differentiation that can persist even when patients are in long-term remission [10]. Thus, little or no repair of lytic lesions occurs in the vast majority of patients with MM, although there have been anecdotal reports of healing of bone lesions in patients receiving bortezomib-based therapy. However, once a patient's bone density is below the fracture threshold, the patient continues to be at an increased risk of fracture and experience persistent bone pain.

A multiplicity of osteoclast stimulating factors are produced by MM cells and induced by MM cells in the bone marrow microenvironment [10]. These factors include MM cell production of Rank ligand, a highly potent osteoclast-stimulating factor, or induction of Rank ligand production by marrow stromal cells and osteocytes in the MM microenvironment. Furthermore, production of MIP-1 α by MM cells, interleukin 3 production by both MM cells and T-lymphocytes in the MM microenvironment, and IL-6 production by marrow stromal cells, osteoclasts, and other cells in the bone microenvironment also occur [10]. In addition, osteoclastic bone resorption and increased osteoclast numbers enhance the growth of MM cells. This process has been described as the vicious cycle hypothesis, in which MM cells induce osteoclastic bone resorption, and the bone resorption process releases growth factors, such as IGF1 and TGF-beta from bone matrix, which in turn stimulate the growth of MM cells (Fig. 31.2). In addition, MM cells induce polarization of T cells in the tumor microenvironment, which reverses the ratio of Th17 to Th1 T cells to 10:1 com-

P.H. Wiernik et al. (eds.), *Neoplastic Diseases of the Blood*, DOI 10.1007/978-3-319-64263-5_31

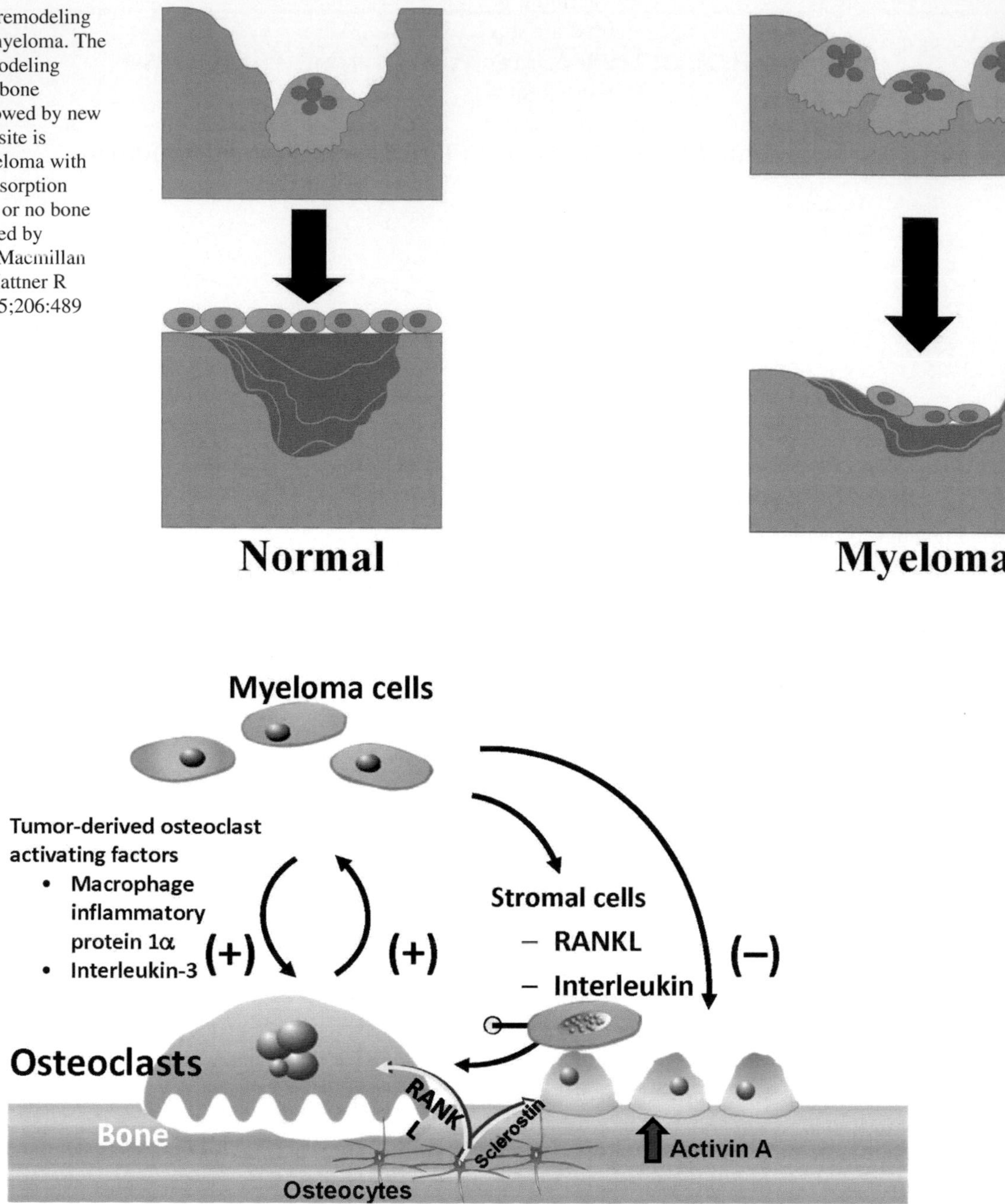

Fig. 31.1 Bone remodeling is uncoupled in myeloma. The normal bone-remodeling process in which bone resorption is followed by new bone at the same site is uncoupled in myeloma with increased bone resorption followed by little or no bone formation. Adapted by permission from Macmillan Publishers Ltd: Hattner R et al. Nature. 1965;206:489

Fig. 31.2 Reciprocal interactions between myeloma cells and bone microenvironment contribute to progression of myeloma. Myeloma cells colonize the marrow and some of the cells engage the endosteal niche and become dormant, while other cells remain active myeloma cells. Active myeloma cells produce factors and induce factors by cells in the bone microenvironment to increase osteoclast formation and resorption. The increased bone resorption in turn releases growth factors from bone matrix to stimulate the growth of myeloma cells. Myeloma cells also suppress osteoblast differentiation to block new bone formation. In addition, myeloma cells directly interact with osteocytes in the bone matrix and these interactions increase myeloma cell growth and osteoclast formation as well as block osteoblast differentiation. Finally, osteoclastic resorption also releases dormant myeloma cells to become active myeloma cells, further contributing to myeloma progression. Adapted from Roodman GD. N Engl J Med. 2004;350(16):1655–1664. Copyright © 2004 Massachusetts Medical Society. Reprinted with permission

pared to the normal ratio of 1:10. Th17 cells produce IL17 that induces dendritic cell differentiation toward the osteoclast lineage, as well as enhance induction of Rank ligand.

MM cells, osteoclasts, and marrow stromal cells in the microenvironment also produce angiogenic factors that further increase the growth of MM cells [11]. In addition, the increased numbers of osteoclasts directly support MM growth. Yaccoby and coworkers demonstrated that primary MM cells from patients can be passaged over feeder layers of osteoclasts for long periods of time [12]. Abe and coworkers found that osteoclasts support the growth of primary MM cells through the production of IL-6 and osteopontin [13].

Finally, direct interactions between osteoclasts and osteocytes enhance bidirectional Notch signaling between the cells to increase the growth of MM cells, induce osteocyte apoptosis, and increase production of sclerostin and Rank ligand by osteocytes that suppresses osteoblast differentiation and stimulates osteoclastogenesis [14]. In addition, osteoclasts produce Annexin II, BAFF, and April that support MM cell growth [15, 16].

Recently, osteoclastic bone resorption has also been shown to play an important role in activating dormant MM cells in the MM microenvironment to active MM cells. Activation of dormant MM cells results in increased tumor burden, bone destruction, and distant colonization of bones. Lawson et al. recently showed by intravital imaging that treatment of mice with Rank ligand increases osteoclast numbers and decreases the numbers of dormant MM cells colonizing the osteoblast niche [17]. Thus, osteoclasts play multiple roles in progression of MM, including activation of dormant MM cells, bone destruction that results in release of matrix-bound growth factors to stimulate tumor growth, and enhancement of MM growth by factors derived from osteoclasts.

Studies in preclinical models of MM found that blocking osteoclastic bone resorption decreases tumor burden in addition to bone destruction [18]. However, until recently this phenomenon has not been demonstrated in patients. The MM IX trial showed that treating newly diagnosed MM patients with zoledronate, a potent bisphosphonate that blocks osteoclastic bone resorption, rather than with clodronate, a weaker bisphosphonate, enhances survival of MM patients. This increase in survival occurred regardless if the patients had detectable bone disease at diagnosis [19]. However, the greatest benefit in survival was seen in patients with detectable bone disease. Based on preclinical and clinical studies, the International Myeloma Working Group (IMWG) guidelines now support targeting osteoclastic bone resorption in all patients with MM [20].

Osteoblast Suppression in Myeloma

As noted above, bone formation is markedly suppressed in patients with MM and persists even when the MM is under excellent control. This explains why bone scans, which measure reactive bone formation, frequently under-represent bone disease in MM patients, making bone scans inappropriate for imaging bone disease in MM patients [21]. Multiple factors produced by MM cells or induced by MM cells in the MM microenvironment block osteoblast precursor differentiation to mature osteoblasts. A large number of inhibitors of osteoblast differentiation have been identified in MM patients, including TNFα, MIP-1 α, IL-3, activin A, sclerostin, DKK1, hepatocyte growth factor, TGF-beta, and IL7 [22]. All these factors can directly suppress osteoblast differentiation and are potential therapeutic targets for treating MM bone disease (see below). However, none of these factors can explain why osteoblast suppression persists in patients even in the absence of MM cells. The mechanisms responsible for the long-term suppression of osteoblast differentiation in MM are just beginning to be understood. D'Souza and all demonstrated that epigenetic changes in the Runx2 promoter in pre-osteoblasts, the master gene controlling osteoblast differentiation, are induced by MM cells [23]. These changes in the Runx2 promoter result from induction of Gfi1 in pre-osteoblastic marrow stromal cells exposed to MM cells. Gfi1 acts as a transcriptional repressor of Runx2 and blocks osteoblast differentiation. Increased expression of Gfi1 persists in marrow stromal cells from MM patients, even when the stromal cells are passaged for long periods of time in the absence of MM cells. Furthermore, knockdown of Gfi1 in marrow stromal cells from MM patients allows them to undergo osteoblast differentiation. These insights into the mechanisms responsible for long-term suppression of osteoblast differentiation have provided potential new therapeutic targets for repairing bone lesions in MM patients. Furthermore, Li and coworkers reported that mature osteoblasts could suppress MM cell growth through the production of decorin [24]. These results suggest that in addition to repairing bone lesions, inducing osteoblast differentiation may also suppress the growth of MM cells in patients.

Imaging of Myeloma Bone Disease

Imaging of MM bone disease has become increasingly important with the development of new criteria for the diagnosis of active MM. These criteria include presence of at least one lytic lesion detected by conventional radiography, whole-body low-dose CT or PET/CT, or presence of more than one focal bone marrow lesion greater than or equal to 5 mm on MRI studies [25]. Skeletal surveys have been the gold standard for detecting MM bone disease. The lesions appear as punched-out lytic bone lesions with the absence of reactive new bone formation and can occur in any bone. However, conventional radiographs are relatively insensitive for detecting bone disease in MM, since more than 30% of bone must be removed before a lesion is detectable. Conventional radiographs are also not useful for following disease progression or response to therapy, because lytic lesions rarely heal in these patients and enumerating new lesions can frequently be difficult in patients with extensive bone disease. In addition, it is often difficult to distinguish between osteoporotic and MM-induced vertebral fractures. Finally, skeletal surveys take a great deal of time to perform, which can be difficult for patients who have severe bone pain.

Low-dose whole-body CT has been recently shown to be superior to conventional radiographs for detecting osteolytic lesions in MM patients, and is especially useful for detecting lesions in the spine or pelvis [26]. Low-dose whole-body CT can take less than 5 min to perform, and has the advantage that it can also demonstrate extraosseous lesions. Because of these advantages, low-dose whole-body CT is becoming the standard screening method for MM bone disease in Europe. However, although low-dose whole-body CT exposes the patients to a higher dose of radiation than standard skeletal surveys, the higher resolution and speed of the examination outweigh the disadvantages. Many experts predict that low-dose whole-body CT will replace skeletal surveys as the new gold standard for detecting MM bone disease [26].

Magnetic resonance imaging (MRI) is also more sensitive than standard skeletal radiographs for detecting MM bone disease, and also detects bone marrow infiltration by MM cells. A large study from the University of Arkansas showed that MRI detected focal lesions in 74% of MM patients, compared to 56% of patients who were examined with whole-body radiographs [27]. MRI is particularly useful for distinguishing between asymptomatic smoldering MM and symptomatic MM. Patients who were thought to have smoldering MM but had more than one focal lesion on MRI had a 70% probability of progression to active MM within 2 years [28]. These results form the basis for adding the presence of more than one focal criteria on MRI to the updated criteria for active MM [25]. The International Myeloma Working Group recommends, at a minimum, MRI examination of the spine and pelvis as part of the evaluation for smoldering MM, if whole-body MRI cannot be done [29]. However, MRI limited to the spine and pelvis will not detect lesions in the peripheral skeleton that occur in 10% of patients who present with focal lesions [30].

PET/CT is a very useful albeit expensive imaging technique for assessing MM bone disease. PET detects the hypermetabolic activity of MM cells in both intraosseous and extramedullary sites, while CT detects bone-destructive lesions. PET/CT has a similar sensitivity to that of MRI, and is better than MRI at detecting bony lesions. More importantly, PET/CT can be used to assess response to therapy [31]. Further, the presence of extramedullary lesions or an SUV Max greater than 4.21 on a PET/CT performed at diagnosis, persistence of FDG uptake following autologous stem cell transplantation for MM, or detection of extramedullary disease are all associated with a poor prognosis for patients. However, it is unclear if PET/CT or MRI is better for determining if patients with solitary plasmacytoma have disease restricted to one site or multiple sites. PET/CT is also useful for following patients with non-secretory MM [32]. However, PET/CT may also detect false-positive findings in patients following radiotherapy or infections.

Treatment of MM Bone Disease

The landmark studies of Berenson and coworkers in 1996 demonstrated that the nitrogen- containing bisphosphonate, pamidronate, decreased skeletal related events (surgery to bone, fractures, radiation to bone, and spinal cord compression) and bone pain in patients with MM bone disease [33]. Pamidronate and zoledronic acid are the cornerstone of treatment for MM bone disease. Bisphosphonates are non-hydrolyzable pyrophosphate analogues that block osteoclastic bone resorption and inhibit osteoclast formation through their capacity to inhibit protein prenylation by inhibiting farnesyl diphosphate synthase required for normal osteoclast activity [34]. Pamidronate is usually administered as a 90 mg intravenous infusion over 2 h, while its more potent analogue, zoledronic acid, is administered as 4 mg intravenously over 15 min. Both bisphosphonates have similar efficacy for treating MM bone disease and are routinely given every 3–4 weeks. Bisphosphonates are very safe drugs and their major toxicity is their potential deleterious effects on renal function. Therefore, serum creatinine levels must be measured prior to infusion. If creatinine levels in patients receiving these agents increase more than 10% from their baseline values, pamidronate or zoledronic acid should be withheld until the serum creatinine returns to within 10% of the previous baseline value. In patients who present with impaired renal function, the infusion time for pamidronate can be increased or the dose of zoledronate can be reduced, since renal toxicity of bisphosphonates is related to peak dose [35]. In patients who present with severe renal failure, initial therapy with bortezomib-based regimens should be started prior to initiation of bisphosphonate therapy (see below).

Multiple organizations have developed guidelines for use of bisphosphonates in MM. Each of these guidelines state that bisphosphonates can be given intravenously every 3–4 weeks for patients with MM bone disease that is identified by plain radiographs or MRI. More recent IMWG recommendations for treatment of MM-related bone disease state that bisphosphonate therapy should be considered for all patients with MM, regardless of the presence of osteolytic bone disease by conventional radiography [20]. These recommendations are based on the results of the MM IX trial that compared clodronate to zoledronic acid therapy in more than 1000 newly diagnosed patients receiving treatment for MM (see above). This study found that patients receiving zoledronate achieved a 5-month survival benefit compared to patients receiving clodronate [19]. This survival advantage occurred regardless if the patient had demonstrable bone disease at diagnosis. A subsequent secondary analysis of this study showed that the major impact on survival occurred in patients with bone disease [36]. However, it's unclear how long patients should continue to receive bisphosphonate therapy. This question became a major concern with the recognition that some MM patients receiving bisphosphonates develop bisphosphonate-associated osteonecrosis of the jaw (BRONJ). This complication of bisphosphonate therapy was first recognized by Marx et al. [37]. The occurrence of

BRONJ is usually dependent on the duration and dose of bisphosphonate therapy, undergoing invasive dental procedures, age of the patient, and treatment with glucocorticoids. BRONJ occurs more frequently in patients receiving zoledronate than pamidronate [37]. Because of concern for development of BRONJ, most guidelines recommend treatment with bisphosphonates for approximately 2 years, unless active MM persists, and then stopping or increasing the interval between administration of bisphosphonates should be considered. However, with the regular institution of close dental monitoring, dental prophylaxis, and performing most dental procedures prior to initiating bisphosphonate therapy, the incidence of BRONJ has markedly decreased.

Another question that often occurs is should bisphosphonate therapy should be stopped prior to invasive dental procedures. The American Dental Association recently recommended not stopping bisphosphonates or other bone-targeted agents when patients undergo dental procedures, and states that the decision to withhold bisphosphonate therapy should be based primarily on the patient's risk of developing a skeletal related event [38]. In contrast, the IMWG recommends stopping bisphosphonates for 90 days before and after invasive dental procedures, such as tooth extraction, dental implants, and surgery to the jaw [20].

Several studies assessed if bone resorption markers are useful for determining the interval between bisphosphonate administration in patients with MM bone disease. Patel and coworkers found in patients who had received bisphosphonate therapy for at least a year and had stable disease that the level of bone resorption markers could be used to determine when to administer bisphosphonate therapy [39]. However, other studies show that bone resorption markers are not sufficiently sensitive to guide bisphosphonate therapy [40]. Importantly, the MM IX trial demonstrated that extending bisphosphonate treatment beyond 2 years continued to have beneficial effects on skeletal related events [36]. However, only small numbers of patients received long-term bisphosphonate therapy in that study. Another consideration with bisphosphonate therapy is whether bisphosphonate therapy can be restarted in patients who developed BRONJ. A retrospective analysis of over 100 MM patients demonstrated that about 50% of patients who developed BRONJ healed their lesions and 50% of those who restarted bisphosphonates did not develop new lesions [41]. These results suggest that patients who have active MM and have healed their osteonecrosis of the jaw can receive bisphosphonate therapy but should be monitored closely for a reoccurrence of BRONJ.

In addition to bisphosphonates, denosumab, a human monoclonal antibody that targets Rank ligand, has been developed, and potently inhibits osteoclast formation and bone resorption. Multiple large phase 3 studies of denosumab versus zoledronate treatment for patients with bone metastasis found that denosumab has either a non-inferior or a superior effect on skeletal related events compared with zoledronate, and patients treated with denosumab who had breast cancer bone metastasis had a survival advantage [42]. A large phase 3 study compared denosumab to zoledronic acid treatment in patients with bone metastasis that did not have prostate cancer or breast cancer, and also included 200 MM patients. This study found a similar decrease in skeletal related events in the MM patients with either treatment, but a post hoc analysis found a decreased survival for MM patients receiving denosumab [43]. Further analysis of this trial found that the baseline characteristics of the MM patients receiving zoledronic acid or denosumab were not balanced, and that the patients receiving zoledronic acid treatment had more early withdrawals from the study compared to those treated with denosumab [43]. A large phase 3 study comparing denosumab to zoledronic acid treatment in newly diagnosed patients with MM bone disease has just been completed, and the results of this trial should be reported soon. It is important to note that the incidence of ONJ is similar in patients receiving denosumab or zoledronic acid so that similar dental screening, routine dental prophylaxis, and follow-up are also required for patients receiving denosumab. Finally, neither denosumab nor zoledronic acid increases bone formation in patients with MM, so there is still a great need for bone anabolic agents that can increase bone formation and are safe for MM patients.

Recently, several agents have been developed to enhance bone formation in patients with MM. These include an antibody to DKK1, BHQ880, and sotatercept, an activin receptor antagonist [22]. A phase 1B clinical trial of anti-DKK1 in patients with MM did not show any benefit for MM bone disease [44], although the anti-DKK1 did show some bone anabolic effects in a phase 2 trial of patients with smoldering MM. No anti-MM activity was found in MM patients or smoldering MM patients receiving anti-DKK1 therapy. Sotatercept is in clinical trial for MM but can also increase hemoglobin levels significantly [45]. Thus, its utility as a bone anabolic agent of MM is still unclear. Most recently an anti-sclerostin antibody has been developed and is in clinical trial for patients with osteoporosis [46]. Anti-sclerostin antibody had potent bone anabolic effects and was well tolerated by the patients. Preclinical studies demonstrated that anti-sclerostin antibody treatment of murine models of MM can increase bone formation and may affect tumor burden. Several agents used to treat MM also have effects on bone. Bortezomib has been reported to have bone anabolic effects in patients with MM whose MM responded to bortezomib therapy [47], and transient increases in alkaline phosphatase activity have been shown in patients receiving bortezomib therapy. In addition there have been anecdotal reports of bone healing in patients receiving bortezomib-based therapies [48]. Furthermore, in preclinical studies, immunomodulatory agents such as pomalidomide can block osteoclast differentiation [47]. Finally, the role of parathyroid hormone as an anabolic agent for MM bone disease remains unclear. Several groups reported the presence of the PTH receptor 1 on MM cells and found that parathyroid hormone-related protein, which activates the PTH receptor, can increase MM cell growth [49]. Other investigators failed to demonstrate PTH receptors on MM cells and preclinical studies have shown an anabolic effect of PTH in SCID-hu mouse model of MM [50].

Radiation Therapy and Surgery for Myeloma Bone Disease

Radiation therapy is frequently used to treat painful bone lesions in myeloma. However, it must be used sparingly because of its myelosuppressive effects. Thus, radiation therapy is used primarily to treat painful lesions, impending fracture and spinal cord compression [20]. Similarly, vertebroplasty and kyphoplasty are used to treat painful vertebral fractures in patients with myeloma [51]. In a randomized study for painful vertebral fractures in patients with myeloma, kyphoplasty was shown to be superior to conservative management, so that kyphoplasty is currently recommended by the IMWG guidelines.

Thromboprophylaxis for Myeloma Patients

Patients with MM have an increased risk of a thrombotic event during the course of their disease. In the original clinical trial of thalidomide for treatment of patients with MM, a 30% incidence of DVT was reported in patients receiving thalidomide [52]. Subsequent studies using combination chemotherapy regimens containing thalidomide also found a high rate of deep venous thrombosis (DVT) in these patients. Lenalidomide and pomalidomide are also associated with increased risk of DVT [52]. These results led to the development of thromboprophylaxis guidelines for patients receiving immunomodulatory agents [6]. These guidelines suggest that patients should receive thromboprophylaxis for at least the first four cycles of immunomodulatory agent-based therapy because the risk of DVT or pulmonary embolism (PE) is greatly increased during that time. The type of DVT prophylaxis is based on individual risk factors (e.g., age, obesity immobilization, history of DVT). Patients who have no or only one risk factor should receive prophylaxis with low-dose or standard-dose aspirin (81–325 mg per day) and patients with two or more risk factors should receive low-molecular-weight heparin or the equivalent or full-dose warfarin therapy to maintain the INR at 2–3. A recent abstract at the American society of clinical oncology found that the risk of VTE persistently changes throughout the disease process [53]. Lipe and coworkers found that VTE can occur in MM patients at a median time from diagnosis of 952 days, much longer than the IMWG guidelines recommend for thromboprophylaxis. Importantly, Lipe et al. found that of 60% of patients at high risk for thrombosis, only 16% ever received the recommended prophylactic therapy. These results suggest that VTE may occur later in MM than was previously thought, and that guidelines for thromboprophylaxis in MM may need to be adjusted. Finally, the use of erythropoiesis-stimulating agents (ESAs) also increases the risk of thrombosis in patients with MM. Katodritou and coworkers reported that ESAs reduced survival in MM patients compared to patients not receiving ESAs (and increased the risk of thrombosis in patients with MM) [54]. Thus, ESAs should be used with caution in patients with MM.

Neuropathy in Myeloma

Neurological complications in MM range from peripheral neuropathy to compression of the nerve roots or spinal cord. Compression of the nerve roots and spinal cord is an oncological emergency and can result from compression by vertebral and extramedullary plasmacytomas, respectively. Early recognition and treatment of spinal cord or nerve root compression are more important than the type of treatment in improving outcomes.

Radiculopathy

Compression of the nerve root by vertebral plasmacytomas, neuroforaminal stenosis, or vertebral fracture usually presents with back pain and a unilateral radiculopathy that may progress to sensory loss and weakness. At least 5% of MM patients suffer from spinal cord or cauda equina compression, and MM is responsible for 15% of hospitalization for malignant spinal cord compression [55]. Spinal cord compression often presents with progressively worsening back pain and may have a symmetric radiculopathy. The thoracic cord is most commonly affected and is associated with a sensory-level deficit. Bowel and bladder dysfunction is a late complication of spinal cord compression and is often preceded by symmetric pain and weakness. Unilateral complaints are rare but may be seen with lateralized cord compression. Complete spinal MRI with contrast is the preferred method of evaluating spinal cord compression, as CT does not clearly demonstrate the spinal cord or epidural space. Immediate treatment with corticosteroids, followed by radiation therapy, is the mainstay of treatment. MRI screening of MM patients for cord compression has not been found to be beneficial for detecting spinal cord compression [56].

Clinically detectable peripheral neuropathy is uncommon in MM at diagnosis and presents as a mild and slowly progressive symmetric neuropathy. Occurrence rates vary from 2% [5] to approximately 50% [57] of patients. Peripheral neuropathy in MM is often caused by accompanying amyloidosis or chemotherapy, and is a major presenting feature of POEMS syndrome. Cranial nerve involvement is rare and is usually a sign of progressive disease. Chemotherapy-induced peripheral neuropathy is a serious and potentially reversible side effect of treatment. The dose and duration of treatment are commonly affected by the neurotoxic profiles of these medications, which in severe cases may result in discontinuation of treatment. The clinical history and neurological examination are crucial for distinguishing CIPN from neuropathic involvement from direct nerve compression by MM. Neuropathy is a frequent complication of thalidomide- and bortezomib-based therapies.

Thalidomide is a potent antiangiogenic therapy that has been used for MM since 1998. Severe peripheral neuropathy occurs in approximately 30% of patients who were treated with doses of thalidomide greater than 200 mg/day [58]. Thalidomide-induced peripheral neuropathy presents as a symmetric distal loss of light touch and temperature that is painful. The neurotoxic effects of thalidomide are cumulative and dose dependent. In approximately 60% of patients, neuropathy results in lowering the dose or discontinuation of treatment [59]. Reduced starting doses of thalidomide of 100 mg/day for patients greater than 75 years old, and 200 mg/day for patients less than 75 years old, have reduced the incidence of severe peripheral neuropathy to less than 10%. However, there has been an overall increase in the incidence of mild-to-moderate peripheral neuropathy at these thalidomide doses. Although peripheral neuropathy is partially reversible with discontinuation of thalidomide, the long-term reversibility of neuropathy with discontinuation of thalidomide requires further long-term studies [60, 61]. The pathogenesis of thalidomide-induced peripheral neuropathy is poorly understood but antiangiogenic and inflammatory insults to the dorsal root ganglia may be the cause. This may explain the reduced sensory nerve action potentials with relative sparing of compound motor action potentials found in thalidomide-treated patients [62]. Other neurotoxic side effects of thalidomide include tremor (in up to 30%) and somnolence.

Bortezomib-associated peripheral neuropathy was recognized as an early side effect in the initial phase I trials. The incidence of bortezomib-induced peripheral neuropathy (BIPN) in phase II and phase III trials was 30–64%, and occurred in up to 46% of patients treated for newly diagnosed MM [62, 63]. BIPN is a subacute predominately sensory neuropathy of the feet and hands that is often painful. Small unmyelinated fibers are affected, causing prominent neuropathic pain in 25–80% of cases [64]. BIPN occurs in 21% and 37% of patients at the onset of treatment at doses of 1.0 mg/m^2, and 1.3 mg/m^2, respectively. The severity typically plateaus by the fifth cycle, with an approximate cumulative dose of 30 mg/m^2 [65]. The pathogenesis of BIPN remains unclear. The involvement of satellite and Schwann cells in BIPN in animal models supports the involvement of the dorsal root ganglia in the pathogenesis of the pain. Although the autonomic nervous system is also innervated by unmyelinated fibers, it is very rarely affected. The clinical presentation of a symmetric distal peripheral neuropathy with a temporal correlation to recent bortezomib treatment is suggestive of BIPN. Electrodiagnostic studies can provide objective evidence to aid in the diagnosis. However, the diagnosis can usually be made clinically. The neurologic examination is very important for distinguishing the cause of peripheral neuropathy. If signs of motor weakness are present, nerve root compression is more likely, since BIPN is primarily a sensory neuropathy. In patients with BIPN, nerve conduction studies show reduced sensory and motor action potentials, with mild slowing of the distal sensory and motor nerve velocities with increased distal motor latencies.

Bortezomib neurotoxicity is a potentially reversible complication that must be recognized early. Currently, there is no accepted proven treatment for BIPN. The mainstay of treatment remains bortezomib dose modification or discontinuation and neuropathic pain medication. Subcutaneous administration of bortezomib has dramatically reduced the incidence of neuropathy, and newer proteasome antagonists (carfilzomib and ixazomib) are less neurotoxic and better tolerated. Severe peripheral neuropathy was reported in less than 1% of patients in phase II trials of carfilzomib who were treated previously with bortezomib [66, 67]. There is a lack of evidence to support prevention of BIPN with neuroprotective agents [65].

Neurologic involvement is a hallmark of POEMS syndrome, a rare osteoscerotic form of MM, and is a major criterion for diagnosis. Approximately 50% of patients present with a distal symmetric neuropathy that ascends proximally. Eventually the vast majority of POEMS patients suffer from prominent sensorimotor neuropathy. Severe neuropathy has been reported in up to 76% of patients [68, 69]. Ocular involvement is common in approximately 2/3 of patients. Papilledema occurs in approximately half of those patients, and patients with papilledema have a worse prognosis [70]. There is also an increased risk of thromboembolic disease and cerebral infarction in POEMS patients. In a retrospective cohort study of 208 POEMS patients 19 (9%) developed cerebral infarction at a relatively young age [71]. The risk of cerebral infarction increased with the degree of thrombocytosis, and of plasma cell proliferation in the BM was also associated with increased stroke risk [71]. Electrodiagnostic studies are important to distinguish neuropathy due to POEMS from CIDP; in contrast to CIDP, prominent axonal loss in the lower limbs rather than slow conduction of the distal nerve segments with conduction block occurs with POEMS. Polyneuropathy is commonly the initial presenting symptom of POEMS with up to 60% of patients with POEMS initially misdiagnosed with CIDP. Thus, distinguishing between CIDP and POEMS is critically important for treatment and prognosis. Nerve conduction studies in POEMS show predominate slowing of the nerve trunk when compared to distal nerve involvement.

Renal Dysfunction in Multiple Myeloma

The characteristic M paraprotein in MM, specifically the light-chain component, is nephrotoxic to the kidney, and frequently the kidney is the major target organ in MM. Up to 50% of patients have evidence of renal impairment at the time of diagnosis and about 10–15% of patients require renal replacement therapy [72]. Multiple studies found that renal impairment alone is a strong negative predictor of overall survival (OS) [4, 73]. In one study, the difference in median OS between patients with and without renal impairment was as high as 8.6 vs. 34.5 months ($P < 0.001$) The same study also showed markedly improved OS if renal impairment was reversible [4]. The Nordic MM study group also found that severity of renal impairment was a determinant of OS MM [73]. Hypercalcemia, lower proteinuria (<1 g/day), and low serum creatinine were positive prognostic factors. Thus, early detection of MM-induced kidney disease is extremely important.

The IMWG defines renal injury as either an elevation of serum creatinine >2 mg/dL or a reduced creatinine clearance (CrCl) of <40 mL/min/1.73m^2, due to MM [74]. CrCl should be assessed using the Modification of Diet in Renal Disease (MDRD) formula or the Chronic Kidney Disease Epidemiology Collaboration (CKD-EPI) equation as these most accurately predict the clearance obtained from inulin-based glomerular filtration rate (GFR) estimation [75, 76]. The CKD-EPI group further suggests that an equation based on creatinine and cystatin C, which also reflects tumor burden, is more accurate, but this remains to be validated in larger studies [75]. The use of eGFR should be restricted to stable patients and not for those presenting with an acute kidney injury (AKI). RIFLE (Risk, Injury, Failure, Loss and End-Stage Kidney Disease) criteria and Acute Kidney Injury Network classification should be used for assessing the severity of AKI [77].

Initial Diagnostic Workup of Renal Injury in Myeloma

All patients with symptomatic MM should have an initial laboratory panel that includes serum creatinine, GFR estimation, electrolytes, serum free light chains (SFLC), and 24-h urine collection for proteinuria and urine electrophoresis. The presence of selective proteinuria composed almost entirely of light chains can be attributed to myeloma cast nephropathy (MCN), whereas the presence of significant albuminuria suggests alternative diagnoses that require further investigation [78]. A renal biopsy should be considered to exclude monoclonal immunoglobulin deposition disease, amyloidosis, or other underlying causes of renal impairment in the presence of nonselective proteinuria [78–80]. If amyloidosis is strongly suspected, a fat pad aspirate should be done prior to kidney biopsy, since a diagnosis of amyloidosis can be obtained in about 70% of cases with the less invasive procedure [80].

Pathogenesis of Myeloma Kidney Disease

Free light chains circulating as monomers (predominantly K, 25KD) or dimers (predominantly λ, 50KD) are freely filtered by the glomerulus. In the proximal tubule cells (PTC) they are reabsorbed by receptor-mediated endocytosis [81]. This glycoprotein receptor cubilin-mediated endocytosis incites a proinflammatory response that induces release of IL-6, IL-8, and monocyte chemoattractant protein 1 (MCP-1) via activation of nuclear factor kappa light-chain enhancer of activated B-cells (NF-kB) in the PTC [82]. Similar to other proteinuric diseases, excess light chains induce factors that promote interstitial injury and fibrosis, as well as direct DNA injury and induction of apoptosis [83].

Once the PTC is injured, LCs overflow into the distal lumen and interact with the Tamm-Horsfall protein (THP) secreted by the thick ascending limb (TAL). This leads to formation of the MM cast that is responsible for the presentation of MCN. The variability in cast formation by this interaction can be explained by the variation in the complementarity-determining region 3 (CDR3) of different LCs [84]. While urinary light chains are required for the formation of casts, the type or quantity of LC does not correlate with the severity of cast formation. Urinary LC quantity, however, is predictive of response to therapy and risk for renal failure. Tubular solute composition and flow rates are other factors that also influence cast formation. Obstructed tubules in turn induce an intense inflammatory response probably related to urine leak into the interstitium [85].

Common Patterns of Renal Insufficiency in Myeloma

Myeloma cast nephropathy (MCN) is the most common histologic finding with autopsy studies reporting rates between 30 and 50% of all MM patients with renal failure [86–88]. MCN almost always occurs in the presence of high free LC burden and typically when serum FLC levels are >100 mg/dL [74, 89]. Almost all MM patients with significant renal impairment will also have high urine FLC levels [90]. The serum and urine FLC levels can be prognostic indicators in MCN [91, 92]. The hallmark of MCN is tubular obstruction due to formation of LC casts, as described previously, from the interaction of Tamm-Horsfall protein (THP) and monoclonal LCs. Factors that can influence formation of casts include urinary concentration of THP, sodium, calcium, pH, urine flow rate, and diuretic use [85].

MCN typically presents with acute renal failure; however, oliguric AKI is a feature in about half of the cases even with very high levels of serum creatinine [93]. The progression of AKI is rapid [94], with volume depletion and hypercalcemia being the most common precipitating factors. Other common risk factors for AKI MM include use of IV contrast media, presence of infection, and nonsteroidal anti-inflammatory drugs (NSAIDs) used for bone pain. One of the initial indicators for MCN is the presence of heavy proteinuria that is disproportionate to the albuminuria detected on a urine dipstick. The median amount of proteinuria is about 2 g/24 h and is almost exclusively Bence Jones protein with albuminuria contributing <10%.

Early identification of MCN is essential for the treatment of MCN since delay in decreasing light-chain burden is associated with lower kidney recovery rates [92]. Treatment is focused on elimination of the precipitating agent and rapid reduction of the paraprotein. This can be achieved with chemotherapy or extracorporeal removal via therapeutic plasma exchange (TPE). While renal replacement therapy (RRT) may be required in certain cases, the indication for initiation of RRT is similar to other AKI states. Role of TPE in the management of MCN and reduction of FLC burden remains controversial. Three randomized controlled trials have published conflicting results [95–97]. The largest trial showed no benefit but was limited by the absence of histologic diagnosis of MCN. A meta-analysis of the three trials showed higher rates of dialysis independence at 6 months for patients when TPE was combined with chemotherapy but no change in overall survival with use of TPE [98]. Arguments against using TPE include the absence of FLC monitoring in previous randomized trials and introduction of newer chemotherapeutic agents with high response rates that did not significantly improve with addition of TPE [99, 100].

The role of high-cutoff hemodialysis (HCO-HD) in treatment of patients with renal insufficiency is being evaluated in two large randomized controlled trials: EuLITE study (European Trial of Free Light Chain Removal by Extended Hemodialysis in Cast Nephropathy; NCT00700531) and the French MYRE study (Studies in Patients with MM and Renal Failure Due To MM Cast Nephropathy; NCT01208818). Both these trials include patients on a bortezomib-based regimen. A prior study examining the use of HCO-HD in combination with chemotherapy in 67 MM patients showed encouraging results, with a sustained reduction in FLCs by day 12 in 67% of patients and dialysis independency in 63% [101]. However, sustained reduction in FLC requires effective chemotherapy. The choice of regimen is oftentimes guided by the presence of renal failure and nonrenally cleared drugs like bortezomib and thalidomide are preferred.

General Principles of Treatment Renal Insufficiency in Myeloma

Initial treatment should include administration of intravenous fluids to achieve high urine, reduction of calcium levels in patients with hypercalcemia, treatment of infection, and avoidance of nephrotoxic agents. However, there is no established role for urine alkalization in treatment of RI [102]. Bisphosphonates can be used for hypercalcemia; however, pamidronate and zoledronic acid should be avoided in patients with CrCl <30 mL/min. Pamidronate has been associated with development of collapsing variant of focal and segmental glomerulosclerosis [103], whereas zoledronic acid is associated with development of ATN [104]. Denosumab may be helpful in this subgroup with close monitoring of serum calcium levels. The role of mechanical treatments, which include therapeutic plasma exchange (TPE) or high-cutoff hemodialysis (HCO-HD), in treatment of MM is limited to MM cast nephropathy (MCN) (see above).

Systemic chemotherapy should be started immediately to reduce FLC burden and provides the best chance of renal recovery, with bortezomib in combination with dexamethasone usually employed [72]. Bortezomib-based therapy has significantly higher rates of renal recovery (≥partial renal response) compared to thalidomide- or lenalidomide-based regimens (77% vs. 55% vs. 43%, respectively) in a large retrospective analysis of 133 patients [105]. Carfilzomib, a second-generation proteasome inhibitor, has shown good safety and efficacy when used in patients with RI, and progression-free survival was better with carfilzomib when compared to bortezomib [106]. High-dose corticosteroids (equivalent to dexamethasone 160 mg or greater over 4 days) can be effective for rapid recovery of renal function regardless of the initial chemotherapy regimen [105]. High-dose steroids should be used in the initial month of therapy for MM. Thalidomide can be used in renal insufficiency without dose adjustment; however there have been reports of hyperkalemia in patients receiving dialysis [107, 108]. The renal recovery rates with use of thalidomide have been as high as 75% in newly diagnosed MM and up to 60% in patients with relapse/refractory disease [105, 107, 109].

Lenalidomide requires dose adjustment in renal insufficiency and response to treatment is not as robust. Autologous stem cell transplant (ASCT) can be used in MM even in presence of severe RI requiring dialysis but requires dose adjustment of the high-dose melphalan [110]. RI at the time of transplantation, however, is associated with higher risk of transplant-related mortality (4% vs. <1%) [110, 111].

AL Amyloidosis

Amyloidosis represents the most common glomerular lesion in MM. AL amyloidosis is a systemic disease with deposition of congophilic fibrils in soft tissue. The fibrils are composed of light chains (AL), heavy chains (AH), or intact immunoglobulins (ALH) [112]. AL amyloidosis is the most common subtype accounting for >95% of cases. Autopsy studies report rates of 5–15% for AL amyloidosis [86–88]. MM is diagnosed in <10% of cases of AL amyloidosis. About 50% of patients present with renal failure. Proteinuria is present in >70% of the cases while about a fourth of the cases present with nephrotic syndrome [113]. As opposed to MCN, the proteinuria is predominantly albumin [78]. Rarely, amyloidosis will present with renal dysfunction in the absence of proteinuria as in vascular limited amyloidosis or diabetes insipidus. Kidney involvement can at times be the only presentation of amyloidosis. A fat pad biopsy can provide a diagnosis in about 70% of cases, whereas the remaining will require kidney biopsy [78]. Kidney response in amyloidosis is predictive of OS [114, 115]. Kidney transplantation can be considered in combination with chemotherapy and ASCT as one of the therapeutic options in patients with AL amyloidosis [116].

Kidney Transplantation in Myeloma

Kidney transplantation is challenging in patients with MM since the transplantation and ensuing use of immunosuppressive medications are thought to portend a high risk for disease recurrence and infections. Most centers require a treatment-free remission period of 3–5 years. The initial lesion can be predictive of graft survival and recurrence. Patients with MCN have a lower risk of graft recurrence if MM stays in remission [117]. In patients with AL amyloidosis, specifically those without significant cardiac involvement, kidney transplantation in combination with chemotherapy and ASCT has shown favorable outcomes [116]. Renal transplantation in patients with MIDD is not recommended unless complete response is noted, as recurrence rates are about 80% in patients who do not have a complete response to treatment [118].

Conclusion

Thus, supportive care for MM patients becomes increasingly important, if MM patients are to enjoy a higher quality of life. MM patients are living longer, receiving more intensive therapy, and are potentially curable.

References

1. Ludwig H, Miguel JS, Dimopoulos MA, Palumbo A, Garcia Sanz R, Powles R, et al. International Myeloma Working Group recommendations for global myeloma care. Leukemia. 2014;28(5):981–92.
2. ACS. 2016. http://www.cancer.org/cancer/multiplemyeloma/detailedguide/multiple-myeloma-key-statistics
3. Greenberg AJ, Rajkumar SV, Therneau TM, Singh PP, Dispenzieri A, Kumar SK. Relationship between initial clinical presentation and the molecular cytogenetic classification of myeloma. Leukemia. 2014;28(2):398–403.
4. Blade J, Fernandez-Llama P, Bosch F, Montoliu J, Lens XM, Montoto S, et al. Renal failure in multiple myeloma: presenting features and predictors of outcome in 94 patients from a single institution. Arch Intern Med. 1998;158(17):1889–93.
5. Dispenzieri A, Kyle RA. Neurological aspects of multiple myeloma and related disorders. Best Pract Res Clin Haematol. 2005;18(4):673–88.
6. Palumbo A, Rajkumar SV, Dimopoulos MA, Richardson PG, San Miguel J, Barlogie B, et al. Prevention of thalidomide- and lenalidomide-associated thrombosis in myeloma. Leukemia. 2008;22(2):414–23.
7. Melton LJ 3rd, Kyle RA, Achenbach SJ, Oberg AL, Rajkumar SV. Fracture risk with multiple myeloma: a population-based study. J Bone Miner Res. 2005;20(3):487–93.
8. Saad F, Lipton A, Cook R, Chen YM, Smith M, Coleman R. Pathologic fractures correlate with reduced survival in patients with malignant bone disease. Cancer. 2007;110(8):1860–7.
9. Kumar SK, Dispenzieri A, Lacy MQ, Gertz MA, Buadi FK, Pandey S, et al. Continued improvement in survival in multiple myeloma: changes in early mortality and outcomes in older patients. Leukemia. 2014;28(5):1122–8.
10. Roodman GD. Pathogenesis of myeloma bone disease. Leukemia. 2009;23(3):435–41.
11. Cackowski FC, Anderson JL, Patrene KD, Choksi RJ, Shapiro SD, Windle JJ, et al. Osteoclasts are important for bone angiogenesis. Blood. 2010;115(1):140–9.
12. Yaccoby S, Wezeman MJ, Henderson A, Cottler-Fox M, Yi Q, Barlogie B, et al. Cancer and the microenvironment: myeloma-osteoclast interactions as a model. Cancer Res. 2004;64(6):2016–23.
13. Abe M, Hiura K, Wilde J, Shioyasono A, Moriyama K, Hashimoto T, et al. Osteoclasts enhance myeloma cell growth and survival via cell-cell contact: a vicious cycle between bone destruction and myeloma expansion. Blood. 2004;104(8):2484–91.
14. Delgado-Calle J, Anderson J, Cregor MD, Hiasa M, Chirgwin JM, Carlesso N, et al. Bidirectional notch signaling and osteocyte-derived factors in the bone marrow microenvironment promote tumor cell proliferation and bone destruction in multiple myeloma. Cancer Res. 2016;76(5):1089–100.
15. Alexandrakis MG, Roussou P, Pappa CA, Messaritakis I, Xekalou A, Goulidaki N, et al. Relationship between circulating BAFF serum levels with proliferating markers in patients with multiple myeloma. Biomed Res Int. 2013;2013:389579.
16. An G, Acharya C, Feng X, Wen K, Zhong M, Zhang L, et al. Osteoclasts promote immune suppressive microenvironment in multiple myeloma: therapeutic implication. Blood. 2016;128:1590–603.

17. Lawson MA, McDonald MM, Kovacic N, Hua Khoo W, Terry RL, Down J, et al. Osteoclasts control reactivation of dormant myeloma cells by remodelling the endosteal niche. Nat Commun. 2015;6:8983.
18. Croucher PI, De Hendrik R, Perry MJ, Hijzen A, Shipman CM, Lippitt J, et al. Zoledronic acid treatment of 5T2MM-bearing mice inhibits the development of myeloma bone disease: evidence for decreased osteolysis, tumor burden and angiogenesis, and increased survival. J Bone Miner Res. 2003;18(3):482–92.
19. Morgan GJ, Child JA, Gregory WM, Szubert AJ, Cocks K, Bell SE, et al. Effects of zoledronic acid versus clodronic acid on skeletal morbidity in patients with newly diagnosed multiple myeloma (MRC Myeloma IX): secondary outcomes from a randomised controlled trial. Lancet Oncol. 2011;12(8):743–52.
20. Terpos E, Morgan G, Dimopoulos MA, Drake MT, Lentzsch S, Raje N, et al. International Myeloma Working Group recommendations for the treatment of multiple myeloma-related bone disease. J Clin Oncol. 2013;31(18):2347–57.
21. Dimopoulos M, Terpos E, Comenzo RL, Tosi P, Beksac M, Sezer O, et al. International myeloma working group consensus statement and guidelines regarding the current role of imaging techniques in the diagnosis and monitoring of multiple Myeloma. Leukemia. 2009;23(9):1545–56.
22. Roodman GD. Osteoblast function in myeloma. Bone. 2011;48(1):135–40.
23. D'Souza S, del Prete D, Jin S, Sun Q, Huston AJ, Kostov FE, et al. Gfi1 expressed in bone marrow stromal cells is a novel osteoblast suppressor in patients with multiple myeloma bone disease. Blood. 2011;118(26):6871–80.
24. Li X, Pennisi A, Yaccoby S. Role of decorin in the antimyeloma effects of osteoblasts. Blood. 2008;112(1):159–68.
25. Rajkumar SV. Updated diagnostic criteria and staging system for multiple myeloma. Am Soc Clin Oncol Educ Book. 2016;35:e418–23.
26. Wolf MB, Murray F, Kilk K, Hillengass J, Delorme S, Heiss C, et al. Sensitivity of whole-body CT and MRI versus projection radiography in the detection of osteolyses in patients with monoclonal plasma cell disease. Eur J Radiol. 2014;83(7):1222–30.
27. Regelink JC, Minnema MC, Terpos E, Kamphuis MH, Raijmakers PG, Pieters-van den Bos IC, et al. Comparison of modern and conventional imaging techniques in establishing multiple myeloma-related bone disease: a systematic review. Br J Haematol. 2013;162(1):50–61.
28. Hillengass J, Fechtner K, Weber MA, Bauerle T, Ayyaz S, Heiss C, et al. Prognostic significance of focal lesions in whole-body magnetic resonance imaging in patients with asymptomatic multiple myeloma. J Clin Oncol. 2010;28(9):1606–10.
29. Kyle RA, Durie BG, Rajkumar SV, Landgren O, Blade J, Merlini G, et al. Monoclonal gammopathy of undetermined significance (MGUS) and smoldering (asymptomatic) multiple myeloma: IMWG consensus perspectives risk factors for progression and guidelines for monitoring and management. Leukemia. 2010;24(6):1121–7.
30. Bauerle T, Hillengass J, Fechtner K, Zechmann CM, Grenacher L, Moehler TM, et al. Multiple myeloma and monoclonal gammopathy of undetermined significance: importance of whole-body versus spinal MR imaging. Radiology. 2009;252(2):477–85.
31. Zamagni E, Tacchetti P, Terragna C, Cavo M. Multiple myeloma: disease response assessment. Expert Rev Hematol. 2016;9:831–7.
32. Lonial S, Kaufman JL. Non-secretory myeloma: a clinician's guide. Oncology (Williston Park). 2013;27(9):924–8. 30
33. Berenson JR, Lichtenstein A, Porter L, Dimopoulos MA, Bordoni R, George S, et al. Efficacy of pamidronate in reducing skeletal events in patients with advanced multiple myeloma. Myeloma Aredia Study Group. N Engl J Med. 1996;334(8):488–93.
34. Russell RG, Xia Z, Dunford JE, Oppermann U, Kwaasi A, Hulley PA, et al. Bisphosphonates: an update on mechanisms of action and how these relate to clinical efficacy. Ann N Y Acad Sci. 2007;1117:209–57.
35. Silbermann R, Roodman GD. Current controversies in the management of myeloma bone disease. J Cell Physiol. 2016;231(11):2374–9.
36. Morgan GJ, Davies FE, Gregory WM, Szubert AJ, Bell SE, Drayson MT, et al. Effects of induction and maintenance plus long-term bisphosphonates on bone disease in patients with multiple myeloma: the Medical Research Council Myeloma IX Trial. Blood. 2012;119(23):5374–83.
37. Marx RE, Sawatari Y, Fortin M, Broumand V. Bisphosphonate-induced exposed bone (osteonecrosis/osteopetrosis) of the jaws: risk factors, recognition, prevention, and treatment. J Oral Maxillofac Surg. 2005;63(11):1567–75.
38. Hellstein JW, Adler RA, Edwards B, Jacobsen PL, Kalmar JR, Koka S, et al. Managing the care of patients receiving antiresorptive therapy for prevention and treatment of osteoporosis: executive summary of recommendations from the American Dental Association Council on Scientific Affairs. J Am Dent Assoc. 2011;142(11):1243–51.
39. Patel CG, Yee AJ, Scullen TA, Nemani N, Santo L, Richardson PG, et al. Biomarkers of bone remodeling in multiple myeloma patients to tailor bisphosphonate therapy. Clin Cancer Res. 2014;20(15):3955–61.
40. Coleman RE, Major P, Lipton A, Brown JE, Lee KA, Smith M, et al. Predictive value of bone resorption and formation markers in cancer patients with bone metastases receiving the bisphosphonate zoledronic acid. J Clin Oncol. 2005;23(22):4925–35.
41. Badros A, Terpos E, Katodritou E, Goloubeva O, Kastritis E, Verrou E, et al. Natural history of osteonecrosis of the jaw in patients with multiple myeloma. J Clin Oncol. 2008;26(36):5904–9.
42. Gul G, Sendur MA, Aksoy S, Sever AR, Altundag K. A comprehensive review of denosumab for bone metastasis in patients with solid tumors. Curr Med Res Opin. 2016;32(1):133–45.
43. Raje N, Vadhan-Raj S, Willenbacher W, Terpos E, Hungria V, Spencer A, et al. Evaluating results from the multiple myeloma patient subset treated with denosumab or zoledronic acid in a randomized phase 3 trial. Blood Cancer J. 2016;6:e378.
44. Iyer SP, Beck JT, Stewart AK, Shah J, Kelly KR, Isaacs R, et al. A Phase IB multicentre dose-determination study of BHQ880 in combination with anti-myeloma therapy and zoledronic acid in patients with relapsed or refractory multiple myeloma and prior skeletal-related events. Br J Haematol. 2014;167(3):366–75.
45. Abdulkadyrov KM, Salogub GN, Khuazheva NK, Sherman ML, Laadem A, Barger R, et al. Sotatercept in patients with osteolytic lesions of multiple myeloma. Br J Haematol. 2014;165(6):814–23.
46. Feurer E, Chapurlat R. Emerging drugs for osteoporosis. Expert Opin Emerg Drugs. 2014;19(3):385–95.
47. Roodman GD. Bone building with bortezomib. J Clin Invest. 2008;118(2):462–4.
48. Mohty M, Malard F, Mohty B, Savani B, Moreau P, Terpos E. The effects of bortezomib on bone disease in patients with multiple myeloma. Cancer. 2014;120(5):618–23.
49. Cafforio P, Savonarola A, Stucci S, De Matteo M, Tucci M, Brunetti AE, et al. PTHrP produced by myeloma plasma cells regulates their survival and pro-osteoclast activity for bone disease progression. J Bone Miner Res. 2014;29(1):55–66.
50. Zangari M, Berno T, Yang Y, Zeng M, Xu H, Pappas L, et al. Parathyroid hormone receptor mediates the anti-myeloma effect of proteasome inhibitors. Bone. 2014;61:39–43.
51. Berenson J, Pflugmacher R, Jarzem P, Zonder J, Schechtman K, Tillman JB, et al. Balloon kyphoplasty versus non-surgical fracture management for treatment of painful vertebral body compression fractures in patients with cancer: a multicentre, randomised controlled trial. Lancet Oncol. 2011;12(3):225–35.
52. Fotiou D, Gerotziafas G, Kastritis E, Dimopoulos MA, Terpos E. A review of the venous thrombotic issues associated with multiple myeloma. Expert Rev Hematol. 2016;9(7):695–706.

53. Lipe B, Baker H, Weckbaugh B, Webb C, Brown A, Mahnken J, et al. Validation of a thrombosis risk assessment model in patients with newly diagnosed multiple myeloma. ASCO Meeting Abstracts. 2016;34(Suppl. 15):8055.
54. Katodritou E, Verrou E, Hadjiaggelidou C, Gastari V, Laschos K, Kontovinis L, et al. Erythropoiesis-stimulating agents are associated with reduced survival in patients with multiple myeloma. Am J Hematol. 2008;83(9):697–701.
55. Mak KS, Lee LK, Mak RH, Wang S, Pile-Spellman J, Abrahm JL, et al. Incidence and treatment patterns in hospitalizations for malignant spinal cord compression in the United States, 1998–2006. Int J Radiat Oncol Biol Phys. 2011;80(3):824–31.
56. Wight J, Stillwell A, Morris E, Grant B, Lai HC, Irving I. Screening whole spine magnetic resonance imaging in multiple myeloma. Intern Med J. 2015;45(7):762–5.
57. Silberman J, Lonial S. Review of peripheral neuropathy in plasma cell disorders. Hematol Oncol. 2008;26(2):55–65.
58. Glasmacher A, Hahn C, Hoffmann F, Naumann R, Goldschmidt H, Lilienfeld-Toal M, et al. A systematic review of phase-II trials of thalidomide monotherapy in patients with relapsed or refractory multiple myeloma. Br J Haematol. 2006;132(5):584–93.
59. Kocer B, Sucak G, Kuruoglu R, Aki Z, Haznedar R, Erdogmus NI. Clinical and electrophysiological evaluation of patients with thalidomide-induced neuropathy. Acta Neurol Belg. 2009;109(2):120–6.
60. Rajkumar SV, Rosinol L, Hussein M, Catalano J, Jedrzejczak W, Lucy L, et al. Multicenter, randomized, double-blind, placebo-controlled study of thalidomide plus dexamethasone compared with dexamethasone as initial therapy for newly diagnosed multiple myeloma. J Clin Oncol. 2008;26(13):2171–7.
61. Hulin C, Facon T, Rodon P, Pegourie B, Benboubker L, Doyen C, et al. Efficacy of melphalan and prednisone plus thalidomide in patients older than 75 years with newly diagnosed multiple myeloma: IFM 01/01 trial. J Clin Oncol. 2009;27(22):3664–70.
62. Jongen JLM, Broijl A, Sonneveld P. Chemotherapy-induced peripheral neuropathies in hematological malignancies. J Neurooncol. 2015;121(2):229–37.
63. Dimopoulos MA, Mateos M-V, Richardson PG, Schlag R, Khuageva NK, Shpilberg O, et al. Risk factors for, and reversibility of, peripheral neuropathy associated with bortezomib-melphalan-prednisone in newly diagnosed patients with multiple myeloma: subanalysis of the phase 3 VISTA study. Eur J Haematol. 2010;86(1):23–31.
64. Corso A, Mangiacavalli S, Varettoni M, Pascutto C, Zappasodi P, Lazzarino M. Bortezomib-induced peripheral neuropathy in multiple myeloma: A comparison between previously treated and untreated patients. Leuk Res. 2010;34(4):471–4.
65. Rampen AJ, Jongen JL, van Heuvel I, Scheltens-de Boer M, Sonneveld P, van den Bent MJ. Bortezomib-induced polyneuropathy. Neth J Med. 2013;71(3):128–33.
66. Richardson PG, Briemberg H, Jagannath S, Wen PY, Barlogie B, Berenson J, et al. Frequency, characteristics, and reversibility of peripheral neuropathy during treatment of advanced multiple myeloma with bortezomib. J Clin Oncol. 2006;24(19):3113–20.
67. Ceresa C, Avan A, Giovannetti E, Geldof AA, Avan A, Cavaletti G, et al. Characterization of and protection from neurotoxicity induced by oxaliplatin, bortezomib and epothilone-B. Anticancer Res. 2014;34(1):517–23.
68. Dispenzieri A. POEMS syndrome: update on diagnosis, risk-stratification, and management. Am J Hematol. 2015;90(10):951–62.
69. Nasu S, Misawa S, Sekiguchi Y, Shibuya K, Kanai K, Fujimaki Y, et al. Different neurological and physiological profiles in POEMS syndrome and chronic inflammatory demyelinating polyneuropathy. J Neurol Neurosurg Psychiatry. 2012;83(5):476–9.
70. Cui R, Yu S, Huang X, Zhang J, Tian C, Pu C. Papilloedema is an independent prognostic factor for POEMS syndrome. J Neurol. 2013;261(1):60–5.
71. Dupont SA, Dispenzieri A, Mauermann ML, Rabinstein AA, Brown RD. Cerebral infarction in POEMS syndrome: incidence, risk factors, and imaging characteristics. Neurology. 2009;73(16):1308–12.
72. Dimopoulos MA, Terpos E, Chanan-Khan A, Leung N, Ludwig H, Jagannath S, et al. Renal impairment in patients with multiple myeloma: a consensus statement on behalf of the International Myeloma Working Group. J Clin Oncol. 2010;28(33):4976–84.
73. Knudsen LM, Hjorth M, Hippe E. Renal failure in multiple myeloma: reversibility and impact on the prognosis. Nordic Myeloma Study Group. Eur J Haematol. 2000;65(3):175–81.
74. Dimopoulos MA, Sonneveld P, Leung N, Merlini G, Ludwig H, Kastritis E, et al. International Myeloma Working Group recommendations for the diagnosis and management of myeloma-related renal impairment. J Clin Oncol. 2016;34(13):1544–57.
75. Inker LA, Schmid CH, Tighiouart H, Eckfeldt JH, Feldman HI, Greene T, et al. Estimating glomerular filtration rate from serum creatinine and cystatin C. N Engl J Med. 2012;367(1):20–9.
76. Masson I, Flamant M, Maillard N, Rule AD, Vrtovsnik F, Peraldi MN, et al. MDRD versus CKD-EPI equation to estimate glomerular filtration rate in kidney transplant recipients. Transplantation. 2013;95(10):1211–7.
77. Srisawat N, Hoste EE, Kellum JA. Modern classification of acute kidney injury. Blood Purif. 2010;29(3):300–7.
78. Leung N, Gertz M, Kyle RA, Fervenza FC, Irazabal MV, Eirin A, et al. Urinary albumin excretion patterns of patients with cast nephropathy and other monoclonal gammopathy-related kidney diseases. Clin J Am Soc Nephrol. 2012;7(12):1964–8.
79. Dimopoulos MA, Terpos E. Renal insufficiency and failure. Hematology Am Soc Hematol Educ Program. 2010;2010:431–6.
80. Merlini G, Palladini G. Differential diagnosis of monoclonal gammopathy of undetermined significance. Hematology Am Soc Hematol Educ Program. 2012;2012:595–603.
81. Batuman V, Verroust PJ, Navar GL, Kaysen JH, Goda FO, Campbell WC, et al. Myeloma light chains are ligands for cubilin (gp280). Am J Physiol. 1998;275(2 Pt 2):F246–54.
82. Sengul S, Zwizinski C, Simon EE, Kapasi A, Singhal PC, Batuman V. Endocytosis of light chains induces cytokines through activation of NF-kappaB in human proximal tubule cells. Kidney Int. 2002;62(6):1977–88.
83. Pote A, Zwizinski C, Simon EE, Meleg-Smith S, Batuman V. Cytotoxicity of myeloma light chains in cultured human kidney proximal tubule cells. Am J Kidney Dis. 2000;36(4):735–44.
84. Ying WZ, Sanders PW. Mapping the binding domain of immunoglobulin light chains for Tamm-Horsfall protein. Am J Pathol. 2001;158(5):1859–66.
85. Hill GS, Morel-Maroger L, Mery JP, Brouet JC, Mignon F. Renal lesions in multiple myeloma: their relationship to associated protein abnormalities. Am J Kidney Dis. 1983;2(4):423–38.
86. Ivanyi B. Frequency of light chain deposition nephropathy relative to renal amyloidosis and Bence Jones cast nephropathy in a necropsy study of patients with myeloma. Arch Pathol Lab Med. 1990;114(9):986–7.
87. Kapadia SB. Multiple myeloma: a clinicopathologic study of 62 consecutively autopsied cases. Medicine. 1980;59(5):380–92.
88. Oshima K, Kanda Y, Nannya Y, Kaneko M, Hamaki T, Suguro M, et al. Clinical and pathologic findings in 52 consecutively autopsied cases with multiple myeloma. Am J Hematol. 2001;67(1):1–5.
89. Hutchison CA, Bradwell AR, Cook M, Basnayake K, Basu S, Harding S, et al. Treatment of acute renal failure secondary to multiple myeloma with chemotherapy and extended high cut-off hemodialysis. Clin J Am Soc Nephrol. 2009;4(4):745–54.
90. Drayson M, Begum G, Basu S, Makkuni S, Dunn J, Barth N, et al. Effects of paraprotein heavy and light chain types and free light chain load on survival in myeloma: an analysis of patients receiving conventional-dose chemotherapy in Medical Research Council UK multiple myeloma trials. Blood. 2006;108(6):2013–9.

91. Hutchison C, Sanders PW. Evolving strategies in the diagnosis, treatment, and monitoring of myeloma kidney. Adv Chronic Kidney Dis. 2012;19(5):279–81.
92. Hutchison CA, Cockwell P, Stringer S, Bradwell A, Cook M, Gertz MA, et al. Early reduction of serum-free light chains associates with renal recovery in myeloma kidney. J Am Soc Nephrol. 2011;22(6):1129–36.
93. Rota S, Mougenot B, Baudouin B, De Meyer-Brasseur M, Lemaitre V, Michel C, et al. Multiple myeloma and severe renal failure: a clinicopathologic study of outcome and prognosis in 34 patients. Medicine. 1987;66(2):126–37.
94. Winearls CG. Acute myeloma kidney. Kidney Int. 1995;48(4):1347–61.
95. Clark WF. Correction: Plasma exchange when myeloma presents as acute renal failure. Ann Intern Med. 2007;146(6):471.
96. Johnson WJ, Kyle RA, Pineda AA, O'Brien PC, Holley KE. Treatment of renal failure associated with multiple myeloma. Plasmapheresis, hemodialysis, and chemotherapy. Arch Intern Med. 1990;150(4):863–9.
97. Zucchelli P, Pasquali S, Cagnoli L, Ferrari G. Controlled plasma exchange trial in acute renal failure due to multiple myeloma. Kidney Int. 1988;33(6):1175–80.
98. Yu X, Gan L, Wang Z, Dong B, Chen X. Chemotherapy with or without plasmapheresis in acute renal failure due to multiple myeloma: a meta-analysis. Int J Clin Pharmacol Ther. 2015;53(5):391–7.
99. Burnette BL, Leung N, Rajkumar SV. Renal improvement in myeloma with bortezomib plus plasma exchange. N Engl J Med. 2011;364(24):2365–6.
100. Kastritis E, Anagnostopoulos A, Roussou M, Gika D, Matsouka C, Barmparousi D, et al. Reversibility of renal failure in newly diagnosed multiple myeloma patients treated with high dose dexamethasone-containing regimens and the impact of novel agents. Haematologica. 2007;92(4):546–9.
101. Hutchison CA, Heyne N, Airia P, Schindler R, Zickler D, Cook M, et al. Immunoglobulin free light chain levels and recovery from myeloma kidney on treatment with chemotherapy and high cut off haemodialysis. Nephrol Dial Transplant. 2012;27(10):3823–8.
102. Analysis and management of renal failure in fourth MRC myelomatosis trial. MRC working party on leukaemia in adults. Br Med J (Clin Res Ed). 1984;288(6428):1411–6.
103. Markowitz GS, Appel GB, Fine PL, Fenves AZ, Loon NR, Jagannath S, et al. Collapsing focal segmental glomerulosclerosis following treatment with high-dose pamidronate. J Am Soc Nephrol. 2001;12(6):1164–72.
104. Markowitz GS, Fine PL, Stack JI, Kunis CL, Radhakrishnan J, Palecki W, et al. Toxic acute tubular necrosis following treatment with zoledronate (Zometa). Kidney Int. 2003;64(1):281–9.
105. Dimopoulos MA, Roussou M, Gkotzamanidou M, Nikitas N, Psimenou E, Mparmparoussi D, et al. The role of novel agents on the reversibility of renal impairment in newly diagnosed symptomatic patients with multiple myeloma. Leukemia. 2013;27(2):423–9.
106. Dimopoulos MA, Moreau P, Palumbo A, Joshua D, Pour L, Hajek R, et al. Carfilzomib and dexamethasone versus bortezomib and dexamethasone for patients with relapsed or refractory multiple myeloma (ENDEAVOR): a randomised, phase 3, open-label, multicentre study. Lancet Oncol. 2016;17(1):27–38.
107. Fakhouri F, Guerraoui H, Presne C, Peltier J, Delarue R, Muret P, et al. Thalidomide in patients with multiple myeloma and renal failure. Br J Haematol. 2004;125(1):96–7.
108. Harris E, Behrens J, Samson D, Rahemtulla A, Russell NH, Byrne JL. Use of thalidomide in patients with myeloma and renal failure may be associated with unexplained hyperkalaemia. Br J Haematol. 2003;122(1):160–1.
109. Tosi P, Zamagni E, Tacchetti P, Ceccolini M, Perrone G, Brioli A, et al. Thalidomide-dexamethasone as induction therapy before autologous stem cell transplantation in patients with newly diagnosed multiple myeloma and renal insufficiency. Biol Blood Marrow Transplant. 2010;16(8):1115–21.
110. San Miguel JF, Lahuerta JJ, Garcia-Sanz R, Alegre A, Blade J, Martinez R, et al. Are myeloma patients with renal failure candidates for autologous stem cell transplantation? Hematol J. 2000;1(1):28–36.
111. Lee CK, Zangari M, Barlogie B, Fassas A, van Rhee F, Thertulien R, et al. Dialysis-dependent renal failure in patients with myeloma can be reversed by high-dose myeloablative therapy and autotransplant. Bone Marrow Transplant. 2004;33(8):823–8.
112. Leung N, Nasr SH, Sethi S. How I treat amyloidosis: the importance of accurate diagnosis and amyloid typing. Blood. 2012;120(16):3206–13.
113. Kyle RA, Gertz MA. Primary systemic amyloidosis: clinical and laboratory features in 474 cases. Semin Hematol. 1995;32(1):45–59.
114. Leung N, Dispenzieri A, Lacy MQ, Kumar SK, Hayman SR, Fervenza FC, et al. Severity of baseline proteinuria predicts renal response in immunoglobulin light chain-associated amyloidosis after autologous stem cell transplantation. Clin J Am Soc Nephrol. 2007;2(3):440–4.
115. Leung N, Glavey SV, Kumar S, Dispenzieri A, Buadi FK, Dingli D, et al. A detailed evaluation of the current renal response criteria in AL amyloidosis: is it time for a revision? Haematologica. 2013;98(6):988–92.
116. Herrmann SM, Gertz MA, Stegall MD, Dispenzieri A, Cosio FC, Kumar S, et al. Long-term outcomes of patients with light chain amyloidosis (AL) after renal transplantation with or without stem cell transplantation. Nephrol Dial Transplant. 2011;26(6):2032–6.
117. Heher EC, Spitzer TR, Goes NB. Light chains: heavy burden in kidney transplantation. Transplantation. 2009;87(7):947–52.
118. Leung N, Lager DJ, Gertz MA, Wilson K, Kanakiriya S, Fervenza FC. Long-term outcome of renal transplantation in light-chain deposition disease. Am J Kidney Dis. 2004;43(1):147–53.

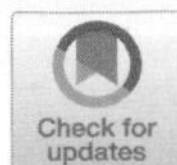

32 POEMS Syndrome

Angela Dispenzieri

Introduction

POEMS syndrome is a rare paraneoplastic syndrome due to an underlying plasma cell disorder. The acronym, which was coined by Bardwick in 1980 [1], refers to several, but not all, of the features of the syndrome: polyradiculoneuropathy, organomegaly, endocrinopathy, monoclonal plasma cell disorder, and skin changes. Other important features not included in the POEMS acronym include papilledema, extravascular volume overload, sclerotic bone lesions, thrombocytosis/ erythrocytosis (P.E.S.T.), elevated vascular endothelial growth factor (VEGF) levels, a predisposition towards thrombosis, and abnormal pulmonary function tests. There is a Castleman disease variant of POEMS syndrome that may be associated with a clonal plasma cell disorder. Other names of the POEMS syndrome that are less frequently used are osteosclerotic myeloma, Takatsuki syndrome, Crow-Fukase syndrome, and PEP syndrome [2, 3]. A national survey conducted in Japan in 2003 showed a prevalence of approximately 0.3 per 100,000 [4].

The pathogenesis of the syndrome is not understood. Distinctive presenting characteristics of the syndrome that differentiate POEMS syndrome from standard multiple myeloma (MM) include the following: (1) dominant symptoms have little to nothing to do with bone pain, extremes of bone marrow infiltration by plasma cells, or renal failure; (2) dominant symptoms are typically neuropathy, endocrine dysfunction, and volume overload; (3) VEGF levels are high; (4) sclerotic bone lesions are present in the majority of cases; (5) overall survival is typically superior; and (6) lambda clones predominate [5]. VEGF is the cytokine that correlates best with disease activity, although it is likely not the driving force of the disease based on the mixed results seen with anti-VEGF therapy [6]. Little is known about the plasma cells in POEMS syndrome except that more than 95% of the time they are lambda light chain restricted with restricted immunoglobulin light-chain variable gene usage (*IGLV1*) [7, 8].

Diagnosis of POEMS Syndrome

The diagnosis is made based on a composite of clinical and laboratory features. The most notable symptoms include the constellation of neuropathy and any of the following: monoclonal protein (especially lambda light chain); thrombocytosis; anasarca; or papilledema. All the features of the acronym are not required to make the diagnosis (Table 32.1). A good history and physical examination followed by appropriate testing—most notably radiographic assessment of bones [9], measurement of VEGF [10–14], and careful analysis of a bone marrow biopsy [15]—can differentiate this syndrome from other conditions like chronic inflammatory polyradiculoneuropathy (CIDP), monoclonal gammopathy of undetermined significance (MGUS) neuropathy, and immunoglobulin light-chain amyloid neuropathy. Figure 32.1 demonstrates several classic findings among patients with POEMS syndrome.

A. Dispenzieri, M.D.
Division of Hematology and Internal Medicine, Mayo Clinic, 200 First Street SW, Rochester, MN 55905, USA

Mayo Medical School, Rochester, MN 55905, USA
e-mail: dispenzieri.angela@mayo.edu

P.H. Wiernik et al. (eds.), *Neoplastic Diseases of the Blood*, DOI 10.1007/978-3-319-64263-5_32

Table 32.1 Criteria for the diagnosis of POEMS syndrome[a]

		% Affected[b]
Mandatory major criteria (both required)	1. Polyradiculoneuropathy (typically demyelinating)	100
	2. Monoclonal plasma cell disorder (almost always λ)	100[c]
Other major criteria (one required)	3. Castleman disease[d]	11–25
	4. Sclerotic bone lesions	27–97
	5. Vascular endothelial growth factor elevation[e]	
Minor criteria (one required)	6. Organomegaly (splenomegaly, hepatomegaly, or lymphadenopathy)	45–85
	7. Extravascular volume overload (edema, pleural effusion, or ascites)	29–87
	8. Endocrinopathy (adrenal, thyroid,[f] pituitary, gonadal, parathyroid, pancreatic[f])	67–84
	9. Skin changes (hyperpigmentation, hypertrichosis, glomeruloid hemangiomata, plethora, acrocyanosis, flushing, white nails)	68–89
	10. Papilledema	29–64
	11. Thrombocytosis/polycythemia[g]	54–88
Other symptoms and signs	Clubbing, weight loss, hyperhidrosis, pulmonary hypertension/restrictive lung disease, thrombotic diatheses, diarrhea, low vitamin B_{12} values	

POEMS polyneuropathy, organomegaly, endocrinopathy, M-protein, skin changes

[a]The diagnosis of POEMS syndrome is confirmed when both of the mandatory major criteria, one of the three other major criteria, and one of the six minor criteria are present

[b]Summary of frequencies of POEMS syndrome features based on largest retrospective series [2, 3, 16–18, 27]

[c]Takasuki and Nakanishi series are included even though only 75% of patients had a documented plasma cell disorder.

[d]There is a Castleman disease variant of POEMS syndrome that occurs *without* evidence of a clonal plasma cell disorder that is not accounted for in this table. This entity should be considered separately

[e]A plasma VEGF level of 200 pg/mL is 95% specific and 68% sensitive for a POEMS syndrome [14]

[f]Because of the high prevalence of diabetes mellitus and thyroid abnormalities, this diagnosis alone is not sufficient to meet this minor criterion

[g]Approximately 50% of patients will have bone marrow changes that distinguish it from a typical MGUS or myeloma bone marrow

*Reproduced with permission from Dispenzieri, A., How I treat POEMS syndrome. Blood, 2012. **119**(24): p. 5650–8*

Clinical and Laboratory Presentation

The peripheral neuropathy is the dominant characteristic [2, 3, 16–18], and it is ascending, symmetrical, and affecting both sensation and motor function [19]. In our experience, pain may be a dominant feature in about 10–15% of patients, and in one report as many as 76% of patients had painful neuropathy [4, 20]. Nerve conduction studies in patients with POEMS syndrome show slowing of nerve conduction that is more predominant in the intermediate than distal nerve segments as compared to CIDP, and there is more severe attenuation of compound muscle action potentials in the lower than upper limbs [4, 21, 22]. In contrast to CIDP, conduction block is rare [4, 22]. The conduction findings suggest that demyelination is predominant in the nerve trunk rather than the distal nerve terminals, and axonal loss is predominant in the lower limb nerves [4]. Axonal loss is greater in POEMS syndrome than it is in CIDP [22]. The nerve biopsy is not specific, but uncompacted myelin lamellae, endothelial cytoplasmic enlargement, opening of the tight junctions between endothelial cells and presence of many pinocytic vesicles adjacent to the cell membranes, and absence of macrophage-associated demyelination have been described [23, 24]. As compared to CIDP, POEMS syndrome demonstrates more axonal degeneration and epineurial neovascularization but less endoneurial inflammation and onion-bulb formation [25].

Depending on the series, 45–85% of patients will have any combination of splenomegaly, hepatomegaly, and/or lymphadenopathy. Lymph nodes may appear reactive or reveal frank Castleman disease or merely "Castleman's disease-like" changes. Between 11 and 30% of POEMS patients with documented clonal plasma cell disorder also have documented Castleman disease or Castleman-like histology [6]. Among individuals with POEMS who undergo lymph node biopsy, about 50% show angiofollicular hyperplasia typical of Castleman disease [3, 18], and 84% are of these are hyaline vascular type [18]. Only those with peripheral neuropathy AND a plasma cell clone should be classified as standard POEMS syndrome; without both, patients can be classified as Castleman disease variant of POEMS if they have other POEMS features [26].

Endocrinopathy is a central but poorly understood feature of POEMS. In one series [27], approximately 84% of patients had a recognized endocrinopathy, with hypogonadism as the most common endocrine abnormality, followed by thyroid

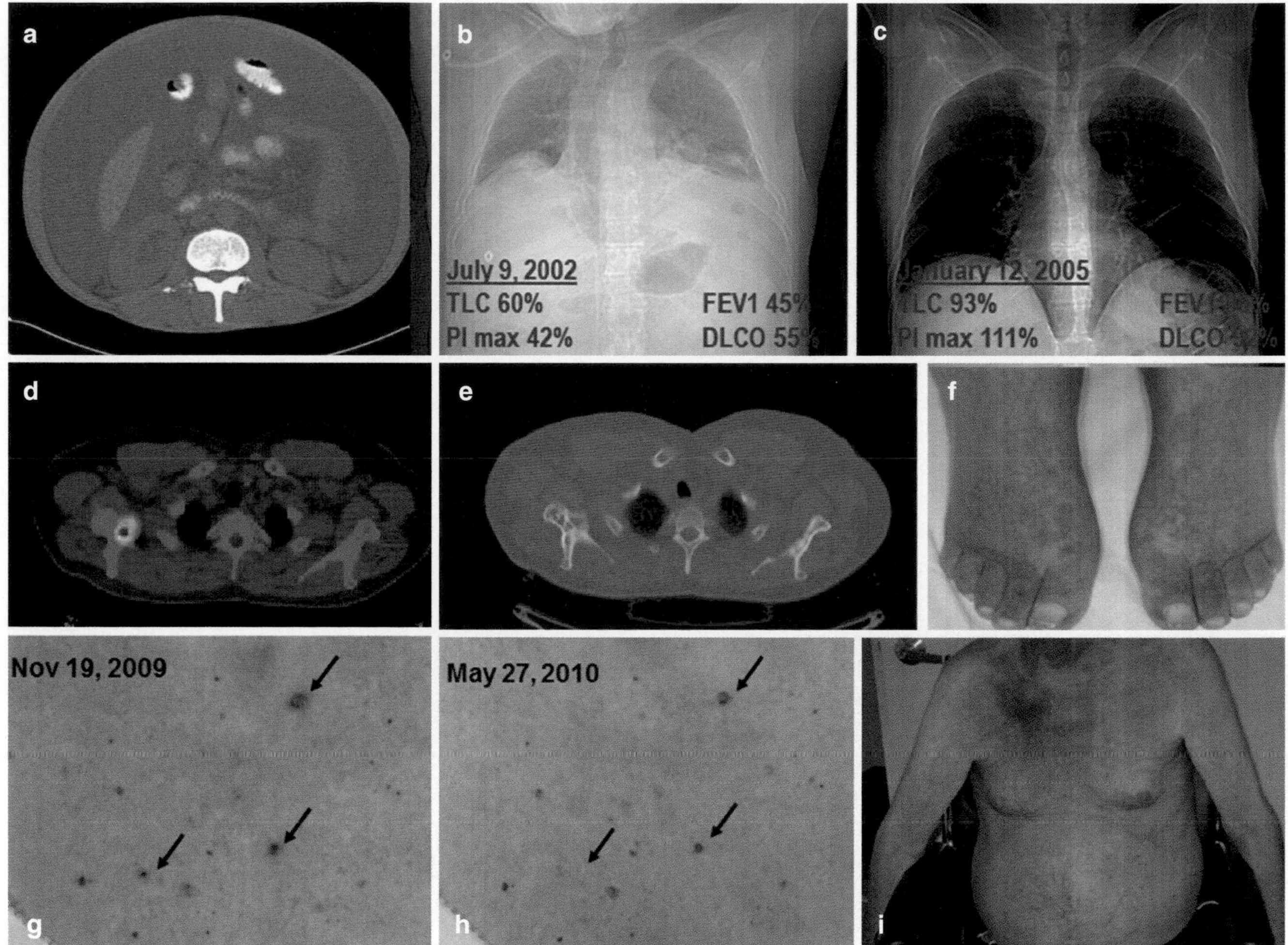

Fig. 32.1 Classic findings of POEMS syndromes. *Reproduced with permission from Dispenzieri, A., How I treat POEMS syndrome. Blood, 2012.* ***119****(24): p. 5650–8.* (**a**) Massive ascites and lipodystrophy. (**b**) Chest radiograph and pulmonary function test results demonstrating reduced lung volumes due to neuromuscular weakness, small effusions, and reduced diffusing capacity of carbon monoxide. (**c**) Improved chest radiograph and pulmonary function tests 2.5 years after ASCT (same patient as **h**). (**d**) Fusion CT PET of mixed lytic/sclerotic lesion in right scapula. (**e**) Bone windows of CT of mixed lytic/sclerotic lesion in right scapula. (**f**) Hyperemia of extremities and white nails. (**g**) Outcropping of cherry angiomata at diagnosis. (**h**) Shrinkage and disappearance of cherry angiomata after radiation to solitary osteosclerotic lesion right femur. (**i**) Plasmacytoma right scapula with overlying erythema as well as gynecomastia, muscle wasting, and ascites. Also present but unrelated is florid tinea corporis due to chronic steroid used for the incorrect diagnosis of CIDP

abnormalities, glucose metabolism abnormalities, and lastly adrenal insufficiency. The majority of patients have evidence of multiple endocrinopathies in the four major endocrine axes (gonadal, thyroid, glucose, and adrenal). Gynecomastia may be present on physical examination.

The characteristic skin changes include hyperpigmentation, a recent outcropping of hemangioma, hypertrichosis, dependent rubor and acrocyanosis, white nails, sclerodermoid changes, facial lipodystrophy, flushing, or clubbing [6]. Rarely calciphylaxis is also seen.

Papilledema is present in at least one-third of patients [28]; the majority of these patients do not have specific symptoms relating to this finding but a minority will report blurred vision, diplopia, or ocular pain. Peripheral edema, ascites, and effusions are the symptoms and signs that cause the next most morbidity after the peripheral neuropathy. The manifestations of extravascular overload occur in 29–87% of patients with POEMS syndrome and are not typically associated with severe hypoalbuminemia. Severe third spacing can lead to worsening renal function. Serum creatinine levels are normal in most cases, but serum cystatin C, which is a surrogate marker for renal function, is high in 71% of patients [29]. In a series from China, 22% of patients had a creatinine clearance (CrCl) of less than 60 mL/min including 8% with a CrCl of less than 30 mL/min; 10% had microhematuria [30]. The renal histologic findings are diverse with membranoproliferative features and evidence of endothelial injury being most common [31].

Finding the monoclonal plasma cell disorder can sometimes be a challenge. In one series, only 53% of patients had a positive protein electrophoresis, with another 31% being immunoelectrophoresis positively only, and 16% had their clone discovered only by either bone marrow biopsy or biopsy of a plasmacytoma, i.e., bone lesion [17]. The CBC is notable for an absence of cytopenias. Nearly half of patients will have thrombocytosis or erythrocytosis [17]. In a series from China, 26% of patients had anemia, which the authors attributed to impaired renal function [18]. Their series was enriched with Castleman disease cases (25%), which may have also contributed to this unprecedentedly high rate of anemia.

The bone marrow biopsy reveals megakaryocyte hyperplasia and megakaryocyte clustering in 54% and 93% of cases, respectively [15]. These megakaryocyte findings are reminiscent of a myeloproliferative disorder, but *JAK2* V617F mutation is uniformly absent. One-third of patients do not have clonal plasma cells on their iliac crest biopsy. These are the patients who present with a solitary or "multiple solitary plasmacytomas." The median percent of plasma cells observed is less than 5%. Immunohistochemical staining is more sensitive than is six-color flow since the former provides information on bone marrow architecture, which is key in making the diagnosis in nearly half of cases. In our study of 67 pretreatment bone marrow biopsies from patients with POEMS syndrome, lymphoid aggregates were found in 49% of cases. Of these, there was plasma cell rimming in all but one; and of these 32 cases, 31 were clonal lambda and 1 was kappa. This finding was not seen in bone marrows from normal controls or from patients with MGUS, multiple myeloma, or amyloidosis. Overall, only 8/67 (12%) of POEMS cases had normal iliac crest bone marrow biopsies, i.e., no detectable clonal plasma cells, no plasma cell-rimmed lymphoid aggregates, and no megakaryocyte hyperplasia.

Osteosclerotic lesions occur in approximately 95% of patients, and can be confused with benign bone islands, aneurysmal bone cysts, non-ossifying fibromas, and fibrous dysplasia [3, 17]. Some lesions are densely sclerotic, while others are lytic with a sclerotic rim, while still others have a mixed soap-bubble appearance. Occasionally patients have a lytic lesion without any evident sclerosis. Bone windows of CT body images are often very informative [32], often even more so than FDG uptake, which can be variable and most useful when there is an obvious lytic component to the bone lesion.

Plasma and serum levels of VEGF are markedly elevated in patients with POEMS [14, 33, 34] and correlate with the activity of the disease [10, 11, 14, 34]. The principal isoform of VEGF expressed is VEGF165 [10]. VEGF levels are independent of M-protein size [10]. IL-1β, TNF-α, IL-6, and IL-12 levels are often also increased [35]. Serum VEGF levels are 10–50 times higher plasma levels of VEGF [36]. Our group has demonstrated that a plasma VEGF level of 200 pg/mL had a specificity of 95% with a sensitivity of 68% in support of a diagnosis of POEMS syndrome.

Respiratory complaints are usually limited given patients' neurologic status impairing their ability to induce cardiovascular challenges [37]. The pulmonary manifestations are protean, including pulmonary hypertension, restrictive lung disease, impaired neuromuscular respiratory function, and impaired diffusion capacity of carbon monoxide, but improve with effective therapy [18, 37, 38]. Pulmonary hypertension has been reported to occur in 27% of unselected patients with POEMS syndrome [39]. Nail clubbing is seen in about 4–49% of cases [3, 37].

Patients are at increased risk for arterial and/or venous thromboses during their course, with nearly 20% of patients experiencing one of these complications [5, 40]. Ten percent of patients present with a cerebrovascular event, most commonly embolic or vessel dissection and stenosis [41]. Thrombocytosis and increased bone marrow infiltration are associated with risk for cerebrovascular accidents [41]. Aberrations in the coagulation cascade have been implicated in POEMS syndrome, but are not usually clinically apparent [24].

Treatment of Poems Syndrome

Despite the relationship between disease response and dropping levels of VEGF, the most experience with successful outcomes has been associated with directing therapy at the underlying clonal plasma cell disorder rather than solely targeting VEGF with anti-VEGF antibodies. The treatment algorithm is based on the extent of the plasma cell infiltration (Fig. 32.2). The approach to therapy differs based on whether there is bone marrow involvement as determined by blind iliac crest sampling [42].

The course of POEMS syndrome is usually chronic with an estimated 10-year survivorship rate of 77–79% [43, 44] and of more than 90% for those who undergo ASCT [17, 37, 44]. The number of POEMS features does not affect survival [5, 16]. Baseline risk factors for inferior survival have included fingernail clubbing, extravascular volume overload—i.e., effusions, edema, and ascites [17]—low serum albumin [44], coexistent Castleman disease [18], and respiratory symptoms [37]. In a recent publication from China of 362 patients, factors associated with inferior survival were age (40% of patients HR 4.1 [95%CI 1.4, 11.8]), pulmonary hypertension (20%, HR 4.0 [95%CI 1.4, 11,0]), pleural effusion (40%; HR 3.8 [95%CI 1.2, 11.8]), and eGFR <30 mL/min/1.73 m^2 (6%; HR 8.2 [95%CI 2.2, 31.2]).

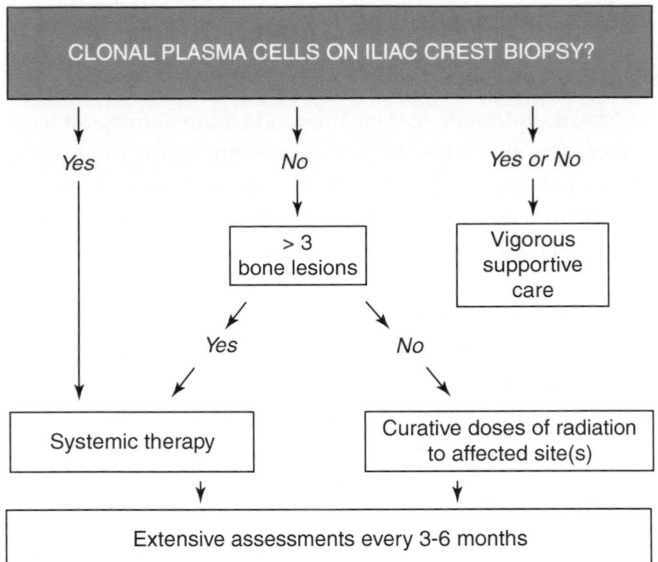

Fig. 32.2 Algorithm for the treatment of POEMS syndrome. *Reproduced with permission from Dispenzieri, A., How I treat POEMS syndrome. Blood, 2012.* ***119****(24): p. 5650–8*

Management of POEMS Syndrome Without Disseminated Bone Marrow Involvement

In the case of patients with an isolated bone lesion without clonal plasma cells found on iliac crest biopsy, radiation is the recommended therapy as it is in the case of a more straightforward solitary plasmacytoma of bone. Not only does radiation to an isolated (or even two or three isolated) lesion(s) improve the symptoms of POEMS syndrome over the course of 3–36 months, but it can also be curative.

Management of POEMS Syndrome with Disseminated Bone Marrow Involvement

Typically, once there is disseminated disease identified, systemic therapy is recommended with the caveat that large bony lesions with a significant lytic component may require adjuvant radiation therapy [42]. Decisions about adjuvant radiation should be made on a case-by-case basis, and typically not until a minimal of 6 months after completing chemotherapy. There is a lag between completion of successful therapy and neurologic response, often with no discernible improvement until 6 months after completion of therapy. Maximal response is not seen until 2–3 years hence. Other features like anasarca, papilledema, and even skin changes typically improve sooner. Optimal FDG-PET response may also lag by 6–12 months.

Table 32.2 Activity of therapy for the treatment of POEMS syndrome

Regimen	Outcome
Radiation	50–70% of patients have significant clinical improvement
Melphalan-dexamethasone	81% hematologic response rate; 100% with some neurologic improvement
Corticosteroids	50% of patients have significant clinical improvement
Cyclophosphamide-dexamethasone	At least 50% of patients have significant improvement
ASCT	100% of surviving patients have significant clinical improvement
Thalidomide-dexamethasone	Reported responses in 12 patients, but not recommended as first line due to risk of neuropathy. Additional 25 patients treated in randomized trial with crossover revealed improved VEGF and motor function [49]
Lenalidomide-dexamethasone	Reported responses in majority of patients (more than 60 patients reported)
Bortezomib	Used as single agent ($n = 1$), with dexamethasone ($n = 2$), with cyclophosphamide and dexamethasone ($n = 1$), and with doxorubicin and dexamethasone ($n = 1$). Reported responses in all
Bevacizumab	Two out of three using it as single agent died within weeks; one improved. Two other patients using it as "salvage" improved, but relapsed and died despite continued therapy, normal VEGF at 3.5 and 5.5 years. Six other cases of use with or after other alkylator-based therapy yielded one death and four patients with improvement

Modified from Dispenzieri [6]

Since there is a paucity of clinical trials among patients with POEMS syndrome [6], treatment recommendations are largely based on case series and anecdote. The treatment armamentarium is borrowed from other plasma cell disorders. Table 32.2 summarizes regimens and observed outcomes. Corticosteroids may provide symptomatic improvement, but response duration is limited. The most experience has been with alkylator-based therapy, either low dose or high dose with peripheral blood stem cell transplant. The first prospective clinical trial to treat POEMS syndrome was reported from China [45]. Thirty-one patients were treated with 12 cycles of melphalan and dexamethasone and 81% of patients achieved hematologic response, 100% had VEGF response, and 100% had at least some improvement in neurologic status. At 21 months, 100% were progression free and alive. Personal experience and retrospective reports of the use of cyclophosphamide-based therapy is effective [42].

High-dose alkylator with peripheral blood stem cell transplant is also quite effective, but selection basis may confound these reports [6]. Case series suggest that 100% of patients achieve at least some neurologic improvement. Doses of melphalan ranging from 140 to 200 mg/m^2 have been used, with the lower doses used for sicker patients. Of the 59 patients with POEMS syndrome treated at the Mayo Clinic Rochester, progression-free survival was 98%, 94%, and 75% at 1, 2, and 5 years, respectively [46]. Symptomatic progressions were rare, whereas radiographic and VEGF progressions were most common. Treatment-related morbidity and mortality can be minimized by recognizing and treating an engraftment-type syndrome characterized by fevers, rash, diarrhea, weight gain, and respiratory symptoms and signs that occur anytime between days 7 and 15 post-stem cell infusion [47]. In a recent EBMT series, engraftment syndrome was reported in 23% of patients. Survival figures were comparable to that seen in the Mayo series [48].

There is one randomized trial for patients with POEMS syndrome. Misawa and colleagues conducted a randomized, double-blind, placebo-controlled phase 2/3 trial for patients with POEMS syndrome who were not candidates for ASCT [49]. Twenty-five patients were randomized to either daily thalidomide plus 4 days of dexamethasone every 4 weeks or placebo and 4 days of dexamethasone for 24 weeks; thereafter all patients received open-label, single-agent thalidomide for 48 weeks. Patients treated with thalidomide had higher rates of VEGF reduction, greater change in summated muscle test scores, and smaller changes in SF-36 QoL physical function and physical scores. Not surprisingly, side effects including sinus bradycardia, constipation, and mild sensory neuropathy were more frequent in patients treated with thalidomide.

Lenalidomide has also yielded favorable results, seemingly with fewer side effects. The French have reported in abstract form their results of a Phase 2 study of lenalidomide and dexamethasone for 2 cycles as neoadjuvant therapy preceding radiation or high-dose therapy or as primary therapy as 9 cycles followed by 12 cycles of single-agent lenalidomide [50]. They treated 27 patients: 10 pre-radiation therapy; 8 pre-ASCT; and 9 primary therapy. Although follow-up is short, the authors report that several patients had rapid neurological response, no patient had died, and one patient had progressed. These results are similar to case reports and case series [51–53]. In the largest case series of 20 patients [53], all patients responded, but 4 patients relapsed 3–10 months after the end of treatment. Another retrospective case series of 12 patients with relapsed or refractory POEMS syndrome treated with lenalidomide and dexamethasone reported a 2-year PFS and OS of 92% [54]. A systematic review of lenalidomide use in patients with POEMS has been published [55], which estimates a 1- and 2-year PFS of 92 and 42% using lenalidomide. Given the intrinsic risk patients with POEMS syndrome have for thrombosis, it is imperative that at least an aspirin be used for prophylaxis. The use of low-molecular-weight heparin or warfarin should be balanced against fall risk.

Like thalidomide and lenalidomide, bortezomib can have anti-VEGF and anti-TNF effects. Enthusiasm for thalidomide and bortezomib should be tempered by the high rate of peripheral neuropathy induced by these drugs. Bortezomib use has been reported in a handful of patients, with favorable results, especially those with severe ascites [6]. Although an anti-VEGF strategy is appealing, the results with bevacizumab have been mixed. Most of these reports include patients who had also received either radiation or alkylator during and/or predating the bevacizumab had benefit [42].

Both our experience and the literature would support that single-agent IV IG or plasmapheresis is not helpful. Other treatments like interferon-alpha, tamoxifen, trans-retinoic acid, ticlopidine, argatroban, and strontium-89 have been reported as having activity mostly as single-case reports.

Managing Symptoms of Disease

Attention to supportive care is imperative. Orthotics, physical therapy, and CPAP all play an important role in patients' recovery. Ankle foot orthotics can increase mobility and reduce falls. Physical therapy reduces the risk for permanent contractures and leads to improved function both in the long and short terms. For those with severe neuromuscular weakness, CPAP and/or biBAP provides better oxygenation and potentially reduces the risk complications associated with hypoventilation like pulmonary infection and pulmonary hypertension.

Monitoring Response

Patients must be followed carefully on a quarterly basis tracking the status of deficits comparing these to baseline [46]. VEGF responses may occur as soon as 3 months [56], but they can be delayed. VEGF is an imperfect marker since discordance between disease activity and response has been reported [57], so trends rather than absolute values should direct therapeutic decisions. Serum M-protein responses by protein electrophoresis, immunofixation electrophoresis, or serum immunoglobulin free light chains also pose a challenge. The size of the M-protein is typically small making standard multiple myeloma response criteria inapplicable in most cases. In addition, patients can derive very significant clinical benefit in the absence of an M-protein response [45, 47]. Finally, despite the fact that the immunoglobulin free light chains are elevated in 90% of POEMS patients, the ratio is normal in all but 18% [29], making the test of limited value for patients with POEMS syndrome.

Conclusion

POEMS syndrome is a rare disorder. There is much to be learned about the pathogenesis of the disease. From a practical standpoint, however, one of the biggest challenges is that diagnosis is often delayed, which results in increased morbidity. Hematologic, clinical, VEGF, and PET scan responses can be achieved with a multitude of therapies, but there are no randomized data to determine which therapies are best in terms of rapid, deepest, and most durable responses. If the diagnosis is made too late, patients may be left with some extent of irreversible nerve damage, so neurologists and hematologists should be vigilant of POEMS in their differential diagnosis of patients with lambda-restricted plasma cell disorder, peripheral neuropathy, and other POEMS syndrome features.

References

1. Bardwick PA, Zvaifler NJ, Gill GN, Newman D, Greenway GD, Resnick DL. Plasma cell dyscrasia with polyneuropathy, organomegaly, endocrinopathy, M protein, and skin changes: the POEMS syndrome. Report on two cases and a review of the literature. Medicine. 1980;59(4):311–22.
2. Takatsuki K, Sanada I. Plasma cell dyscrasia with polyneuropathy and endocrine disorder: clinical and laboratory features of 109 reported cases. Jpn J Clin Oncol. 1983;13(3):543–55.
3. Nakanishi T, Sobue I, Toyokura Y, Nishitani H, Kuroiwa Y, Satoyoshi E, et al. The Crow-Fukase syndrome: a study of 102 cases in Japan. Neurology. 1984;34(6):712–20.
4. Nasu S, Misawa S, Sekiguchi Y, Shibuya K, Kanai K, Fujimaki Y, et al. Different neurological and physiological profiles in POEMS syndrome and chronic inflammatory demyelinating polyneuropathy. J Neurol Neurosurg Psychiatry. 2012;83(5):476–9.
5. Dispenzieri A. POEMS syndrome. Blood Rev. 2007;21(6):285–99.
6. Dispenzieri A. POEMS syndrome: update on diagnosis, risk-stratification, and management. Am J Hematol. 2015;90(10): 951–62.
7. Soubrier M, Labauge P, Jouanel P, Viallard JL, Piette JC, Sauvezie B. Restricted use of Vlambda genes in POEMS syndrome. Haematologica. 2004;89(4):ECR02.
8. Nakaseko C, Abe D, Takeuchi M, Takeda Y, Tanaka H, Oda K, et al. Restricted oligo-clonal usage of monoclonal immunoglobulin {lambda} light chain germline in POEMS syndrome. ASH Annual Meeting Abstracts. 2007;110(11):2483.
9. Alberti MA, Martinez-Yelamos S, Fernandez A, Vidaller A, Narvaez JA, Cano LM, et al. 18F-FDG PET/CT in the evaluation of POEMS syndrome. Eur J Radiol. 2010;76(2):180–2.
10. Watanabe O, Maruyama I, Arimura K, Kitajima I, Arimura H, Hanatani M, et al. Overproduction of vascular endothelial growth factor/vascular permeability factor is causative in Crow-Fukase (POEMS) syndrome. Muscle Nerve. 1998;21(11):1390–7.
11. Scarlato M, Previtali SC, Carpo M, Pareyson D, Briani C, Del Bo R, et al. Polyneuropathy in POEMS syndrome: role of angiogenic factors in the pathogenesis. Brain. 2005;128(8):1911–20.
12. Nobile-Orazio E, Terenghi F, Giannotta C, Gallia F, Nozza A. Serum VEGF levels in POEMS syndrome and in immune-mediated neuropathies. Neurology. 2009;72(11):1024–6.
13. Briani C, Fabrizi GM, Ruggero S, Torre CD, Ferrarini M, Campagnolo M, et al. Vascular endothelial growth factor helps differentiate neuropathies in rare plasma cell dyscrasias. Muscle Nerve. 2010;43(2):164–7.
14. D'Souza A, Hayman SR, Buadi F, Mauermann M, Lacy MQ, Gertz MA, et al. The utility of plasma vascular endothelial growth factor levels in the diagnosis and follow-up of patients with POEMS syndrome. Blood. 2011;118(17):4663–5.
15. Dao LN, Hanson CA, Dispenzieri A, Morice WG, Kurtin PJ, Hoyer JD. Bone marrow histopathology in POEMS syndrome: a distinctive combination of plasma cell, lymphoid and myeloid findings in 87 patients. Blood. 2011;117(24):6438–44.
16. Soubrier MJ, Dubost JJ, Sauvezie BJ. POEMS syndrome: a study of 25 cases and a review of the literature. French Study Group on POEMS Syndrome. Am J Med. 1994;97(6):543–53.
17. Dispenzieri A, Kyle RA, Lacy MQ, Rajkumar SV, Therneau TM, Larson DR, et al. POEMS syndrome: definitions and long-term outcome. Blood. 2003;101(7):2496–506.
18. Li J, Zhou DB, Huang Z, Jiao L, Duan MH, Zhang W, et al. Clinical characteristics and long-term outcome of patients with POEMS syndrome in China. Ann Hematol. 2011;90(7):819–26.
19. Kelly JJ Jr, Kyle RA, Miles JM, Dyck PJ. Osteosclerotic myeloma and peripheral neuropathy. Neurology. 1983;33(2):202–10.
20. Koike H, Iijima M, Mori K, Yamamoto M, Hattori N, Watanabe H, et al. Neuropathic pain correlates with myelinated fibre loss and cytokine profile in POEMS syndrome. J Neurol Neurosurg Psychiatry. 2008;79(10):1171–9.
21. Kelly JJ Jr. The electrodiagnostic findings in peripheral neuropathy associated with monoclonal gammopathy. Muscle Nerve. 1983;6(7):504–9.
22. Mauermann ML, Sorenson EJ, Dispenzieri A, Mandrekar J, Suarez GA, Dyck PJ. Uniform demyelination and more severe axonal loss distinguish POEMS syndrome from CIDP. J Neurol Neurosurg Psychiatry. 2012;83(5):480–6.
23. Arimura K. [Increased vascular endothelial growth factor (VEGF) is causative in Crow-Fukase syndrome] [Japanese]. Rinsho Shinkeigaku [Clin Neurol]. 1999;39(1):84–5.
24. Saida K, Kawakami H, Ohta M, Iwamura K. Coagulation and vascular abnormalities in Crow-Fukase syndrome. Muscle Nerve. 1997;20(4):486–92.
25. Piccione EA, Engelstad J, Dyck PJ, Mauermann ML, Dispenzieri A, Dyck PJ. Nerve pathologic features differentiate POEMS syndrome from CIDP. Acta Neuropathol Commun. 2016;4(1):116.
26. Dispenzieri A. POEMS syndrome: 2011 update on diagnosis, risk-stratification, and management. Am J Hematol. 2011;86(7):591–601.
27. Ghandi GY, Basu R, Dispenzieri A, Basu A, Montori V, Brennan MD. Endocrinopathy in POEMS syndrome: the Mayo Clinic experience. Mayo Clin Proc. 2007;82(7):836–42.
28. Kaushik M, Pulido JS, Abreu R, Amselem L, Dispenzieri A. Ocular findings in patients with polyneuropathy, organomegaly, endocrinopathy, monoclonal gammopathy, and skin changes syndrome. Ophthalmology. 2011;118(4):778–82.
29. Stankowski-Drengler T, Gertz MA, Katzmann JA, Lacy MQ, Kumar S, Leung N, et al. Serum immunoglobulin free light chain measurements and heavy chain isotype usage provide insight into disease biology in patients with POEMS syndrome. Am J Hematol. 2010;85(6):431–4.
30. Ye W, Wang C, Cai QQ, Cai H, Duan MH, Li H, et al. Renal impairment in patients with polyneuropathy, organomegaly, endocrinopathy, monoclonal gammopathy and skin changes syndrome: incidence, treatment and outcome. Nephrol Dial Transplant. 2015:gfv261.
31. Sanada S, Ookawara S, Karube H, Shindo T, Goto T, Nakamichi T, et al. Marked recovery of severe renal lesions in POEMS syndrome with high-dose melphalan therapy supported by autologous blood stem cell transplantation. Am J Kidney Dis. 2006;47(4):672–9.
32. Glazebrook K, Guerra Bonilla FL, Johnson A, Leng S, Dispenzieri A. Computed tomography assessment of bone lesions in patients with POEMS syndrome. Eur Radiol. 2015;25(2):497–504.

33. Watanabe O, Arimura K, Kitajima I, Osame M, Maruyama I. Greatly raised vascular endothelial growth factor (VEGF) in POEMS syndrome [letter]. Lancet. 1996;347(9002):702.
34. Soubrier M, Dubost JJ, Serre AF, Ristori JM, Sauvezie B, Cathebras P, et al. Growth factors in POEMS syndrome: evidence for a marked increase in circulating vascular endothelial growth factor. Arthritis Rheum. 1997;40(4):786–7.
35. Kanai K, Sawai S, Sogawa K, Mori M, Misawa S, Shibuya K, et al. Markedly upregulated serum interleukin-12 as a novel biomarker in POEMS syndrome. Neurology. 2012;79(6):575–82.
36. Tokashiki T, Hashiguchi T, Arimura K, Eiraku N, Maruyama I, Osame M. Predictive value of serial platelet count and VEGF determination for the management of DIC in the crow-Fukase (POEMS) syndrome. Intern Med. 2003;42(12):1240–3.
37. Allam JS, Kennedy CC, Aksamit TR, Dispenzieri A. Pulmonary manifestations in patients with POEMS syndrome: a retrospective review of 137 patients. Chest. 2008;133(4):969–74.
38. Lesprit P, Godeau B, Authier FJ, Soubrier M, Zuber M, Larroche C, et al. Pulmonary hypertension in POEMS syndrome: a new feature mediated by cytokines. Am J Respir Crit Care Med. 1998;157(3):907–11.
39. Li J, Tian Z, Zheng HY, Zhang W, Duan MH, Liu YT, et al. Pulmonary hypertension in POEMS syndrome. Haematologica. 2013;98(3):393–8.
40. Lesprit P, Authier FJ, Gherardi R, Belec L, Paris D, Melliere D, et al. Acute arterial obliteration: a new feature of the POEMS syndrome? Medicine. 1996;75(4):226–32.
41. Dupont SA, Dispenzieri A, Mauermann ML, Rabinstein AA, Brown RD Jr. Cerebral infarction in POEMS syndrome: incidence, risk factors, and imaging characteristics. Neurology. 2009;73(16):1308–12.
42. Dispenzieri A. How I treat POEMS syndrome. Blood. 2012;119(24):5650–8.
43. Wang C, Huang XF, Cai QQ, Cao XX, Duan MH, Cai H, et al. Prognostic study for overall survival in patients with newly diagnosed POEMS syndrome. Leukemia. 2017;31(1):100–6.
44. Kourelis TV, Buadi FK, Kumar SK, Gertz MA, Lacy MQ, Dingli D, et al. Long-term outcome of patients with POEMS syndrome: an update of the Mayo Clinic experience. Am J Hematol. 2016;91(6):585–9.
45. Li J, Zhang W, Jiao L, Duan MH, Guan HZ, Zhu WG, et al. Combination of melphalan and dexamethasone for patients with newly diagnosed POEMS syndrome. Blood. 2011;117(24):6445–9.
46. D'Souza A, Lacy M, Gertz M, Kumar S, Buadi F, Hayman S, et al. Long-term outcomes after autologous stem cell transplantation for patients with POEMS syndrome (osteosclerotic myeloma): a single-center experience. Blood. 2012;120(1):56–62.
47. Dispenzieri A, Lacy MQ, Hayman SR, Kumar SK, Buadi F, Dingli D, et al. Peripheral blood stem cell transplant for POEMS syndrome is associated with high rates of engraftment syndrome. Eur J Haematol. 2008;80(5):397–406.
48. Cook G, Iacobelli S, van Biezen A, Ziagkos D, LeBlond V, Abraham J, et al. High-dose therapy and autologous stem cell transplantation in patients with POEMS syndrome: a retrospective study of the Plasma Cell Disorder sub-committee of the Chronic Malignancy Working Party of the European Society for Blood & Marrow Transplantation. Haematologica. 2017;102(1):160–7.
49. Misawa S, Sato Y, Katayama K, Nagashima K, Aoyagi R, Sekiguchi Y, et al. Safety and efficacy of thalidomide in patients with POEMS syndrome: a multicentre, randomised, double-blind, placebo-controlled trial. Lancet Neurol. 2016;15(11):1129–37.
50. Jaccard A, Lazareth A, Karlin L, Choquet S, Frenzel L, Garderet L, et al. A prospective phase II trial of Lenalidomide and dexamethasone (LEN-DEX) in POEMS syndrome. Blood. 2014;124(21):36.
51. Vannata B, Laurenti L, Chiusolo P, Sora F, Balducci M, Sabatelli M, et al. Efficacy of lenalidomide plus dexamethasone for POEMS syndrome relapsed after autologous peripheral stem-cell transplantation. Am J Hematol. 2012;87(6):641–2.
52. Dispenzieri A, Klein CJ, Mauermann ML. Lenalidomide therapy in a patient with POEMS syndrome. Blood. 2007;110(3):1075–6.
53. Royer B, Merlusca L, Abraham J, Musset L, Haroche J, Choquet S, et al. Efficacy of lenalidomide in POEMS syndrome: a retrospective study of 20 patients. Am J Hematol. 2013;88(3):207–12.
54. Cai QQ, Wang C, Cao XX, Cai H, Zhou DB, Li J. Efficacy and safety of low-dose lenalidomide plus dexamethasone in patients with relapsed or refractory POEMS syndrome. Eur J Haematol. 2015;95(4):325–30.
55. Zagouri F, Kastritis E, Gavriatopoulou M, Sergentanis TN, Psaltopoulou T, Terpos E, et al. Lenalidomide in patients with POEMS syndrome: a systematic review and pooled analysis. Leuk Lymphoma. 2014;55(9):2018–23.
56. Kuwabara S, Misawa S, Kanai K, Suzuki Y, Kikkawa Y, Sawai S, et al. Neurologic improvement after peripheral blood stem cell transplantation in POEMS syndrome. Neurology. 2008;71(21):1691–5.
57. Goto H, Nishio M, Kumano K, Fujimoto K, Yamaguchi K, Koike T. Discrepancy between disease activity and levels of vascular endothelial growth factor in a patient with POEMS syndrome successfully treated with autologous stem-cell transplantation. Bone Marrow Transplant. 2008;42(9):627–9.

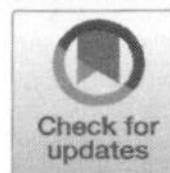

Waldenstrom's Macroglobulinemia

33

Steven P. Treon, Giampaolo Merlini, and Meletios Dimopoulos

Background

Waldenstrom's macroglobulinemia (WM) is a lymphoid neoplasm resulting from the accumulation, predominantly in the marrow, of a clonal population of lymphocytes, lymphoplasmacytic cells, and plasma cells, which secrete a monoclonal immunoglobulin (Ig) M [1]. WM corresponds to lymphoplasmacytic lymphoma (LPL) as defined in the Revised European-American Lymphoma (REAL) and World Health Organization classification systems [2, 3]. Most cases of LPL are WM; less than 5% of cases are IgA-secreting, IgG-secreting, or nonsecreting LPL.

Epidemiology

The age-adjusted incidence rate of WM is 3.4 per 1 million among males and 1.7 per 1 million among females in the United States. It increases in incidence geometrically with age [4, 5]. The incidence rate is higher among Americans of European descent. African-American descendants represent approximately 5% of all patients.

Genetic factors play a role in the pathogenesis of WM. Approximately 20% of WM patients are of Ashkenazi-Jewish ethnic background [6]. Familial disease has been reported commonly, including multigenerational clustering of WM and other B-cell lymphoproliferative diseases [6–9]. Approximately 28% of 924 sequential patients with WM presenting to a tertiary referral center had a first- or second-degree relative with either WM or another B-cell disorder [6]. Familial clustering of WM with other immunologic disorders, including hypogammaglobulinemia and hypergammaglobulinemia (particularly polyclonal IgM), autoantibody production (particularly to the thyroid), and manifestation of hyperactive B cells, has also been reported in relatives without WM [6, 9]. Increased expression of the *BCL-2* gene with enhanced survival has been observed in B cells from familial patients and their family members [9].

The role of environmental factors is uncertain, but chronic antigenic stimulation from infections and certain drug or chemical exposures have been considered but have not reached a level of scientific certainty. Hepatitis C virus (HCV) infection was implicated in WM causality in some series, but in a study of 100 consecutive WM patients in whom serologic and molecular diagnostic studies for HCV infection were performed no association was found [10–12].

Pathogenesis

Nature of the WM Clone

Examination of the B-cell clone(s) found in the bone marrow of WM patients reveals a range of differentiation from small lymphocytes with large focal deposits of surface immunoglobulins to lymphoplasmacytic cells and to mature plasma cells that contain intracytoplasmic IgM (Fig. 33.1) [13]. Circulating clonal B cells are often detectable in patients with WM, though lymphocytosis is uncommon [14, 15]. WM cells express the monoclonal IgM, and some clonal cells also express surface IgD [16]. The characteristic immunophenotypic profile of WM lymphoplasmacytic cells includes the expression of the pan B-cell markers CD19, CD20 (including FMC7), CD22, and CD79 [16, 17]. Expression of CD5, CD10, and CD23 can be present in 10–20% of cases, and their presence does not exclude the diagnosis of WM [18]. In addition, multiparameter flow

S.P. Treon, M.D., Ph.D. (✉)
Department of Medicine, Harvard Medical School, Dana Farber Cancer Institute, 450 Brookline Avenue, Boston, MA 02215, USA
e-mail: steven_treon@dfci.harvard.edu

G. Merlini, M.D.
Department of Medicine, Center for Research and Treatment of Systematic Amyloidoses, University of Pavia, University Hospital Policlinico San Matteo, Viale Golgi 19, Pavia 27100, Italy

M. Dimopoulos, M.D.
Department of Experimental Therapeutics, University of Athens, 80 Vas. Sofias Avenue, Athens 11528, Greece

P.H. Wiernik et al. (eds.), *Neoplastic Diseases of the Blood*, DOI 10.1007/978-3-319-64263-5_33

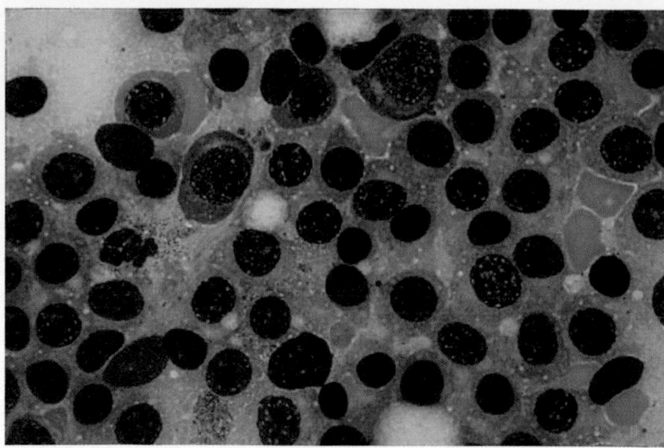

Fig. 33.1 Marrow film from a patient with Waldenstrom's macroglobulinemia. Note infiltrate of mature lymphocytes, lymphoplasmacytic cells, and plasma cells (*used with permission from Marvin J. Stone, MD*)

cytometric analysis has also identified CD25 and CD27 as being characteristic of the WM clone, and that a CD22^{dim}/CD25^{+}/CD27^{+}/IgM^{+} population can be observed among clonal B lymphocytes in IgM MGUS patients who ultimately progressed to WM [19].

Somatic mutations in immunoglobulin genes are present with increased frequency of nonsynonymous versus silent mutations in complement-determining regions along with somatic hypermutation, thereby supporting a post-germinal center derivation for the WM B-cell clone in most patients [20, 21]. A strong preferential usage of VH3/JH4 gene families without intraclonal variation, and without evidence for any isotype-switched transcripts, has also been shown [22, 23]. Taken together, these data support an IgM^{+} and/or IgM^{+}IgD^{+} memory B-cell origin for most cases of WM.

In contrast to myeloma plasma cells, no recurrent translocations have been described in WM, which can help to distinguish IgM myeloma cases that often exhibit t11;14 translocations from WM [24, 25]. Despite the absence of IgH translocations, recurrent chromosomal abnormalities are present in WM cells. These include deletions in chromosome 6q21–23 in 40–60% of WM patients, with concordant gains in 6p in 41% of 6q-deleted patients [26–29]. In a series of 174 untreated WM patients, 6q deletions, followed by trisomy 18, 13q deletions, 17p deletions, trisomy 4, and 11q deletions, were observed [29]. Deletion of 6q and trisomy 4 were associated with adverse prognostic markers in this series. As 6q deletions represent the most recurrent cytogenetic finding in WM cases, there has been great interest in identifying the region of minimal deletion and possible target genes within this region. Two putative gene candidates within this region include TNFAIP3, a negative regulator of nuclear factor kappa B signaling (NFκB), and PRDM1, a master regulator of B-cell differentiation [28, 30]. The removal of an NFκB-negative regulator is of particular interest as the phosphorylation and translocation of NFκB into the nucleus are crucial events for WM cell survival [31]. The success of proteasome inhibitor therapy in WM has been postulated to occur because the degradation of negative regulators of NFκB such as the inhibitor of kappa B (IκB) is blocked [32, 33].

Mutation in MYD88

A highly recurrent somatic mutation (MYD88^{L265P}) was first identified in WM patients by whole-genome sequencing (WGS), and confirmed by multiple studies through Sanger sequencing and/or allele-specific polymerase chain reaction assays [34–39]. MYD88^{L265P} is expressed in 90–95% of WM cases when more sensitive allele-specific PCR has been employed using both CD19-sorted and unsorted bone marrow (BM) cells [35–39]. By comparison, MYD88^{L265P} was absent in myeloma samples, including IgM myeloma, and was expressed in a small subset (6–10%) of MZL patients, who surprisingly have WM-related features [35–37, 40]. By polymerase chain reaction assays, 50–80% of IgM MGUS patients also express MYD88^{L265P}, and expression of this mutation was associated with increased risk for malignant progression [35–37, 41]. The presence of MYD88^{L265P} in IgM MGUS patient suggests a role for this mutation as an early oncogenic driver, and other mutations and/or copy number alterations leading to abnormal gene expression are likely to promote disease progression [28].

The impact of MYD88^{L265P} to growth and survival signaling in WM cells has been addressed in several studies (Fig. 33.2). Knockdown of MYD88 decreased survival of MYD88^{L265P}-expressing WM cells, whereas survival was enhanced by knock-in of MYD88^{L265P} versus wild-type MYD88 [42]. The discovery of a mutation in MYD88 is of significance given its role as an adaptor molecule in Toll-like receptor (TLR) and interleukin-1 receptor (IL-1R) signaling [43]. All TLRs except for TLR3 use MYD88 to facilitate their signaling. Following TLR or IL-1R stimulation, MYD88 is recruited to the activated receptor complex as a homodimer which then complexes with IRAK4 and activates IRAK1 and IRAK2 [44–46]. Tumor necrosis factor receptor-associated factor 6 is then activated by IRAK1 leading to NF-κB activation via IκBα phosphorylation [47]. Use of inhibitors of MYD88 pathway led to decreased IRAK1 and IκBα phosphorylation, as well as survival of MYD88^{L265P}-expressing WM cells. These observations are of particular relevance to WM since NF-κB signaling is important for WM growth and survival [31]. Bruton's tyrosine kinase (BTK) is also activated by MYD88^{L265P} [42]. Activated BTK co-immunoprecipitates with MYD88 that could be abrogated by use of a BTK kinase inhibitor, and overexpression of MYD88^{L265P} but

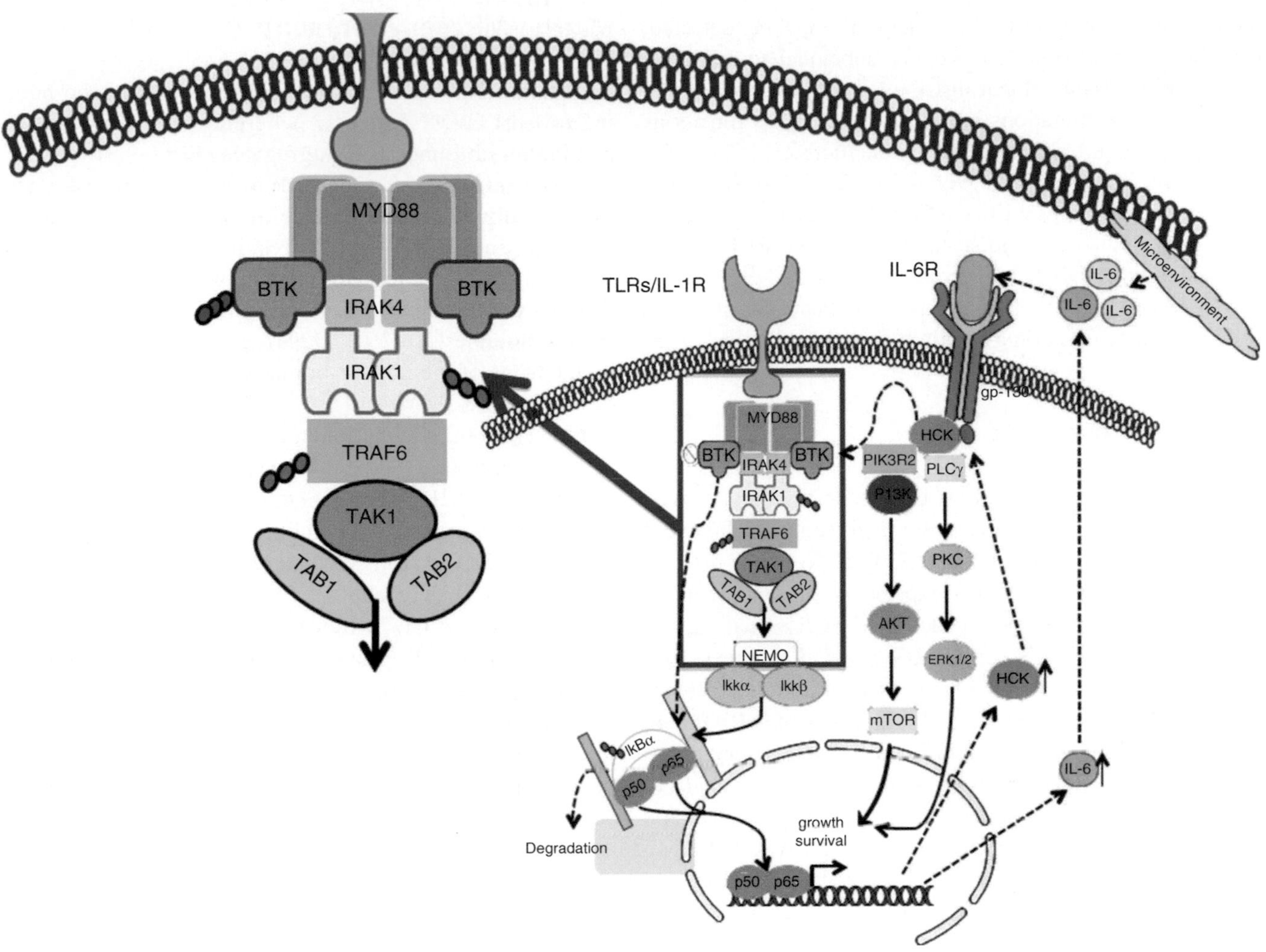

Fig. 33.2 MYD88-activating mutations are highly prevalent in patients with Waldenstrom's macroglobulinemia and trigger multiple growth and survival pathways. Activated MYD88 triggers NF-kB through BTK and IRAK1/IRAK4, as well as HCK that activates BTK, AKT, and ERK

not wild-type (WT) MYD88 triggers BTK activation. Knockdown of MYD88 by lentiviral transfection or use of a MYD88 homodimerization inhibitor also abrogated BTK activation in MYD88^{L265P}-mutated WM cells. MYD88 also triggers HCK, a SRC family member that regulates AKT and ERK survival signaling, and also activates BTK itself [48]. Rarely, non-L265P-activating mutations in WM may also occur, and Sanger sequencing of the entire MYD88 gene should be considered in patients suspected of having WM in whom PCR testing for MYD88^{L265P} is negative [49].

CXCR4 WHIM Mutations

The second most common somatic mutation after MYD88^{L265P} revealed by whole-genome sequencing was found in the C-terminus of the CXCR4 receptor. These mutations are present in 30–35% of WM patients, and impact serine phosphorylation sites that regulate CXCR4 signaling by its only known ligand SDF-1a (CXCL12) [28, 50–52]. The location of somatic mutations found in the C-terminus of CXCR4 in WM is similar to that observed in the germline of patients with WHIM (warts, hypogammaglobulinemia, infections, and myelokathexis) syndrome, a congenital immunodeficiency disorder characterized by chronic noncyclic neutropenia [53]. Patients with WHIM syndrome exhibit impaired CXCR4 receptor internalization following SDF-1a stimulation, which results in persistent CXCR4 activation and myelokathexis [54].

In WM patients, two classes of CXCR4 mutations occur in the C-terminus. These include non-sense (CXCR4$^{WHIM/NS}$) mutations that truncate the distal 15–20 amino acid region, and frameshift (CXCR4$^{WHIM/FS}$) mutations that compromise a region of up to 40 amino acids in the C- terminal domain [28, 50]. Non-sense and frameshift mutations are almost equally divided among WM patients with CXCR4 somatic mutations, and over 30 different types of CXCR4^{WHIM} mutations have been identified in WM patients [28, 50]. In some patients multiple $CXCR^{WHIM}$ mutations may be detected. $CXCR4^{WHIM}$ mutations are usually subclonal to MYD88, with highly variable clonal distribution [55]. The subclonal nature of these mutations suggests that CXCR4 mutations were likely acquired after MYD88 mutations.

Preclinical studies with WM cells engineered to express nonsense and frameshift $CXCR4^{WHIM}$-mutated receptors have shown enhanced and sustained AKT and ERK signaling following SDF-1a relative to $CXCR4^{WT}$, as well as increased cell migration, adhesion, growth and survival, and drug resistance (including ibrutinib) in WM cells [56, 57].

Other Somatic Events

Many copy number alterations have been revealed in WM patients that impact growth and survival pathways. Frequent loss of HIVEP2 (80%) and TNAIP3 (50%) genes that are negative regulators of NFkB expression, as well as LYN (70%) and IBTK (40%) that modulate BCR signaling, has been revealed by WGS [28]. WGS has also revealed common defects in chromatin remodeling with somatic mutations in ARID1A present in 17%, and loss of ARID1B in 70% of WM patients. Both ARID1A and ARID1B are members of the SWI/SNF family of proteins, and are thought to exert their effects via p53 and CDKN1A regulation. TP53 is mutated in 7% of sequenced WM genomes, while PRDM2 and TOP1 that participate in TP53-related signaling are deleted in 80% and 60% of WM patients, respectively [28]. Taken together, somatic events that contribute to impaired DNA damage response are also common in WM.

Impact of WM Genomics on Clinical Presentation

The importance of MYD88 and CXCR4 mutations in the clinical presentation of WM patients was recently reported. Significantly higher BM disease involvement, serum IgM levels, and symptomatic disease requiring therapy, including hyperviscosity syndrome, were observed in those patients with $MYD88^{L265P}CXCR4^{WHIM/NS}$ mutations [50]. Patients with $MYD88^{L265P}CXCR4^{WHIM/FS}$ or $MYD88^{L265P}CXCR4^{WT}$ had intermediate BM and serum IgM levels; those with $MYD88^{WT}CXCR4^{WT}$ showed the lowest BM disease burden. Fewer patients with $MYD88^{L265P}$ and $CXCR4^{WHIM/FS\ or\ NS}$ compared to $MYD88^{L265P}CXCR4^{WT}$ presented with adenopathy, further delineating differences in disease tropism based on CXCR4 status. Despite the more aggressive presentation associated with $CXCR4^{WHIM/NS}$ genotype, risk of death was not impacted by CXCR4 mutation status. Risk of death was found to be tenfold higher in patients with $MYD88^{WT}$ versus $MYD88^{L265P}$ genotype [50].

Marrow Microenvironment

Increased numbers of mast cells are found in the bone marrow of WM patients, wherein they are usually admixed with tumor cell aggregates (Fig. 33.3) [13, 17, 55]. The role of mast cells in WM has been investigated in one study wherein coculture of primary autologous or mast cell lines with WM LPC resulted in dose-dependent WM cell proliferation and/or tumor colony formation, through CD40 ligand (CD40L) signaling [58]. WM cells release soluble CD27 (sCD27) which may be triggered by cleavage of membrane-bound CD27 by matrix metalloproteinase 8 (MMP8) [59]. sCD27 levels are elevated in the serum of WM patients, and follow disease burden in mice engrafted with WM cells, as well as in WM patients [61]. sCD27 triggers the upregulation of CD40L as well as a proliferation-inducing ligand (APRIL) on mast cells derived from WM patients, as well as mast cell lines through its receptor CD70. Modeling in mice engrafted with a CD70-blocking antibody shows inhibition of tumor cell growth suggesting that WM cells require a microenvironmental support system for their growth and survival [60]. High levels of CXCR4 and very late antigen-4 (VLA-4) have also been observed in WM cells [61]. In blocking experiments studies, CXCR4 was shown to support migration of WM cells, while VLA-4 contributed to adhesion of WM cells to bone marrow stromal cells [61].

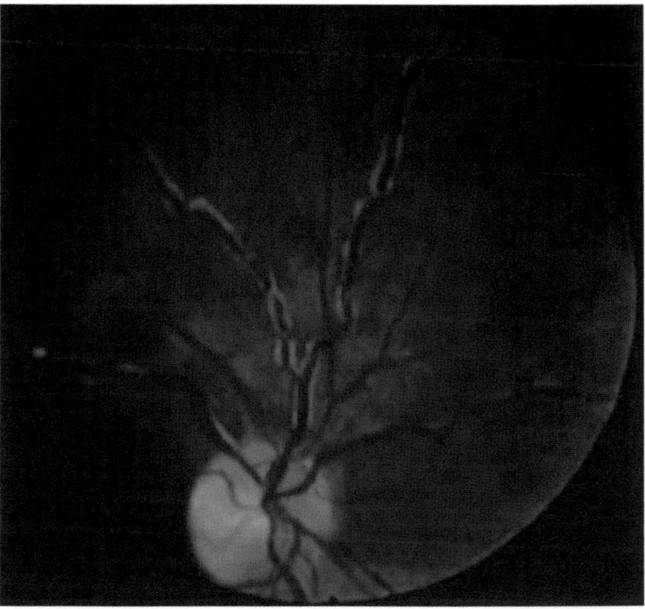

Fig. 33.3 Funduscopic examination of a patient with Waldenstrom's macroglobulinemia with hyperviscosity-related changes, including dilated retinal vessels, hemorrhages, and "venous sausaging." The white material at the edge of the veins may be cryoglobulin (*used with permission from Marvin J. Stone, MD*)

Clinical Features

Table 33.1 presents the clinical and laboratory findings at the time of diagnosis of WM in one large institutional study [15]. Unlike most indolent lymphomas, splenomegaly and lymphadenopathy are uncommon (≤15%). Purpura is frequently associated with cryoglobulinemia and in rare circumstances with light-chain (AL) amyloidosis. Hemorrhagic and neuropathic manifestations are multifactorial (see "IgM-Related Neuropathy" below). The morbidity associated with WM is caused by the concurrence of two main components: tissue infiltration by neoplastic cells and, importantly, the physicochemical and immunologic properties of the monoclonal IgM. As shown in Table 33.2, the monoclonal IgM can produce clinical manifestations through several different mechanisms related to its physicochemical properties, nonspecific interactions with other proteins, antibody activity, and tendency to deposit in tissues [62–64].

Morbidity Mediated by the Effects of IGM

Hyperviscosity Syndrome

The increased plasma IgM levels lead to blood hyperviscosity and its complications [65]. The mechanisms behind the marked increase in the resistance to blood flow and the resulting impaired transit through the microcirculatory system are complex [65–68]. The main determinants are (1) a high concentration of monoclonal IgMs, which may form aggregates and may bind water through their carbohydrate component, and (2) their interaction with blood cells. Monoclonal IgM increases red cell aggregation (rouleaux formation) and red cell internal viscosity

Table 33.1. Clinical and laboratory findings for 356 consecutive newly diagnosed patients with Waldenstrom's macroglobulinemia [14]

	Median	Range	Normal reference range
Age (years)	58	32–91	NA
Gender (male/female)	215/141		NA
Marrow involvement (% of area on slide)	30	5–95	NA
Adenopathy (% of patients)	15		NA
Splenomegaly (% of patients)	10		NA
IgM (mg/dL)	2620	270–12,400	40–230
IgG (mg/dL)	674	80–2770	700–1600
IgA (mg/dL)	58	6–438	70–400
Serum viscosity (cp)	2.0	1.1–7.2	1.4–1.9
Hematocrit (%)	35	17–45	35–44
Platelet count ($\times 10^9$/L)	275	42–675	155–410
White cell count ($\times 10^9$/L)	6.4	1.7–22	3.8–9.2
β_2-M (mg/dL)	2.5	0.9–13.7	0–2.7
LDH (U/mL)	313	61–1701	313–618

β_2M β_2-microglobulin, *cp* centipoise, *LDH* lactic dehydrogenase, *NA* not applicable
Source: Data from patients seen at the Dana Farber Cancer Institute, Boston, MA

Table 33.2 Physicochemical and immunological properties of the monoclonal IGM protein in Waldenstrom's macroglobulinemia [62–64]

Properties of IgM monoclonal protein	Diagnostic condition	Clinical manifestations
Pentameric structure	Hyperviscosity	Headaches, blurred vision, epistaxis, retinal hemorrhages, leg cramps, impaired mentation, intracranial hemorrhage
Precipitation on cooling	Cryoglobulinemia (type I)	Raynaud phenomenon, acrocyanosis, ulcers, purpura, cold urticaria
Autoantibody activity to myelin-associated glycoprotein, ganglioside M_1, sulfatide moieties on peripheral nerve sheaths	Peripheral neuropathies	Sensorimotor neuropathies, painful neuropathies, ataxic gait, bilateral foot drop
Autoantibody activity to IgG	Cryoglobulinemia (type II)	Purpura, arthralgia, renal failure, sensorimotor neuropathies
Autoantibody activity to red blood cell antigens	Cold agglutinins	Hemolytic anemia, Raynaud phenomenon, acrocyanosis, livedo reticularis
Tissue deposition as amorphous aggregates	Organ dysfunction	Skin: Bullous skin disease, papules, Schnitzler syndrome
		Gastrointestinal: Diarrhea, malabsorption, bleeding
		Kidney: Proteinuria, renal failure (light-chain component)
Tissue deposition as amyloid fibrils (light-chain component most commonly)	Organ dysfunction	Fatigue, weight loss, edema, hepatomegaly, macroglossia, organ dysfunction of involved organs (heart, kidney, liver, peripheral sensory, and autonomic nerves)

while reducing red cell deformability. The presence of cryoglobulins contributes to increasing blood viscosity, as well as to the tendency to induce erythrocyte aggregation. Serum viscosity is proportional to IgM concentration up to 30 g/L, and then increases sharply at higher levels. Increased plasma viscosity may also contribute to inappropriately low erythropoietin production, which is the major reason for anemia in these patients [68]. Renal synthesis of erythropoietin is inversely correlated with plasma viscosity. Clinical manifestations are related to circulatory disturbances that can be best appreciated by ophthalmoscopy, which shows distended and tortuous retinal veins, hemorrhages, and papilledema (Fig. 33.4) [69]. Symptoms usually occur when the monoclonal IgM concentration exceeds 50 g/L or when serum viscosity is >4.0 centipoises (cp), but there is individual variability, with some patients showing no evidence of hyperviscosity even at 10 cp [65]. The most common symptoms are oronasal mucosal bleeding, visual disturbances because of retinal bleeding, and dizziness that rarely may lead to stupor or coma. Heart failure can be aggravated, particularly in the elderly, owing to increased blood viscosity, expanded plasma volume, and anemia. Inappropriate red cell transfusion can exacerbate hyperviscosity and may precipitate cardiac failure.

Cryoglobulinemia

The monoclonal IgM can behave as a cryoglobulin in up to 20% of patients, and is usually type I and asymptomatic in most cases [15, 65, 70]. Cryoprecipitation is mainly dependent on the concentration of monoclonal IgM; for this reason plasmapheresis or plasma exchange is commonly effective in this condition. Symptoms result from impaired blood flow in small vessels and include Raynaud phenomenon, acrocyanosis, and necrosis of the regions most exposed to cold, such as the tip of the nose, ears, fingers, and toes (Fig. 33.5); malleolar ulcers; purpura; and cold urticaria. Renal manifestations are infrequent. Mixed cryoglobulins (type II) consisting of IgM-IgG complexes may be associated with hepatitis C infections [70].

Autoantibody Activity

Monoclonal IgM may exert its pathogenic effects through specific recognition of autologous antigens, the most notable being nerve constituents, immunoglobulin determinants, and red blood cell antigens.

IgM-Related Neuropathy

IgM-related peripheral neuropathy is common in WM patients, with estimated prevalence rates of 5–40% [71–73]. Approximately 8% of idiopathic neuropathies are associated with a monoclonal gammopathy, with a preponderance of IgM (60%) followed by IgG (30%) and IgA (10%) [74, 75]. The nerve damage is mediated by diverse pathogenetic mechanisms: (1) IgM antibody activity toward nerve constituents causing demyelinating polyneuropathies; (2) endoneurial granulofibrillar deposits of IgM without antibody activity, associated with axonal polyneuropathy; (3) occasionally by tubular deposits in the endoneurium associated with IgM cryoglobulin; and, rarely, (4) by amyloid deposits or by neoplastic cell infiltration of nerve structures [73, 76].

Half of the patients with IgM neuropathy have a distinctive clinical syndrome that is associated with antibodies against a minor 100-kDa glycoprotein component of nerve known as the myelin-associated glycoprotein (MAG). Anti-MAG antibodies are generally monoclonal IgMκ, and usually also exhibit reactivity with other glycoproteins or glycolipids that share antigenic determinants with MAG [77–79]. The anti–MAG-related neuropathy is typically distal and symmetrical,

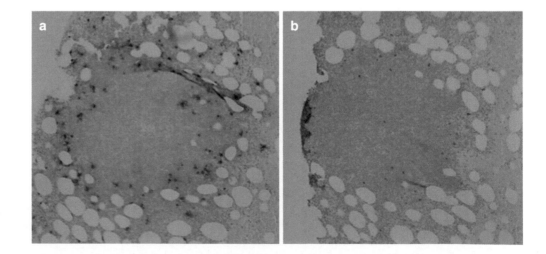

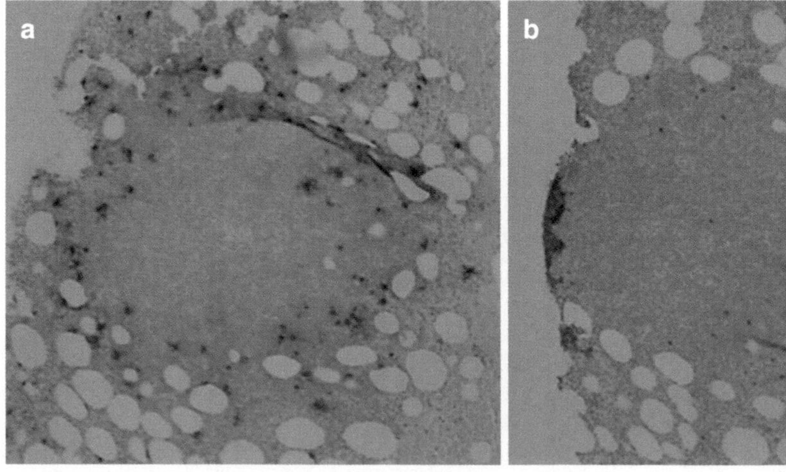

Fig. 33.4 Cryoglobulinemia manifesting with severe acrocyanosis in a patient with Waldenstrom's macroglobulinemia before (**a**) and following warming and plasmapheresis (**b**)

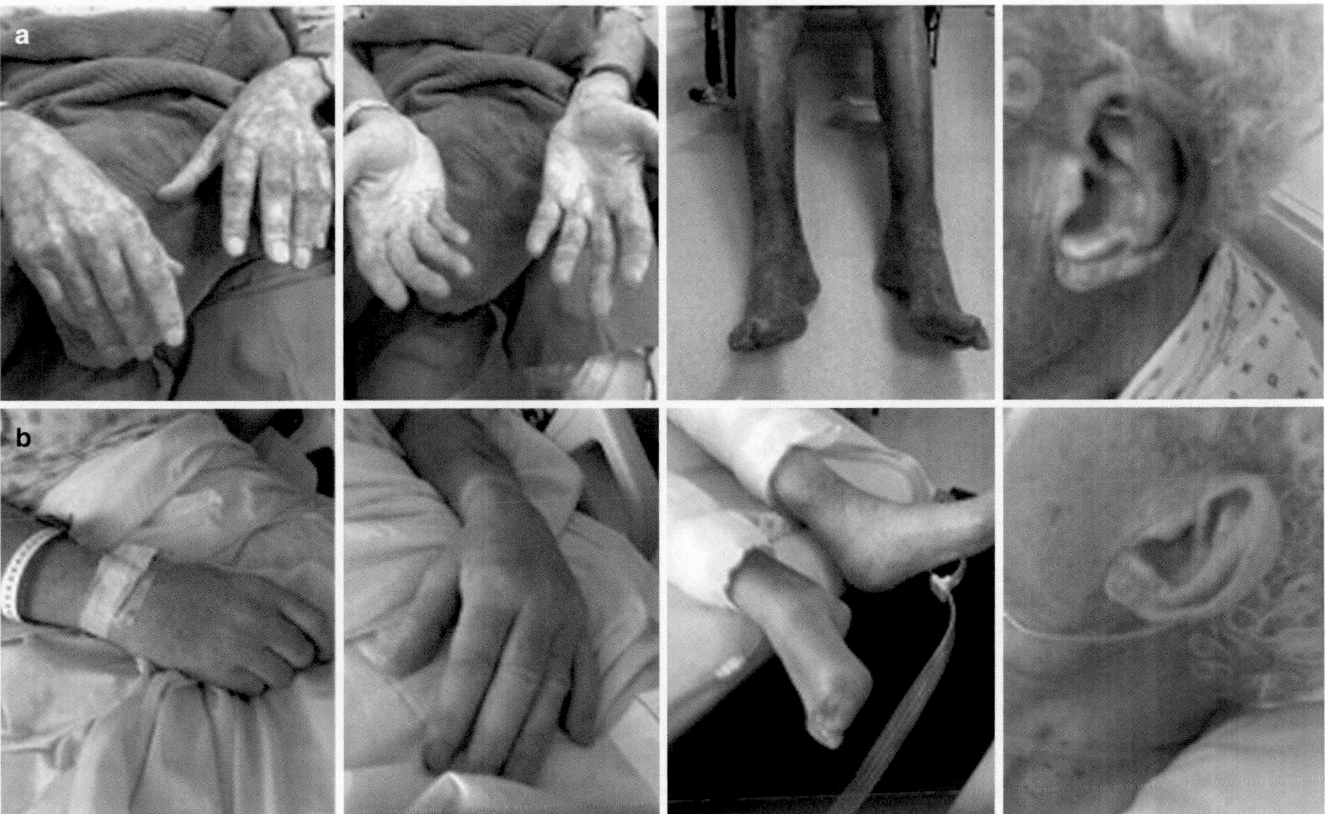

Fig. 33.5 Marrow clot section. (**a**) Tryptase-staining mast cells surrounding a nodule of lymphoplasmacytic cells in a patient with Waldenstrom's macroglobulinemia. (**b**) Mast cells in the same section exhibit strong CD40 ligand signaling, which has been shown to support (at least in part) the growth and survival of lymphoplasmacytic cells

affecting both motor and sensory functions; it is slowly progressive with a long period of stability [72, 80]. Most patients present with sensory complaints (paresthesias, aching discomfort, dysesthesias, or lancinating pains), imbalance, and gait ataxia, owing to lack of proprioception and leg muscle atrophy in advanced stage. Patients with predominantly demyelinating sensory neuropathy in association with monoclonal IgM to gangliosides with disialosyl moieties, such as GD1b, GD3, GD2, GT1b, and GQ1b have also been reported [81, 82]. Anti-GD1b and anti-GQ1b antibodies were associated with sensory ataxic neuropathy. These antiganglioside monoclonal IgMs present core clinical features of chronic ataxic neuropathy sometimes with ophthalmoplegia and/or red blood cell cold-agglutinating activity. The disialosyl epitope is also present on red blood cell glycophorins, thereby accounting for the red cell cold agglutinin activity of anti-Pr2 specificity [83, 84]. Monoclonal IgM proteins that bind to gangliosides with a terminal trisaccharide moiety, including ganglioside M_2 (GM_2) and GalNac-GD1A, are associated with chronic demyelinating neuropathy and severe sensory ataxia, unresponsive to glucocorticoids [85]. Antiganglioside IgM proteins may also cross-react with lipopolysaccharides of *Campylobacter jejuni*, whose infection is known to precipitate the Miller-Fisher syndrome, a variant of the Guillain-Barré syndrome [86]. Thus, molecular mimicry may play a role in this condition. Antisulfatide monoclonal IgM proteins, associated with sensory-sensorimotor neuropathy, have been detected in 5% of patients with IgM monoclonal gammopathy and neuropathy [87]. Motor neuron disease has been reported in patients with WM and monoclonal IgM with anti-GM_1 and sulfoglucuronyl paragloboside activity [88]. Polyneuropathy, organomegaly, endocrinopathy, M-protein, and skin changes (the POEMS syndrome) are rare in patients with WM [89].

Cold Agglutinin Hemolytic Anemia

Monoclonal IgM may have cold agglutinin activity; that is, it can recognize specific red cell antigens at temperatures below 37 °C, producing chronic hemolytic anemia. This disorder occurs in <10% of WM patients and is associated with cold agglutinin titers greater than 1:1000 in most cases [90]. The monoclonal component is usually an IgMκ and reacts most commonly with red cell I/i antigens, resulting in complement fixation and activation [91, 92]. Mild-to-moderate chronic hemolytic anemia can be exacerbated after cold exposure. Hemoglobin usually remains above 70 g/L. The hemolysis is usually extravascular, mediated by removal of C3b-opsonized red cells by the mononuclear phagocyte system, primarily in the liver. Intravascular hemolysis from complement destruction of red blood cell membrane is infrequent. The agglutination of red cells in the skin circulation also causes Raynaud syndrome, acrocyanosis, and livedo reticularis. Macroglobulins with the properties of both cryoglobulins and cold agglutinins with anti-Pr specificity can occur. These properties may have as a common basis the binding of the sialic acid-containing carbohydrate present on red blood cell glycophorins and on Ig molecules. Several other macroglobulins with antibody activity toward autologous antigens (i.e., phospholipids, tissue and plasma proteins) and foreign ligands have also been described.

IgM Tissue Deposition

The monoclonal protein can deposit in several tissues as amorphous aggregates. Linear deposition of monoclonal IgM along the skin basement membrane is associated with bullous skin disease [93]. Amorphous IgM deposits in the dermis result in IgM storage papules on the extensor surface of the extremities, referred to as macroglobulinemia cutis [94]. Deposition of monoclonal IgM in the lamina propria and/or submucosa of the intestine may be associated with diarrhea, malabsorption, and gastrointestinal bleeding [95, 96]. Kidney involvement is less common and less severe in WM than in myeloma, probably because the amount of light chain excreted in the urine is generally lower in WM than in myeloma and because of the absence of contributing factors, such as hypercalcemia. Urinary cast nephropathy, however, has occurred in WM [97]. On the other hand, the IgM macromolecule is more susceptible to being trapped in the glomerular loops where ultrafiltration presumably contributes to its precipitation, forming subendothelial deposits of aggregated IgM proteins that occlude the glomerular capillaries [98]. Mild and reversible proteinuria may result and most patients are asymptomatic. The deposition of monoclonal light chain as fibrillar amyloid deposits (AL amyloidosis) is uncommon in patients with WM [99]. Clinical expression and prognosis are similar to those of other AL amyloidosis patients with involvement of heart (44%), kidneys (32%), liver (14%), lungs (10%), peripheral or autonomic nerves (38%), and soft tissues (18%). The incidence of cardiac and pulmonary involvement is higher in patients with monoclonal IgM than with other immunoglobulin isotypes. The association of WM with reactive amyloidosis has been documented rarely [100, 101]. Simultaneous occurrence of fibrillary glomerulopathy, characterized by glomerular deposits of wide noncongophilic fibrils and amyloid deposits, has been described [102].

Manifestations Related to Tissue Infiltration by Neoplastic Cells

Tissue infiltration by neoplastic cells is uncommon but can involve various organs and tissues, including the liver, spleen, lymph nodes, lungs, gastrointestinal tract, kidneys, skin, eyes, and central nervous system.

Lung

Pulmonary involvement in the form of masses, nodules, diffuse infiltrate, or pleural effusions is uncommon; the overall incidence of pulmonary and pleural findings is approximately 4% [103–105]. Cough is the most common presenting symptom, followed by dyspnea and chest pain. Chest radiographic findings include parenchymal infiltrates, confluent masses, and effusions.

Gastrointestinal Tract

Malabsorption, diarrhea, bleeding, or obstruction may indicate involvement of the gastrointestinal tract at the level of the stomach, duodenum, or small intestine [106–109].

Renal System

In contrast to myeloma, infiltration of the kidney interstitium with lymphoplasmacytoid cell can occur in WM, and renal or perirenal masses are not uncommon [110, 111].

Skin

The skin can be the site of dense lymphoplasmacytic infiltrates, similar to those seen in the liver, spleen, and lymph nodes, forming cutaneous plaques and, rarely, nodules [112]. Chronic urticaria and IgM gammopathy are the two cardinal features of the Schnitzler syndrome, which is not usually associated initially with clinical features of WM, although evolution to WM is not uncommon [113]. Thus, close follow-up of these patients is important.

Joints

Invasion of articular and periarticular structures by WM malignant cells is rarely reported [114].

Eye

The neoplastic cells can infiltrate the periorbital structures, lacrimal gland, and retro-orbital lymphoid tissues, resulting in ocular nerve palsies [115, 116].

Central Nervous System

Direct infiltration of the central nervous system by monoclonal lymphoplasmacytic cells as infiltrates or as tumors constitutes the rarely observed Bing-Neel syndrome, characterized clinically by confusion, memory loss, disorientation, and motor dysfunction. The diagnosis and management of Bing-Neel syndrome are reviewed in 117.

Laboratory Findings

Blood Abnormalities

Anemia is the most common finding in patients with symptomatic WM and is caused by a combination of factors: decrease in red cell survival, impaired erythropoiesis, moderate plasma volume expansion, hepcidin production leading to iron reutilization defect, and blood loss from the gastrointestinal tract [15, 118, 119]. Blood films are usually normocytic and normochromic, and rouleaux formation is often pronounced. Mean red cell volume may be elevated spuriously owing to erythrocyte aggregation. In addition, the hemoglobin estimate can be inaccurate, that is, falsely high, because of interaction between the monoclonal protein and the diluent used in some automated analyzers [120]. Leukocyte and platelet counts are usually within the reference range at presentation, although patients may occasionally present with severe thrombocytopenia. Monoclonal B-lymphocytes expressing surface IgM and late-differentiation B-cell markers are uncommonly detected in blood by flow cytometry. A raised erythrocyte sedimentation rate is almost always present and may be the first clue to the presence of the macroglobulinemia. The clotting abnormality detected most frequently is prolongation of thrombin time. AL amyloidosis should be suspected in all patients with nephrotic syndrome, cardiomyopathy, hepatomegaly, or peripheral neuropathy. Diagnosis requires the demonstration of green birefringence under polarized light of amyloid deposits stained with Congo red.

Marrow Findings

Central to the diagnosis of WM is the demonstration, by trephine biopsy, of marrow infiltration by a lymphoplasmacytic cell population characterized by small lymphocytes with evidence of plasmacytoid and plasma cell maturation (Fig. 33.1) [1, 13]. The pattern of marrow infiltration may be diffuse, interstitial, or nodular, usually with an intertrabecular pattern of infiltration. A solely paratrabecular pattern of infiltration is unusual and should raise the possibility of follicular lymphoma [1]. The marrow cell immunophenotype should be confirmed by flow cytometry and/or immunohistochemistry. The cell immunoprofile $sIgM^{+}CD19^{+}CD20^{+}CD22^{+}CD79^{+}$ is characteristic of WM [13, 120, 121]. Up to 20% of cases may express either CD5, CD10, or CD23 [18]. In these cases, chronic lymphocytic leukemia and mantle cell lymphoma should be excluded. "Intranuclear" periodic acid-Schiff–positive inclusions (Dutcher-Fahey bodies) [122] consisting of IgM deposits in the perinuclear space, and sometimes in intranuclear vacuoles, may be seen occasionally in lymphoid cells. An increased number of mast cells, usually in association with the lymphoid aggregates, is commonly found, and their presence may help in differentiating WM from other B-cell lymphomas (see Fig. 33.3) [13]. $MYD88^{L265P}$ testing of bone marrow samples has been incorporated into many clinical laboratories, and may help in clarifying the diagnosis of WM from other IgM-secreting entities [34–38]. The use of peripheral blood B cells may also permit determination of $MYD88^{L265P}$ status by allele-specific polymerase chain reaction assays, particularly in untreated WM patients. CXCR4 mutation testing may also be useful in patients being considered for ibrutinib therapy (discussed below).

Immunologic Abnormalities

High-resolution electrophoresis combined with immunofixation of serum and urine is recommended for identification and characterization of the IgM monoclonal protein. The light chain of the monoclonal IgM is κ in 75–80% of patients. More than one M-component may be present. The concentration of the serum monoclonal protein is very variable but in most cases lies within the range of 15–45 g/L. Densitometry should be adopted to determine IgM levels for serial evaluations because nephelometry is unreliable and shows large laboratory variation. The presence of cold agglutinins or cryoglobulins may affect determination of IgM levels and, therefore, testing for cold agglutinins and cryoglobulins should be performed at diagnosis. If present, subsequent serum samples should be analyzed at 37 °C for determination of serum monoclonal IgM level. Although Bence Jones proteinuria is frequently present, it exceeds 1 g/24 h in only 3% of cases. Whereas IgM levels are elevated in WM patients, IgA and IgG levels are most often depressed and do not recover after successful treatment [123].

Serum Viscosity

Because of its large size (almost 1,000,000 daltons), most IgM molecules are retained within the intravascular compartment and can exert an undue effect on serum viscosity [65]. Serum viscosity can be measured if the patient has signs or symptoms of hyperviscosity syndrome, though levels often slow to be resulted and erratic due to a lack of standardization in many clinical laboratories [15]. As such, serum IgM levels may be more expedient and relied upon. Patients typically become symptomatic at serum viscosity levels of 4.0 centipoise and above that relates to serum IgM levels above 6000 mg/dL [124, 125]. Patients may be symptomatic at lower serum viscosity and IgM levels, and in these patients cryoglobulins may be present. Recurring nosebleeds, headaches, and visual disturbances are common symptoms in patients with symptomatic hyperviscosity [15]. Funduscopy is an important indicator of clinically relevant hyperviscosity. Among the first clinical signs of hyperviscosity are the appearance of peripheral and midperipheral dot- and blot-like hemorrhages in the retina, which are best appreciated with indirect ophthalmoscopy and scleral depression [69]. In more severe cases of hyperviscosity, dot-, blot-, and flame-shaped hemorrhages can appear in the macular area along with markedly dilated and tortuous veins with focal constrictions resulting in "venous sausaging," as well as papilledema (Fig. 33.4).

Imaging

Magnetic resonance imaging (MRI) of the spine in conjunction with computed tomography (CT) of the abdomen and pelvis is useful in evaluating the disease status [126]. Marrow involvement can be documented by MRI studies of the spine in more than 90% of patients; CT of the abdomen and pelvis demonstrates enlarged nodes in approximately 20% of WM patients at diagnosis but may be higher at relapse [126].

Lymph Node Biopsy

Lymph node biopsy may show preserved architecture or replacement by infiltration of neoplastic cells with lymphoplasmacytoid, lymphoplasmacytic, or polymorphous cytologic patterns. Testing for MYD88 mutations may help.

Treatment

Initiating Treatment

As part of the Second International Workshop on Waldenstrom's macroglobulinemia, a consensus panel was organized to recommend criteria for the initiation of therapy in patients with WM [127]. The panel recommended that initiation of therapy should not be based on the IgM level per se, as this may not correlate with the clinical manifestations of WM. The consensus panel did, however, agree that initiation of therapy is appropriate for patients with constitutional symptoms, such as recurrent fever, night sweats, fatigue as a consequence of anemia, or weight loss. Progressive symptomatic lymphadenopathy and/or splenomegaly provide additional reasons to begin therapy. Anemia with a hemoglobin value of $\leq$10 g/dL or a platelet count of $\leq 100 \times 10^9$/L owing to marrow infiltration also justifies treatment. Certain complications, such as hyperviscosity syndrome, symptomatic sensorimotor peripheral neuropathy, systemic amyloidosis, renal insufficiency, or symptomatic cryoglobulinemia, may also be indications for therapy [15, 127].

Initial Therapy

The International Workshops on Waldenström's Macroglobulinemia have also formulated consensus recommendations for both initial therapy and therapy for refractory disease based on the best available evidence. The most recent recommendations emerged from the Eighth International Workshop on WM [128]. Individual patient considerations, including the presence of cytopenias, need for more rapid disease control, age, and candidacy for autologous transplant therapy, should be taken into account in making the choice of the drugs to use. For patients who are candidates for autologous stem cell transplantation, which typically is reserved for those patients younger than 70 years of age, the panel recommended that exposure to alkylating agents or nucleoside analogues should be limited. The use of nucleoside analogues should be approached cautiously in WM patients as there appears to be an increased risk for the development of disease transformation as well as myelodysplasia and acute myelogenous leukemia.

Oral Alkylating Agents

Oral alkylating drugs, alone and in combination therapy with glucocorticoids, have been extensively evaluated in the treatment of WM. Chlorambucil has been administered on both a continuous (i.e., daily-dose schedule) and an intermittent schedule. Patients receiving chlorambucil on a continuous schedule typically receive 0.1 mg/kg per day, whereas on the intermittent schedule patients typically receive 0.3 mg/kg for 7 days, every 6 weeks. In a prospective randomized study, no significant difference in the overall response rate between these schedules was observed [129], although the median response duration was greater for patients receiving intermittent- versus continuous-dose chlorambucil (46 versus 26 months). Despite the favorable median response duration in this study for use of the intermittent schedule, no difference in the median overall survival was observed. Moreover, an increased incidence for development of myelodysplasia and acute myelogenous leukemia with the intermittent (3 of 22 patients) versus the continuous (0 of 24 patients) chlorambucil schedule prompted the preference for use of continuous chlorambucil dosing. The use of glucocorticoids in combination with alkylating agent therapy has also been explored. Chlorambucil (8 mg/m^2) plus prednisone (40 mg/m^2) given orally for 10 days, every 6 weeks, resulted in a major response (i.e., reduction of IgM by more than 50%) in 72% of patients [130]. Alkylating agent regimens employing melphalan and cyclophosphamide in combination with glucocorticoids have also been examined [131, 132]. This approach produced slightly higher overall response rates and response durations, although the benefit of these more complex regimens over chlorambucil remains to be demonstrated. Pretreatment factors associated with shorter survival in the entire population of patients receiving single-agent chlorambucil were age older than 60 years, male sex, hemoglobin less than 10 g/dL, leukocytes less than 4 × 10^9/L, and platelets less than 150 × 10^9/L. Organomegaly, signs of hyperviscosity, renal failure, monoclonal IgM level, blood lymphocytosis, and percentage of marrow lymphoid cells were not significantly correlated with survival [133]. Additional factors to be taken into account in considering alkylating agent therapy for patients with WM include necessity for more rapid disease control given the slow response, as well as consideration for preserving stem cells in patients who are candidates for autologous stem cell transplantation therapy. A large randomized study showed an inferior response rate and time to progression in WM patients receiving chlorambucil versus fludarabine, as well as a higher incidence of secondary malignancies in the former. Neutropenia was however more pronounced in those patients on fludarabine [134].

Nucleoside Analogue Therapy

Cladribine administered as a single agent by continuous intravenous infusion, by 2-h daily infusion, or by subcutaneous bolus injections for 5–7 days has resulted in major responses in 40–90% of patients who received primary therapy, whereas in the previously treated patients, responses have ranged from 38 to 54% [135–141]. Median time to achievement of response in responding patients following cladribine ranged from 1.2 to 5 months. The overall response rate with daily infusion of fludarabine, administered mainly on 5-day schedules, in previously untreated and treated patients ranged from 38 to 100% and 30 to 40%, respectively [142–147], similar to the responses to cladribine. Median time to achievement of response for fludarabine (3–6 months) was also similar to cladribine. In general, response rates and durations of responses have been greater for patients receiving nucleoside analogues as initial therapy, although in several studies in which both untreated and previously treated patients were enrolled, no difference in the overall response rate was reported.

Myelosuppression commonly occurs following prolonged exposure to either of the nucleoside analogues. A sustained decrease in both CD4+ and CD8+ T lymphocytes, measured 1 year following initiation of therapy, is notable [135–137]. Treatment-related mortality as a consequence of myelosuppression and/or opportunistic infections attributable to immunosuppression occurred in up to 5% of all treated patients in some series with nucleoside analogues.

Factors predicting for a better response to nucleoside analogues include younger age at start of treatment (<70 years), higher pretreatment hemoglobin (>95 g/L), higher platelet count (>75 × 10^9/L), disease relapsing off therapy, and a long interval between first-line therapy and initiation of a nucleoside analogue in relapsing patients [135, 140, 146]. There are limited data on the use of an alternate nucleoside analogue in previously treated patients among whom disease relapsed or who had resistance when not on cladribine or fludarabine therapy [148, 149]. Three of four (75%) patients responded to cladribine after progression following an unmaintained remission to fludarabine, whereas only one of ten (10%) with disease resistant to fludarabine responded to cladribine [148]. A response in two of six patients (33%) and disease stabilization in the remaining patients to fludarabine, in spite of an inadequate response or progressive disease, following cladribine therapy has been reported [149].

Harvesting autologous blood stem cells succeeded on the first attempt in 14 of 15 patients who did not receive nucleoside analogue therapy as compared to 2 of 6 patients who received a nucleoside analogue [150]. A sevenfold increase in transformation to an aggressive lymphoma and a threefold increase in the development of myelodysplasia or acute myelogenous leukemia were observed among patients who received a nucleoside analogue versus other therapies for their WM [151]. A meta-analysis of several trials in which patients were treated with nucleoside analogues in WM patients, included patients who had previously received an alkylating agent, and showed a crude incidence of approximately 8% for development of disease transformation and of approximately 5% for development of myelodysplasia or acute myelogenous leukemia [152]. None of the risk factors—that is, gender, age, family history of WM, or B-cell malignancies, typical markers of tumor burden and prognosis, type of nucleoside analogue therapy (cladribine versus fludarabine), time from diagnosis to nucleoside analogue use, nucleoside analogue treatment as primary or salvage therapy, or treatment with an oral alkylator (i.e., chlorambucil)—predicted for the occurrence of transformation or development of myelodysplasia or acute myelogenous leukemia in patients treated with a nucleoside analogue [152].

CD20-Directed Antibody Therapy

Rituximab is a chimeric monoclonal antibody that targets CD20, a widely expressed antigen on lymphoplasmacytic cells in WM [153]. Several retrospective and prospective studies have indicated that rituximab, when used at standard doses (i.e., 4-weekly infusions of 375 mg/m^2), induced major responses in approximately 30% of previously treated and untreated patients [154, 155]. Even patients who achieved minor responses benefited from rituximab by improved hemoglobin and platelet counts, and reduction of lymphadenopathy and/or splenomegaly [154]. The median time to treatment failure in these studies was found to range from 8 to 27+ months. Patients on an extended rituximab schedule consisting of 4-weekly courses at 375 mg/m^2 per week, repeated 3 months later by another 4-week course, have demonstrated major response rates of approximately 45%, with time to progression estimates of 16+ to 29+ months [156, 157].

In many WM patients, a transient increase or flare of the serum IgM may occur immediately following initiation of rituximab treatment [156, 158, 159]. Such an increase does not herald treatment failure and most patients will return to their baseline serum IgM level by 12 weeks. Some patients continue to show a prolonged increase in IgM despite an apparent reduction in their marrow tumor cells. However, patients with baseline serum IgM levels of >50 g/dL or serum viscosity of >3.5 cp may be particularly at risk for a hyperviscosity-related event and plasmapheresis should be considered in these patients in advance of rituximab therapy [158]. Because of the decreased likelihood of response in patients with higher IgM levels, as well as the possibility that serum IgM and blood viscosity levels may abruptly rise, rituximab monotherapy should not be used as sole therapy for the treatment of patients at risk for hyperviscosity symptoms [128, 156, 157].

Time to response after rituximab is slow and exceeds 3 months on the average. The time to best response in one study was 18 months [157]. Patients with baseline serum IgM levels of <60 g/dL are more likely to respond, regardless of the underlying marrow involvement by tumor cells [156, 157]. An analysis of 52 patients who were treated with single-agent rituximab found that the objective response rate was significantly lower in patients who had either low serum albumin (<35 g/L) or a serum monoclonal protein greater than 40 g/L. [160] The presence of both adverse prognostic factors was associated with a short time to progression (3.6 months). Patients who had normal serum albumin and relatively low serum monoclonal protein levels derived a substantial benefit from rituximab with a time to progression exceeding 40 months.

A correlation between polymorphisms at position 158 in the FcγRIIIa receptor (CD16), an activating Fc receptor on important effector cells that mediate antibody-dependent cell-mediated cytotoxicity, and rituximab response was observed in WM patients [161]. Individuals may encode either the amino acid valine or phenylalanine at position 158 in the FcγRIIIa receptor. WM patients who carried the valine amino acid (either in a homozygous or in a heterozygous pattern) had a fourfold higher major response rate (i.e., 50% decline in serum IgM levels) to rituximab versus those patients who expressed phenylalanine in a homozygous pattern.

Proteasome Inhibitors

Both bortezomib and carfilzomib have been evaluated in prospective studies in patients with WM, though the latter only in combination therapy (discussed below). In a retrospective study, ten patients with refractory or relapsed WM were treated with bortezomib administered intravenously at a dose of 1.3 mg/m^2 on days 1, 4, 8, and 11 in a 21-day cycle for a total of four cycles. Most patients had been exposed to all active agents for WM and eight patients had received three or more regimens. Six of these patients achieved a partial response which occurred at a median of 1 month. The median time to progression in the responding patients is expected to exceed 11 months. Peripheral neuropathy occurred in three patients and one patient developed severe paralytic ileus in this series [162]. In a prospective study among 27 relapsed or refractory patients who received up to eight cycles of bortezomib at 1.3 mg/m^2 on days 1, 4, 8, and 11, median serum IgM levels declined significantly from 4.7 g/dL to 2.1 g/dL [32]. The overall response rate was 85%, with 10 and 13 patients achieving a minor (<25%) and major (<50%) decrease in IgM level. Responses occurred at a median of 1.4 months. The median time to progression for all responding patients in this study was 7.9 (range: 3–21.4+) months, and the most common grade III/IV toxicities were sensory neuropathies (22.2%), leukopenia (18.5%), neutropenia (14.8%), dizziness (11.1%), and thrombocytopenia (7.4%). Sensory neuropathies resolved or improved in nearly all patients following cessation of therapy. Twenty-seven patients with both untreated (44%) and previously treated (56%) disease received bortezomib, utilizing the standard schedule until they either demonstrated progressive disease or two cycles beyond a complete response or stable disease [163]. The overall response rate was 78%, with major responses observed in 44% of patients. Sensory neuropathy occurred in 20 patients following 2–4 cycles of therapy. Among the 20 patients developing a neuropathy, 14 showed resolution or improvement 2–13 months after therapy.

Combination Therapies

Because rituximab is not myelosuppressive, its combination with chemotherapy has been explored. A regimen of rituximab, cladribine, and cyclophosphamide used in 17 previously untreated patients resulted in a partial response in 94% of WM patients, including a complete response in 18% [161]. No patient had relapsed with a median follow-up of

21 months. The combination of rituximab and fludarabine used in 43 patients of whom 32 (75%) were previously untreated led to an overall response rate of 95.3%, with 83% of patients achieving a major response (i.e., 50% reduction in disease burden) [165]. The median time to progression was 51.2 months in this series, and was longer for those patients who were previously untreated and for those achieving a very good partial remission (i.e., 90% reduction in disease) or better. Hematologic toxicity was common: grade 3 neutropenia and thrombocytopenia observed in 27 and 4 patients, respectively. Two deaths occurred in this study from pneumonia. Secondary malignancies including transformation to aggressive lymphoma and development of myelodysplasia or acute myelogenous leukemia were observed in six patients in this series. The addition of rituximab to fludarabine and cyclophosphamide has also been explored in previously treated patients, of whom four of five patients had a response [166]. In another combination study, rituximab along with pentostatin and cyclophosphamide given to 13 patients with untreated and previously treated WM or lymphoplasmacytic lymphoma resulted in a major response in 77% of patients [167]. The combination of rituximab, dexamethasone, and cyclophosphamide was used as primary therapy to treat 72 patients with WM in whom a major response was observed in 74% of patients in this study, and the 2-year progression-free survival was 67% [168]. Therapy was well tolerated, although one patient died of interstitial pneumonia.

Two studies have examined cyclophosphamide, doxorubicin, vincristine, and prednisone (CHOP) in combination with rituximab (R-CHOP). In a randomized trial involving 69 patients, most of whom had WM, the addition of rituximab to CHOP resulted in a higher overall response rate (94% versus 67%) and median time to progression (63 versus 22 months) in comparison to patients treated with CHOP alone [169]. R-CHOP was also used in 13 WM patients, 10 of whom had relapsed or refractory disease [170]. Among 13 evaluable patients, 10 patients achieved a major response (77%), including 3 complete and 7 partial remissions. Two other patients achieved a minor response. In a retrospective study of symptomatic WM patients who received either R-CHOP; rituximab, cyclophosphamide, vincristine, and prednisone (R-CVP) or cyclophosphamide, prednisone, and rituximab (R-CP) and were similar in most pretreatment variables, the overall response rates to therapy were comparable among all three treatment groups—R-CHOP (96%), R-CVP (88%), and R-CP (95%)—although there was a trend for more complete remissions among patients treated with R-CVP and R-CHOP [171]. Adverse events attributed to therapy showed a higher incidence for neutropenic fever and treatment-related neuropathy for R-CHOP and R-CVP versus R-CP. The results of this study suggest that in WM, the use of R-CP may provide analogous treatment responses to more intense cyclophosphamide-based regimens while minimizing treatment-related complications. The extended alkylator bendamustine has also been evaluated in combination with rituximab in both untreated and previously treated WM patients. A randomized study by the German STiL Group examined bendamustine plus rituximab (Benda-R) versus R-CHOP in patients with untreated, indolent B-cell lymphomas including WM [172]. Patients with WM in this study showed similar overall responses (96% versus 94%), though progression-free survival was significantly longer (69 versus 29 months) in patients who received Benda-R versus R-CHOP. Treatment was also better tolerated in patients receiving Benda-R. In the relapsed or refractory setting, an overall response rate of 83% was observed with bendamustine in combination with a CD20 monoclonal antibody [173]. The median time to progression was 13 months in this study. Prolonged myelosuppression was more common in patients who received prior nucleoside analogues.

The use of two cycles of oral cyclophosphamide along with subcutaneous cladribine to 37 patients with previously untreated WM led to a partial response in 84% of patients and the median duration of response was 36 months [164]. Fludarabine in combination with intravenous cyclophosphamide resulted in partial responses in 6 of 11 (55%) WM patients with either primary refractory disease or who had relapsed on treatment [174]. The combination of fludarabine plus cyclophosphamide was also evaluated in 49 patients, 35 of whom were previously treated. Seventy-eight percent of the patients achieved a response, and the median time to treatment failure was 27 months [175]. Hematological toxicity was frequent, and three patients died of treatment-related toxicities. Two important findings in this study were the development of acute leukemia in two patients, histologic transformation to diffuse large B-cell lymphoma in one patient, and two cases of solid malignancies (prostate and melanoma), as well as failure to mobilize stem cells in four of six patients.

The combination of bortezomib, dexamethasone, and rituximab (BDR) as primary therapy in 23 patients with WM resulted in an overall response rate of 96%, and a major response rate of 83% [176]. Maintenance therapy with BDR was used in this study. The incidence of grade 3 neuropathy was approximately 30%, and led to discontinuance of bortezomib in 60% of patients on BDR. An increased incidence of herpes zoster was also observed prompting the prophylactic use of antiviral therapy. The median progression-free survival in this study was 66 months, and resolution of treatment-related neuropathy to at least grade 1 or less was observed in most (13/16; 81%) of the patients with prolonged follow-up [177].

Alternative schedules for administration of bortezomib (i.e., once weekly at higher doses) in combination with rituximab in patients with WM have achieved overall response rates of 80–90% [178, 179]. The European Myeloma Network (EMN) recently showed that transitioning bortezomib from twice-weekly intravenous dosing during the first cycle to weekly administration thereafter reduced grade 3 neuropathy to under 10% in patients treated with BDR [180]. Overall, treatment was well tolerated and the overall response rate was 85% that included 68% major responders. The median PFS in this study was 43 months [181]. While subcutaneous bortezomib is also used to decrease the risk of treatment-related neuropathy with bortezomib, no formal studies addressing the safety and efficacy of subcutaneous bortezomib use in WM have been reported.

Carfilzomib is a proteasome inhibitor that is associated with a low risk of treatment-related peripheral neuropathy. The combination of carfilzomib with rituximab and dexamethasone (CaRD) was evaluated in WM patients [33]. Carfilzomib was administered intravenously at 20 mg/m^2 (cycle 1), and then 36 mg/m^2 (cycles 2–6), together with dexamethasone (20 mg) on days 1, 2, 8, and 9 as part of a 21-day cycle. As part of this regimen, rituximab 375 mg/m^2 was given on days 2 and 9 every 21 days. Maintenance therapy was given 8 weeks following induction therapy with intravenous carfilzomib (36 mg/m^2) and dexamethasone (20 mg) administered on days 1 and 2 and rituximab 375 mg/m^2 on day 2 every 8 weeks for up to eight cycles. Overall response rate with this regimen was 87% with major responses observed in 68% of patients, and was not impacted by MYD88^{L265P} or CXCR4^{WHIM} mutation status. With a median follow-up of 15.4 months, 20 patients remained progression free. Grade ≥2 toxicities included asymptomatic hyperlipasemia (41.9%), reversible neutropenia (12.9%), and cardiomyopathy in one patient (3.2%) with multiple risk factors. Treatment-related neuropathy occurred in one patient (3.2%) that was grade 2. Declines in serum IgA and IgG were common, and some patients required intravenous gamma globulin therapy for recurring sinus and bronchial infections.

Novel Therapeutics

The use of ibrutinib was recently approved by the United States Food and Drug Administration and the European Medicines Agency for the treatment of symptomatic patients with WM. Ibrutinib targets BTK and HCK, both targets of ibrutinib that are transactivated by MYD88^{L265P} [42, 48]. In a multicenter study that examined the role of ibrutinib in previously treated (median two prior therapies, 40% refractory) WM patients, the overall response rate was 91% [182]. Patients on this study received 420 mg a day of ibrutinib by mouth. Post-therapy, median serum IgM levels declined from 3610 to 880 mg/dL; hemoglobin rose from 10.5 to 13.8 g/dL, and bone marrow involvement declined from 60 to 25%. Decreased or resolved adenopathy was observed in 60% of patients with extramedullary disease, and five of nine patients with IgM-related PN had symptomatic improvement. At a median of 37 months of follow-up, the median progression-free and overall survival was 68% and 90%, respectively. Major responses were absent in patients with wild-type MYD88, and slower response kinetics were observed in those patients who were both MYD88 and CXCR4 mutated. Major response rates were also lower in those patients with CXCR4 mutations (62%) versus those with wild-type CXCR4 (92%). Grade ≥2 treatment-related toxicities included neutropenia (25%) and thrombocytopenia (14%) that were more common in heavily pretreated patients; atrial fibrillation associated with a prior history of arrhythmia (5%); and bleeding associated with procedures and marine oil supplements (3%). Serum IgA and IgG levels were unchanged following treatment with ibrutinib, and treatment-related infections were infrequent. A multicenter trial also examined the activity of ibrutinib in rituximab-refractory WM patients who had a median of four prior therapies. The overall response rate in this study was 90%, with major responses observed in 71% of patients. With a median follow-up of 18 months, the median progression-free and overall survival was 86 and 97% [183]. Delays in serum IgM and hemoglobin responses were observed among MYD88-mutated patients with CXCR4 mutations, versus those who were wild-type for CXCR4. One patient with wild-type MYD88 did not respond. A clinical study of the CXCR4 antagonist ulocuplumab with ibrutinib is being initiated in symptomatic WM patients with CXCR4 mutations.

Everolimus is an oral inhibitor of the mTOR pathway that is active in WM. A multicenter study examined everolimus in 60 previously treated patients that showed an ORR of 73%, with 50% of patients attaining a major response [184]. The median progression-free survival in this study was 21 months. Grade 3 or higher related toxicities were observed in 67% of patients with cytopenias constituting the most common toxicity. Pulmonary toxicity occurred in 5% of patients, and dose reductions due to toxicity occurred in 52% of patients. A clinical trial examining the activity of everolimus in 33 previously untreated patients with WM has also been reported that included serial bone marrow biopsies in response assessment [185]. The ORR in this study was 72%, including partial or better responses in 60% of patients. Among genotyped patients, nonresponders associated with wild-type MYD88 and mutated CXCR4 status. Median time to response was 4 weeks. Discordance between serum IgM levels and bone marrow disease burden was remarkable. The median time to progression was 21 months for all patients, and 33 months for major responders. Discontinuation of everolimus led to rapid serum IgM rebound in seven patients and symptomatic hyperviscosity in two patients. Toxicity led to treatment discontinuation in 27% of patients, including 18% for pneumonitis which appeared more pronounced versus previously treated WM patients.

Maintenance Therapy

The outcome of rituximab-naïve patients who were either observed or received maintenance rituximab categorical responses was examined in a large retrospective study [186]. Categorical responses improved after induction therapy in 42% of patients who received maintenance rituximab versus 10% in patients on observation. Additionally, both progression-free (56.3 versus. 28.6 months) and overall survival (>120 versus 116 months) were longer in patients who received maintenance rituximab. Improved progression-free survival was evident despite previous treatment status, induction with rituximab alone or in combination therapy. Best serum IgM response was also lower, and hematocrit higher in those patients who received maintenance rituximab. Among patients who received maintenance rituximab therapy, an increased number of infectious events, predominantly grade 1 or 2 sinusitis and bronchitis, were observed, along with lower serum IgA and IgG levels. A prospective study examining the role of maintenance rituximab has also been initiated by the German STiL group [187]. In this study, patients received up to six cycles of bendamustine and rituximab, and responders randomized to either observation or maintenance rituximab every 2 months for 2 years. Enrollment for this study is complete, and response outcome for maintenance rituximab therapy is awaited.

High-Dose Therapy and Stem Cell Transplantation

The European Bone Marrow Transplant Registry reported the largest experience for both autologous and allogeneic SCT in WM [188, 189]. Among 158 WM patients receiving an autologous SCT, which included primarily relapsed or refractory patients, the 5-year progression-free and overall survival rate was 39.7% and 68.5%, respectively [188]. Non-relapse mortality at 1 year was 3.8%. Chemorefractory disease and the number of prior lines of therapy at time of the autologous SCT were the most important prognostic factors for progression-free and overall survival. In the allogeneic SCT experience from the EBMT, the long-term outcome of 86 WM patients was reported [189]. A total of 86 patients received allograft by either myeloablative or reduced-intensity conditioning. The median age of patients in this series was 49 years, and 47 patients had three or more previous lines of therapy. Eight patients failed prior to autologous SCT. Fifty-nine patients (68.6%) had chemotherapy-sensitive disease at the time of allogeneic SCT. Non-relapse mortality at 3 years was 33% for patients receiving a myeloablative transplant, and 23% for those who received reduced-intensity conditioning. The overall response rate was 75.6%. The relapse rates at 3 years were 11% for myeloablative, and 25% for reduced-intensity conditioning recipients. Five-year progression-free and overall survival for WM patients who received a myeloablative allogeneic SCT were 56% and 62%, and for patients who received reduced-intensity conditioning were 49% and 64%, respectively. The occurrence of chronic graft-versus-host disease was associated with improved progression-free survival, and suggested the existence of a clinically relevant graft-versus-WM effect in this study.

Response Criteria in Waldenstrom's Macroglobulinemia

Table 33.3 summarizes the response categories and criteria for progressive disease in WM based on the most recent consensus recommendations [190]. The term "overall response" is used to characterize all responses, including minor

Table 33.3 Summary of consensus response criteria for Waldenstrom's macroglobulinemia [190]

Complete response	CR	Absence of serum monoclonal IgM protein by immunofixation
		Normal serum IgM level
		Complete resolution of extramedullary disease, i.e., lymphadenopathy/splenomegaly if present at baseline
		Morphologically normal bone marrow aspirate and trephine biopsy
Very Good Partial Response	VGPR	Monoclonal IgM protein is detectable
		90% reduction in serum IgM level from baseline, or normalization of serum IgM level
		Complete resolution of extramedullary disease, i.e., lymphadenopathy/splenomegaly if present at baseline
		No new signs or symptoms of active disease
Partial Response	PR	Monoclonal IgM protein is detectable
		≥50% but <90% reduction in serum IgM level from baseline
		Reduction in extramedullary disease, i.e., lymphadenopathy/splenomegaly if present at baseline
		No new signs or symptoms of active disease
Minor response	MR	Monoclonal IgM protein is detectable
		≥25% but <50% reduction in serum IgM level from baseline
		No new signs or symptoms of active disease
Stable disease	SD	Monoclonal IgM protein is detectable
		<25% reduction and <25% increase in serum IgM level from baseline
		No progression in extramedullary disease, i.e., lymphadenopathy/splenomegaly
		No new signs or symptoms of active disease
Progressive disease	PD	>25% increase in serum IgM level from lowest nadir (requires confirmation) and/or progression in clinical features attributable the disease

responses. "Major responses" only include partial, very good partial, and complete responses. The attainment of very good partial or complete responses is associated with improved progression-free survival [165, 176, 180, 188, 191]. Response assessments in WM rely primarily on serum IgM or IgM paraprotein levels, though complete responses require disappearance of the IgM monoclonal protein, and resolution of bone marrow and/or extramedullary WM disease [190]. An important concern with the use of IgM as a surrogate marker of disease is that it can fluctuate, independent of tumor cell killing with some agents. By way of example, rituximab can induce a flare in serum IgM levels, whereas everolimus, bortezomib, and ibrutinib can suppress IgM levels independent of tumor cell killing in some patients, a finding referred to as IgM discordance [32, 156, 158, 159, 182, 185, 192]. Moreover, with selective B-cell-depleting agents such as rituximab and alemtuzumab, residual IgM-producing plasma cells are spared and continue to persist, thus potentially skewing the relative response and assessment to treatment [193]. Soluble CD27 levels have been investigated as an alternative surrogate marker in WM given their correlation with WM disease burden, and may remain a faithful marker of disease in patients experiencing a rituximab-related IgM flare, as well as after plasmapheresis [194]. The use of quantitative allele-specific polymerase chain reaction assays to assess serial MYD88^{L265P} burden in WM patients is also under investigation [35, 37, 195].

Course and Prognosis

WM typically presents as an indolent disease. The presence of 6q deletions may have prognostic significance, but does not appear to impact overall survival [29, 196, 197]. Age is an important prognostic factor (>65 years) [198–200], but is influenced by comorbidities. Anemia that reflects both marrow involvement and serum level of the IgM monoclonal protein (because of the impact of IgM on intravascular fluid retention) has emerged as a strong adverse prognostic factor with hemoglobin levels of <9 to 12 g/dL associated with decreased survival in several series [145, 198–200]. Other cytopenias also may be significant predictors of survival, and the number of cytopenias in a given patient has been proposed as a prognostic factor [199]. Serum albumin levels have also correlated with survival in some studies in WM patients [199, 200]. Elevated serum β_2-microglobulin levels (>3–3.5 g/dL) have also shown strong prognostic correlation in WM [145, 200, 201]. Several scoring systems have been proposed based on these analyses (Table 33.4), including the WM International Prognostic Scoring System (WM IPSS) which incorporates five adverse covariates: advanced age (>65 years), hemoglobin less than or equal to 11.5 g/dL, platelet count less than or equal to 100 × 10^9/L, beta2-microglobulin more than 3 mg/L, and serum monoclonal protein concentration more than 7.0 g/dL [202]. Among

Table 33.4 Prognostic scoring systems in Waldenstrom's macroglobulinemia

Study	Adverse prognostic factors	Number of groups	Survival
Gobbi et al. [198]	Hgb <9 g/dL	0–1 prognostic factors	Median: 48 months
	Age > 70 years	2–4 prognostic factors	Median: 80 months
	Weight loss		
	Cryoglobulinemia		
Morel et al. [199]	Age ≥ 65 years	0–1 prognostic factors	5 years: 87% of patients
	Albumin <4 g/dL	2 prognostic factors	5 years: 62%
	Number of cytopenias:	3–4 prognostic factors	5 years: 25%
	Hgb <12 g/dL		
	Platelets <150 × 10^9/L		
	WBC <4 × 10^9/L		
Dhodapkar et al. [147]	β_2M ≥ 3 g/dL	β_2M < 3 mg/dL + Hgb ≥12 g/dL	5 years: 87% of patients
	Hgb <12 g/dL	β_2M < 3 mg/dL + Hgb <12 g/dL	5 years: 63%
	IgM <4 g/dL	β_2M ≥ 3 mg/dL + IgM ≥4 g/dL	5 years: 53%
		β_2M ≥ 3 mg/dL + IgM <4 g/dL	5 years: 21%
Application of international staging system criteria for myeloma to WM Dimopoulos et al. [200]	Albumin ≤3.5 g/dL	Albumin ≥3.5 g/dL + β_2M < 3.5 mg/dL	Median: NR
	β_2M ≥ 3.5 mg/L	Albumin ≤3.5 g/dL + β_2M < 3.5 or	Median: 116 months
		β_2M 3.5–5.5 mg/dL	Median: 54 months
		β_2M > 5.5 mg/dL	
International Prognostic Scoring System for WM Morel et al. [202]	Age > 65 year	0–1 prognostic factors (excluding age)	5 years: 87% of patients
	Hgb <11.5 g/dL	2 prognostic factors (or age > 65 years)	5 years: 68%
	Platelets <100 × 10^9/L	3–5 prognostic factors	5 years: 36%
	β_2M > 3 mg/L		
	IgM >7 g/dL		

β_2M β_2-microbloulin, *Hgb* hemoglobulin, *NR* not reported, *WBC* white blood cell count

537 WM patients evaluated in the development of WM IPSS, low-risk patients (27%) presented with no or one of the adverse characteristics and advanced age, intermediate-risk patients (38%) with two adverse characteristics or only advanced age, and high-risk patients (35%) with more than two adverse characteristics. Five-year survival rates for these patients were 87%, 68%, and 36%, respectively. Importantly, the WM IPSS retained its prognostic significance in subgroups defined by age, treatment with alkylating agent, and nucleoside analogues. Recent data from the Surveillance, Epidemiology, and End Results (SEER) database involving 7744 WM patients showed that the relative survival of WM patients has improved over time [203]. Patients diagnosed during 2001–2010 had higher 5-year (78% versus 67%) and 10-year (66% versus 49%) relative survival rates versus patients diagnosed during 1980–2000. A Greek study that included 345 patients with WM failed to show any overall or cause-specific survival improvement in recent years, though the study might have been underpowered to detect any expected benefit [204]. However, a Swedish study of 1555 patients diagnosed with WM between 1980 and 2005 showed that the 5-year relative survival rate improved from 57% in 1980–1985 to 78% in 2001–2005 [205].

References

1. Owen RG, Treon SP, Al-Katib A, et al. Clinicopathological definition of Waldenström's macroglobulinemia: consensus panel recommendations from the second international workshop on Waldenström's macroglobulinemia. Semin Oncol. 2003;30:110.
2. Harris NL, Jaffe ES, Stein H, et al. A revised European-American classification of lymphoid neoplasms: a proposal from the international lymphoma study group. Blood. 1994;84:1361.
3. Harris NL, Jaffe ES, Diebold J, et al. The World Health Organization classification of neoplastic diseases of the hematopoietic and lymphoid tissues. Report of the Clinical Advisory Committee meeting, Airlie House, Virginia, November, 1997. Ann Oncol. 1999;10:1419.
4. Groves FD, Travis LB, Devesa SS, et al. Waldenström's macroglobulinemia: incidence patterns in the United States, 1988–1994. Cancer. 1998;82:1078.
5. Herrinton LJ, Weiss NS. Incidence of Waldenström's macroglobulinemia. Blood. 1993;82:3148.
6. Hanzis C, Ojha RP, Hunter Z, et al. Associated malignancies in patients with Waldenstrom's macroglobulinemia and their kin. Clin Lymphoma Myeloma Leuk. 2011;11:88.
7. Bjornsson OG, Arnason A, Gudmunosson S, et al. Macroglobulinaemia in an Icelandic family. Acta Med Scand. 1978;203:283.
8. Renier G, Ifrah N, Chevailler A, et al. Four brothers with Waldenström's macroglobulinemia. Cancer. 1989;64:1554.
9. Ogmundsdottir HM, Sveinsdottir S, Sigfusson A, et al. Enhanced B cell survival in familial macroglobulinaemia is associated with increased expression of Bcl-2. Clin Exp Immunol. 1999;117:252.
10. Santini GF, Crovatto M, Modolo ML, et al. Waldenström macroglobulinemia: a role of HCV infection? Blood. 1993;82:2932.
11. Silvestri F, Barillari G, Fanin R, et al. Risk of hepatitis C virus infection, Waldenström's macroglobulinemia, and monoclonal gammopathies. Blood. 1996;88:1125.
12. Leleu X, O'Connor K, Ho A, et al. Hepatitis C viral infection is not associated with Waldenström's macroglobulinemia. Am J Hematol. 2007;82:83.
13. Swerdlow SH, Campo E, Harris NL, et al. WHO classification of tumours of haematopoietic and lymphoid tissues. 4th ed. Lyon: IARC Press; 2008.
14. Smith BR, Robert NJ, Ault KA. In Waldenstrom's macroglobulinemia the quantity of detectable circulating monoclonal B lymphocytes correlates with clinical course. Blood. 1983;61:911.
15. Treon SP. How I treat Waldenstrom's macroglobulinemia. Blood. 2009;114:2375.
16. Preud'homme JL, Seligmann M. Immunoglobulins on the surface of lymphoid cells in Waldenström's macroglobulinemia. J Clin Invest. 1972;51:701.
17. San Miguel JF, Vidriales MB, Ocio E, et al. Immunophenotypic analysis of Waldenstrom's macroglobulinemia. Semin Oncol. 2003;30:187.
18. Hunter ZR, Branagan AR, Manning R, et al. CD5, CD10, and CD23 expression in Waldenstrom's macroglobulinemia. Clin Lymphoma. 2005;5:246.
19. Paiva B, Montes MC, García-Sanz R, et al. Multiparameter flow cytometry for the identification of the Waldenström's clone in IgM MGUS and Waldenström's Macroglobulinemia: new criteria for differential diagnosis and risk stratification. Leukemia. 2013;28:166.
20. Wagner SD, Martinelli V, Luzzatto L. Similar patterns of V kappa gene usage but different degrees of somatic mutation in hairy cell leukemia, prolymphocytic leukemia, Waldenstrom's macroglobulinemia, and myeloma. Blood. 1994;83:3647.
21. Aoki H, Takishita M, Kosaka M, Saito S. Frequent somatic mutations in D and/or JH segments of Ig gene in Waldenström's macroglobulinemia and chronic lymphocytic leukemia (CLL) with Richter's syndrome but not in common CLL. Blood. 1995;85:1913.
22. Shiokawa S, Suehiro Y, Uike N, Muta K, Nishimura J. Sequence and expression analyses of mu and delta transcripts in patients with Waldenström's macroglobulinemia. Am J Hematol. 2001;68:139.
23. Sahota SS, Forconi F, Ottensmeier CH, et al. Typical Waldenstrom macroglobulinemia is derived from a B-cell arrested after cessation of somatic mutation but prior to isotype switch events. Blood. 2002;100:1505.
24. Ackroyd S, O'Connor SJM, Owen RG. Rarity of IgH translocations in Waldenström macroglobulinemia. Cancer Genet Cytogenet. 2005;163:77.
25. Avet-Loiseau H, Garand R, Lode L, Robillard N, Bataille R. 14q32 translocations discriminate IgM multiple myeloma from Waldenstrom's macroglobulinemia. Semin Oncol. 2003;30:153.
26. Braggio E, Keats JJ, Leleu X, et al. High-resolution genomic analysis in Waldenström's macroglobulinemia identifies disease-specific and common abnormalities with marginal zone lymphomas. Clin Lymphoma Myeloma. 2009;9:39.
27. Schop RF, Kuehl WM, Van Wier SA, et al. Waldenström macroglobulinemia neoplastic cells lack immunoglobulin heavy chain locus translocations but have frequent 6q deletions. Blood. 2002;100:2996.
28. Hunter ZR, Xu L, Yang G, et al. The genomic landscape of Waldenstom's Macroglobulinemia is characterized by highly recurring MYD88 and WHIM-like CXCR4 mutations, and small somatic deletions associated with B-cell lymphomagenesis. Blood. 2014;123:1637.
29. Nguyen-Khac F, Lambert J, Chapiro E, et al. Chromosomal aberrations and their prognostic value in a series of 174 untreated patients with Waldenstrom's macroglobulinemia. Haematologica. 2013;98:649.
30. Braggio E, Keats JJ, Leleu X, et al. Identification of copy number abnormalities and inactivating mutations in two negative regulators of nuclear factor-kappaB signaling pathways in Waldenstrom's macroglobulinemia. Cancer Res. 2009;69:3579.

31. Leleu X, Eeckhoute J, Jia X, et al. Targeting NF-kappaB in Waldenstrom macroglobulinemia. Blood. 2008;111:5068.
32. Treon SP, Hunter ZR, Matous J, et al. Multicenter clinical trial of bortezomib in relapsed/refractory Waldenstrom's macroglobulinemia: results of WMCTG trial 03-248. Clin Cancer Res. 2007;13:3320.
33. Treon SP, Tripsas CK, Meid K, et al. Carfilzomib, rituximab and dexamethasone (CaRD) is active and offers a neuropathy-sparing approach for proteasome-inhibitor based therapy in Waldenstrom's macroglobulinemia. Blood. 2014;124:503.
34. Treon SP, Xu L, Yang G, et al. MYD88 L265P somatic mutation in Waldenstrom's macroglobulinemia. N Engl J Med. 2012;367:826.
35. Xu L, Hunter Z, Yang G, et al. MYD88 L265P in Waldenstrom macroglobulinemia, immunoglobulin M monoclonal gammopathy, and other B-cell lymphoproliferative disorders using conventional and quantitative allele-specific polymerase chain reaction. Blood. 2013;121:2051.
36. Varettoni M, Arcaini L, Zibellini S, et al. Prevalence and clinical significance of the MYD88 L265P somatic mutation in Waldenstrom macroglobulinemia, and related lymphoid neoplasms. Blood. 2013;121:2522.
37. Jiménez C, Sebastián E, Del Carmen Chillón M, et al. MYD88 L265P is a marker highly characteristic of, but not restricted to, Waldenström's macroglobulinemia. Leukemia. 2013;27:1722.
38. Poulain S, Roumier C, Decambron A, et al. MYD88 L265P mutation in Waldenstrom's macroglobulinemia. Blood. 2013;121:4504.
39. Ansell SM, Hodge LS, Secreto FJ, et al. Activation of TAK1 by MYD88 L265P drives malignant B-cell growth in Non-Hodgkin lymphoma. Blood Cancer J. 2014;4:e183. https://doi.org/10.1038/bcj.2014.4.
40. Ngo VN, Young RM, Schmitz R, Jhavar S, Xiao W, Lim KH, et al. Oncogenically active MYD88 mutations in human lymphoma. Nature. 2011;470:115.
41. Landgren O, Staudt L. MYD88 L265P somatic mutation in IgM MGUS. N Engl J Med. 2012;367:2255.
42. Yang G, Zhou Y, Liu X, Xu L, Cao Y, Manning RJ, et al. A mutation in MYD88 (L265P) supports the survival of lymphoplasmacytic cells by activation of Bruton tyrosine kinase in Waldenstrom macroglobulinemia. Blood. 2013;122:1222.
43. Watters T, Kenny EF, O'Neill LAJ. Structure, function and regulation of the Toll/IL-1 receptor adaptor proteins. Immunol Cell Biol. 2007;85:411.
44. Cohen L, Henzel WJ, Baeuerie PAIKAP. Is a scaffold protein of the IkappaB kinase complex. Nature. 1998;395:292.
45. Loiarro M, Gallo G, Fanto N, et al. Identification of critical residues of the MYD88 death domain involved in the recruitment of downstream kinases. J Biol Chem. 2009;284:28093.
46. Lin SC, Lo YC, Wu H. Helical assembly in the MYD88-IRAK4-IRAK2 complex in TLR/IL-1R signaling. Nature. 2010;465:885.
47. Kawagoe T, Sato S, Matsushita K, et al. Sequential control of Toll-like receptor dependent responses by IRAK1 and IRAK2. Nat Immunol. 2008;9:684.
48. Yang G, Buhrlage SJ, Tan L, et al. HCK is a survival determinant transactivated by mutated MYD88, and a direct target of ibrutinib. Blood. 2016;127:3237.
49. Treon SP, Xu L, Hunter ZR. MYD88 mutations and response to ibrutinib in Waldenstrom's macroglobulinemia. N Engl J Med. 2015;373:584.
50. Treon SP, Cao Y, Xu L, et al. Somatic mutations in MYD88 and CXCR4 are determinants of clinical presentation and overall survival in Waldenstrom macroglobulinemia. Blood. 2014;123:2791.
51. Roccaro A, Sacco A, Jiminez C, et al. C1013G/CXCR4 acts as a driver mutation of tumor progression and modulator of drug resistance in lymphoplasmacytic lymphoma. Blood. 2014;123:4120.
52. Stephanie Poulain S, Roumier C, Doye E, et al. Genomic landscape of CXCR4 mutations in Waldenstrom's macroglobulinemia. Clin Cancer Res. 2016;22(6):1480–8.
53. Busillo JM, Amando S, Sengupta R, et al. Site-specific phosphorylation of CXCR4 is dynamically regulated by multiple kinases and results in differential modulation of CXCR4 signaling. J Biol Chem. 2010;285:7805.
54. Dotta L, Tassone L, Badolato R. Clinical and genetic features of warts, Hypogammaglobulinemia, infections and Myelokathexis (WHIM) syndrome. Curr Mol Med. 2011;11:317.
55. Xu L, Hunter ZR, Tsakmaklis N, et al. Clonal architecture of CXCR4 WHIM-like mutations in Waldenström macroglobulinaemia. Br J Haematol. 2016;172:735.
56. Cao Y, Hunter ZR, Liu X, et al. The WHIM-like CXCR4S338X somatic mutation activates AKT and ERK, and promotes resistance to ibrutinib and other agents used in the treatment of Waldenstrom's macroglobulinemia. Leukemia. 2015;29:169–76. https://doi.org/10.1038/leu.2014.
57. Cao Y, Hunter ZR, Liu X, et al. CXCR4 WHIM-like frameshift and nonsense mutations promote ibrutinib resistance but do not supplant MYD88 L265P directed signaling in Waldenstrom macroglobulinaemia cells. Br J Haematol. 2015;168:701.
58. Tournilhac O, Santos DD, Xu L, et al. Mast cells in Waldenstrom's macroglobulinemia support lymphoplasmacytic cell growth through CD154/CD40 signaling. Ann Oncol. 2006;17:1275.
59. Zhou Y, Liu X, Xu L, et al. Matrix metalloproteinase-8 is overexpressed in Waldenström's macroglobulinemia cells, and specific inhibition of this metalloproteinase blocks release of soluble CD27. Clin Lymphoma Myeloma Leuk. 2011;11:172.
60. Ho AW, Hatjiharissi E, Ciccarelli BT, et al. CD27-CD70 interactions in the pathogenesis of Waldenstrom macroglobulinemia. Blood. 2008;112:4683.
61. Ngo HT, Leleu X, Lee J, et al. SDF-1/CXCR4 and VLA-4 interaction regulates homing in Waldenstrom macroglobulinemia. Blood. 2008;112:150.
62. Merlini G, Farhangi M, Osserman EF. Monoclonal immunoglobulins with antibody activity in myeloma, macroglobulinemia and related plasma cell dyscrasias. Semin Oncol. 1986;13:350.
63. Farhangi M, Merlini G. The clinical implications of monoclonal immunoglobulins. Semin Oncol. 1986;13:366.
64. Marmont AM, Merlini G. Monoclonal autoimmunity in hematology. Haematologica. 1991;76:449.
65. Mackenzie MR, Babcock J. Studies of the hyperviscosity syndrome. II: Macroglobulinemia. J Lab Clin Med. 1975;85:227.
66. Gertz MA, Kyle RA. Hyperviscosity syndrome. J Intensive Care Med. 1995;10:128.
67. Kwaan HC, Bongu A. The hyperviscosity syndromes. Semin Thromb Hemost. 1999;25:199.
68. Singh A, Eckardt KU, Zimmermann A, et al. Increased plasma viscosity as a reason for inappropriate erythropoietin formation. J Clin Invest. 1993;91:251.
69. Menke MN, Feke GT, McMeel JW, et al. Hyperviscosity-related retinopathy in Waldenström's macroglobulinemia. Arch Ophthalmol. 2006;124:1601.
70. Stone MJ. Waldenström's macroglobulinemia: hyperviscosity syndrome and cryoglobulinemia. Clin Lymphoma Myeloma. 2009;9:97.
71. Dellagi K, Dupouey P, Brouet JC, et al. Waldenström's macroglobulinemia and peripheral neuropathy: a clinical and immunologic study of 25 patients. Blood. 1983;62:280.
72. Nobile-Orazio E, Marmiroli P, Baldini L, et al. Peripheral neuropathy in macroglobulinemia: incidence and antigen-specificity of M proteins. Neurology. 1987;37:1506.
73. Treon SP, Hanzis C, Ioakimidis L, et al. Clinical characteristics and treatment outcome of disease-related peripheral neuropathy

in Waldenstrom's macroglobulinemia (WM). J Clin Oncol. 2010;Suppl 15, Abstract 8114:28.
74. Nemni R, Gerosa E, Piccolo G, Merlini G. Neuropathies associated with monoclonal gammopathies. Haematologica. 1994;79:557.
75. Ropper AH, Gorson KC. Neuropathies associated with paraproteinemia. N Engl J Med. 1998;338:1601.
76. Vital A. Paraproteinemic neuropathies. Brain Pathol. 2001;11:399.
77. Latov N, Braun PE, Gross RB, et al. Plasma cell dyscrasia and peripheral neuropathy: identification of the myelin antigens that react with human paraproteins. Proc Natl Acad Sci U S A. 1981;78:7139.
78. Chassande B, Leger JM, Younes-Chennoufi AB, et al. Peripheral neuropathy associated with IgM monoclonal gammopathy: correlations between M-protein antibody activity and clinical/electrophysiological features in 40 cases. Muscle Nerve. 1998;21:55.
79. Weiss MD, Dalakas MC, Lauter CJ, et al. Variability in the binding of anti-MAG and anti-SGPG antibodies to target antigens in demyelinating neuropathy and IgM paraproteinemia. J Neuroimmunol. 1999;95:174.
80. Latov N, Hays AP, Sherman WH. Peripheral neuropathy and anti-MAG antibodies. Crit Rev Neurobiol. 1988;3:301.
81. Dalakas MC, Quarles RH. Autoimmune ataxic neuropathies (sensory ganglionopathies): are glycolipids the responsible autoantigens? Ann Neurol. 1996;39:419.
82. Eurelings M, Ang CW, Notermans NC, et al. Antiganglioside antibodies in polyneuropathy associated with monoclonal gammopathy. Neurology. 2001;57:1909.
83. Ilyas AA, Quarles RH, Dalakas MC, et al. Monoclonal IgM in a patient with paraproteinemic polyneuropathy binds to gangliosides containing disialosyl groups. Ann Neurol. 1985;18:655.
84. Willison HJ, O'Leary CP, Veitch J, et al. The clinical and laboratory features of chronic sensory ataxic neuropathy with anti-disialosyl IgM antibodies. Brain. 2001;124:1968.
85. Lopate G, Choksi R, Pestronk A. Severe sensory ataxia and demyelinating polyneuropathy with IgM anti-GM2 and GalNAc-GD1A antibodies. Muscle Nerve. 2002;25:828.
86. Jacobs BC, O'Hanlon GM, Breedland EG, et al. Human IgM paraproteins demonstrate shared reactivity between Campylobacter jejuni lipopolysaccharides and human peripheral nerve disialylated gangliosides. J Neuroimmunol. 1997;80:23.
87. Nobile-Orazio E, Manfredini E, Carpo M, et al. Frequency and clinical correlates of antineural IgM antibodies in neuropathy associated with IgM monoclonal gammopathy. Ann Neurol. 1994;36:416.
88. Gordon PH, Rowland LP, Younger DS, et al. Lymphoproliferative disorders and motor neuron disease: an update. Neurology. 1997;48:1671.
89. Pavord SR, Murphy PT, Mitchell VE. POEMS syndrome and Waldenström's macroglobulinaemia. J Clin Pathol. 1996;49:181.
90. Crisp D, Pruzanski W. B-cell neoplasms with homogeneous cold-reacting antibodies (cold agglutinins). Am J Med. 1982;72:915.
91. Pruzanski W, Shumak KH. Biologic activity of cold-reacting autoantibodies (first of two parts). N Engl J Med. 1977;297:538.
92. Pruzanski W, Shumak KH. Biologic activity of cold-reacting autoantibodies (second of two parts). N Engl J Med. 1977;297:583.
93. Whittaker SJ, Bhogal BS, Black MM. Acquired immunobullous disease: a cutaneous manifestation of IgM macroglobulinaemia. Br J Dermatol. 1996;135:283.
94. Daoud MS, Lust JA, Kyle RA, Pittelkow MR. Monoclonal gammopathies and associated skin disorders. J Am Acad Dermatol. 1999;40:507.
95. Gad A, Willen R, Carlen B, et al. Duodenal involvement in Waldenström's macroglobulinemia. J Clin Gastroenterol. 1995;20:174.
96. Case records of the Massachusetts General Hospital. Weekly clinicopathological exercises. Case 3–1990. A 66-year-old woman with Waldenström's macroglobulinemia, diarrhea, anemia, and persistent gastrointestinal bleeding. N Engl J Med. 1990;322:183.
97. Isaac J, Herrera GA. Cast nephropathy in a case of Waldenström's macroglobulinemia. Nephron. 2002;91:512.
98. Morel-Maroger L, Basch A, Danon F, et al. Pathology of the kidney in Waldenström's macroglobulinemia. Study of sixteen cases. N Engl J Med. 1970;283:123.
99. Gertz MA, Kyle RA, Noel P. Primary systemic amyloidosis: a rare complication of immunoglobulin M monoclonal gammopathies and Waldenström's macroglobulinemia. J Clin Oncol. 1993;11:914.
100. Moyner K, Sletten K, Husby G, Natvig JB. An unusually large (83 amino acid residues) amyloid fibril protein AA from a patient with Waldenström's macroglobulinaemia and amyloidosis. Scand J Immunol. 1980;11:549.
101. Gardyn J, Schwartz A, Gal R, et al. Waldenström's macroglobulinemia associated with AA amyloidosis. Int J Hematol. 2001;74:76.
102. Dussol B, Kaplanski G, Daniel L, et al. Simultaneous occurrence of fibrillary glomerulopathy and AL amyloid. Nephrol Dial Transplant. 1998;13:2630.
103. Rausch PG, Herion JC. Pulmonary manifestations of Waldenström macroglobulinemia. Am J Hematol. 1980;9:201.
104. Fadil A, Taylor DE. The lung and Waldenström's macroglobulinemia. South Med J. 1998;91:681.
105. Kyrtsonis MC, Angelopoulou MK, Kontopidou FN, et al. Primary lung involvement in Waldenström's macroglobulinaemia: report of two cases and review of the literature. Acta Haematol. 2001;105:92.
106. Kaila VL, el Newihi HM, Dreiling BJ, et al. Waldenström's macroglobulinemia of the stomach presenting with upper gastrointestinal hemorrhage. Gastrointest Endosc. 1996;44:73.
107. Yasui O, Tukamoto F, Sasaki N, et al. Malignant lymphoma of the transverse colon associated with macroglobulinemia. Am J Gastroenterol. 1997;92:2299.
108. Rosenthal JA, Curran WJ Jr, Schuster SJ. Waldenström's macroglobulinemia resulting from localized gastric lymphoplasmacytoid lymphoma. Am J Hematol. 1998;58:244.
109. Recine MA, Perez MT, Cabello-Inchausti B, et al. Extranodal lymphoplasmacytoid lymphoma (immunocytoma) presenting as small intestinal obstruction. Arch Pathol Lab Med. 2001;125:677.
110. Veltman GA, van Veen S, Kluin-Nelemans JC, et al. Renal disease in Waldenström's macroglobulinaemia. Nephrol Dial Transplant. 1997;12:1256.
111. Moore DF Jr, Moulopoulos LA, Dimopoulos MA. Waldenström macroglobulinemia presenting as a renal or perirenal mass: clinical and radiographic features. Leuk Lymphoma. 1995;17:331.
112. Mascaro JM, Montserrat E, Estrach T, et al. Specific cutaneous manifestations of Waldenström's macroglobulinaemia. A report of two cases. Br J Dermatol. 1982;106:17.
113. Schnitzler L, Schubert B, Boasson M, et al. Urticaire chronique, lésions osseuses, macroglobulinémie IgM: Maladie de Waldenström? Bull Soc Fr Dermatol Syphiligr. 1974;81:363.
114. Roux S, Fermand JP, Brechignac S, et al. Tumoral joint involvement in multiple myeloma and Waldenström's macroglobulinemia—report of 4 cases. J Rheumatol. 1996;23:2175.
115. Orellana J, Friedman AH. Ocular manifestations of multiple myeloma, Waldenström's macroglobulinemia and benign monoclonal gammopathy. Surv Ophthalmol. 1981;26:157.
116. Ettl AR, Birbamer GG, Philipp W. Orbital involvement in Waldenström's macroglobulinemia: ultrasound, computed tomography and magnetic resonance findings. Ophthalmologica. 1992;205:40.
117. Minnema MC, Kimby E, D'Sa S, et al. Guideline for the diagnosis, treatment and response criteria for Bing-Neel syndrome. Haematologica. 102:43–51. https://doi.org/10.3324/haematol.2016.147728. Epub 2016 Oct 6.

118. Ciccarelli BT, Patterson CJ, Hunter ZR, et al. Hepcidin is produced by lymphoplasmacytic cells and is associated with anemia in Waldenström's Macroglobulinemia. Clin Lymphoma Myeloma Leuk. 2011;11:160.
119. Treon SP, Tripsas C, Ciccarelli BT, Manning RJ, Patterson CJ, Sheehy P, Hunter ZR. Patients with Waldenstrom macroglobulinemia commonly present with iron deficiency and those with severely depressed transferrin saturation levels show response to parenteral iron administration. Clin Lymphoma Myeloma Leuk. 2013;13:241.
120. Owen RG, Barrans SL, Richards SJ, et al. Waldenström macroglobulinemia. Development of diagnostic criteria and identification of prognostic factors. Am J Clin Pathol. 2001;116:420.
121. Feiner HD, Rizk CC, Finfer MD, et al. IgM monoclonal gammopathy/Waldenström's macroglobulinemia: a morphological and immunophenotypic study of the bone marrow. Mod Pathol. 1990;3:348.
122. Dutcher TF, Fahey JL. The histopathology of macroglobulinemia of Waldenström. J Natl Cancer Inst. 1959;22:887.
123. Hunter ZR, Manning RJ, Hanzis C, et al. IgA and IgG hypogammaglobulinemia in Waldenstrom's macroglobulinemia. Haematologica. 2010;95:470.
124. Stone MJ, Bogen SA. Evidence-based focused review of management of hyperviscosity syndrome. Blood. 2012;119:2205.
125. Menke MN, Treon SP. Hyperviscosity syndrome. In: Sekeres M, Kalaycio M, Bolwell B, editors. Clinical malignant hematology. New York: McGraw Hill; 2007. p. 937–41.
126. Moulopoulos LA, Dimopoulos MA, Varma DG, et al. Waldenström macroglobulinemia: MR imaging of the spine and CT of the abdomen and pelvis. Radiology. 1993;188:669.
127. Kyle RA, Treon SP, Alexanian R, et al. Prognostic markers and criteria to initiate therapy in Waldenström's macroglobulinemia: consensus panel recommendations from the second international workshop on Waldenström's macroglobulinemia. Semin Oncol. 2003;30:116.
128. Leblond V, Kastritis E, Advani R, et al. Treatment recommendations for Waldenström macroglobulinemia from the eighth international workshop on WM. Blood. 2016;128:1321.
129. Kyle RA, Greipp PR, Gertz MA, et al. Waldenström's macroglobulinaemia: a prospective study comparing daily with intermittent oral chlorambucil. Br J Haematol. 2000;108:737.
130. Dimopoulos MA, Alexanian R. Waldenström's macroglobulinemia. Blood. 1994;83:1452.
131. Petrucci MT, Avvisati G, Tribalto M, et al. Waldenström's macroglobulinaemia: results of a combined oral treatment in 34 newly diagnosed patients. J Intern Med. 1989;226:443.
132. Case DC Jr, Ervin TJ, Boyd MA, Redfield DL. Waldenström's macroglobulinemia: long-term results with the M-2 protocol. Cancer Investig. 1991;9(1):1.
133. Facon T, Brouillard M, Duhamel A, et al. Prognostic factors in Waldenström's macroglobulinemia: a report of 167 cases. J Clin Oncol. 1993;11:1553.
134. Leblond V, Johnson S, Chevret S, et al. Results of a randomized trial of chlorambucil versus fludarabine for patients with Waldenstrom macroglobulinemia, marginal zone lymphoma, or lymphoplasmacytic lymphoma. J Clin Oncol. 2013;31:301.
135. Dimopoulos MA, Kantarjian H, Weber D, et al. Primary therapy of Waldenström's macroglobulinemia with 2-chlorodeoxyadenosine. J Clin Oncol. 1994;12:2694.
136. Delannoy A, Ferrant A, Martiat P, et al. 2-Chlorodeoxyadenosine therapy in Waldenström's macroglobulinaemia. Nouv Rev Fr Hematol. 1994;36:317.
137. Fridrik MA, Jager G, Baldinger C, et al. First-line treatment of Waldenström's disease with cladribine. Ann Hematol. 1997;74:7.
138. Liu ES, Burian C, Miller WE, Saven A. Bolus administration of cladribine in the treatment of Waldenström macroglobulinaemia. Br J Haematol. 1998;103:690.
139. Hellmann A, Lewandowski K, Zaucha JM, et al. Effect of a 2-hour infusion of 2-chlorodeoxyadenosine in the treatment of refractory or previously untreated Waldenström's macroglobulinemia. Eur J Haematol. 1999;63:35.
140. Betticher DC, Hsu Schmitz SF, Ratschiller D, et al. Cladribine (2-CDA) given as subcutaneous bolus injections is active in pretreated Waldenström's macroglobulinaemia. Swiss Group for Clinical Cancer Research (SAKK). Br J Haematol. 1997;99:358.
141. Dimopoulos MA, Weber D, Delasalle KB, et al. Treatment of Waldenström's macroglobulinemia resistant to standard therapy with 2-chlorodeoxyadenosine: identification of prognostic factors. Ann Oncol. 1995;6:49.
142. Dimopoulos MA, O'Brien S, Kantarjian H, et al. Fludarabine therapy in Waldenström's macroglobulinemia. Am J Med. 1993;95:49.
143. Foran JM, Rohatiner AZ, Coiffier B, et al. Multicenter phase II study of fludarabine phosphate for patients with newly diagnosed lymphoplasmacytoid lymphoma, Waldenström's macroglobulinemia, and mantle-cell lymphoma. J Clin Oncol. 1999;17:546.
144. Thalhammer-Scherrer R, Geissler K, Schwarzinger I, et al. Fludarabine therapy in Waldenström's macroglobulinemia. Ann Hematol. 2000;79:556.
145. Dhodapkar MV, Jacobson JL, Gertz MA, et al. Prognostic factors and response to fludarabine therapy in patients with Waldenström macroglobulinemia: results of United States intergroup trial (Southwest Oncology Group S9003). Blood. 2001;98:41.
146. Zinzani PL, Gherlinzoni F, Bendandi M, et al. Fludarabine treatment in resistant Waldenström's macroglobulinemia. Eur J Haematol. 1995;54:120.
147. Leblond V, Ben Othman T, Deconinck E, et al. Activity of fludarabine in previously treated Waldenström's macroglobulinemia: a report of 71 cases. Groupe Cooperatif Macroglobulinemie. J Clin Oncol. 1998;16:2060.
148. Dimopoulos MA, Weber DM, Kantarjian H, et al. 2-Chlorodeoxyadenosine therapy of patients with Waldenström macroglobulinemia previously treated with fludarabine. Ann Oncol. 1994;5:288.
149. Lewandowski K, Halaburda K, Hellmann A. Fludarabine therapy in Waldenström's macroglobulinemia patients treated previously with 2-chlorodeoxyadenosine. Leuk Lymphoma. 2002;43:361.
150. Popat U, Saliba R, Thandi R, et al. Impairment of filgrastim-induced stem cell mobilization after prior lenalidomidein patients with multiple myeloma. Biol Blood Marrow Transplant. 2009;15:718.
151. Leleu XP, Manning R, Soumerai JD, et al. Increased incidence of transformation and myelodysplasia/acute leukemia in patients with Waldenström macroglobulinemia treated with nucleoside analogs. J Clin Oncol. 2009;27:250.
152. Leleu X, Tamburini J, Roccaro A, et al. Balancing risk versus benefit in the treatment of Waldenström's macroglobulinemia patients with nucleoside analogue based therapy. Clin Lymphoma Myeloma. 2009;9:71.
153. Treon SP, Kelliher A, Keele B, et al. Expression of serotherapy target antigens in Waldenström's macroglobulinemia: therapeutic applications and considerations. Semin Oncol. 2003;30:248.
154. Treon SP, Agus DB, Link B, et al. CD20-directed antibody-mediated immunotherapy induces responses and facilitates hematologic recovery in patients with Waldenström's macroglobulinemia. J Immunother. 2001;24:272.
155. Gertz MA, Rue M, Blood E, et al. Multicenter phase 2 trial of rituximab for Waldenström macroglobulinemia (WM): an Eastern Cooperative Oncology Group Study (E3A98). Leuk Lymphoma. 2004;45:2047.
156. Dimopoulos MA, Zervas C, Zomas A, et al. Treatment of Waldenström's macroglobulinemia with rituximab. J Clin Oncol. 2002;20:2327.

157. Treon SP, Emmanouilides C, Kimby E, et al. Extended rituximab therapy in Waldenström's macroglobulinemia. Ann Oncol. 2005;16:132.
158. Treon SP, Branagan AR, Hunter Z, et al. Paradoxical increases in serum IgM and viscosity levels following rituximab in Waldenström's macroglobulinemia. Ann Oncol. 2004;15:1481.
159. Ghobrial IM, Fonseca R, Greipp PR, et al. Initial immunoglobulin M "flare" after rituximab therapy in patients with Waldenström macroglobulinemia: an Eastern Cooperative Oncology Group Study. Cancer. 2004;101:2593.
160. Dimopoulos MA, Anagnostopoulos A, Zervas C, et al. Predictive factors for response to rituximab in Waldenström's macroglobulinemia. Clin Lymphoma. 2005;5:270.
161. Treon SP, Hansen M, Branagan AR, et al. Polymorphisms in FcγRIIIA (CD16) receptor expression are associated with clinical responses to rituximab in Waldenström's macroglobulinemia. J Clin Oncol. 2005;23:474.
162. Dimopoulos MA, Anagnostopulos A, Kyrtsonis MC, et al. Treatment of relapsed or refractory Waldenström's macroglobulinemia with bortezomib. Haematologica. 2005;90:1655.
163. Chen CI, Kouroukis CT, White D, et al. Bortezomib is active in patients with untreated or relapsed Waldenström's macroglobulinemia: a phase II study of the National Cancer Institute of Canada Clinical Trials Group. J Clin Oncol. 2007;25:1570.
164. Weber DM, Dimopoulos MA, Delasalle K, et al. 2-chlorodeoxyadenosine alone and in combination for previously untreated Waldenström's macroglobulinemia. Semin Oncol. 2003;30:243.
165. Treon SP, Branagan AR, Ioakimidis L, et al. Long term outcomes to fludarabine and rituximab in Waldenström's macroglobulinemia. Blood. 2009;113:3673.
166. Tam CS, Wolf MM, Westerman D, et al. Fludarabine combination therapy is highly effective in first-line and salvage treatment of patients with Waldenström's macroglobulinemia. Clin Lymphoma Myeloma. 2005;6:136.
167. Hensel M, Villalobos M, Kornacker M, et al. Pentostatin/cyclophosphamide with or without rituximab: an effective regimen for patients with Waldenström's macroglobulinemia/lymphoplasmacytic lymphoma. Clin Lymphoma Myeloma. 2005;6:131.
168. Dimopoulos MA, Anagnostopoulos A, Kyrtsonis MC, et al. Primary treatment of Waldenström's macroglobulinemia with dexamethasone, rituximab and cyclophosphamide. J Clin Oncol. 2007;25:3344.
169. Buske C, Hoster E, Dreyling MH, et al. The addition of rituximab to front-line therapy with CHOP (R-CHOP) results in a higher response rate and longer time to treatment failure in patients with lymphoplasmacytic lymphoma: results of a randomized trial of the German Low-Grade Lymphoma Study Group (GLSG). Leukemia. 2009;23:153.
170. Treon SP, Hunter Z, Branagan A. CHOP plus rituximab therapy in Waldenström's macroglobulinemia. Clin Lymphoma Myeloma. 2005;5:273.
171. Ioakimidis L, Patterson CJ, Hunter ZR, et al. Comparative outcomes following CP-R, CVP-R and CHOP-R in Waldenström's macroglobulinemia. Clin Lymphoma Myeloma. 2009;9:62.
172. Rummel M, Niederle N, Maschmeyer G, et al. Bendamustine plus rituximab versus CHOP plus rituximab as first-line treatment for patients with indolent and mantle-cell lymphomas: an open-label, multicentre, randomised, phase 3 non-inferiority trial. Lancet. 2013;381:1203–10.
173. Treon SP, Hanzis C, Tripsas C, et al. Bendamustine therapy in patients with relapsed or refractory Waldenstrom's macroglobulinemia. Clin Lymphoma Myeloma Leuk. 2011;211:133–5.
174. Dimopoulos MA, Hamilos G, Efstathiou E, et al. Treatment of Waldenström's macroglobulinemia with the combination of fludarabine and cyclophosphamide. Leuk Lymphoma. 2003;44:993.
175. Tamburini J, Levy V, Chateilex C, et al. Fludarabine plus cyclophosphamide in Waldenström's macroglobulinemia: results in 49 patients. Leukemia. 2005;19:1831.
176. Treon SP, Ioakimidis L, Soumerai JD, et al. Primary therapy of Waldenström's macroglobulinemia with bortezomib, dexamethasone and rituximab. J Clin Oncol. 2009;27:3830.
177. Treon SP, Meid K, Gustine J, et al. Long-term outcome of a prospective study of Bortezomib, dexamethasone and rituximab (BDR) in previously untreated, symptomatic patients with Waldenstrom's macroglobulinemia. Blood. 2015;126(23):Abstract 1833.
178. Ghobrial IM, Matous J, Padmanabhan S, et al. Phase II trial of combination of bortezomib and rituximab in relapsed and/or refractory Waldenström's macroglobulinemia. Blood. 2008;112:832.
179. Agathocleous A, Rohatiner A, Rule S, et al. Weekly versus twice weekly bortezomib given in conjunction with rituximab in patients with recurrent follicular lymphoma, mantle cell lymphoma, and Waldenström macroglobulinemia. Br J Haematol. 2010;151:346.
180. Dimopoulos MA, García-Sanz R, Gavriatopoulou M, et al. Primary therapy of Waldenstrom macroglobulinemia (WM) with weekly bortezomib, low-dose dexamethasone, and rituximab (BDR): long-term results of a phase 2 study of the European Myeloma Network (EMN). Blood. 2013;122:3276.
181. Gavriatopoulou M, Garcia-Sanz R, Kastritis E, et al. BDR in newly diagnosed patients with WM: final analysis of a phase 2 study after a minimum follow up of 6 years. Blood. 2017;129(4):456.
182. Treon SP, Tripsas CK, Meid K, et al. Ibrutinib in previously treated patients with Waldenström's macroglobulinemia. N Engl J Med. 2015;372(15):1430.
183. Dimopoulos MA, Trotman J, Tedeschi A, et al. Single agent ibrutinib in rituximab-refractory patients with Waldenström's macroglobulinemia: results from a multicenter, open-label phase 3 substudy (iNNOVATETM). Lancet Oncol. 2016;18(2):241.
184. Ghobrial IM, Witzig TE, Gertz M, et al. Long-term results of the phase II trial of the oral mTOR inhibitor everolimus (RAD001) in relapsed or refractory Waldenstrom macroglobulinemia. Am J Hematol. 2014;89(3):237.
185. Treon SP, Tripsas CK, Meid K, et al. Prospective, multicenter study of everolimus as primary therapy in Waldenstrom's macroglobulinemia. Clin Cancer Res. 1822:2016. https://doi.org/10.1158/1078-0432.122.
186. Treon SP, Hanzis C, Manning RJ, et al. Maintenance rituximab is associated with improved clinical outcome in rituximab naïve patients with Waldenstrom's Macroglobulinemia who respond to a Rituximab containing regimen. Br J Haematol. 2011;154:357.
187. Rummel MJ, Lerchenmüller C, Greil R, et al. Bendamustine-rituximab induction followed by observation or rituximab maintenance for newly diagnosed patients with Waldenström's Macroglobulinemia: results from a prospective, randomized, multicenter study (StiL NHL 7-2008). Blood. 2012;120(21):Abstract 2739.
188. Kyriakou C, Canals C, Sibon D, et al. High-dose therapy and autologous stem-cell transplantation in Waldenstrom macroglobulinemia: the lymphoma working Party of the European Group for blood and marrow transplantation. J Clin Oncol. 2010;28:2227.
189. Kyriakou C, Canals C, Cornelissen JJ, et al. Allogeneic stem-cell transplantation in patients with Waldenström macroglobulinemia: report from the lymphoma working Party of the European Group for blood and marrow transplantation. J Clin Oncol. 2010;28:4926.
190. Owen RG, Kyle RA, Stone MJ, et al. Response assessment in Waldenstrom macroglobulinemia. Br J Haematol. 2013;160(2):171.
191. Treon SP, Yang G, Hanzis C, et al. Attainment of complete/very good partial response following rituximab based therapy is an important determinant to progression-free survival and is impacted by polymorphisms in FCGR3A in Waldenstrom macroglobulinaemia. Br J Haematol. 2011;154:223.

192. Strauss SJ, Maharaj L, Hoare S, et al. Bortezomib therapy in patients with relapsed or refractory lymphoma: potential correlation of in vitro sensitivity and tumor necrosis factor alpha response with clinical activity. J Clin Oncol. 2006;24:2105.
193. Varghese AM, Rawstron AC, Ashcroft J, et al. Assessment of bone marrow response in Waldenström's macroglobulinemia. Clin Lymphoma Myeloma. 2009;9:53.
194. Ciccarelli BT, Yang G, Hatjiharissi E, et al. Soluble CD27 is a faithful marker of disease burden and is unaffected by the rituximab induced IgM flare, as well as plasmapheresis in patients with Waldenström's macroglobulinemia. Clin Lymphoma Myeloma. 2009;9:56.
195. Xu L, Hunter ZR, Yang G, et al. Detection of MYD88 L265P in peripheral blood of patients with Waldenström's macroglobulinemia and IgM monoclonal gammopathy by allele-specific PCR. Leukemia. 2014;28(8):1698.
196. Ocio EM, Schop RF, Gonzalez B, et al. 6q deletion in Waldenström macroglobulinemia is associated with features of adverse prognosis. Br J Haematol. 2007;136(1):80.
197. Chang H, Qi C, Trieu Y, et al. Prognostic relevance of 6q deletion in Waldenström's macroglobulinemia: a multicenter study. Clin Lymphoma Myeloma. 2009;9(1):36.
198. Gobbi PG, Bettini R, Montecucco C, et al. Study of prognosis in Waldenström's macroglobulinemia: a proposal for a simple binary classification with clinical and investigational utility. Blood. 1994;83:2939.
199. Morel P, Monconduit M, Jacomy D, et al. Prognostic factors in Waldenström macroglobulinemia: a report on 232 patients with the description of a new scoring system and its validation on 253 other patients. Blood. 2000;96:852.
200. Dimopoulos M, Gika D, Zervas K, et al. The international staging system for multiple myeloma is applicable in symptomatic Waldenström's macroglobulinemia. Leuk Lymphoma. 2004;45:1809.
201. Anagnostopoulos A, Zervas K, Kyrtsonis M, et al. Prognostic value of serum beta 2-microglobulin in patients with Waldenström's macroglobulinemia requiring therapy. Clin Lymphoma Myeloma. 2006;7:205.
202. Morel P, Duhamel A, Gobbi P, et al. International prognostic scoring system for Waldenström macroglobulinemia. Blood. 2009;113:4163.
203. Castillo JJ, Olszewski A, Cronin AM, et al. Survival trends in Waldenstrom macroglobulinemia: an analysis of the surveillance, epidemiology and end results database. Blood. 2014;123:3999.
204. Kastritis S, Kyrtsonis MC, Hatjiharissi E, et al. No significant improvement in the outcome of patients with Waldenstrom macroglobulinemia treated over the last 25 years. Am J Hematol. 2011;86:479.
205. Kristinsson SY, Eloranta S, Dickman PW, et al. Patterns of survival in lymphoplasmacytic lymphoma/Waldenstrom macroglobulinemia: a population based study of 1,555 patients diagnosed in Sweden from 1980 to 2005. Am J Hematol. 2013;88:60.

34 Plasma Cell Leukemia

Nisha S. Joseph and Sagar Lonial

Introduction

Plasma cell leukemia (PCL) is a rare and aggressive variant of multiple myeloma that comprises roughly 1% of all myeloma cases [1]. This unique plasma cell dyscrasia is characterized by an increased number of circulating plasma cells in the peripheral blood. It can either arise de novo, as is the case in primary plasma cell leukemia (pPCL), or alternatively as a transformed leukemic phase in an end-stage previously diagnosed case of myeloma.

PCL was first described in 1906 by Professor Gluzinski and Dr. Reichenstein at the University Hospital of Lemberg, now located in present-day western Ukraine [2]. The authors reported a case of a 47-year-old male presenting with bone pain, a palpable chest wall mass, anemia, and splenomegaly. Diagnostic workup revealed elevated urine protein and immature plasma cells on the peripheral blood smear. Plasma cells were elevated at 91% in the blood, and the patient was subsequently diagnosed with multiple myeloma and "leucaemia lymphatica plasmocellularis." He was treated with arsenic-based compounds with an initial reprieve in symptoms; however the patient eventually succumbed to his disease and passed away within 6 months. Unfortunately, despite the significant progress we have seen in multiple myeloma, the prognosis of PCL has not changed much since its initial discovery.

Though the myeloma community has experienced significant advancements and progress in outcomes with the advent of novel therapeutic agents such as bortezomib and lenalidomide, followed by high-dose therapy (HDT) and autologous stem cell transplantation (ASCT), unfortunately the same success has not yet been achieved in PCL. Historically, the use of conventional chemotherapeutics such as alkylating agents, anthracyclines, and steroids in PCL has proven ineffective. The prognosis remains poor, with even worse outcomes observed in patients with sPCL. Utilization of HSCT has improved survival, but still has not achieved lasting results. With such significant success of novel agents in MM, this area warrants further exploration in PCL. The literature in this subject area is limited and our knowledge base is mainly restricted to findings from small retrospective studies and case reports. Furthermore, these studies often do not differentiate between pPCL and sPCL or between younger and older patients, making extrapolation of data to the clinical setting difficult. In this chapter, we review the clinical presentation and diagnostic evaluation of plasma cell leukemia, review the data available to date about optimal treatment options for PCL, as well as discuss future directions in research for this challenging disease.

N.S. Joseph, M.D. • S. Lonial, M.D. (✉)
Department of Hematology and Medical Oncology, Winship Cancer Institute, Emory University School of Medicine, 1365 Clifton Rd, Building C, Room 4004, Atlanta 30322, GA, USA
e-mail: sloni01@emory.edu

Epidemiology

The epidemiology of PCL is very similar to that of multiple myeloma. The median age of diagnosis is 67. Primary PCL (pPCL) is more common than secondary PCL (sPCL), accounting for 60–70% of cases. Per the SEER database that surveyed patients between the years of 1973 and 2004, 291 patients with PCL were identified out of the 49,000 multiple myeloma patient in sum making the incidence of PCL 0.6%. There were no significant differences between gender, age, or race as compared with myeloma patients. Of note, this database did not distinguish between primary and secondary PCL [3].

Clinical Presentation

The clinical presentation of PCL is also very similar to that seen in patients with myeloma and leukemia. As in myeloma, many patients present with renal insufficiency, anemia, hypercalcemia, and bone pain associated with lytic lesions;

P.H. Wiernik et al. (eds.), *Neoplastic Diseases of the Blood*, DOI 10.1007/978-3-319-64263-5_34

similarly, as seen in patients with leukemia, PCL patients often present with coagulopathy, cytopenias, and hepatosplenomegaly. Other physical exam findings can include lymphadenopathy, pleural effusions, and neurologic symptoms secondary to CNS involvement. Compared with multiple myeloma, patients presenting with pPCL are more likely to have an aggressive presentation including increased tumor burden, extramedullary disease, renal involvement, and cytopenias [3].

Diagnosis

The diagnostic criteria for PCL are not clearly defined or universally agreed upon, but the diagnostic workup for a suspected case of PCL is essentially the same for that of multiple myeloma and would include peripheral blood smear, a bone marrow aspirate and biopsy, serum and urine protein electrophoresis, free light chain assay, skeletal survey, as well as chemistry panel, complete blood count with differential, and β2-microglobulin. Additional imaging and diagnostic tests such as lumbar puncture, cross-sectional imaging, or PET-CT may also be needed depending on symptoms and potential concern for extramedullary involvement. On physical examination, particular attention should be paid to bone pain, neurologic symptoms, and pleural effusions (Table 34.1).

The diagnosis of PCL must include an absolute plasma cell count $>2 \times 10^9$/L in addition to greater than 20% circulating plasma cells of the white blood cell differential in the peripheral blood. On review of a peripheral blood smear, detection of circulating plasma cells can often be difficult morphologically as the appearance of the plasma cell can vary depending on the stage of maturity. Commonly, flow cytometry is used to confirm the diagnosis and identify the malignant clone of plasma cells. As with myeloma cells, CD138 and CD38 are often expressed whereas CD19 and CD20 are absent, and unlike myeloma, CD56 is often not expressed [4, 5].

Table 34.1 Initial diagnostic workup for plasma cell leukemia

Complete medical history and physical exam
Peripheral blood smear
Laboratory studies
CBC with differential
Comprehensive Metabolic Panel (BUN, Cr, electrolytes, Ca, Albumin)
LDH
Quantitative immunoglobulins (IgG, IgM, IgA)
β-2 microglobulin
Serum protein electrophoresis/immunofixation
Urine protein electrophoresis/immunofixation
Serum free light chain assay
Bone marrow aspirate and biopsy
Flow cytometry
FISH (t(4;14), t(14;16), t(11;14), del13, del 17p, 1 gains)
Lumbar puncture (CNS symptoms)
Imaging (As indicated)
MRI
CT scan
PET-CT

Bone marrow aspiration with biopsy is part of the diagnostic workup for pPCL for morphology and cytogenetic analysis by FISH. In PCL, pathologic review often shows an elevated number of monoclonal plasma cells with extensive infiltration of the marrow and high proliferation index. Of note, the median plasma cell percentage is higher in pPCL than in myeloma [6]. Additionally, biologic differences are seen between the myeloma plasma cell and the plasma cell seen in PCL. In PCL, malignant cells proliferate in the bone marrow as in myeloma; however these cells have an increased capacity for release into the peripheral circulation due to different expression of adhesion markers, namely NCAM (neural cell adhesion molecule/CD56) and LFA-1 (leukocyte function-associated antigen-1). Additionally, there is different expression of chemokine receptors and other genetic abnormalities that allow even more pronounced independent growth, evasion of immune detection, and prevention of apoptosis [6]. These genetic abnormalities are also seen in myeloma cells, though they tend to accumulate throughout the progression from MGUS to symptomatic myeloma, whereas in PCL, they are present at the onset. These differences may explain the extramedullary disease seen in PCL and superior evasion from immune surveillance.

Cytogenetic testing is routinely done in plasma cell dyscrasias as part of risk stratification and more recently for staging purposes. Analysis is focused on high-risk mutations such as del(17p13), del(13q), del(1p21), and amp(1q21) as well as translocations t(11;14), t(14;16), t(4;14), and t(14;20). Heavy gene translocations and hyperdiploidy are both significant oncogenic events key in the transformation to a malignant plasma cell and are seen in PCL as well. There are no distinguishable genetic features seen in PCL as compared to myeloma, but the same high-risk mutations seen in myeloma tend to occur at higher rates. Hyperdiploidy, conversely, is only found in up to 8.8% of pPCL cases whereas it is seen in ~50% of myeloma cases. This same trend is seen in sPCL, although hyperdiploidy is seen at an even higher rate (~17%) [6–9]. IgH translocations occur at a significantly higher rate in pPCL. The most commonly seen translocation in PCL is t(11;14) which used to be thought of as a favorable prognosticator in myeloma and is now more likely to be a neutral finding; however in PCL, t(11;14) is associated with an unfavorable prognosis. The translocations t(4;14) and t(14;16) associated with poor risk in myeloma are seen in both primary and secondary PCL but at higher frequencies [3]. In PCL, an increased incidence of monosomy 13 (86% versus 26%) and a decreased incidence of trisomy 6 and monosomy 9 are seen. Additionally, it is more common to have a complex karyotype.

The differential diagnosis should include diagnoses that would also be defined by abnormal circulating cells like leukemias/lymphomas, though this can easily be distinguished with flow cytometry. It is also imperative to exclude a reactive polyclonal plasmacytosis that can be seen with bacterial or viral infections, autoimmune disorders, and serum sickness. A polyclonal plasmacytosis can be ruled out by confirming light-chain restriction on immunofixation.

Treatment

There have only been two prospective randomized trials conducted to date and these were conducted quite recently. Most of our information regarding optimal treatment in PCL is drawn from small retrospective studies and case reports; thus we have limited evidence-based data on which to base treatment decisions. For initial cytoreduction, in younger fit patients, historically aggressive chemotherapeutic regimens such as VAD and VDT-PACE were favored followed by ASCT versus chemotherapy alone in transplant-ineligible patients [10]. In the era of novel therapeutics, efforts have focused on utilization of these agents, namely lenalidomide and bortezomib (Table 34.2). These agents have shown to provide benefit but not as pronounced as in myeloma. Nevertheless, utilization of immunomodulatory agents and proteasome inhibitors has become standard of care in PCL.

Lenalidomide

The first prospective trial evaluating the optimal initial treatment in pPCL was conducted by Musto et al. and specifically studied the efficacy of lenalidomide in combination with low-dose dexamethasone in newly diagnosed pPCL. The study selected newly diagnosed pPCL patients with a performance status of 0–2, who then received lenalidomide 25 mg daily for 21 days with oral dexamethasone 40 mg given on days 1, 8, 15, and 22 on a 28-day cycle. After completion of four cycles, transplant-ineligible patients continued on with four additional cycles followed by maintenance lenalidomide at 10 mg daily on days 1–21 of a 28-day cycle until evidence of relapsed disease. Transplant-eligible patients proceeded to ASCT following four cycles of lenalidomide and dexamethasone. Patients who did not respond or progressed on initial treatment were taken off study. On intention-to-treat analysis, the overall response rate was 73.9%, and at a median follow-up of 34 months, median PFS and median overall survival were 14 and 28 months, respectively. Additionally, in evaluating the role of ASCT in treatment, PFS and OS were 27 months and not reached, respectively, in the cohort who underwent ASCT in comparison to PFS and OS of 2 and 12 months, respectively, for those patients who were transplant ineligible. Important conclusions from this study include demonstration of lenalidomide and dexamethasone as a valid frontline therapy in pPCL, as well as the important role consolidative ASCT may play as part of the larger treatment plan [11].

Bortezomib

There have been several studies that supported bortezomib-containing regimens followed by auto-SCT. Bortezomib has been shown to quickly reduce tumor volume and reverse

Table 34.2 Induction regimens for plasma cell leukemia

				Best response					
Author, year	*N*	Regimen	Median f/u	PR	VGPR	CR	PFS (m)	OS (m)	ORR
Musto, 2014	23	Rd	34 months	8 (34.7%)	6 (26.1%)	3 (13%)	14 months	28 months	73.90%
Royer, 2016	40	PAD versus VCD	28.7 months	9 (23%)	10 (26%)	4 (10%)	15.1 months	36.3 months	69%
D'Arena, 2012	29	BBR	24 months	12 (41%)	3 (10%)	8 (28%)			79%
Pagano, 2011	73	Vel ± Thal		18 (25%)		22 (30%)		12.6 months	
Katodritou, 2014	42	BBR	51 months	69%	27.50%			13 months	55%
Musto, 2007	12	BBR	21 months	5 (42%)	4 (33%)	2 (17%)	8 months	12 months	92%

PAD pegylated doxorubicin and oral dexamethasone, *VCD* bortezomib, oral cyclophosphamide, and oral dexamethasone, *BBR* bortezomib-based regimens, *Vel* bortezomib, *Thal* thalidomide end-organ damage, namely renal dysfunction. It has also been shown to overcome the negative implication of high-risk mutations such as del17p and t(4;14) [6].

The first prospective trial to date investigating the utilization of bortezomib-based regimens (BBR) in PCL was a prospective phase two clinical trial conducted by the IFM in 2016. The aim of the study was to evaluate the efficacy of induction regimens combining both standard chemotherapy with bortezomib in conjunction with HDT and autologous stem cell transplant followed by immunomodulatory agent and/or proteasome inhibitor maintenance versus a second allogeneic transplant [12]. Forty patients were enrolled and age 70 or younger and were treated with four alternating cycles of VAD and VCD followed by ASCT. Younger, fit patients then underwent a consolidative reduced-intensity allogeneic transplant, and the remainder of patients underwent a second ASCT followed by maintenance with RVD (lenalidomide, bortezomib, and dexamethasone) for 1 year. At a median follow-up of 28.7 months, the median PFS was 15.1 months and median overall survival was 36.3 months. The overall response rate to bortezomib-containing induction was 69%. This was the first prospective trial in PCL that demonstrated that bortezomib-containing induction regimens followed by transplant led to better response rates and improved PFS.

There have been several retrospective analyses published regarding use and efficacy of bortezomib-based regimens in PCL. The largest multicenter retrospective study comes from the Italian GIMEMA working group that focused on 29 patients with pPCL who received bortezomib in varying combination regimens with other therapeutics such as dexamethasone, thalidomide, doxorubicin, melphalan, prednisone, vincristine, or cyclophosphamide. The overall response rate was ORR 79%, with 38% of subjects achieving a VGPR or better. At a median follow-up time of 24 months, 55% of these patients were living and three-quarters of these patients were in remission. The most lasting results were seen in those who had undergone HSCT following induction. Additionally, improvement in renal function was seen in 10 of the 11 patients who had presented initially with renal failure, highlighting the benefit of bortezomib particularly in those with renal dysfunction at diagnosis [13].

Another multicenter retrospective study analyzed 128 patients with plasma cell leukemia, 73 of which were classified as primary plasma cell leukemia, from January 2000 to December 2008. In this group of patients who were treated with either alkylators, anthracycline-based regimens, or bortezomib/thalidomide used as additional or single agents, it was concluded that those patients receiving thalidomide or bortezomib as first-line therapy experienced and increased duration of response by 79% [14].

Katodritou and colleagues conducted another retrospective study with the purpose of examining the efficacy of bortezomib-based regimens in 42 PCL patients, 25 with pPCL, and 17 with sPCL. BBR were given to 29 of the patients, and 6 of the 25 patients with pPCL underwent ASCT. Response rates, being defined as a PR or better, were higher in patients treated with BBR (69% versus 30.8% in those that were treated with other regimens). The ORR of pPCL treated with BBR was 88.9%, which was the highest ORR seen in the varying cohorts. With a median follow-up of 51 months, median overall survival of the BBR group was 13 versus 2 months. Between the pPCL and sPCL, median overall survival differed by 18 and 7 months. Of note, improved response rates were seen regardless of ASCT and showed treatment of PCL with BBR induces better response rates [15].

Finally, another retrospective study done by the Italian group examined patients with either primary or secondary PCL who were treated with BBR either alone or in combination with other therapies. Twelve patients were included, three of whom received bortezomib as frontline treatment, and the remaining nine patients received bortezomib after 1–4 prior lines of treatment. Important findings included an overall response rate of 92% with 50% of patients achieving VGPR or better. The median PFS and median overall survival after bortezomib were 8 and 12 months, respectively [16].

The role of immunomodulatory agents and proteasome inhibitors in PCL is promising and needs to be further explored. Additionally, combinations of these agents, which have only been studied in small patient samples, have potential and call for further study as well.

Role of Transplant

In 1983, Dr. Mcelwain and Dr. Powell in the United Kingdom first described the use of melphalan 140 mg/m^2 in a patient with pPCL, and impressively, the patient lived for 30 months after therapy [17]. HDT followed by ASCT has become the standard of care in multiple myeloma, but its role is not as well defined in PCL. Prospective randomized trials to date of HCT have excluded PCL patients. There are some case reports that have noted improved outcomes and long-term responses with ASCT/allo-SCT. The following are some of the more significant studies published regarding the role of HCT in PCL, which suggest that HCT have a role in PCL treatment; however it becomes difficult to draw definitive conclusions given the lack of randomization and no comparison of allogeneic versus autologous transplantation.

The largest retrospective study to date reviewing the role of HCT in PCL was conducted by the European Group for

Blood and Marrow Transplantation. The study identified 272 pPCL patients and compared outcomes following autologous stem cell transplant with over 20,000 myeloma patients between the years of 1980 and 2006 [18]. The median PFS following transplant of PCL versus myeloma patients was 14.3 months versus 27.4 months, and the medial overall survival was 25.7 months versus 62.3 months, respectively. Significantly improved outcomes were seen in myeloma patients, and there was higher transplant-related mortality seen in the pPCL group as well.

The Center for International Blood and Marrow Transplant Research (CIBMTR) led another large retrospective study published in 2012. Of 147 patients with pPCL, 97 underwent autologous transplant and 50 underwent allogeneic HCT. Significant findings include the following: a median PFS of 34%, median overall survival at 3 years was 64% versus 39%, and relapse rate at 3 years was 61% versus 38% in the autologous group versus allogeneic group, respectively. Though the relapse rate was significantly lower with allogeneic transplant, transplant-related mortality was significantly higher (41% versus 5% in the autologous transplant cohort). Given better OS with autologous transplant in light of increased mortality associated with allogeneic transplant, this study supported use of ASCT with improved outcomes and decreased toxicities [19].

Another multicenter retrospective analysis performed by Pagano et al. looked at 73 patients with pPCL. In those patients who had undergone HSCT, they experienced longer overall survival and duration of response at 83.1 and 25.8 months, respectively, in contrast to 9.1 and 7.3 months seen in non-transplanted patients. Impressively, this analysis revealed an increase in mean overall survival by 69% and duration of response by 88%; however though this study supported use of HSCT, it unfortunately did not differ between autologous and allogeneic transplantation.

Prognosis

In general, the prognosis for PCL remains poor. These dismal outcomes are likely attributable to the increased incidence of the same high-risk mutations seen in myeloma, namely del17p, t(14;16), and t(4;14). As in myeloma, these mutations are noted to be of high risk due to the more aggressive nature and higher proliferative rate of these malignant cells. Mean overall survival is less than 1 year, and even worse in those patients with secondary PCL in the context of relapsed/refractory multiple myeloma. There has been modest improvement in outcomes with incorporation of ASCT in conjunction with novel agents. This is best demonstrated by a registry study including 445 patients which shows improved median survival from decade to decade, particularly when entering the early 2000s which encompasses the time period when novel agents were introduced in myeloma. Median survival through the decades trended as follows: from 1973 to 1995 median overall survival was 5 months, from 1996 to 2000 median overall survival was 6 months, from 2001 to 2005 median overall survival was 4 months, and then notably from 2006 to 2009 median overall survival improved to 12 months [20]. The most significant improvement has been seen in older patients, with early mortality decreasing from rate of 26 to 15% since the 1970s. Additional prognostic value can be drawn from patient's response to treatment. In those whose disease does not respond to initial therapy, prognosis is generally only a few months. Response to induction is defined as at least 50% reduction in circulating plasma cells within the first 10 days of treatment or complete clearance within 1 month [21].

Future Directions

There continues to be significant advances and study of novel therapeutics for multiple myeloma, and this provides the opportunity for continued study in the PCL subset. There are numerous ongoing clinical trials, some of which include study of efficacy of newer proteasome inhibitors (carfilzomib and ixazomib), peptide vaccines, second-generation immunomodulatory agent pomalidomide in combination with ixazomib, and the kinesin spindle inhibitor ARRY-520, among several others (Table 34.3). Future areas for exploration also include investigating monoclonal antibodies elotuzumab and daratumumab and utility of CAR T-cells. Of note, a new phase two prospective trial for pPCL being conducted by the European Myeloma Network is currently under way. The study looks at the use of carfilzomib in combination with lenalidomide and dexamethasone (KRD), followed by autologous transplant, then a second autologous transplant versus a non-myeloablative allogeneic transplant, and finally maintenance therapy with carfilzomib and lenalidomide. The findings of this study are eagerly anticipated and will provide further insight into the efficacy of these newer agents.

Table 34.3 Future directions for therapy in PCL: current therapeutic options being actively studied in clinical trials for PCL as single-agent and/or combination regimens

Carfilzomib (second-generation proteasome inhibitor)
Ixazomib (third-generation proteasome inhibitor)
Pomalidomide (second-generation immunomodulatory agent)
Peptide vaccines
CAR T-Cells
Venetoclax (BCL-2 inhibitor)
ARRY-520 (kinesin spindle inhibitor)
Elotuzumab, daratumumab (monoclonal antibodies)

References

1. Albarracin F, Fonseca R. Plasma cell leukemia. Blood Rev. 2011;25(3):107–12.
2. Gluzinski A, Reichenstein M. Myeloma und leucaemia lymphatica plasmocellularis. Wien Klin Wochenschr. 1906;121(5):749–57.
3. Ramsingh G, et al. Primary plasma cell leukemia: a surveillance, epidemiology, and end results database analysis between 1973 and 2004. Cancer. 2009;115(24):5734–9.
4. Ioannou MG, et al. Immunohistochemical evaluation of 95 bone marrow reactive plasmacytoses. Pathol Oncol Res. 2009;15(1):25–9.
5. Craig FE, Foon KA. Flow cytometric immunophenotyping for hematologic neoplasms. Blood. 2008;111(8):3941–67.
6. van de Donk NW, et al. How I treat plasma cell leukemia. Blood. 2012;120(12):2376–89.
7. Tiedemann RE, et al. Genetic aberrations and survival in plasma cell leukemia. Leukemia. 2008;22(5):1044–52.
8. Jimenez-Zepeda VH, Neme-Yunes Y, Braggio E. Chromosome abnormalities defined by conventional cytogenetics in plasma cell leukemia: what have we learned about its biology? Eur J Haematol. 2011;87(1):20–7.
9. Chang H, et al. Genetic aberrations including chromosome 1 abnormalities and clinical features of plasma cell leukemia. Leuk Res. 2009;33(2):259–62.
10. Rajkumar SV. Multiple myeloma: 2012 update on diagnosis, risk-stratification, and management. Am J Hematol. 2012;87(1):78–88.
11. Musto P, et al. Lenalidomide and low-dose dexamethasone for newly diagnosed primary plasma cell leukemia. Leukemia. 2014;28(1):222–5.
12. Royer B, et al. Bortezomib, doxorubicin, cyclophosphamide, dexamethasone induction followed by stem cell transplantation for primary plasma cell leukemia: a prospective phase II study of the Intergroupe Francophone du Myelome. J Clin Oncol. 2016;34(18):2125–32.
13. D'Arena G, et al. Frontline chemotherapy with bortezomib-containing combinations improves response rate and survival in primary plasma cell leukemia: a retrospective study from GIMEMA Multiple Myeloma Working Party. Ann Oncol. 2012;23(6):1499–502.
14. Pagano L, et al. Primary plasma cell leukemia: a retrospective multicenter study of 73 patients. Ann Oncol. 2011;22(7):1628–35.
15. Katodritou E, et al. Treatment with bortezomib-based regimens improves overall response and predicts for survival in patients with primary or secondary plasma cell leukemia: analysis of the Greek myeloma study group. Am J Hematol. 2014;89(2):145–50.
16. Musto P, et al. Efficacy and safety of bortezomib in patients with plasma cell leukemia. Cancer. 2007;109(11):2285–90.
17. McElwain TJ, Powles RL. High-dose intravenous melphalan for plasma-cell leukaemia and myeloma. Lancet. 1983;2(8354):822–4.
18. Drake MB, et al. Primary plasma cell leukemia and autologous stem cell transplantation. Haematologica. 2010;95(5):804–9.
19. Mahindra A, et al. Hematopoietic cell transplantation for primary plasma cell leukemia: results from the Center for International Blood and Marrow Transplant Research. Leukemia. 2012;26(5):1091–7.
20. Gonsalves WI, et al. Trends in survival of patients with primary plasma cell leukemia: a population-based analysis. Blood. 2014;124(6):907–12.
21. Dimopoulos MA, et al. Primary plasma cell leukaemia. Br J Haematol. 1994;88(4):754–9.

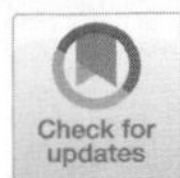

Prognosis of Myeloma/Genetics of Myeloma

35

Sébastien Robiou-Du-Pont, Jill Corre, and Hervé Avet-Loiseau

Multiple myeloma (MM) is a very heterogeneous disease. This heterogeneity is observed at all the levels: clinical, biological, and molecular. This heterogeneity translates in extremely variable length of survival, from a few weeks to more than 15 years, and even cure. MM is probably the cancer for which the highest number of prognostic parameters have been described. These prognostic factors can be divided in three parts: related to the patient's conditions, related to disease burden, and related to the tumor clone itself.

Prognostic Parameters

Patient's Conditions

The first parameter is age. As for many diseases, patients diagnosed at an earlier age display a better outcome. Several factors contribute to this survival variability. Older patients more frequently present comorbidities (cardiac, renal, pulmonary, hepatic) which could prevent the optimal delivery of therapy. Another major parameter is related to the treatment schema. It has been shown that high-dose melphalan, with autologous stem cell rescue, improved at least the progression free survival (PFS), and even overall survival (OS). However, this intensive approach is not feasible in the oldest population. Historically, the cutoff has been set at 65 years of age. With the improvement of patients' condition, it is now currently set at 70 years. All these parameters translate in a shorter OS in elderly patients, in the 5–6 years range.

S. Robiou-Du-Pont, Ph.D.
UGM—CRCT Team 13, Toulouse University Hospital—IUCT, 1, Avenue Irène Joliot-Curie, Toulouse 31059, France

J. Corre, Pharm.D., Ph.D.
Hematological Laboratory, UGM, University Hospital, IUC, 1, Avenue Irène Joliot-Curie, Toulouse 31000, France

H. Avet-Loiseau, M.D., Ph.D. (✉)
Laboratoire UGM, IUC-Oncopole,
1, Avenue Irene Joliot-Cutie, 31059 Toulouse, France
e-mail: avet-loiseau.h@chu-toulouse.fr

Tumor Burden

As in many cancers, the clinical stage is associated with outcome. In MM, this fact has been shown by Durie and Salmon [1]. Their staging system correlated with the tumor burden, even if this system is currently abandoned for prognosis assessment. The tumor burden is reflected, at least partially, by the serum β2-microglobulin level [2]. This protein is expressed at the surface of the malignant plasma cells, and is shed by proteases, and released in the serum. The outcome is linearly correlated with the β2-microglobulin levels, the highest levels being associated with the shortest survivals. This serum level is also correlated with renal function, since the protein is eliminated via the kidney. Whether the level of β2-microglobulin is prognostic in case of renal failure is still a matter of debate. β2-Microglobulin level is the basis of the International Staging System (ISS), in association with the serum albumin level (Table 35.1) [3]. This system divides the patients in three groups, with very significant differences in both PFS and OS, independently of age and treatment approach. Other parameters have been linked to the tumor burden, and especially the bone marrow involvement. Even though the mechanisms of anemia and thrombocytopenia are probably very complex in MM, it has been clearly shown that both factors were associated with a shorter OS [4].

Table 35.1 International staging system

ISS 1	β2m < 3.5 mg/L and Albumin ≥35 g/L
ISS 2	All other cases
ISS 3	β2m > 5.5 mg/L

β2m = β2-microglobulin

P.H. Wiernik et al. (eds.), *Neoplastic Diseases of the Blood*, DOI 10.1007/978-3-319-64263-5_35

Tumor Clone

Several characteristics of the tumor clone are associated with outcome. First, extra-medullary localizations are clearly associated with shorter survival. This is particularly obvious in the case of primary plasma cell leukemias, with a median OS of less than two years [5]. The causes of these extra-medullary developments are poorly understood, and might be related to the default of bone marrow homing factors expression. The second parameter is the tumor proliferation. It can be evaluated by the plasma cell labeling index (assessed by flow cytometry), or by conventional cytogenetics [6, 7]. High proliferation correlates with shorter survival. But the most important prognostic factor is certainly genetics, meaning the chromosomal/molecular abnormalities observed in the tumor plasma cells.

Genetics

Myeloma is characterized by many chromosomal changes [8]. Even though conventional karyotypes are often normal (because of the low proliferative index of the tumor plasma cells), analyses based on SNP array did show that the large majority of patients present chromosomal changes, with usually complex molecular karyotypes. Multiple myeloma can be divided in two groups based on ploidy, i.e., hyperdiploidy and non-hyperdiploidy. Hyperdiploidy is observed in at least 50% of the patients, with a nonrandom gain of specific chromosomes, i.e., chromosomes 3, 5, 7, 9, 11, 15, 19, and 21 [9]. The causes of these nonrandom gains are currently totally unknown. Non-hyperdiploidy is characterized by usual more complex karyotypes, displaying many structural abnormalities (partial gains and losses), with a specific enrichment of 14q32 translocations (60–70% of the cases). These 14q32 translocations systematically involve the *IGH* gene at 14q32, with several chromosomal partners. The most frequent partners are *CCND1* at 11q13 (15–20% of the patients) [10], *MMSET* and *FGFR3* at 4p16 (12–15% of the patients) [11], and *MAF* at 16q23 (3% of the patients) [12]. These specific translocations are due to errors during the physiological class switch and hypermutation processes. What is unknown so far is the specificity of the partners.

Many other chromosomal changes have been identified, including monosomy 13, gain of 1q, and losses of the 1p, 8p, 14q, 16q, and 17p regions. At the molecular level, frequent rearrangements of the *MYC* locus have been described. Recent exome sequencing studies revealed another level of heterogeneity [13–16]. No specific gene mutation has been observed. The most frequently mutated genes were *KRAS* (~20%), *NRAS* (~15%), *DIS3*, *TP53*, *BRAF*, and many others. Compared with other hematopoietic tumors, and especially with leukemias, MM present a high number of mutations. In contrast, if compared with solid tumors, the mutation load is low.

Prognostic Impact of Chromosomal Abnormalities

Many of the chromosomal changes observed in the tumor plasma cells are associated with specific outcomes (Table 35.2). Very few "good risk" abnormalities have been described, in contrast to "high-risk" changes. Most of these prognostic values have been described with old treatment strategies, and have to be reevaluated in the context of novel therapies.

High-Risk Features

The first chromosomal abnormality associated with a shorter PFS and OS has been del(13q14) [17]. Actually, this chromosomal loss is mainly due to chromosome 13 monosomies. Further studies did show that monosomy 13 does not present an intrinsic prognostic value [4]. The shorter PFS and OS observed in old studies were in fact related to the frequent association of monosomy 13 with the specific t(4;14) and del(17p) (80% of those cases).

The loss of part of the chromosome 17 short arm has been associated with very dismal outcome [18]. The minimal target region is currently unknown, even though all the studies did focus on the 17p13 region, and more specifically on the *TP53* gene. The *TP53* gene is a tumor suppressor gene, and per se, has to be mutated on the second allele to display its oncogenic properties. Several studies did address this issue, and none of them did show a systematic mutation on the remaining allele [14, 19], in contrast to what has been observed in chronic lymphoid leukemia or diffuse large B-cell lymphoma. In the 30–50% of the cases presenting a *TP53* mutation, *TP53* is probably the target gene. In the 50–70% remaining cases, other gene(s) are probably the cause of the prognostic impact of del(17p) losses. A recent study in a mouse model of leukemia/lymphoma did suggest that the loss of several genes in the *TP53* vicinity is associated with tumorigenesis [20]. This paradigm has to be dem-

Table 35.2 Prognostic value of cytogenetic abnormalities

t(4;14)	High Risk
Del(17p)	High Risk
1q gain	High Risk
Del(1p32)	High Risk
Trisomy 3	Good Risk
Trisomy 5	Good Risk
Trisomy 21	High Risk

onstrated in MM. However, all the cases of del(17p) (7–10% of the patients) are associated with a poor outcome, independently of *TP53* mutations. This poor outcome is not related to lower response to therapy, but to a shorter PFS. Recent clinical studies in relapse patients with novel proteasome inhibitors such as carfilzomib and ixazomib did show that this prognostic impact might be overcome, at least partially [21, 22]. This important finding has to be confirmed in the frontline setting, but may lead to a new paradigm in the therapeutic strategy for these specific patients. One hot topic is the relationship between the prognostic impact and the size of clone harboring the deletion. It has been suggested that the deletion is impacting the survival only if present in the major subclone [4]. This issue is currently evaluated.

The second important prognostic parameter is the translocation t(4;14). The target gene on chromosome 14 is *IGH*. This gene is targeted in many B-cell malignancies, but in contrast to the other translocations, the t(4;14) is peculiar since it disrupts two genes on chromosome 4: *FGFR3* and *MMSET* [11]. The *FGFR3* gene is displaced on chromosome 14, leading to its overexpression in a classical mechanism. In contrast, the *MMSET* gene remains on chromosome 4, and is upregulated through a novel fusion gene, *Eμ-MMSET*. The most important event is probably this latter one, for at least two reasons: (1) in 1/3 of the patients presenting the t(4;14), *FGFR3* is lost through an unbalanced translocation [23], and (2) the prognostic impact of the translocation is the same, independently of the translocation configuration [24]. The *MMSET* gene is a methyl-transferase, and its upregulation leads to a chromatin configuration modification, that may modify the expression of many target genes. Observed in 12–15% of the patients, the prognostic value of t(4;14) has been clearly shown in the context of old drugs [4]. Since the availability of proteasome inhibitors such as bortezomib, its prognostic impact is more questionable. Several studies did show that bortezomib may partially overcome this impact [25], and this fact has been recently confirmed in studies using second generation proteasome inhibitors such as carfilzomib and ixazomib [21, 22].

Other factors have been shown to negatively impact the prognosis. Extra-copies of the chromosome 1 long arm (1q gains) are observed in about 1/3 of the patients, and have been shown to be associated with a shorter survival [26]. However, the prognostic value of 1q gains seems to be lower than del(17p) or t(4;14). Since in the large majority of the cases the whole 1q is gained, it is difficult to find a single target gene which could drive the prognosis. The chromosome 1 does also drive the prognosis through deletions of the short arm (del(1p)). Several regions can be involved, but the most important seems to be the 1p32 region, targeting the *FAF1* and/or *CDKN2C* genes [27]. These del(1p32) are observed in 7–8% of the patients, and are associated with a dismal outcome.

Table 35.3 Revised-international staging system

R-ISS 1	ISS 1 *and* no high-risk cytogenetics *and* LDH = Normal
R-ISS 2	All other cases
R-ISS 3	ISS 3 *and* [high-risk cytogenetics *or* LDH > Normal]

High-risk cytogenetics = del(17p), or t(4;14), or t(14;16)

Good/Standard Risk Features

Some studies did suggest that hyperdiploidy may be associated with a better outcome. However, these studies were based on conventional cytogenetics, and so the results are restricted to patients presenting a proliferative disease. Two studies did address the issue of the impact of trisomies in the high-risk patients, with totally opposite results [28, 29]. A third study based on SNP array did show that only some specific trisomies (chromosome 3 and 5) improve the outcome of high-risk features. In contrast, another trisomy (chromosome 21) worsens the prognosis [30].

In conclusion, cytogenetics is probably the most important prognostic parameter in MM. But all the abnormalities should be analyzed more globally, some high-risk changes could become standard risk if combined with some trisomies. A first attempt has been proposed by IMWG with the R-ISS (Revised-International Staging System), which combines ISS with chromosomal abnormalities (Table 35.3) [31]. In the future, global analyses including ISS and multiparametric genetic analyses may contribute to define high risk more precisely, but also good and standard risk groups.

Prognostic Impact of Gene Expression Profiling

Besides the chromosomal changes, MM is also characterized by abnormalities in the gene expression profiles (GEP) . In 2006, the Arkansas group proposed a MM classification based on similarities of GEP [32]. This classification is mostly driven by the chromosomal changes, i.e., 14q32 translocations and hyperdiploidy. Two other subgroups, corresponding to "proliferation" and "bone disease" were identified. This molecular classification has been partially confirmed by a study by the HOVON group [33]. The "low bone disease" group was not confirmed. In contrast, three other groups were identified: one group enriched by "myeloid" genes (that could be related to plasma cell sorting problems), one group characterized by overexpression of cancer testis antigen genes, and finally a group defined by overexpression of positive regulators of the NFκB pathway. However, these classifications, based on gene expression, were not translated into prognostic subgroups. Different studies based on GEP did identify a high-risk group [33–35]. Of note, these different prognostic models, based on variable number of genes, do not share any common gene. Whether these discrepancies are due to different algorithms to identify the high-risk signatures, or to differences in the treatments used in the training cohort is still unresolved.

Prognostic Impact of Next Generation Sequencing

Next generation sequencing (NGS) has been used to analyze the different mutations present in the tumor plasma cells. At least four studies based on exome sequencing have been published, with a total of more than 700 patients analyzed [13–15, 36]. So far, preliminary results are rather disappointing, without the identification of significant group of patients who would present a good or poor prognosis. All these studies describe subclonality, but none of them did show that this process can be useful in either prognostic assessment, or adaptation of treatment strategies. Whether the number of mutations per patient is prognostic is still unresolved.

Conclusions

The assessment of prognosis in patients with MM is mandatory at diagnosis. The most important variables are age, ISS, and cytogenetic changes, summarized in the R-ISS. In the future, the development of multiparametric systems will probably enable to improve this assessment.

References

1. Salmon SE, Durie BG. Cellular kinetics in multiple myeloma. A new approach to staging and treatment. Arch Intern Med. 1975;135:131–8.
2. Bataille R, Durie BG, Grenier J. Serum beta2 microglobulin and survival duration in multiple myeloma: a simple reliable marker for staging. Br J Haematol. 1983;55:439–47.
3. Greipp PR, San Miguel J, Durie BG, Crowley JJ, Barlogie B, Bladé J, et al. International staging system for multiple myeloma. J Clin Oncol. 2005;23:3412–20.
4. Avet-Loiseau H, Attal M, Moreau P, Charbonnel C, Garban F, Hulin C, et al. Genetic abnormalities and survival in multiple myeloma: the experience of the Intergroupe Francophone du Myélome. Blood. 2007;109:3489–95.
5. Avet-Loiseau H, Roussel M, Campion L, Leleu X, Marit G, Jardel H, et al. Cytogenetic and therapeutic characterization of primary plasma cell leukemia: the IFM experience. Leukemia. 2012;26:158–9.
6. Greipp PR, Lust JA, O'Fallon WM, Katzmann JA, Witzig TE, Kyle RA. Plasma cell labeling index and beta 2-microglobulin predict survival independent of thymidine kinase and C-reactive protein in multiple myeloma. Blood. 1993;81:3382–7.
7. Barlogie B, Pineda-Roman M, van Rhee F, Haessler J, Anaissie E, Hollmig K, et al. Thalidomide arm of Total Therapy 2 improves complete remission duration and survival in myeloma patients with metaphase cytogenetic abnormalities. Blood. 2008;112:3115–21.
8. Carrasco DR, Tonon G, Huang Y, Zhang Y, Sinha R, Feng B, et al. High-resolution genomic profiles define distinct clinicopathogenetic subgroups of multiple myeloma patients. Cancer Cell. 2006;9:313–25.
9. Smadja NV, Bastard C, Brigaudeau C, Leroux D, Fruchart C. Hypodiploidy is a major prognostic factor in multiple myeloma. Blood. 2001;98:2229–38.
10. Fonseca R, Blood EA, Oken MM, Kyle RA, Dewald GW, Bailey RJ, et al. Myeloma and the t(11;14)(q13;q32): evidence for a biologically defined unique subset of patients. Blood. 2002;99:3735–41.
11. Chesi M, Nardini E, Brents LA, Schröck E, Ried T, Kuehl WM, et al. Frequent Translocation t(4;14)(p16.3;q32.3) in multiple myeloma is associated with increased expression and activating mutations of fibroblast growth factor receptor 3. Nat Genet. 1997;16:260–4.
12. Hurt EM, Wiestner A, Rosenwald A, Shaffer AL, Campo E, Grogan T, et al. Overexpression of *c-maf* is a frequent oncogenic event in multiple myeloma that promotes proliferation and pathological interactions with bone marrow stroma. Cancer Cell. 2004;5:191–9.
13. Chapman MA, Lawrence MS, Keats JJ, Cibulskis K, Sougnez C, Schinzel AC, et al. Initial genome sequencing and analysis of multiple myeloma. Nature. 2011;471:467–72.
14. Bolli N, Avet-Loiseau H, Wedge DC, Van Loo P, Alexandrov LB, Martincorena I, et al. Heterogeneity of genomic evolution and mutational profiles in multiple myeloma. Nat Commun. 2014;5:2997.
15. Lohr JG, Stojanov P, Carter SL, Cruz-Gordillo P, Lawrence MS, Auclair D, et al. Widespread genetic heterogeneity in multiple myeloma: implications for targeted therapy. Cancer Cell. 2014;25:91–101.
16. Walker BA, Wardell CP, Murison A, Boyle EM, Begum DB, Dahir NM, et al. APOBEC family mutational signatures are associated with poor prognosis translocations in multiple myeloma. Nat Commun. 2015;6:1–11.
17. Facon T, Avet-Loiseau H, Guillerm G, Moreau P, Geneviève F, Zandecki M, et al. Chromosome 13 abnormalities identified by FISH analysis and serum beta2-microglobulin produce a powerful myeloma staging system for patients receiving high dose therapy. Blood. 2001;97:1566–71.
18. Chang H, Qi C, Yi QL, Reece D, Stewart AK. *p53* gene deletion detected by fluorescence in situ hybridization is an adverse prognostic factor for patients with multiple myeloma following autologous stem cell transplantation. Blood. 2005;105:358–60.
19. Lode L, Eveillard M, Trichet V, Soussi T, Wuilleme S, Richebourg S, et al. Mutations in TP53 are exclusively associated with del(17p) in multiple myeloma. Haematologica. 2010;95:1973–6.
20. Liu Y, Chen C, Xu Z, Scuoppo C, Rillahan CD, Gao J, et al. Deletions linked to TP53 loss drive cancer through p53-independent mechanisms. Nature. 2016;531:471–5.
21. Stewart AK, Rajkumar SV, Dimopoulos MA, Masszi T, Špička I, Oriol A, et al. Carfilzomib, lenalidomide, and dexamethasone for relapsed multiple myeloma. N Engl J Med. 2015;372:142–52.
22. Moreau P, Masszi T, Grzasko N, Bahlis NJ, Hansson M, Pour L, et al. Oral ixazomib, lenalidomide, and dexamethasone for multiple myeloma. N Engl J Med. 2016;374:1621–34.
23. Santra M, Zhan F, Tian E, Barlogie B, Shaughnessy J. A subset of multiple myeloma harboring the t(4;14)(p16;q32) translocation lacks FGFR3 expression but maintains an IGH/MMSET fusion transcript. Blood. 2003;101:2374–6.
24. Hebraud B, Magrangeas F, Cleynen A, Lauwers-Cances V, Chretien ML, Hulin C, et al. Role of additional chromosomal changes in the prognostic value of t(4;14) and del(17p) in multiple myeloma: the IFM experience. Blood. 2015;125:2095–100.
25. Avet-Loiseau H, Leleu X, Roussel M, Moreau P, Guerin-Charbonnel C, Caillot D, et al. Bortezomib plus dexamethasone induction improves outcome of patients with t(4;14) myeloma but not outcome of patients with del(17p). J Clin Oncol. 2010;28:4630–4.

26. Hanamura I, Stewart JP, Huang Y, Zhan F, Santra M, Sawyer JR, et al. Frequent gain of chromosome band 1q21 in plasma-cell dyscrasias detected by fluorescence in situ hybridization: incidence increases from MGUS to relapsed myeloma and is related to prognosis and disease progression following tandem stem-cell transplantation. Blood. 2006;108:1724–32.
27. Hebraud B, Leleu X, Lauwers-Cances V, Roussel M, Caillot D, Marit G, et al. Deletion of the 1p32 region is a major independent prognostic factor in young patients with myeloma: The IFM experience on 1195 patients. Leukemia. 2014;28:675–9.
28. Kumar S, Fonseca R, Ketterling RP, Dispenzieri A, Lacy MQ, Gertz MA, et al. Trisomies in multiple myeloma: impact on survival in patients with high-risk cytogenetics. Blood. 2012;119:2100–5.
29. Pawlyn C, Melchor L, Murison A, Wardell CP, Brioli A, Boyle EM, et al. Coexistent hyperdiploidy does not abrogate poor prognosis in myeloma with adverse cytogenetics and may precede *IGH* translocations. Blood. 2015;125:831–40.
30. Chretien ML, Corre J, Lauwers-Cances V, Magrangeas F, Cleynen A, Yon E, et al. Understanding the role of hyperdiploidy in myeloma prognosis: which trisomies really matter? Blood. 2015;126:2713–9.
31. Palumbo A, Avet-Loiseau H, Oliva S, Lokhorst HM, Goldschmidt H, Rosinol L, et al. Revised international staging system for multiple myeloma: a report from International Myeloma Working Group. J Clin Oncol. 2015;33:2863–9.
32. Zhan F, Huang Y, Colla S, Stewart JP, Hanamura I, Gupta S, et al. The molecular classification of multiple myeloma. Blood. 2006;108:2020–8.
33. Broyl A, Hose D, Lokhorst H, de Knegt Y, Peeters J, Jauch A, et al. Gene expression profiling for molecular classification of multiple myeloma in newly diagnosed patients. Blood. 2010. https://doi.org/10.1182/blood-2009-12-261032.
34. Decaux O, Lodé L, Magrangeas F, Charbonnel C, Gouraud W, Jézéquel P, et al. Prediction of survival in multiple myeloma based on gene-expression profiles revealed cell cycle and chromosomal instability signatures in high-risk patients and hyperdiploid signatures in low-risk patients. J Clin Oncol. 2008;26:4798–805.
35. Shaughnessy JD, Zhan F, Burrington BE, Huang Y, Colla S, Hanamura I, et al. A validated gene expression model of high-risk multiple myeloma is defined by deregulated expression of genes mapping to chromosome 1. Blood. 2007;109:2276–84.
36. Walker BA, Boyle EM, Wardell CP, Murison A, Begum DB, Dahir NM, et al. Mutational spectrum, copy number changes, and outcome: results of a sequencing study of patients with newly diagnosed myeloma. J Clin Oncol. 2015;33:3911–20.

Immunoglobulin Light Chain Amyloidosis (AL)

36

Morie A. Gertz, Francis K. Buadi, Taimur Sher, and Angela Dispenzieri

History

"The term 'lardaceous change' has … come more into use chiefly through the instrumentality of the Vienna School… The term 'lardaceous changes' … has but very little to do with these tumors, and rather refers to things, upon which the old writers … who are better connoisseurs in bacon than our friends in Vienna, would hardly have bestowed such a name [1]… The appearance of such organs … are said to look like bacon, bears … a much greater resemblance to wax and I have, therefore, now for a long time … made use of the term waxy change… These structures … are the simple action of iodine … assume just as blue a color as vegetable start…"

In this publication by Rudolph Virchow [2], he decides that amyloid must be made of starch. The iodine reaction turning amyloid deposits blue is a throwback to high school chemistry when iodine will stain the open face of a potato blue, documenting it as starch. At the same time, Prof. Virchow directly insults his chief competitor of the day, Rokitansky, who had previously written about lardaceous changes because of the greasy texture the liver of an amyloid patient would have and implies that the Viennese School is incapable of distinguishing amyloid from bacon, reflecting the intense competitive nature of two leaders during the age of medical discovery.

M.A. Gertz, M.D. (✉) • F.K. Buadi, M.D.
Department of Hematology, Mayo Clinic, Rochester, MN, USA
e-mail: Gertz.morie@mayo.edu

T. Sher, M.D.
Division of Hematology and Internal Medicine, Mayo Clinic, Jacksonville, FL, USA

A. Dispenzieri, M.D.
Division of Hematology and Internal Medicine, Mayo Clinic, Rochester, MN, USA

Mayo Medical School, Rochester, MN, USA

The term "amyloid" was first used in 1838 by Schleiden to describe a normal constituent of plants. Virchow, in 1858, gave a lecture entitled, "Amyloid Degeneration." Virchow's conclusion that amyloid substance was starch continues today, where amyloid means amyl-like or starch-like. In 1859, Friedreich, Nikolau, and Kekule indicated that the waxy spleen described by Virchow did not contain starch and that the deposits were derived from protein.

Budd analyzed the liver of a patient with amyloidosis and found it was not lardaceous. Wilks described a 52-year-old patient that had lardaceous change that was unrelated to any secondary cause and may have been the first description of AL. Schmiedeberg, in 1920, indicated that amyloid was composed of amino acids and strongly resembled the composition of serum globulin. In 1922, Bennhold first used Congo red as a specific stain. Five years later, Divry and Florkin reported green birefringence under polarized light when amyloid-laden brain from an Alzheimer's patient was stained with Congo red. In 1931, Magnus-Levy postulated that Bence-Jones proteins were a precursor of the amyloid substance and noted that there was a relationship between amyloid, Bence-Jones protein, and multiple myeloma. Cohen and Calkins published in 1959 that, under electron microscopy, all forms of amyloid were fibrils of indefinite length but a constant width of 9.5 nm [3]. Apitz claimed that amyloid in tissues was analogous to the excretion of light chain proteins by the kidneys and coined the term "paraprotein" to describe monoclonal immunoglobulins. Isobe and Osserman, in 1974, published that Bence-Jones proteins had a direct role in the pathogenesis of AL [4]. In 1968, Eanes and Glenner reported by X-ray diffraction [5] that amyloid proteins formed an alternate three-dimensional configuration of a beta-pleated sheet [6] unlike the normal alpha-helical configuration of proteins. Amyloid proteins are highly resistant to solvents, and the first amyloid extraction relied on this insolubility by repeated centrifugations in saline where the supernatant, containing all the soluble compounds, would be

P.H. Wiernik et al. (eds.), *Neoplastic Diseases of the Blood*, DOI 10.1007/978-3-319-64263-5_36

discarded, and the residual pellet contained all the amyloid and could be suspended in distilled water. Amyloid was first purified in 1968 [7]. The first sequence of an immunoglobulin light chain amyloid was reported in 1970 as the N-terminal fragment of the immunoglobulin light chain.

Introduction

Amyloid is a vague term that describes a group of disorders that have only one thing in common, and that is the deposition of protein fibrils composed of protofibrils. The clinical presentation depends on the organ involved and the protein subunit structure of the amyloid protein. These heterogenous disorders are classed together because they share common tinctorial properties of an amorphous eosinophilic deposit when stained with hematoxylin and eosin, and distinct binding to the cotton-wool dye, Congo red, in the sine qua non of green birefringence when viewed under polarized light [8]. Congo red is an imperfect stain insofar as there is a measurable false-positive rate either due to trapping of dye in thick sections or the misinterpretation of white birefringence as green and points out the importance of having positive and negative controls whenever amyloid is diagnosed.

The immunoglobulin fragments that compose AL amyloidosis are thermodynamically unstable and will demonstrate misfolding into the β-pleated sheet configuration [9]. It is possible to synthetically create amyloid fibrils by pepsin digestion of monoclonal immunoglobulin light chains.

Injection into mice of purified immunoglobulin light chains from the urine of patients with multiple myeloma does not produce any pathologic deposits. However, when light chains extracted from the urine of patients with amyloidosis are injected into mice, amyloid deposits do develop, reflecting the importance of [10] the amino acid structure of the immunoglobulin light chain in predisposing to misfolding into an amyloid configuration. Amyloid associated with the λ6 subgroup of light chains is virtually always associated with amyloidosis, and nearly 60% of patients with light chain amyloidosis have a λ light chain compared to only one-third of patients that have multiple myeloma [11].

As part of the standard evaluation of light chain amyloidosis, a bone marrow is routinely performed. Patients that fulfill criteria for multiple myeloma with >10% plasma cells or have myeloma-associated CRAB criteria (hypercalcemia, cast nephropathy, anemia due to marrow infiltration or bone lesions) have a shortened survival when compared with patients with light chain amyloidosis and <10% plasma cells, and this has important therapeutic implications with regard to systemic chemotherapy [12]. Renal insufficiency in amyloidosis is not due to cast formation in the tubule but due to progressive destruction of the glomerular basement membrane and loss of glomeruli associated with long-standing proteinuria that results in tubular atrophy [13].

Amyloidosis does not appear to be neoplastic, although it is clonal. Monitoring of the bone marrow over time in a patient with amyloidosis does not show the proliferative characteristics that myeloma patients have where, left untreated, the bone marrow plasma cell percentage rises over time [14]. In light chain amyloidosis, the disorder is far more static. Moreover, although patients with light chain amyloidosis have a high frequency of t(11;14), high-risk features such as seen in multiple myeloma such as -17p, t(4;14), or t(14;16) are lacking [15]. If multiple myeloma is not present at the time of diagnosis, it will subsequently develop in <1% of patients. Even in those patients that have a high proportion of plasma cells in the bone marrow, the cause of death is generally amyloid-related organ failure and not the typical problems associated with end-stage myeloma such as pancytopenia and infection [16, 17].

Amyloidosis is thought to occur in approximately eight patients per million per year and is approximately one-fifth as common as multiple myeloma [18]. Although recent estimates are not available, since the current incidence of multiple myeloma in the United States is 24,000 new patients per year, it is reasonable to speculate that the number of new patients with light chain amyloidosis is approximately 5000 annually. Translocations of the immunoglobulin heavy chain locus located on chromosome 14, band 14q32, have been reported in 55% of patients with light chain amyloidosis. Cyclin D1 overexpression accounts for 76% of all IgH translocations [19].

Symptoms and Signs of Amyloidosis

The most common symptoms associated with amyloidosis are weight loss, fatigue, edema, dyspnea on exertion, and paresthesias [20]. Unfortunately, these common symptoms of AL are nonspecific and are generally not helpful in determining when the diagnosis should be suspected and when to launch an investigation. Extreme weight loss usually results in a futile search for metastatic malignancy [21]. Fatigue, which can be related to early cardiac or renal involvement, can be quite subtle since the restrictive cardiomyopathy is usually associated with a normal ejection fraction and a cardiac etiology may be overlooked. Reduced filling, seen in the heart during diastole, will result in a decline in systolic blood pressure, but it is often difficult to associate this with the presence of an infiltrative cardiomyopathy [22]. Typically, patients with cardiac amyloid have normal coronary arteries; and not infrequently, coronary angiography is performed, and the patient's symptoms are interpreted as being noncardiac in origin [23].

Lightheadedness and orthostatic syncope occurs in a significant proportion of patients [24]. Patients that have significant proteinuria and hypoalbuminemia lose oncotic effect, and serum will, therefore, transude from the intravascular space into the extravascular, extracellular space. This results in contraction in the intravascular volume and can lead to orthostatic hypotension. Diuretics used to manage the edema that patients with hypoalbuminemia have will frequently result in further hypotension and reduced renal blood flow and resultant rise in serum creatinine level. When these patients undergo echocardiography, it is common to see thickening of the walls, which is often interpreted as hypertrophy, which is then considered a reflection of untreated hypertension or workload hypertrophy, since valvular insufficiency is often seen on echocardiography [25].

Occasional patients will have autonomic failure as the cause of their orthostatic hypotension. This is generally associated with peripheral neuropathy and other signs of autonomic dysfunction, such as upper intestinal dysmotility with pseudo-obstruction and vomiting or lower intestinal dysmotility with alternating obstipation and intractable diarrhea [26]. Since the symptoms associated with light chain amyloidosis are often vague, clinicians may rely on the signs of amyloidosis to lead to a diagnosis. Unfortunately, the signs, which are highly specific, are quite insensitive. The classic pinch or periorbital purpura (Fig. 36.1) seen with amyloidosis is seen in <20% of patients [27]. Clues are that the purpura tends to stop at the nipple line; can be periorbital or petechiae on the eyelids; and can be seen on the webbing of the neck, malar regions, and upper chest. These purpura have been misinterpreted as being senile purpura in an elderly population. Hepatomegaly is present in only 10% of patients and is rarely over 5 cm below the right costal margin. Splenomegaly and splenic rupture are rarely seen [28].

Macroglossia is the most specific finding of amyloidosis (Fig. 36.2). Patients can be misdiagnosed as tongue cancer, acromegaly, and hypothyroidism [29]. Tongue enlargement with submandibular indentations, due to pressure on the lower row of teeth, is quite specific for immunoglobulin light chain amyloidosis and, virtually, is never seen in AA or TTR amyloidosis. Tongue enlargement, however, is seen in only approximately 10% of patients and is very easy to overlook unless massive and interferes with the patient's ability to swallow or concomitant sleep apnea when supine. Tongue enlargement is associated with bilateral enlargement of the submandibular salivary glands. Dry mouth can be seen and can be misdiagnosed as Sjögren syndrome [30].

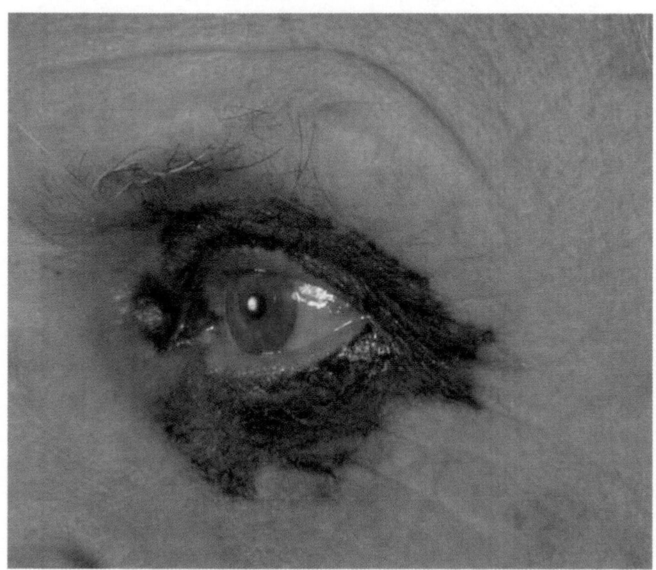

Fig. 36.1 Periorbital purpura in amyloidosis

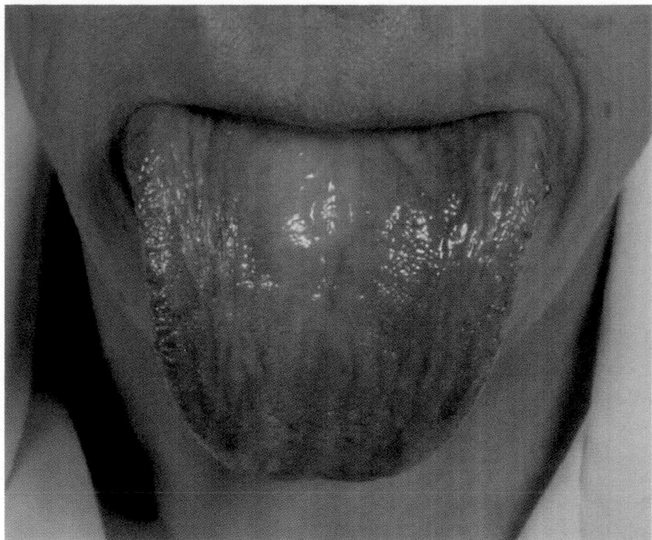

Fig. 36.2 Enlarged tongue in an AL amyloidosis patient

Occasional patients have diffuse small vessel amyloidosis that can cause calf, jaw [31], or buttock claudication with exertion and is difficult to distinguish from pseudoclaudication related to spinal stenosis. A rare patient will have coronary arteriolar amyloid deposits that will result in exertional angina [32]. A very rare finding is periarticular amyloid deposition leading to the shoulder-pad sign (Fig. 36.3), which represents pseudohypertrophy of the shoulder joint. As a consequence, if one waits for the signs of amyloidosis to develop, the majority of patients will be overlooked [33].

Diagnosis of Amyloidosis

The diagnosis of amyloidosis is best suspected when patients fulfill one of the five following criteria [34] (Fig. 36.4):

1. Diastolic heart failure, heart failure with preserved ejection fraction, or infiltrative cardiomyopathy
2. Nephrotic range proteinuria in a nondiabetic
3. Unexplained hepatomegaly with alkaline phosphatase elevation with no history of malignancy
4. A progressive demyelinating peripheral neuropathy with paresthesias that is generally painless
5. A patient presenting to the hematologist with "atypical" multiple myeloma where fatigue and edema are the

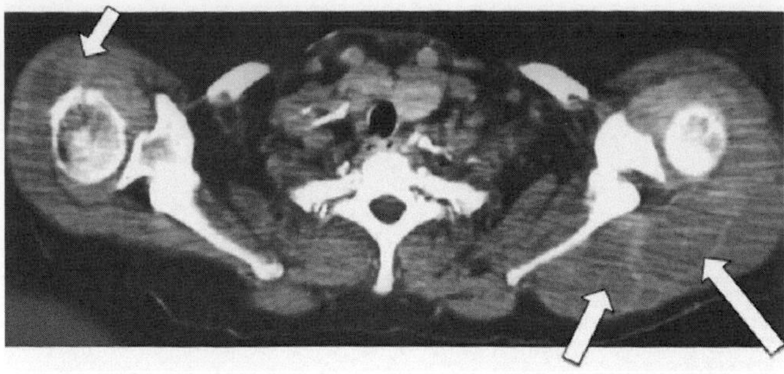

Fig. 36.3 CT scan of the shoulder showing periarticular infiltration (shoulder pad sign)

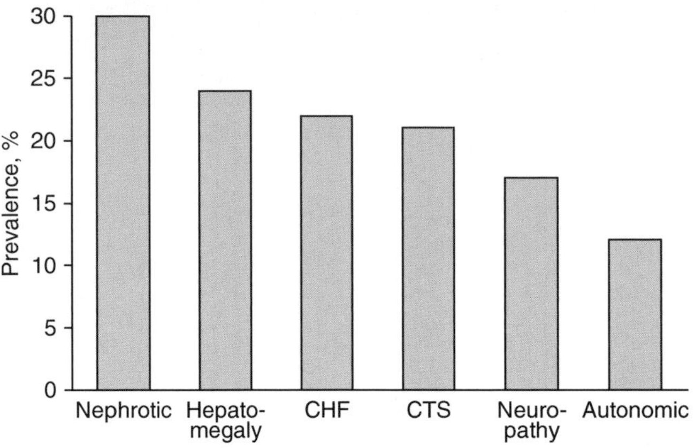

Fig. 36.4 Prevalence of clinical syndromes in AL

presenting symptoms rather than the classical CRAB criteria of anemia, renal insufficiency, or bone disease

In patients that present with any of these symptoms, the first screening should be immunofixation of the serum and an immunoglobulin free light chain assay [35]. Nearly all patients with immunoglobulin light chain amyloidosis will have an abnormal involved free light chain or the presence of a monoclonal protein on serum immunofixation. A positive result would be a powerful clue to the origin of the patient's symptoms and is quite sensitive with only 1% of amyloid patients failing to have a monoclonal protein [36]. The test is specific since only 3% of the adult population will have an incidental monoclonal gammopathy of undetermined significance. Using sensitive techniques, whether immunohistochemistry or flow cytometry of the bone marrow, a clonal population of plasma cells can be demonstrated [37]. All patients with a monoclonal gammopathy of undetermined significance that have any symptoms of dyspnea or fatigue should have the urine screened and should be screened with cardiac biomarkers to exclude the possibility of an infiltrative cardiomyopathy [38].

A clonal population of plasma cells is observed in virtually all patients with AL, even when the marrow percentage of plasma cells is 1–2% [39]. The amyloid deposits of light chain amyloidosis are derived, usually, from a fragment of the immunoglobulin light chain variable region. The source of this light chain (which averages approximately 12 kDa or half the molecular weight of a normal intact immunoglobulin light chain) is the clonal plasma cell population. An immunoglobulin free light chain assay is important for screening any patients with dyspnea, neuropathy, and proteinuria. Serum immunofixation will fail to detect a monoclonal light chain in nearly a quarter of patients. The light chain levels are low in AL, and a high percentage of the light chain passes through the glomerular basement membrane into the urine, and there is no discernible monoclonal peak in the serum [40]. The immunoglobulin free light chain assay is ten times more sensitive than serum immunofixation, capable of detecting levels as low as 2 mg/dL; where serum protein electrophoresis detects peaks of 200 mg/dL, and the estimated sensitivity of immunofixation is 20 mg/dL [41].

The plasma cells in patients with light chain amyloidosis are λ in nearly 70% of patients. If a patient with known amyloidosis does not have a monoclonal protein in the serum, polyclonal bone marrow plasma cells, and normal levels of immunoglobulin free light chain, the amyloidosis should be considered either localized or, if systemic, it should be considered an inherited or acquired form of non-AL until proven otherwise [42].

All forms of amyloid contain approximately 15% glycoprotein by weight, consisting of amyloid P component. Mass spectroscopic analysis identifies P component in all amyloid deposits [43]. The function of amyloid P component remains unknown, but no human has ever been described lacking amyloid P component, suggesting it performs a vital function. Outside of the United States, imaging with I123-labeled amyloid P component can be used to identify amyloid deposits in vivo [44]. Patients that have high amyloid burdens have shorter survival. P component is also a potential target of antibody therapy as will be described in the treatment section [45].

Serialized imaging with P component has been used to assess response and progression to therapeutic interventions [46]. P component scanning is incapable of distinguishing among the various forms of amyloid deposits. The heart cannot be imaged with the P component scan, and kidneys are not well seen. The correlation between imaging findings and the extent of organ dysfunction assessed biochemically is not good. However, the diagnostic sensitivity of SAP scintigraphy for AL amyloidosis is 90% [47].

Biopsy Proof of Amyloidosis

At the time of diagnosis, amyloidosis is widespread, and extensive involvement of microvessels is characteristic. As a consequence, it is possible to biopsy nearly any site to obtain a diagnosis. Although biopsy of an affected organ (such as heart, kidney, liver, and nerve) will yield a diagnosis, the widespread nature of the disorder allows one to establish a histologic diagnosis noninvasively. Biopsy of the skin [48], subcutaneous fat, bone marrow [49], and gingiva [50] are highly sensitive and easily accessible (Fig. 36.5). Fine needle aspiration of the fat will yield a diagnosis in 75% of patients [51], but a trial comparing subcutaneous fat aspiration with surgical biopsy demonstrated a higher yield with surgical biopsy [52]. Biopsy of these less-invasive sites reduces the risk of bleeding that has been reported with liver and kidney biopsies. Endoscopic biopsy of the stomach, jejunum, and colon will also yield a diagnosis in nearly 95% of patients, usually localized to submucosal blood vessels [53]. Endoscopy can be performed then as an outpatient, and the risk of GI hemorrhage is quite small. Labial salivary gland biopsy has been reported for its ability to diagnose amyloidosis noninvasively [54].

The specificity of a subcutaneous fat aspirate is 99%, and the false-positive rate is 1%. Concordance between pathologists is 95%, and the tissue is suitable for mass spectroscopic analysis of the amyloid deposits [55]. At our center, trained nurses perform both the subcutaneous fat aspiration and the bone marrow biopsy as a single procedure that allows two samples to be submitted for analysis and an overall sensitivity to detect amyloidosis of 85%. A bone marrow is required to estimate the percentage of plasma cells, and it is convenient to do both procedures at a single setting. Caution is required when interpreting the Congo red stain because of the risk of false-positives [56]. Rectal biopsy specimens [57] with amyloid have been misinterpreted as collagenous colitis. As a screening technique in our laboratories, the myocardial biopsies are stained with sulfated Alcian blue; and in our peripheral nerve laboratory, crystal violet screening is used subsequently confirmed with Congo red [58].

Identifying the Type of Amyloid

Once amyloid has been recognized by a pathologist on tissue section, classification of the type of amyloid is required. Immunohistochemical staining with commercial antisera has been promoted as a highly sensitive technique. There are major drawbacks with the use of antibody-mediated techniques to identify amyloid deposits [59] (Fig. 36.6). Since the immunoglobulin protein in light chain amyloidosis is only a fragment of the immunoglobulin light chain, constant portions may be deleted [60]. Most commercial antisera identify light chains by binding to the constant region, and with the deletion of constant immunoglobulin fragment the epitope cannot be recognized [61]. Moreover, one characteristic of the light chains in amyloid is misfolding of the light chain, which can result in suppression of the epitopes that commercial antisera recognize buried within the misfolded protein [62]. As a consequence, particularly for immunoglobulin light chain amyloidosis, immunohistochemistry lacks sensitivity. It has been repeatedly demonstrated that immunohistochemistry is an excellent technique for the recognition of both TTR and AA amyloidosis. Unfortunately, there are over a dozen recognized forms of amyloidosis, which include

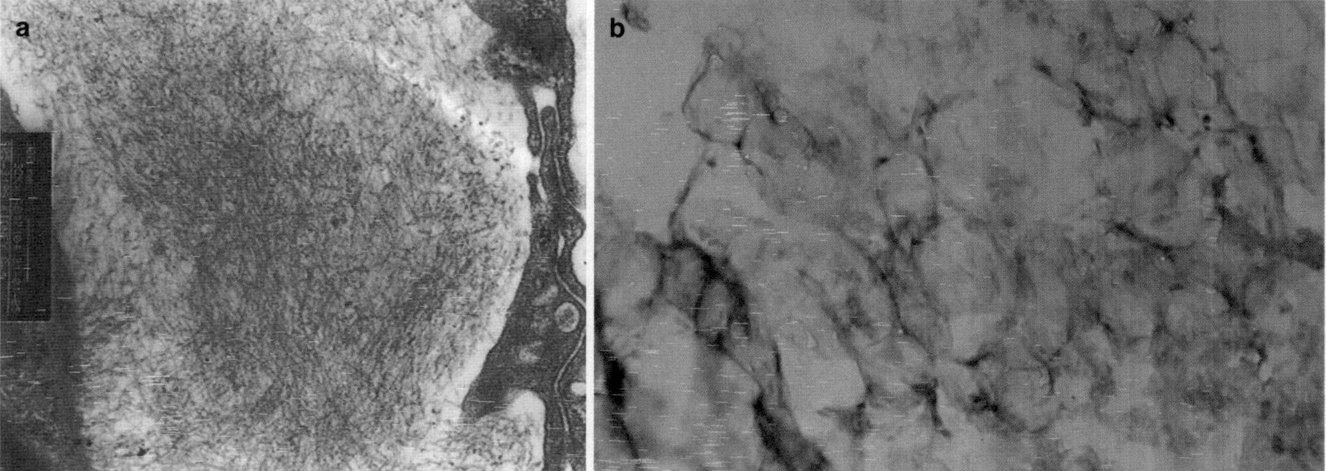

Fig. 36.5 (**a**) Electronic micrograph of amyloid fibrils (published from the prior book chapter). (**b**) Congo red stained fat aspiration

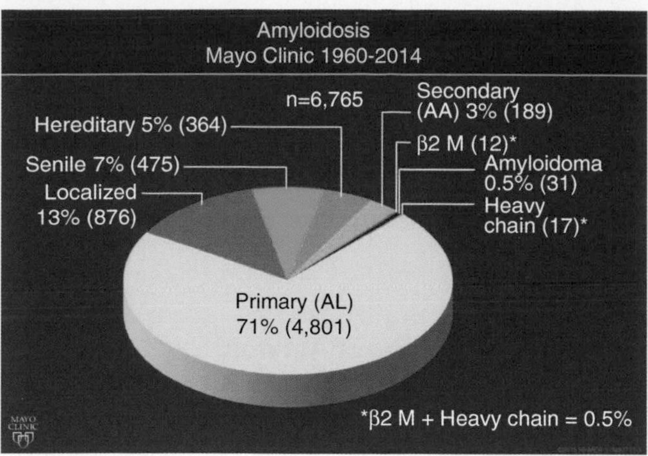

Fig. 36.6 Amyloid type seen at Mayo Clinic

apolipoprotein, lysozyme, insulin, gelsolin, etc. [63]. Most laboratories are not adequately configured to perform immunohistochemical studies for all forms of amyloidosis. Currently, the gold standard for the identification of amyloid deposits is laser capture microdissection mass spectroscopic analysis of the amyloid deposits [64]. Sequencing of the proteome and subsequent comparison with a library of protein sequences is virtually 100% sensitive in identifying the primary structure of the amyloid protein subunit [65] (Table 36.1). LCMS is also capable of identifying other proteins such as apolipoprotein E, serum amyloid P, and vitronectin, which are common in amyloid deposits and validate that the deposit is indeed amyloid [43]. Using this technique, we have demonstrated that 38% of amyloid deposits are not of immunoglobulin light chain origin, and an increasing number of new proteins have been identified, including Alect2, keratin, A-fibrinogen, and A-atrial natriuretic factor [66].

One of the great dangers in clinical practice reflects the high prevalence of monoclonal gammopathies in the serum of the elderly, ranging from 3% prevalence at age 70 years to 5% at age 90 years. This is the same population that has a high incidence of wild-type TTR cardiac amyloidosis. Therefore, the finding of classic amyloidosis in the heart of an elderly male that has a monoclonal protein does not necessarily indicate cardiac AL amyloidosis. A tissue specimen is required in order to exclude wild-type TTR amyloidosis, and mass spectroscopy is well suited to make this distinction [8, 67].

Distinguishing Localized and Systemic Amyloidosis

Even when mass spectroscopic analysis demonstrates immunoglobulin light chain as the primary protein subunit of the amyloid deposits, it does not prove that it is systemic. There are a number of localized forms of AL amyloidosis that can involve skin, bladder, larynx, and gastrointestinal tract and not be evidence of a systemic syndrome [68–70]. Supportive evidence in these instances is the absence of a monoclonal protein in serum and urine, a normal immunoglobulin free light chain assay, and failure to find a clonal population of plasma cells in the bone marrow. At Mayo Clinic, nearly 16% of patients seen with amyloidosis have localized disease. Amyloidosis involving the renal pelvis [71], ureter, bladder [72], and urethra can present with hematuria, unilateral renal obstruction, mimicking colic, or imaging findings that would be suggestive of ureteral and bladder carcinoma, respectively. Patients with tracheobronchial amyloidosis will present with hoarseness, poor vocal cord movement, and occasional stridor. Patients with genitourinary and tracheobronchial amyloid do not benefit from systemic therapy and need to be treated locally.

Table 36.1 Types of amyloid identified in tissues

Amyloid subtype	Percentage
AL (light chain)	61.7
ATTR (familial or wild type)	24.5
AA (secondary)	3.7
ALECT-2 (renal)	3.6
A Ins (localized insulin)	1.1
Keratin (cutaneous)	0.9
A Apo 1 (inherited)	0.7
AH (heavy chain)	0.7
A Fib (hereditary renal)	0.6

Pulmonary nodules that have all the characteristics of a solitary malignancy can represent localized nodular amyloidosis [73]. These deposits are AL in origin, are unassociated with a systemic light chain disorder, and do not require therapy.

Cutaneous deposits of amyloid are usually found to represent keratin [74] deposits and are 1% of all amyloid proteins analyzed at Mayo Clinic. These lesions cause pruritus but are not at risk of developing a systemic form of amyloidosis. Localized amyloidosis has also been described in the conjunctiva [75]. Management is by an oculoplastic surgeon. Conjunctival amyloid can often be confused with conjunctival lymphoma. Carpal tunnel syndrome is seen in 15% of patients with light chain amyloidosis, but there is a separate syndrome of localized carpal tunnel amyloidosis, which has been demonstrated to be composed of TTR [76]. Men who have wild-type TTR cardiac amyloidosis have a history of carpal tunnel syndrome in nearly 50% [58]. Trace amounts of amyloid can be found in the cartilage of the hip and the knee and represent incidental findings. There is also a form of localized atrial amyloidosis that is composed of atrial natriuretic factor and contributes to atrial arrhythmias but is not associated with systemic cardiac amyloidosis with ventricular dysfunction [77]. Whenever amyloidosis is detected, exclusion of localized amyloid that does not require chemotherapy is essential. Amyloid deposits found in the cardiac ventricle, kidney, and liver virtually always represent systemic AL amyloidosis even if only a single organ is involved.

Systemic Forms of Amyloidosis that Are Not Immunoglobulin Light Chain in Origin

The clinical presentation of systemic non-AL amyloidosis involving nerve, kidney, and heart are not distinguishable from light chain amyloidosis. Patients with renal amyloidosis can be composed of light chains, Alect2, fibrinogen-Aα, or be a manifestation of AA amyloid [78]. In all instances, there is proteinuria or renal insufficiency. Most patients with light chain, AA and fibrinogen amyloid present with nephrotic range proteinuria. Patients with Alect2 actually have modest degrees of amyloid deposition with significant elevations in serum creatinine, and histology shows preferential deposition in the tubular and interstitial regions of the kidney [79]. Apolipoprotein amyloid, also an inherited form of amyloid preferentially involving the kidney, presents with creatinine elevation and only modest degrees of proteinuria in the range of 1 g/24 h [63].

The differential diagnosis of systemic cardiac amyloid is AL amyloid; mutant TTR amyloid, formerly known as familial amyloid cardiomyopathy; and wild-type TTR cardiac amyloid, formerly known as senile cardiac amyloid or senile systemic amyloid [80]. Mutant TTR amyloidosis has echocardiographic features similar to AL amyloidosis but is 90% men, usually over the age of 60 years, with a high incidence of associated carpal tunnel syndrome [81]. The extent of amyloid infiltration seen on echocardiography is usually greater than that in AL, suggesting that the fibrils of TTR amyloid are less toxic to the myocardium [82]. It is not unusual to see an interventricular septal thickness of 20 mm in TTR amyloidosis, where this would be unusual in AL amyloidosis. Increased recognition has led to a surge in the diagnosis of wild-type TTR amyloidosis as the willingness of cardiologists to biopsy the heart in older individuals is increasing and as new investigational therapies become available. Wild-type TTR amyloidosis also has a much better prognosis than light chain amyloidosis [83], with survivals of 5–7 years, compared with AL amyloidosis of 1–2 years. Recently, it has been demonstrated that radionuclide scanning with either technetium pyrophosphate [84] or technetium DPD [85] is quite specific for TTR amyloidosis. The finding of a compatible echocardiogram with restrictive cardiomyopathy and poor filling with a positive technetium imaging scan (Fig. 36.7 PYP or DPD) is diagnostic of TTR amyloidosis and is a useful distinguishing feature.

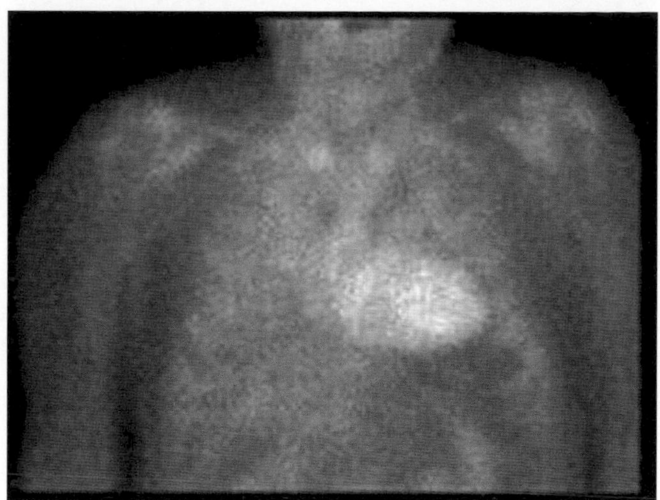

Fig. 36.7 PYP scan of TTR amyloidosis

Amyloidosis and the Heart

The heart is the most important organ to be involved with amyloidosis and drives the prognosis. Amyloid is deposited extracellularly and results in the thickened and noncompliant left ventricle that is seen on echocardiography and magnetic resonance imaging [86]. Because systolic function is preserved until late in the course and cardiomegaly is not seen on a chest radiograph, it is easy to misattribute the thickening to a more common systemic illness such as hypertension or valvular disease. Coronary angiography is typically normal. The median septal thickness for patients with immunoglobulin light chain amyloidosis is 14 mm (normal <11) [87]. Thickening of the septum has also been misattributed to asymmetric septal hypertrophy. The finding of a monoclonal protein in a patient with "hypertrophic cardiomyopathy" or "hypertensive cardiomyopathy" should lead to an evaluation for amyloidosis [88]. Doppler studies on echocardiography are quite useful in demonstrating the restriction to inflow and the rapid rise in diastolic filling pressures characteristic of the restrictive physiology of amyloidosis [22]. Wall thickness and fractional shortening are predictive of survival in this disease [89]. The recent introduction of strain echocardiography allows measurement of a rate at which the myocardial wall shortens; normal is −18% or less (−20% normal). Amyloid is characterized by rises (−15%, −12%, etc.) and is shown to predict survival in patients with amyloidosis [90]. Patients with amyloidosis of the heart can develop atrial thrombi, which can be a potential source of arterial embolization and stroke [91]. There is a high incidence of supraventricular rhythm disturbances that are resistant to ablation therapy [92]. There is a high incidence of sudden death [93], and nearly 30% of patients with cardiac amyloidosis die within the first 2 months of recognition [94]. There is a rare syndrome of intramural coronary arteriolar amyloidosis. These patients present with classic anginal symptoms with normal extramural coronary arteries seen after angiography [95].

A particular area of misdiagnosis is in elderly African-American men, 3% of whom carry a mutation for TTR V122I [96]. The finding of cardiac amyloidosis in an African-American male necessitates mass spectroscopic analysis of the deposits due to the high prevalence of this form of inherited TTR amyloidosis. The echocardiographic features of these forms of amyloidosis are indistinguishable, and all are positive for Congo red, necessitating careful analysis of the amyloid protein subunit.

There is increasing recognition of wild-type TTR cardiac amyloidosis, formerly known as senile systemic amyloid and senile cardiac amyloid. These patients have the same echocardiographic features as other patients with cardiac amyloid but tend to be older, nearly 90% are men, nearly half have associated carpal tunnel syndrome, and renal involvement is conspicuously absent [97]. The severity of the heart failure is less for the extent of infiltration identified by echocardiography, and median survival is longer than that in cardiac AL. These patients do not benefit from systemic chemotherapy, and the mechanism by which a normal protein, such as TTR, preferentially deposits in the myocardium of elderly men remains unknown. In an observational study, patients with mutant TTR amyloid had a survival of 25.6 months inferior to those with wild-type TTR amyloidosis at 43 months. In a subsequent analysis of 272 patients with wild-type TTR, the mean age was 77; 89% were men and the median survival was 3.5 years. We have seen rare patients with wild-type TTR amyloid under the age of 60. So the overlap is quite substantial, and age alone cannot be used as a distinguishing feature. The clinical spectrum of wild-type TTR amyloidosis is quite broad. It is the obligation of the hematologist to ensure that these patients are not inappropriately administered cytotoxic chemotherapy [98].

The mechanism whereby immunoglobulin light chains and amyloid produce cardiac dysfunction is not well understood [99]. Light chains produce oxidative stress, cellular dysfunction, and apoptosis in adult cardiac myocytes through activation of p38 mitogen-activated protein kinase [100, 101]. The presentation of cardiac amyloidosis is heart failure with a preserved ejection fraction [58]. Again, hypertrophy, asymmetric septal hypertrophy, and hypertrophic cardiomyopathy have all been incorrectly diagnosed in patients with light chain cardiac amyloidosis. The electrocardiogram in light chain amyloidosis is neither sensitive nor specific. Low voltage is found in only 46%, a pseudo-infarct in 47%, and 16%, despite infiltration, had EKG findings that met criteria for LVH [102]. Since this is a diastolic disorder, ejection fraction remains normal until advanced disease onset. The standard for evaluating cardiac amyloidosis is the echocardiogram, showing increased wall thickness, left ventricular outflow obstruction, peak systolic tissue velocity, abnormal systolic strain, and abnormal systolic strain rate compared with patients without amyloidosis [103]. Doppler imaging is used to detect impaired left ventricular diastolic filling. In 249 consecutive patients, strain rate imaging predicted mortality and was independent of age and New York Heart Association class as well as cardiac biomarkers [104]. Not all patients with cardiac amyloid have thickening of the ventricular walls; 36% of patients in one trial had a left ventricular wall thickness of ≤12 mm with a median survival of 2 years [105].

Radionuclide imaging serum amyloid P component will bind to all forms of amyloid and will demonstrate deposits but not in the heart. Technetium 99 M derivatives, including pyrophosphate and DPD [106], are capable of binding to TTR cardiac amyloid and are a useful test to distinguish AL from ATTR amyloidosis. Technetium DPD is primarily used in Europe, and Technetium PYP [84] is primarily used in the United States. Carbon 11-PIB with PET scanning has been used to study amyloidosis affecting the heart after it was shown to be effective in diagnosing Alzheimer's plaques; this is ongoing [107].

Cardiac Magnetic Resonance Imaging

MRI is an effective technique when cardiac amyloidosis is suspected. It shows ventricular wall thickening, ventricular wall mass, and a characteristic late gadolinium enhancement [108, 109] (Fig. 36.8). The use of gadolinium in patients

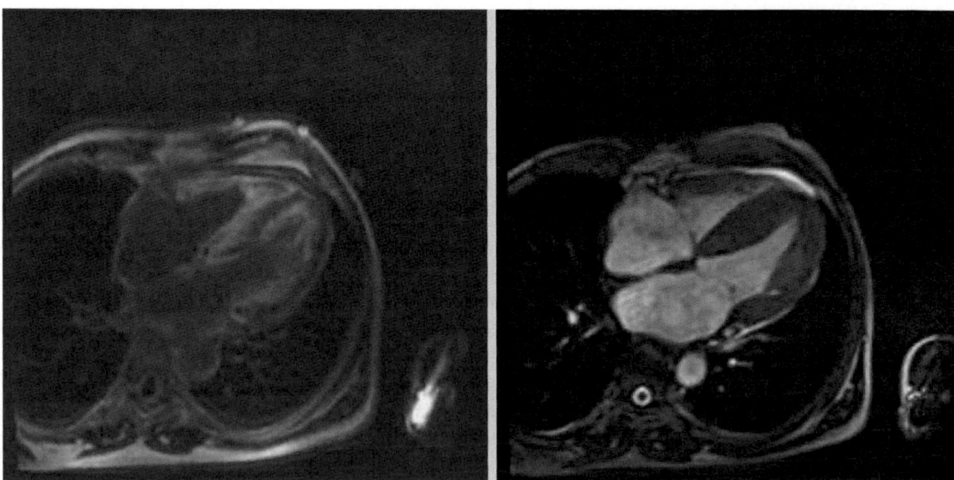

Fig. 36.8 MRI of heart showing amyloid

with renal amyloid is unwise because they are at risk of developing late systemic fibrosis [110]. Cardiac MRI can identify 91% of patients with restrictive filling patterns. Expansion of the extracellular space indicative of amyloid deposition in the heart results in circumferential late shortening of the endocardium and thickening of the myocardial wall. Diffuse transmural late gadolinium enhancement correlates with interstitial amyloid infiltration and correlates with other clinical indicators such as New York Heart Association class and left ventricular wall thickness.

Biomarkers

Although echocardiogram and cardiac magnetic resonance imaging has been a standard for diagnosis for nearly three decades, there are issues of interobserver variability and reproducibility so that serial changes of the echocardiogram over time have not been validated as being predictive of survival. Serum biomarkers that indicate myocyte injury (troponin) or left atrial stress (N-terminal propeptide of B natriuretic peptide (NT-proBNP)) are more reproducible and have been incorporated into systems designed both to stage and predict outcomes in patients with amyloidosis [16, 111].

The symptoms of cardiac amyloidosis are nonspecific. Poor diastolic filling, low left ventricular end-diastolic volume, and reduced cardiac output result in reduction in systolic blood pressure. Levels of troponin T and NT-proBNP can be used in conjunction with the immunoglobulin free light chain level to determine patient's stage and median survival and can be used to predict early [112] mortality with autologous stem cell transplantation [113]. The main cause of death in patients with all forms of light chain amyloidosis (whether hepatic, renal, or peripheral nerve) is cardiac involvement with subsequent heart failure or sudden death. In a multivariable model of over 800 patients with AL amyloidosis, the concentration of cardiac troponin T and NT-proBNP independently predicted overall survival. The cutoffs were NT-proBNP > or < 332 ng/mL and troponin T of 0.035 μg/L. By assigning one point for each, patients could have both normal, one abnormal, or both abnormal, resulting in three stages [114]. It has subsequently been demonstrated that the DFLC is prognostic as is the percentage of plasma cells in the bone marrow and whether the patient has multiple myeloma in the bone marrow or any CRAB criteria, all of which shorten the survival in patients with light chain amyloidosis [12].

The new system has four stages, where one point is assigned for a cardiac troponin T level > or < 0.025 μg/L, an NT-proBNP level ≥ 1800 ng/L, and a clonal free light chain burden >18 mg/dL. Investigators at University College London Amyloid Center have further refined stage 3 into stage 3A (BNP between 1800 and 8500) and stage 3B (all features of stage 3 with an NT-proBNP > 8500) [115]. This results in four (or five) stages. The median survival in the Mayo system for the four stages, respectively, is 94.1, 40.3, 14, and 5.6 months (Table 36.2).

Table 36.2 Amyloid staging system [112]

1 Point each for:
dFLC >18 mg/dL
cTnT >0.025 ng/mL
NT-proBNP >1800 pg/mL
Median survivals: 0 = 94.1; 1 = 40.3; 2 = 14; 3 = 5 months

Renal Amyloidosis

In a patient with nephrotic range proteinuria, measurement of immunoglobulin free light chains, if abnormal, will rapidly narrow the possibilities into myeloma cast nephropathy, Randall light chain deposition disease, light chain amyloidosis, and cryoglobulinemia [116]. In most instances, the finding of light chains in the serum and in the urine will obviate the need for renal biopsy since biopsy of the fat and bone marrow will usually demonstrate the presence of amyloid without having to proceed with the risks of renal biopsy. It is important that all patients with proteinuria have immunofixation performed of the serum, urine, and a free light chain assay. The kidneys are affected in nearly 40% of patients with AL amyloidosis; and for nondiabetic adults with nephrotic range proteinuria, amyloid is 12% of renal biopsy specimens. If one looks at all renal biopsy specimens that are performed, amyloid represents 2.8%. A recent system looking at the initial urinary protein and the serum creatinine at diagnosis is useful for predicting the risk of dialysis (see Table 36.3) [117]. The amount of urinary protein has no impact on overall survival, which is driven by the presence or absence of cardiac involvement.

Two-thirds of AL patients with immunoglobulin light chain amyloidosis have detectable light chains in the urine or in the serum. Monoclonal light chain proteins are more common when the urinary protein loss is high. Symptomatically, the massive proteinuria leads to hypoalbuminemia, and the decline in oncotic pressure results in progressive edema, requiring diuretics. However, diuretics often will further

Table 36.3 Renal staging system [117]

Proteinuria >5 g/24 h
eGFR <50 mL/min
Risk at dialysis at 3 years:
Both favorable: 0–4%
Both unfavorable: 60–85%
1 Unfavorable: 30%

decrease intravascular volume, which can result in significant hypotension and decline in renal vascular blood flow, with resultant rise in the serum creatinine level. Approximately one-third of our patients have an antecedent history of a marked change in the level of serum cholesterol, and the rapid rise in cholesterol is a manifestation of the evolving nephrotic syndrome. In our experience, the median time from diagnosis of nephrotic syndrome to dialysis was 14 months [118]. After initiation of dialysis, the median survival time was 8 months, with patients usually succumbing to cardiac involvement. There does not appear to be any reported differences between hemodialysis and peritoneal dialysis in terms of outcome [119]. Effective chemotherapy will reduce urinary protein loss and slow the progression to end-stage renal disease and ultimately improve survival [120]. Concomitant cardiac amyloidosis makes dialysis quite difficult to complete because of hypotension with each dialysis run. There is no correlation between the amount of amyloid in the glomerulus and the extent of urinary protein loss. The urinary sediment is rather benign with fat or fatty acid crystals, but the sediment is not inflammatory or nephritic. Occasionally, amyloid patients will present with adult Fanconi syndrome with crystalline deposits in the proximal tubules and resultant urinary loss of uric acid, phosphorus, amino acids, and potassium. Immunotactoid glomerulopathy can be confused with light chain amyloidosis, but the majority of patients with immunotactoid fibrils in the kidney do not have an associated plasma cell dyscrasia [43]. The fibrils seen by electron microscopy in immunotactoid glomerulopathy do not stain with Congo red. Randall light chain deposition disease is very hard to distinguish from light chain amyloidosis. However, light chain deposition disease rarely involves liver, heart, and nerves [121, 122].

Therapy

Supportive Care Treatment for Amyloidosis

For both cardiac and renal amyloidosis, the mainstay is diuretic therapy. Diuretic therapy can be complicated because so many patients have orthostatic hypotension and intravascular volume contraction due to their hypoalbuminemia. Diuretic therapy can raise the creatinine level and lower the systolic blood pressure. Our cardiologists appear to have a preference for torsemide over furosemide as having better bioavailability for patients; and for those patients in whom loop diuretics fail to control edema, the addition of Metolazone in doses from 2.5 mg QOD to 5 mg BID can be beneficial but can be complicated with relatively severe hypokalemia. Patients that develop orthostatic syncope are often treated with fludrocortisone or midodrine. The latter is complicated by severe supine hypertension.

Cardiac arrhythmias are a common problem in patients with amyloidosis; and clearly, if syncope can be documented to be related to severe bradycardia or supraventricular tachyarrhythmia that results in poor filling in between beats, a permanent pacemaker can be placed [123]. There is no evidence that afterload reduction with ACE or ARBS is of any benefit for patients with cardiac amyloidosis, and it has been our observation that patients tolerate these medications poorly and symptomatically feel worse. Moreover, because of poor diastolic filling, many of these patients require a rapid heart rate to maintain their stroke volume. As a result, artificially lowering a rapid heart rate with beta blockers can result in a decline in cardiac output and symptomatic deterioration in patients. Our cardiologists tend to avoid the use of beta blockers in amyloidosis patients [51].

There is data to suggest that an implantable defibrillator can be of benefit in patients for whom ventricular fibrillation has been diagnosed or those with recurrent syncope that cannot be attributed to orthostatic hypotension [93, 124] and is likely to be related to high-grade cardiac arrhythmias [125]. Digoxin is relatively contraindicated in the management of amyloid heart disease because there has been a previously reported high prevalence of sudden cardiac death. However, there are instances where it can be used to increase AV nodal blockade and reduce the heart rate in patients with rapid ventricular response. Calcium channel blockers have been reported to precipitate congestive heart failure and are best avoided in the management of these patients.

A small number of patients with cardiac amyloidosis have been reported with a left ventricular assist device as both destination therapy and as a bridge to transplantation. The numbers are too small to actually determine the appropriate role of a left ventricular assist device [126].

Cardiac transplantation has been used at multiple centers for amyloid, but major problems exist [127]. Systemic chemotherapy is clearly required. Without chemotherapy, one can expect recurrence of amyloid into the allografted heart [128]. Virtually all reported outcomes suggest that patients with heart transplant for amyloid do not do as well as patients with cardiomyopathy. As long as organ availability remains an issue, the question arises for every amyloid patient that gets a heart, which patient did not get a heart? Different centers have different philosophies about chemotherapy either before or after cardiac transplant. On one side, systemic chemotherapy is given before cardiac transplant in order to ensure chemotherapy sensitivity and the ability to control light chains. The downside of this is patients with advanced cardiac failure who are candidates for heart transplants do not tolerate significant amounts of systemic chemotherapy, and a real test of the ability to control the plasma cell dyscrasia cannot be accomplished. Unfortunately, delaying chemotherapy until after a heart transplant runs the risk that patients will be chemotherapy nonresponsive after they have received an allografted heart, and this raises major challenges in trying to prevent recurrence. The Mayo Clinic standard has been to give patients an allografted heart followed by an autologous stem cell transplant [129]; and if there is persistent disease, use bortezomib-based chemotherapy as part of consolidation [130]. Cardiac transplantation does not bring up any major technical problems compared with patients receiving an allograft for cardiomyopathy, but outcomes will not be favorable without treatment of the underlying plasma cell dyscrasia [131]. Between May 1992 and November 2012, 178 adult patients referred for cardiac transplant for amyloidosis were evaluated; 78 did not complete evaluation, 94 completed evaluation, and 38 were considered ineligible primarily because of extracardiac amyloidosis, which we consider exclusion criteria for transplant; 56 were listed for transplant and 31 received transplant, 22 of whom had AL amyloidosis. The overall survival of the patients was a median of approximately 4 years with 20% alive at 10 years. Survival following heart transplant of amyloid patients was 81.6% and at 5 years, 48%. This compares with non-amyloid patients who have a 1- and 5-year survival of 93.4 and 83.6, respectively [132]. Chemotherapy and/or stem cell transplant following a heart transplant may significantly improve survival and needs ongoing study. The role of cardiac transplant in AL amyloidosis remains uncertain. Other groups have performed cardiac transplantation reported through the UNOS database, and 69 patients were reported in aggregate with 5 operative deaths and 29 late deaths and 9 deaths attributed to amyloid-related complications. The 5 patients had sequential cardiac and stem cell transplantation; 2 died of progressive amyloid 33 and 90 months after heart transplant; 1 patient actually had an allogeneic bone marrow transplant. In the United Kingdom, 24 patients with amyloid heart disease were reported with cardiac transplantation, 17AL [133]. One-, two-, and five-year survival rate was 86%, 86%, and 64%, respectively. Progression of amyloid systemically contributed to increased mortality.

Supportive care for renal amyloidosis includes hemodialysis for those patients who go onto end-stage renal disease, but their outcomes are inferior related to the high proportion of patients that have concomitant cardiac amyloidosis. Renal transplantation has also been performed for these patients [134]. The majority at Mayo Clinic receive a living related kidney because of the long wait for a cadaver donor [135]. These patients also require systemic chemotherapy because amyloid deposits in the transplanted kidney are well reported [136]. In a report of 45 patients who underwent kidney transplantation, the 3-year survival rate was 51%, with recurrent amyloid in the transplanted kidney detected in four. The estimated recurrence rate of amyloid at 1 year after transplant was 20%. No specific predictors of recurrence were identified. Sequential living donor renal transplant and autologous stem cell transplant is feasible. We have reported eight such patients with six long-term survivors.

Chemotherapy Treatment for Light Chain Amyloidosis

The primary therapy currently available for the treatment of light chain amyloidosis is plasma cell-directed therapy. Therapies are capable of destroying the underlying plasma cell clone responsible for the synthesis of the immunoglobulin light chains. These chains ultimately become resistant to catabolic breakdown and subsequently misfold into the amyloid configuration. Alkylator and steroid therapy remains one of the viable options for the treatment of amyloidosis, but none of the available regimens have been subjected to rigorous phase III randomized clinical trials [87]. The first use of alkylating agents dates back to 1972. The use of high-dose, alkylating-agent chemotherapy followed by autologous stem cell transplantation dates back over 20 years [137]. The ultimate goal of therapy is not reduction of the M component the way it is in multiple myeloma where response depth is a prediction of improved survival. In light chain amyloidosis, the goal of plasma cell-directed chemotherapy is to eventually invoke an organ response with improved cardiac, renal, or hepatic function. Because response to chemotherapy is time-dependent and there is a lag time between a hematologic response and an organ response, there are a number of patients that will succumb due to advanced organ failure before sufficient time elapses to allow for reducing the burden of toxic circulating light chains. The first alkylator combination was melphalan and prednisone, and two phase III trials have been performed using colchicine as the comparator arm that showed benefit [138]. Unfortunately, the majority of patients failed to achieve a hematologic response; and as in multiple myeloma, the doublet of melphalan and prednisone has been relegated to historical interest only. Early patients treated with melphalan and prednisone have clear-cut organ regression and improvement with SAP scintigraphy demonstration of a reduction in amyloid deposits.

The Mayo Clinic experience with melphalan and prednisone reported an objective hematologic response rate of 18%. Moreover, patients presenting with a serum creatinine >3 mg/dL were nonresponders and destined to go on to dialysis-dependent renal failure. The best responses were seen in renal amyloid nephrotic syndrome, but patients with amyloid cardiomyopathy can definitely respond; and melphalan and prednisone can be dose-adjusted so that it can be administered to virtually any patient of any age with any degree of cardiac or renal dysfunction [139]. Although only a few patients actually respond to melphalan, when they do, median survival is as long as 89 months. For melphalan-based therapy, it can be a challenge to know when to abandon the therapy since organ responses can be delayed. A trial of bortezomib-based chemotherapy and melphalan-dexamethasone failed to demonstrate a survival advantage for the bortezomib arm [140]. Even in the era of melphalan and prednisone, 10-year survivors were regularly seen, almost all responders to alkylating-agent chemotherapy. Predictors of poor outcome, as in all trials of amyloid, include heart failure, age, serum creatinine, and percentage bone marrow plasma cells. When melphalan-prednisone was compared to colchicine, median survival in the melphalan-prednisone arm was 17 months compared to 8.5 months. These short survivals are a reflection both of the late diagnosis commonly seen with melphalan treatment of amyloidosis as well as the relatively low frequency with which response was achieved. Melphalan, particularly with prolonged exposure, has a significant risk of MDS or ANLL. In a series of 153 closely followed patients exposed only to melphalan, ten ultimately developed therapy-related MDS or ANLL [141]; eight of the ten showed classic cytogenetic features, which include hypodiploidy, deletion of chromosome 5, or deletion of chromosome 7. The actuarial risk for developing myelodysplasia at 42 months was 21%, reflecting the small proportion of long-term survivors. Today, melphalan is rarely given for longer than 12 months; and with the multiple alternatives available, reexposure to melphalan is uncommon, and rates of MDS that we are currently seeing are approximately 1%.

Approximately 10 years ago, melphalan-prednisone was supplanted with melphalan and high-dose dexamethasone [142]. Most patients were selected on the basis of stem cell transplant ineligibility. In an original trial of 46 patients, a hematologic response was seen in 67%, with an organ response in 33%, where hematologic response was the most powerful predictor of organ response [143]. This oral regimen had only a 4% all-cause mortality at day-100 and resulted in resolution of cardiac failure in 6 of 32 patients, with a median time to response of 4.5 months. In a follow-up trial of 93 patients, complete hematologic responses were seen in 24%, and improvement in amyloid-related organ failure was seen in 45%, with a 2-year event-free survival of 52%. In this trial, heart failure and β2 microglobulin levels predicted adverse outcome and durable reversal of amyloid-related organ dysfunction. Since patients on chemotherapy trials of amyloidosis are usually cared for at a trial center, there is inherent referral bias with regard to the outcomes, which is not reflective of the real-world experience.

Stem Cell Transplantation for the Management of Amyloidosis

Since the first report of five patients receiving high-dose therapy with stem cell transplant for the treatment of patients with amyloidosis, hundreds of articles have been published, demonstrating the benefits of stem cell transplantation in this disorder [144]. In multiple myeloma, patients tend to have unhealthy bone marrow but tend to have preserved vital organ function. Unfortunately, in patients with amyloidosis, comorbidities associated with cardiac failure, hypoalbuminemia, renal insufficiency, and chronic hepatic dysfunction lead to major complications after the administration of high-dose melphalan. The visceral organ dysfunction, which is always part of amyloidosis, has resulted in early mortality rates reported as high as 10% [145]. A mortality level this high was previously acceptable when the number of standard-dose chemotherapeutic alternatives was small but would not be considered an acceptable mortality rate in an era when multiple alternatives to transplantation exist. Most centers collect stem cells in amyloidosis without mobilizing chemotherapy. Although the majority of patients can be collected with growth factor alone, there has been an increasing tendency to give plerixafor [146] to enhance peripheral blood stem cell collection [147]. Patients with amyloid have a tendency to retain a good deal of fluid during filgrastim mobilization of peripheral blood stem cells [148, 149]. Although many centers incorporate plerixafor on a routine basis, our policy is to measure the peripheral blood CD34 on day-5; and if it is <10, we would begin plerixafor that evening and initiate collections the following morning. We dose plerixafor at 0.24 mg/kg when the creatinine clearance is >50; and for patients with a creatinine clearance <50, we reduce the dose to 0.16 mg/kg, and we never exceed a maximum dose of 24 mg. Even using this regimen, we find a high proportion of patients that still retain fluid; and in up to 20%, stem cell transplant would be delayed while we use diuretics to restore their weight to the pre-mobilization level.

We have successfully reduced the transplant-related mortality rate to 1.1% [150] and continue to see good outcomes, including patients with cardiac amyloidosis before the onset of advanced congestive heart failure. Our hematologic and cardiac response rates are now approaching 66% and 41%, and hematologic response is directly connected to survival. We have reported our 10-year results and survival in patients who have received transplants and it is 43% [151]. At Boston University Medical Center, 10-year survival has been reported to be 53%, with mortality rates of 4–7%.

Currently, we are excluding patients from stem cell transplant who have an NT-proBNP level > 8500 or a systolic blood pressure < 90, suggesting that the extent of cardiac failure makes high-dose chemotherapy excessively toxic. Overall, we find 20–25% of all patients eligible for transplant. We are now seeing complete posttransplant responses of 39%. The most important predictor of survival is Mayo stage. The most important predictor of outcome, however, is maximal hematologic response. Some patients improve long before it would be considered possible for amyloid to be removed from the organ. This is particularly the case with cardiac amyloid and does suggest that immunoglobulin light chains have a direct toxicity to the heart, and this has been verified in isolated mouse muscle studies and in a *C. elegans* model of contractility [152]. Occasional second courses of high-dose chemotherapy can be administered in those patients that had a durable first response. Induction chemotherapy plays an important role in the treatment of amyloidosis. In a prospective randomized study recently published, albeit small, the use of induction chemotherapy followed by transplant resulted in a better overall survival than transplant alone. Unfortunately, this trial was not stratified for the percentage of plasma cells in the bone marrow at the time of diagnosis and randomization. A recent review of the ABMTR registry identified 1536 patients with AL transplanted at 134 centers. The overall survival and early mortality were analyzed in three time cohorts: 1995–2000, 2001–2006, and 2007–2012. When available, both hematologic and renal response data was included. This trial showed that all-cause mortality at day-100 declined from 20% to 5%, with a 5-year overall survival improvement from 55% to 77% [145]. In the cohort study from 2007 to 2012, hematologic response to transplantation improved, and the renal response rate was 32%. This trial reported that centers that performed more than four AL transplants per year had superior outcomes, suggesting experience matters, and familiarity with myeloma transplant is not a surrogate for amyloidosis experience. In a multivariable analysis, cardiac AL was associated with the highest mortality and worst progression-free and overall survival. Higher doses of melphalan were associated with a reduced risk of relapse, although patients who received lower doses of melphalan are generally older and have greater degrees of cardiac and renal insufficiency. A creatinine of 2 mg was associated with a poorer overall survival [145].

In an observational trial of GCSF and plerixafor, the combination produced a higher total CD34 yield and a greater proportion of CD34 cells collected on the first day of apheresis. Four patients were mobilization failures with G but none with G and plerixafor, and patients who received plerixafor actually had a lower weight gain of 0.5 kg vs. 3.2 kg. The number of apheresis sessions, the number of hospitalization days, and cardiac arrhythmias were similar. This trial suggests that the up-front use of plerixafor results in a superior stem cell mobilization compared with G alone [153].

The British Amyloidosis Center reported on 90 patients who had undergone autologous stem cell transplantation over a 9-year period (38% as part of initial therapy). The responses, as measured by complete and very good partial response rates, were thought to be superior to those reported with low-dose chemotherapy. Renal responses were noted in 33% and liver responses in 7%; and out of 17 patients evaluable for a cardiac response, a cardiac response was seen in 6 (35%). The median progression-free survival was approximately 4 years, supporting the use of stem cell transplantation and its ability to produce deep and durable responses [154].

Oregon Health Sciences University reported on 31 patients receiving autologous stem cell transplant, including patients who were pretreated and those who had received prior induction chemotherapy; 13 patients proceeded directly to transplant after diagnosis, 12 received a bortezomib-containing regimen before transplant, and 6 had other variable induction therapies prior to transplant. The all-cause, day-100 mortality was 9.6%, and the hematologic and organ response rates were 77% and 58%, respectively. The median time to hematologic response after transplant was shorter in the group that received bortezomib induction, 3 vs. 14 months. The overall cardiac response rate was 60% (100% in those pretreated with bortezomib and 43% in those without induction treatment). The 3-year progression-free and overall survival was 66% and 73%, and they concluded that bortezomib-based induction was well tolerated both in patients with and without cardiac involvement and could be considered as part of the initial therapy of amyloidosis [155].

The European HOVON German Cooperative Group for the treatment of amyloidosis conducted a phase II trial evaluating three courses of vincristine, doxorubicin, and dexamethasone, followed by an autologous transplant; and 69 patients were transplanted between November 2000 and January 2006. After long-term follow-up of 115 months, the median survival of all patients was 96 months from registration and, for the transplanted patients, 120 months from the date of transplant. Therapy-related mortality was 12%. Four patients died during vincristine, doxorubicin, and dexamethasone, and two additional patients of the remaining 57 (or approximately 4%) died following high-dose melphalan. A two-step approach consisting of less toxic induction therapy followed by high-dose melphalan may result in extended overall survival [156].

The Mayo Clinic Group has now completed stem cell transplantations on a total of 663 patients. The profound effect of NT-proBNP on outcome is given in the figure where survival is split at the level of NT-proBNP of 1800 pg/mL (Fig. 36.9).

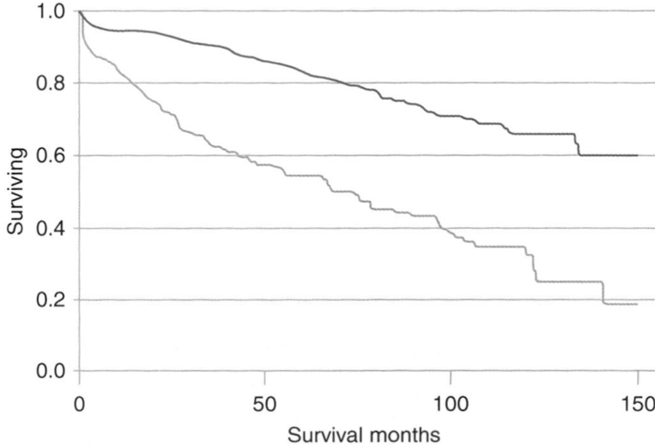

Fig. 36.9 Survival after stem cell transplantation stratified by NT-proBNP ≥ 1000 ng/mL. *Blue line*: NT-proBNP < 1000 ng/mL; *orange line*: NT-proBNP ≥ 1000 ng/mL

There is no reliable phase III data that demonstrates a survival advantage for stem cell transplantation. The only published phase III trial was plagued with poor patient selection and a very high therapy-related mortality [157]. Patients with AL, however, are highly selected for transplant. They are younger, have fewer organs involved, and will not have advanced heart failure. Therefore, concluding that stem cell transplantation is superior to conventional chemotherapy is not possible. The experience of most amyloid experts remains that if the patient is eligible for stem cell transplantation, they should be referred for therapy. Our current policy is to offer induction chemotherapy for those patients that have >10% plasma cells in the bone marrow. However, if the percentage of plasma cells is well below the threshold for multiple myeloma, then we are comfortable in going directly to stem cell transplantation and following the policy of Memorial Hospital in New York that uses bortezomib consolidation after transplant for those that have not, as yet, achieved a complete response [158].

Immunomodulatory Drugs

Thalidomide, lenalidomide, and, most recently, pomalidomide have been introduced for the treatment of immunoglobulin light chain amyloidosis, and all have shown significant activity. In the first thalidomide trial of amyloidosis, 16 patients had dose escalations to 300 mg/day. At this dose, treatment was poorly tolerated, and a high proportion had to abandon therapy before they had an opportunity to develop an organ response [159]. In a report of 12 patients with light chain amyloidosis treated with thalidomide, nine had severe drug-related toxicity and a median treatment exposure of only 72 days [160].

In Great Britain, thalidomide was combined with cyclophosphamide, thalidomide, and dexamethasone at only 100 mg/day, and 31% still had to discontinue therapy, although the hematologic response rate was 55%, and the treatment-related mortality was only 4%. Bradycardia can be seen in as many as 26% of patients. Therefore, care is required when this is administered to patients with cardiac amyloidosis [161]. A recent joint European study compared outcomes of bortezomib-based regimens with thalidomide-based regimens, and this retrospective multicenter review suggested that risk-adjusted bortezomib regimens were better than IMID-based regimens [162].

The second-generation immunomodulatory drug, lenalidomide, has a much better safety and toxicity profile in patients with amyloidosis [163]. It has been used with dexamethasone as well as with cyclophosphamide. The usual maximum-tolerated dose of lenalidomide is approximately 15 mg/day, but it can produce a response rate of 58%, 42 complete, with a 2-year overall survival of 81%. As with thalidomide, prophylaxis against venous thromboembolism is required. A combination of cyclophosphamide, lenalidomide, and dexamethasone is safe. No comparative trials exist to determine if it offers advantages to the doublet alone. Lenalidomide has been reported to increase the level of NT-proBNP and can actually aggravate heart failure; and the dose should not exceed 15 mg daily. The discontinuation rate of lenalidomide is high within the first three cycles. Skin rash, fatigue, and myelosuppression remain common. In a study of lenalidomide and dexamethasone in patients who failed melphalan and bortezomib, two (8%) died prior to first-response evaluation, 50% experienced grade 3 or greater toxicity, and the hematologic response rate overall was 41%. The median overall survival was 14 months. When cyclophosphamide was added in doses of 100 mg/day, the hematologic response rate was 55%. Lenalidomide was associated with fatigue and fluid retention. When amyloidosis, refractory to both melphalan and bortezomib, was treated with lenalidomide and dexamethasone, 24 patients were enrolled; 19 were refractory to thalidomide, two died before response evaluation, and the adverse event rate was 50%. Survival was shorter in patients with an elevated troponin and in those patients diagnosed <18 months before treatment initiation. Hematologic response rate was 41%, with a median overall survival of 14 months [164].

Melphalan and dexamethasone have been combined with lenalidomide; and in a phase I dose escalation, an MTD of 15 mg was achieved. Melphalan dose for amyloid patients was scaled back due to their frailty at 0.17 mg/kg/day for 4 days. In this trial, dexamethasone was given in a little-used schedule of 40 mg on days 1–4 every 28 days. All patients received low-molecular-weight heparin for DVT prophylaxis; 26 patients were evaluable, and 6 deaths were seen. The complete response rate was 42%, PR rate was 9 of 26, and an overall response rate was 58%, with 50% organ responses, a 54% event-free survival of 2 years, and an overall survival of 81% at 2 years [165].

When melphalan, dexamethasone, and lenalidomide was used in advanced cardiac amyloidosis, 25 patients were enrolled at a dose of 0.18 mg/kg/day for 4 days and dexamethasone 40 mg once weekly with lenalidomide 10 mg/day. Early cardiac deaths were seen in 42% of patients, arrhythmias in 33%, and the hematologic response rate was 58%. Overall survival at 1 year was 58%, but cardiac response rate was only 9%; and the median overall survival for patients with heart failure was 1.75 months [166].

Lenalidomide, dexamethasone, and cyclophosphamide were given to patients for 12 cycles, two-thirds of whom had no prior therapy. The MTD for lenalidomide was 15 mg, and the MTD for cyclophosphamide was 100 mg/day. The PR rate was 55%, the CR was 8%, and four of five prior bortezomib patients responded. In 6-month survivors, the organ response rate was 40%, and the 2-year overall survival rate was 41%. A trial in newly diagnosed amyloidosis with cyclophosphamide, lenalidomide, and dexamethasone ended up enrolling a total of 41 patients. The ≥VGPR rate was 43%. Organ responses were seen in 23 heart, 23 kidney, and 4 liver patients. The overall and progression-free survival in those patients who achieved a PR or better was highly significant ($p < 0.001$).

Bortezomib-Based Chemotherapy for AL Amyloidosis

Eighteen patients, including seven who had relapsed or progressed, were treated with bortezomib and dexamethasone; 94% had a hematologic response, 44% complete, five patients (28%) had a response of at least one affected organ, first establishing activity of bortezomib in amyloid [167]. Our report on bortezomib in 20 patients with active clonal disease despite prior therapy, including thalidomide, was reported. Three (15%) achieved completed hematologic response, and a further 13 (65%) achieved a partial response, but 75% experienced toxicity, requiring discontinuation in 40% [168]. The first published study of weekly and twice-weekly bortezomib that was prospective reported hematologic responses in 50% of 30 evaluable patients, including 20% complete responses with a median time to response of 1.2 months with no difference between once-week and twice-weekly bortezomib [169]. A multicenter survey on the use of bortezomib across Europe reported on 94 patients from three centers. Previously untreated patients had a 47% complete response rate, and a 1-year survival was 76% with the NT-proBNP independently associated with survival [170]. In a series of 26 patients treated with bortezomib and dexamethasone, 69% received it as first-line therapy. The overall response rate was reported at 54%, with 31% hematologic complete responses. Median progression-free and overall survival was 5 and 18 months, respectively, but not reached in complete-response patients [171]. Bortezomib has also been used following autologous stem cell transplant as back-end consolidation for patients who do not achieve a complete response and was demonstrated to eradicate clonal disease at 12 months post stem cell transplantation. Consolidation with bortezomib achieves high stringent complete response rates [158]. An update of the original phase I-II trial conducted in Canada showed 1-year hematologic progression-free rates of 72.2 and 74.6 in patients receiving weekly and twice-weekly bortezomib. Organ responses included 29% renal and 13% cardiac [172].

The combination of cyclophosphamide, bortezomib, and dexamethasone was administered to 17 patients; a response was seen in 16 (94%), 71% achieving a complete hematologic response, and 24% a partial response. Three patients originally not eligible for stem cell transplantation became eligible, and this has become the standard of care at Mayo Clinic [173]. Bortezomib has also been combined with cyclophosphamide and dexamethasone, and the patients who received this at initial therapy had complete response rates of 65% with a 2-year progression-free survival of 66.5% and an overall survival at 2 years of 97.7% [174]. A confirmatory trial of cyclophosphamide, bortezomib, and dexamethasone as first-line treatment reported an overall response rate of 93% with 59% achieving a very good partial or complete response with no grade III-IV peripheral neuropathy [175]. Induction therapy with bortezomib and dexamethasone followed by autologous stem cell transplantation resulted in better outcomes than patients who went directly to stem cell transplantation without bortezomib therapy, achieving statistically significant improvement in overall survival at 24 months (95% vs. 69.4%) [176].

Bortezomib, cyclophosphamide, and dexamethasone have also been shown to be effective in high-risk cardiac amyloidosis (Mayo Clinic stage III). The overall response rate in this cohort was 68%. The estimated 1-year survival was 57%, 40% dying on therapy. Although unable to save the poorest-risk patients, bortezomib, cyclophosphamide, and dexamethasone achieved a high number of hematologic and cardiac responses [177]. Bortezomib has been combined with melphalan and prednisolone in the treatment of newly diagnosed AL amyloidosis. Among 19 patients enrolled in the trial, 16 (84%) had a hematologic response, including 37% complete responses with cardiac and renal responses in 44% and 33%, respectively [178]. In a matched-case control study of melphalan and dexamethasone with or without bortezomib, a higher rate of complete responses was observed with bortezomib (42% vs. 19%), but this did not result in a survival improvement for the overall population [140]. Induction bortezomib followed by high-dose melphalan and autologous stem cell transplantation was reported in 12 patients. The day-100 treatment-related mortality was 9.6%. Hematologic and organ response rates in the entire cohort were 77% and 58%, respectively. Overall cardiac response rate was 60%. The 3-year progression-free and overall survival rates were 66% and 73% [155]. A matched comparison of cyclophosphamide, bortezomib, dexamethasone with cyclophosphamide, thalidomide, and dexamethasone reported that the bortezomib-containing combination improved depth of response and resulted in a superior progression-free survival, supporting its use as opposed to a thalidomide-based therapy [161]. Translocation 11;14 is associated with a poorer outcome in patients treated with bortezomib-based regimens. The reason for this negative impact of this translocation remains uncertain [15]. Bortezomib-based induction for transplant and eligible amyloidosis has resulted in a significant improvement to allow patients to undergo transplant; and in one trial, 8 of 24 initially transplant-ineligible patients became eligible, 7 of whom achieved sustained hematologic response 33 months posttransplant [179]. An update of long-term outcomes after bortezomib therapy of patients reported a median survival of 47 months in patients treated with bortezomib. Bortezomib was associated with improved 1-year survival compared to lenalidomide therapy (81% vs. 56%) [162]. A European collaborative report of cyclophosphamide, bortezomib, and dexamethasone reported 230 patients treated with front-line cyclophosphamide, bortezomib, and dexamethasone. Overall hematologic response rate was 60%, cardiac responses in 17%, and renal responses in 25% [180]. Induction therapy with bortezomib followed by bortezomib and melphalan conditioning for autologous stem cell transplantation was applied to 27 patients, and 100% hematologic responses were seen, 37 very good partial responses; and with a median follow-up of 36 months, median overall and progression-free survival had not been reached [181].

Seventy-three consecutive unselected patients were treated with first-line bortezomib-based induction. Hematologic responses were seen in 77%, including 33% very good partial responses. First-line bortezomib resulted in favorable response and survival [182]. In conclusion, it appears that bortezomib is the single most active agent available for the treatment of amyloidosis. A current randomized phase III trial looking at the oral proteasome inhibitor, ixazomib, is underway.

Antibodies

Anti-plasma-cell-directed chemotherapy does nothing to address established amyloid deposits. Three monoclonal antibodies are currently being tested for efficacy in the treatment of amyloidosis. The 11-1F antibody is currently undergoing clinical testing for efficacy. A second antibody against serum amyloid P component has been shown to improve the amount of amyloid in the liver and spleen and has resulted in improved ultrasound characteristics of the liver. Finally, the Neotope antibody has been given to 27 patients who no longer required anti-plasma-cell chemotherapy; and of 14 cardiac evaluable patients, 57% met the criteria for cardiac response; and of 15 renal evaluable patients, 60% met the criteria for renal response. This antibody, NEOD001, is now undergoing a global phase III trial [183].

Conclusion

Light chain amyloidosis needs to be considered in the differential diagnosis of patients with nondiabetic nephrotic range proteinuria, unexplained fatigue or heart failure with preserved ejection fraction, a progressive peripheral neuropathy associated with a monoclonal protein, or atypical multiple myeloma. Screening involves serum and urine immunofixation and an immunoglobulin free light chain assay. Most patients can have the diagnosis established via biopsy of the bone marrow and subcutaneous fat. Visceral organ biopsy is rarely needed. The prognosis is determined by the DFLC, the levels of cardiac biomarkers, troponin and BNP. Therapy includes high-dose chemotherapy; and for patients ineligible for high-dose chemotherapy, bortezomib appears to be the single most active agent (Fig. 36.10). Combinations of bortezomib and the inclusion of monoclonal antibodies are the subject of further studies.

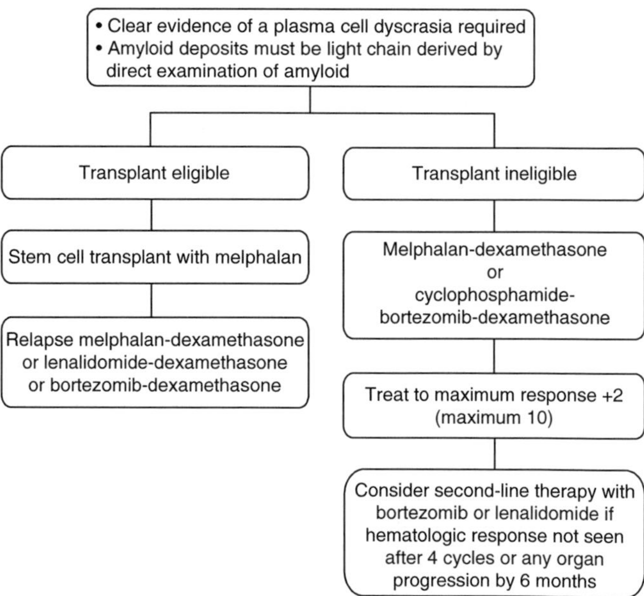

Fig. 36.10 Algorithm for amyloidosis therapy

References

1. Buxbaum JN, Linke RP. A molecular history of the amyloidoses. J Mol Biol. 2012;421(2–3):142–59. https://doi.org/10.1016/j.jmb.2012.01.024.
2. Unsal C, Paydas S, Gonlusen G. Cholestasis and renal failure in a patient with secondary amyloidosis. Ren Fail. 2002;24(6):863–6.
3. Cohen AS, Calkins E. Electron microscopic observations on a fibrous component in amyloid of diverse origins. Nature. 1959;183(4669):1202–3.
4. Isobe T, Osserman EF. Patterns of amyloidosis and their association with plasma-cell dyscrasia, monoclonal immunoglobulins and Bence-Jones proteins. N Engl J Med. 1974;290(9):473–7. https://doi.org/10.1056/NEJM197402282900902.
5. Eanes ED, Glenner GG. X-ray diffraction studies on amyloid filaments. J Histochem Cytochem. 1968;16(11):673–7.
6. Desai HV, Aronow WS, Peterson SJ, Frishman WH. Cardiac amyloidosis: approaches to diagnosis and management. Cardiol Rev. 2010;18(1):1–11. https://doi.org/10.1097/CRD.0b013e3181bdba8f.
7. Kaplan B, Murphy CL, Ratner V, Pras M, Weiss DT, Solomon A. Micro-method to isolate and purify amyloid proteins for chemical characterization. Amyloid. 2001;8(1):22–9.
8. Fernandez de Larrea C, Verga L, Morbini P, et al. A practical approach to the diagnosis of systemic amyloidoses. Blood. 2015;125(14):2239–44. https://doi.org/10.1182/blood-2014-11-609883.
9. Blancas-Mejia LM, Tischer A, Thompson JR, et al. Kinetic control in protein folding for light chain amyloidosis and the differential effects of somatic mutations. J Mol Biol. 2014;426(2):347–61. https://doi.org/10.1016/j.jmb.2013.10.016.
10. Wall JS, Paulus MJ, Gleason S, Gregor J, Solomon A, Kennel SJ. Micro-imaging of amyloid in mice. Methods Enzymol. 2006;412:161–82.
11. Pelaez-Aguilar AE, Rivillas-Acevedo L, French-Pacheco L, et al. Inhibition of light chain 6aJL2-R24G amyloid fiber formation associated with light chain amyloidosis. Biochemistry. 2015;54(32):4978–86. https://doi.org/10.1021/acs.biochem.5b00288.
12. Kourelis TV, Kumar SK, Gertz MA, et al. Coexistent multiple myeloma or increased bone marrow plasma cells define equally high-risk populations in patients with immunoglobulin light chain amyloidosis. J Clin Oncol. 2013;31(34):4319–24. https://doi.org/10.1200/JCO.2013.50.8499.
13. Huang X, Wang Q, Jiang S, Chen W, Zeng C, Liu Z. The clinical features and outcomes of systemic AL amyloidosis: a cohort of 231 Chinese patients. Clin Kidney J. 2015;8(1):120–6. https://doi.org/10.1093/ckj/sfu117.
14. Hasserjian RP, Goodman HJ, Lachmann HJ, Muzikansky A, Hawkins PN. Bone marrow findings correlate with clinical outcome in systemic AL amyloidosis patients. Histopathology. 2007;50(5):567–73. https://doi.org/10.1111/j.1365-2559.2007.02658.x.
15. Bochtler T, Hegenbart U, Kunz C, et al. Translocation t(11;14) is associated with adverse outcome in patients with newly diagnosed AL amyloidosis when treated with bortezomib-based regimens. J Clin Oncol. 2015;33(12):1371–8. https://doi.org/10.1200/JCO.2014.57.4947.
16. Dispenzieri A, Gertz MA, Kumar SK, et al. High sensitivity cardiac troponin T in patients with immunoglobulin light chain amyloidosis. Heart. 2014;100(5):383–8. https://doi.org/10.1136/heartjnl-2013-304957.
17. Zhou P, Hoffman J, Landau H, Hassoun H, Iyer L, Comenzo RL. Clonal plasma cell pathophysiology and clinical features of disease are linked to clonal plasma cell expression of cyclin D1 in systemic light-chain amyloidosis. Clin Lymphoma Myeloma Leuk. 2012;12(1):49–58. https://doi.org/10.1016/j.clml.2011.09.217.
18. Kazmi M. AL amyloidosis. Medicine. 2013;41(5):299–301. https://doi.org/10.1016/j.mpmed.2013.03.006.
19. Warsame R, Kumar SK, Gertz MA, et al. Abnormal FISH in patients with immunoglobulin light chain amyloidosis is a risk factor for cardiac involvement and for death. Blood Cancer J. 2015;5:e310. https://doi.org/10.1038/bcj.2015.34.
20. Sher T, Hayman SR, Gertz MA. Treatment of primary systemic amyloidosis (AL): role of intensive and standard therapy. Clin Adv Hematol Oncol. 2012;10(10):644–51.
21. Caccialanza R, Palladini G, Klersy C, et al. Nutritional status independently affects quality of life of patients with systemic immunoglobulin light-chain (AL) amyloidosis. Ann Hematol. 2012;91(3):399–406. https://doi.org/10.1007/s00277-011-1309-x.
22. Buss SJ, Emami M, Mereles D, et al. Longitudinal left ventricular function for prediction of survival in systemic light-chain amyloidosis: incremental value compared with clinical and biochemical markers. J Am Coll Cardiol. 2012;60(12):1067–76. https://doi.org/10.1016/j.jacc.2012.04.043.
23. Tsai SB, Seldin DC, Wu H, O'Hara C, Ruberg FL, Sanchorawala V. Myocardial infarction with "clean coronaries" caused by amyloid light-chain AL amyloidosis: a case report and literature review. Amyloid. 2011;18(3):160–4. https://doi.org/10.3109/13506129.2011.571319.
24. Matsuda M, Gono T, Morita H, Katoh N, Kodaira M, Ikeda S. Peripheral nerve involvement in primary systemic AL amyloidosis: a clinical and electrophysiological study. Eur J Neurol. 2011;18(4):604–10. https://doi.org/10.1111/j.1468-1331.2010.03215.x.
25. Amin HZ, Mori S, Sasaki N, Hirata K. Diagnostic approach to cardiac amyloidosis. Kobe J Med Sci. 2014;60(1):E5–E11.
26. Hafner J, Ghaoui R, Coyle L, Burke D, Ng K. Axonal excitability in primary amyloidotic neuropathy. Muscle Nerve. 2015;51(3):443–5. https://doi.org/10.1002/mus.24508.
27. Agarwal A, Chang DS, Selim MA, Penrose CT, Chudgar SM, Cardones AR. Pinch purpura: a cutaneous manifestation of systemic amyloidosis. Am J Med. 2015;128(9):e3–4. https://doi.org/10.1016/j.amjmed.2015.04.008.
28. Skok P, Knehtl M, Ceranic D, Glumbic I. Splenic rupture in systemic amyloidosis - case presentation and review of the literature. Z Gastroenterol. 2009;47(3):292–5. https://doi.org/10.1055/s-2008-1027628.
29. Tsourdi E, Darr R, Wieczorek K, et al. Macroglossia as the only presenting feature of amyloidosis due to MGUS. Eur J Haematol. 2014;92(1):88–9. https://doi.org/10.1111/ejh.12163.
30. Perlat A, Decaux O, Gervais R, Rioux N, Grosbois B. Systemic light chain amyloidosis and Sjogren syndrome: an uncommon association. Amyloid. 2009;16(3):181–2. https://doi.org/10.1080/13506120903090692.
31. Audemard A, Boutemy J, Galateau-Salle F, Macro M, Bienvenu B. AL amyloidosis with temporal artery involvement simulates giant-cell arteritis. Joint Bone Spine. 2012;79(2):195–7. https://doi.org/10.1016/j.jbspin.2011.09.007.
32. Mesquita T, Chorao M, Soares I, Mello e Silva A, Abecasis P. Primary amyloidosis as a cause of microvascular angina and intermittent claudication. Rev Port Cardiol. 2005;24(12):1521–31.

33. M'Bappe P, Grateau G. Osteo-articular manifestations of amyloidosis. Best Pract Res Clin Rheumatol. 2012;26(4):459–75. https://doi.org/10.1016/j.berh.2012.07.003.
34. Lousada I, Comenzo RL, Landau H, Guthrie S, Merlini G. Light chain amyloidosis: patient experience survey from the amyloidosis research consortium. Adv Ther. 2015;32(10):920–8. https://doi.org/10.1007/s12325-015-0250-0.
35. Gerth J, Sachse A, Busch M, et al. Screening and differential diagnosis of renal light chain-associated diseases. Kidney Blood Press Res. 2012;35(2):120–8. https://doi.org/10.1159/000330715.
36. Akar H, Seldin DC, Magnani B, et al. Quantitative serum free light chain assay in the diagnostic evaluation of AL amyloidosis. Amyloid. 2005;12(4):210–5. https://doi.org/10.1080/13506120500352339.
37. Filipova J, Rihova L, Vsianska P, et al. Flow cytometry in immunoglobulin light chain amyloidosis: short review. Leuk Res. 2015;39(11):1131–6. https://doi.org/10.1016/j.leukres.2015.07.002.
38. Chaulagain CP, Comenzo RL. New insights and modern treatment of al amyloidosis. Curr Hematol Malig Rep. 2013;8(4):291–8. https://doi.org/10.1007/s11899-013-0175-0.
39. Paiva B, Vidriales MB, Perez JJ, et al. The clinical utility and prognostic value of multiparameter flow cytometry immunophenotyping in light-chain amyloidosis. Blood. 2011;117(13):3613–6. https://doi.org/10.1182/blood-2010-12-324665.
40. Mollee P, Tate J, Pretorius CJ. Evaluation of the N latex free light chain assay in the diagnosis and monitoring of AL amyloidosis. Clin Chem Lab Med. 2013;51(12):2303–10. https://doi.org/10.1515/cclm-2013-0361.
41. Radovic V. Recommendations for use of free light chain assay in monoclonal gammopathies. J Mol Biol. 2010;29(1):1–8. https://doi.org/10.2478/v10011-009-0034-7.
42. Monge M, Chauveau D, Cordonnier C, et al. Localized amyloidosis of the genitourinary tract: report of 5 new cases and review of the literature. Medicine (Baltimore). 2011;90(3):212–22. https://doi.org/10.1097/MD.0b013e31821cbdab.
43. Sethi S, Theis JD, Vrana JA, et al. Laser microdissection and proteomic analysis of amyloidosis, cryoglobulinemic GN, fibrillary GN, and immunotactoid glomerulopathy. Clin J Am Soc Nephrol. 2013;8(6):915–21. https://doi.org/10.2215/CJN.07030712.
44. Glaudemans AW, Slart RH, Noordzij W, Dierckx RA, Hazenberg BP. Utility of 18F-FDG PET(/CT) in patients with systemic and localized amyloidosis. Eur J Nucl Med Mol Imaging. 2013;40(7):1095–101. https://doi.org/10.1007/s00259-013-2375-1.
45. Richards DB, Cookson LM, Berges AC, et al. Therapeutic clearance of amyloid by antibodies to serum amyloid P component. N Engl J Med. 2015;373(12):1106–14. https://doi.org/10.1056/NEJMoa1504942.
46. Wechalekar AD, Offer M, Gillmore JD, Hawkins PN, Lachmann HJ. Cardiac amyloidosis, a monoclonal gammopathy and a potentially misleading mutation. Nat Clin Pract Cardiovasc Med. 2009;6(2):128–33. https://doi.org/10.1038/ncpcardio1423.
47. Hazenberg BP, van Rijswijk MH, Lub-de Hooge MN, et al. Diagnostic performance and prognostic value of extravascular retention of 123I-labeled serum amyloid P component in systemic amyloidosis. J Nucl Med. 2007;48(6):865–72. https://doi.org/10.2967/jnumed.106.039313.
48. Lee DD, Huang CY, Wong CK. Dermatopathologic findings in 20 cases of systemic amyloidosis. Am J Dermatopathol. 1998;20(5):438–42.
49. Miyazaki K, Kawai S, Suzuki K. Abdominal subcutaneous fat pad aspiration and bone marrow examination for the diagnosis of AL amyloidosis: the reliability of immunohistochemistry. Int J Hematol. 2015;102(3):289–95. https://doi.org/10.1007/s12185-015-1827-8.
50. Bogov B, Lubomirova M, Kiperova B. Biopsy of subcutaneus fatty tissue for diagnosis of systemic amyloidosis. Hippokratia. 2008;12(4):236–9.
51. Desport E, Bridoux F, Sirac C, et al. Al amyloidosis. Orphanet J Rare Dis. 2012;7:54. https://doi.org/10.1186/1750-1172-7-54.
52. Sanchorawala V, Seldin DC. AL amyloidosis: who, what, when, why, and where. Oncology (Williston Park). 2012;26(2):164–166, 169.
53. Tokoro C, Inamori M, Sekino Y, et al. Localized primary AL amyloidosis of the colon without other GI involvement. Gastrointest Endosc. 2011;74(4):925–926; discussion 927. https://doi.org/10.1016/j.gie.2011.06.022.
54. Suzuki T, Kusumoto S, Yamashita T, et al. Labial salivary gland biopsy for diagnosing immunoglobulin light chain amyloidosis: a retrospective analysis. Ann Hematol. 2016;95(2):279–85. https://doi.org/10.1007/s00277-015-2549-y.
55. Gertz MA, Dispenzieri A, Sher T. Pathophysiology and treatment of cardiac amyloidosis. Nat Rev Cardiol. 2015;12(2):91–102. https://doi.org/10.1038/nrcardio.2014.165.
56. Chee CE, Lacy MQ, Dogan A, Zeldenrust SR, Gertz MA. Pitfalls in the diagnosis of primary amyloidosis. Clin Lymphoma Myeloma Leuk. 2010;10(3):177–80. https://doi.org/10.3816/CLML.2010.n.027.
57. Bayer-Garner IB, Smoller BR. AL amyloidosis is not present as an incidental finding in cutaneous biopsies of patients with multiple myeloma. Clin Exp Dermatol. 2002;27(3):240–2.
58. Mohammed SF, Mirzoyev SA, Edwards WD, et al. Left ventricular amyloid deposition in patients with heart failure and preserved ejection fraction. JACC Heart Fail. 2014;2(2):113–22. https://doi.org/10.1016/j.jchf.2013.11.004.
59. Satoskar AA, Efebera Y, Hasan A, et al. Strong transthyretin immunostaining: potential pitfall in cardiac amyloid typing. Am J Surg Pathol. 2011;35(11):1685–90. https://doi.org/10.1097/PAS.0b013e3182263d74.
60. Alim MA, Yamaki S, Hossain MS, et al. Structural relationship of kappa-type light chains with AL amyloidosis: multiple deletions found in a VkappaIV protein. Clin Exp Immunol. 1999;118(3):344–8.
61. Olsen KE, Sletten K, Westermark P. The use of subcutaneous fat tissue for amyloid typing by enzyme-linked immunosorbent assay. Am J Clin Pathol. 1999;111(3):355–62.
62. Takeda S, Takazakura E, Haratake J, Hoshii Y. Light chain deposition disease detected by antisera to a variable region of the kappa1 light chain subgroup. Nephron. 1998;80(2):162–5.
63. Pinney JH, Lachmann HJ, Sattianayagam PT, et al. Renal transplantation in systemic amyloidosis-importance of amyloid fibril type and precursor protein abundance. Am J Transplant. 2013;13(2):433–41. https://doi.org/10.1111/j.1600-6143.2012.04326.x.
64. Dasari S, Theis JD, Vrana JA, et al. Proteomic detection of immunoglobulin light chain variable region peptides from amyloidosis patient biopsies. J Proteome Res. 2015;14(4):1957–67. https://doi.org/10.1021/acs.jproteome.5b00015.
65. Vrana JA, Theis JD, Dasari S, et al. Clinical diagnosis and typing of systemic amyloidosis in subcutaneous fat aspirates by mass spectrometry-based proteomics. Haematologica. 2014;99(7):1239–47. https://doi.org/10.3324/haematol.2013.102764.
66. Said SM, Sethi S, Valeri AM, et al. Characterization and outcomes of renal leukocyte chemotactic factor 2-associated amyloidosis. Kidney Int. 2014;86(2):370–7. https://doi.org/10.1038/ki.2013.558.
67. Collins AB, Smith RN, Stone JR. Classification of amyloid deposits in diagnostic cardiac specimens by immunofluorescence. Cardiovasc Pathol. 2009;18(4):205–16. https://doi.org/10.1016/j.carpath.2008.05.004.
68. Kobayashi T, Roberts J, Levine J, Degrado J. Primary bladder amyloidosis. Intern Med. 2014;53(21):2511–3.

69. Ozyigit LP, Kiyan E, Okumus G, Yilmazbayhan D. Isolated laryngo-tracheal amyloidosis presenting as a refractory asthma and longstanding hoarseness. J Asthma. 2009;46(3):314–7. https://doi.org/10.1080/02770900802660956.
70. Cowan AJ, Skinner M, Seldin DC, et al. Amyloidosis of the gastrointestinal tract: a 13-year, single-center, referral experience. Haematologica. 2013;98(1):141–6. https://doi.org/10.3324/haematol.2012.068155.
71. Tsujioka Y, Jinzaki M, Tanimoto A, et al. Radiological findings of primary localized amyloidosis of the ureter. J Magn Reson Imaging. 2012;35(2):431–5. https://doi.org/10.1002/jmri.22858.
72. Hosseini A, Ploumidis A, Adding C, Wiklund NP. Radical surgery for treatment of primary localized bladder amyloidosis: could prostate-sparing robot-assisted cystectomy with intracorporeal urinary diversion be an option? Scand J Urol. 2013;47(1):72–5. https://doi.org/10.3109/00365599.2012.693539.
73. Grogg KL, Aubry MC, Vrana JA, Theis JD, Dogan A. Nodular pulmonary amyloidosis is characterized by localized immunoglobulin deposition and is frequently associated with an indolent B-cell lymphoproliferative disorder. Am J Surg Pathol. 2013;37(3):406–12. https://doi.org/10.1097/PAS.0b013e318272fe19.
74. Chang YT, Liu HN, Wang WJ, Lee DD, Tsai SF. A study of cytokeratin profiles in localized cutaneous amyloids. Arch Dermatol Res. 2004;296(2):83–8. https://doi.org/10.1007/s00403-004-0474-3.
75. Ray M, Tan AW, Thamboo TP. Atypical presentation of primary conjunctival amyloidosis. Can J Ophthalmol. 2012;47(1):e2–4. https://doi.org/10.1016/j.jcjo.2011.08.009.
76. Sueyoshi T, Ueda M, Jono H, et al. Wild-type transthyretin-derived amyloidosis in various ligaments and tendons. Hum Pathol. 2011;42(9):1259–64. https://doi.org/10.1016/j.humpath.2010.11.017.
77. Esplin BL, Gertz MA. Current trends in diagnosis and management of cardiac amyloidosis. Curr Probl Cardiol. 2013;38(2):53–96. https://doi.org/10.1016/j.cpcardiol.2012.11.002.
78. von Hutten H, Mihatsch M, Lobeck H, Rudolph B, Eriksson M, Rocken C. Prevalence and origin of amyloid in kidney biopsies. Am J Surg Pathol. 2009;33(8):1198–205. https://doi.org/10.1097/PAS.0b013e3181abdfa7.
79. Mereuta OM, Theis JD, Vrana JA, et al. Leukocyte cell-derived chemotaxin 2 (LECT2)-associated amyloidosis is a frequent cause of hepatic amyloidosis in the United States. Blood. 2014;123(10):1479–82. https://doi.org/10.1182/blood-2013-07-517938.
80. Patel KS, Hawkins PN. Cardiac amyloidosis: where are we today? J Intern Med. 2015;278(2):126–44. https://doi.org/10.1111/joim.12383.
81. Dubrey S, Ackermann E, Gillmore J. The transthyretin amyloidoses: advances in therapy. Postgrad Med J. 2015;91(1078):439–48. https://doi.org/10.1136/postgradmedj-2014-133224.
82. Quarta CC, Solomon SD, Uraizee I, et al. Left ventricular structure and function in transthyretin-related versus light-chain cardiac amyloidosis. Circulation. 2014;129(18):1840–9. https://doi.org/10.1161/CIRCULATIONAHA.113.006242.
83. Benson MD, Breall J, Cummings OW, Liepnieks JJ. Biochemical characterisation of amyloid by endomyocardial biopsy. Amyloid. 2009;16(1):9–14. https://doi.org/10.1080/13506120802676914.
84. Bokhari S, Castano A, Pozniakoff T, Deslisle S, Latif F, Maurer MS. (99m)Tc-pyrophosphate scintigraphy for differentiating light-chain cardiac amyloidosis from the transthyretin-related familial and senile cardiac amyloidoses. Circ Cardiovasc Imaging. 2013;6(2):195–201. https://doi.org/10.1161/CIRCIMAGING.112.000132.
85. Longhi S, Bonfiglioli R, Obici L, et al. Etiology of amyloidosis determines myocardial 99mTc-DPD uptake in amyloidotic cardiomyopathy. Clin Nucl Med. 2015;40(5):446–7. https://doi.org/10.1097/RLU.0000000000000741.
86. Gertz MA. Immunoglobulin light chain amyloidosis: 2014 update on diagnosis, prognosis, and treatment. Am J Hematol. 2014;89(12):1132–40. https://doi.org/10.1002/ajh.23828.
87. Lebovic D, Hoffman J, Levine BM, et al. Predictors of survival in patients with systemic light-chain amyloidosis and cardiac involvement initially ineligible for stem cell transplantation and treated with oral melphalan and dexamethasone. Br J Haematol. 2008;143(3):369–73. https://doi.org/10.1111/j.1365-2141.2008.07327.x.
88. Dinwoodey DL, Skinner M, Maron MS, Davidoff R, Ruberg FL. Light-chain amyloidosis with echocardiographic features of hypertrophic cardiomyopathy. Am J Cardiol. 2008;101(5):674–6. https://doi.org/10.1016/j.amjcard.2007.10.031.
89. Cappelli F, Baldasseroni S, Bergesio F, et al. Echocardiographic and biohumoral characteristics in patients with AL and TTR amyloidosis at diagnosis. Clin Cardiol. 2015;38(2):69–75. https://doi.org/10.1002/clc.22353.
90. Modesto KM, Dispenzieri A, Cauduro SA, et al. Left atrial myopathy in cardiac amyloidosis: implications of novel echocardiographic techniques. Eur Heart J. 2005;26(2):173–9. https://doi.org/10.1093/eurheartj/ehi040.
91. Hausfater P, Costedoat-Chalumeau N, Amoura Z, et al. AL cardiac amyloidosis and arterial thromboembolic events. Scand J Rheumatol. 2005;34(4):315–9. https://doi.org/10.1080/03009740510015203.
92. Finocchiaro G, Merlo M, Pinamonti B, et al. Long term survival in patients with cardiac amyloidosis. Prevalence and characterisation during follow-up. Heart Lung Circ. 2013;22(8):647–54. https://doi.org/10.1016/j.hlc.2013.01.010.
93. Patel KS, Hawkins PN, Whelan CJ, Gillmore JD. Life-saving implantable cardioverter defibrillator therapy in cardiac AL amyloidosis. BMJ Case Rep. 2014;2014. https://doi.org/10.1136/bcr-2014-206600.
94. Kumar SK, Gertz MA, Lacy MQ, et al. Recent improvements in survival in primary systemic amyloidosis and the importance of an early mortality risk score. Mayo Clin Proc. 2011;86(1):12–8. https://doi.org/10.4065/mcp.2010.0480.
95. Soma K, Takizawa M, Uozumi H, et al. A case of ST-elevated myocardial infarction resulting from obstructive intramural coronary amyloidosis. Int Heart J. 2010;51(2):134–6.
96. Connors LH, Prokaeva T, Lim A, et al. Cardiac amyloidosis in African Americans: comparison of clinical and laboratory features of transthyretin V122I amyloidosis and immunoglobulin light chain amyloidosis. Am Heart J. 2009;158(4):607–14. https://doi.org/10.1016/j.ahj.2009.08.006.
97. Nakagawa M, Sekijima Y, Tojo K, Ikeda S. High prevalence of ATTR amyloidosis in endomyocardial biopsy-proven cardiac amyloidosis patients. Amyloid. 2013;20(2):138–40. https://doi.org/10.3109/13506129.2013.790809.
98. Chau EM, Cheung SC, Chow SL, Fu KH. Nonsecretory immunoglobulin-derived amyloidosis of the heart: diagnosis by immunohistochemistry of the endomyocardium. Clin Cardiol. 1997;20(5):494–6.
99. Guan J, Mishra S, Shi J, et al. Stanniocalcin1 is a key mediator of amyloidogenic light chain induced cardiotoxicity. Basic Res Cardiol. 2013;108(5):378. https://doi.org/10.1007/s00395-013-0378-5.
100. Migrino RQ, Hari P, Gutterman DD, et al. Systemic and microvascular oxidative stress induced by light chain amyloidosis. Int J Cardiol. 2010;145(1):67–8. https://doi.org/10.1016/j.ijcard.2009.04.044.
101. Ando Y, Nyhlin N, Suhr O, et al. Oxidative stress is found in amyloid deposits in systemic amyloidosis. Biochem Biophys Res Commun. 1997;232(2):497–502.
102. Suresh R, Grogan M, Maleszewski JJ, et al. Advanced cardiac amyloidosis associated with normal interventricular septal

thickness: an uncommon presentation of infiltrative cardiomyopathy. J Am Soc Echocardiogr. 2014;27(4):440–7. https://doi.org/10.1016/j.echo.2013.12.010.

103. Bellavia D, Pellikka PA, Dispenzieri A, et al. Comparison of right ventricular longitudinal strain imaging, tricuspid annular plane systolic excursion, and cardiac biomarkers for early diagnosis of cardiac involvement and risk stratification in primary systematic (AL) amyloidosis: a 5-year cohort study. Eur Heart J Cardiovasc Imaging. 2012;13(8):680–9. https://doi.org/10.1093/ehjci/jes009.

104. Koyama J, Falk RH. Prognostic significance of strain Doppler imaging in light-chain amyloidosis. JACC Cardiovasc Imaging. 2010;3(4):333–42. https://doi.org/10.1016/j.jcmg.2009.11.013.

105. Grogan M, Dispenzieri A. Natural history and therapy of AL cardiac amyloidosis. Heart Fail Rev. 2015;20(2):155–62. https://doi.org/10.1007/s10741-014-9464-5.

106. Perugini E, Guidalotti PL, Salvi F, et al. Noninvasive etiologic diagnosis of cardiac amyloidosis using 99mTc-3,3-diphosphono-1,2-propanodicarboxylic acid scintigraphy. J Am Coll Cardiol. 2005;46(6):1076–84. https://doi.org/10.1016/j.jacc.2005.05.073.

107. Antoni G, Lubberink M, Estrada S, et al. In vivo visualization of amyloid deposits in the heart with 11C-PIB and PET. J Nucl Med. 2013;54(2):213–20. https://doi.org/10.2967/jnumed.111.102053.

108. Rivera RJ, Vicenty S. Cardiac manifestations of amyloid disease. Bol Asoc Med P R. 2008;100(4):60–70.

109. Fontana M, Pica S, Reant P, et al. Prognostic value of late gadolinium enhancement cardiovascular magnetic resonance in cardiac amyloidosis. Circulation. 2015;132(16):1570–9. https://doi.org/10.1161/CIRCULATIONAHA.115.016567.

110. Barison A, Aquaro GD, Pugliese NR, et al. Measurement of myocardial amyloid deposition in systemic amyloidosis: insights from cardiovascular magnetic resonance imaging. J Intern Med. 2015;277(5):605–14. https://doi.org/10.1111/joim.12324.

111. Dispenzieri A, Gertz MA, Saenger A, et al. Soluble suppression of tumorigenicity 2 (sST2), but not galactin-3, adds to prognostication in patients with systemic AL amyloidosis independent of NT-proBNP and troponin T. Am J Hematol. 2015;90(6):524–8. https://doi.org/10.1002/ajh.24001.

112. Kumar S, Dispenzieri A, Lacy MQ, et al. Revised prognostic staging system for light chain amyloidosis incorporating cardiac biomarkers and serum free light chain measurements. J Clin Oncol. 2012;30(9):989–95. https://doi.org/10.1200/JCO.2011.38.5724.

113. Gertz MA, Lacy MQ, Dispenzieri A, et al. Refinement in patient selection to reduce treatment-related mortality from autologous stem cell transplantation in amyloidosis. Bone Marrow Transplant. 2013;48(4):557–61. https://doi.org/10.1038/bmt.2012.170.

114. Dispenzieri A, Gertz MA, Buadi F. What do I need to know about immunoglobulin light chain (AL) amyloidosis? Blood Rev. 2012;26(4):137–54. https://doi.org/10.1016/j.blre.2012.03.001.

115. Wechalekar AD, Schonland SO, Kastritis E, et al. A European collaborative study of treatment outcomes in 346 patients with cardiac stage III AL amyloidosis. Blood. 2013;121(17):3420–7. https://doi.org/10.1182/blood-2012-12-473066.

116. Leung N, Glavey SV, Kumar S, et al. A detailed evaluation of the current renal response criteria in AL amyloidosis: is it time for a revision? Haematologica. 2013;98(6):988–92. https://doi.org/10.3324/haematol.2012.079210.

117. Palladini G, Hegenbart U, Milani P, et al. A staging system for renal outcome and early markers of renal response to chemotherapy in AL amyloidosis. Blood. 2014;124(15):2325–32. https://doi.org/10.1182/blood-2014-04-570010.

118. Gertz MA, Leung N, Lacy MQ, et al. Clinical outcome of immunoglobulin light chain amyloidosis affecting the kidney. Nephrol Dial Transplant. 2009;24(10):3132–7. https://doi.org/10.1093/ndt/gfp201.

119. Gude D, Chennemsetty S, Jha R, Narayan G. Primary amyloidosis treated with continuous ambulatory peritoneal dialysis. Saudi J Kidney Dis Transpl. 2012;23(6):1285–7. https://doi.org/10.4103/1319-2442.103578.

120. Dember LM, Sanchorawala V, Seldin DC, et al. Effect of dose-intensive intravenous melphalan and autologous blood stem-cell transplantation on al amyloidosis-associated renal disease. Ann Intern Med. 2001;134(9 Pt 1):746–53.

121. Melmed GM, Fenves AZ, Stone MJ. Urinary findings in renal light chain-derived amyloidosis and light chain deposition disease. Clin Lymphoma Myeloma. 2009;9(3):234–8. https://doi.org/10.3816/CLM.2009.n.046.

122. Lachmann HJ. Paraprotein-related renal disease and amyloid. Medicine. 2007;35(9):512–5. https://doi.org/10.1016/j.mpmed.2007.06.005.

123. Sayed RH, Rogers D, Khan F, et al. A study of implanted cardiac rhythm recorders in advanced cardiac AL amyloidosis. Eur Heart J. 2015;36(18):1098–105. https://doi.org/10.1093/eurheartj/ehu506.

124. Mori M, Kitagawa T, Sasaki Y, et al. Long-term survival of a patient with multiple myeloma-associated severe cardiac AL amyloidosis after implantation of a cardioverter-defibrillator. Rinsho Ketsueki. 2014;55(4):450–5.

125. Lin G, Dispenzieri A, Kyle R, Grogan M, Brady PA. Implantable cardioverter defibrillators in patients with cardiac amyloidosis. J Cardiovasc Electrophysiol. 2013;24(7):793–8. https://doi.org/10.1111/jce.12123.

126. Spiliopoulos S, Koerfer R, Tenderich G. A first step beyond traditional boundaries: destination therapy with the SynCardia total artificial heart. Interact Cardiovasc Thorac Surg. 2014;18(6):855–6. https://doi.org/10.1093/icvts/ivu065.

127. Gray Gilstrap L, Niehaus E, Malhotra R, et al. Predictors of survival to orthotopic heart transplant in patients with light chain amyloidosis. J Heart Lung Transplant. 2014;33(2):149–56. https://doi.org/10.1016/j.healun.2013.09.004.

128. Varr BC, Liedtke M, Arai S, Lafayette RA, Schrier SL, Witteles RM. Heart transplantation and cardiac amyloidosis: approach to screening and novel management strategies. J Heart Lung Transplant. 2012;31(3):325–31. https://doi.org/10.1016/j.healun.2011.09.010.

129. Kamble RT. Orthotopic heart transplant facilitated autologous hematopoietic stem cell transplantation in light-chain amyloidosis. Methodist Debakey Cardiovasc J. 2012;8(3):17–8.

130. Estep JD, Bhimaraj A, Cordero-Reyes AM, Bruckner B, Loebe M, Torre-Amione G. Heart transplantation and end-stage cardiac amyloidosis: a review and approach to evaluation and management. Methodist Debakey Cardiovasc J. 2012;8(3):8–16.

131. Dey BR, Chung SS, Spitzer TR, et al. Cardiac transplantation followed by dose-intensive melphalan and autologous stem-cell transplantation for light chain amyloidosis and heart failure. Transplantation. 2010;90(8):905–11. https://doi.org/10.1097/TP.0b013e3181f10edb.

132. Lacy MQ, Dispenzieri A, Hayman SR, et al. Autologous stem cell transplant after heart transplant for light chain (al) amyloid cardiomyopathy. J Heart Lung Transplant. 2008;27(8):823–9. https://doi.org/10.1016/j.healun.2008.05.016.

133. Gillmore JD, Goodman HJ, Lachmann HJ, et al. Sequential heart and autologous stem cell transplantation for systemic AL amyloidosis. Blood. 2006;107(3):1227–9.

134. Bansal T, Garg A, Snowden JA, McKane W. Defining the role of renal transplantation in the modern management of multiple myeloma and other plasma cell dyscrasias. Nephron Clin Pract. 2012;120(4):c228–35. https://doi.org/10.1159/000341760.

135. Herrmann SM, Gertz MA, Stegall MD, et al. Long-term outcomes of patients with light chain amyloidosis (AL) after renal transplantation with or without stem cell transplantation. Nephrol Dial Transplant. 2011;26(6):2032–6. https://doi.org/10.1093/ndt/gfr067.

136. Casserly LF, Fadia A, Sanchorawala V, et al. High-dose intravenous melphalan with autologous stem cell transplantation in AL amyloidosis-associated end-stage renal disease. Kidney Int. 2003;63(3):1051–7.
137. Comenzo RL, Steingart RM, Cohen AD. High-dose melphalan versus melphalan plus dexamethasone for AL amyloidosis. N Engl J Med. 2008;358(1):92; author reply 92–93
138. Rajkumar SV, Dispenzieri A, Kyle RA. Monoclonal gammopathy of undetermined significance, Waldenstrom macroglobulinemia, AL amyloidosis, and related plasma cell disorders: diagnosis and treatment. Mayo Clin Proc. 2006;81(5):693–703. https://doi.org/10.4065/81.5.693.
139. Palladini G, Russo P, Nuvolone M, et al. Treatment with oral melphalan plus dexamethasone produces long-term remissions in AL amyloidosis. Blood. 2007;110:787–8. https://doi.org/10.1182/blood-2007-02-076034.
140. Palladini G, Milani P, Foli A, et al. Melphalan and dexamethasone with or without bortezomib in newly diagnosed AL amyloidosis: a matched case-control study on 174 patients. Leukemia. 2014;28(12):2311–6. https://doi.org/10.1038/leu.2014.227.
141. Gertz MA, Lacy MQ, Lust JA, Greipp PR, Witzig TE, Kyle RA. Long-term risk of myelodysplasia in melphalan-treated patients with immunoglobulin light-chain amyloidosis. Haematologica. 2008;93(9):1402–6. https://doi.org/10.3324/haematol.12982.
142. Palladini G, Milani P, Foli A, et al. Oral melphalan and dexamethasone grants extended survival with minimal toxicity in AL amyloidosis: long-term results of a risk-adapted approach. Haematologica. 2014;99(4):743–50. https://doi.org/10.3324/haematol.2013.095463.
143. Merlini G, Wechalekar AD, Palladini G. Systemic light chain amyloidosis: an update for treating physicians. Blood. 2013;121(26):5124–30. https://doi.org/10.1182/blood-2013-01-453001.
144. Sanchorawala V, Sun F, Quillen K, Sloan JM, Berk JL, Seldin DC. Long-term outcome of patients with AL amyloidosis treated with high-dose melphalan and stem cell transplantation: 20-year experience. Blood. 2015;126(20):2345–7. https://doi.org/10.1182/blood-2015-08-662726.
145. D'Souza A, Dispenzieri A, Wirk B, et al. Improved outcomes after autologous hematopoietic cell transplantation for light chain amyloidosis: a center for international blood and marrow transplant research study. J Clin Oncol. 2015;33(32):3741–9. https://doi.org/10.1200/JCO.2015.62.4015.
146. Dunn D, Vikas P, Jagasia M, Savani BN. Plerixafor in AL amyloidosis: improved graft composition and faster lymphocyte recovery after auto-SCT in patient with end-stage renal-disease. Bone Marrow Transplant. 2012;47(8):1136–7. https://doi.org/10.1038/bmt.2011.226.
147. Dhakal B, D'Souza A, Arce-Lara C, et al. Superior efficacy but higher cost of plerixafor and abbreviated-course G-CSF for mobilizing hematopoietic progenitor cells (HPC) in AL amyloidosis. Bone Marrow Transplant. 2015;50(4):610–2. https://doi.org/10.1038/bmt.2014.318.
148. Comenzo RL, Michelle D, LeBlanc M, et al. Mobilized CD34+ cells selected as autografts in patients with primary light-chain amyloidosis: rationale and application. Transfusion. 1998;38(1):60–9.
149. Bashir Q, Langford LA, Parmar S, Champlin RE, Qazilbash MH. Primary systemic amyloid light chain amyloidosis decompensating after filgrastim-induced mobilization and stem-cell collection. J Clin Oncol. 2011;29(4):e79–80. https://doi.org/10.1200/JCO.2010.31.4161.
150. Leung N, Slezak JM, Bergstralh EJ, et al. Acute renal insufficiency after high-dose melphalan in patients with primary systemic amyloidosis during stem cell transplantation. Am J Kidney Dis. 2005;45(1):102–11.
151. Cordes S, Dispenzieri A, Lacy MQ, et al. Ten-year survival after autologous stem cell transplantation for immunoglobulin light chain amyloidosis. Cancer. 2012;118(24):6105–9. https://doi.org/10.1002/cncr.27660.
152. Diomede L, Rognoni P, Lavatelli F, et al. A caenorhabditis elegans-based assay recognizes immunoglobulin light chains causing heart amyloidosis. Blood. 2014;123(23):3543–52. https://doi.org/10.1182/blood-2013-10-525634.
153. Dhakal B, Strouse C, D'Souza A, et al. Plerixafor and abbreviated-course granulocyte colony-stimulating factor for mobilizing hematopoietic progenitor cells in light chain amyloidosis. Biol Blood Marrow Transplant. 2014;20(12):1926–31. https://doi.org/10.1016/j.bbmt.2014.08.002.
154. Venner CP, Gillmore JD, Sachchithanantham S, et al. Stringent patient selection improves outcomes in systemic light-chain amyloidosis after autologous stem cell transplantation in the upfront and relapsed setting. Haematologica. 2014;99(12):e260–3. https://doi.org/10.3324/haematol.2014.108191.
155. Scott EC, Heitner SB, Dibb W, et al. Induction bortezomib in al amyloidosis followed by high dose melphalan and autologous stem cell transplantation: a single institution retrospective study. Clin Lymphoma Myeloma Leuk. 2014;14(5):424–430. e421. https://doi.org/10.1016/j.clml.2014.02.003.
156. Hazenberg BP, Croockewit A, van der Holt B, et al. Extended follow up of high-dose melphalan and autologous stem cell transplantation after vincristine, doxorubicin, dexamethasone induction in amyloid light chain amyloidosis of the prospective phase II HOVON-41 study by the Dutch-Belgian co-operative trial Group for Hematology Oncology. Haematologica. 2015;100(5):677–82. https://doi.org/10.3324/haematol.2014.119198.
157. Jaccard A, Moreau P, Leblond V, et al. High-dose melphalan versus melphalan plus dexamethasone for AL amyloidosis. N Engl J Med. 2007;357(11):1083–93. https://doi.org/10.1056/NEJMoa070484.
158. Landau H, Hassoun H, Rosenzweig MA, et al. Bortezomib and dexamethasone consolidation following risk-adapted melphalan and stem cell transplantation for patients with newly diagnosed light-chain amyloidosis. Leukemia. 2013;27(4):823–8. https://doi.org/10.1038/leu.2012.274.
159. Dispenzieri A, Lacy MQ, Rajkumar SV, et al. Poor tolerance to high doses of thalidomide in patients with primary systemic amyloidosis. Amyloid. 2003;10(4):257–61. https://doi.org/10.3109/13506120309041743.
160. Seldin DC, Choufani EB, Dember LM, et al. Tolerability and efficacy of thalidomide for the treatment of patients with light chain-associated (AL) amyloidosis. Clin Lymphoma. 2003;3(4):241–6.
161. Venner CP, Gillmore JD, Sachchithanantham S, et al. A matched comparison of cyclophosphamide, bortezomib and dexamethasone (CVD) versus risk-adapted cyclophosphamide, thalidomide and dexamethasone (CTD) in AL amyloidosis. Leukemia. 2014;28(12):2304–10. https://doi.org/10.1038/leu.2014.218.
162. Kastritis E, Roussou M, Gavriatopoulou M, et al. Long-term outcomes of primary systemic light chain (AL) amyloidosis in patients treated upfront with bortezomib or lenalidomide and the importance of risk adapted strategies. Am J Hematol. 2015;90(4):E60–5. https://doi.org/10.1002/ajh.23936.
163. Dispenzieri A, Lacy MQ, Zeldenrust SR, et al. The activity of lenalidomide with or without dexamethasone in patients with primary systemic amyloidosis. Blood. 2007;109(2):465–70. https://doi.org/10.1182/blood-2006-07-032987.
164. Palladini G, Russo P, Foli A, et al. Salvage therapy with lenalidomide and dexamethasone in patients with advanced AL amyloidosis refractory to melphalan, bortezomib, and thalidomide. Ann Hematol. 2012;91(1):89–92. https://doi.org/10.1007/s00277-011-1244-x.

165. Moreau P, Jaccard A, Benboubker L, et al. Lenalidomide in combination with melphalan and dexamethasone in patients with newly diagnosed AL amyloidosis: a multicenter phase 1/2 dose-escalation study. Blood. 2010;116(23):4777–82. https://doi.org/10.1182/blood-2010-07-294405.
166. Dinner S, Witteles W, Afghahi A, et al. Lenalidomide, melphalan and dexamethasone in a population of patients with immunoglobulin light chain amyloidosis with high rates of advanced cardiac involvement. Haematologica. 2013;98(10):1593–9. https://doi.org/10.3324/haematol.2013.084574.
167. Kastritis E, Anagnostopoulos A, Roussou M, et al. Treatment of light chain (AL) amyloidosis with the combination of bortezomib and dexamethasone. Haematologica. 2007;92(10):1351–8. https://doi.org/10.3324/haematol.11325.
168. Wechalekar AD, Lachmann HJ, Offer M, Hawkins PN, Gillmore JD. Efficacy of bortezomib in systemic AL amyloidosis with relapsed/refractory clonal disease. Haematologica. 2008;93(2):295–8. https://doi.org/10.3324/haematol.11627.
169. Reece DE, Sanchorawala V, Hegenbart U, et al. Weekly and twice-weekly bortezomib in patients with systemic AL amyloidosis: results of a phase 1 dose-escalation study. Blood. 2009;114(8):1489–97. https://doi.org/10.1182/blood-2009-02-203398.
170. Kastritis E, Wechalekar AD, Dimopoulos MA, et al. Bortezomib with or without dexamethasone in primary systemic (light chain) amyloidosis. J Clin Oncol. 2010;28(6):1031–7. https://doi.org/10.1200/JCO.2009.23.8220.
171. Lamm W, Willenbacher W, Lang A, et al. Efficacy of the combination of bortezomib and dexamethasone in systemic AL amyloidosis. Ann Hematol. 2011;90(2):201–6. https://doi.org/10.1007/s00277-010-1062-6.
172. Reece DE, Hegenbart U, Sanchorawala V, et al. Efficacy and safety of once-weekly and twice-weekly bortezomib in patients with relapsed systemic AL amyloidosis: results of a phase 1/2 study. Blood. 2011;118(4):865–73. https://doi.org/10.1182/blood-2011-02-334227.
173. Mikhael JR, Schuster SR, Jimenez-Zepeda VH, et al. Cyclophosphamide-bortezomib-dexamethasone (CyBorD) produces rapid and complete hematologic response in patients with AL amyloidosis. Blood. 2012;119(19):4391–4. https://doi.org/10.1182/blood-2011-11-390930.
174. Venner CP, Lane T, Foard D, et al. Cyclophosphamide, bortezomib, and dexamethasone therapy in AL amyloidosis is associated with high clonal response rates and prolonged progression-free survival. Blood. 2012;119(19):4387–90. https://doi.org/10.1182/blood-2011-10-388462.
175. Shah G, Kaul E, Fallo S, et al. Bortezomib subcutaneous injection in combination regimens for myeloma or systemic light-chain amyloidosis: a retrospective chart review of response rates and toxicity in newly diagnosed patients. Clin Ther. 2013;35(10):1614–20. https://doi.org/10.1016/j.clinthera.2013.08.015.
176. Huang X, Wang Q, Chen W, et al. Induction therapy with bortezomib and dexamethasone followed by autologous stem cell transplantation versus autologous stem cell transplantation alone in the treatment of renal AL amyloidosis: a randomized controlled trial. BMC Med. 2014;12(1):1–10. https://doi.org/10.1186/1741-7015-12-2.
177. Jaccard A, Comenzo RL, Hari P, et al. Efficacy of bortezomib, cyclophosphamide and dexamethasone in treatment-naive patients with high-risk cardiac AL amyloidosis (Mayo Clinic stage III). Haematologica. 2014;99(9):1479–85. https://doi.org/10.3324/haematol.2014.104109.
178. Lee JY, Lim SH, Kim SJ, et al. Bortezomib, melphalan, and prednisolone combination chemotherapy for newly diagnosed light chain (AL) amyloidosis. Amyloid. 2014;21(4):261–6. https://doi.org/10.3109/13506129.2014.960560.
179. Cornell RF, Zhong X, Arce-Lara C, et al. Bortezomib-based induction for transplant ineligible AL amyloidosis and feasibility of later transplantation. Bone Marrow Transplant. 2015;50(7):914–7. https://doi.org/10.1038/bmt.2015.73.
180. Palladini G, Sachchithanantham S, Milani P, et al. A European collaborative study of cyclophosphamide, bortezomib, and dexamethasone in upfront treatment of systemic AL amyloidosis. Blood. 2015;126(5):612–5. https://doi.org/10.1182/blood-2015-01-620302.
181. Sanchorawala V, Brauneis D, Shelton AC, et al. Induction therapy with bortezomib followed by bortezomib-high dose melphalan and stem cell transplantation for light chain amyloidosis: results of a prospective clinical trial. Biol Blood Marrow Transplant. 2015;21(8):1445–51. https://doi.org/10.1016/j.bbmt.2015.04.001.
182. Gatt ME, Hardan I, Chubar E, et al. Outcomes of light-chain amyloidosis patients treated with first-line bortezomib: a collaborative retrospective multicenter assessment. Eur J Haematol. 2016;96(2):136–43. https://doi.org/10.1111/ejh.12558.
183. Gertz MA, Landau H, Comenzo RL, et al. First-in-human phase i/ii study of neod001 in patients with light chain amyloidosis and persistent organ dysfunction. J Clin Oncol. 2016;34(10):1097–103. https://doi.org/10.1200/JCO.2015.63.6530.